SEVENTEENTH EDITION

Williams Obstetrics

SEVENTEENTH EDITION

Williams
Obstetrics

Jack A. Pritchard, M.D.

Gillette Professor, Department of Obstetrics and Gynecology
University of Texas Southwestern Medical School
University of Texas Health Science Center at Dallas, Texas

Paul C. MacDonald, M.D.

Professor, Departments of Obstetrics and Gynecology and Biochemistry
University of Texas Southwestern Medical School
Director of the Cecil H. and Ida Green Center for Reproductive Biology Sciences
University of Texas Health Science Center at Dallas, Texas

Norman F. Gant, M.D.

Professor, Department of Obstetrics and Gynecology
University of Texas Southwestern Medical School
University of Texas Health Science Center at Dallas, Texas

APPLETON-CENTURY-CROFTS/Norwalk, Connecticut

0-8385-9733-5

Our knowledge in the clinical sciences is constantly changing. As new information becomes available, changes in treatment and in the use of drugs become necessary. The authors and the publisher of this volume have taken care to make certain that the doses of drugs and schedules of treatment are correct and compatible with the standards generally accepted at the time of publication. The reader is advised to consult carefully the instruction and information material included in the package insert of each drug or therapeutic agent before administration. This advice is especially important when using new or infrequently used drugs.

86 87 88 89 / 10 9 8 7 6 5 4 3

Prentice-Hall International, Inc., London
Prentice-Hall of Australia, Pty. Ltd., Sydney
Prentice-Hall Canada, Inc.
Prentice-Hall of India Private Limited, New Delhi
Prentice-Hall of Japan, Inc., Tokyo
Prentice-Hall of Southeast Asia (Pte.) Ltd., Singapore
Whitehall Books Ltd., Wellington, New Zealand
Editora Prentice-Hall do Brasil Ltda., Rio de Janeiro

Library of Congress Cataloging in Publication Data

Williams J. Whitridge (John Whitridge), 1866–1931.
    Williams Obstetrics.

    Includes bibliographies and index.
    1. Obstetrics.   I. Pritchard, Jack A., 1921–
II. MacDonald, Paul C., 1930–   III. Gant, Norman F.
IV. Title.   [DNLM: 1. Obstetrics. WQ 100 W724w]
RG524.W7 1985   618.2   84-14448
ISBN 0-8385-9733-5

Design: Jean M. Sabato-Morley

PRINTED IN THE UNITED STATES OF AMERICA

This, the seventeenth edition of Williams Obstetrics,
*is dedicated to all Departmental Chairmen, who face the
difficult task of providing for the expansion and
exploitation of knowledge of human reproduction and for
the application of that knowledge to the needs of
society, especially the unborn and newborn,
irrespective of socioeconomic status.*

Contents

Preface

Quality of life for the mother and her infant is our most important concern. Happily, we live and work in an era in which the fetus is established as our second patient with many rights and privileges comparable to those previously achieved only after birth. It remains a most exciting time and we welcome you again to join us in the exciting venture of optimal human reproduction.

The revisions and additions incorporated in this edition are many. For example, there are 151 new figures. Profound advances in the molecular biology of human reproduction have been made since publication of our previous edition and these changes are reflected in extensive revision and additions, especially in those chapters concerned with endocrinology of human reproduction and the biochemistry and physiology of human parturition.

The voluminous literature concerned with clinical aspects of maternal–fetal medicine that has become available since the previous edition has also been carefully reviewed and cited frequently. At the same time the cumulative experiences provided by the very large obstetric service at Parkland Memorial Hospital have served as source material for some specific recommendations concerning the management of a variety of obstetric problems. However, such recommendations, which are based on our own extensive personal obstetric experiences, should *not* be interpreted as being the only treatment regimen that would favorably influence the outcome of the affected pregnancy. More than likely, quite different approaches that have been or will be rec-

ommended by others will also serve to optimize pregnancy outcome in many instances. In other words we have provided *a* proven method of management which is not necessarily the only way of providing effective treatment.

While the information presented in this edition has been substantially increased, improvement in design and typography have enabled us to maintain the desirable feature of legibility without sacrificing transportability.

The magnitude of effort that has been expended on this major revision involved the participation of a large number of people in the Department of Obstetrics and Gynecology to whom we are most grateful. Included among the many individuals are Dr. F. Gary Cunningham, Dr. Rigoberto Santos, and Dr. Kenneth Leveno. Another colleague, Dr. Linette Casey, provided invaluable scientific and technical assistance. Mr. Tom Sims again provided elegant art work. We also express our thanks to Dr. Richard Voet of the Department of Pathology. David Stires and Robin Millay of Appleton-Century-Crofts have been most supportive.

Last, but certainly not least, the contributions of Lynne McDonnell and Signe Pritchard must be acknowledged. Lynne McDonnell demonstrated emphatically that the hand can be quicker than the eye by her skilled use of the displaywriter to prepare essentially all of the text. Signe Pritchard effectively stimulated the authors to complete their contributions with reasonable promptness and then efficiently collated the seemingly infinite number of parts that make up this book. Thank you all!

SEVENTEENTH EDITION

Williams Obstetrics

1
Obstetrics in Broad Perspective

Definition

Obstetrics* is the branch of medicine that deals with parturition, its antecedents, and its sequels. It is concerned principally, therefore, with the phenomena and management of pregnancy, labor, and the puerperium, in both normal and abnormal circumstances.

In a broader sense, obstetrics is concerned with reproduction of a society. Obstetric care, when appropriately practiced, should promote health and well-being, both physical and mental, among couples and their offspring and help them develop healthy attitudes toward sex, family life, and the place of the family in society. Obstetrics is concerned with all the physiologic, psychologic, and social factors that profoundly influence both the quantity and the quality of human reproduction. The problems of population growth are the natural heritage of obstetrics. The vital statistics of the nation, published monthly by the National Center for Health Statistics, attest to society's concern with the charge of this specialty.

The word *obstetrics* is derived from the Latin term *obstetrix,* meaning midwife. The etymology of obstetrix, however, is obscure. Most dictionaries connect it with the verb *obstare,* which means *to stand by* or *in front of.* The rationale of this derivation is that the midwife stood by or in front of the parturient. This etymology has long been attacked by some etymologists who believed that the word was originally *adstetrix* and that the *ad* had been changed to *ob.* In that case, obstetrix would mean *the woman assisting the parturient.* The fact that on certain inscriptions *obstetrix* is also spelled *opstetrix* has led to the conjecture that it was derived from *ops* (*aid*) and *stare,* meaning *the woman rendering aid.* According to Temkin,† the most likely interpretation is that obstetrix meant *the woman who stood by the parturient.* Whether it alluded merely to the midwife's standing in front of or near the parturient or whether

---

* Oxford English Dictionary. Oxford at the Clarendon Press, 1933. The statements about the history of the term obstetrics, *as well as the definition of obstetrics as stated in the first sentence of this chapter, were obtained chiefly from this source.*

† Previous communication. Dr. Owsei Temkin, Associate Professor of the History of Medicine, Johns Hopkins University School of Medicine, graciously devoted time to a study of the etymology of the word obstetrics, *and the comments cited were entirely his.*

it carried the additional connotation of rendering aid is not clear.

The term *obstetrics* is of relatively recent usage. The Oxford English Dictionary gives the earliest example from a book published in 1819, indicating that in 1828 it was necessary to apologize for the use of the word *obstetrician.* Kindred terms, however, are much older. For example, *obstetricate* occurs in English works published as early as 1623; *obstetricatory,* in 1640; *obstetricious,* in 1645; and *obstetrical,* in 1775. These terms were often used figuratively. As an example of such usage, the adjective *obstetric* appears in Pope's *Dunciad* (1742) in the famous couplet:

> There all the Learn'd shall at the labour stand,
> and Douglas lend his soft, obstetric hand.

The much older term *midwifery* was used instead of *obstetrics* until the latter part of the nineteenth century in both the United States and Great Britain. It is derived from the Middle English *mid,* meaning *with,* and *wif,* meaning wife in the sense of a *woman.* The term *midwife* was used as early as 1303, and *midwifery,* in 1483. In England today, the term *midwifery* carries the same connotation as obstetrics, and the two words are used synonymously.

Aims of Obstetrics

The transcendent objective of obstetrics is that every pregnancy be wanted and culminate in a healthy mother and a healthy baby. Obstetrics strives to minimize the number of women and infants who die as a result of the reproductive process or who are left physically, intellectually, or emotionally injured therefrom. Obstetrics is concerned further with the number and spacing of children so that both mother and offspring, indeed all the family, may enjoy optimal physical and emotional well-being. Finally, obstetrics strives to analyze and influence the social factors that impinge on reproductive efficiency.

Vital Statistics

To aid in the reduction of the number of mothers and infants who die as the result of pregnancy and labor, it is important to know how many such deaths occur in this country each year and in what circumstances. To try to help evaluate these data correctly, a variety of events concerned with pregnancy outcomes have been defined by various agencies:

- *Birth.* This is the complete expulsion or extraction from the mother of a fetus irrespective of whether or not the umbilical cord has been cut or the placenta is attached. In many states fetuses weighing less than 500 g usually are not considered as births, but rather as abortions, for purposes of perinatal vital statistics. In the absence of a birth weight, a body length of 25 cm, crown to heel, is usually equated with 500 g. Twenty weeks gestational age, that is, from the last menstrual period, has been commonly considered to be equivalent to 500 g fetal weight; however, a 500-g fetus is more likely to be 22 weeks gestational age, or 20 weeks ovulation or fertilization age.
- *Birth Rate.* The number of births per 1000 population is the birth rate, or crude birth rate.
- *Fertility Rate.* This important term refers to the number of live births per 1000 female population aged 15 through 44 years.
- *Live Birth.* Whenever the infant at or after birth breathes spontaneously or shows any other sign of life such as heart beat or definite spontaneous movement of voluntary muscles, a live birth is recorded.
- *Stillbirth.* None of the above signs of life are present at or after birth.
- *Neonatal Death.* Early neonatal death refers to death of a live-born infant during the first 7 days of life. Late neonatal death refers to death after 7 but before 29 days of life.
- *Stillbirth Rate.* This rate expresses the number of stillborn infants per 1000 infants born.
- *Fetal Death Rate.* This term is synonymous with stillbirth rate.
- *Neonatal Mortality Rate.* This rate refers to the number of neonatal deaths per 1000 live births.
- *Perinatal Mortality Rate.* This rate is defined as the number of fetal deaths (stillbirths) plus neonatal deaths per 1000 total births.
- *Low Birth Weight.* If the first weight obtained after birth is 2500 g or less, low birth weight is identified.
- *Term Infant.* An infant born any time after 37 completed weeks of gestation through 41 completed weeks of gestation (260 to 287 days) has been defined by some to be a term infant. Such a definition implies that birth at any time within this period is optimal whereas birth before or afterward is not. Such an implication is not warranted. Some infants born between 37 and 38 weeks are at risk of functional prematurity; for example, the development of respiratory distress in the newborn infant of a diabetic mother (see Chapter 28, p. 600). Moreover, any risk to the fetus

that might be imposed by remaining in utero until 42 weeks rather than 41 weeks does not appear to be appreciable. Consequently, there is no good reason for distorting the range for term birth to 3 weeks below the mean of 40 weeks but only 1 week beyond the mean. Therefore, it is our opinion that a term infant is better defined as one who is born no earlier than 38 weeks but not later than 42 weeks of gestation (see Chapter 37, p. 745).
- *Preterm or Premature Infant.* An infant born before 37 completed weeks has been so classified, although born before 38 completed weeks would seem more appropriate for reasons stated above.
- *Postterm Infant.* An infant born at 42 weeks gestational age or more has been appropriately classified, by some, at least, as being postterm.
- *Abortus.* A fetus or embryo removed or expelled from the uterus during the first half of gestation (20 weeks or less), or weighing less than 500 g, or measuring less than 25 cm is also referred to as an abortus.
- *Direct Maternal Death.* Death of the mother resulting from obstetric complications of the pregnancy state, labor, or puerperium, and from interventions, omissions, incorrect treatment, or a chain of events resulting from any of the above is considered a direct maternal death. (Example: exsanguination from rupture of uterus.)
- *Indirect Maternal Death.* An obstetric death not directly due to obstetric causes but resulting from previously existing disease, or a disease that developed during pregnancy, labor, or the puerperium, but which was aggravated by the maternal physiologic adaptation to pregnancy, is classified as an indirect maternal death. (Example: mitral stenosis.)
- *Nonmaternal Death.* Death of the mother resulting from accidental or incidental causes in no way related to the pregnancy may be classified as a nonmaternal death. (Example: death from an airplane crash.)
- *Maternal Death Rate or Mortality.* This rate refers to number of maternal deaths that occur as the result of the reproductive process per 100,000 live births. (Note: this rate is calculated per *one hundred thousand* live births and not per *one thousand.*)
- *Reproductive Mortality.* Deaths resulting from the use of contraceptive techniques to avoid pregnancy plus deaths that are the consequence of pregnancy provide the basis for this rate, expressed as number of deaths per 100,000 women.

The Birth Rate and Fertility Rate. One index of the need for obstetric personnel and facilities is the number of births each year. Additional indices are the birth rate and the fertility rate. From these data, particularly the fertility rate, the expected number of births in future years can be estimated.

TABLE 1-1. MATERNAL MORTALITY IN THE UNITED STATES 1935–1982

Maternal Deaths		Rate Per 100,000 Live Births		
Year	Number	Total	White	Other
1935	12,544	582.1	530.6	945.7
1940	8,876	376.0	319.8	773.5
1945	5,668	107.2	172.1	454.8
1950	2,960	83.3	61.1	221.6
1955	1,901	47.0	32.8	130.3
1960	1,579	37.1	26.0	97.9
1965	1,189	31.6	21.0	83.7
1970	803	21.5	14.4	55.9
1975	403	12.8	9.1	29.0
1980	334	9.2	6.7	19.8
1982*	330	8.9	—	—

* Provisional.

In 1983, there were 3.61 million live births in the United States, a very slight reduction from the previous year. The fertility rate in 1983 was 66.9, also a very slight reduction.

Maternal Mortality. Maternal deaths per 100,000 live births have decreased remarkably in the past half century. There were only 330 maternal deaths reported in 1982 in the United States or 8.9 per 100,000 live births. By way of comparison, in 1935 there were 12,544 maternal deaths, or 582.1 per 100,000 live births! Values for intervening years are presented in Table 1-1.

The nearly threefold difference in maternal mortality rates that exists between white and black women appears to result primarily from social and economic factors, such as a relative lack of skilled personnel and appropriate facilities at delivery, lack of antepartum care, lack of family planning services, faulty health education, and perhaps dietary deficiencies and poor hygiene. As these unfavorable social and economic conditions are improved, the racial difference in the maternal death rates will doubtless decrease.

The maternal mortality rate varies also with the age of the mother. In all races, the remarkable increase in mortality with advancing age is probably best explained on the basis of an intrinsic maternal factor. The increasing frequency of hypertension with advancing years and the greater tendency to uterine hemorrhage contribute significantly to the elevation of the mortality rate. Advanced age and high parity act independently to increase the risk of childbearing, but their effects are usually additive. In the actual analysis of cases, it is difficult to dissociate these two factors.

Common Causes of Maternal Mortality. Hemorrhage, hypertension that is either induced or aggravated by pregnancy, and infection still account for most maternal deaths. In Texas, for example, direct maternal deaths occurring in more recent years were attributable to hemorrhage in 36 percent of all fatalities, hypertensive disorders of pregnancy in 24 percent, and infection in 21 percent (Harrison, 1982). The causes of obstetric hemor-

rhage are multiple: postpartum hemorrhage, bleeding in association with abortion, bleeding from rupture of the fallopian tube (ectopic pregnancy), bleeding as the result of abnormal placental location or separation (placenta previa and abruptio placentae), and bleeding from rupture of the uterus. Hypertension induced or aggravated by pregnancy, occurring in about 6 or 7 percent of gravid women, is accompanied commonly by edema and proteinuria (preeclampsia), and in some severe cases by convulsions and coma (eclampsia). Puerperal infection of the genital tract usually originates as metritis, which sometimes undergoes extension to cause pelvic and abdominal abscesses, peritonitis, thrombophlebitis, bacteremia, septicemia, and distant foci of infection. Details of the origin, prevention, and treatment of these conditions form a considerable portion of the subject matter of obstetrics.

Reasons for Decline in Maternal Mortality Rate. Many factors and agencies are responsible for the dramatic fall in the maternal death rate in this country over the past 50 years. Obviously, there has been a general improvement in medical practice. The widespread use of blood transfusion and antibiotics and the maintenance of fluid, electrolyte, and acid–base balance in the serious complications of pregnancy and labor have materially changed obstetric practice. Equally important is the development of widespread obstetric training and continuing educational programs, which have provided more and better qualified specialists.

Obstetrics is unique in that no other branch of medicine is subject to such careful public scrutiny. Not only are births a matter of public record, but maternal and perinatal deaths are examined by municipal, state, and national health authorities. In many areas, local medical or obstetric and gynecologic societies also examine such deaths, and mortality conferences are frequently conducted as part of the continuing medical education of the obstetrician.

The sine qua non of good work in any field is well-trained personnel, but they could not have achieved the excellent results had there not been a great expansion in facilities for good obstetric care. Despite increased facilities, there remain areas in the United States where obstetric services are woefully inadequate, particularly in rural areas and in some of our large inner cities.

From the viewpoint of safer care during labor, the outstanding advance of the past 50 years has been the great increase in the proportion of hospital deliveries. As recently as 1940, only three out of five white births took place in hospitals; this figure now is 99 percent. Hospital births not only mean better facilities but imply care by individuals specially trained in obstetrics and perinatology.

Reproductive Mortality. In more recent years, as the national mortality rate decreased markedly, some deaths were occurring as the consequence of a great increase in the use of various contraceptive techniques. The sum of the mortalities from pregnancy and from the use of these

TABLE 1-2. REPRODUCTIVE MORTALITY IN THE UNITED STATES BY CAUSE—1955 AND 1975

| | Estimated Number of Deaths | | | | | | | |
| | Pregnancy Related | | | Contraception Related | | | | |
Year	Ectopic Pregnancy	Abortion	Other Deaths	OC*	IUD*	Steri- lization	Total Deaths	Reproductive Mortality Rate†
1955	139	485	2,065	—	—	14	2,703	7.8
1975	50	49	428	452	6	14	999	2.1

* OC indicates oral contraceptives; IUD, intrauterine device (neither used in 1955).
† Rate per 100,000 women.
(*From Sachs and co-workers, 1982.*)

techniques to prevent pregnancy has been termed reproductive mortality. Data provided by Sachs and co-workers (1982) are presented in Table 1-2. In spite of the innovation and widespread use of oral contraceptives and intrauterine devices accompanied by a marked increase in surgical sterilization, the number of deaths from contraception was slight compared to the decrease in maternal mortality.

Perinatal Mortality. The sum of stillbirths and neonatal deaths is the perinatal mortality. The perinatal death rate has fallen by nearly 50 percent in the past 25 years (Table 1-3). Currently, there are somewhat more than 100 perinatal deaths for every maternal death. With the current very low incidence of maternal deaths, perinatal loss rates not only are a better index of the level of obstetric care, but also give a valid indication of an equally important datum, the infant morbidity. To some extent, the total perinatal loss is correlated with the age and parity of the mother. The rates tend to be highest for the first born of very young women and births of the order of six and over.

Factors Affecting the Stillbirth Rate. One half or more of perinatal deaths are stillbirths. Stillbirths tend to decline as the quality of care during and throughout pregnancy improves. Some deaths could be avoided by better prenatal care, proper hospitalization, and, at times, deliberate delivery remote from term when the intrauterine environment has become hostile. In a proportion of deaths in utero, unfortunately, there may be no obvious explanation.

Neonatal Deaths. In 1977, for the first time in the United States, there were fewer neonatal deaths than fetal deaths (stillbirths). Nearly half of the neonatal deaths occur in the first day of life. The number of deaths during those 24 hours exceeds that from the second month to the completion of the first year. The causes of this wastage during the neonatal period are numerous, but low birth weight is a common event in neonatal fatalities. The proportion of infants of low birth weight differs among ethnic groups, ranging from about 50 per 1000 for white mothers to approximately 100 per 1000 for black mothers. The interracial difference in the

rates of low birth weight accounts for the major difference in neonatal mortality between these two groups. Social and environmental factors probably weigh more heavily than race, however, in the cause of this difference.

As well as deaths, low birth weight has contributed appreciably to infant morbidity and for a large fraction of the neurologic and intellectual deficits that are tragic individually and costly to society. Why some women go into labor prematurely is one of the great unsolved problems of obstetrics.

The second most common cause of neonatal death is injury to the central nervous system. Here the word *injury* is used in its broad sense to indicate both cerebral injury resulting from hypoxia in utero or soon after birth and traumatic injury to the brain during labor and delivery. Some of these deaths might be prevented by more judicious management of labor. An important cause of neonatal death is congenital malformation.

The Birth Certificate. Statutes in all 50 states and the District of Columbia require that a birth certificate be completed for every birth and submitted promptly to the local registrar. After the birth has been duly registered, notification is sent to the parents of the child and a complete report is forwarded to the National Center for Health Statistics in Washington.

There are many reasons why the complete and ac-

TABLE 1-3. PERINATAL MORTALITY IN THE UNITED STATES 1950–1980

| | Perinatal | | Fetal | | Neonatal | |
Year	Number	Ratio†	Number	Ratio	Number	Ratio*
1950	141,117	39.7	68,262	19.2	72,855	20.5
1955	146,504	36.2	69,153	17.1	77,351	19.1
1960	148,213	34.8	68,480	16.1	79,733	18.7
1965	127,278	33.9	60,859	16.2	66,419	17.7
1970	109,240	29.3	52,961	14.2	56,279	15.1
1975	70,212	22.3	33,796	10.7	36,416	11.6
1977	65,913	19.6	33,053	9.9	32,860	9.8
1980	63,971	17.7	33,353	9.2	30,618	8.5
1983	—	—	—	—	—	7.4

* Deaths per 1000 live births; neonatal deaths up to 28 days.
† Deaths per 1000 births.

curate registration of births is essential. Certification of the facts of birth is needed as evidence of age, citizenship, and family relationships. Moreover, the data they provide are of immeasurable importance to all agencies (social, public health, demographic, or obstetrics) dealing with human reproduction. For instance, the data presented in the foregoing paragraphs were culled almost entirely from information published by the National Center for Health Statistics on the basis of birth certificates; they represent, furthermore, only a small fraction of the information obtainable from that source. *Hence, the prompt and accurate completion of this certificate after each birth is not only a legal duty but a contribution to the broad field of obstetric knowledge.*

Obstetrics and Other Branches of Medicine

Obstetrics is a multifaceted subject, with close and numerous relations to other branches of medicine. It is so intimately related to the kindred subject of gynecology that obstetrics and gynecology are generally regarded as one specialty. Gynecology deals with the physiology and the pathology of the female reproductive organs in the nonpregnant state, whereas obstetrics deals with the pregnant state in the broadest sense. Correct differential diagnosis in either obstetrics or gynecology entails an intimate acquaintance with the clinical syndromes met in both; in addition, the methods of examination and many operative techniques are common to both disciplines. It is therefore obligatory that every obstetrician be experienced in gynecology, and vice versa.

The scope of intrauterine diagnosis and treatment has broadened remarkably (see Chapter 14 and elsewhere). This, as well as the concern of obstetrics with the newborn infant, has brought the subject into close relation with pediatrics and given rise to the concept of perinatology. The boundaries between obstetrics and neonatology are not sharp, but rather overlap to the benefit of the fetus and infant. Even in metropolitan centers, emergency deliveries often impose on the obstetrician the management of the newborn during the most critical hours of life. The obstetrician must possess expertise, therefore, in the management of the infant at this time as well as before birth.

Since pregnant and nonpregnant women are subject to the same diseases, the obstetrician commonly encounters and therefore must be knowledgeable about a variety of diseases in pregnant women. As emphasized in Chapter 28, the clinical picture presented by some of these disorders is altered greatly during pregnancy and the immediate puerperium; conversely, these diseases affect the course of gestation.

Obstetrics is intimately related to the preclinical sciences. As pointed out in Chapter 24, the study of spontaneous abortion, for example, depends on knowledge of anomalous development of the early embryo and trophoblasts. Abortion may also involve hormonal defects, which condition would link the subjects of obstetrics and endocrinology. Abortion may result from chromosomal

defects, and such a condition would forge a link to cytogenetics. The concept of Rh isoimmunization has shown how immunologic factors may interfere with the successful outcome of pregnancy, but in turn, by appropriate immunotherapy, be successfully prevented, as emphasized in Chapter 38. Obstetrics and general pathology meet closely in the rapidly developing field of perinatal pathology. Other important relations of obstetrics to preclinical sciences include: microbiology, in the study of maternal and fetal infections—bacterial, viral, and other; biochemistry and physiology, in relation to myriad events including labor; and pharmacology, in the action and metabolism of drugs in the mother and in the fetus and newborn infant. The numerous applications of the preclinical sciences to problems of human reproduction are evident in the relatively short but remarkable history of the National Institute of Child Health and Human Development.

Obstetrics is related also to certain fields that are not strictly medical. Since nutritional requirements are altered by pregnancy, obstetrics requires knowledge of the science of nutrition. In studies of fetal malformation, genetics is obviously of importance. Since the mother–child relationship is the basis of the family unit, the obstetrician is continually dealing with psychologic and sociologic problems. Economics play a prominent role in obstetrics since health care has become quite expensive, and especially so when those who provide it have little concern for costs. In addition, obstetrics has important legal aspects, especially in regard to the increasing number of malpractice suits.

Obstetrics, the Mother, and Her Family

In spite of the remarkable record of safety for the hospitalized expectant mother and her fetus-infant that has been achieved in recent years (Tables 1-1 and 1-3), there has evolved a small but quite vocal group of dissidents made up of former parturients, their partners, and those who would attempt to provide care during home delivery. Hopefully, those complaints about hospitalization, for which there are real bases, can be resolved short of sacrificing the safety that can be provided by appropriately hospitalizing for delivery the mother and especially her fetus-infant.

There is no question that some individuals who collaborate in the effort to provide optimal in-hospital care for the mother and the fetus-infant have not necessarily been as considerate of the pregnant mother and her family as they should have been. The expectant mother has been commonly treated as if she were seriously ill, even when she was quite healthy. All too often she has been forced to conform to a common pathway of care that stripped her of most of her individuality and much of her dignity. Niceties of surroundings have not been provided; instead, hospital austerity has prevailed. Hospital administrators have tended not to seek her business, claiming they lost money on obstetrics, or to accept her and her fetus only when full payment could be guaranteed. In recent years, obstetricians, for many good reasons, have worked mostly in groups; as a consequence, about the time of delivery—the ultimate event in the minds of the mother and her family—there may have been either a "changing of the obstetric guard" or the obstetrician created the appearance of wanting to hurry the labor and delivery since he or she would soon be "going off." The same picture has been presented by the nurses and other personnel intimately involved in providing care for the mother and fetus-infant. Too often the expectant mother has felt that her fate and the fate of her baby were dependent not so much on skilled personnel but upon a mysterious electronic gadget that appeared to possess inherently some great power that prevailed above all others. Fortunately, appropriate applications of medical science do not require that excellent care be a dehumanizing ordeal. Excellent obstetric care and the many benefits that accrue can be provided in a hospital setting that, at the same time, is enjoyed by the mother and family, and is acceptable economically to all parties involved.

The Future

Although the recent decline in the maternal mortality rate has been enormous, the millennium is neither here nor close by. If the nonwhite mortality rate were reduced to the level of that of the white by providing equal care, and if the white deaths considered preventable by many mortality studies were prevented, approximately two thirds of these mothers' lives could be saved each year. Maternal mortality affects most seriously the socially and economically deprived. Many of these deaths result from sheer lack of adequate facilities, including lack of properly distributed units for antepartum care, lack of suitable hospital arrangements, and lack of readily avail-

able blood. Others are caused by errors of management by the obstetric personnel. Errors of omission include failure to provide antepartum care, failure to follow the woman and fetus carefully throughout labor and the early puerperium, and failure to obtain appropriate consultation. Among errors of commission, trauma at delivery still looms large.

These several deficiencies in maternity care must obviously be corrected if maternal and perinatal mortality rates are to be brought to the irreducible minimum. They can and doubtless will be lowered to that level by the same methods that have proved efficacious in the past: more and better trained personnel and more and better equipped facilities that are readily available to all pregnant women and their fetuses and newborn infants.

The concept of the right of every child to be physically, mentally, and emotionally "well-born" is fundamental to human dignity. If obstetrics is to play a role in its realization, the specialty must maintain and even extend its role in the control of population.

The right to be "well-born" in its broadest sense is simply incompatible with unrestricted fertility (Chapter 40). Yet our knowledge of all the forces operative in the fluctuation and control of population growth is still rudimentary. This concept of obstetrics as a social as well as a biologic science impels us to accept a responsibility unprecedented in American medicine.

REFERENCES

Harrison EE Jr: Why do pregnant women die? Dallas Med J (Sept–Oct):242, 1982
Sachs BP, Layde PM, Rubin GL, Rochat RW: Reproductive mortality in the United States. JAMA 247:2789, 1982

2
The Anatomy of the Reproductive Tract of Women

The organs of reproduction of women are classified according to those that are external and those that are internal. The external organs and the vagina serve for copulation; the internal organs provide for ovulation, a site of ovum fertilization and blastocyst transport, implantation, and thence development and birth of the fetus.

EXTERNAL GENERATIVE ORGANS

The *pudenda,* or the external organs of generation, are commonly designated the *vulva,* which includes all structures visible externally from the pubis to the perineum, that is, the mons pubis, the labia majora and minora, the clitoris, hymen, vestibule, urethral opening, and various glandular and vascular structures (Fig. 2-1).

Mons Pubis

The mons pubis, or mons veneris, is the fat-filled cushion that lies over the anterior surface of the symphysis pubis. After puberty, the skin of the mons pubis is covered by curly hair that forms the *escutcheon.* Generally, the distribution of pubic hair differs in the two sexes. In women, it is distributed in a triangular area, the base of which is formed by the upper margin of the symphysis, and a few hairs are distributed downward over the outer surface of the labia majora. In men, the escutcheon is not so well circumscribed, hairs from the pubic area grow in a region that extends upward toward the umbilicus and downward and inward over the inner surface of the thighs.

Labia Majora

There are two rounded folds of adipose tissue that are covered with skin, and that extend downward and backward from the mons pubis; these are the labia majora. Among adult women, these structures vary somewhat in appearance, principally according to the amount of fat that is contained within these tissues. Embryologically, the labia majora are homologous with the scrotum of

men. The round ligaments terminate at the upper borders of the labia majora. After repeated childbearing, the labia majora are less prominent, and in old age usually begin to shrivel. Ordinarily, these structures are 7 to 8 cm in length, 2 to 3 cm in width, and 1 to 1.5 cm in thickness, and are somewhat tapered at the lower extremities. In children and nulliparous women, the labia majora usually lie in close apposition and thereby completely conceal the underlying tissues, whereas in multiparous women, the labia majora may gape widely (Fig. 2-1). The labia majora are continuous directly with the mons pubis above and merge into the perineum posteriorly, at a site where these structures are joined medially to form the *posterior commissure.*

Before puberty, the outer surface of each labium majus is similar to that of the adjacent skin, but after puberty each is covered with hair. In nulliparous women, the inner surface is moist and resembles a mucous membrane, whereas in multiparous women, the inner surface becomes more skinlike, but is not covered with hair. The labia majora are richly supplied with sebaceous glands. Beneath the skin, there is a layer of dense connective tissue that is rich in elastic fibers and adipose tissue, but is nearly void of muscular elements. Unlike the squamous epithelium of the vagina and cervix, in parts of the vulvar skin there are epithelial appendages. Beneath the skin, there is a mass of fat, which provides the bulk of the volume of the labium; this adipose tissue is supplied with a plexus of veins that, as the result of external injury, may rupture to create a hematoma.

Labia Minora

Two flat reddish folds of tissue are visible when the labia majora are separated; these structures are the labia minora, or nymphae, structures that join at the upper extremity of the vulva. Among women, the labia minora vary greatly in size and shape. In nulliparous women, the labia minora usually are not visible behind the non-separated labia majora, whereas in multiparous women, it is common for the labia minora to project beyond the labia majora.

Each labium minus is a thin fold of tissue that,

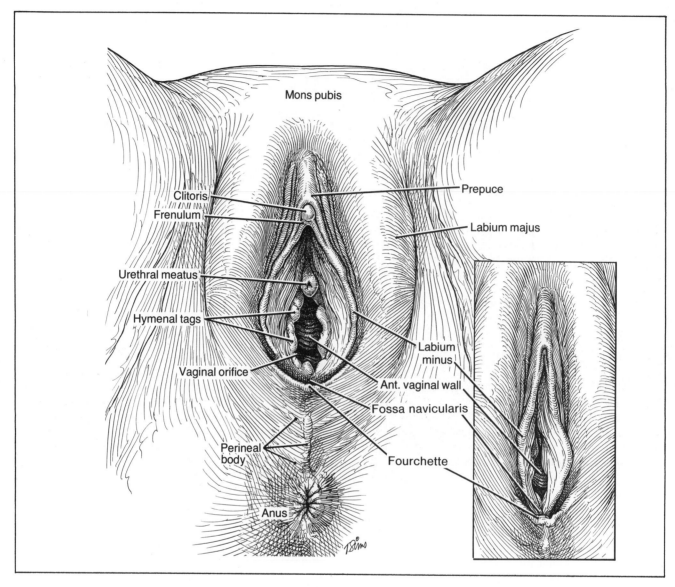

Figure 2-1. External organs of reproduction of women. The lower anterior vaginal wall is visible through the labia minora. In nulliparous women, the vaginal orifice is not so readily visible (*inset*) because of the close apposition of the labia minora.

when protected, is moist and reddish in appearance and thus is similar to that of a mucous membrane. These structures, however, are covered by stratified squamous epithelium into which numerous papillae project. There are no hair follicles in the labia minora but there are many sebaceous follicles and, occasionally, a few sweat glands. The interior of the labial folds is comprised of connective tissue in which there are many vessels and some smooth muscular fibers, as is the case in typical erectile structures. These structures are extremely sensitive and are supplied with a variety of nerve endings.

The tissues of the labia minora converge superiorly where each is divided into two lamellae, the lower pair of which fuse to form the *frenulum of the clitoris,* and

the upper pair merges to form the *prepuce* of the clitoris. Inferiorly, the labia minora extend to approach the midline as low ridges of tissue that fuse to form the *fourchet* that is readily visible in nulliparous women; in multiparous women, however, the labia minora usually are imperceptibly contiguous with the labia majora.

Clitoris

The clitoris, the homologue of the penis, is a small, cylindrical, erectile body that is located near the superior extremity of the vulva. This organ projects downward between the branched extremities of the labia minora, which, as stated, converge to form the prepuce and frenulum of the clitoris. The clitoris is comprised of a glans, a body (corpus), and two crura. The glans is made up of spindle-shaped cells, and in the body there are two corpora cavernosa, in the walls of which are smooth muscle fibers. The long, narrow crura arise from the inferior surface of the ischiopubic rami and fuse just below the middle of the pubic arch to form the body of the clitoris.

Rarely does the clitoris exceed 2 cm in length, even in a state of erection; and, it is bent sharply by traction that is exerted by the labia minora. As a result, the free end of the clitoris is pointed downward and inward toward the vaginal opening. The glans, which rarely exceeds 0.5 cm in diameter, is covered by stratified squamous epithelium that is richly supplied with nerve endings and is, therefore, extremely sensitive to touch. The vessels of the erectile clitoris are connected with the vestibular bulbs; the clitoris is believed to be one, if not the principal, erogenous organ of women.

Kranz (1958) studied the nerve supply of the external genitalia; in the labia majora, as well as the labia minora and clitoris, he found that there is a delicate network of free nerve endings, the fibers of which terminate in small knoblike thickenings in or adjacent to the cells. These nerve endings are encountered more frequently in the papillae than elsewhere; moreover, tactile discs also are found in abundance in these areas. The number of genital corpuscles, which are considered the main structures that are mediators of erotic sensation, vary considerably. These structures are distributed sparsely and randomly in the labia majora deep in the corium, but in the labia minora there are a great number of these corpuscles, particularly in the prepuce and skin that overlies the glans clitoris.

Vestibule

The vestibule is an almond-shaped area that is enclosed by the labia minora laterally and extends from the clitoris above to the fourchet below. The vestibule is the functionally mature female structure of the urogenital sinus of the embryo; in the mature state it usually is perforated by six openings: the urethra, the vagina, the ducts of the Bartholin glands, and, at times, the ducts of the paraurethral glands, also called Skene ducts and glands (Fig. 2-2). The posterior portion of the vestibule between the fourchet and the vaginal opening is called the *fossa navicularis*. Rarely is it observed except in nulliparous women, since usually it is obliterated as the result of childbirth.

Related to the vestibule are the *major vestibular glands,* i.e., the *Bartholin glands* (Fig. 2-2). These are a pair of small compound glands that are about 0.5 to 1 cm in diameter; each is situated beneath the vestibule on either side of the vaginal opening. The Bartholin glands lie under the constrictor muscle of the vagina and sometimes are found to be covered partially by the vestibular bulbs. The gland ducts are 1.5 to 2 cm long and open on the sides of the vestibule just outside the lateral margin of the vaginal orifice. The small lumina of the glands or-

dinarily admit only the finest of probes. At times of sexual arousal, mucoid material is secreted from these glands. The ducts sometimes harbor gonococci, or other bacteria, that may gain access to the gland, and cause suppuration and a Bartholin gland abscess.

Urethral Opening

The lower two thirds of the urethra lies immediately above the anterior vaginal wall and terminates externally in the urethral meatus. The urethral meatus is in the midline of the vestibule, 1 to 1.5 cm below the pubic arch, and a short distance above the vaginal opening; usually it is puckered in appearance. The orifice of the urethra appears as a vertical slit, which can be distended to 4 or 5 mm in diameter. Ordinarily, the *paraurethral ducts* open on the vestibule on either side of the urethra, but occasionally open on the posterior wall of the urethra just inside the meatus (Fig. 2-2). These ducts are of small caliber, about 0.5 mm in diameter, and of variable length. In the United States, the paraurethral ducts generally are known as Skene ducts.

Vestibular Bulbs

Beneath the mucous membrane of the vestibule on either side are the vestibular bulbs, which are almond-shaped aggregations of veins, 3 to 4 cm long, 1 to 2 cm wide, and 0.5 to 1 cm thick. These bulbs lie in close apposition to the ischiopubic rami and are partially covered by the ischiocavernosus and constrictor vaginae muscles. The lower terminations of the vestibular bulbs usually are at about the middle of the vaginal opening; and, anteriorly, these bulbs extend upward toward the clitoris.

Embryologically, the vestibular bulbs correspond to the anlage of the corpus spongiosum of the penis. The vestibular bulbs of women, during childbirth, usually are pushed up beneath the pubic arch; since the posterior ends partially encircle the vagina, however, these structures are liable to injury and rupture, which may give rise to a hematoma of the vulva or else to profuse hemorrhage.

Vaginal Opening and Hymen

The vaginal opening is in the lower portion of the vestibule and varies considerably in size and shape among women. In virginal women, it most often is hidden entirely by the overlapping labia minora, and when exposed, it usually appears almost completely closed by the membranous hymen.

Among women there are marked differences in shape and consistency of the hymen. This tissue is comprised mainly of connective tissue, both elastic and collagenous. Both the outer and inner surfaces are covered by stratified squamous epithelium. Connective tissue papillae are more numerous on the vaginal surface and at the free edge. According to Mahran and Saleh (1964),

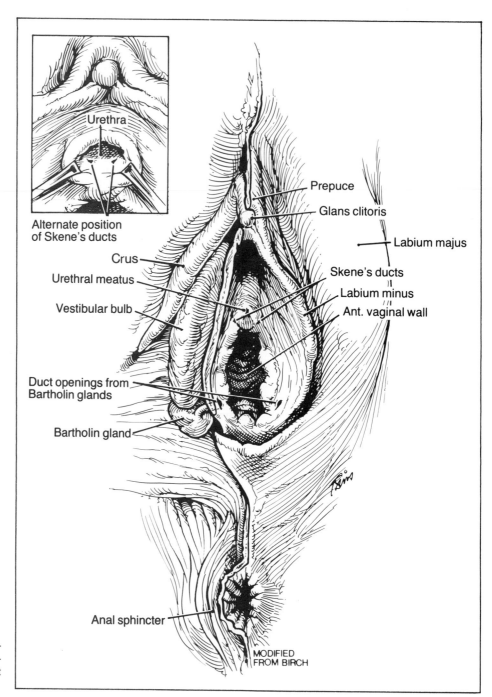

Urethra

Alternate position
of Skene's ducts

Crus

Urethral meatus

Vestibular bulb

Duct openings from
Bartholin glands

Bartholin gland

Anal sphincter

Prepuce

Glans clitoris

Labium majus

Skene's ducts

Labium minus

Ant. vaginal wall

MODIFIED
FROM BIRCH

Figure 2-2. The external genitalia with the skin and subcutaneous tissue removed from the right side.

there are no glandular or muscular elements in the hymen and it is not richly supplied with nerve fibers.

In the newborn, the hymen is very vascular and redundant; in pregnant women, the epithelium is thick and the tissue is rich in glycogen; after menopause, the epithelium of the hymen is thin and focal cornification may develop. In adult virginal women, the hymen is a membrane of various thickness that surrounds the vaginal opening more or less completely; among virginal women, the aperture of the hymen varies in diameter from that of a pinpoint to a caliber that admits the tip of one or

even two fingers. The hymenal opening usually is crescentic or circular, but occasionally may be cribriform, septate, or fimbriated. As the fimbriated type of hymen in virginal women may be mistaken for one that has been penetrated during intercourse, it is wise to exercise caution when making definite statements with regard to "rupture" of the hymen.

As a rule, the hymen is torn at several sites during first coitus, usually in the posterior portion. The edges of the torn tissue soon cicatrize, and the hymen becomes divided permanently into two or more portions that are separated by narrow sulci that extend down to its base. The extent to which rupture occurs varies with the structure of the hymen and the extent to which it is distended. Although commonly it is believed that rupture of the hymen is accompanied by bleeding, this is not the case or else is not evident in all women. Occasionally with hymenal rupture, however, there may be profuse bleeding. Rarely, the hymenal membrane may be very resistant to penetration or perforation and surgical incision of the tissue may be necessary before coitus can be accomplished.

The changes in the hymen that are brought about by coitus are occasionally of medico-legal importance, especially in instances of alleged rape, in which the physician is called upon to examine the victim and to testify concerning the physical findings. In virgins who are examined a few hours after the alleged sexual attack, the finding of fresh hymenal lacerations or abrasions, or the finding of bleeding points on the hymen constitute corroborative evidence of recent vaginal penetration, possibly by intercourse. The absence of such findings is of no significance, however, since the hymen may not be lacerated even with repeated coitus in a short time period. In fact, many cases of pregnancy have been reported in women in whom the hymen did not appear to have been "ruptured."

As a rule, the changes produced in the hymen by childbirth are readily recognizable. After the puerperium, several cicatrized nodules of various sizes are formed, the tissue remnants of the hymen, the *myrtiform caruncles*.

Imperforate hymen, a rare lesion, is a condition in which the vaginal orifice is occluded completely, causing retention of the menstrual discharge.

Vagina

The vagina is a tubular, musculomembranous structure that extends from the vulva to the uterus; the vagina is interposed anteriorly and posteriorly between the urinary bladder and the rectum (Fig. 2-3). The vagina is an organ of many functions: the excretory canal of the uterus, through which uterine secretions and menstrual flow escape; the female organ of copulation; and, part of the birth canal at the time of childbirth. The upper portion of the vagina in women arises from the müllerian ducts; the lower portion is formed from the urogenital sinus. Anteriorly, the vagina is in contact with the bladder and urethra, from which it is separated by connective tissue that often is referred to as the vesicovaginal septum. Posteriorly, that is, between the lower portion of the vagina and the rectum, there are

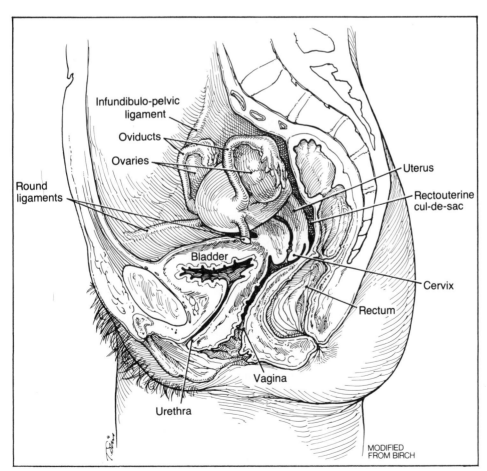

Infundibulo-pelvic ligament

Oviducts

Ovaries

Round ligaments

Bladder

Uterus

Rectouterine cul-de-sac

Cervix

Rectum

Vagina

Urethra

MODIFIED FROM BIRCH

Figure 2-3. Sagittal section of the pelvis of an adult woman that is illustrative of relations of pelvic viscera.

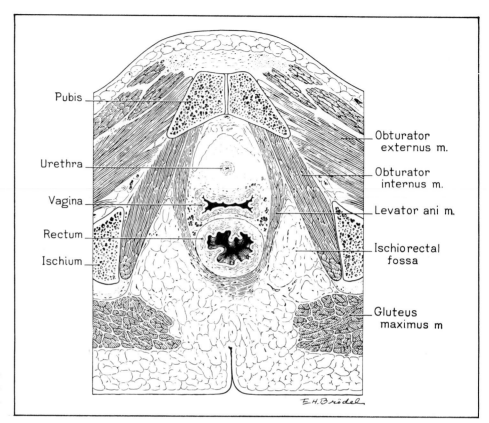

Figure 2-4. Cross-section of the pelvis of an adult woman; the H-shaped lumen of the vagina is apparent (m. = muscle).

similar tissues that, together, form the rectovaginal septum. Usually, the upper one fourth of the vagina is separated from the rectum by the rectouterine pouch, or, as it is sometimes called, the cul-de-sac of Douglas.

Normally, the anterior and posterior walls of the vagina lie in contact with only a slight space that intervenes between the lateral margins. Thus, when not distended, the vaginal canal on transverse section is H-shaped (Fig. 2-4). The vagina can be distended markedly, a characteristic that is most evident during childbirth.

The upper end of the vagina is the termination of a vault into which the lower portion of the uterine cervix projects. The vaginal vault is subdivided into the anterior, posterior, and two lateral fornices. Since the vagina is attached higher up on the posterior wall than on the anterior wall of the cervix, the depth of the posterior fornix is appreciably greater than the anterior. The lateral fornices are intermediate in depth. The fornices are of considerable clinical importance since the internal pelvic organs usually can be palpated through the thin walls of the fornices. Moreover, by way of the posterior fornix, there usually is provided ready surgical access to the peritoneal cavity. Among women, the vagina varies considerably in length. Commonly, the anterior and posterior vaginal walls are, respectively, 6 to 8 cm, and 7 to 10 cm in length.

Prominent longitudinal ridges project into the va-

ginal lumen from the midlines of both the anterior and posterior walls. In nulliparous women, these numerous transverse ridges, or *rugae,* extend outward from, and almost at right angles to, the longitudinal vaginal ridges. The rugae gradually recede as the lateral walls are approached. The rugae are such as to form a corrugated surface, which is not present before menarche and is one that gradually becomes obliterated after repeated childbirth and after menopause. In elderly multiparous women, the vaginal walls often are smooth.

The mucosa of the vagina (Fig. 2-5) is comprised of noncornified stratified squamous epithelium. Beneath the epithelium there is a thin fibromuscular coat; usually, there is an inner circular layer and an outer longitudinal layer of smooth muscle that can be identified. There is a thin layer of connective tissue that overlies the mucosa and the muscularis, one that is rich in blood vessels, and one in which there are a few small lymphoid nodules. The mucosa and muscularis are attached very loosely to the underlying connective tissue, and, by surgical means, these tissues are easily dissected free. Some argument remains as to whether this connective tissue, which sometimes is referred to as perivaginal endopelvic fascia, is a definite fascial plane in the strict anatomic sense.

Normally, glands are not present in the vagina. In parous women, however, fragments of stratified epithelium, which sometimes give rise to cysts, are occasionally embedded in the vaginal connective tissue. These va-

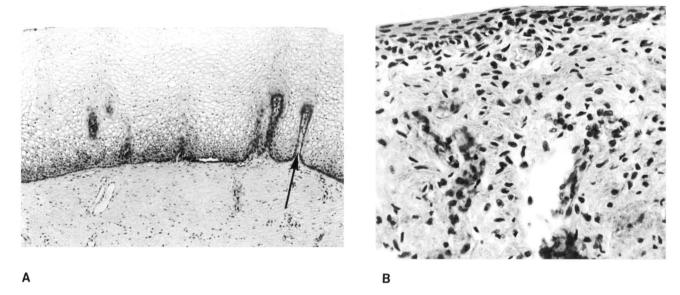

A   B

Figure 2-5. A. Photomicrograph of the vagina of an adult woman that is characterized by noncornified, thick, stratified squamous epithelium; note that epithelial appendages are not present. Arrow is pointed to a papilla. **B.** Photomicrograph of typical thin vaginal epithelium of a prepubertal girl.

ginal inclusion cysts are not glands; rather, these are remnants of mucosal tags that were buried during the repair of vaginal lacerations after childbirth. Other cysts that are lined by columnar or cuboidal epithelium may be found; these are believed to be derived from embryonic remnants.

From early in infancy until after menopause, there is a considerable amount of glycogen in the cells of the superficial layer of the vaginal mucosa. By examination of cells that are exfoliated from the vaginal epithelium, one can identify the various hormonal events of the ovarian cycle.

In nonpregnant women, the vagina is kept moist by a small amount of secretion from the uterus. During pregnancy, there is copious vaginal secretion, which normally consists of a curdlike product of exfoliated epithelium and bacteria, which is markedly acidic. Bacilli are the predominant bacteria of the vagina during pregnancy, although cocci also are found. The acidic reaction is attributable to the presence of lactic acid, which arises from the metabolism of glycogen from the cells in the mucosa by Lactobacilli. The pH of the vaginal secretion varies with the nature of the ovarian hormones that are secreted. Before puberty, the pH of the secretions of the vagina varies between 6.8 and 7.2, whereas in adult women it is well below this, and typically ranges from 4.0 to 5.0.

There is an abundant vascular supply to the vagina; the upper third is supplied by the cervicovaginal branches of the uterine arteries, the middle third by the inferior vesical arteries, and the lower third by the middle hemorrhoidal and internal pudendal arteries. There is an extensive venous plexus that immediately sur-

rounds the vagina, vessels from which follow the course of the arteries; eventually, these veins empty into the hypogastric veins. For the most part, the lymphatics from the lower third of the vagina, along with those of the vulva, drain into the inguinal lymph nodes, those from the middle third into the hypogastric nodes, and those from the upper third into the iliac nodes. The vaginas of women, according to Krantz (1958), are devoid of any special nerve endings (genital corpuscles); occasionally, however, free nerve endings are found in the papillae.

The Perineum

The many structures that make up the perineum are illustrated in Figure 2-6. Most of the support of the perineum is provided by the pelvic and urogenital diaphragms. The *pelvic diaphragm* consists of the levator ani muscles plus the coccygeus muscles posteriorly and the fascial coverings of these muscles. The levator ani muscles form a broad muscular sling that originates from the posterior surface of the superior rami of the pubis, from the inner surface of the ischial spine, and between these two sites, from the obturator fascia. The muscle fibers are inserted in several locations as follow: around the vagina and rectum to form efficient functional sphincters for each; into a raphe in the midline between the vagina and rectum; into a midline raphe below the rectum; and, into the coccyx. The *urogenital diaphragm* is positioned external to the pelvic diaphragm, i.e., in the triangular area between the ischial tuberosities and the symphysis pubis. The urogenital diaphragm is comprised of the deep transverse perineal

14

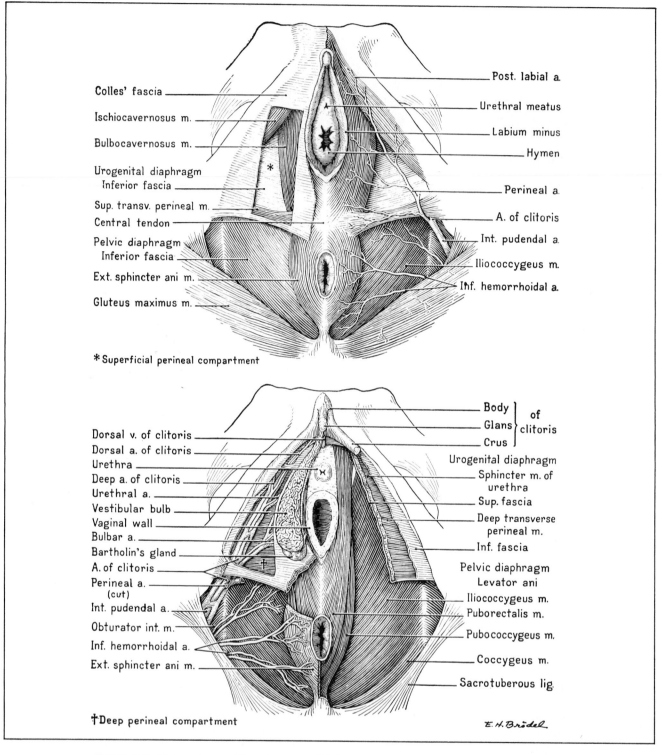

Colles' fascia

Ischiocavernosus m.

Bulbocavernosus m.

Urogenital diaphragm
Inferior fascia

Sup. transv. perineal m.

Central tendon

Pelvic diaphragm
Inferior fascia

Ext. sphincter ani m.

Gluteus maximus m.

Post. labial a.

Urethral meatus

Labium minus

Hymen

Perineal a.

A. of clitoris

Int. pudendal a.

Iliococcygeus m.

Inf. hemorrhoidal a.

*Superficial perineal compartment

Dorsal v. of clitoris

Dorsal a. of clitoris

Urethra

Deep a. of clitoris

Urethral a.

Vestibular bulb

Vaginal wall

Bulbar a.

Bartholin's gland

A. of clitoris

Perineal a.
(cut)

Int. pudendal a.

Obturator int. m.

Inf. hemorrhoidal a.

Ext. sphincter ani m.

Body ⎤
Glans ⎬ of clitoris
Crus ⎦

Urogenital diaphragm

Sphincter m. of urethra

Sup. fascia

Deep transverse perineal m.

Inf. fascia

Pelvic diaphragm
Levator ani

Iliococcygeus m.

Puborectalis m.

Pubococcygeus m.

Coccygeus m.

Sacrotuberous lig.

†Deep perineal compartment

E. H. Brödel

Figure 2-6. The perineum. The more superficial components are illustrated above and the deeper structures below (m. = muscle; a. = artery; lig. = ligament; Int. = internal; Ext. = external; Inf. = inferior).

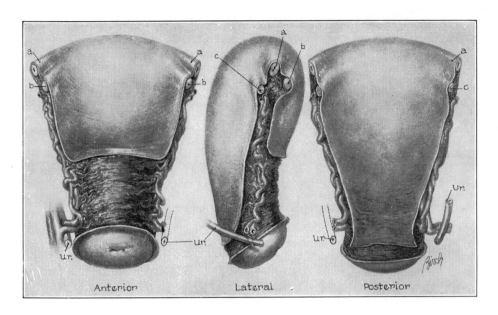

Figure 2-7. Anterior, right lateral, and posterior views of the uterus of an adult woman; a, oviduct; b, round ligament; c, ovarian ligament; Ur. = ureter.

muscles, the constrictor of the urethra, and the internal and external fascial coverings.

Perineal Body

The median raphe of the levator ani, which is positioned between the anus and the vagina, is reinforced by the central tendon of the perineum, on which converge the bulbocavernosus muscles, the superficial transverse perineal muscles, and the external anal sphincter. These structures, which contribute to the perineal body and provide much of the support for the perineum, often are lacerated during delivery unless an adequate episiotomy is made at an appropriate time (Chapter 17, p. 347).

INTERNAL GENERATIVE ORGANS

Uterus

The uterus is a muscular organ that is covered, partially, by peritoneum, or serosa. The cavity of the uterus is lined by the endometrium. During pregnancy, the uterus serves for reception, implantation, retention, and nutrition of the conceptus, which it then expels during labor.

Anatomic Relationships. The uterus of the nonpregnant woman is situated in the pelvic cavity between the bladder anteriorly and the rectum posteriorly. The inferior portion, i.e., the cervix, projects into the vagina. Almost the entire posterior wall of the uterus is covered by serosa, or peritoneum, the lower portion of which forms the anterior boundary of the *rectouterine cul-de-sac,* or pouch of Douglas. Only the upper portion of the anterior wall of the uterus is so covered (Fig. 2-7). The lower portion is united to the posterior wall of the bladder by a well-defined but normally loose layer of connective tissue (Figs. 2-3, 2-8).

Size and Shape. The uterus is a structure that resembles a flattened pear in shape (Figs. 2-7, 2-8) and consists of two major but unequal parts: an upper triangular portion, i.e., the *body* (or *corpus*) and a lower, cylindric, or fusiform portion, i.e., the *cervix*. The anterior surface of the body of the uterus is almost flat, whereas the posterior surface is distinctly convex. The oviducts, or fallopian tubes, emerge from the *cornua* of the uterus at the junction of the superior and lateral margins. The convex upper segment between the points of insertion of the fallopian tubes is called the *fundus uteri*. The lateral margins extend from the cornua on either side to the pelvic floor. Laterally, the portion of the uterus below the insertion of the fallopian tubes is not covered directly by peritoneum, but it is the site of the attachments of the broad ligaments.

Among women, there are marked variations in size and shape of the uterus that vary with age and parity. Before puberty, the organ varies in length from 2.5 to 3.5 cm. The uterus of adult nulliparous women is from 6 to 8 cm in length as compared with 9 to 10 cm in multiparous women (Fig. 2-8). Uteri of nonparous and parous women also differ considerably in weight; normally, the former weighs from 50 to 70 g, and the latter weighs 80 g or somewhat more (Langlois, 1970). The relationship between the length of the body of the uterus and that of the cervix likewise varies widely. In the young girl, the body of the uterus is only half as long as the cervix; in nulliparous women, the two are about equal in length; in multiparous women, the cervix is only a little more than one third of the total length of the organ (Fig. 2-8).

The great bulk of the body of the uterus, but not the cervix, is comprised of muscle. The inner surface of the anterior and posterior walls of the uterus lie almost in contact; the cavity between these walls forms a mere slit (Figs. 2-8, 2-9). The cervical canal is fusiform and is open at each end by small apertures, i.e., the *internal os* and the *external os*. On frontal section, the cavity of the

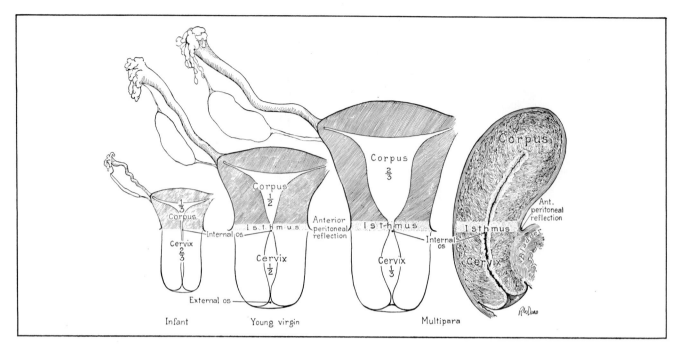

Figure 2-8. Comparison of the size of uteri of prepubertal girls and adult nonparous and parous women by frontal and sagittal sections.

body of the uterus is triangular, whereas that of the cervix is fusiform in shape. The margins of the uteri of women who have borne children become concave instead of convex, and hence the triangular appearance of the uterine cavity is less pronounced. After menopause, the size of the uterus decreases as a consequence of atrophy of the myometrium and the endometrium also is atrophic.

The *isthmus* (Fig. 2-8) is of special obstetric significance because, in pregnancy, it is essential to the formation of the lower uterine segment (see Chapter 15, p. 308).

Uterine Cervix

The cervix is the specialized portion of the uterus that is below the isthmus. Anteriorly, the upper boundary of the cervix, the internal os, corresponds, approximately, to the level at which the peritoneum is reflected upon the bladder.

The cervix is divided by the attachment of the vagina into vaginal and supravaginal portions. The supravaginal segment on its posterior surface is covered by peritoneum. Laterally, it is attached to the cardinal ligaments; and, anteriorly, it is separated from the overlying bladder by loose connective tissue. The external os is located at the lower extremity of the vaginal portion of the cervix, i.e., the *portio vaginalis.*

Among women, the external os of the cervix varies greatly in appearance; before childbirth, it is a small, regular, oval opening; after childbirth, the orifice is converted into a transverse slit that is divided such that there are the so-called anterior and posterior lips of the

cervix. If the cervix were torn deeply during delivery, it might heal in such a manner that it appears to be irregular, nodular, or stellate. These changes are sufficiently characteristic to permit an examiner to ascertain with some certainty whether a given woman has borne children by vaginal delivery (Figs. 2-10, 2-11).

The cervix is composed of some smooth muscle fibers, but predominantly of collagenous tissue plus elastic tissue and blood vessels. The transition from the primarily collagenous tissue of the cervix to the primarily muscular tissue of the body of the uterus, although gen-

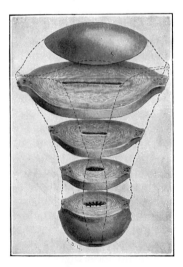

Figure 2-9. Reconstruction of the uterus to illustrate the shape of the uterine cavity.

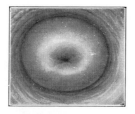

Figure 2-10. Cervical external os of a nonparous woman.

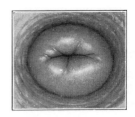

Figure 2-11. Cervical external os of a parous woman.

erally abrupt, may be gradual, and may extend over as much as 10 mm. The results of studies by Danforth and colleagues (1960) are suggestive that the physical properties of the cervix are determined, in large measure, by the state of the connective tissue, and that during pregnancy and labor the remarkable ability of the cervix to dilate is the result of dissociation of collagen. Buckingham and co-workers (1965) quantified the amount of muscle and collagen in the tissue of the cervix of women. In the normal cervix, the proportion of muscle is, on average, about 10 percent, whereas in "incompetent" cervices, the proportion of muscle is appreciably greater.

Characteristically, the mucosa of the cervical canal, although embryologically a direct continuation of the endometrium, is differentiated in such a way that the appearance of sections through the canal are reminiscent of a honeycomb. The mucosa is composed of a single layer of very high, columnar epithelium that rests upon a thin basement membrane. The oval nuclei are situated near the base of the columnar cells, the upper portions of which appear to be rather clear because of the content of mucus. These cells are supplied abundantly with cilia.

There are numerous cervical glands that extend from the surface of the endocervical mucosa directly into the subjacent connective tissue; since there is no submucosa as such, these glands furnish the thick, tenacious secretion of the cervical canal. If the ducts of the cervical glands are occluded, retention cysts may form, which are a few millimeters in diameter, the so-called *nabothian follicles* or *nabothian cysts.*

Normally, the squamous epithelium of the vaginal portion of the cervix and the columnar epithelium of the cervical canal form a sharp line of division very near the external os, i.e., the squamo-columnar junction. In response to inflammation or trauma, however, the stratified epithelium may extend gradually up the cervical canal and come to line the lower third, or occasionally even the lower half, of the canal. This change is more marked in the cervices of multiparous women, in whom the lips of the cervix often are everted. Uncommonly, the two varieties of epithelium abut on the vaginal portion outside the external os, as in *congenital ectropion.*

Changes in the characteristics of the cervical mucosa are dependent upon the variations in the hormonal patterns of the ovarian cycle, as discussed in Chapter 4 (p. 72).

Body of the Uterus

The wall of the body of the uterus is composed of three layers: the serosal, the muscular, and the mucosal. The serosal layer is formed by the peritoneum that covers the uterus, and to which it is firmly adherent except at sites just above the bladder and at the lateral margins where the peritoneum is deflected in a manner to form the broad ligaments.

Endometrium. The innermost portion of the uterus, or mucosal layer, that lines the uterine cavity in nonpregnant women, is the *endometrium*. It is a thin, pink, velvet-like membrane, which on close examination is found to be perforated by a large number of minute openings; these are the ostia of the uterine glands. Because of the repetitive cyclic changes that occur during the reproductive years of a woman's life, the endometrium normally varies greatly in thickness and measures from 0.5 mm to as much as 5 mm. The endometrium is comprised of surface epithelium, glands, and interglandular mesenchymal tissue in which there are numerous blood vessels.

The epithelium of the endometrial surface is comprised of a single layer of closely packed, high columnar, ciliated cells. During much of the endometrial cycle, the oval nuclei are situated in the lower portions of the cells but not so near the base as in the endocervix.

Cilia have been demonstrated in the cells of the endometria of many mammals; the ciliated cells are located in discrete patches, whereas secretory activity appears to be limited to nonciliated cells. The ciliary current in both the fallopian tubes and the uterus is in the same direction and extends downward from the fimbriated end of the tubes toward the external os.

The tubular *uterine glands* are invaginations of the epithelium, which, in the resting state, are reminiscent of the fingers of a glove. The glands extend through the entire thickness of the endometrium to the myometrium, which is occasionally penetrated for a short distance. Histologically, the inner glands resemble the epithelium of the surface and are lined by a single layer of columnar, partially ciliated epithelium that rests upon a thin basement membrane. The glands secrete a thin alkaline fluid that serves to keep the uterine cavity moist (see Figs. 4-3, 4-4).

In the classic monograph of Hitschmann and Adler, published in 1908, it was reported that the endometrium undergoes constant, hormonally controlled changes dur-

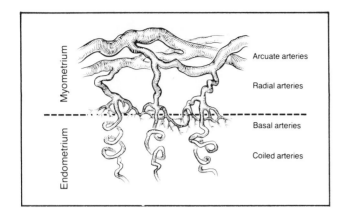

Figure 2-12. Stereographic representation of myometrial and endometrial arteries in the macaque. Above are shown parts of myometrial arcuate arteries from which myometrial radial arteries course toward the endometrium. Below are shown the larger endometrial coiled arteries and the smaller endometrial basal arteries. (*From Okkels and Engle: Acta Pathol Microbiol Scand 15:150, 1938.*)

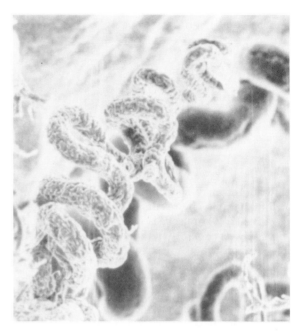

Figure 2-13. Corrosion cast of the complexly branching endometrial capillary network of the upper compact layer of a Rhesus monkey on the 25th day of the menstrual cycle × 400. (*From Ferenczy and Richart: Female Reproductive System: Dynamics of Scan and Transmission Electron Microscopy. New York, Wiley, 1974.*)

ing each ovarian cycle. These three fundamental phases—*menstrual, proliferative (follicular)*, and *secretory (luteal)*—are discussed in detail in Chapter 4 in the section on menstruation. In brief, immediately after menstruation the endometrium is normally quite thin, and the tubular glands are well separated. Thereafter, the endometrium rapidly increases in thickness and, before the next menses, usually contains many convoluted or sacculated glands. After menopause, the endometrium is atrophic: the epithelium flattens, the glands gradually disappear, and the interglandular tissue becomes more fibrous.

The connective tissue of the endometrium, between the surface epithelium and the myometrium, is a mesenchymal stroma. Immediately after menstruation, the stroma is comprised of closely packed cells with oval and spindle-shaped nuclei, around which there is very little cytoplasm. When separated by edema, the cells appear to be stellate, with cytoplasmic processes that branch to form anastomoses. These cells are packed more closely around the glands and blood vessels than elsewhere. Several days before menstruation, the stromal cells usually become larger and more vesicular, like decidual cells; and, at the same time, there is a diffuse leukocytic infiltration.

The vascular architecture of the endometrium is of signal importance in the phenomena of menstruation and pregnancy. Arterial blood is transported to the uterus by way of the uterine and ovarian arteries. As the arterial branches penetrate the uterine wall obliquely inward and reach its middle third, these vessels ramify in a plane that is parallel to the surface and thence these vessels are named the *arcuate arteries*. Radial branches extend from the arcuate arteries at right angles toward the endometrium. The endometrial arteries are comprised of *coiled* or *spiral arteries*, which are a continua-

tion of the radial arteries, and *basal arteries*, which branch from the radial arteries at a sharp angle, as illustrated in Figures 2-12 and 2-13. The coiled arteries supply most of the midportion and all of the superficial third of the endometrium. It has been shown by several criteria that the walls of these vessels are responsive, i.e., sensitive, to the action of hormones, especially by vasoconstriction, and thus probably serve an important role in the mechanism(s) of menstruation as described in Chapter 4 (p. 68). The straight basal endometrial arteries are smaller in both caliber and length than are the coiled vessels. These vessels extend only into the basal layer of the endometrium, or at most a short distance into the middle layer, and are not responsive to hormonal action.

Myometrium. The major portion of the uterus, i.e., the myometrium, is comprised of bundles of smooth muscle that are united by connective tissue in which there are many elastic fibers. According to Schwalm and Dubrauszky (1966), the number of muscle fibers of the uterus progressively diminishes caudally such that in the cervix, muscle is only 10 percent of the tissue mass. In the inner wall of the body of the uterus, there is relatively more muscle than in the outer layers, and in the anterior and posterior walls, there is more muscle than in the lateral walls. During pregnancy, the myometrium, through hypertrophy primarily, increases greatly but there is no significant change in the muscle content of the cervix. The anatomic changes that occur in the myometrium during pregnancy are presented in detail in Chapter 9.

Ligaments of the Uterus

The broad, the round, and the uterosacral ligaments extend from either side of the uterus. The *broad ligaments* are comprised of two winglike structures that extend from the lateral margins of the uterus to the pelvic walls and thereby divide the pelvic cavity into anterior and posterior compartments. Each broad ligament consists of a fold of peritoneum in which there are enclosed various structures and of which there are superior, lateral, inferior, and medial margins. The inner two thirds of the superior margin form the *mesosalpinx,* to which the oviducts, i.e., fallopian tubes, are attached. The outer third of the superior margin of the broad ligament, which extends from the fimbriated end of the oviduct to the pelvic wall, forms the *infundibulopelvic ligament* (suspensory ligament of the ovary), through which the ovarian vessels traverse.

At the lateral margin of each broad ligament, the peritoneum is reflected onto the side of the pelvis. The base of the broad ligament, which is quite thick, is con-

tinuous with the connective tissue of the pelvic floor. The densest portion—referred to as the *cardinal ligament,* the transverse cervical ligament, or Mackenrodt ligament—is composed of connective tissue that medially is united firmly to the supravaginal portion of the cervix. In the base of the broad ligament, the uterine vessels and the lower portion of the ureter are enclosed.

A vertical section through the uterine end of the broad ligament is triangular; the uterine vessels are found within its broad base (Fig. 2-14). In its lower part, it is widely attached to the connective tissues that are adjacent to the cervix, i.e., the *parametrium.* The upper part is comprised of three folds that, in turn, nearly cover the oviduct, the utero-ovarian ligament, and the round ligament.

The *round ligaments* extend on either side from the lateral portion of the uterus; these ligaments arise somewhat below and anterior to that of the origin of the oviducts. Each round ligament is located in a fold of peritoneum that is continuous with the broad ligament and extends outward and downward to the inguinal canal, through which it passes to terminate in the upper portion of the labium majus. In nonpregnant women, the round ligament varies from 3 to 5 mm in diameter, and

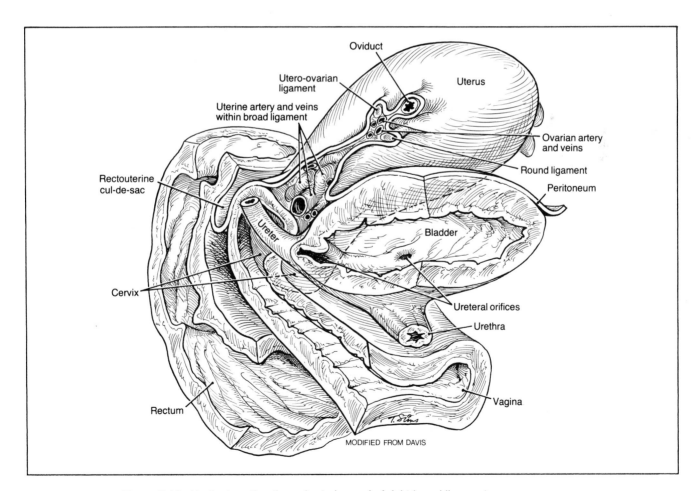

Figure 2-14. Vertical section through uterine end of right broad ligament.

is comprised of smooth muscle cells that are continuous directly with those of the uterine wall and a certain amount of connective tissue. The round ligament corresponds, embryologically, to the gubernaculum testis of men. During pregnancy, the round ligaments undergo considerable hypertrophy and increase appreciably in both length and diameter.

Each *uterosacral ligament* extends from an attachment posterolaterally to the supravaginal portion of the cervix to encircle the rectum, and thence insert into the fascia over the second and third sacral vertebrae. The uterosacral ligaments are comprised of connective tissue and some smooth muscle and are covered by peritoneum. These ligaments form the lateral boundaries of the rectouterine cul-de-sac, or pouch of Douglas, and are of some importance in retaining the body of the uterus in its usual anterior position by traction that is exerted posteriorly upon the cervix.

Position. When nonpregnant women are standing upright, the body of the uterus most often is almost horizontal and is flexed somewhat anteriorly and the fundus is resting upon the bladder, whereas the cervix is directed backward toward the tip of the sacrum with the external os approximately at the level of the ischial spines. The position of the body of the uterus is variable as a function of the degree of distension of the bladder or rectum or both.

Normally, the uterus is a partially mobile organ; whereas the cervix is anchored, the body of the uterus is free to move in the anteroposterior plane. Therefore, posture and gravity are factors that influence the position of the uterus.

Blood Vessels. The vascular supply of the uterus is derived principally from the uterine and ovarian arteries. The uterine artery, a main branch of the hypogastric artery (Fig. 2-15A–G), descends for a short distance, enters the base of the broad ligament, and makes its way medially to the side of the uterus. In so doing, it crosses anterior to the ureter, as described subsequently. Immediately adjacent to the supravaginal portion of the cervix, the uterine artery is divided into two main branches. The smaller cervicovaginal artery supplies blood to the lower portion of the cervix and the upper portion of the vagina. The main branch turns abruptly upward and extends thereafter as a highly convoluted vessel that traverses along the margin of the uterus; a branch of considerable size extends to the upper portion of the cervix and numerous other branches penetrate the body of the uterus. Just before the main branch of the uterine artery reaches the oviduct, it is divided into three terminal branches: fundal, tubal, and ovarian. The ovarian branch of the uterine artery anastomoses with the terminal branch of the ovarian artery; the tubal branch makes its way through the mesosalpinx and supplies part of the blood supply to the oviduct; the fundal branch is distributed to the uppermost portion of the uterus.

About 2 cm lateral to the cervix, the uterine artery crosses over the ureter, as shown in Figures 2-7, 2-15, and 2-16. The proximity of the uterine artery and uterine vein to the ureter at this point is of great surgical significance because, during hysterectomy, the ureter may be injured or ligated in the process of clamping and ligating the uterine vessels.

The *ovarian artery,* a direct branch of the aorta, enters the broad ligament through the infundibulopelvic ligament. At the ovarian hilum, it is divided into a number of smaller branches that enter the ovary, whereas the main stem of the ovarian artery traverses the entire length of the broad ligament very near the mesosalpinx and makes its way to the upper portion of the lateral margin of the uterus, where it anastomoses with the ovarian branch of the uterine artery. There are numerous additional communications among the arteries on both sides of the uterus.

When the uterus is in a contracted state, the lumina of its veins, which are in abundance, are collapsed; however, in injected specimens the greater part of the uterine wall appears to be occupied by dilated venous sinuses. On either side, the arcuate veins unite to form the *uterine vein,* which empties into the hypogastric vein and thence into the common iliac vein.

Some of the blood from the upper part of the uterus and blood from the ovary and upper part of the broad ligament is collected by several veins that, within the broad ligament, form the large *pampiniform plexus,* the vessels from which terminate in the ovarian vein. The right ovarian vein empties into the vena cava, whereas the left ovarian vein empties into the left renal vein.

Lymphatics. The endometrium is abundantly supplied with lymphatics, but true lymphatic vessels are confined largely to the basal layer. The lymphatics of the underlying myometrium are increased in number toward the serosal surface and form an abundant lymphatic plexus just beneath it, especially on the posterior wall of the uterus and, to a lesser extent, on the anterior wall.

The lymphatics from the various segments of the uterus drain into several sets of lymph nodes. Those from the cervix terminate mainly in the hypogastric nodes, which are situated near the bifurcation of the common iliac vessels between the external iliac and hypogastric arteries. The lymphatics from the body of the uterus are distributed to two groups of nodes. One set of vessels drains into the hypogastric nodes; the other set, after joining certain lymphatics from the ovarian region, terminates in the periaortic lymph nodes.

Innervation. The nerve supply is derived principally from the sympathetic nervous system, but also partly from the cerebrospinal and parasympathetic systems. The parasympathetic system is represented on either side by the pelvic nerve, which is comprised of a few fibers that are derived from the second, third, and fourth sacral nerves; it loses its identity in the cervical ganglion of Frankenhaüser. The sympathetic system enters the

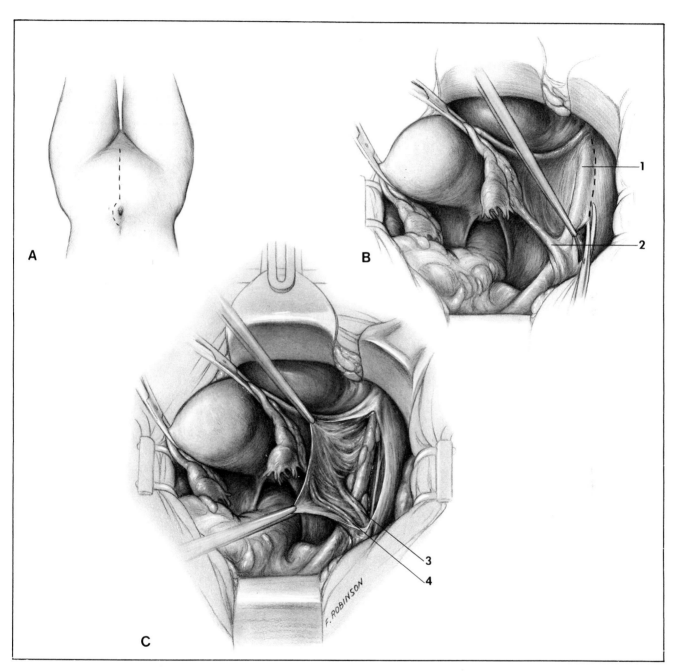

Figure 2-15 (A–C). Illustrated are the pelvic viscera as seen through a long midline incision **(A)** made in the lower abdomen. **B.** Retractors have been placed to spread the abdominal incision. The small intestine and omentum that overlie the pelvic contents have been displaced from the operative field. The oviducts, utero-ovarian ligaments, and round ligaments have been clamped bilaterally at their origin immediately adjacent to the uterus. Peritoneum just lateral to the right external iliac artery (1) is incised and the right infundibulopelvic ligament (2) is tensed by pulling the uterus to the left. **C.** The right broad ligament has been opened laterally. The right ureter (3) is now visible as it crosses the iliac vessels at the pelvic brim and courses medially and downward towards the cervix and bladder. The right ovarian artery and vein (4) are visible after dissection of the infundibulopelvic ligament.

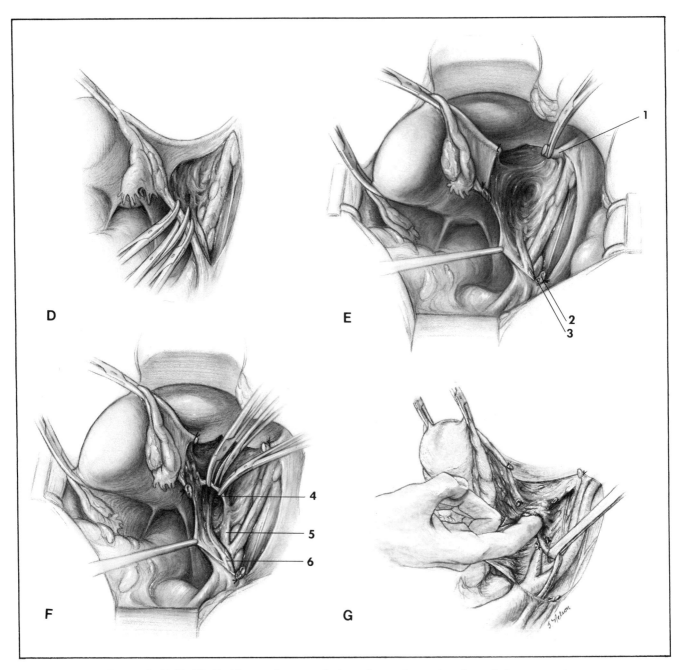

Figure 2-15 (D–G). D. The ovarian vessels have been clamped and are being severed. (From Nelson JH Jr. Atlas of Radical Pelvic Surgery, 2nd ed. New York, Appleton, 1977, p. 131.) **E.** The round ligament (1) and the ovarian vessels (2) have been ligated and severed. More of the ureter is visible (3). **F.** The origin of the right uterine artery (4) from the right hypogastric artery (5) is illustrated. Note the ureter (6) coursing beneath the uterine artery (4) just lateral to the junction of the cervix and body of the uterus. **G.** The operator's finger is in the paracervical ureteral tunnel through the right cardinal ligament just lateral to the supravaginal portion of the cervix. The ureter is being retracted laterally. (*From Nelson JH Jr. Atlas of Radical Pelvic Surgery, 2nd ed. New York, Appleton, 1977, p. 133.*)

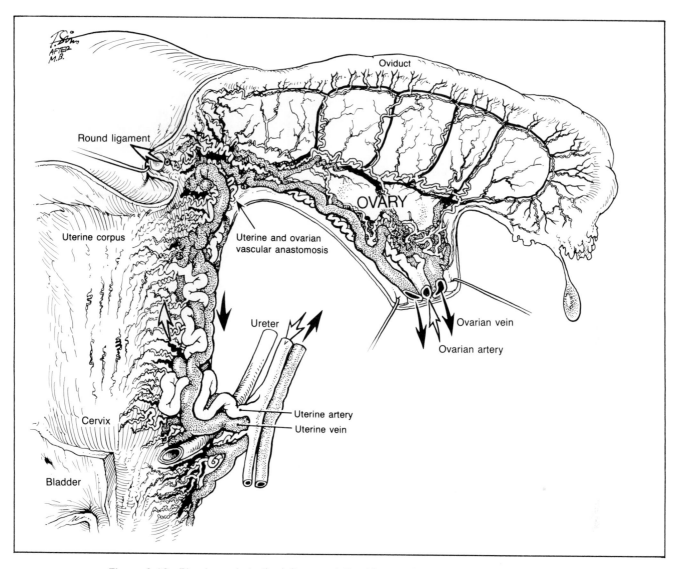

Figure 2-16. Blood supply to the left ovary, left oviduct, and the left side of the uterus. The ovarian and uterine vessels anastomose freely. Note the uterine artery and vein crossing over the ureter that lies immediately adjacent to the cervix.

pelvis by way of the hypogastric plexus that arises from the aortic plexus just below the promontory of the sacrum. After descending on either side, it also enters the uterovaginal plexus of Frankenhaüser, which is comprised of ganglia of various sizes, but particularly of a large ganglionic plate that is situated on either side of the cervix and just above the posterior fornix in front of the rectum.

Branches from these plexuses supply the uterus, bladder, and upper part of the vagina and are comprised of both myelinated and nonmyelinated fibers. Some of these fibers terminate freely between the muscular fibers, whereas others accompany the arteries into the endometrium.

In the eleventh and twelfth thoracic nerve roots, there are sensory fibers from the uterus that transmit the painful stimuli of uterine contractions to the central

nervous system of women. The sensory nerves from the cervix and upper part of the birth canal pass through the pelvic nerves to the second, third, and fourth sacral nerves, whereas those from the lower portion of the birth canal pass primarily through the pudendal nerve (Chapter 18).

Oviducts

The oviducts, or fallopian tubes, extend from the uterine cornua to a site near the ovaries and provide access for the ova to the uterine cavity. The oviducts vary from 8 to 14 cm in length, are covered by peritoneum, and the lumen is lined by mucous membrane. Each fallopian tube is divided into an *interstitial portion, isthmus, ampulla,* and *infundibulum.* The interstitial portion is embodied within the muscular wall of the uterus. Its course

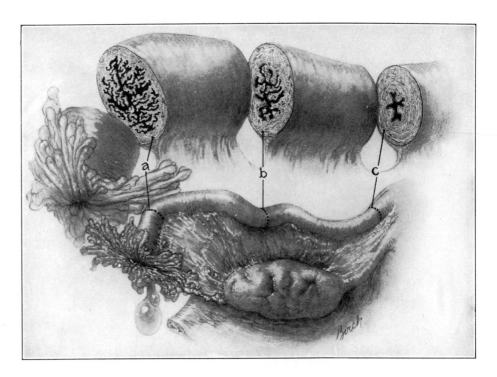

Figure 2-17. The oviduct of an adult woman with cross-sectioned illustrations of the gross structure of the epithelium in several portions: a, infundibulum; b, ampulla; c, isthmus.

is roughly obliquely upward and outward from the uterine cavity. The isthmus, or the narrow portion of the tube that adjoins the uterus, passes gradually into the wider, i.e., lateral portion, or *ampulla*. The *infundibulum,* or fimbriated extremity, is the funnel-shaped opening of the distal end of the fallopian tube (Fig. 2-17). The oviduct varies considerably in thickness; the narrowest portion of the isthmus measures from 2 to 3 mm in diameter and the widest portion of the ampulla measures between 5 to 8 mm. The oviduct is surrounded completely by peritoneum except at the attachment of the mesosalpinx.

The fimbriated end of the infundibulum opens into the abdominal cavity. One projection, the *fimbria ovarica,* which is considerably longer than the other fimbriae, forms a shallow gutter that approaches or reaches the ovary.

The musculature of the fallopian tube is arranged, in general, in two layers, an inner circular and an outer longitudinal layer. In the distal portion of the oviduct, the two layers are less distinct and, near the fimbriated extremity, are replaced by an interlacing network of muscular fibers. The tubal musculature undergoes rhythmic contractions constantly, the rate of which varies with the hormonal changes of the ovarian cycle. The greatest frequency and intensity of contractions is reached during transport of ova and are slowest and weakest during pregnancy.

The fallopian tube is lined by a mucous membrane, the epithelium of which is composed of a single layer of columnar cells, some of them ciliated and others secretory. The ciliated cells are most abundant at the fimbriated extremity; elsewhere, these cells are found in discrete patches. There are differences in the proportions of these two types of cells in different phases of the ovarian cycle. Since there is no submucosa, the epithelium is in close contact with the underlying muscle. In the tubal mucosa, there are cyclic histologic changes similar to, but much less striking than, those of the endometrium. The postmenstrual phase is characterized by a low epithelium that rapidly increases in height. During the follicular phase, the cells are taller, the ciliated elements are broad, with nuclei near the margin, and the nonciliated cells are narrow, with nuclei nearer the base. During the luteal phase, the secretory cells enlarge, project beyond the ciliated cells, and the nuclei are extruded. During the menstrual phase, these changes are even more marked. Changes in the fallopian tubes during late pregnancy and in the puerperium include the development of a low mucosa, plugging of the capillaries with leukocytes, and a decidual reaction.

The mucosa of the oviducts is arranged in longitudinal folds that are more complex toward the fimbriated end; consequently, the appearance of the lumen varies from one portion of the tube to another. On cross sections through the uterine portion, four simple folds are found that form a figure that resembles a Maltese cross. The isthmus is more complex; in the ampulla, the lumen is occupied almost completely by the arborescent mucosa, which consists of very complicated folds (Figs. 2-17, 2-18).

The current produced by the tubal cilia is such that the direction of flow is toward the uterine cavity; indeed, minute foreign bodies that are introduced into the abdominal cavities of animals may eventually appear in the vagina after these are transported through the tubes and the cavity of the uterus. Tubal peristalsis also is believed

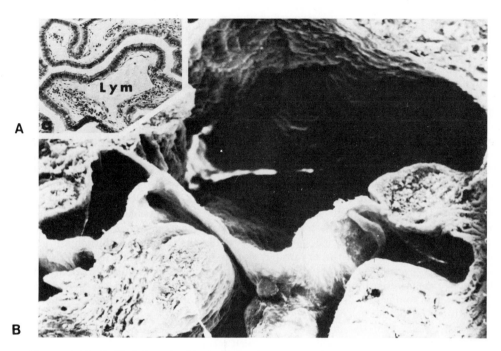

Figure 2-18. A. Fimbriae of oviduct. At the time of ovulation, the lymphatic vessels (Lym) in the lamina propria of the fimbria become greatly distended by the rapid accumulation of lymph. The dilatation of the lymphatic vasculature in the fimbriated end is believed to contribute to the fimbrial "erection" in grasping the ovary as follicles rupture at the time of ovulation (H & E stain, × 30). **B.** Fimbria of oviduct. Scanning electron micrograph of greatly dilated, labyrinthine lymphatic channels at the time of ovulation × 200. (*From Ferenczy and Richart: Female Reproductive System: Dynamics of Scan and Transmission Electron Microscopy. New York, Wiley, 1974.*)

to be an extraordinarily important factor in transport of the ovum.

The tubes are richly supplied with elastic tissue, blood vessels, and lymphatics. Sympathetic innervation of the tubes is extensive, in contrast to parasympathetic innervation. The role of these nerves in tubal function is poorly understood (Hodgson and Eddy, 1975).

Diverticula may extend occasionally from the lumen of the tube for a variable distance into the muscular wall and reach almost to the serosa. These diverticula may serve a role in the development of ectopic pregnancy (Chapter 22).

Pertinent gross anatomic, histologic, and ultrastructural information about the human oviduct is well summarized by Woodruff and Pauerstein (1969).

Embryologic Development of the Uterus and Oviducts. The uterus and the tubes arise from the müllerian ducts, which first appear near the upper pole of the urogenital ridge in the fifth week of development in embryos that are 10 to 11 mm long. This ridge is comprised of the mesonephros, the gonad, and associated ducts. The first indication of the development of the müllerian duct is a thickening of the coelomic epithelium at about the level of the fourth thoracic segment. This thickening becomes the fimbriated extremity (infundibulum) of the fallopian tube, which invaginates and grows

caudally to form a slender tube at the lateral edge of the urogenital ridge. In the sixth week of embryonic life, the growing tips of the two müllerian ducts approach each other in the midline and reach the sinus 1 week later (embryos of 30 mm). At that time, a fusion of the two müllerian ducts is begun at the level of the inguinal crest, or gubernaculum (primordium of the round ligament), to form a single canal. Thus, the upper ends of the müllerian ducts produce the oviducts and the fused parts give rise to the uterus. The uterine lumen from the fundus to the vagina is completed during the third month of fetal life. According to Koff (1933), the vaginal canal is not patent throughout its entire length until the sixth month of fetal life.

The Ovaries

The ovaries are almond-shaped organs, the functions of which are the development and extrusion of ova and the synthesis and secretion of steroid hormones. Among women, the ovaries vary considerably in size. During the childbearing years, the ovaries are 2.5 to 5 cm in length, 1.5 to 3 cm in breadth, and 0.6 to 1.5 cm in thickness. After menopause, the size of the ovary is diminished remarkably.

Normally, the ovaries are situated in the upper part of the pelvic cavity and rest in a slight depression on the lateral wall of the pelvis between the divergent external iliac and hypogastric vessels—the ovarian fossa of Waldeyer. When women are standing, the long axes of the ovaries are almost vertical, but become horizontal when women are supine. The position of the ovaries, however, is subject to marked variation, and it is rare to find both ovaries at exactly the same level.

The lateral surface of the ovary is in contact with the ovarian fossa whereas the medial surface is facing the uterus. The margin of the ovary that is attached to the mesovarium is more or less straight and is designated as the hilum, whereas the free margin is convex and is directed backward and inward toward the rectum.

The ovary is attached to the broad ligament by the *mesovarium*. The *utero-ovarian ligament* extends from the lateral and posterior portion of the uterus, just beneath the tubal insertion, to the uterine, i.e., the lower pole, of the ovary. Usually, it is several centimeters long and 3 to 4 mm in diameter. It is covered by peritoneum and is made up of muscle and connective tissue fibers that are continuous with those of the uterus. The *infundibulopelvic* or *suspensory ligament of the ovary* extends from the upper, or tubal, pole to the pelvic wall (Fig. 2-15B); through it course the ovarian vessels and nerves.

The exterior surface of the ovary varies in appearance with age. In young women, the organ is smooth, with a dull white surface through which glisten several small, clear follicles. As the woman grows older, the ovaries become more corrugated; in elderly women, the exterior surfaces may be convoluted markedly.

The general structure of the ovary can be studied best in cross sections, in which two portions may be distinguished, the *cortex* and the *medulla*. The cortex, or outer layer, varies in thickness with age and becomes thinner with advancing years. It is in this layer that the ova and graafian follicles are located. The cortex of the ovary is composed of spindle-shaped connective tissue cells and fibers, among which there are scattered primordial and graafian follicles that are in various stages of development. As the woman grows older, the follicles become less numerous. The outermost portion of the cortex, which is dull and whitish, is designated as the *tunica albuginea;* on its surface, there is a single layer of cuboidal epithelium, the germinal epithelium of Waldeyer.

The medulla, or central portion, of the ovary is composed of loose connective tissue that is continuous with that of the mesovarium. There are a large number of arteries and veins in the medulla and a small number of smooth muscle fibers that are continuous with those in the suspensory ligament; the muscle fibers may be functional in movements of the ovary.

Both sympathetic and parasympathetic nerves are supplied to the ovaries. The sympathetic nerves are derived, in large part, from the ovarian plexus that accompanies the ovarian vessels; a few are derived from the plexus that surrounds the ovarian branch of the uterine artery. The ovary is richly supplied with non-myelinated nerve fibers, which, for the most part, accompany the blood vessels. These are merely vascular nerves, whereas others form wreaths around normal and atretic follicles, and these give off many minute branches that have been traced up to, but not through, the membrana granulosa.

Development of the Ovary. The developmental changes in the human urogenital system have been described in ovaries from the third gestational week after conception to maturity. At first, the changes in the gonads are the same in both sexes. The earliest sign of a gonad is one that appears on the ventral surface of the embryonic kidney at a site between the eighth thoracic and fourth lumbar segments at about 4 weeks. As illustrated in Figure 2-19, the coelomic epithelium is thickened, and clumps of cells are seen to bud off into the underlying mesenchyme. This circumscribed area of the coelomic epithelium often is called the *germinal epithelium.* By the fourth to sixth week, however, there are many large ameboid cells in this region that have migrated into the body of the embryo from the yolk sac; these cells have been recognized in this region as early as the third week. These *primordial germ cells* are distinguishable by a large size and certain morphologic and cytochemical features. They react strongly in tests for alkaline phosphatase (McKay, Robinson, and Hertig, 1949), and are recognizable even after repeated divisions. Primordial germ cells have been studied in many animals. If they are destroyed before migration begins or prevented from reaching the genital area, a "gonad" that is lacking germ cells will develop.

When the primordial germ cells reach the genital area, some enter the germinal epithelium and others mingle with the groups of cells that proliferate from it or lie in the mesenchyme. By the end of the fifth week, rapid division of all these types of cells results in development of a prominent *genital ridge.* The ridge projects into the body cavity medially to a fold in which there are the mesonephric (wolffian) and the müllerian ducts (Fig. 2-20A–E). Since the growth of the gonad at the surface is more rapid, it enlarges centrifugally. By the seventh week (Figs. 2-19, 2-20), it is separated from the mesonephros except at the narrow central zone, the future hilum, where the blood vessels enter. At that time, the sexes can be distinguished since the testes can be recognized by well-defined radiating strands of cells (sex cords). These cords are separated from the germinal epithelium by mesenchyme that is to become the tunica albuginea. The sex cords, which consist of large germ cells and smaller epithelioid cells that are derived from the germinal epithelium, develop into the seminiferous tubules and tubuli reti. The rete, probably derived from mesonephric elements, establishes connection with the mesonephric tubules that develop into the epididymis (Fig. 2-20). The mesonephric ducts become the vas deferens.

In the female, the germinal epithelium continues to proliferate for a much longer time. The groups of cells

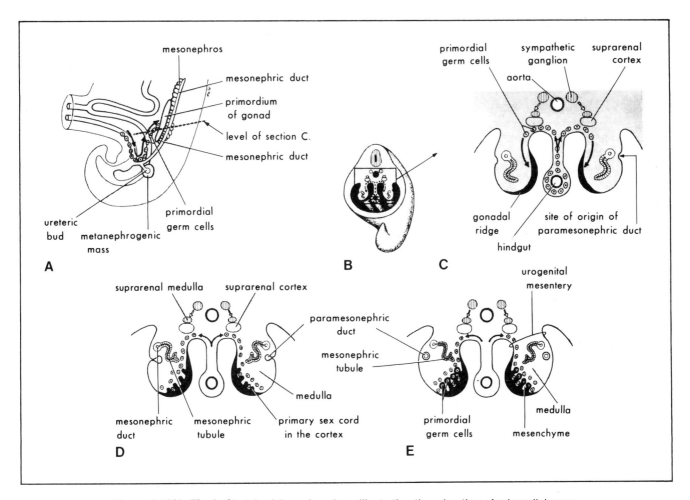

Figure 2-19(A–E). **A.** Sketch of 5-week embryo illustrating the migration of primordial germ cells. **B.** Three-dimensional sketch of the caudal region of a 5-week embryo showing the location and extent of the gonadal ridges on the medial aspect of the urogenital ridges. **C.** Transverse section showing the primordium of the adrenal glands, the gonadal ridges, and the migration of primordial germ cells. **D.** Transverse section through a 6-week embryo showing the primary sex cords and the developing paramesonephric ducts. **E.** Similar section at later stage showing the indifferent gonads and the mesonephric and paramesonephric ducts. (*From Moore K: The Developing Human. Philadelphia, Saunders, 1983.*)

thus formed lie at first in the region of the hilum. As connective tissue develops between them, these appear as sex cords. These give rise to the medullary cords and persist for variable times (Forbes, 1942). By the third month, medulla and cortex are defined, as illustrated in Figure 2-20. The bulk of the organ is comprised of cortex, a mass of crowded germ and epithelioid cells that show some signs of grouping, but there are no distinct cords as in the testis. Strands of cells extend from the germinal epithelium into the cortical mass, and mitoses are numerous. The rapid succession of mitoses soon reduces the size of the germ cells to the extent that these no longer are differentiated clearly from the neighboring cells; now, these cells are called *oogonia*. Some of the oogonia in the medullary region soon are distinguishable by a series of peculiar nuclear changes. Large masses of nuclear chromatin appear, very different from the chro-

mosomes of the oogonial divisions. This change marks the beginning of *synapsis,* which involves interactions between pairs of chromosomes that are derived originally from father and mother. Various stages of synapsis soon can be seen throughout the cortex; since similar changes occur in adjacent cells, groups (or "nests") appear. During one stage of synapsis, the chromatin is massed at one side of the nucleus, and the cytoplasm becomes highly fluid. Unless the in vitro preservation is prompt and perfect, these cells appear to be degenerating. Such artifacts frequently have been misinterpreted as evidence of widespread degeneration among oogonia.

By the fourth month, some germ cells, again in the medullary region, having passed through synapsis, begin to enlarge. These are called *primary oocytes* (Fig. 2-21) at the beginning of the phase of growth that continues

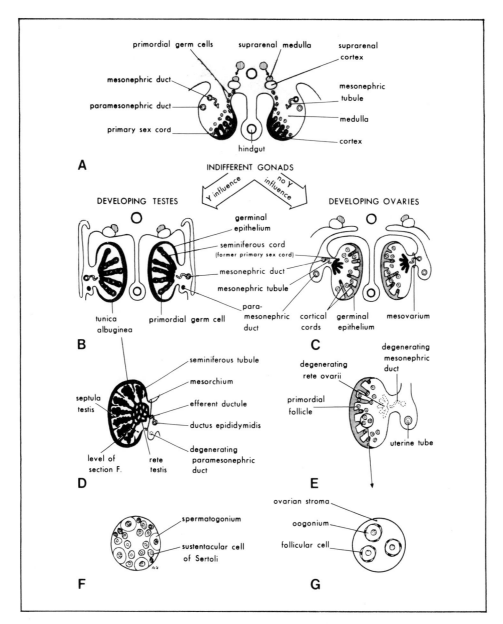

Figure 2-20(A–G). Schematic sections illustrating the differentiation of the indifferent gonads into testes or ovaries. **A.** Six weeks, showing the indifferent gonads that are comprised of an outer cortex and an inner medulla. **B.** Seven weeks, showing testes developing under the influence of a Y chromosome. Note that the primary sex cords have become seminiferous cords and that they are separated from the surface epithelium by the tunica albuginea. **C.** Twelve weeks, showing ovaries beginning to develop in the absence of Y chromosome influence. Cortical cords have extended from the surface epithelium, displacing the primary sex cords centrally into the mesovarium, where they form the rudimentary rete ovarii. **D.** Testis at 20 weeks, showing the rete testis and the seminiferous tubules derived from the seminiferous cords. An efferent ductule has developed from a mesonephric tubule, and the mesonephric ducts has become the duct of the epididymis. **E.** Ovary at 20 weeks, showing the primordial follicles formed from the cortical cords. The rete ovarii derived from the primary sex cords and the mesonephric tubule and duct are regressing. **F.** Section of a seminiferous tubule from a 20-week fetus. Note that no lumen is present at this stage and that the seminiferous epithelium is comprised of two kinds of cells. **G.** Section from the ovarian cortex of a 20-week fetus showing three primordial follicles. (*From Moore K: The Developing Human. Philadelphia, Saunders, 1983.*)

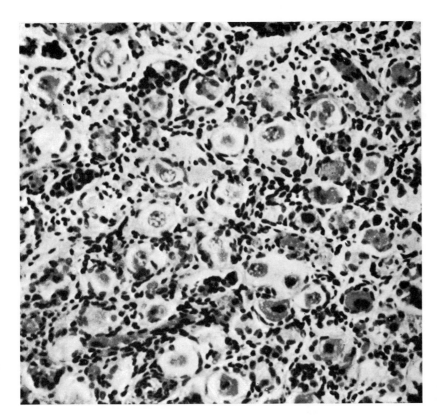

Figure 2-21. Ovary of newborn girl. Numerous primordial follicles are shown.

until maturity is reached. During this period of cell growth, many oocytes undergo degeneration, both before and after birth. The primary oocytes soon become surrounded by a single layer of flattened *follicle* cells that were derived originally from the germinal epithelium (see Fig. 3-5). These structures are now called *primordial follicles* and are first seen in the medulla and later in the cortex. Some follicles begin to grow even before birth and some are believed to persist in the cortex almost unchanged until menopause.

By 8 months of gestation, the ovary has become a long, narrow, lobulated structure that is attached to the body wall along the line of the hilum by the *mesovarium,* in which lies the *epoophoron.* At that stage of development, the germinal epithelium has been separated for the most part from the cortex by a band of connective tissue (tunica albuginea), which is absent in many small areas where strands of cells, usually referred to as cords of Pflüger, are in contact with the germinal epithelium. Among these cords are cells believed by many investigators to be oogonia that have come to resemble the other epithelial cells as a result of repeated mitoses. In the underlying cortex, there are two distinct zones. Superficially, there are nests of germ cells in synapsis, interspersed with Pflüger cords and strands of connective tissue. In the deeper zone, there are many groups of germ cells in synapsis, as well as primary oocytes, prospective follicular cells, and a few primordial follicles. In addition, there are numerous, but scattered, degenerating cells, although this zone is well vascularized. Such cellular degeneration is present regularly at

certain stages in various rapidly growing regions of normal embryos.

At term, the various types of ovarian cells in the human female fetus may still be found. In some cases, there are vesicular follicles in the medulla, which are all doomed to early degeneration.

Microscopic Structure of Ovary. From the first stages of its development until after the menopause, the ovary undergoes constant change. The number of oocytes at the onset of puberty has been estimated variously at 200,000 to 400,000 (see Chapter 3, p. 33). Since only one ovum ordinarily is cast off during each ovarian cycle, it is evident that a few hundred ova suffice for purposes of reproduction. The mode by which the others disappear is discussed in the section dealing with the corpus luteum and follicular atresia (see Chapter 3, p. 48).

Mossman and co-workers (1964), in an attempt to clarify the terminology of glandular elements of ovaries of adult women, distinguished interstitial, thecal, and luteal cells. The interstitial glandular elements are formed from cells of the theca interna of degenerating or atretic follicles; the thecal glandular cells are formed from the theca interna of ripening follicles; and, the true luteal cells are derived from the granulosa cells of ovulated follicles and from the undifferentiated stroma that surround them.

The huge store of primordial follicles at birth is exhausted gradually during the time of sexual maturation. Block (1952) found that there is a gradual decline from a mean of 439,000 oocytes in girls under 15 years to a mean of 34,000 in women over the age of 36. Öhler (1951) and others have refuted the concept of continued oogenesis after birth in higher mammals, which include women.

In the young girl, the greater portion of the ovary is comprised of the cortex, which is filled with large numbers of closely packed primordial follicles. Those nearest the central portion of the ovary are at the most advanced stages of development. In young women, the cortex is relatively thinner but still contains a large number of primordial follicles that are separated by bands of connective tissue cells in which there are spindle-shaped or oval nuclei. Each primordial follicle is comprised of an oocyte and its surrounding single layer of epithelial cells, which are small and flattened, spindle-shaped, and somewhat sharply differentiated from the still smaller and spindly cells of the surrounding stroma (Fig. 2-21).

The oocyte is a large, spherical cell in which there is clear cytoplasm and a relatively large nucleus that is located near the center of the ovum. In the nucleus, there is one large and several smaller nucleoli, and numerous masses of chromatin. The diameter of the smallest oocytes in the ovaries of adult women averages 0.033 mm, and that of the nuclei, 0.020 mm.

Embryologic Remnants

The *parovarium,* which can be found in the scant loose connective tissue within the broad ligament in the vicinity of the mesosalpinx, comprises a number of narrow vertical tubules that are lined by ciliated epithelium. These tubules connect at the upper ends with a longitudinal duct that extends just below the oviduct to the lateral margin of the uterus, where ordinarily it ends blindly near the internal os, but, infrequently, it may extend laterally down the vagina to the level of the hymen. This canal, the remnant of the wolffian (mesonephric) duct in women, is called the *Gartner duct.* The parovarium, also a remnant of the wolffian duct, is homologous, embryologically, with the caput epididymis in men. The cranial portion of the paraovarium is the *epoophoron* or organ of Rosenmüller; the caudal portion, or *paroophoron,* is a group of vestigial mesonephric tu-

bules that lie in or around the broad ligament. It is homologous, embryologically, with the paradidymis of men. Usually, the paroophoron in adult women disappears; but, on occasion, macroscopic cysts are formed from these remnants.

REFERENCES

Block E: Quantitative morphological investigation of the follicular system in women. Acta Anat 14:108, 1952

Buckingham JC, Buethe RA Jr, Danforth DN: Collagen-muscle ratio in clinically normal and clinically incompetent cervices. Am J Obstet Gynecol 91:232, 1965

Danforth DN, Buckingham JC, Roddick JW Jr: Connective tissue changes incident to cervical effacement. Am J Obstet Gynecol 80:939, 1960

Forbes TR: On the fate of the medullary cords of the human ovary. Contrib Embryol 30:9, 1942

Hitschmann F, Adler L: The structure of the endometrium of the sexually mature woman. Mschr Geburtsh Gynaek 27:1, 1908

Hodgson BJ, Eddy CA: The autonomic nervous system and its relationship to tubal ovum transport—A reappraisal. Gynecol Invest 6:161, 1975

Koff AK: Development of the vagina in the human fetus. Contrib Embryol 24:59, 1933

Krantz KE: Innervation of the human vulva and vagina. Obstet Gynecol 13:382, 1958

Langlois PL: The size of the normal uterus. J Reprod Med 4:220, 1970

Mahran M, Saleh AM: The microscopic anatomy of the hymen. Anat Rec 149:313, 1964

McKay DG, Robinson D, Hertig AT: Histochemical observations on granulosa cell tumors, thecomas and fibromas of the ovary. Am J Obstet Gynecol 58:625, 1949

Mossman HW, Koering MJ, Ferry D Jr: Cyclic changes in interstitial gland tissue of the human ovary. Am J Anat 115:235, 1964

Öhler I: Contribution to the knowledge of the ovarian epithelium and its relationship to oogenesis. Acta Anat 12:1, 1951

Schwalm H, Dubrauszky V: The structure of the musculature of the human uterus-muscles and connective tissue. Am J Obstet Gynecol 94:391, 1966

Woodruff JD, Pauerstein CJ: The Fallopian Tube. Baltimore, Williams and Wilkins, 1969

3

The Human Ovary and Ovulation

Presented in this chapter are some of the exciting new findings of a number of talented investigators who have identified the fail-safe systems of the ovary, brain, and pituitary that ensure dependable functions of the ovary without the requirement of a "delicate balance." Such a "delicate balance" has been claimed in the past to describe the molecular events that result in ovulation at cyclic intervals. Whereas only a few of us will become students of the molecular events that serve to embody fail-safe systems for the virtual guarantee of cyclic ovulation, we all can become expert in the management of the reproductive physiology and pathophysiology of women. Certainly, the regulation of the ovarian cycle—that is, the predictable alterations in hormone production and cyclic extrusion of a single ovum at approximately 1-month intervals—is the rule and not the exception. If this were not the case, the population explosion in the world would not constitute such an enormous problem. It is true that some women are, on occasion, anovulatory—and a few are permanently so—but this event is extremely rare compared with the reverse, that is, the regular, predictable, cyclic repetition of the ovarian cycle and the morphologic changes in reproductive tissues that are attendant of this synchronous event.

SIGNIFICANCE OF REGULAR MENSES

The obstetrician–gynecologist commonly must assume the role of endocrinologist, but as such has a significant advantage over his internist colleagues who are obliged to deal with endocrine abnormalities in men. This is so because a detailed knowledge of the physiologic events that accompany the ovarian cycle and the clinical manifestations of abnormalities thereof are sensitive guides to the endocrine milieu of women. Specifically, the occurrence of spontaneous, predictable menses at reasonable intervals is strong evidence for the occurrence of ovulation. Moreover, if such menses are associated with some degree of discomfort, which may vary from only a prodroma of impending menstruation to that of severe dysmenorrhea, the likelihood of cyclic ovulation is even more assured. We do not subscribe to the thesis that regular, predictable menses occur with any frequency in anovulatory women (excepting those that are artificially produced by exogenous steroid compounds). For these reasons, two equations can be formulated: (1) cyclic,

predictable, spontaneous menses = ovulation; (2) ovulation = normal sex hormone production.

For women who are ovulatory, therefore, it can be assumed with considerable confidence that the production of pituitary gonadotropins, both follicle-stimulating hormone (FSH) and luteinizing hormone (LH), as well as estrogens, androgens, and progesterone, is appropriate. Such a history is of more value than many hundreds of dollars worth of endocrine tests. For this reason, a thorough and carefully obtained menstrual history is both of real and potential value. Consider the woman, for example, who experiences regular, cyclic, predictable onset of menstruation, but who sustains abnormal bleeding thereafter. Such a woman almost invariably will have some organic disease of the uterus to account for the abnormal bleeding. At the same time, except in women over 40 years of age, the occurrence of unpredictable uterine bleeding, that is, unpredictable in onset, amount, or duration of bleeding, which usually is painless, is most often the result of chronic anovulation or undiagnosed pregnancy rather than organic uterine disease.

For these reasons, as well as the requirement of ovulation for pregnancy, this chapter and the next are devoted to a consideration of the integrated and synchronized phenomena that involve the ovary and endometrium of nonpregnant women during each ovarian cycle of their reproductive years. Teleologically, the purpose of the ovarian cycle is to provide an ovum for fertilization, whereas that of the endometrial cycle is to establish a suitable site in which a fertilized ovum, i.e., the blastocyst, can implant and develop. Since the endometrial changes are regulated by the ovarian hormones, the two cycles are intimately, but not precisely, related in time.

Although both the ovarian and menstrual cycles customarily are considered to extend from the first day of one menstrual period to the first day of the next menstrual period, it is likely that the succeeding ovarian cycle, in the context of follicular maturation preparatory to the next ovulation, begins prior to the succeeding menstruation. The typical human menstrual cycle is said to be 28 days, although 29 to 30 days is more usual, and variations are common and normal (see Table 4-2).

The history of the study of the regulation of the ovarian cycle and its hormones is not dissimilar to that of the investigations of many other reproductive processes. From a very simplistic, but at the same time

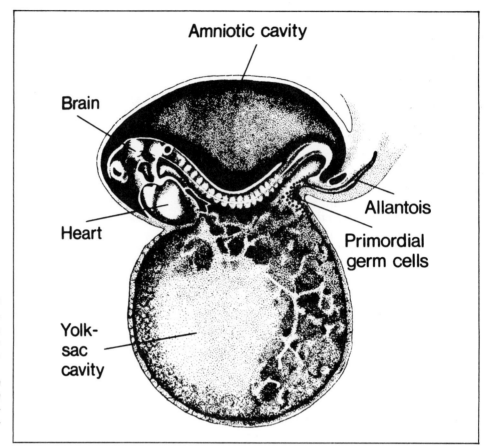

Figure 3-1. Reconstruction of 24-day human embryo in its amnion. The primordial germ cells (*black dots*) are grouped at the top of the yolk sac and in the ventral wall of the developing hindgut. (*From Baker. In Austin and Short (eds): Primordial Germ Cells in Germ Cells and Fertilization. Cambridge, Cambridge University Press, 1978.*)

quite sophisticated interpretation of events—namely, that the pituitary served as the "master gland"—we have marched, sometimes "majestically backward," through a host of hypotheses. Many of these were meritorious and were supported by data that, although convincing at the time, were obviously incomplete. Perhaps, the pervading theory of the preceding few decades was one in which it was envisioned that the brain—and in particular specialized functions of the hypothalamus— served as the central processing site for receipt of and thence transmittal of signals that controlled the function of the anterior pituitary. The release of small peptides into hypophysial–portal blood was and is now considered to be of paramount importance in the hypothalamic regulation of anterior pituitary release of gonadotropins.

"Fail-Safe" Systems

In the past decade, many investigators have guided our thinking to a consideration of internal control mechanisms that may constitute the fail-safe systems so important in the successful maintenance of cyclic ovarian function. We know that the levels of various hormones in blood at any given stage of the ovarian cycle vary widely among women and even in a given woman from one cycle to the next. Yet, the sine qua non of perfection in ovarian function, viz., ovulation is accomplished. It is recognized that the nature of the molecular events that are controlled by these fail-safe systems are of such real and potential importance that new, descriptive, and even somewhat romantic terms now are used to describe some of the putative agents, e.g., folliculostatin and cybernins, gonadocrinins, and gonadostatins.

EMBRYOGENESIS OF OVARY, OVA, AND FOLLICLE

The march that encompasses a parade of events that lead to the development of the mature graafian follicle begins early in embryonic development. Baker (1978) states with considerable conviction that, "One of the most important concepts in reproductive physiology is that the definitive germ cells—the eggs and spermatozoa—are derived solely from the primitive sex cells (that are) found early in embryonic development." He goes on to say that there is "a continuity of the germ-cell line from embryo to adult." As Baker again emphasizes, "there is overwhelming evidence in support of the classical view of the continuity of the germ-cell line. . ." but no evidence for "the transformation of epithelial (somatic) cells into those of the germinal line."

About 3 weeks after conception, the germ cells in the human fetus are localized in the epithelium of the yolk sac near the developing allantois (Baker, 1978, Fig. 3-1). Thereafter, these germ cells migrate to the connec-

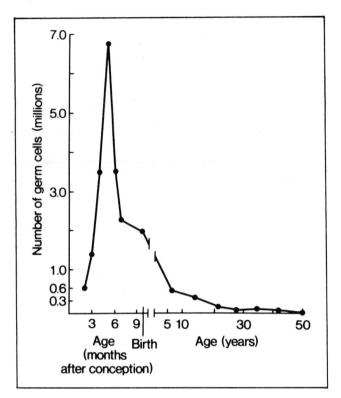

Figure 3-2. Changes in the total population of germ cells in the human ovary with increasing age. (*From Baker: Am J Obstet Gynecol 110:746, 1978.*)

tive tissue of the hindgut and thence progressively to the gonadal primordia or ridges (Fig. 2-19). The number of germ cells is believed to increase by mitosis. There may be a substance (telopheron) that directs the anatomic migration of the germ cell to the genital ridge. The exact means by which germ cells migrate is not fully defined; amoeboid activity, chemotactic substances, and lytic enzyme activities all may be involved. Even movement by way of blood with "hone-in" mechanisms to the gonad may be involved (Baker, 1978). Generally, the germ cells remain in the cortex if the presumptive gonad is to be an ovary. The differentiation of the fetal female gonad is late when compared with that of the male. The ovary is different from the testis in that it fails to assume the recognizable appearance of an ovary by an appointed time in development. The number of germ cells in developing ovaries, by mitosis, changes rapidly during gestational development (Fig. 3-2).

After a definitive number of mitoses, the oogonia are transformed into oocytes—at this time, prophase, which is the first of two meiotic divisions, is entered (Baker, 1978); thereafter, there are no new oocytes formed. Therefore, as oogonia are eliminated from the ovary—before birth primarily—the population of germ cells only can be reduced in number.

Prodigality—as Baker states—is the "keynote" in the early history of the germ cells, that is, the oogonia. Yet, if this were true of ova, consider the extraordinary

extent of prodigality in the case of spermatogoonia when more than a billion may be ejaculated in a single copulation.

The lifetime history of germ cell maturation, loss, atresia, development, and ovulation is recapitulated in Figure 3-2, which is reproduced, in large measure, from data assembled by Baker.

There is no reliable evidence in support of the proposition that ova normally are formed in the human after birth. It has been estimated that there are 600,000 oogonia in the ovaries of female fetuses at 2 months gestation and 6,800,000 at 5 months gestation. Degeneration occurs thereafter and 2,000,000 are found at birth, but only 400,000 in prepubertal girls (Baker, 1972, Fig. 3-2). Before puberty, mature graafian follicles are found only in the deeper portions of the cortex. Later, however, mature follicles also develop in the superficial portions of the ovary. During each cycle, one follicle makes its way to the surface, and there it appears as a transparent vesicle that may vary from a few to 10 or 12 mm in diameter. As the follicle approaches the surface of the ovary, the wall becomes thinner and is supplied more abundantly with vessels (Fig. 3-3), except in the most prominent projecting portion, which appears almost bloodless. This avascular locus is designated as the *stigma,* the site of the follicle where rupture is to occur.

Folliculogenesis

After formation of the oocytes in the early primordial follicles, these cells are surrounded by flattened epithelial-like cells (Fig. 3-4). As folliculogenesis progresses, the follicular cells proliferate and become cuboidal (Figs. 3-5, 3-6) and then commence to secrete a fluid that accumulates, ultimately, into one large pool—and an antrum is formed. Ovarian stromal cells differentiate to form the theca externa and theca interna (Figs. 3-5, 3-6). This stage of follicular development appears to proceed in a manner that is independent of gonadotropin action. Hereafter, an integrated set of metabolic events appear to be necessary for complete maturation of the follicle, i.e., the dominant follicle that is destined to be the source of the ovum to be ovulated in a given cycle. Thereafter, as folliculogenesis proceeds, there is an orderly and progressive sequence of hormonally responsive and operative events that permit and facilitate the final stages in the maturation of the dominant follicle in preparation for ovulation.

During this time of folliculogenesis, two major functions emerge: (1) a gonadotropin hormone-receptor adenylate cyclase coupling system and (2) a cell-contact system for intercellular communication (Albertini, 1980). It is recognized that not only do gonadotropins serve to stimulate and to activate the enzymatic processes of the cells of the follicles, but estradiol-17β, synthesized within the granulosa cells, also may act to alter gonadotropin receptor content and serve to stimulate growth and development of gap junctions in preantral follicles. The great majority of vesicular follicles, including all of those

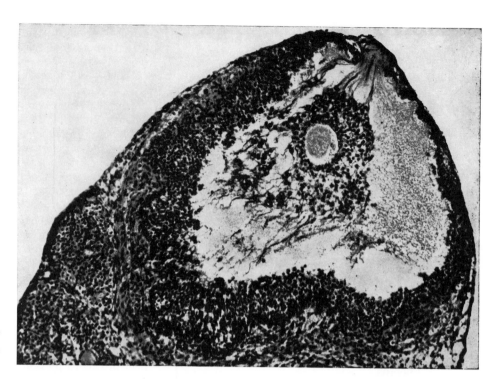

Figure 3-3. Rat ovary just prior to ovulation. (*Courtesy of Dr. Richard J. Blandau.*)

before puberty, undergo degeneration at various stages of formation (Baker, 1978, Fig. 3-2).

As follicular maturation progresses, the order of events is as follows: (1) increase in size of the oocyte; (2) alteration in granulosa cells from flat to cuboidal, followed by replication; and (3) formation of the zona pellucida (Baker, 1978). The zona pellucida is a clear, mucoid band that envelops the ovum and persists until after the fertilized ovum reaches the uterus (Figs. 3-7, 3-8). Thereafter, the theca interna is vascularized and is surrounded by the theca externa (Figs. 3-9, 3-10). As the follicle increases in size, there is a disproportionate increase in the size of the follicle compared with that of the ovum (Fig. 3-11).

During any ovarian cycle, 20 or more follicles may embark on the processes that appear to be on the road to ovulation. We know little, in fact nothing, of how these few of so many thousand are chosen, let alone how 1 of these 20 or so follicles becomes the dominant or chosen *one!*

TOWARD THE DEVELOPMENT OF THE GRAAFIAN FOLLICLE

Mature Graafian Follicle

The mature follicle is known as a *graafian follicle,* after the Dutch anatomist, de Graaf, who described this structure in 1677. The follicular cells, or granulosa cells, that immediately surround the ovum, constitute the *cumulus oophorus* or *discus proligerus,* a group of granulosa cells that project into the now abundant follicular fluid in the antrum of the mature follicle. As the graafian follicle grows, the stromal cells that surround it enlarge and the capillary net about these cells becomes closer and forms the theca interna (Fig. 3-10), which is a cellular site of synthesis of steroids, likely C_{19}-steroids, and in particular androstenedione. In the cells of the theca interna, lipid droplets develop; after ovulation these cells persist and lie immediately adjacent to the enlarged follicular cells that are now called the granulosa lutein cells. The results of measurements of diameters of ova in sections of a well-preserved ovary are indicative that although the ovum grows slowly during the development of the graafian follicle, the volume of the ovum increases about 40-fold before maturity is completed. The nucleus, however, increases in size only about threefold during this period. The large increase in cytoplasm is accompanied by the accumulation of nutrients such as yolk granules.

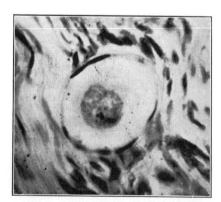

Figure 3-4. Primordial follicle from ovary of an adult woman.

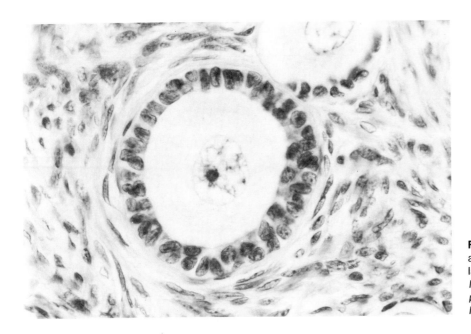

Figure 3-5. An early growing follicle in an ovary of a 4-year-old girl. A theca layer begins to form. (*From Peters: In Midgley and Sadler (eds): Some Aspects of Early Follicular Development. New York, Raven, 1979.*)

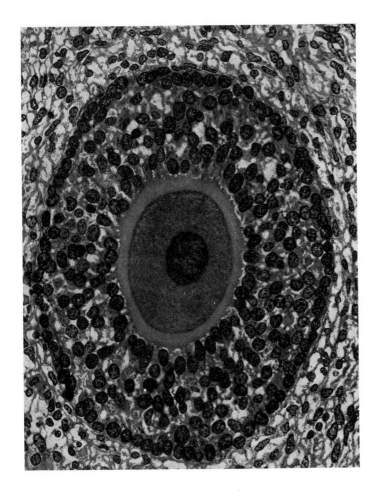

Figure 3-6. Developing follicle.

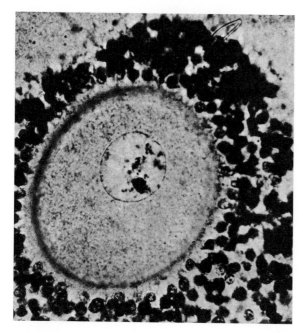

Figure 3-7. Human oocyte from a large graafian follicle. (*Courtesy of Carnegie Laboratory.*)

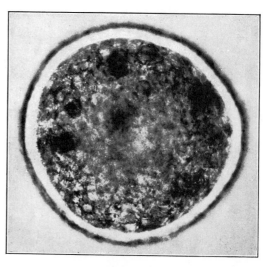

Figure 3-8. Human ovum washed from tube. Fresh specimen, surrounded by semitransparent zona pellucida, consists largely of lipoid masses. Ovum measured 0.136 mm in the living state. (*Carnegie Collection No. 6289, Dr. WH Lewis.*)

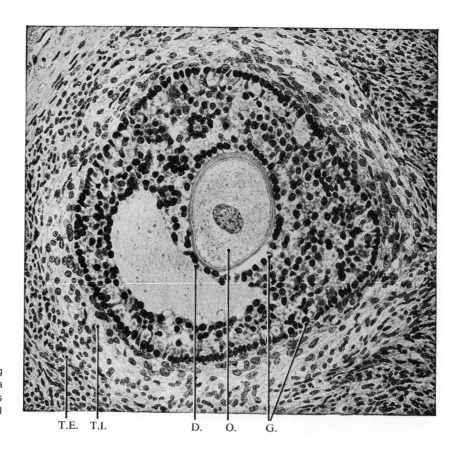

Figure 3-9. Graafian follicle approaching maturity. T.E. = theca externa; T.I. = theca interna; D. = discus proligerus (cumulus oophorus); O. = ovum; G. = granulosa cell layer.

T.E.　T.I.　D.　O.　G.

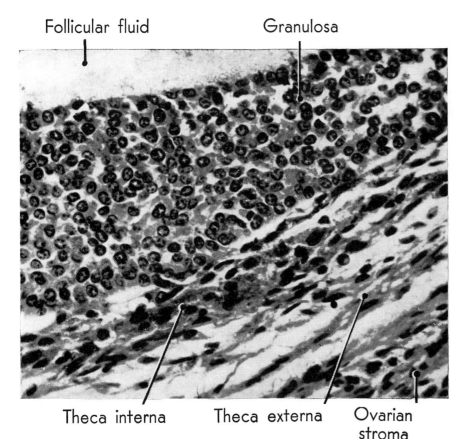

Follicular fluid   Granulosa

Theca interna   Theca externa   Ovarian stroma

Figure 3-10. Section through the wall of a mature graafian follicle.

From the outside inward, the mature graafian follicle is comprised of (1) a layer of specialized connective tissue, the theca folliculi, (2) an epithelial lining, the membrana granulosa, (3) the ovum, and (4) the liquor folliculi. The theca folliculi is comprised of an outer layer of cells, the theca externa, and an inner layer, the theca interna. The theca externa is comprised of ordinary ovarian stroma that is arranged concentrically about the follicle, but the connective tissue cells of the theca interna are modified greatly.

Almost as soon as the primordial follicle begins to develop, mitotic figures appear in the cells of the surrounding stroma, considerable multiplication of cells occurs, and these cells become distinctly larger than those of the surrounding connective tissue. As the follicle increases in size, these cells, i.e., the *theca lutein cells,* accumulate lipid and a yellowish pigment, and this gives rise to a granular appearance. Simultaneously, a striking increase in the vascularity and the number of lymphatic spaces of the theca develops.

Before ovulation, the theca cells are separated from the granulosa cells by a highly polymerized membrane. It is possible that luteinizing hormone may act to depolymerize this membrane at about the time of ovulation and thus allow vascularization of the granulosa cells to take place.

The epithelial lining of the follicle, or membrana granulosa, is one that consists of several layers of small polygonal or cuboidal cells in which there are round,

darkly staining nuclei; the larger the follicle, the fewer the number of layers. At one time, the membrana granulosa is much thicker than elsewhere, and a mound is formed in which the ovum is included, i.e., the cumulus oophorus (discus proligerus).

The follicle is filled with a clear, proteinaceous fluid,

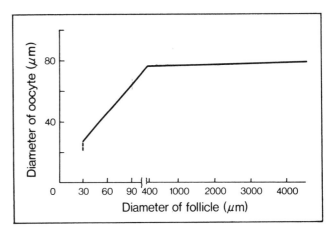

Figure 3-11. Growth of the oocyte and follicle in the human ovary. First the oocyte alone enlarges, then both grow at a corresponding pace; finally, growth is restricted almost entirely to the follicle. (*From Baker: In Austin and Short (eds): Primordial Germ Cells and Fertilization. Cambridge, Cambridge University Press, 1978.*)

the liquor folliculi, or follicular fluid. The usual fat stains are not taken up by the granulosa cells until the stage of preovulatory swelling, a time of rapid growth that commences about 24 hours before ovulation and apparently is related to the onset of, or preparation for, the secretion of progesterone.

Maturation of Ovum

The human ovum, as it approaches maturity, is barely visible to the naked eye when brightly illuminated on a dark background. According to Hartman (1929) and Allen and co-workers (1930), the average diameter of the mature human ovum is 0.133 mm.

If the nearly mature ovum is examined in the follicular fluid or in physiologic saline, the structures that can be distinguished in and about it are as follows: (1) a surrounding corona radiata; (2) a zona pellucida; (3) a perivitelline space; (4) a small clear zone of protoplasm; (5) a broad, finely granulated zone of protoplasm; (6) a central, deutoplasmic zone; (7) the nucleus, or germinal vesicle, within it a germinal spot; and, if appropriately stained, (8) many small spheroidal mitochondria. The ovum is free to rotate within the zona pellucida even though the outer vitelline membrane of the ovum appears to be applied closely to it. After fertilization, shrinkage of the ovum results in its complete separation from the zona pellucida as it floats in the perivitelline fluid. During growth, the oocyte accumulates deutoplasm (yolk granules). Before ovulation, the ovum, in the living state, is transparent with a faint yellowish tinge. There also are larger lipoid granules, which in preserved material appear to surround the nucleus (germinal vesicle). Numerous mitochondria are distributed through the cytoplasm. The spherical nucleus is located near the center of the oocyte; and, in it, there is a large nucleolus and sparsely distributed chromatin. Shortly before ovulation, the nucleus migrates toward the periphery, and meiosis is reinitiated. At the completion of the first and second meiotic divisions, the number of chromosomes in the oocyte is halved, and two polar bodies are formed: the first before ovulation and the second after penetration of the oocyte by a spermatozoan. Both polar bodies are extruded into the perivitelline space.

The mechanisms that control meiosis and, consequently, the formation of polar bodies are defined more clearly in Chapter 5. After mitosis ceases, which occurs usually before the seventh month of gestation, the oogonia become primary oocytes. Characteristically, such cells have entered prophase of the first meiotic division. The primary oocytes continue through various stages of prophase (lepotene, zygotene, pachytene), until arrested in diplotene. By 6 months gestational age, all oocytes have either reached diplotene or else have become atretic. These primary oocytes remain in diplotene until shortly before ovulation unless these also undergo atresia. The factors responsible for arresting oocytes in diplotene are not defined; at the time of arrest, however, oocytes are encircled by a layer of follicle cells; the hypothesis has evolved that the follicle acts to inhibit

meiosis in some way. The hypothesis that there is a follicular source of inhibition is supported by the fact that meiosis is reinitiated under one of two conditions: (1) after gonadotropic stimulation or (2) after removal of the ovum from the follicle and culture in vitro in the absence of gonadotropins. The nature of the inhibitor has been postulated variously as a lack of oxygen, as steroids, and more recently as protein (Chapter 5). In accordance with the inhibition theory, gonadotropins act to overcome the inhibition by direct action on the oocyte or else by indirect action through the follicular cells. There may be more than one inhibitor, since smaller oocytes will mature only to metaphase I in vitro, and oocytes progress only as far as metaphase II unless fertilization occurs. Yet another possibility exists, according to Baker (1978), which is that the so-called inhibition is in reality a stage in development and that the resumption of meiosis is dependent on the proper interaction among gonadotropins, follicle cells, and oocytes.

Ovarian follicles develop throughout childhood and occasionally attain considerable size, but normally do not rupture at this time, instead these undergo atresia in situ. The relative rates of increase in oocyte size and follicular size with maturation are considerably different (Fig. 3-11). Even in adult women, many follicles that reach a diameter of 5 mm or more undergo atresia. Usually, only one of a group of enlarging follicles continues to grow and to produce a normal mature egg that is extruded by ovulation. The mechanisms that normally limit maturation and ovulation to only one of the enlarging follicles has not been defined and this phenomenon continues to constitute one of the major enigmas of ovarian physiology.

Molecular Events Involved in the Final Stages of Follicular Maturation and Ovulation

The characteristic cyclicity of secretion of estradiol-17β and progesterone, as well as that of the C_{19}-steroids, androstenedione, dehydroisoandrosterone, and testosterone, by the ovaries of young women is regulated by mechanisms that are considerably different with respect to C_{18}- and C_{21}-steroids as compared with those of the C_{19}-steroids. It now is clear that a variety of molecular events in the theca and granulosa cells of the ovaries of women are subject to regulatory processes that involve actions of gonadotropins and steroids as well. It is recognized that follicular maturation can proceed, in the absence of pituitary hormone guidance, to the preantral stage of development and even to replication of granulosa cells to a finite point, i.e., four-cell layer thickness. Beyond this stage, however, gonadotropin and most likely steroids produced in response to gonadotropin action are required for full expression of follicular maturation and responsiveness. Since the integrated actions of gonadotropins upon the cells of the follicles and those of the steroids produced within the follicles appear to be a requisite part of follicular maturation, it seems prudent to consider the two processes as those that act with some degree of simultaneity. In order to do so, it now seems apparent that the two-cell hypothesis, with respect to follicular steroidogenesis, is in all likelihood an exact description of the incredible synchrony that exists between theca cells and granulosa cells. This synchrony results in a coordinated biosynthetic schemata that results in the appropriate, rhythmical production of steroids that facilitate, characterize, and seemingly are imperative to the fulfillment of the destiny of the chosen follicle—ovulation.

FSH acts to increase the activity in granulosa cells to aromatize C_{19}-steroids. This activity is believed to be mediated by an increase in adenylate cyclase activity and by "androgens" that act in an as-yet undefined manner to increase aromatase activity. But more than that, estradiol-17β synthesized by the dominant follicle also appears to act to increase the follicular cell actions of FSH to enhance LH responsiveness. The stimulation of aromatase activity by cyclic-AMP is probably mediated by cyclic-AMP-dependent phosphorylation of a number of cellular proteins, an increase in the rate of transcription of specific genes that encode for aromatase protein(s), or an increase in the rate of translation of existing messenger RNAs. It is only after FSH-priming that cells become competent to LH action. This is believed to be the result of FSH-induced LH receptors and, perhaps, FSH-induced prolactin receptors. Thus, FSH appears to act to induce the activation of aromatase activity, as well as LH and prolactin receptors.

We now must enter into a consideration of the "two-cell hypothesis." LH is known to act to increase cholesterol side-chain cleavage enzyme activity, which is believed to be the rate-limiting step in steroidogenesis in many steroidogenic tissues, and in thecal cells to increase the activities of 17α-hydroxylase and 17,20-lyase activities, enzymes important, indeed crucial, to the formation of C_{19}-steroids, that is, androgen-like compounds such as dehydroisoandrosterone, androstenedione, and testosterone.

THECA-GRANULOSA CELL COOPERATIVITY IN ESTRADIOL-17β SYNTHESIS

The Two-Cell Hypothesis Revisited

Approximately two decades ago, a new, or revised, hypothesis was championed by Ryan and Smith (1959), with respect to the mechanism of steroid production in the ovary, and, in particular, the maturing follicle. The validity of that hypothesis is now supported, for the most part by new and in some cases seemingly unrelated data. Heretofore, there appeared to be many confusing and inexplicable findings, both clinical and biochemical, with respect to the cyclic production of steroid hormones by the ovary. Consider the following: some ovarian tumors, it seemed, secreted androgens, whereas others that appeared to share a similar histogenic origin, seemed to secrete estrogens, and yet other, apparently identical tumors were associated with clinical evidence of both feminization and virilization. For these reasons, it

was assumed—erroneously, in retrospect—that a given tumor may secrete estrogen, androgen, or both.

Extraglandular Hormone Formation

We now know that these heretofore inexplicable findings can be explained by extragonadal formation of hormones from prehormones secreted by ovarian tumors. For example, a common secretory product of the ovarian stroma and certain ovarian tumors is the C_{19}-steroid, androstenedione. This compound is commonly, but perhaps incorrectly, referred to as an androgen. Strictly speaking, androstenedione may, per se, have little or *no* intrinsic androgenic activity. Its chemical structure, however, is very similar to that of the potent androgen, testosterone. Androstenedione, however, in a variety of extraglandular sites, is converted to the estrogen, estrone, and to the androgen, testosterone. On average, 1.5 percent of androstenedione is converted, in extraglandular sites, to estrone, whereas 5 percent of androstenedione is converted to testosterone. Yet, it should be remembered that, physiologically, estrogen is produced in microgram quantities, whereas androgen is produced in milligram amounts. Thus, if a modest increase in the production of prehormone, androstenedione, occurred during times of anovulation or else with an ovarian tumor, estrogenic manifestations in that woman may prevail. Even though the extent of conversion of androstenedione to estrone is only one third that of the conversion of androstenedione to testosterone, 10 to 100 times more androgen is required, in the physiologic range, to exert maximal biologic effects. If somewhat more androstenedione were produced, the clinical manifestations could encompass both feminization and masculinization. On the other hand, if large amounts of androstenedione are produced, the large amounts of extraglandularly produced testosterone will act to impede estrogen action, and, thus, the clinical manifestations will appear to be exclusively those of virilization. Thus the multipotential of all ovarian cells to produce both estrogens and androgens appears to be invalid.

Steroid Production in Isolated Cell Types

At first glance, it appears reasonable that an evaluation of the potential of each cell type of the ovary to produce a variety of steroids would be a rational approach to a dissection of the molecular events involved in ovarian steroidogenesis. This has proven not to be the case for several reasons. Granulosa cells can be isolated and maintained in culture. Strange, if not inexplicable, events accompany the maintenance of granulosa cells in culture; importantly, seemingly spontaneous luteinization of such cells occur in culture.

We have known for many years that, ultimately, cholesterol must be the precursor of all steroid hormones. What we did not consider, until recently, was that the source of cholesterol for a given steroidogenic cell may differ. Together with the pioneering studies of Brown and colleagues (1979), who demonstrated that many extrahepatic tissues assimilate cholesterol by up-take and processing of circulating lipoproteins, it was soon demonstrated that similar processes are applicable to the assimilation of cholesterol for steroidogenesis in endocrine glands and placenta. The specific type and source of cholesterol utilized by a given gland, however, varies widely among species and perhaps within a given cell type of a given gland in a single species. By way of example, utilization of cholesterol by the corpus luteum for progesterone biosynthesis is among the most diverse. Consider the following: In the rabbit, cholesterol is synthesized in the corpus luteum de novo, i.e., from 2-carbon fragments such as acetate. In the rat, however, circulating high-density lipoprotein (HDL) is used as the cholesterol source. In women, however, there is little de novo synthesis of cholesterol in the corpus luteum; HDL is not assimilated by human granulosa cells, but rather, low-density lipoprotein (LDL) is the almost exclusive source of cholesterol for progesterone biosynthesis. The molecular weight of LDL is approximately 3,000,000. If we recall that follicular granulosa cells are not vascularized, it is apparent that a precursor source of cholesterol becomes extraordinarily important in the mechanisms that provide for full luteinization and optimal progesterone biosynthesis. Let us consider the extremes. In women, there is very limited capacity for the de novo synthesis of cholesterol in granulosa cells, and these cells do not utilize HDL as a source of cholesterol. In the follicular fluid that surrounds the avascular granulosa cells,

there is little or no LDL. Thus, it is obvious that little or no steroidogenesis by way of utilization of cholesterol could proceed in this unique environment. This is the case. Prior to ovulation, there is little progesterone produced by the granulosa cells of women. On the other hand, if granulosa cells obtained from the follicles of women are placed in culture, these cells luteinize and respond to appropriate trophic stimuli by producing progesterone in large amounts. It must be remembered, however, that the culture medium that bathes these cells contains serum—and thus LDL, a lipoprotein not present in follicular fluid, but the one known to be used specifically for a source of cholesterol in human granulosa cells is provided in this serum for steroid formation. Thus, the "spontaneous" luteinization and thence the biosynthesis of progesterone by granulosa cells of women may be attributable, in part, to the availability to these cells of a utilizable source of cholesterol, viz., LDL.

HDL is present in follicular fluid of the developing ovarian follicles of women; we presume that the considerable difference in molecular weights of HDL and LDL is accountable for the absence of LDL in follicular fluid. It may be a moot point in women, however, since HDL is not a utilizable source of cholesterol for the granulosa cells. Yet, consider the fact that HDL can be used by steroidogenic tissues of the rat, a considerable species difference in precursor source and availability for corpus luteum progesterone biosynthesis. Before addressing this

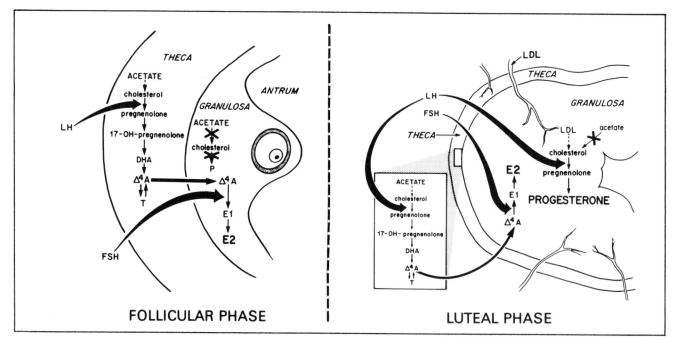

Figure 3-12. A. Relation between theca and granulosa cells in estradiol-17β (E2) production. Androstenedione (Δ⁴A) is synthesized by way of pregnenolone and dehydroisoandrosterone (DHA) formation in theca cells. Note that LH stimulates the formation of pregnenolone by increasing side chain cleavage of cholesterol. Aromatization occurs in granulosa cells to give E2 by way of estrone (E1). The aromatization of androstenedione is stimulated by FSH. Progesterone (P, Prog) synthesis from plasma low-density lipoprotein (LDL) occurs in granulosa cells. Testosterone (T) also is synthesized in the ovary.

issue, however, let us consider the other extreme, namely, progesterone biosynthesis in the corpus luteum of the rabbit, an induced ovulator. In this species, all progesterone production by the corpora lutea can be accounted for from the utilization of progesterone synthesized de novo; namely, in the rabbit, circulating lipoprotein is not necessary for optimum progestin biosynthesis. We suggest that these considerations may be of extraordinary importance in the evaluation of putative ovarian cybernins. The in vitro alteration of cholesterol availability may affect, in a profound manner, the processes that are involved in luteinization in a species-specific manner that is dependent upon the capacity of the granulosa cells of the ovarian follicles of that species to synthesize cholesterol or else to utilize that cholesterol that may or may not be available from follicular fluid.

As is the case in many studies of physiologic events in the human, there is an entity, abetalipoproteinemia, that affects women and is of particular utility in defining the origin of steroids in the ovaries of women. We have put forward the proposition of others that there is cooperativity in the follicular, that is, theca-granulosa cell production of estradiol-17β (Fig. 3-12A). We also proposed that the corpus luteum of women is almost absolutely dependent upon plasma LDL as a source of cholesterol for precursor for progesterone biosynthesis. Recently, the steroid levels in a presumably ovulatory woman with abetalipoproteinemia were

described. In such a woman, there is no LDL; hence the term, abetalipoproteinemia. As illustrated in Figure 3-12B, there appears to be cyclic ovarian function, i.e., midcycle LH surge, appropriate levels of FSH and LH, cyclicity, *but no progesterone!* These findings are strongly supportive of the proposition that de novo cholesterol synthesis in theca can be sufficient to support the biosynthesis of C_{19}-steroids that are secreted by and transported by way of follicular fluid to the granulosa cells for follicular estradiol-17β production that is characteristic of cyclic estrogen biosynthesis during the ovarian cycle. On the other hand, in this woman, there was no post-LH surge in progesterone secretion. We take this as evidence that the granulosa cells are dependent nearly exclusively upon LDL as the cholesterol precursor for progesterone biosynthesis. Thus, the two-cell hypothesis seems to be complete. We cannot disregard the potential of theca cells to utilize LDL-cholesterol; nevertheless, from the findings in the case of the woman with abetalipoproteinemia presented, it seems likely that sufficient de novo synthesis of cholesterol can proceed in theca to provide adequate quantities of androstenedione for granulosa cell estradiol-17β synthesis.

OVULATION

As the graafian follicle grows to a size of 10 to 12 mm in diameter, in response to the hormonal mechanisms described subsequently and demonstrated schematically on page 36, it gradually reaches the surface of the ovary and ultimately protrudes above it. Necrobiosis of the overlying tissues, rather than pressure within the follicle, is the principal factor that causes follicular rupture. The cells at the exposed tip of the follicle float away at the site of the pale stigma so that the region becomes transparent. The thinnest clear area then bursts, and the follicular liquid and the ovum surrounded by the zona pellucida and corona radiata are extruded at the time of ovulation. The actual rupture of the follicle is not explosive; the discharge of the ovum together with the zona pellucida and attached follicular cells takes not more than 2 to 3 minutes, and in the rabbit at least, it is expedited by the separation, just before rupture, of the ovum with the surrounding granulosa cells (corona radiata) from the follicular wall as the result of accumulation of fluid in the cumulus; hence, the ovum floats freely in the liquor. Strickland and Beers (1979) demonstrated that the granulosa cells produce plasminogen activator. The extracellular level of this enzyme is correlated closely with ovulation, and the activity of the enzyme is modulated by the action of gonadotropins, cyclic nucleotides, and prostaglandins. Further, by the action of this enzyme on plasminogen, which is present in follicular fluid, plasmin, a proteolytic enzyme that has been shown to weaken the follicular wall (Beers, 1975), is generated.

Excellent motion pictures of the process of ovulation in the rat have been obtained by Richard Blandau and others. In Figures 3-3 and 3-13, two frames from these

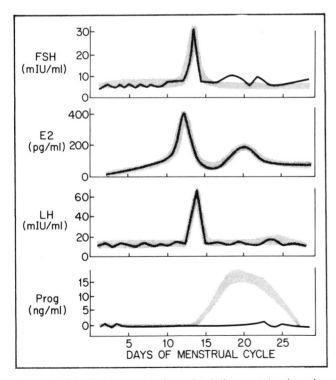

Figure 3-12. B. Hormones throughout the menstrual cycle. The shaded areas represent mean values noted in normal ovulatory women. The solid lines represent those values measured in a woman with abetalipoproteinemia. (*Adapted from Illingworth: Proc Natl Acad Sci USA 79:6685, 1982.*)

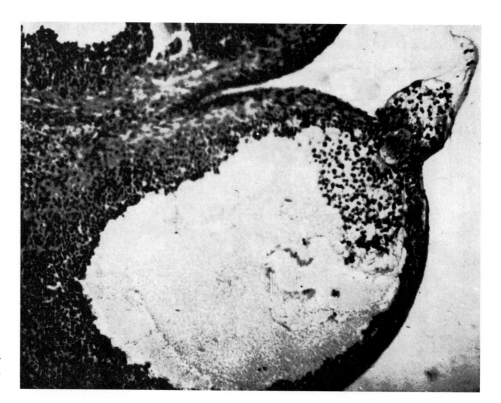

Figure 3-13. Moment of ovulation in the rat. (*Courtesy of Dr. Richard J. Blandau.*)

movies are illustrated. The follicle is shown just before ovulation and the expulsion of the ovum also is shown. In the first (Fig. 3-3), the stigma is clearly visible, whereas in the second (Fig. 3-13) the actual expulsion of the ovum is illustrated. In Figure 3-14, there is presented a scanning electron micrograph of an oocyte and the follicle of a mouse at the time of ovulation.

Time of Ovulation

The exact time of ovulation in the cycle is of the utmost importance for several reasons. First, since the life-span of both the spermatozoa and the unfertilized ovum are limited, fertilization must take place within hours after ovulation if conception is to occur in that cycle. In some

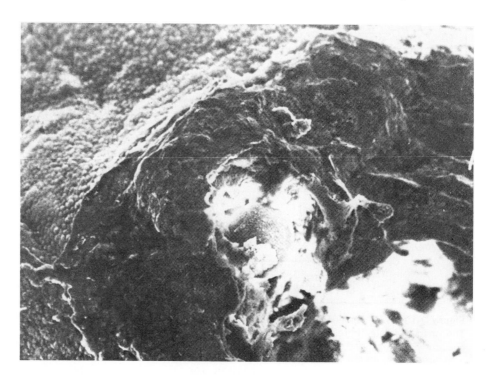

Figure 3-14. Scanning electron micrograph of an oocyte and the follicle of a mouse at the time of ovulation. (*From Motta and Hafez (eds): Biology of the Mouse Ovary. The Hague, Martinus Nijhoff, 1980.*)

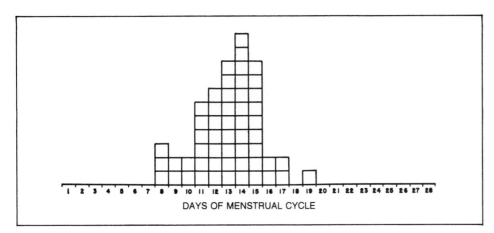

Figure 3-15. Day of ovulation in 54 women calculated from the apparent age of the corpus luteum. Each block represents an observation of one woman.

infertile couples, detection of the time of ovulation and appropriate adjustment of the time of coitus are important considerations in therapy. Importantly, for couples who use the "rhythm method" to avoid conception, coitus should be limited to that part of the cycle several days removed from the time of ovulation, or the "safe period." Ovulation usually marks approximately the midpoint of both the ovarian and menstrual cycles. The period from the first day of menstrual bleeding to ovulation is designated as the proliferative phase of the menstrual cycle. The proliferative phase encompasses roughly the first half of the menstrual cycle; the *postovulatory phase* is known as the secretory phase.

Various methods have been used in attempts to determine the time of ovulation in women. Allen and colleagues (1930) recovered mature unfertilized ova from the fallopian tube on the 12th, 15th, and 16th days of the cycle, and concluded that ovulation occurs approximately on day 14 of a 28-day menstrual cycle. Other indirect methods by which to ascertain the time of ovulation are the examination of fertilized ova and evaluation of the changes that have taken place at the site of the ruptured follicle. By use of these techniques, it has been demonstrated that, although ovulation frequently

occurs between the 12th and 16th days of the cycle, there is considerable variation in the timing of ovulation. It is not uncommon for ovulation to take place at any time between the 8th and 20th days, as illustrated in Figure 3-15. *The time of ovulation bears a closer temporal relation to the onset of the next menstrual period than to the previous menses.* Ovulation usually occurs approximately 14 days before the first day of the succeeding menstrual bleeding.

Signs and Symptoms of Ovulation

On or about the day of ovulation, as many as 25 percent of women experience lower abdominal discomfort on the involved side. This so-called *Mittelschmerz* is believed to be caused by peritoneal irritation by follicular fluid or blood that escapes from the ruptured follicle. The symptoms rarely occur during every cycle.

A useful means of detecting ovulation is by documentation of a shift in basal body temperature from a relatively constant lower level during the follicular or preovulatory phase to a somewhat higher level early in the luteal or postovulatory phase, as illustrated in Figure 3-16. Most likely, ovulation occurs just before or during

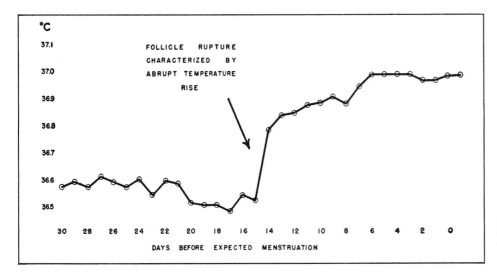

Figure 3-16. Basal temperature shift characteristic of rupture of follicle (*From Palmer: Obstet Gynecol Survey 4:1, 1949.*)

the shift in temperature. The increase in the basal body temperature is caused by the thermogenic action in brain of progesterone. A similar thermal response can be induced by the injection of progesterone into a castrated woman. The rise in basal body temperature, therefore, may be evidence for the development of a corpus luteum and the secretion of progesterone. Extensive luteinization of the granulosa, however, may occur in a follicle that still contains an ovum (luteinized follicle or entrapped ovum). Such an event is believed to be one cause of a short luteal phase and, thereby, infertility.

Other Tests for Ovulation

During the follicular phase, the cervical mucus increases in amount; near the time of ovulation, the appearance of the cervical mucus changes from opaque to clear. At this time, the viscosity of the mucus decreases considerably and it can be drawn into long threads with considerable elastic recoil (*Spinnbarkeit*). Also at this time, when the cervical mucus is spread on a glass slide and allowed to dry, it undergoes marked arborization, or "ferning," because of its content of sodium chloride (see Fig. 4-6, and p. 72). These changes in cervical mucus become maximal at about the time of ovulation. Unfortunately, these cyclic changes in cervical mucus offer no proof of ovulation, but, in normal circumstances, are those that herald the augmented secretion of estrogen that is unopposed by progesterone. Similar changes in cervical mucus may be induced in castrated women by the administration of appropriate doses of estrogen. After ovulation, the changes in the mucus regress; the arborization of dried mucus is lost and a beaded, or "cellular," pattern develops (Fig. 4-7).

As discussed in Chapter 4, there are numerous characteristic morphologic changes that take place in the endometrium after the formation of the corpus luteum and the secretion of progesterone. Since ovulation is nearly always associated with these changes, the demonstration of a well-developed secretory endometrium is strong evidence that ovulation has occurred during that cycle.

An increase in plasma levels of progesterone in a nonpregnant woman is additional evidence that luteinization of a follicle and, very likely, ovulation have taken place. Convenient, rapid, and inexpensive methods for the quantification of progesterone in serum by protein displacement or radioimmunoassay techniques are now readily available. These tests are extremely valuable, but not absolutely definitive, in reaching a presumptive conclusion that ovulation has occurred. Generally, plasma progesterone measurements have replaced the measurement of urinary pregnanediol as a reflection of progesterone secretion.

Many other tests, which range from detection of altered symptoms or physical findings to biochemical or biophysical changes, have been proposed for detecting ovulation. Most of these have been reviewed by Speck (1959). There is still, however, no accurate test that can be conducted easily by women to warn them of impending ovulation. The striking increase in LH secretion that gives rise to the preovulatory LH surge is the most predictable endocrine event that precedes ovulation. It is conceivable that this "surge" could be monitored by sensitive and specific immunoassay techniques in order to predict more precisely that ovulation was imminent provided that the time to complete the test were sufficiently short. Such a technique would have great utility in problems of infertility, and possibly as yet undefined advantages in the prevention of pregnancy.

CORPUS LUTEUM FORMATION

Normally, the corpus luteum forms in the ovary at the site of the ruptured follicle immediately after ovulation (Fig. 3-17A). It is colored by a golden pigment, from which it derives its name, which means "yellow body." Microscopically, it has been observed that the corpus luteum undergoes four stages of development and demise: proliferation, vascularization, maturity, and regression.

When the mature graafian follicle ruptures, the ovum, follicular liquid, and a considerable portion of the surrounding granulosa are discharged. The collapsed walls of the empty follicle form convolutions about the blood-filled cavity (Fig. 3-17B). The remaining granulosa cells appear polyhedral, with round, vesicular nuclei, and frothy cytoplasm. There are many large lacunae that contain extravasated blood but, initially, no blood vessels. The theca interna is invaginated, and its vascular channels are greatly dilated. Endothelial sprouts from the vessels penetrate the granulosa and the hemorrhagic cavity of the ruptured follicle. Hertig (1964) described the K cells (Fig. 3-18) that can be recognized in the mature graafian follicle as stellate cells in which there is deeply eosinophilic, homogenous cytoplasm. During the proliferative stage, strands of K cells, which migrate from the theca, extend into the membrana granulosa to a position as far as the central coagulum.

In the stage of vascularization (that soon follows ovulation), the blood-filled cavity of the ruptured follicle undergoes rapid organization. Grossly, the central coagulum appears pale gray with only a few hemorrhagic foci. Microscopically, there are fibroblasts, but no capillaries, within the coagulum. Elsewhere in the granulosa layer, dilated capillaries are conspicuous. As the stage of vascularization of the corpus luteum progresses to maturity, there is vacuolation in the periphery of the luteinized cells that originate from granulosa; this finding is suggestive that the luteinized cells are physiologically active. The theca interna cells also are vacuolated; when stained for lipid, many more coarse droplets are present in the theca interna cells than in the granulosa lutein cells. The K cells continue to constitute a prominent portion of the corpus luteum cell mass at that stage and also contain lipid, as well as alkaline phosphatase activity in great amounts. The mature corpus luteum is usually 1 to 3 cm in diameter but occasionally may occupy a third or more of the entire ovary. At this stage, the corpus luteum characteristically is bright yellow.

Regressive changes occur in the corpus luteum, oc-

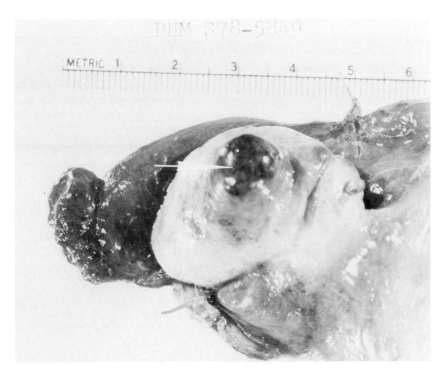

Figure 3-17. A. Arrow points to an intact corpus luteum of early pregnancy. (*Courtesy of Dr. R. Vogt.*)

casionally as early as the 23rd day of the menstrual cycle. These changes become progressively more marked, up to the onset of menstruation, until the central coagulum has been obliterated by connective tissue, and blood pigment has been removed by leukocytes. There is no further capillary proliferation; the nuclei of the granulosa lutein cells become pale, and vacuolization of the peripheral cytoplasm decreases as coarse lipid droplets accumulate. The theca cells can be seen only in widely separated clumps. The K cells develop hyperchromatic nuclei, and the cellular outlines almost disappear. There is a progressive loss of lipid-staining material throughout the entire corpus luteum. Before menstruation, complete regression of the corpus luteum takes place. If fertilization does not take place, the corpus luteum is destined to be a *corpus luteum of menstruation.* If fertilization does take place, a *corpus luteum of pregnancy* is initiated, presumably by the ac-

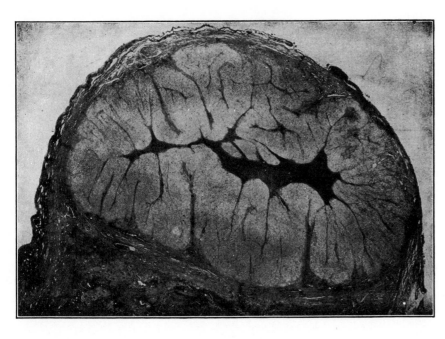

Figure 3-17. B. Corpus luteum of pregnancy (Low power; see also Fig. 3-19.)

"K" cell   Theca lutein   Lutein cells

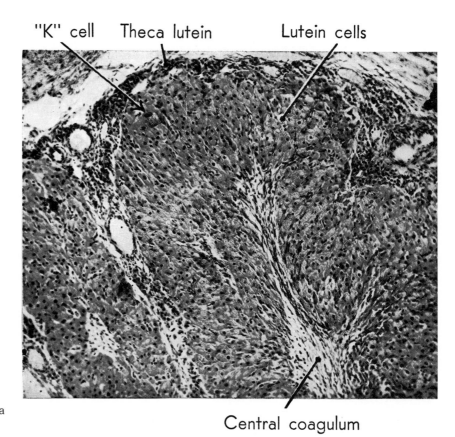

Figure 3-18. Section through the wall of a mature corpus luteum of menstruation.

Central coagulum

tion of chorionic gonadotropin, and the degenerative changes that otherwise would occur are postponed (Fig. 3-19).

Ultrastructure of the Corpus Luteum of Menstruation

Adams and Hertig (1969) described the ultrastructure of human corpora lutea obtained approximately 2, 3, 5, 11, and 15 days after ovulation. The day 5 (menstrual cycle day 19) corpus luteum, compared with younger, differentiating and with older, regressing specimens, is one in which ultrastructural characteristics that are consistent with maximal secretion of progesterone are apparent. In the day 5 luteal cell, there is a peripheral mass of agranular endoplasmic reticulum, which is merged with a large paranuclear Golgi area. Parallel cisternae of granular endoplasmic reticulum are present in the periphery. Lipid droplets and mitochrondria with tubular cristae are numerous in the physiologically active cells, and the complex plasma membranes are suggestive of specialized activities.

Corpus Luteum of Pregnancy

The duration and the function of the corpus luteum of pregnancy are the subjects of much speculation and investigation. The scientific validity of hormonal therapy in the prevention of early abortion after surgical removal

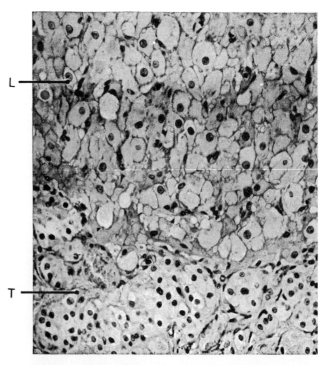

Figure 3-19. Corpus luteum of pregnancy (High power; L = lutein cells; T = theca lutein cells).

of the corpus luteum is dependent on an understanding of the function of this structure.

Hertig (1964) enumerated the morphologic criteria of a very early corpus luteum of pregnancy; these include (1) a surge of hyperplasia from the 23rd to 28th day after the last menstrual period, which results presumably, at least in part, from the stimulus of chorionic gonadotropin, (2) an increasing number of K cells, and (3) the absence of atrophic, ischemic, or regressive changes that are similar to those that appear when menstruation is imminent. The degenerative changes in the corpus luteum are delayed for a variable time but take place most frequently at about 6 months of gestation, although corpora lutea that appear to be normal have been found at term.

Ultrastructure of the Corpus Luteum of Pregnancy.

Adams and Hertig (1969) compared the ultrastructure of human corpora lutea obtained during the 6th, 10th, 16th, and 35th weeks of pregnancy with that of those obtained during the menstrual cycle. In pregnancy, the luteal cell appears to be more highly compartmentalized with a peripheral mass of endoplasmic reticulum and a central area in which mitochondria and Golgi complexes are concentrated. The area that is rich in mitochondria and Golgi complexes extends to the cell surface where microvilli are found that face a vascular space. In certain luteal cells with irregular nuclear membranes, there are vesicular aggregates within the peripheral nucleoplasm or the perinuclear cytoplasm. These nuclear vesicular aggregates and certain spherical bodies may be reflective of prolonged endocrine stimulation and thence secretory exhaustion, which ultimately produce electron-dense cells in which there are pyknotic nuclei.

Crisp and co-workers (1970), in an ultrastructure study, compared the granulosa and theca lutein cells of human corpora lutea. In early pregnancy, granulosa lutein cells may be distinguished from theca lutein cells on the basis of more homogeneous, electronlucent matrix, enlarged pleomorphic mitochondria, abundant endoplasmic reticulum, and several other important ultrastructural features. Furthermore, granulosa lutein cells of early pregnancy may be distinguished from those of the progestational phase of the ovarian cycle by a well-developed endoplasmic reticulum, large spherical mitochondria, more numerous membrane-bound granules, and greater numbers of intercellular canaliculi. These investigators suggested that these differences are a result of the action of chorionic gonadotropin during early gestation. On the basis of morphologic specializations, it seems likely that the corpus luteum secretes, in addition to steroids, a proteinaceous product, i.e., relaxin (see Chapter 3, p. 56).

Function of the Corpus Luteum in Pregnancy

Numerous human pregnancies have succeeded despite early ablation of the corpus luteum. Pratt (1927) reported continuation of pregnancy after an operation was performed as early as the 20th day after the last menstrual period to remove the corpus luteum or about the time of implantation. In a review of cases in which the corpus luteum had been removed early in pregnancy, Hall (1955) reported a rate of abortion of a little greater than 20 percent. He believed that such a rate was not higher than expected after any abdominal surgery that is conducted in the first trimester of pregnancy. In a well-designed study, Tulsky and Koff (1957) removed the corpora lutea from 14 women who requested sterilization and therapeutic abortion. Spontaneous abortion occurred in only two; in the remainder, the pregnancies were terminated by dilatation and curettage; 10 of the 14 women continued to excrete normal quantities of pregnanediol until the conceptus was removed.

The degenerative changes in the corpus luteum of an infertile cycle are delayed by the administration of chorionic gonadotropin. The corpus luteum, of course, secretes progesterone; soon after implantation, however, the human placenta apparently produces enough progesterone to maintain pregnancy. Thus, the corpus luteum, while necessary for implantation in the human, is not required for pregnancy in women beyond the earliest stages of pregnancy.

Inevitably, however, the clinician must face certain therapeutic choices when obliged to remove the corpus luteum in early pregnancy from a woman who wishes to continue that pregnancy. Our choice is the use of a parenteral progestin, for example, 17α-hydroxyprogesterone caproate (Delalutin, 150 mg) when the corpus luteum is removed prior to 10 weeks gestation. We choose 17α-hydroxyprogesterone caproate because (1) the duration of action is predictable; (2) rarely, if ever, does such treatment lead to virilization of a female fetus; and (3) it can be given intramuscularly. Beyond 8 weeks gestation, we administer the progestin only at the time of surgery, if at all. Between 6 and 8 weeks, there may be some merit in a second injection 1 week after surgery.

Corpora Albicantia

In the absence of pregnancy, degenerated lutein cells are rapidly resorbed; within a short time, the corpus luteum is replaced by newly formed connective tissue that resembles closely that of the surrounding ovarian stroma. The structures formed, called corpora albicantia, appear, on cut-section, to be dull and white, somewhat like scar tissue (Fig. 3-20); these are, however, invaded gradually by the surrounding stroma and are broken up into increasingly small hyaline masses, which eventually are completely resorbed. Ultimately, the site of the original follicle is indicated only by an area of slightly thickened connective tissue. In older women, this process may be slower and less complete. In women near the age of menopause, it is not uncommon to find that ovaries are almost filled by scars of various sizes.

Atretic Follicles

Theca lutein cells are admixed somewhat with granulosa lutein cells, but, for the most part, the two cell types are distinctive in appearance. The granulosa lutein cells are larger, more highly vacuolated, and there is a smaller nucleus; the theca lutein cells are somewhat smaller, more deeply stained, and there is a relatively larger nucleus. The theca lutein cells serve a prominent role in the life history of follicles that degenerate without rupture. This process, that is, *follicular atresia,* is particularly pronounced during pregnancy. In this circumstance, after the follicle has attained a certain size, the ovum undergoes cytolysis, while the membrana granulosa degenerates, is cast off into the liquor folliculi, and eventually is resorbed. While these changes are in progress, the theca lutein cells proliferate to form, about the follicle, a tunic many layers thick that frequently becomes yellowish. Eventually, as the follicular fluid disappears, the walls of the follicle collapse and in the theca cells that surround it, there are fatty and hyaline changes. Finally, an irregular hyaline body results that cannot be distinguished from a similar structure that was derived from a corpus luteum.

Atresia is the fate of the vast majority of follicles that develop beyond the primordial stage; the process begins during intrauterine life and continues until after the menopause. Corpora lutea, however, always develop only from the comparatively few follicles, usually one each ovarian cycle, that rupture after reaching maturity. Possibly, one of the functions of the corpus luteum is the obliteration of the spaces left by the ruptured follicles without the formation of cicatricial tissue; thus, the conversion of the entire ovary to scar tissue is prevented.

THE OVARIAN HORMONES

The human ovary produces at least four kinds of hormones—estrogens, progesterone, androgens, and relaxin.

ESTROGENS

Terminology

In 1936, the Council on Pharmacy and Chemistry of the American Medical Association adopted *estrogen* as the collective term for all substances that are capable of producing the typical changes of estrus: enlargement of the uterus, "cornification" of the vaginal epithelium, and mating behavior in immature female animals or in oophorectomized adult female animals. The chemical names of the common estrogens in humans are estradiol-17β, estrone, and estriol.

Discovery

In 1900, Knauer, in a classic study, demonstrated that ovarian transplants prevented atrophy of the uterus in ovariectomized rabbits. Twelve years later, Adler (1912) extracted a substance from ovaries that he found to be the cause of estrus in guinea pigs; and, in 1917, Stockard and Papanicolaou described cyclic variations in the vaginal cells of guinea pigs. This test became a bioassay that enabled Allen and Doisy, in 1923, to isolate a potent estrogen from follicular fluid of ovaries of sows. In 1927, Aschheim and Zondek found that urine of pregnant women was rich in estrogenic substances. With a ready source of crude material and a satisfactory method of bioassay, the way was paved for final chemical identification. Within the next 2 years, Doisy (1929) and Butenandt (1929), almost simultaneously, announced the crystallization from urine of an estrogenic substance that later was designated as *estrone* (Fig. 3-21). In 1930, Browne, while working in Collip's laboratory, isolated the estrogenic steroid *estriol* from placental tissue (Fig. 3-21). It was not until 1936, however, that MacCorquodale and his associates, while working in Doisy's laboratory, crystallized *estradiol-17β* (Fig. 3-21), the most potent growth-promoting factor of these three estrogenic substances.

Chemistry of the Estrogens

The parent hydrocarbon of the estrogens that occur in nature, estrane, is one of an 18-carbon skeleton and differs from the parent compound of the C_{19}-steroid series in that the angular methyl group at position 10 is absent. All the estrogens that have been isolated from human sources are modifications of this basic structure, and, in addition, ring A is characteristically aromatic, as in es-

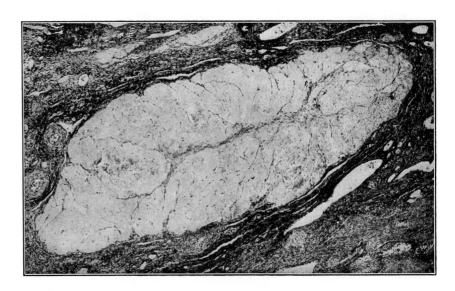

Figure 3-20. Corpus albicans.

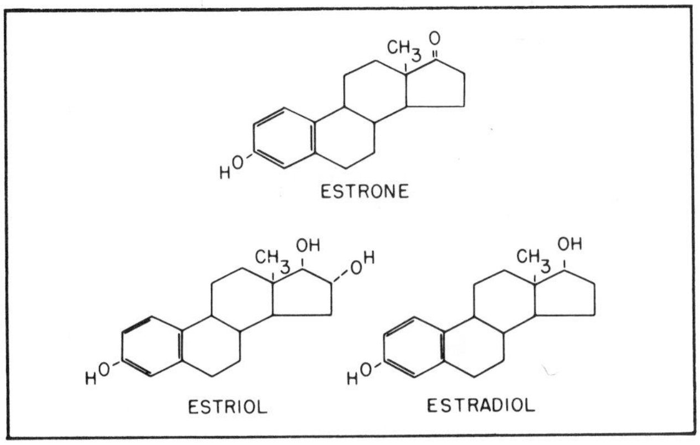

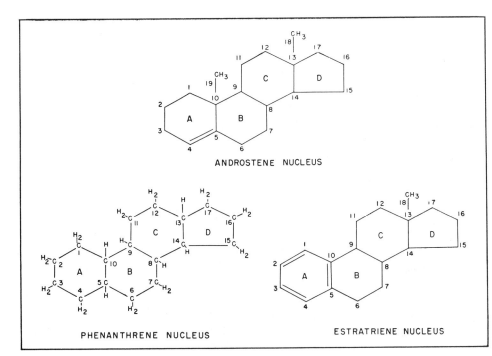

Figure 3-21. Structural formulas of the three important estrogens.

tratriene (Fig. 3-22). Thus, the hydroxyl group at position 3 of the estrogens is phenolic, i.e., weakly acidic. The phenolic structure accounts for the solubility of these compounds in alkali and provides the basis for the separation of these substances from neutral steroids, such as the 17-ketosteroids.

The biosynthesis and metabolism of the classic estrogens—estradiol-17β, estrone, and estriol—have been studied extensively; a large number of additional metabolites, however, have been isolated and characterized from urine of human and various other sources. By the technique of isotope dilution in vivo, it has been shown that most of these metabolites are derived from the classic estrogens, estradiol-17β and estrone. The biologic role, if any, of these metabolites, however, is unknown at present.

In urine, estrogens are present typically in conjugated forms, i.e., linked either to glucuronic acid or to

sulfuric acid, or both; in blood, unconjugated estrogens and estrogen sulfates are present. In nonpregnant women, the estrogen that is present in blood in highest concentration is estrone sulfate.

Catechol Estrogens. The major metabolites of estrone and estradiol-17β are the catechol estrogens. The catechol estrogens are so named because of a hydroxyl function at the C-2 position of the A-ring. Two hydroxyl groups that are ortho to one another in an aromatic ring is a structural feature common to the catecholamines—dopamine, epinepherine, and norepinepherine (Fig. 3-23). Because of this structural similarity, it was suspected that the catechol estrogens may act to modulate the metabolism or action of catecholamines. Impetus for this postulate was gained from the observation that the catechol estrogens have a much greater affinity for the enzyme catechol-O-methyltransferase than do the catecholamines. Catechol-O-methyltransferase catalyzes the conversion of the catecholamines to inactive methyl ether(s) (metanephrine) metabolites.

Sources of Estrogens. The results of the histochemical investigations of Dempsey and Bassett (1943) and of McKay and Robinson (1947) were indicative that the theca cells elaborate estradiol-17β (presently, however, this is not believed to be the case). Additional experimental data that were gathered from studies of implantation of granulosa or theca cells into castrated animals were suggestive that endocrine activity was associated only with the transplanted thecal cells. Furthermore, ovarian irradiation that resulted in destruction of the granulosa and proliferation of the theca allowed a persistence of estrogenic activity. Observations of experimentally produced ovarian tumors were indicative that

Figure 3-22. Theoretical structural nuclei from which the estrogens and androgens are derived.

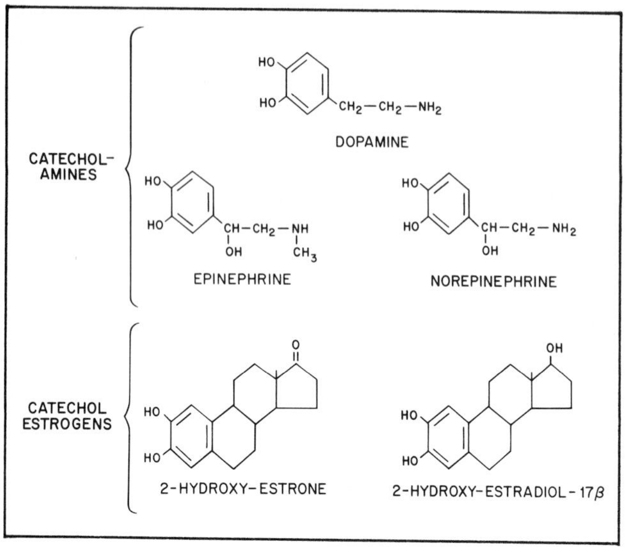

Figure 3-23. Structural similarities between catecholamines and catechol estrogens.

the thecal component of the granulosa cell tumor, rather than the granulosa component, secreted estrogens. The conversion of C_{19}-steroids to estrogens, however, an enzymatic process referred to as aromatization, is demonstrable in isolated granulosa cells in vitro. Presently, the relative contribution of each of the cellular elements of the follicle to total estradiol-17β production by the ovary is not known, nor is it known if such contributions may be profoundly different in the follicular and luteal phases of the ovarian cycle. This issue, however, is discussed in greater detail in Chapter 5. The theca cells are considered to be the principal site of formation of C_{19}-steroids in the developing follicle, but the granulosa cells of the corpus luteum are enzymatically competent to produce estrogens from the C_{19}-steroid precursors and may serve as a quantitatively significant source of estradiol-17β during the follicular and luteal phases of the ovarian cycle.

In addition, estrogens in the plasma and urine of nonpregnant women are derived from yet another source. The existence of an extraglandular source of estrogen now is established. This extraglandular estrogen is derived from the conversion of plasma androstenedione to estrone (MacDonald and co-workers, 1967). Indeed, extraglandular estrogen production constitutes the principal mechanism for estrogen formation in prepubertal children, in postmenopausal women, and in men. In young adult men, estrogen is derived largely from extraglandular sources by the conversion of plasma androstenedione and plasma testosterone. A small amount of estradiol-17β is secreted directly by the testes in normal men. In young women, extraglandular estrogen production is principally the result of the formation of estrone, in many extraglandular tissue sites, from the aromatization of plasma androstenedione. The plasma prehor-

mone, androstenedione, originates by direct secretion from both the adrenal cortices and the ovaries. In young women, approximately 3 to 4 mg of androstenedione enter the blood each day from these two sources of direct secretion. Approximately 1.5 percent of this androstenedione is converted, in extraglandular sites, to the product hormone, estrone. Thus, in young women, the extraglandular estrogen (i.e., estrone) production rate amounts to 40 to 60 μg of estrone per day. In certain anovulatory women with excessive production of androstenedione, usually of ovarian origin, the extraglandular formation of estrone may be increased by the increased availability of the plasma androstenedione substrate. Indeed, in such women, extraglandular estrone may be the principal source of estrogen formation. In normal ovulatory women, however, the fluctuating secretion of estradiol-17β by the ovary is additive to the extraglandular estrogen production, and total estrogen production in such women is the sum of its formation by these two mechanisms.

Biosynthetic Pathways of Estrogen Formation in the Ovary. Through the work of numerous investigators, many of the steps involved in ovarian biosynthesis of estrogens have been elucidated. These steps are illustrated in Figure 3-24, in which several noteworthy features of this biosynthetic system are shown.

First, incubation of ovarian tissue with simple precursors such as acetate or cholesterol results in the formation of estrogen (Ryan and Smith, 1959). Unlike the placenta, therefore (see Chapter 7), the ovary does not require circulating C_{19}-steroid precursors for the biosynthesis of estrogens, but, rather, in the ovary there is the capacity for estrogen synthesis de novo.

Second, several investigators have demonstrated that at least two separate pathways for the synthesis of estradiol-17β may be operative in the human ovary. One proceeds by way of androstenedione and testosterone in the biosynthesis of estradiol-17β; the other may proceed by way of $\triangle^5$-3β-hydroxysteroid intermediates, namely pregnenolone, 17α-hydroxy pregnenolone, and dehydroisoandrosterone in the synthesis of estradiol-17β. Ryan (1959) speculated that the two pathways may have a cellular separation in the ovary. It is possible that the $\triangle^5$-3β-hydroxy pathway is preferred in the theca cells, whereas the $\triangle^4$-3-ketone pathway may be utilized principally in corpus luteum, which is known to be a rich source of 3β-hydroxysteroid dehydrogenase, the enzyme that catalyzes the conversion of $\triangle^5$-3β-hydroxysteroids to the $\triangle^4$-3-ketone moieties. It is quite possible, of course, that the synthetic capacities of the two cellular types differ quantitatively, rather than qualitatively, so that an absolute division of enzymatic capacities is not demonstrable by in vitro techniques. It must be recalled that androstenedione is the precursor of estrogen biosynthesis by way of either pathway.

Third, as stated, both proposed pathways of ovarian estrogen synthesis proceed through "androgenic," i.e., daily production rates of estradiol-17β have been calculated from the amount of dilution by endogenously produced hormone of an intravenously administered radiolabeled tracer dose of estradiol-17β. The extent to which endogenous hormone dilutes the administered tracer is estimated by determining the specific activity of a urinary metabolite, for example, estradiol-17β glucuronoside. Employing this experimental design, Goering and Herrmann (1964) found that the production rate of estradiol-17β during the immediate premenstrual and postmenstrual phases of the cycle was about 50 μg per 24 hours, but rose to 150 to 300 μg per 24 hours at the time of ovulation. These results are in good agreement with estimates made by indirect techniques. From studies of measurements of estradiol-17β in plasma, it appears that the secretory rate of estradiol-17β may reach 600 to 1000 μg per 24 hours just prior to the LH surge at midcycle. Levels this high are not detected by urinary techniques, since these methods are those that are reflective of the "average" daily production over the 3- to 5-day period of urine collections.

These isotope dilution studies as well as those that involve direct sampling of ovarian venous blood also have provided results that are supportive of the view that the principal estrogen that is the secretory product of the ovary is estradiol-17β, which, in turn, is the precursor of multiple urinary metabolites. Fishman and co-workers (1960) demonstrated that estradiol-17β that is introduced into the circulation is converted quickly to estrone. Although intravenously administered estrone also is converted to estradiol-17β, this transformation proceeds at a much slower rate. Gurpide and associates (1963) found that more than 90 percent of intravenously administered isotope-labeled estradiol-17β is metabolized by way of estrone, whereas 50 percent of intravenously administered radioactive estrone is metabolized by way of estradiol-17β. The conversion of plasma estradiol-17β to plasma estrone and of plasma estrone to plasma estradiol-17β, however, is considerably less than 90 and 50 percent, respectively. Namely, only 15 percent of estradiol-17β appears in plasma as estrone, whereas only 5 percent of estrone appears in plasma as estradiol-17β. The reason for the differences as measured by urinary and plasma methods is that there is further metabolism of the estrogen product in the tissue sites of conversion prior to reentry of the product into plasma. Estradiol-17β, for example, may be converted in a tissue site to estrone, but the estrone formed may be metabolized further, irreversibly, e.g., to estrone glucuronoside, prior to reentry into blood.

Estrogens in Biologic Fluids. The estrogens that circulate in blood are principally sulfuric acid conjugates, whereas the metabolites found in urine are principally glucuronic acid conjugates. Only a small fraction of the total amount of estrogens produced is excreted in the urine. (The combined concentration of estradiol-17β, estrone, and estriol in 24 hours of urine is equal to about 15 percent of the estradiol-17β and estrone produced

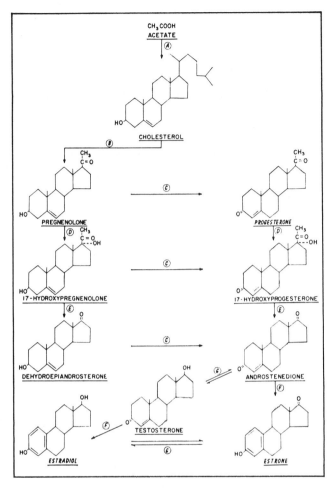

Figure 3-24. Pathway of steroid biosynthesis in the ovary. A. formation of sterol from acetate. B. cleavage of cholesterol side chain—converts C27 to C21 compound. C. 3β-hydroxysteroid dehydrogenase and Δ4-Δ5-isomerase reaction. D. 17α-hydroxylation. E. cleavage of side chain—converts C21 to C19 compounds. F. aromatizing reaction. G. 17β-hydroxysteroid dehydrogenase (reversible). (*From Smith and Ryan: Am J Obstet Gynecol 84:141, 1962.*)

C19-steroid, intermediates, dehydroisoandrosterone, Δ4-androstenedione, and testosterone. Thus, not only is the enzymatic potential of the ovary to produce androgen established, but the secretion of C19-steroids, including testosterone, during the normal ovarian cycle has been demonstrated.

Nature of the Ovarian Secretion of Estrogen. Estimations of the daily "production rate" of estrogen in ovulatory women have been made. This rate is a measure of the total daily production of estrogen, that is, the amount of estrogen produced from all sources. Although the production rate is not a direct determination of ovarian secretion, it does provide a means for the determination of the total amount of estrogen produced both by ovarian secretion (estradiol-17β) and by extraglandular formation from plasma androstenedione (estrone). The

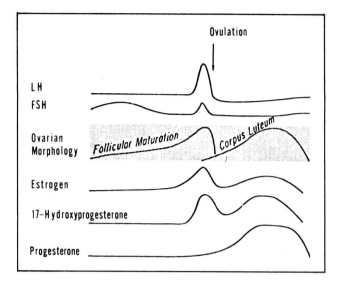

Figure 3-25. Changes in plasma of the various hormones involved in ovulation in women. LH = luteinizing hormone; FSH = follicle-stimulating hormone. (*From Strott, Yoshimi, Ross, Lipsett: J Clin Endocrinol Metab 29:1166, 1969.*)

each day.) Substantial amounts of estrogens have been identified in the feces.

Frank and associates (1932) first noted the tendency toward a biphasic curve of estrogen excretion in urine, with one peak at or near the time of ovulation and a second peak during the midluteal phase. During the 4 or 5 days before the next menstrual period, the excretion of estrogens declines rapidly. A similar pattern has been identified for the levels of estrogens in plasma, as shown in Figure 3-25.

Actions of the Estrogens

Estradiol-17β may be regarded as a growth hormone with selective affinity for tissues derived from the müllerian ducts, namely the fallopian tubes, the endometrium, the myometrium, the cervix, and the vagina. Jensen and Jacobson (1962), and others, have shown that whereas only a small amount of a physiologic dose of estradiol-17β can be found in an estrogen-growth-responsive tissue, the tissues derived from müllerian ducts are those with a much greater capacity to "incorporate and retain estradiol-17β (but not estrone) for a prolonged (period of) time" than are other tissues, such as liver, kidney, and skeletal muscle.

The developmental role, if any, of estrogens in sexual differentiation remains to be ascertained. Jost (1953) and others have shown that the male sex hormone, testosterone, is necessary for the development of the wolffian ducts into the male internal genitalia as well as the differentiation of the genital tubercle into the male external genitalia. Moreover, yet another fetal testicular secretory product—a protein of seminiferous tubule (sertoli cell) origin—causes regression of the müllerian ducts—hence the name *müllerian duct regression factor*

or substance. It has been assumed, by inference, that the female sex hormone is unnecessary in the embryo for the proper development of the müllerian ducts, although by no means has this been demonstrated satisfactorily. It is likely, however, that in the absence of the testis the müllerian ducts and the genital tubercle differentiate along female lines, that is, no positive stimulus is necessary.

At puberty, the effects of estrogens are apparent in the development of the adult habitus of women. Cornification of the vaginal epithelium is achieved and the uterus attains the adult size and configuration. The ratio of the size of the body of the uterus to that of the cervix changes from 1 to 1 to the adult ratio of 2 to 1. In addition to the production of these end-organ responses, estrogens also act to influence the actions of other endocrine glands and the action of other hormones.

Effects on Uterus. It has been demonstrated convincingly that estrogens act on the uterus by way of at least two mechanisms. One of these is through a system that involves a receptor in cytosol of uterine tissue that provides for the concentration of estradiol-17β in the cytosol and the subsequent translocation to the nucleus of the estrogen–receptor complex. After a conformational change, this complex elicits DNA transcription that is followed by messenger RNA translation and thence protein synthesis. Additionally, Szego and Davis (1969) have shown that estradiol-17β will evoke, within 15 seconds of administration, an increase in the uterine concentration of cyclic AMP, a so-called second messenger, which apparently results from an interaction of trophic hormone and inner cell membrane adenylate cyclase system. No doubt, many other metabolic effects of estrogens at other sites within the uterine cell will be defined ultimately.

The spiral arteries respond to the growth stimulus of estrogens even more actively than the rest of the endometrium; as a result, the tips of these vessels grow progressively to approach the epithelial surface.

Effects on Cervix. In addition, estrogens affect the activity of the cervical epithelium in such a manner that the cervical mucus increases in quantity and pH, attains a clear fluid state, and is penetrated more rapidly by spermatozoa. Microscopically, the dried mucus is characterized by the formation of a "fern," as discussed on page 72.

Effects on Vagina. Estrogens produce thickening of the vaginal epithelium. In castrated women, estrogens cause a change in the vaginal epithelium from a structure that is only two or three cells thick to a membrane that is densely packed with compressed cells.

Effects on Fallopian Tubes. Estrogens stimulate growth of the fallopian tubes and appear to influence the activity of the tubal musculature. In experimental animals, tubal contractions become maximal at estrus. The dependence of these contractions on estrogens is indi-

cated by the disappearance of contractions after ovariectomy and the restoration thereof by the administration of estrogens.

Effects on Breasts. The administration of estrogens to the immature or ovariectomized animal, in which the mammary glands are rudimentary or atrophic, causes an extension of the ducts comparable to that seen in the sexually mature, nulliparous animal. The type of growth varies in different species. In women and in the monkey, partial lobule–alveolar growth is induced, as is ductal development by estrogen. In other animals, the action of estrogens is solely on the ducts, and the action of progesterone is necessary for the proliferation of the lobule–alveolar system.

Effects on Other Endocrine Organs. Estrogens suppress the secretion of follicle-stimulating hormone (FSH) by the pituitary, as demonstrated by Frank and Salmon (1935) who showed that the elevated urinary FSH titer found in menopausal or ovariectomized women could be lowered by the administration of estrogens. The actual pituitary content of FSH was lower after estrogen administration; this finding is indicative that the effect was not just the result of secretory suppression and increased glandular storage. In women, estrogens trigger the release of luteinizing hormone (LH), which, in turn, brings about ovulation in a mature ovarian follicle.

Effects on Ovary. Bradbury (1961) demonstrated that there is a direct action of estrogenic hormones on ovarian tissue per se. Estradiol-17β, by a local effect, stimulates the growth of the ovarian follicle even in the absence of FSH and thereby potentiates the response to gonadotropins. This action of estrogen on the follicle may account for the almost exponential rise in estradiol-17β secretion and concentration in blood just prior to the LH "surge."

Effects on Skeletal System. In immature animals and in humans estrogens promote linear growth of bone and then epiphyseal closure.

PROGESTERONE

During the postovulatory phase of the ovarian cycle, progesterone is secreted by the corpus luteum.

Definition

Progesterone is a specific, biologically active steroid that produces progestational changes in the uterus of suitably estrogen-prepared immature or ovariectomized animals.

Discovery.
Prenant, in 1898, first suggested that the corpus luteum was an organ of internal secretion. Fraenkel, in 1910, demonstrated that the corpus luteum in the rabbit was necessary for the maintenance of pregnancy. In the same year,

Bouin and Ancel (1910) described the histology of the progestational endometrium and thereby provided the foundation upon which Corner and Allen (1929) established their classic method of bioassay of progesterone, one that enabled them, in 1928, to isolate from sows' ovaries the hormone that they named "progestin" to indicate its specific role in gestation. Somewhat later, when Butenandt (1930) characterized progesterone as a steroid, he suggested that the chemical nature be indicated in the nomenclature by the suffix "sterone." Thus, the term *progesterone* arose from the combination of the two words.

Butenandt (1930) described a urinary steroid excreted in large amounts during pregnancy, pregnanediol. The significance of pregnanediol, however, was not recognized until 1937, when Venning demonstrated a correlation between the rate of excretion of pregnanediol in the urine and the presence of endogenous or exogenous progesterone. She demonstrated that pregnanediol, which is excreted as the sodium salt of pregnanediol glucuronoside, was a metabolite of progesterone. Previously, only minute amounts of progesterone had been isolated directly from the corpus luteum or from the blood of the ovarian vein. No metabolites of progesterone had yet been identified, and, therefore, no means of monitoring the secretion of progesterone was available.

Chemistry of Progesterone

Progesterone, the principal hormone secreted by the corpus luteum, is a derivative of the 21-carbon skeleton, pregnane. In addition to the 2-carbon side chain at carbon 17, in progesterone there is a ketone group at carbon 20 and a $\triangle^4$-3-ketone configuration in ring A, a characteristic that is common to a number of hormonally active steroids. Progesterone and two compounds that are closely related structurally, that is, 20α- and 20β-dihydroprogesterone, have been isolated from the corpus luteum, ovarian vein blood, the placenta, and the adrenal. Progesterone is found in peripheral venous blood, but little is found in the urine or feces.

Metabolism of Progesterone

In the human, the major urinary metabolite of progesterone is pregnanediol. Dorfman, Ross, and Shipley (1948) found pregnanolone in the urine after administration of progesterone; the "allo" forms of both pregnanolone and pregnanediol also are recoverable in substantially smaller amounts. The liver has been identified as a major site of conversion of progesterone to these metabolites.

From the results of a number of studies, however, it is known that progesterone is a preferred substrate for the ubiquitous and metabolically important enzyme, 5α-reductase; thus, progesterone is a competitive inhibitor of 5α-reductase (Massa and Martini, 1971). It is this enzyme that also catalyzes the conversion of testosterone to dihydrotestosterone, a compound that, in turn, is one that modulates androgenic effects in certain androgen-responsive end-organs. Moreover, based on the results of some studies, it seems possible that progesterone may exert definitive biologic action through its conversion to 5α-dihydroprogesterone in some tissues. Recently, it has been shown that there are considerable amounts of 5α-dihydroprogesterone in the blood of pregnant women (Milewich and co-workers, 1975). The exact source of this compound and the biologic significance of this finding are not yet clear.

From the results of histologic studies of the endometrium that were conducted by Jones, Wade, and Goldberg (1952) it is known that glandular cells that are rich in glycogen are low in alkaline phosphatase, an enzyme that decreases greatly when large amounts of progesterone are given. These investigators also found that progesterone blocks the formation of high-energy phosphate bonds in compounds in hepatic mitochrondria of the rat, and thereby the production of glycogen is favored.

Progesterone and Metabolites in Blood and Urine.

In the blood of ovulatory women, the maximum concentration of progesterone and metabolites thereof are attained about 1 week after ovulation. About 65 percent of injected radiolabeled progesterone can be recovered as metabolites in the urine and feces, with 20 percent in the urine, and 45 percent in the bile or feces. In the urine, half of the radioactive metabolites are excreted as pregnanediol, 10 to 20 percent as pregnanolone, and a small amount as other metabolites. The metabolites of progesterone in the bile are from pregnanediol (50 to 60 percent), pregnanolone (30 to 40 percent), and other unidentified, that is, more polar (i.e., water-soluble) metabolites (about 10 percent). In women with normal ovarian cycles, the peak excretion of pregnanediol occurs on the 20th and 21st days of the menstrual cycle. Excretion of pregnanediol usually declines and may be almost absent by 2 days before menstruation.

These findings are correlated well with the progesterone determinations in the corpus luteum of menstruation that were conducted by Hoffman (1948); he found the first measurable quantity of progesterone was on the 14th day of the menstrual cycle. The levels increased to maximal values by the 16th day and remained elevated until the 24th day of the cycle, after which time there was a gradual decline until the onset of menstruation. The rate of secretion of progesterone by the mid-luteal phase corpus luteum has been estimated to be 25 to 50 mg per day. This is the highest rate of steroid secretion per unit weight of tissue of any endocrine organ!

Actions of Progesterone

The more profound effects of progesterone that are recognized thus far include the following: conversion of proliferative endometrium to secretory endometrium and thence to decidua; inhibition of the contractility of smooth muscle, especially of the uterus; stimulation of natriuesis and, in turn, increased aldosterone production; and, stimulation of the respiratory center and increased respiratory rate. More recently, it has been shown by

several investigators that small amounts of progesterone that are given to castrated or postmenopausal women who previously had been given an estrogen lead to a sudden, but transient, rise in circulating luteinizing hormone. The thermogenic effects of progesterone have been discussed previously.

Effects on Endometrium.

A major function of progesterone is an action to prepare the endometrium for blastocyst implantation and maintenance of pregnancy. The classic progestational changes in the endometrium were described by Hitschmann and Adler (1908) and were described in detail later by Noyes, Hertig, and Rock (1950). In the properly estrogen-primed endometrium, progesterone acts to produce manifold evidences of secretory activity. The tubular endometrial glands that are characteristic of the preovulatory phase are converted into tortuous structures. Subnuclear vacuoles, in the epithelial cells, are the first histologic evidence of a progesterone effect on endometrial gland secretion. These vacuoles increase in size and thereafter migrate toward the luminal margin of the cell, and finally allow for secretion to pour into the lumens of the glands. If these same glandular epithelial cells are suitably stained, glycogen can be demonstrated at about the time that vacuolization first appears. Thereafter, glycogen steadily increases in amount until shortly before menstruation; the alkaline phosphatase activity, however, appears to become maximal around the time of ovulation. The stroma becomes edematous, and the constituent cells undergo hypertrophy with an increased amount of cytoplasm. If stimulation persists, the stromal cells form sheets of decidual cells; these characteristic histologic, cytochemical, and ultrastructural changes are considered further in Chapter 4.

The normal menstrual flow occurs from the endometrium that is deprived of progesterone. The amount of progesterone necessary to produce the typical endometrial effects is influenced by the previous estrogenic stimulation as well as the duration of the stimulation by progesterone and the continuity of the amount of progesterone produced. Progesterone (10 mg) given intramuscularly daily for 7 days produces minimal secretory glandular changes. The level for vascular response, however, seems to be lower than that for the glandular reaction, since half this dose may produce withdrawal bleeding in the absence of any demonstrable glandular progestational effect. To prevent menstruation, as the corpus luteum regresses, it is necessary to give large amounts of progesterone, 100 to 250 mg daily in divided doses. With these amounts of progesterone, menstruation can be delayed for 10 to 14 days or longer.

Maintenance of Pregnancy.

The progestational endometrium, with the deposition of glycogen that occurs in response to the action of progesterone, furnishes proper nutritive conditions for the nidation and support of the fertilized ovum. If, because of a deficiency of progesterone secretion, the endometrial bed degenerates, the products of conception implanted therein are aborted. In several animal species, for example, the rat and rabbit, the presence of the corpus luteum seems to be necessary throughout pregnancy, as its removal at any stage of gestation causes abortion. The classic studies of Corner and Allen have shown that ovariectomy in the pregnant rabbit or destruction of all the corpora lutea before the last few days of its gestational period regularly causes abortion. By administering an extract of sow's corpora lutea, Corner and Allen (1929) were able to maintain pregnancy to term (32 days, approximately) in rabbits that were ovariectomized shortly after mating.

The ability of women to carry pregnancy to completion in the absence of the corpus luteum in no way indicates that progesterone is unnecessary for the maintenance of pregnancy. The placenta, which normally produces progesterone and estrogen in large quantities throughout much of pregnancy, is able to synthesize these hormones even at a very early stage in gestation in quantities sufficient to maintain gestation.

Effects on Uterine Motility. Knaus (1926) concluded that, in rabbits, progesterone acts on both endometrium and myometrium. He demonstrated that there was decreased spontaneous uterine activity and complete inhibition of the response to the oxytocic hormone in the postovulatory phase of the ovarian cycle during the time of transportation, implantation, and early development of the fertilized ovum. He found that progesterone also inhibited spontaneous contractility and the response in the human uterus to posterior pituitary extracts. Csapo (1954) found, by use of isolated muscle strips, that progesterone acted to decrease the electrochemical gradient and could inhibit myometrial functions in the presence of a complete actomyosin and adenosine triphosphate system. The decrease in the electrochemical gradient causes the muscle to be insensitive to oxytocin, epinephrine, acetylcholine, and histamine.

Effects on Oviducts. From histologic studies, it was shown that, to a degree, the tubal mucosa undergoes cyclic changes. During the luteal phase, it undergoes changes that are indicative of secretory activity. This interpretation is substantiated by Joël's observation (1939) that the content of glycogen and ascorbic acid in the human tubal mucosa is greatest during the luteal phase. This has been demonstrated in the rabbit by Westman and co-workers (1931) and by Caffier (1938). Cyclic variations in the activity of the tubal musculature also have been ascribed to progesterone. There are rhythmic contractions, whose amplitude is greatest at the height of the follicular phase and least during the luteal phase of the cycle; the relative quiescence in the latter phase, which is attributed to the action of progesterone, may play an important part in transport of the fertilized ovum to the uterine cavity. A very specific action of progesterone on the chick oviduct, the elaboration of avidin, has been demonstrated by the elegant studies of O'Malley and co-workers (1970).

Effects on Cervix. The cervix produces different types of mucus during various phases of the cycle. After ovulation, the secretions are scanty, viscid, full of leukocytes, impermeable to spermatozoa, and do not form a fern pattern after drying. These characteristics presumably are the effect primarily of progesterone that counteracts estrogen action.

Effects on Ovulation. Hertz, Meyer, and Spielman (1937) demonstrated that progesterone caused the copulatory response in the guinea pig. In women, however, progesterone is produced after ovulation.

Effects on Breasts. Progesterone is largely responsible for the acinar and lobular development that occurs during the luteal phase of the ovarian cycle, after action of estrogens on the ductal epithelium. Progesterone plus estrogens, by dual action, are capable of bringing about complete mammary development, estrogens acting principally on the ductal system and progesterone on the lobular alveolar apparatus. Progesterone also apparently inhibits the action of prolactin in α-lactalbumin synthesis. This action is apparently an explanation for the enigma of the failure of lactation during pregnancy when prolactin levels are greater than those found in puerperal women. Upon delivery of the placenta and the removal of the source of the massive progesterone production, the inhibitory effect of progesterone on the breast is removed and lactation can proceed under the influence of prolactin, insulin, and cortisol.

Effects on Other Endocrine Systems. Progesterone will not suppress the pituitary production of FSH, according to Greep and Jones (1950), and is ineffective in the relief of menopausal vasomotor symptoms. Salhanick and associates (1952) thought that progesterone might suppress the secretion of luteinizing hormone, but this point is still debated.

Thermogenic Effects. The induction of an increase in the basal body temperature by progesterone has been used to identify luteal function.

Synthetic Progestins. Several synthetic steroid compounds with various degrees of progesteronelike activities are used in clinical medicine, especially when combined with estrogens, as in oral contraceptives (see Chapter 40).

ANDROGENS

The human ovary is enzymatically capable of synthesizing dehydroisoandrosterone, androstenedione, and testosterone. Evidence obtained by isolation of steroids from incubations of ovarian tissue, analysis of ovarian venous blood, and measurements of secretory rates before and after adrenal suppression are indicative that the normal ovary secretes dehydroisoandrosterone, androstenedione, and testosterone. Androstenedione levels in blood from the ovarian vein increase sharply in the late follicular phase, decrease slightly during the early luteal phase, and then increase again (Baird and co-workers, 1974). In normal ovulatory women, plasma androstenedione originates from both adrenal and ovarian secretion. Dehydroisoandrosterone and its sulfate ester are derived principally from adrenal secretion. Testosterone, on the other hand, is derived primarily from the extraglandular conversion of androstenedione to testosterone; a lesser amount of testosterone arises by direct ovarian secretion. During the premenopausal years, women produce approximately 300 μg of testosterone per day, one half to two thirds of which originates by the extraglandular conversion from the plasma prehormone, androstenedione. Thus, androstenedione represents a plasma prehormone for conversion at extraglandular sites not only to estrogen but also to the biologically important androgen, testosterone.

RELAXIN

In a recent review, Bryant-Greenwood (1982) chose to entitle her manuscript, "Relaxin as a New Hormone." She pointed out that whereas relaxin was first discovered by Frederick Hisaw (1926), the hormone fell into disrepute for nearly 4 decades. There were many reasons, as Bryant-Greenwood noted, for the neglect of relaxin research. Hisaw demonstrated that relaxin acted to effect separation of the symphysis pubis in certain experimental animals. Crude preparations of porcine relaxin were made available for use in women and these preparations were promoted, transiently, as a means to arrest premature labor. In the course of administration of these compounds, some obstetricians were struck by the apparent association of relaxin treatment and subsequent cervical ripening. Thus, some physicians began to use relaxin preparations to effect cervical ripening prior to the induction of labor in women in whom the cervix was believed to be unfavorable to the induction of labor. Thus, to many, relaxin became, if not a subject of ridicule, a matter of considerable confusion. The question posed was, "How can we use a compound to arrest labor that appears to be more effective in acting to bring about the first physical changes that we associate with parturition, that is, softening of the uterine cervix?" But as is so often the case in biomedical research, confusion reigns when one assesses physiologic or biochemical responses to putative compounds before these are adequately purified and characterized.

Bryant-Greenwood (1982) suggests that we may now be well back on the right track in the investigations of relaxin and that more properly this agent should be considered as a hormone of the reproductive tract of women with "potential significance in the remodeling of collagen." Now, the amino acid sequences of relaxins of a number of species are known and the rat relaxin gene has been cloned. There are considerable analogies be-tween the structure of relaxin and those of insulin and insulinlike growth factors.

By use of a relaxin-specific radiolabeled DNA synthetic probe, Hudson and associates (1981) demonstrated that the greatest concentration of relaxin messenger RNA was found in the corpora lutea of pregnant rats. It may be that the corpus luteum is the principal site of synthesis of relaxin in species that are dependent upon the corpus luteum for maintenance of pregnancy, for example, the rat and pig. In other species, for example, the cow and guinea pig, there is little relaxin detectable in the corpora lutea in pregnancy. Relaxin is also produced and stored in the corpus luteum of pregnant women.

The uterus is believed to be a target tissue for relaxin and, in some species, not only in the guinea pig, a site also of relaxin synthesis, probably in the endometrium. In women, it is believed that placenta and decidua are sources of relaxin, albeit in much smaller amounts than that produced by the corpus luteum. On the other hand, the placenta may be the principal source of relaxin in the pregnant mare.

Ordinarily, maximal effects of relaxin are demonstrable in the estrogen-primed animal. There appear to be two primary effects of relaxin. One effect is acute, that is, relaxation of myometrium, but the other is long-term, namely, the remodeling of collagen.

Myometrial receptors for relaxin have been demonstrated and the number of such receptors is highly dependent upon the estrogen status of the animal. Oxytocin and prostaglandin $F_{2\alpha}$ will act to override the myometrial quiescense induced by relaxin but much less effectively so in the estrogen-primed myometrium. Interestingly, prolactin acts to antagonize the effects of relaxin on estrogen-primed uteri.

A number of investigators have demonstrated that relaxin acts to induce cervical softening without the induction of a change in tensile strength. Initial studies have been conducted in near-term pregnant women to ascertain if relaxin would act to induce cervical softening. Although preliminary in nature, the results of these studies are encouraging. A prepartum surge in circulating relaxin levels, however, is not demonstrable.

PITUITARY GONADOTROPIC HORMONES

The importance of the pituitary gland in the sexual cycle was first appreciated from the results of studies on hypophysectomized animals that were conducted by Philip Smith (1927). Fluhmann, in 1929, contributed to our early clinical understanding of gonadotropin secretion when he discovered large amounts of pituitary gonadotropin in the blood of postmenopausal women. In 1931, Fevold, Hisaw, and Leonard demonstrated that this pituitary gonadotropic fraction actually contained two active components, FSH and LH. In 1939, investigators at the Evans Laboratory in Berkeley, California and those at the Squibb Biological Research Laboratory, directed by Van Dyke, described almost simultaneously the chemical separation and identification of these substances. These findings made possible experiments with relatively pure hormones and provided for further elucidation of the physiologic activity of the pituitary gonadotropins.

The next major contribution in the control of the ovarian cycle by the pituitary hormones came from Harris (1952), who appreciated the importance of the hypophysial portal system, a series of blood vessels along the pituitary stalk that serve as a communication system between the hypothalamic centers and the pituitary. Wislocki (1938) showed that the blood flow in this system was principally from the hypothalamus to the anterior pituitary gland rather than in the reverse direction. The results of other studies are indicative that changes in the hypothalamus are responsible for the onset of puberty, rather than maturation of the ovary or the pituitary, both of which are capable of adult function at birth if properly stimulated.

Follicle Stimulating Hormone

FSH, when administered to hypophysectomized immature female rats, causes growth of the follicle, development of the antrum of the follicle, and an increase in ovarian weight. FSH is essential for the production of estrogen by the ovary: however, the metabolic fate of FSH is largely unknown. It appears to be excreted partly in the urine in much the same form in which it is secreted by the pituitary.

Although FSH was one of the first gonadotropic hormones to be identified, it was one of the last to be isolated in pure form; it is a readily water-soluble glycoprotein; and, the isoelectric point of the hormone isolated from pituitary of swine is pH 4.8. The carbohydrate fraction of the hormone includes mannose and hexosamine.

FSH usually is detectable in the blood and urine of children, but the levels begin to increase at about 11 years of age. Just prior to puberty, the levels of gonadotropins increase principally at night and primarily during times of sleep. During the normal menstrual cycle, before ovulation, the levels of FSH remain relatively constant or change only slightly until just prior to ovulation, when the levels rise somewhat. By the time of ovulation, any previous increase in the FSH level has receded to near baseline levels. During the remainder of the ovarian cycle, FSH levels are low but rise again very slightly just prior to menstruation (Figs. 3-25, 3-26). The rise in plasma FSH levels just before ovulation is coincident with an increase in luteinizing hormone (the LH "surge"), the magnitude of which is much greater than is that of FSH.

After the menopause, when the secretion of estrogens by the ovary is negligible or absent, the levels of FSH in plasma and the amount excreted in the urine are increased greatly. Administration of an estrogen lowers markedly, but does not abolish, the secretion of FSH by the pituitary of postmenopausal women.

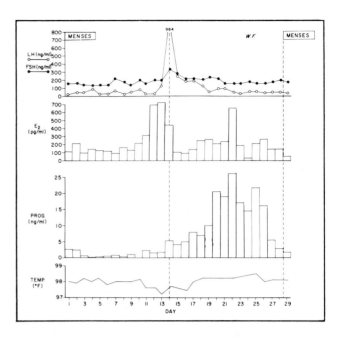

Figure 3-26. Plasma levels throughout the menstrual cycle of the hormones involved in ovulation. LH = luteinizing hormone; FSH = follicle-stimulating hormone; E₂ = estradiol; Prog., = progesterone; Temp. = basal body temperature; ng = nanogram; pg = picogram. (*From VandeWiele and associates: Recent Prog Horm Res 126:63, 1970.*)

Luteinizing Hormone

LH also is referred to as interstitial cell-stimulating hormone. LH acts to restore the interstitial cells in the ovary of hypophysectomized mature female rats and acts also to stimulate androgen secretion by testicular interstitial cells of hypophysectomized mature male rats.

An electrophoretically pure preparation of LH was obtained from pituitary glands of sheep and swine in 1939; the fractions obtained from these sources have slightly different chemical characteristics. LH, like FSH, is a water-soluble glycoprotein.

According to Yussman and Taymor (1970), the LH levels in plasma rise sharply 12 to 24 hours before the estimated time of ovulation and a maximum is reached about 8 hours later. These investigators also noted that FSH follows a similar but less marked pattern of response. Plasma progesterone levels were found by them to increase after the rise in LH. Therefore, even though progesterone, in small doses, has been demonstrated to trigger LH release, the evidence is that in the normal ovarian cycles of women, significant amounts of circulating progesterone are not present until after the LH "surge."

Estradiol-17β, in sufficient quantities, will act to trigger the release of LH. Moreover, estradiol-17β, in plasma, has been found to reach a maximal level at, or more likely just before, the time of the increase of LH release. VandeWiele and associates (1970) treated mature rats with an antibody to estradiol-17β and thereby successfully blocked the commonly recognized end-organ responses to estrogen and also prevented LH release and ovulation. Treatment with a synthetic estrogen, stilbestrol, however, which is not inhibited by antibodies to estradiol-17β, restored ovulation. The results obtained by VandeWiele and co-workers with antiestradiol were in sharp contrast to those obtained with antibodies to progesterone. Although progesterone antibodies blocked the recognized end-organ response to progesterone, these antibodies did not prevent the discharge of LH or ovulation. Thus, a rise in circulating estrogen appears to be the important stimulus for the preovulatory LH surge.

Luteotropic Hormones

Even in the rat, there does not appear to be a single luteotropic hormone. Instead, luteinizing hormone, follicle-stimulating hormone, and estrogens as well as prolactin all appear to be required for normal function of the corpus luteum in the rat.

VandeWiele and associates (1970) studied corpus luteum function in women who previously had undergone hypophysectomy. Ovulation and corpus luteum formation were induced by giving repeated injections of FSH and then LH (Fig. 3-27). In one woman, the dose of LH, all given in 1 day, was sufficient to simulate the normal LH surge that occurs just before ovulation. There were increases, initially, in estrogens and progesterone in the plasma, but these were not sustained. Within 5 days, the levels of estrogens and progesterone then became very low; and, on the sixth day after injection of the LH, the patient menstruated. These results were duplicated in other women who received LH for only 1 day. The studies were then repeated, but the injection of LH was con-

tinued daily. Progesterone and estrogens were detectable in the plasma until the onset of menstruation, viz., 17 days after LH treatment was commenced. VandeWiele and associates (1970) were not able to prolong the life of the corpus luteum by giving LH in an attempt to delay the onset of menstruation much beyond the normal time of about 14 to 15 days. One woman conceived during the course of these studies; she subsequently gave birth to quintuplets who survived. These investigators concluded that LH is essential to maintain the normal life-span of the corpus luteum, but that the life-span of the corpus luteum cannot be prolonged for more than a few days by the action of LH.

Luteolytic factors, the activities of which depend in some species on the presence of a uterus, have been suggested on the basis of the results of experiments in several animals, including sheep, sow, and guinea pig. No proof of a uterine luteolytic factor in women, however, has yet been provided.

Prolactin

There is no evidence from results of experiments in women that prolactin serves as a luteotropic hormone. Indeed, from measurements of prolactin there is no clear-cut pattern of prolactin concentrations that can be related to the events of the ovarian cycle. There is episodic secretion of prolactin, but increased plasma concentrations of prolactin in women have been observed during sleep. Interestingly, thyrotropin-releasing hormone (TRH) is known to cause a significant increase in the secretion of prolactin in the human. This finding may explain, in part, the previously inexplicable occurrence of galactorrhea in hypothyroid women and the occurrence of galactorrhea that occurs together with sexual precocity in hypothyroid girls. The physiologic role(s) of prolactin in the human is yet to be defined. Historically, as well as phylogenetically, prolactin occupies a crucial role in many species in salt and water metabolism, lipid metabolism, renal function, and glucose metabolism; it also has a significant influence upon the kinetics of a host of important enzyme reactions. Nonetheless, the importance of prolactin in human health and disease, except for lactation, is largely undefined.

In addition to the possible role of TRH in eliciting prolactin secretion by the pituitary, direct and indirect evidence has been obtained for the existence of a prolactin-inhibitory factor (PIF) of hypothalamic origin. Moreover, a close relationship between the apparent activity of prolactin inhibitory factor and that of luteinizing hormone releasing hormone (LHRH) have been described. Thus, with increasing activity of LHRH and PIF, the net result is an increase in secretion of gonadotropins and a decrease in prolactin secretion. Conversely, with decreasing levels of LHRH and decreasing levels of PIF, the net result is a decrease in gonadotropin secretion and an increase in prolactin secretion. This combination of events is frequently observed in clinical medicine; the result is the common triad of amenorrhea, estrogen defi-

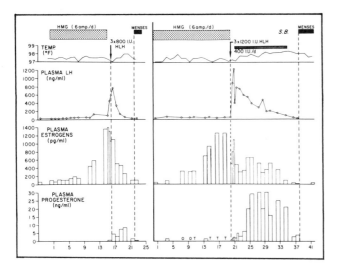

Figure 3-27. Induction of ovulation in a woman without a pituitary by giving human menopausal gonadotropin (hMG) for 14 days followed by human luteinizing hormone (hLH). LH = luteinizing hormone; FSH = follicle-stimulating hormone; ng = nanogram; pg = picogram. (*From VandeWiele and associates: Recent Prog Horm Res 126:63, 1970.*)

ciency, and galactorrhea. This state is commonly induced by a number of drugs that either inhibit the synthesis of catecholamines, for example, dopamine, or else act to deplete the brain concentration of such agents, for example, certain tranquilizers and reserpine. Presently, there is considerable evidence that is supportive of the view that *dopamine* is PIF.

NEUROHUMORAL CONTROL

Anterior pituitary function is under neurohumoral control. Humoral agents, now called releasing factors or hormones, are liberated from nerve endings of the hypothalamic tracts into the capillaries that empty into the portal vessels in the median eminence. The releasing factors are then carried through the hypophysial–portal circulation to the anterior pituitary (Porter and associates, 1973).

During the past decade, considerable evidence has accumulated for the existence of distinct releasing factors for each of the hormones secreted by the anterior pituitary. The releasing factors all appear to be peptides of rather low molecular weight. Two of these, TRH and LHRH, have been identified and synthesized, and, more recently, from ovine hypothalami, corticotropin releasing factor (CRF) has been isolated and identified (Vale, 1981). In addition, there are factors (hormones) that originate in the hypothalamus that inhibit the secretion of anterior pituitary hormones; for example, PIF (dopamine) inhibits the secretion of prolactin, and somatostatin inhibits the secretion of growth hormone.

During the past two decades, our views of the control of pituitary hormone release and subsequent ovarian response has altered materially. For a time, the possibility was considered that the anterior pituitary was principally under the control of the brain through a series of events that led to the production of hypophysiotrophic substances that traversed the long portal vessels and were conveyed in the blood to the sinusoids of the anterior pituitary. In turn, it was envisioned that the activity of the ovary, principally through the secretion of estradiol-17β, influenced brain function in this regard, and thus the ovarian follicle was considered to control, in part, its own fate. The massive increase in concentration of estradiol-17β, for example, at midovarian cycle, precedes, and is believed to elicit, the midcycle LH surge. Thus, the ovary could signal the brain when a follicle became mature enough to respond to a significant increase in LH, the result being ovulation. Although this formulation of the sequence of events still has considerable merit, it is clear that the interaction between the ovary, brain, and pituitary is considerably more complex. Porter and associates (1976), for example, have shown that there is no direct relationship between the concentration of LHRH in the portal blood and the rate of secretion of LH by the pituitary. The LH-to-LHRH molecular secretory ratio in diestrous female rats was found to be 53 whereas the LH-to-LHRH molecular secretory ratio

in castrated females was 1300. Thus, it is apparent that either a considerable increase in gain is effected with an increase in LHRH secretion or that the hormones that are elaborated by the ovaries significantly influence pituitary responsiveness, or both. In this regard, Yen (1972, 1974) and others have demonstrated that LH response to administered LHRH in women is augmented considerably by endogenous or exogenously administered estrogens.

OVARIAN CYCLE FAIL-SAFE SYSTEM

At the beginnning of this chapter, we put forward the proposition that the events of the ovarian cycle were not subject to a delicate balance but rather were protected by fail-safe systems that serve to ensure proper ovarian function in the face of considerable variation in particular components. These systems, which include internal and external control systems, are potentially of extraordinary importance in the guarantee of successful ovarian function. Heretofore, we have considered, somewhat naively, that gonadotropins of the anterior pituitary act on the ovary, and that steroids produced by the ovary (i.e., the follicles) act upon the brain, and possibly pituitary as well, to establish a system of internal control. If this were the case—and the entire case—then surely a delicate balance would exist. But now, there is considerable evidence in favor of the proposition that ovarian function is subject to internal as well as external control modifications.

Folliculostatin

The term *folliculostatin* was coined to indicate a substance in follicular fluid that is defined as one that specifically regulates the secretion of FSH. As early as 1932, McCullagh described the presence in testes of a water-soluble compound that acted to suppress FSH levels; the substance was designated *inhibin*. Later, a similarly acting substance was demonstrated in follicular fluid. Thus, initially there were inhibin-M (male, i.e., from testis) and inhibin-F (female, i.e., from follicular fluid) since it was not then (or now) known if these two FSH inhibitors were identical. Marder, Channing, and Schwartz (1977) and Lorenzen, Channing, and Schwartz (1979) first used the term folliculostatin and since that time the term has gained popularity.

There were many reasons to believe that a nonsteroidal gonadal substance acted to regulate FSH. For some time, it has been known that gonadotropin releasing hormone (GnRH) or luteinizing hormone releasing hormone (LHRH) from the hypothalamus acts to stimulate the anterior pituitary release of both FSH and LH. Yet, there is not necessarily synchrony between the rates of secretion of FSH and LH. For example, bilateral ovariectomy is followed by a striking rise in plasma FSH that is not totally prevented by estradiol-17β treatment. After castration of long standing, both FSH and LH levels are elevated. Treatment of such castrates with estrogens brings about a lowering of LH, but not of FSH, to basal levels. Indeed, Uilenbroek and associates (1978) have provided convincing evidence from cleverly conducted in vivo experiments that the ovary secretes a substance with specific FSH-suppressing activity.

Indeed, it has been shown that folliculostatin (void of steroid contamination) acts to suppress blood levels of FSH with no effect on LH levels. Moreover, this action of folliculostatin to suppress FSH appears to be independent of other hormonal events in that exogenously administered folliculostatin causes suppression of FSH levels on any day of the ovarian cycle. From the results of many and varied studies, there is convincing evidence that folliculostatin acts in a manner to suppress FSH secretion specifically.

Folliculostatin is a substance that may exert its action in a number of ways. Franchimont and colleagues (1981) have presented evidence that folliculostatin acts at the level of the pituitary to decrease FSH biosynthesis. LH release, however, also is reduced in folliculostatin-stimulated pituitary cells. Folliculostatin-induced suppression of FSH synthesis is reversible; nevertheless, folliculostatin does not affect the pituitary synthesis of TSH, prolactin, or growth hormone either in vivo or in vitro.

Other investigators (reviewed by Franchimont and associates, 1981) also have presented evidence in favor of an action of folliculostatin to suppress FSH by an action at the hypothalamus. There also may be an intraovarian action of folliculostatin to inhibit progesterone secretion; these actions, however, are not clearly established since purified folliculostatin is not available.

The cumulative evidence is in favor of the proposition that folliculostatin is produced by the granulosa cells, even by granulosa cells in monolayer culture (Erickson and Hsueh, 1978; Channing and associates, 1980), but not by theca cells (Channing and associates, 1981).

After luteinization of granulosa cells, there appears to be an inverse relationship between the rate of secretion of progesterone and that of folliculostatin (Henderson and Franchimont, 1981). Furthermore, gonadotropins [FSH, LH, or human chorionic gonadotropin (hCG)] do not appear to act to increase folliculostatin synthesis. On the other hand, treatment of granulosa cells with C_{19}-steroids, for example, androstenedione, testosterone, and 5α-dihydrotestosterone, causes a striking increase in folliculostatin synthesis. In this regard, it is important to recall that 5α-dihydrotestosterone cannot be converted to estrogens. Estrogens do not cause an increase in folliculostatin secretion; progesterone, however, acts to inhibit the secretion of folliculostatin in granulosa cells; moreover, luteinized granulosa cells that secrete large quantities of progesterone do not secrete folliculostatin. There appears to be an inverse relationship between the follicular fluid concentrations of estradiol-17β and folliculostatin (Franchimont and colleagues, 1981). From these and other data, it can be speculated that

there also is an inverse relation between follicular size and folliculostatin concentration. These findings, however, may be related more to the concentration of androgens (C_{19}-steroids) since the concentration of the C_{19}-steroids, that is, "androgen-like" precursors, falls (perhaps due to increased aromatization) as the follicle enlarges. Androgens, then, may act in the process of atresia in several ways; this issue is addressed in detail in another section.

Cybernins

A few years ago, the distinguished reproductive biologist and Nobel laureate Roger Guillemin introduced the term *cybernin* to describe a special class of compounds that act to exert profound local effects "in and from cells that are not neurones" (Guillemin, 1981). According to the definition of a hormone, as formulated first by Ernest Henry Starling in 1905, a cybernin is not a hormone. In coining the term cybernin, Guillemin considered the possibility that paracrine might be a satisfactory substitute but ultimately rejected its use because it is an adjective, that is, "paracrine secretory cells" and "paracrine secretion." He also rejected the terms "parahormone" and "parhormone" because "neither was euphonic or easy to pronounce in either French or English, or German for that matter." As defined by Guillemin, "a cybernin is a polypeptide (that is) biosynthesized, processed and released by a cell or group of cells that represents [is] information that will affect the function of another cell or group of cells in the vicinity of the first cell or group of cells."

As defined, Guillemin emphasizes that such compounds as "steroids, prostaglandins, or molecules such as cyclic-AMP" are excluded as cybernins. The term, cybernin, was from the Greek *kurbenetes*, meaning pilot or rudder of a boat, implying the local nature of the command or information involved.

CORPUS LUTEUM LH-RECEPTOR BINDING INHIBITOR

Aqueous extracts of corpora lutea of a number of species are found to contain a substance(s) that inhibits LH binding and it is called LH receptor binding inhibitor (LH-RBI). The amount of LH-RBI in corpora lutea tissue appears to increase as a function of age of the corpus luteum and such a substance is not found in immature rat ovaries, nonluteal ovarian tissue, or in other tissues such as lung, heart, muscle, and testes (Yang and coworkers, 1981). There is indirect evidence in favor of the proposition that LH-RBI inhibits LH binding by association with the LH receptor at a site separate from that occupied by hCG or LH. It also has been demonstrated that LH-RBI acts to inhibit the LH-induced increase in progesterone secretion. There is evidence, however, that there may be more than one form of LH-RBI, that is, one of low and one of high molecular weight. A physiologic role for LH-RBI is not established, and it will be interesting to ascertain if such a substance is important in the regulation of the life-span of the corpus luteum of women.

LUTEINIZATION INHIBITOR

Follicular fluid from immature follicles or from atretic follicles acts to inhibit luteinization of granulosa cells in culture; this putative luteinization inhibitor (LI) is believed to inhibit the accumulation of cyclic-AMP in response to LH treatment and to decrease the secretion of progesterone. The morphologic changes that normally accompany luteinization of granulosa cells is also said to be prevented by LI. Interestingly, LI is not detected in large, preovulatory follicles. These several findings have led to speculation that LI may be important in the regulation of granulosa cell luteinization (Channing and colleagues, 1982).

LUTEINIZATION STIMULATOR

In addition to the claim of the presence of a luteinization inhibitory factor in fluid of small or atretic follicles, evidence has been put forward for the existence in fluid of large follicles (equine) of a substance(s) that stimulates both estrogen and progesterone synthesis by equine granulosa cells in culture (Younglai, 1972). It has been suggested that as the follicle matures, there is a decrease in the concentration of luteinization inhibitor in follicular fluid and an increase in the concentration of a substance that enhances luteinization, namely, luteinization stimulation (LS) (Ledwitz-Rigby and associates, 1977). In view of the presence of both LI and LS activities in follicular fluid, it has been speculated that the ratios of LS/LI in follicular fluid of individual follicles may be important in the modulation of the response of the follicle to gonadotropins. For example, as the follicle matures, a synergistic relationship between LS and LH and FSH may promote LH receptor induction and ovulation, wheras in the absence of sufficient LS, atresia ensues (Channing and colleagues, 1982).

GONADOCRININS

A substance(s) of low molecular weight, that is, < 3500, from rat follicular fluid that stimulates the secretion of both LH and FSH has been demonstrated and referred to as gonadocrinin (Ying and co-workers, 1981). In preliminary studies of the amino acid composition of gonadocrinin, this peptide appears to be distinct from LHRH (Ying and associates, 1981). Gonadocrinin(s) does not stimulate the release of other anterior pituitary hormones such as prolactin, growth hormone, or TSH. The biologic behavior of gonadocrinin is similar to that of LHRH; gonadocrinin, however, is believed to be pro-

duced by granulosa cells, and more mature follicles contain more gonadocrinin activity than do immature follicles.

LH-BINDING STIMULATORY ACTIVITY

In the process of purification of FSH-binding inhibitory (FSH-BI) substance(s), LH-binding stimulatory activity (LH-SA) was observed in some fractions from high-pressure liquid chromatograms. LH-SA was demonstrable in human serum (Reichert and co-workers, 1981).

FSH-BINDING INHIBITORY ACTIVITY

An FSH-binding inhibitory (FSH-BI) activity has been found in bovine follicular fluid and in human and rat serum (Reichert and colleagues, 1981). As in the case of other cybernins believed to be present in follicular fluid, there are both high and low molecular weight substances with FSH-BI activities. FSH-BI inhibits binding of radiolabeled human FSH to membrane preparations of bovine granulosa cells.

EXTRAPITUITARY ACTIONS OF LHRH

The hypothalamic gonadotropin-releasing hormone, variously referred to as gonadotropin releasing hormone (GnRH), and more recently as the luteinizing hormone releasing hormone (LHRH), is known to act in tissue sites other than the anterior pituitary, notably in the gonads of both sexes. Whereas it is unlikely that sufficient LHRH of hypothalamic origin could reach the ovaries or testis to exert a significant biologic effect, this does not rule out the possibility that intragonadally produced LHRH-like substances [e.g., gonadocrinin(s)] or else exogenously administered LHRH or agonists thereof may act to cause profound alterations in gonadal function.

For example, it has been shown that LHRH or potent LHRH agonists in large doses or during chronic administration act to "down regulate" gonadotropin secretion. Thereby a form of "medical castration" can be induced; in so doing it is perceived that a variety of medical benefits may accrue. An elegant review of the subject of "Clinical applications of gonadotropin-releasing hormone and gonadotropin-releasing hormone analogs" was presented recently (Yen, 1983). Yen points out that such diverse disorders as hypogonadotropic hypogonadism, delayed puberty, cryptorchidism, anovulation, precocious puberty, endometriosis, hormone-dependent tumors, ovarian androgen excess, as well as male and female infertility–fertility may be amenable to LHRH treatment, dependent upon dose and means of administration. Thus, it is possible that LHRH may act to "down regulate" pituitary responsiveness or else, by virtue of the induction of large increases in LH secretion, to "down regulate" gonadal response to LH.

As stated earlier, however, there appears to be a third means (at least) by which LHRH or agonists thereof may affect gonadal function, that is, by a direct action on the gonads. An excellent review of these various alternatives was presented by Hsueh and Jones (1981). It has been demonstrated that LHRH inhibits, in granulosa cells of rats, the FSH stimulation of estrogen synthesis, LH, and prolactin receptor formation—but such inhibition was negated when an LHRH antagonist was present in the culture medium. In luteal cells of the rat, LHRH acts to inhibit LH- , prolactin- , or β_2-adrenergic agent-stimulation of progesterone secretion. In rat granulosa cells, LHRH acts to prevent the prolactin-induced increase in LH receptors. By way of contrast, LHRH, like gonadotropins, stimulates follicular prostaglandin formation. LHRH appears to bind with high affinity to membrane preparations of luteinized rat ovarian tissue. The direct action of LHRH on ovarian granulosa cells of women has not been demonstrated unequivocally.

LHRH and agonists do not interfere, directly, with gonadotropin binding; rather there appear to be specific binding sites for LHRH.

Thus, by way of a variety of internal fail-safe control mechanisms, ovulation may be regulated in a manner by which delicate hormonal control is not necessary.

REFERENCES

Adams EC, Hertig AT: Studies on the human corpus luteum: I. Observations on the ultrastructure of development and regression of the luteal cells during the menstrual cycle. J Cell Biol 41:696, 1969

Adams EC, Hertig AT: Studies on the human corpus luteum: II. Observations on the ultrastructure of luteal cells during pregnancy. J Cell Biol 41:716, 1969

Adler L: (Physiology and pathology of ovarian function.) Arch Gynaekol 95:349, 1912

Albertini DF: Structural modifications of the granulosa cell plasma membrane during folliculogenesis. In Motta PM, Hafez ESE (eds): Biology of the Ovary. The Hague, Martinus Nijhoff, 1980

Allen E, Doisy EA: An ovarian hormone: A preliminary report on its localization, extraction, and partial purification, and action on test animals. JAMA 81:819, 1923

Allen E, Pratt JP, Newell QU, Bland LJ: Human tubal ova: Related early corpora lutea and uterine tubes. Contrib Embryol 22:45, 1930

Aschheim S, Zondek B: (Anterior pituitary hormone and ovarian hormone in the urine of pregnant women.) Klin Wochenchr 6:248, 1927

Baird DT, Burger PE, Heavon-Jones GD, Scaramuzzi RJ: The site of secretion of androstenedione in non-pregnant women. J Endocrinol 63:201, 1974

Baker TG: Oogenesis and ovulation. In Austin CR, Short RV (eds): Reproduction in Mammals: I. Germ Cells and Fertilization. Cambridge, Cambridge University Press, 1978

Beers WH: Follicular plasminogen and plasminogen activator

and the effect of plasmin on ovarian follicle wall. Cell 6:379, 1975

Blandau R: Personal communication.

Bouin P, Ancel P: (Research on the function of the corpus luteum.) J Physiol Pathol Gen 12:1, 1910

Bradbury J: Direct action of estrogen on the ovary of the immature rat. Endocrinology 68:115, 1961

Brown MS, Kovanen PT, Goldstein JL: Receptor-mediated uptake of lipoprotein cholesterol and its utilization for steroid synthesis in the adrenal cortex. Rec Prog Horm Res 35:215, 1979

Browne JSL: Further observations on ovary stimulating hormones of placenta. Cited by Collip JB, Can Med Assoc J 22:761, 1930

Bryant-Greenwood GD: Relaxin as a new hormone. Endocr Rev 3:62, 1982

Butenandt A: (On "Progynon," a crystallized female sexual hormone.) Naturwissenschaften 17:879, 1929

Butenandt A: (On pregnanediol, a new steroid derivative from pregnant urine.) Ber Chem Ges 63:659, 1930

Caffier P: (On the hormone influence of the human tubal mucosa and its therapeutic utilization.) Zentralbl Gynaekol 62:1024, 1938

Channing CP, Schaerf FW, Anderson LD, Tsafrir A: Ovarian folicular and luteal physiology. In Greep RO (ed): Reproductive Physiology. III. International Review of Physiology. Baltimore, University Park Press, 1980

Channing CP, Anderson LD, Stone SL, Batta SK: Porcine and human ovarian nonsteroidal follicular regulators. In McKerns KW (ed): Reproductive Processes and Contraception. New York, Plenum, 1981

Channing CP, Anderson LD, Hoover DJ, Kolena J, Osteen KG, Pomerantz SH, Tanaba K: The role of nonsteroidal regulators in control of oocyte and follicular maturation. Rec Prog Horm Res 38:331, 1982

Corner GW, Allen WM: Physiology of the corpus luteum: II. Production of a special uterine reaction (progestational proliferation) by extracts of the corpus luteum. Am J Physiol 88:326, 1929

Crisp TM, Dessouky DA, Denys FR: The fine structure of the human corpus luteum of early pregnancy and during the progestational phase of the menstrual cycle. Am J Anat 127:37, 1970

Csapo AI: The molecular basis of myometrial function and its disorders. In La Prophylaxie en Gynecologie et Obstetrique, Congres International de Gynecologie et Obstetrique. Geneve, Georg, 1954, p 693

De Graaf R: De Mulierum organis generationi inservientibus. Lugd, Batav, 1677, p 161

Dempsey EW, Bassett DL: Observations on the fluorescence, birefringence and histochemistry of the rat ovary during the reproductive cycle. Endocrinology 33:384, 1943

Doisy EA, Veler CD, Thayer S: Folliculin from urine of pregnant women. Am J Physiol 90:329, 1929

Dorfman RI, Ross E, Shipley RA: Metabolism of the steroid hormones: The metabolism of progesterone and ethynyl testosterone. Endocrinology 42:77, 1948

Erickson GF, Hsueh AJW: Stimulation of aromatase activity by follicle stimulating hormone in rat granulosa cells in vivo and in vitro. Endocrinology 102:1275, 1978

Fevold HL, Hisaw FL, Leonard SL: The gonad-stimulating and the luteinizing hormones of the anterior lobe of the hypophysis. Am J Physiol 97:291, 1931

Fishman J, Bradlow HL, Gallagher TF: Oxidative metabolism of estradiol. J Biol Chem 235:3104, 1960

Fluhmann CF: Anterior pituitary hormone in blood of women with ovarian deficiency. JAMA 93:672, 1929

Fraenkel L: (New experiments on the function of the corpus luteum.) Arch Gynaekol 91:705, 1910

Franchimont P, Henderson K, Verhoeven G, Hazee-Hagalstein M-T, Charlet-Renard C, Demoulin A, Bourguignon J-P, Lecomte-Yerna M-J: Inhibin: Mechanisms of action and secretion. In Franchimont P, Channing CP (eds): Intragonadal Regulation of Reproduction. New York, Academic, 1981

Frank RT, Salmon UJ: Effect of administration of estrogenic factor upon hypophyseal hyperactivity in the menopause. Proc Soc Exp Biol Med 33:311, 1935

Frank RT, Goldberger MA, Spielmen F: Utilization and excretion of female sex hormone. Proc Soc Exp Biol Med 29:1229, 1932

Goering RW, Herrmann WL: Estrogen secretion rate studies in normal women. Clin Res 12:115, 197, 1964

Greep RO, Jones IC: Recent Progress in Hormone Research, vol 5. New York, Academic, 1950

Guillemin R: On the word: Cybernin. In Franchimont P, Channing CP (eds): Intragonadal Regulation of Reproduction. New York, Academic, 1981

Hall RE: Removal of the corpus luteum in early pregnancy: A review of the literature and report of 2 cases. Bull Sloane Hosp Women 1:49, 1955

Harris GW: Hypothalamic control of the anterior pituitary gland. CIBA Found Colloq Endocrinol 4:105, 1952

Harris GW: Ovulation. Am J Obstet Gynecol 105:659, 1969

Hartman CG: How large is the mammalian egg? Q Rev Biol 4:581, 1929

Henderson KM, Franchimont P: Regulation of inhibin production by bovine ovarian cells in vitro. J Reprod Fertil 63:431, 1981

Hertig AT: Gestational hyperplasia of endometrium: A morphologic correlation of ova, endometrium, and corpora lutea during early pregnancy. Lab Invest 13:1153, 1964

Hertz R, Meyer RK, Spielman MA: Specificity of progesterone in inducing sexual receptivity in ovariectomized guinea pig. Endocrinology 21:533, 1973

Hisaw FL: Experimental relaxation of the pubic ligament of the guinea pig. Proc Soc Exper Biol 23:661, 1926

Hitschmann F, Adler L: (The structure of the endometrium of sexually mature women with special reference to menstruation.) Monatsschr Geburtshilfe Gynaekol 27:1, 1908

Hoffman F: (On the content of progesterone in the ovary and blood during the cycle.) Geburtshilfe Frauenheilkd 8:723, 1948

Hsueh AJ, Jones PB: Extrapituitary actions of gonadotropin-releasing hormone. Endocrine Rev 2:437, 1981

Hudson P, Haley J, Cronk M, Shine J, Niall HD: Molecular cloning and characterization of DNA sequences coding for rat relaxin. Nature 291:127, 1981

Illingworth DR, Corbin DK, Kemp ED, Keenan EJ: Hormone changes during the menstrual cycle in abetalipoproteinemia: Reduced luteal phase progesterone in a patient with homozygous hypobetalipoproteinemia. Proc Natl Acad Sci USA 79:6685, 1982

Jensen EV, Jacobson HI: Basic guides to the mechanism of estrogen action. Recent Prog Horm Res 18:387, 1962

Jöel K: The glycogen content of the fallopian tubes during the menstrual cycle and during pregnancy. J Obstet Gynaecol Br Emp 46:721, 1939

Jones HW, Wade R, Goldberg B: Phosphate liberation by endometrium in the presence of adenosinetriphosphate. Am J Obstet Gynecol 64:1118, 1952

Jost A: Problems of fetal endocrinology. Recent Prog Horm Res 8:379, 1953

Knauer E: (Ovarian transplantation.) Arch Gynaekol 60:322, 1900

Knaus H: The action of pituitary extract upon the pregnant uterus of the rabbit. J Physiol 61:383, 1926

Ledwitz-Rigby F, Rigby BW, Gay VL, Stetson M, Young J, Channing CP: Inhibitory action of porcine follicular fluid upon granulosa cell luteinization in vitro: Assay and influence of follicular maturation. J Endocrinol 74:175, 1977

Lorenzen JR, Channing CP, Schwartz NB: Partial characterization of FSH suppressing activity (folliculostatin) in porcine follicular fluid using the metestrous rat as an in vitro bioassay model. Biol Reprod 79:635, 1978

MacCorquodale DW, Thayer SA, Doisy EA: The isolation of the principal estrogenic substance of liquor folliculi. J Biol Chem 115:435, 1936

MacDonald PC, Rombaut RP, Siiteri PK: Plasma precursors of estrogen. I. Extent of conversion of plasma Δ^4-androstenedione to estrone in normal males and nonpregnant normal, castrated and adrenalectomized females. J Clin Endocrinol Metab 27:1103, 1967

McCullagh DR: Dual endocrine activity of the testes. Science 76:19, 1932

McKay DG, Robinson D: Observations on fluorescence, birefringence and histochemistry of human ovary during menstrual cycle. Endocrinology 41:378, 1947

Marder ML, Channing CP, Schwartz NB: Suppression of serum follicle stimulating hormone in intact and acutely ovariectomized rats by porcine follicular fluid. Endocrinology 101:1639, 1977

Massa R, Martini L: Interference with the 5α-reductase system. A new approach for developing anti-androgens. Gynecol Invest 2:253, 1971

Milewich L, Gomez-Sanchez C, Madden JD, MacDonald PC: Isolation and characterization of 5α-pregnane-3,20-dione and progesterone in peripheral blood of pregnant women. Measurement throughout pregnancy. Gynecol Invest 6:291, 1975

Noyes RW, Hertig AT, Rock J: Dating the endometrial biopsy. Fertil Steril 1:3, 1950

O'Malley BW, Sherman MR, Toft DO: Progesterone "receptors" in the cytoplasm and nucleus of chick oviduct target tissue. Proc Natl Acad Sci USA 65:501, 1970

Porter JC, Ben-Jonathan N, Oliver C, Eskay RL, Winters AJ: The interrelationship of the CSF, hypophysial portal vessels, and the hypothalamus and their role in the regulation of anterior pituitary function. In Anand Kumar TC (ed): Neuroendocrine Regulation of Fertility. Basel, Karger, 1976

Porter JC, Mical RS, Ben-Jonathan N, Ondo JG: Neurovascular regulation of the anterior hypophysis. Horm Res 29:161, 1973

Pratt JP: Corpus luteum in its relation to menstruation and pregnancy. Endocrinology 11:195, 1927

Prenant A: (On the morphologic importance of the corpus luteum, and its physiologic and possible therapeutic action.) Rev Med Liest 30:385, 1898

Reichert LE Jr, Sanzo MA, Dias JA: Studies on purification and characterization of gonadotropin binding inhibitors and stimulators from human serum and seminal plasma. In Franchimont P, Channing CP (eds): Intragonadal Regulation of Reproduction. New York, Academic, 1981

Ryan KJ: Biological aromatization of steroids. J Biol Chem 234:268, 1959

Ryan KJ: Synthesis of hormones in the ovary. In Grady HG,

Smith DE (eds): The Ovary. Baltimore, Williams & Wilkins, 1963, p 69

Ryan KJ, Smith OW: Biogenesis of estrogens by the human ovary: I. Conversion of acetate-1-C^{14} to estrone and estradiol. J Biol Chem 234:268, 1959

Salhanick HA, Hisaw FL, Zarrow MX: The action of estrogen and progesterone on the gonadotropin content of the pituitary of the monkey. J Clin Endocrinol Metab 12:310, 1952

Smith OW, Ryan KJ: Estrogen in the human ovary. Am J Obstet Gynecol 84:141, 1962

Smith PE: The disabilities caused by hypophysectomy and their repair. JAMA 88:158, 1927

Speck G: The determination of the time of ovulation. Obstet Gynecol Survey 14:798, 1959

Starling EH: On the chemical correlation of the function of the body. Lancet 2:339, 1905

Stockard CR, Papanicolaou GN: The existence of a typical oestrous cycle in the guinea pig, with a study of its histological and physiological changes. Am J Anat 22:225, 1917

Strickland S, Beers WH: Studies of the enzymatic basis and hormonal control of ovulation. In Midgley AR, Sadler WA (eds): Ovarian Follicular Development. New York, Raven, 1979

Strott CA, Yoshimi T, Ross GT, Lipsett MB: Ovarian physiology: Relationship between plasma LH and steroidogenesis by the follicle and corpus luteum; effect of HCG. J Clin Endocrinol Metab 29:1157, 1969

Szego CM, Davis JS: Inhibition of estrogen-induced cyclic AMP elevation in rat uterus: II. By glucocorticoids. Life Sci 8:1109, 1969

Tulsky AS, Koff AK: Some observations on the role of the corpus luteum in early human pregnancy. Fertil Steril 8:118, 1957

Uilenbroek JTJ, Tiller R, deJong FH, Vels F: Specific suppression of follicle-stimulating hormone secretions in gonadectomized male and female rats with intrasplenic ovarian transplants. J Endocrinol 78:399, 1978

Vale W, Spiers J, Rivier C, Rivier J: Characterization of a 41-residue ovine hypothalamic peptide that stimulates secretion of corticotropin and β-endorphin. Science 213:1394, 1981

VandeWiele RL, Bogumil J, Dyrenfurth I, Ferin M, Jewelewicz R, Warran M, Rizkallah T, Mikhail G: Mechanisms regulating the menstrual cycle in women. Recent Prog Horm Res 126:63, 1970

Venning EH, Browne JSL: Urinary excretion of sodium pregnanediol glucuronidate in the menstrual cycle. (An excretion product of progesterone.) Am J Physiol 119:417, 1937

Westman A, Jorpes E, Widstrom G: (Investigation of the mucosa cycle in the uterine tube, its hormonal regulation and the significance of the tubal secretion for vitality of the fertilized eggs.) Acta Obstet Gynecol Scand 11:279, 1931

Wislocki GB: The vascular supply of the hypophysis cerebri of the rhesus monkey and man. Proc A Res Nerv Ment Dis 17:48, 1938

Yang KP, Neira ES, Yen HH, Samaan NA, Wong TS, Ward DN, Channing CP: Corpus luteum LH-receptor binding inhibitor (LH-RBI). In Franchimont P, Channing CP (eds): Intragonadal Regulation of Reproduction. New York, Academic, 1981

Yen SSC, Vandenberg G, Rebar R, Thara Y: Variation of pituitary responsiveness to synthetic LRF during different phases of the menstrual cycle. J Clin Endocrinol Metab 35:931, 1972

Yen SSC, Vandenberg G, Siler TM: Modulation of pituitary responsiveness to LRF by estrogen. J Clin Endocrinol Metab 39:170, 1974

Yen SC: Clinical application of gonadotropin-releasing hormone and gonadotropin-releasing hormone analogs. Fertil Steril 39:257, 1983

Ying S, Ling N, Böhlen P, Guillemin R: Gonadostatins and gonadocrinin: Peptides from the gonads regulating the secretion of gonadotropins. In Jagiello G, Vogel HJ (eds): Bioregulators of Reproduction. New York, Academic, 1981

Younglai EV: The influence of follicular fluid and plasma on steroidogenic activity of equine granulosa cells. J Reprod Fertil 28:95, 1972

Yussman MA, Taymor ML: Serum levels of follicle stimulating hormone and luteinizing hormone and of plasma progesterone related to ovulation by corpus luteum biopsy. J Clin Endocrinol 30:396, 1970

4

The Endometrium and Menstruation: Unique Properties

It is not generally appreciated that in the adult human, few cells or tissues undergo significant replication. Among these few are those of squamous epithelium of skin and vaginal mucosa, the mucosa of the gut, and the endometrium of ovulatory women. The endometrium of women is a remarkable tissue; during a woman's life, the endometrium normally is shed and regenerated no fewer than 400 times. The lifetime cumulative menstrual blood loss associated with normal endometrial shedding is 10 to 20 liters or more, an amount of blood that contains at least three times the total body iron content of the average adult woman. If one assumes that the mass of endometrium attained at midluteal or midsecretory phase (day 20) is 5 g and if this rate of growth were to continue uninterrupted with a doubling time of 20 days, at the end of 1 year the mass of endometrium would be almost 1 ton (Table 4-1).

This unique tissue, the endometrium, has become a model for investigations concerned with an elucidation of the mechanism of action of steroid hormones and other agents, for example, the prostaglandins. The accessibility of human endometrial tissue, together with recently developed techniques that permit the separation of endometrial glandular epithelium from stroma, rightfully have attracted the interest of endocrinologists and molecular biologists who seek to define the molecular nature of hormone action(s) in target tissues.

Estrogen Action

Estradiol-17β acts to promote responses of the endometrium in a manner that now stands as one model for the mechanism of hormone action. Estradiol-17β, biologically the most potent of the naturally occurring estrogens, enters the endometrial cell, apparently by simple diffusion. In the cell, the hormone becomes associated with a cytosolic macromolecule that is characterized by a high affinity, but low capacity, for estradiol-17β and other biologically active estrogens including synthetic estrogens. The estradiol-17β-receptor complex that evolves is translocated, probably after transformational changes, to the nucleus of the cell, where the complex becomes associated with chromatin. The result is a transcriptional

event that brings about synthesis of messenger RNA and, subsequently, protein synthesis. Among the many proteins synthesized are macromolecules that are characterized by high affinity for progesterone, namely, progesterone receptors, as well as additional receptor molecules for estradiol-17β. Thus, among the actions of estradiol-17β on the endometrium are those that provide both for the perpetuation of the cellular milieu in which estrogen can act and for the initiation of events that provide for responses to the actions of progesterone.

Progesterone Action

This hormone also apparently enters the endometrial cell by diffusion and thence becomes associated with receptors with high affinity, but low capacity, for progesterone. The concentration of progesterone receptors is dependent, however, on previous estrogen action. The progesterone-receptor complex is also translocated to the nucleus, but the action initiated therein is strikingly different from that of the estradiol-17β-receptor complex. The progesterone-receptor complex acts to bring about a decrease in the production of estradiol-17β receptor molecules (Tseng and Gurpide, 1975), an action that serves eventually as one means by which progesterone acts to negate the action of estrogen. Progesterone also acts to bring about an increase in the activity of the enzyme *estradiol-17β dehydrogenase,* the enzyme that catalyzes the interconversion of estradiol-17β and estrone. Tseng and Gurpide (1974) have shown that the reaction kinetics of estradiol-17β dehydrogenase in endometrium are such that the formation of estrone, a biologically weaker estrogen than estradiol-17β, is favored. Progesterone also acts to increase sulfurylation of estrogen (Tseng and Liu, 1981), another means of estrogen inactivation. Thus, progesterone can attenuate estrogen action in a number of ways: (1) by reducing the rate of synthesis of estrogen receptors, (2) by bringing about a reduction in the intracellular level of estradiol-17β, and (3) by increasing estrogen inactivation through sulfurylation.

The findings of these important studies also have provided tools for investigators to identify markers of estrogen and progesterone action—tools believed to be

TABLE 4-1. THEORETICAL MASS OF ENDOMETRIUM THAT COULD BE ATTAINED IF NORMAL RATES OF GROWTH IN FIRST 20 DAYS OF MENSTRUAL CYCLE WERE UNINTERRUPTED.*

Theoretical Days (years)	Endometrial Mass	
	(Grams)	(Pounds)
20	5	
40	10	
60	20	
80	40	
100	80	
120	160	0.4
140	320	0.7
160	640	1.4
180 (0.5)	1,280	2.8
200	2,560	5.6
220	5,120	11.0
240	10,240	22.5
260	20,480	45.1
280	40,960	90.0
300	81,920	180.0
320	163,840	360.0
340	327,680	720.0
360	655,360	1440.0
365 (1.0)	819,200	1800.0

* The mathematical equation that is descriptive of this relationship is $z = 2^{x-1}y$, where x is the *number* of doubling times, y is the *mass* of endometrium at the end of one doubling time, and z is the *mass* at the end of x doubling times. Thus, after 180 days, or 9 doubling times, $z = 2^8 \times 5$ g, or 1280 g.

important in the identification of and thence in the management of hormone responsive tumors. For example, a marker of estrogen action in a given tissue (or tumor) is the presence of progesterone receptors. Horwitz and colleagues (1975) have pioneered the delineation of estrogen-responsive breast cancers by showing that tumors in which progesterone receptors are demonstrable are likely to be more responsive to endocrine ablation procedures.

The presence of estradiol-17β dehydrogenase activity also is indicative of progesterone action, and the presence of this enzyme activity in endometrial carcinoma tissue may signal responsiveness, therapeutically, of such tumors to progesterone or related synthetic progestational agents.

Decidua

The human decidua, the specialized endometrium of pregnancy, is produced by prolonged stimulation by progesterone and estrogen and is a tissue of great interest to endocrinologists as well as immunologists. The special relationship that exists between endometrium-decidua and invading trophoblast seemingly defies the laws of transplantation immunology. The success of this unique autograft not only is a curiosity but an event that many investigators believe may hold the solution to the future of successful transplantation surgery and perhaps the control of neoplasia as well.

The mysteries of the human decidua continue to increase. Convincing evidence has been presented by Riddick and co-workers (1979) and Golander and associates (1978), for example, that is supportive of the view that the decidua is the source of prolactin that is found in enormous amounts in the amnionic fluid during human pregnancy. Levels of prolactin of 10,000 ng/ml of amnionic fluid are found during the 20th to 24th week of pregnancy, compared with levels of 150 ng/ml in plasma of near-term pregnant women (Tyson and co-workers, 1972). Thus the human endometrium not only plays a unique role in the physiology of womanhood but constitutes a marvelous model system for study by endocrinologists, molecular biologists, immunologists, oncologists, and lipid biochemists.

THE ENDOMETRIAL CYCLE

The histologic changes that occur in the endometrium during the menstrual cycle are summarized in Figure 4-1; the findings are taken from those of Noyes, Hertig, and Rock (1950). So characteristic are these alterations that an experienced pathologist can accurately "date" an endometrial specimen from its microscopic appearance with respect to the day of the menstrual cycle.

In response to the changes that are evoked by hormone action during each ovulatory ovarian cycle, there are morphologic changes in the endometrium that evolve with such precise regularity that the histologic features of the endometrium can be used to determine the day of the menstrual cycle on which the endometrium was removed. The endocrine changes during the ovarian cycle, as described in Chapter 3, p. 41, are summarized: (1) During the preovulatory, or follicular, phase of the ovarian cycle, estradiol-17β is secreted principally by the dominant follicle in increasing quantities. (2) During the postovulatory, or luteal, phase of the cycle, progesterone, in addition to estradiol-17β, is secreted by the corpus luteum. (3) During the premenstrual phase, the corpus luteum regresses and the rates of secretion of both estradiol-17β and progesterone diminish. Consequent upon these changes in hormone secretion during the ovarian cycle, there are four main stages of the endometrial cycle: (1) postmenstrual reorganization and thence *proliferation* in response to stimulation (direct or indirect) by estradiol-17β; (2) abundant glandular *secretion,* which results from the combined action of estrogen and progesterone; (3) *premenstrual ischemia* and involution; and (4) *menstruation,* which is accompanied by collapse and desquamation of all but the deepest layer of the endometrium. Ultimately, menstruation is the consequence of progesterone withdrawal. The follicular (preovulatory) or proliferative phase, and the postovulatory (luteal) or secretory phase customarily are divided into early and late stages. The normal secretory phase may be subdivided rather finely (almost day by day), by histologic criteria, from shortly after ovulation until the onset of menstruation.

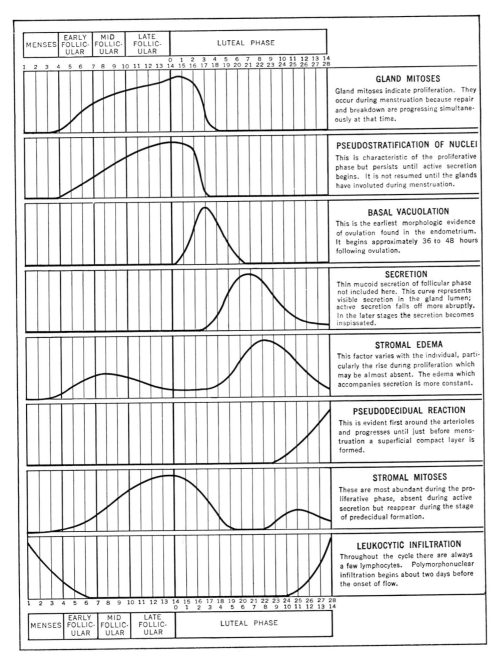

Figure 4-1. Dating of the endometrium according to the day of the menstrual cycle during a hypothetical 28-day ovarian cycle. Correlation of typical morphologic findings. (*From Noyes, Hertig, and Rock: Fertil Steril 1:3, 1950.*) It is notable that the paper in which the day-to-day characteristic changes that occur in endometrium of cyclic women were described was the lead article in the first volume of the journal *Fertility and Sterility*, 35 years ago.

The figure contains the following labelled panels and descriptions:

GLAND MITOSES
Gland mitoses indicate proliferation. They occur during menstruation because repair and breakdown are progressing simultaneously at that time.

PSEUDOSTRATIFICATION OF NUCLEI
This is characteristic of the proliferative phase but persists until active secretion begins. It is not resumed until the glands have involuted during menstruation.

BASAL VACUOLATION
This is the earliest morphologic evidence of ovulation found in the endometrium. It begins approximately 36 to 48 hours following ovulation.

SECRETION
Thin mucoid secretion of follicular phase not included here. This curve represents visible secretion in the gland lumen; active secretion falls off more abruptly. In the later stages the secretion becomes inspissated.

STROMAL EDEMA
This factor varies with the individual, particularly the rise during proliferation which may be almost absent. The edema which accompanies secretion is more constant.

PSEUDODECIDUAL REACTION
This is evident first around the arterioles and progresses until just before menstruation a superficial compact layer is formed.

STROMAL MITOSES
These are most abundant during the proliferative phase, absent during active secretion but reappear during the stage of predecidual formation.

LEUKOCYTIC INFILTRATION
Throughout the cycle there are always a few lymphocytes. Polymorphonuclear infiltration begins about two days before the onset of flow.

Early Proliferative Phase

The endometrium during the early proliferative phase of the menstrual cycle is thin, usually less than 2 mm in depth. Histologically, the glands are narrow, tubular structures that pursue almost a straight course from the surface toward the basal layer. The glandular epithelium is low columnar, and the nuclei are round and basal. In the deeper part of the endometrium, the cells of the stroma are packed rather densely and the nuclei of these cells are deep-staining and small. In the superficial, or reorganizing, layer, the stromal cells are packed more loosely, and the nuclei are more nearly round, more vesicular, and larger than in the deeper layers. Mitotic figures, especially in the glands, are present by the fifth day after the onset of menstruation and mitotic activity is evident until 2 to 3 days after ovulation. Although the blood vessels are numerous and prominent, there is no extravasated blood or lymphocytic infiltration at this stage.

Late Proliferative Phase

The endometrium in the late proliferative phase becomes thicker, as a result of both glandular hyperplasia and an increase in stromal ground substance. The loose stroma is especially prominent superficially, and the glands are separated widely compared with those of the deeper zone, where the glands are crowded and tortuous and the stroma is more dense. Gradually, the glandular epithelium becomes taller and pseudostratified at about the time of ovulation. Day-by-day "dating" of the proliferative phase of the endometrium ordinarily is not possible because of the considerable variation among women. This is due primarily to the fact that, whereas the luteal or secretory (i.e., postovulatory) phase of the cycle among women is remarkably constant in duration, the proliferative or follicular (i.e., preovulatory) phase varies greatly.

Early Secretory Phase

After ovulation, there are changes in endometrial morphology that occur with such regularity as to permit the endometrium to be dated with great precision. The total thickness of the endometrium may decrease slightly because of loss of fluid. During the secretory stage, three zones of the endometrium become well defined: (1) the basal zone, or layer adjacent to the myometrium; (2) the compact zone, or layer immediately beneath the endometrial surface; and, (3) the spongy zone, or layer between the compact and basal layers. Actually, the basal layer undergoes little, if any, histologic alteration during the menstrual cycle, but mitoses are found in the glands. The spongy middle layer consists of a lacy labyrinth with little stroma between the tortuous, serrated glands that characterize the luteal phase. In the compact superficial layer, the glands are more nearly straight and are narrower, but the glandular lumens often are filled with secretions. Edema of the abundant stroma is an important factor in the thickening of the endometrium, but there also is an increase in dry weight.

Late Secretory Phase

The endometrium at this time is extremely vascular, succulent, rich in glycogen; apparently, it is ideally suited for the implantation and growth of the fertilized ovum. The stromal cells, and in particular those around the blood vessels, undergo hypertrophic changes similar to, but less extensive than, those of the true decidua of pregnancy (p. 100). At the time of the cycle that corresponds to implantation, that is, about 1 week after ovulation, the endometrium is 5 to 6 mm thick and the secretory changes preparatory to nidation of the fertilized ovum appear to be maximal.

A further characteristic of the secretory phase is the striking development of the *spiral, or coiled, arteries,* which become much more tortuous. In the compact layer, the arteries branch and the arterioles break up into capillaries within this zone. During the first week of the menstrual cycle, the arterioles extend only about halfway through the endometrium. Since the arterioles lengthen more rapidly than the endometrium thickens, the distal ends of the vessels reach progressively closer to the surface of the endometrium. This unequal growth results in a disproportion between the length of the arterioles and the thickness of the endometrium, and, for this reason, the vessels become coiled increasingly.

Premenstrual Phase

This phase of the cycle encompasses the 2 or 3 days before menstruation and corresponds, in time, to the regression of the corpus luteum and, in turn, to the decline in secretion of progesterone and estrogen. The chief histologic characteristic of the premenstrual phase is infiltration of the stroma by polymorphonuclear or mononuclear leukocytes, by which is imparted a pseudoinflammatory appearance. At the same time, in the superficial zone, the reticular framework of the stroma disintegrates. As a result of the loss of tissue fluid and secretion, the thickness of the endometrium often decreases appreciably during the 2 days before menstruation. In the process of reduction in thickness, the glands and arteries collapse.

Endometrial Ischemia. In a classic study, Markee (1940) observed and thence described the vascular changes that occur before menstruation, as seen in intraocular transplants of endometrium in the rhesus monkey. He found that as the result of the compression of endometrium, the coiling of the arterioles increases markedly. Although the coils are fairly regular earlier in the cycle, just before menstruation they become quite irregular.

Furthermore, Markee demonstrated two entirely different vascular phenomena in endometrial transplants for the few days that precede menstrual bleeding. Beginning 1 to 5 days before the onset of menstruation, there is a period of slowed circulation, or relative stasis, during which vasodilatation may occur. Thereafter, there is a period of vasoconstriction that commences 4 to 24 hours before the extravasation of any blood. The period of stasis is extremely variable and ranges from less than 24 hours to 4 days. It was Markee's opinion that the slowing of the circulation that leads to stasis is caused by the increased resistance to blood flow offered by the coiled arteries. As more coils are added, the blood flow becomes increasingly slower. Another explanation, however, must be invoked for bleeding during anovulatory cycles and for bleeding that follows withdrawal of estrogens, in which circumstances the arteries may be quite simple or relatively uncoiled; in such cases, there may be a more direct mechanism that involves arteriolar vasoconstriction.

Thus, it is envisioned by most authorities that vasoconstriction of the arterioles and coiled arteries precedes the onset of menstrual bleeding by the 4 to 24 hours that correspond to the premenstrual ischemic phase. After the constriction has begun, the superficial one half to two thirds of the endometrium is inadequately supplied with blood during the remainder of that menstrual cycle; the anemic appearance of the functional zone may be striking. When, after a period of constriction, an individual coiled artery relaxes, hemorrhage occurs from that artery or its branches. Then, in sequence, these constricted arteries relax and bleed, the succession of small hemorrhages from individual arterioles or capillaries continuing for a variable time. Although this sequence of vasoconstriction, relaxation, and hemorrhage appears to be well established, the mechanism that actually brings about the escape of blood from the vessels remains an enigma. It is entirely possible that the damage to the walls of the vessels during the period of vasoconstriction results in their rupture when the constricted segment relaxes and the blood flow is resumed.

Dating of the Endometrium by Histologic Criteria.

Benirschke (1978), in an excellent review, has summarized the histologic features of the endometrium that permit accurate dating of endometrium obtained after ovulation. Immediately after ovulation, that is, days 14 to 16 of an idealized 28-day cycle, and presumably in response to the action of progesterone secreted by the developing corpus luteum, characteristic subnuclear glycogen-rich vacuoles develop in the glandular epithelium. By days 17 to 18, the vacuoles have displaced the nuclei toward the middle of the cells and mitoses are rare; by day 18, mitosis has ceased. The migration of vacuoles continues past the nuclei to the luminal surface of the glands and by day 20, near-maximum secretion into the lumen of the glands has transpired. By this time, there are only a few vacuoles that remain in the glandular epithelium. During the early luteal phase of the cycle, mitosis ceases but the glands become more tortuous as the luteal response continues. There are, simultaneously, hormonally induced changes in the stroma—indeed, by days 20 to 21, there is considerable interstitial edema. Predecidualization, a process that consists of an increase in the cytoplasm of stromal cells, is apparent by days 23 to 24—commencing first in cells around the spiral arterioles. Thereafter, the decidual changes extend throughout the stroma. Granulocytes and lymphocytes infiltrate the predecidual secretory endometrium. The premenstrual phase of the endometrial cycle is characterized by a decrease in thickness of the endometrium, extravasation of blood, disassociation, and thence disintegration of stromal cells. In Benirschke's description of these morphologic changes, he points out that "amazingly" at a time when the surface epithelium of the premenstrual endometrium is still intact, there is extensive hemorrhage into and disintegration of the stroma.

The Role of Prostaglandins in Menstruation.

The prostaglandins, a unique class of tissue hormones, are synthesized in the cells in which these substances act or else in nearby cells. Thus, this group of substances are tissue hormones rather than humoral hormones. In most tissues, prostaglandins are degraded rapidly in the tissues of origin or in nearby tissues, as well as in more remote sites, such as the lungs. The prostaglandins or prostaglandinlike substances are synthesized from an essential fatty acid, arachidonic acid. Most often, arachidonic acid is found in tissues in an esterified form, usually in the

sn-2 position of glycerophospholipids. In this esterified form, arachidonic acid *cannot* be converted to prostaglandins. The enzyme, *phospholipase A_2*, catalyzes the hydrolysis of the *sn*-2 fatty acid ester of certain glycerophospholipids to effect the release of free arachidonic acid. Other lipases, which commonly act in concert in a series of reactions, catalyze the hydrolysis of arachidonic acid from other lipid stores. Thus, the rate of release of free arachidonic acid is believed to be the rate-limiting step in the formation of prostaglandins in most tissues. Both endometrium and decidua are richly endowed with prostaglandin synthase activity. It has been shown that the decidua also is enriched with arachidonic acid. The possible role of prostaglandin metabolism in decidua in the initiation of parturition or in the maintenance of labor is discussed in Chapter 15 (p. 300).

A role for prostaglandins in the initiation of menstruation also is envisioned (Casey and co-workers, 1980). Prostaglandins, administered to nonpregnant women, will bring about menstruation. It has been proposed that this action of prostaglandins is mediated by way of the induction of vasoconstriction of the endometrial arterioles. In menstrual blood, there are large amounts of prostaglandins, and prostaglandin administration gives rise to symptoms that mimic those of the dysmenorrhea that is commonly associated with normal ovulatory menses, that is, menses initiated by progesterone withdrawal.

NAD^+-dependent *15-hydroxyprostaglandin dehydrogenase* (PGDH), the enzyme that catalyzes the first reaction in the degradation of prostaglandins, is found in endometrium, principally in the cells of the glandular epithelium (Casey and co-workers, 1980). The specific activity of this enzyme is highest in endometrial tissue obtained during the luteal phase of the cycle, whereas it is barely detectable or absent on days 26 to 28, just before the onset of menses, and on days 1 to 5 of the menstrual cycle (Fig. 4-2). Thus, the specific activity of PGDH in endometrium appears to follow the levels of progesterone. It has been hypothesized that the fall in activity of PGDH as the levels of progesterone fall, and, in turn, the reduced rate of degradation of prostaglandins, may serve to enhance the levels of prostaglandins in the endometrium.

Menstrual Phase

Menstrual bleeding may be of either arterial or venous origin, but the former is predominant. It appears at the outset to result from rhexis of a coiled artery with consequent formation of a hematoma, but occasionally it takes place by leakage through the vessel. When a hematoma forms, the superficial endometrium is distended and then ruptures. Subsequently, fissures develop in the adjacent functional layers, and blood as well as fragments of tissue of various sizes become detached. Although autolysis occurs, as a rule fragments of tissue can be identified in the menstrual tissue in the vagina. Hemorrhage stops when the coiled artery returns to a state of constriction. The changes that accompany partial necro-

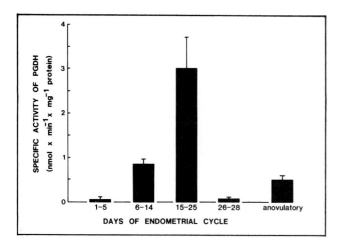

Figure 4-2. Specific activities (mean ± SEM) of NAD^+-dependent 15-hydroxyprostaglandin dehydrogenase (PGDH) in cytosolic fractions of human endometrial tissues obtained on various days of menstrual cycle or from anovulatory women. Days of the menstrual cycle were idealized to that of a 28-day ovulatory cycle for postovulatory samples according to menstrual history, histologic appearance of the endometrium, and serum estradiol-17β and progesterone concentrations on the day of endometrial sampling. (*Data from Casey et al: Prostaglandins 19:115, 1980. Courtesy of Dr. M. L. Casey.*)

sis also serve to seal off the tip of the vessel; and, in the superficial portion, often only the endothelium remains. The endometrial surface is restored, according to Markee (1940), by growth of the flanges, or collars, that form the everted free ends of the uterine glands. These flanges increase in diameter very rapidly, and the continuity of the endometrium is effected by the fusion of the edges of these sheets of thin, migrating cells.

Among the more thorough studies of the process of menstruation are those of McLennan and Rydell (1965) who concluded that loss of endometrial tissue may be less extensive than previous investigators had suggested. In their opinion, regeneration of the uterine surface occurs from the residual spongy layer rather than from the most basal elements.

Ultrastructure. From the findings of the studies of Wynn and associates (1967) and White and Buchsbaum (1973) on the ultrastructure of the endometrium, there is secretion of cytoplasmic components of the endometrial cells into the glandular lumens throughout the menstrual cycle (Figs. 4-3, 4-4). The terms *proliferative* and *secretory,* therefore, are reflective less accurately of the histologic pattern than are the terms *preovulatory* (follicular) and *postovulatory* (luteal).

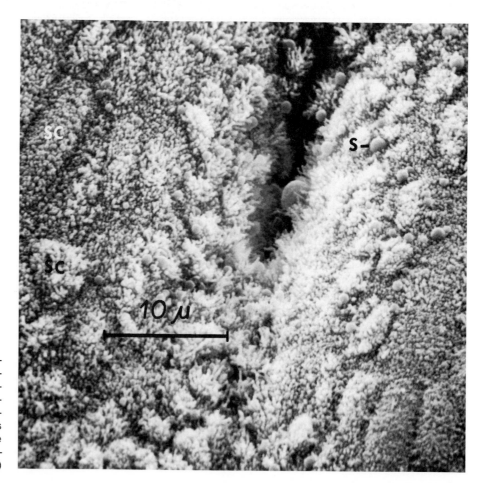

Figure 4-3. Gland ostium and surrounding endometrium in proliferative phase seen by scanning electron microscopy. Many secretory droplets are seen on cell surfaces. Microvilli are prominent on secretory cells (SC) and individual cell margins are identified. (*From White and Buchsbaum: Gynecol Oncol 1:330, 1973.*)

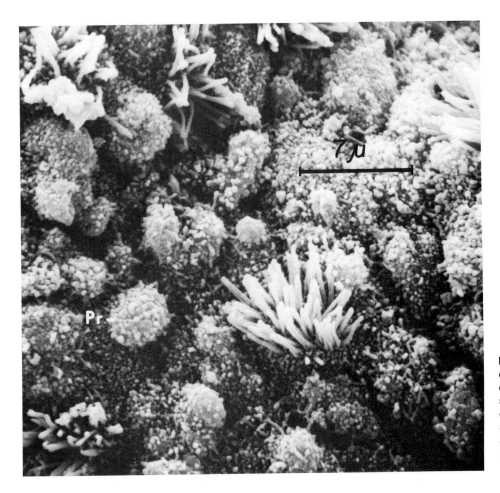

Figure 4-4. Cellular detail for secretory phase endometrium on day 24 of the cycle, demonstrated by scanning electron microscopy. Microvilli are prominent and cellular protuberances (Pr) are evident. (*From White and Buchsbaum: Gynecol Oncol 1:330,1973.*)

The Endometrial Cycle in Retrospect

The correlations of the hormonal events of the ovarian cycle and the morphologic changes of the endometrial cycle and the action of the pituitary gonadotropic hormones are summarized in Table 4-2 and in Figure 4-5. Commonly, we presume incorrectly that the ovarian cycle and the endometrial or menstrual cycles are coincident in time. Thus, again somewhat incorrectly, the follicular phase of the ovarian cycle has been presumed to be absolutely coincident with the proliferative phase of the endometrial or menstrual cycle. At the same time, the terms *luteal phase* and *secretory phase* have been regarded, in terms of the cycle, to be coincident if not synonymous. In fact, the ovarian cycle, as we now understand it, and the menstrual cycle, as we define it (i.e., that cycle that begins on the first day of menses), are not coincident. We now know that follicular recruitment, presumably brought about in part by a modest but significant increase in FSH secretion, commences not with menstruation but a few days before the onset of menses, at a time of maximum regression of the corpus luteum; indeed, that ovarian cycle terminates before the onset of menstruation when the corpus luteum of the succeeding ovarian cycle regresses. Although the cycles are divided into phases for descriptive purposes and for convenience

in description, the changes are continuous throughout an ovulatory cycle. Furthermore, there is considerable individual variation in both the activity of the endocrine glands and in the response of the target organ, the uterus. Secretory changes that resemble closely those of the luteal phase may appear occasionally before ovulation. Although the postovulatory phase of the cycle generally is very close to 14 days in length, the normal follicular phase may vary from 1 to 3 weeks. Finally, whereas the bleeding at the end of a typical ovulatory menstrual cycle is preceded by endometrial ischemia, uterine bleeding, on occasion, may appear at the expected time without prior ovulation, formation of a corpus luteum, or secretion of progesterone. Anovulatory cycles sometimes occur in otherwise apparently normal women, but the incidence is difficult to ascertain because adequate observations of the ovaries are rarely possible. It appears that in some such cycles a follicle enlarges but then becomes cystic and degenerates. In others, no follicles grow beyond a few millimeters throughout an entire cycle. Withdrawal of progesterone, therefore, is not essential for cyclic uterine bleeding. **It is rare, however, for women with persistent anovulation to menstruate regularly unless they are ingesting oral contraceptives.**

At about 27 to 35 days after the first day of the last

menstrual period, there may be bleeding around the site of implantation of the fertilized ovum, an event that results in slight vaginal bleeding that is sometimes mistaken for menses. This "placental sign" (Hartmann, 1932) of bleeding always occurs during pregnancy in the rhesus monkey.

CERVICAL, VAGINAL, AND TUBAL CYCLES

Cervix

Cyclic changes occur in the endocervical glands, especially during the follicular phase of the cycle. During the early follicular phase, the glands are only slightly tortuous and the secretory cells are not very tall. Secretion of mucus is meager. The late follicular phase, however, is characterized by pronounced tortuosity of the glands, deep invagination, tumescence of the epithelium, high columnar cells, and abundant secretion. The connective tissue acquires a looser texture and more extensive vascularization. After ovulation, these characteristics regress.

The secretory activity of the endocervical glands is maximal at about the time of ovulation and is the result of estrogenic stimulation. Only at that time, in most women, is the quality of the cervical mucus such as to permit penetration by spermatozoa. The property of the cervical mucus that permits it to be drawn out in long strands is termed *Spinnbarkeit,* a property of mucus that is maximal at the time of ovulation. The synchronization of the height of secretory activity in the cervical and endometrial cycles is precise and purposeful. In the cervix, where the mucus facilitates passage of the spermatozoa, it occurs just before the ovum is to be released (i.e., at ovulation), a period probably of not more than about 36 to 48 hours. In the endometrium, where the purpose of the highly developed secretory activity seems to be to provide a site favorable for nidation of the fertilized ovum, the changes are maximum about 6 to 7 days later, when the fertilized ovum is ready to implant.

The "Fern Pattern." If cervical mucus is aspirated, spread on a glass slide, allowed to dry for a few minutes, and examined microscopically, characteristic patterns can be discerned that are dependent on the stage of the ovarian cycle and the presence or absence of pregnancy (i.e., progesterone secretion in large amounts). From about the 7th day of the menstrual cycle to about the 18th day, a fern-like pattern of dried cervical mucus is seen (Fig. 4-6); it is sometimes called a process of "arborization" or the "palm leaf pattern." After approximately the 21st day, this fern pattern does not develop, but rather a quite different pattern forms, one that is beaded or cellular in appearance (Fig. 4-7). This beaded pattern usually also is encountered in pregnancy.

TABLE 4-2. IMPORTANT MILESTONES IN THE CORRELATION OF OVARIAN AND ENDOMETRIAL (MENSTRUAL) CYCLES (IDEALIZED 28-DAY CYCLE)

Phase	Menstrual	Early Follicular	Advanced Follicular	Ovulation	Early Luteal	Advanced Luteal	Premenstrual
Days	1–5	6–8	9–13	14	15–19	20–25	26–28
OVARY	Formation of corpus albicans from corpus luteum of preceding cycle. Recruitment of follicles.	Folicular maturation and development of the chosen or dominant follicle.		Ovulation and luteinization of granulosa cells in the ruptured follicle.	Vascularization of granulosa lutein cells and formation of corpus luteum. Follicular atresia.	Mature corpus luteum and continued follicular atresia.	Involution of corpus luteum and initiation of follicular recruitment for the next cycle.
ESTROGEN	Low; derived principally from extra-glandularly produced estrone; little estradiol-17β secretion by the ovary.	Estradiol-17β secretion, principally by granulosa cells of the dominant follicle, increases strikingly, maximal rates being attained just prior to the LH surge.		Immediately after, or coincident with, ovulation, there is an abrupt, indeed, precipitous decline in estradiol-17β secretion.	Gradual and progressive postovulatory rise in estradiol-17β secretion by the corpus luteum.	Maximal rates of postovulatory estradiol-17β secretion are attained; luteal phase estradiol-17β secretion rates, however, are not nearly as great as those observed in the immediate preovulatory phase.	Estradiol-17β secretion declines precipitously and, as during menstruation, the principal estrogen produced is estrone, which is formed in extra-glandular sites.

(continued)

TABLE 4-2. *(Continued)*

Phase	Menstrual	Early Follicular	Advanced Follicular	Ovulation	Early Luteal	Advanced Luteal	Premenstrual
Days	1–5	6–8	9–13	14	15–19	20–25	26–28
PROGESTERONE	Low secretion; there is little secretion of progesterone by the adrenal cortex and the corpus luteum of the preceding ovarian cycle has regressed.	During the follicular phase of the ovarian cycle, progesterone levels remain low. This is due to the fact that human granulosa cells cannot synthesize cholesterol, the obligate precursor of progesterone, but are dependent upon LDL-cholesterol that can be obtained only from the blood after vascularization of the granulosa cells after ovulation.		Progesterone secretion increases steadily as the consequence of the availability of LDL and LH action to effect cholesterol side-chain cleavage.	Progesterone secretion remains high until the end of the advanced luteal phase.		Precipitous decline in progesterone secretion.
ENDOMETRIUM	Menstrual desquamation and early reorganization of endometrial glandular epithelium.	Proliferation of glandular epithelium with many mitoses.	Pseudostratification of nuclei—no secretion, early stromal changes.	Appearance of subnuclear vacuoles that are rich in glycogen.	Migration of vacuoles to the luminal surface; cessation of mitosis. The endometrial glands become very tortuous.	Vacuoles have been secreted and decidualization commences. Stromal edema and enlargement of stromal cells is prominent.	Disruption and disintegration of stromal cells. Leukocyte infiltration and interstitial hemorrhage.
Pituitary Secretion FSH	Continuing decline in FSH levels that had become modestly increased coincident with the decline in steroid secretion by the regressing corpus luteum of the preceding cycle.	FSH secretion is at all times pulsatile in nature but during the proliferative phase of the ovarian cycle, prior to the time of the LH surge at midcycle, FSH levels remain low.		There is a significant surge of FSH secretion, albeit less prominent than that of LH, that heralds the commencement of the ovulatory process.	After the midcycle gonadotropin surge, FSH levels fall abruptly to levels similar to those found during the preovulatory phase of the cycle.		As steroid secretion by the regressing corpus luteum diminishes, there is a modest but significant increase in FSH.
Pituitary Secretion LH	The levels of LH are low and reasonably constant until just prior to ovulation			Coincident with, or just after, the striking increase in estradiol-17β secretion by the dominant follicle, there is a striking increase in LH secretion— the LH "surge."	The levels of LH are low and reasonably constant until just prior to ovulation.		

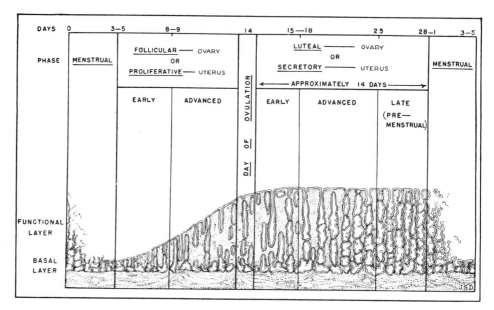

Figure 4-5. Cyclic changes in thickness and in form of glands and arteries of endometrium and the relation of these changes to those of the ovarian cycle.

The crystallization of the mucus, which is necessary for the production of the fern, or arborized pattern, is dependent upon the concentration of electrolytes, principally sodium chloride, in the secretion. In general, a concentration of sodium chloride of 1 percent is required for the full development of a fern pattern; below that concentration, either a beaded pattern or atypical, incomplete arborization is seen.

The concentration of sodium chloride, and, in turn, the presence or absence of the fern pattern, is determined by the response of the cervix to hormonal action. Whereas the cervical mucus is relatively rich in sodium chloride when estrogen, but not progesterone, is being produced, the secretion of progesterone (even without a reduction in the rate of secretion of estrogen) promptly acts to lower the sodium chloride concentration of the mucus, either cervical or nasal, to levels at which ferning will not occur as the specimen dries. During pregnancy, progesterone usually exerts a similar effect, even though the amount of estrogen produced is enormous compared with that produced during a normal ovarian cycle.

Vagina

There is constant desquamation of the superficial cells of the vaginal epithelium. Consequently, the nature of maturity of the cells in the vaginal fluid is reflective to some degree of the changes in the epithelium of the surface of the vagina that occur in response to hormone action. The vaginal epithelium of women, under estrogenic stimulation is characterized by cyclic changes during which the greatest development is reached at the end of the follicular phase. This stage is characterized by enlargement, flattening, and spreading of the superficial cells and by relative leukopenia, whereas in the smear taken in the luteal phase, there is an increase in the number of basophilic cells and leukocytes, as well as irregular grouping of the cells.

CLINICAL ASPECTS OF MENSTRUATION

Menstruation is the normal, periodic, physiologic discharge of blood, mucus, and cellular debris from the uterine mucosa and occurs at more or less regular intervals from menarche to menopause, except during periods of pregnancy and lactation.

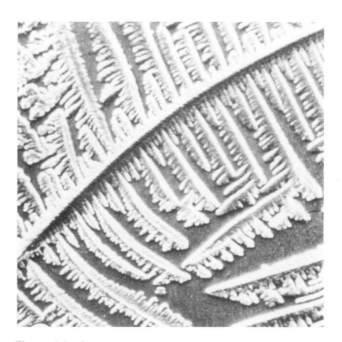

Figure 4-6. Scanning electron microscopy of cervical mucus obtained on day 11 of the menstrual cycle. (*From Zaneveld, Tauber, Port, Propping. Obstet Gynecol 46:424, 1975.*)

The Menarche and Puberty

Historically, the age at which menstruation begins (menarche) has declined steadily until recent years (Fig. 4-8). This decline has ceased in the United States. The average time at which menstruation begins is now between the 12th and 13th years of age, but in a small minority of apparently normal girls, menarche may occur as early as the 10th or as late as the 16th year. The menarche refers specifically to the first menstruation, whereas puberty is a broader term that refers to the entire transitional stage between childhood and sexual maturity. The menarche, hence, is just one sign of puberty.

The Menopause and Climacteric

Menopause is the cessation of menses. There are wide variations in the age at which menopause occurs. About one half of all women cease menstruating between the ages of 45 and 50, about one quarter stop before the age of 45, and another one quarter continue to menstruate until past 50 years of age. The term climacteric is derived from the Greek word that means "rung of a ladder" and bears the same relation to the menopause as the term *puberty* bears to menarche. The climacteric refers to the time in a woman's life known to the laity as the "change of life."

Interval and Duration

Although the *model interval* at which menstruation occurs is considered to be 28 days, there is considerable variation among women, in general, as well as in the cycle lengths of an individual woman. Marked variation in the length of menstrual cycles does not necessarily mean infertility.

Arey (1939), who analyzed 12 different studies, which comprised about 20,000 calendar records from 1500 women, reached the conclusion that there is no evidence of perfect regularity. In a study by Gunn and co-workers (1937) of 479 normal British women, the typical difference between the shortest and longest cycle was 8 or 9 days. In 30 percent of women, it was more than 13 days but in no woman was it fewer than 2 days. Arey found that in an average adult woman, one third of her cycles departed by more than 2 days from the mean of the lengths of her cycles. Arey's analysis of 5322 cycles in 485 normal women was indicative of an average interval of 28.4 days; his finding for the average cycle length in pubertal girls was longer, 33.9 days. Chiazze and associates (1968) analyzed the length of 30,655 menstrual cycles of 2316 women. The mean for all cycles was 29.1 days. For cycles that range from 15 to 45 days, the average length was 28.1 days. The degree of variability was such that only 13 percent of the women experienced cycles that varied in length by fewer than 6 days. Haman (1942) surveyed 2460 cycles in 150 housewives who attended a clinic where special attention was directed to recording accurately the length of the menstrual cycles. Arey's data and those of Haman, the distribution curves of which are superimposed and shown in Figure 4-9, are almost identical

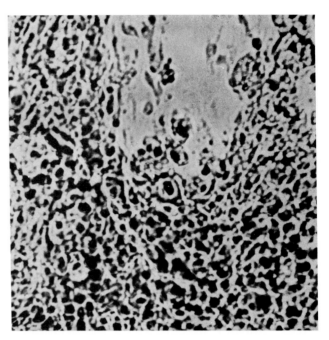

Figure 4-7. Photomicrograph of dried cervical mucus obtained from the cervical canal of a woman pregnant at 32 to 33 weeks. The beaded pattern is characteristic of progesterone action on the endocervical gland mucus composition. (*Courtesy of Dr. J. C. Ullery.*)

Duration and Amount

The duration of menstrual flow also is variable; the usual duration is 4 to 6 days, but lengths between 2 and 8 days may be considered physiologic. In any individual woman, however, the duration of the flow is usually fairly similar from cycle to cycle.

The menstrual discharge consists of shed fragments of endometrium mixed with a variable quantity of blood. Usually the blood is liquid, but if the rate of blood flow is excessive, clots of various size may appear. Considerable attention has been directed to the usual state of incoagulability of menstrual blood. The most logical explanation for its incoagulability is that the blood was coagulated as it was shed, but promptly was liquefied by fibrinolytic activity. In endometrial tissue, there not only are potent thromboplastic properties, which promptly initiate clotting, but also a potent activator of plasminogen to plasmin, which effects prompt lysis of fibrin clots.

At one time, the toxic properties of the menstrual discharge attracted considerable interest. The discharge undoubtedly contains toxic proteins and peptides that most likely arise from proteolytic activity present in the mixture of blood and endometrial tissue fragments but also from bacterial contamination.

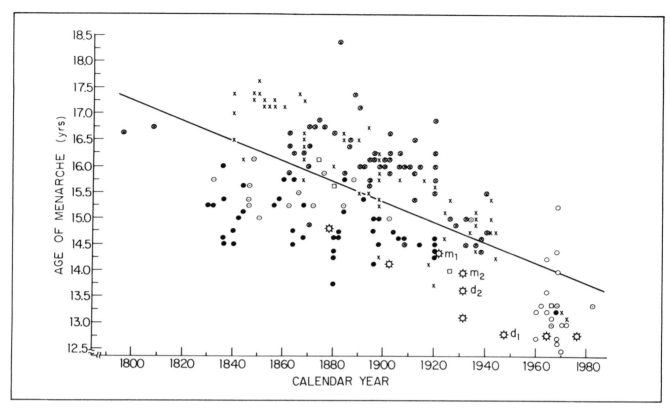

Figure 4-8. Mean or Median Age of Menarche as a Function of Calendar Year from 1790 to 1980. The symbols refer to England (⊙); France (●); Germany (⊗); Holland (□); Scandinavia (X) (Denmark, Finland, Norway, and Sweden); Belgium, Czechoslovakia, Hungary, Italy, Poland (rural), Romania (urban and rural), Russia (15.2 years at an altitude of 2500 m and 14.4 years at 700 m), Spain, and Switzerland (all labeled ✿); and the United States (O , data not included in the regression line). Twenty-seven points for Europe were identical and do not appear on the graph. The regression line cannot, of course, be extended indefinitely. The age of menarche has already leveled off in some European countries, as it has in the United States. (*From Wyshak and Frisch: N Engl J Med 306:1033, 1982.*)

The average amount of blood lost by normal women during a menstrual period has been determined by several groups of investigators, who found it to range from about 25 to 60 ml (Baldwin and associates, 1961; Barker and Fowler, 1936; Hallberg and co-workers, 1966; Hytten and associates, 1964; Millis, 1951). With a normal hemoglobin concentration of 14 g/dl and a hemoglobin iron content of 3.4 mg/g, these volumes of blood contain from 12 to 29 mg of iron and represent a blood loss equivalent of 0.4 to 1.0 mg of iron for every day of the cycle, or from 150 to 400 mg per year. Finch (1959) determined the rate of decrease in the specific activity of the miscible iron of the body for a period of years after the injection of ^{55}Fe to ascertain the rate of loss of iron from the body. In women who menstruated, the iron loss on average was 0.6 mg per day more than the iron loss in men or postmenopausal women. Since the amount of iron that is absorbed from the diet usually is quite limited, this seemingly "negligible" iron loss is important because it contributes further to the low iron stores that are present in the majority of women (Hallberg and co-workers, 1968; Scott and Pritchard, 1967).

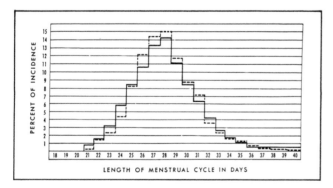

Figure 4-9. Duration of menstrual cycle based on distribution data of Arey (*continuous line*) and Haman (*broken line*). (*Courtesy of Eli Lilly and Co.*)

Changes in Body Weight

It has been reported frequently that about 30 percent of women gain 1 to 3 pounds shortly before the onset of menstruation, an amount of weight that is lost promptly as menstruation begins. Although only a minority of women manifest weight gains, there has been a tendency to regard the increase in weight as a normal characteristic of the cycle that is reflective of the influence of steroid hormones. Actually, the average weight gain is insignificant, perhaps a quarter of a pound, as shown in a statistical study of the question by Chesley and Hellman (1957) and by Golub and associates (1965). It would appear, therefore, that the concept of appreciable premenstrual weight gain, as a physiologic phenomenon, is not valid. Preece and co-workers (1975) could find no consistent change in total body water during the menstrual cycle.

REFERENCES

Arey LB: The degree of normal menstrual irregularity: An analysis of 20,000 calendar records from 1,500 individuals. Am J Obstet Gynecol 37:12, 1939

Baldwin RM, Whalley PJ, Pritchard JA: Measurements of menstrual blood loss. Am J Obstet Gynecol 81:739, 1961

Barker AP, Fowler WM: The blood loss during normal menstruation. Am J Obstet Gynecol 31:979, 1936

Benirschke K: The endometrium. In Yen SSC, Jaffe RB (eds): Reproductive Endocrinology: Physiology, Pathophysiology and Clinical Management. Philadelphia, Saunders, 1978

Casey ML, Hemsell DL, MacDonald PC, Johnston JM: NAD+-dependent 15-hydroxyprostaglandin dehydrogenase activity in human endometrium. Prostaglandins 19:122, 1980

Chesley LC, Hellman LM: Variations in body weight and salivary sodium in the menstrual cycle. Am J Obstet Gynecol 74:582, 1957

Chiazze L, Brayer FT, Macisco JJ, Parker MP, Duffy BJ: The length and variability of the human menstrual cycle. JAMA 203:377, 1968

Finch CA: Body iron exchange in man. J Clin Invest 38:392, 1959

Golander A, Hurley T, Barret J, Hizi A, Handwerger S: Prolactin synthesis by human chorion decidual tissue. A possible source of prolactin in the amniotic fluid. Science 202:311, 1978

Golub LJ, Menduke H, Conly SS Jr: Weight changes in college women during the menstrual cycle. Am J Obstet Gynecol 91:89, 1965

Gunn DL, Jenkin PM, Gunn AL: Menstrual periodicity; statistical observations on a large sample of normal cases. J Obstet Gynaecol Br Emp 44:839, 1937

Hallberg L, Hogdahl A-M, Nilsson L, Rybo G: Menstrual blood loss, a population study: Variation at different ages and attempts to define normality. Acta Obstet Gynecol Scand 45:320, 1966

Hallberg L, Hallgren J. Hollender A, Hogdahl AM, Tibblin G: Occurrence of iron deficiency anemia in Sweden. Symp Swedish Nutri Found 6:19, 1968

Haman JO: The length of the menstrual cycle: A study of 150 normal women. Am J Obstet Gynecol 43:870, 1942

Hartman CG: Studies in the reproduction of the monkey Macaca (Pithecus) rhesus with special reference to menstruation and pregnancy. Contrib Embryol 23:1, 1932

Horwitz KB, McGuire WL, Pearson OH, Segaloff A: Predicting response to endocrine therapy in human breast cancer: A hypothesis. Science 189:726, 1975

Hytten FE, Cheyne GA, Klopper AI: Iron loss at menstruation. J Obstet Gynaecol Br Commw 71:255, 1964

Markee JE: Menstruation in intraocular endometrial transplants in the rhesus monkey. Contrib Embryol 28:219, 1940

McLennan CE, Rydell AH: Extent of endometrial shedding during normal menstruation. Obstet Gynecol 26:605, 1965

Millis J: The iron losses of healthy women during consecutive menstrual cycles. Med J Aust 2:874, 1951

Noyes RW, Hertig AT, Rock J: Dating the endometrial biopsy. Fertil Steril 1:3, 1950

Preece PE, Richards AR, Owen GM, Hughes LE: Mastalgia and total body water. Br Med J 4:498, 1975

Riddick DH, Luciano AA, Kusmik WF, Maslar IA: Evidence of a nonpituitary source of amniotic fluid prolactin. Fertil Steril 31:35, 1979

Scott DE, Pritchard JA: Iron deficiency in healthy young college women. JAMA 199:897, 1967

Tseng L, Gurpide E: Estradiol and 20α-dihydroprogesterone dehydrogenase activities in human endometrium during the menstrual cycle. Endocrinology 94:419, 1974

Tseng L, Gurpide E: Effects of progestins on estradiol receptor levels in human endometrium. J Clin Endocrinol Metab 41:402, 1975

Tseng L, Liu HC: Stimulation of arylsulfotransferase activity by progestins in human endometrium in vitro. J Clin Endocrinol Metab 53:418, 1981

Tyson JE, Hwang P, Guyda H, Friesen HG: Studies of prolactin secretion in human pregnancy. Am J Obstet Gynecol 113:14, 1972

White AJ, Buchsbaum HJ: Scanning electron microscopy of the human endometrium. Gynecol Oncol 1:330, 1973

Wynn RM, Harris JA: Ultrastructural cyclic changes in the human endometrium: I. Normal preovulatory phase. Fertil Steril 18:632, 1967

Wynn RM, Woolley RS: Ultrastructural cyclic changes in the human endometrium: II. Normal postovulatory phase. Fertil Steril 18:721, 1967

5

Gametogenesis and Development of the Ovum

For many decades, our most talented reproductive biologists, physiologists, cytogeneticists, and biochemists have labored diligently to define the molecular events that are essential to successful reproduction. As discussed in Chapters 3 and 4, considerable progress has been made in defining the molecular events that serve to regulate the maturation of the follicle and thence ovulation. Such fundamental information has provided great insight for the development of approaches to the correction or at least the successful treatment of infertility due to anovulation caused by a variety of disorders. The results of these many studies of the mechanisms of control of the ovarian cycle also have provided means of developing effective and principally safe and acceptable means of population control. Many other examples could be given, but those cited are obviously among the important issues that affect, directly or indirectly, every person of the world.

At the same time, generally, while investigations of the regulation of the processes of follicular maturation and ovulation were proceeding with great success, other investigators were pursuing a definition of the molecular events that serve to control the biochemistry of gametogenesis, fertilization, ovum and blastocyst transport, and implantation. Still others were evaluating the role of cervical mucus in sperm penetration and transport, the potential role of spermatozoa capacitation, and the difficult dilemma of antibody formation as a cause of infertility—or even as a means of inducing infertility. Whereas these investigations were proceeding with success at a rate equal to that of the definition of the hormonal regulation of the reproductive processes, the clinical applicability of the knowledge so attained has lagged behind by two to three decades. Clinicians could not keep pace. The reasons for this were multiple, but they revolve principally about the fact that failure of fertilization in women is commonly caused by tubal disease—a transport problem that may be beyond current boundaries of surgical repair. The magnitude, if any, of immunologic infertility has been difficult to define because of the lack of tests of sufficient precision and reliability to address, in a meaningful way, the nature and cause, let alone the prevalence, of the putative problem.

At the time of this writing, however, a new era is emerging. In vitro fertilization of ova of women, with successful pregnancy and birth after reimplantation of the fertilized ovum, is a reality. New tests are being developed to evaluate the nature of infertility in couples in whom previously no cause was found.

As is customarily the case, we still are far behind our veterinarian colleagues, who for years have successfully frozen and preserved sperm from prize males, artificially inseminated many species, developed ova transport systems, succeeded with in vitro fertilization, effected superovulation, and on and on.

Nevertheless, at the time of this writing, the future is bright. All that stands in the way of a new era—one that may hold the promise for the solution to many problems of infertility not previously believed to be treatable—is further development and refinement of technical details. Perhaps (and possibly of greater socio-economic significance for all the world) equally close is the development of new means of population control, the delivery systems for which may be the answer to population control in underdeveloped nations. It is with this optimism that we now can address with renewed enthusiasm the issues of gametogenesis, fertilization, and development, and transport of the fertilized ovum.

GAMETOGENESIS

Primitive germ cells are present in the human embryo by the end of the third week of development. Both *oogenesis,* in the course of which mature ova are formed from primitive oogonia, and *spermatogenesis,* which results in the production of spermatids, share a basic biologic feature of maturation, namely, reduction and division. Such special cellular division, known as *meiosis,* is limited to germ cells. The process of meiosis is characterized by a long and unusual prophase, and involves a process that provides for the exchange of genetic material between homologous chromosomes and the reduction of the *diploid* number of chromosomes, 46, to the *haploid* number, 23. In man, the diploid number of chromosomes is comprised of 44 autosomes and 2 sex

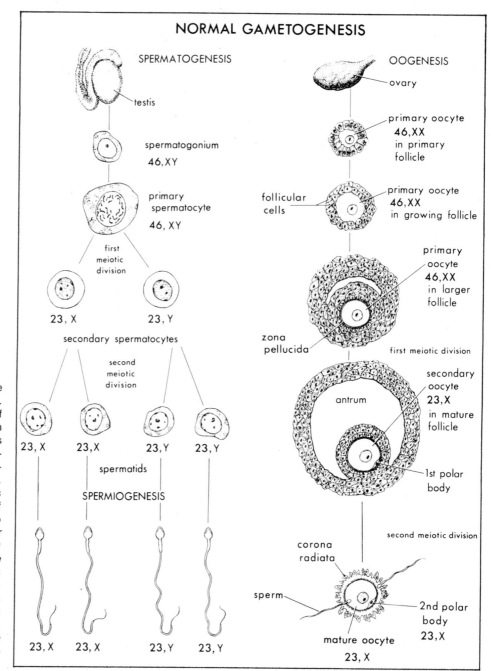

Figure 5-1. Drawings to compare spermatogenesis and oogenesis. The chromosome complement of the germ cells is shown at each stage. The number designates the total number of chromosomes, including the sex chromosome(s) shown after the comma. Note that (1) after the two meiotic divisions, the diploid number of chromosomes, 46, is reduced to the haploid number, 23; (2) *four sperms* form from one primary spermatocyte, whereas only *one* mature oocyte (ovum) results from maturation of a primary oocyte; and, (3) the cytoplasm is conserved during oogenesis to form one large cell, the mature oocyte (ovum). (*From Moore. The Developing Human, 2nd ed. Philadelphia, Saunders, 1977.*)

chromosomes; during meiosis, mature gametes are formed, in each of which there are 22 autosomes and 1 sex chromosome. The diploid number of chromosomes is not restored until fertilization with the union of the ovum and sperm (Fig. 5-1). *Spermatogenesis* is the process that encompasses the final maturational events that lead to production of mature male gametes and is one that involves changes in the shape of the spermatids and the transformation of these cells to spermatozoa. The fact that the mature germ cells are derived directly from primitive cells that may have migrated from the yolk sac to the developing gonads as early as the fifth week of embryonic life, is one that underlies the concept of *continuity of the germ plasm.* In the case of human ova, some germ cells may remain dormant for as long as 50 years.

Meiosis

In all primitive germ cells, that is, *oogonia* and *spermatogonia,* there are a diploid number of chromosomes (46). When these stem cells divide to produce primary oocytes and spermatocytes, each chromosome undergoes replication by splitting longitudinally to form a double-stranded structure. During this typical *mitosis*, one strand of each chromosome enters each daughter cell, and, in this manner, the identical chromosomal components of the parent cells are obtained.

When the primary oocytes and spermatocytes continue maturation to form secondary oocytes and spermatocytes, respectively, however, the meiotic division that ensues is quite different; this is the case in that each of the newly formed cells receives only 23, or the haploid number of chromosomes. The basic difference between meiosis and mitosis is the prolonged prophase in meiosis, in which there is, in meiosis, preliminary pairing of homologous chromosomes before division. During the *leptotene* stage of meiotic prophase, the 46 chromosomes appear as single slender threads; in the next stage, the *zygotene*, the homologous chromosomes are aligned in a parallel manner to one another in *synapsis*, with the formation of 23 bivalent components. Each chromosome then divides longitudinally, except at the *centromere*, and the ensuing *pachytene* stage is comprised of *tetrads* of four chromatids, the shape of which is dependent upon the position of the centromere. At this stage, the chromatids break and thence recombine with strands from the homologous chromosome to effect an exchange of genetic material. During the *diplotene* stage, which follows, the homologous strands separate. During the metaphase of the first meiotic division, the bivalents (two chromatids that comprise each chromosome) become oriented on the spindle; when the cell divides, the members of each pair move toward opposite poles into the daughter cells, which then contain the haploid number of chromosomes, still as chromatid pairs. *The individual chromosomes now are no longer genetically identical with those of the parent cell.* Each secondary oocyte will thus receive 22 autosomes and an X chromosome, and each secondary spermatocyte will receive 22 autosomes and either an X or Y chromosome.

At the second meiotic division, the *dyad* splits at the centromere to form two *monads*, one of which becomes associated with each daughter cell, probably having already undergone a typical mitotic longitudinal replication. The mature ovum (23,X), if fertilized by a spermatozoan with a Y chromosome (23,Y) will produce a male zygote (46,XY), whereas the ovum fertilized by a spermatozoan with an X chromosome (23,X) will produce a female (46,XX).

Biochemistry of Cellular Division. During mitotic interphase, duplication of the chromosomes is accomplished by replication of DNA. The results of autoradiographic studies of the incorporation of tritium-labeled thymidine into chromosomes are indicative that duplication is accomplished by separation of the two original DNA strands of each chromosome and by subsequent synthesis of two new DNA strands. At the next cellular division, each chromatid receives one original and one newly synthesized strand.

Oogenesis

In the sections of Chapters 2 and 3 that deal with the embryology of the ovary, the derivation of the primitive germ cells from the yolk sac and the histogenesis of the granulosal and thecal elements are described. Pinkerton and colleagues (1961) were able to trace the development of the human ovum by use of histochemical techniques that were dependent principally upon the high content of alkaline phosphatase that is characteristic of the germ cells. In the first phase (migration), the germ cells reach the medial slope of the mesonephric ridge where the gonads arise, divide rapidly, and become oogonia; in the second phase (division), the germ cells divide mitotically at a rate that is maximal during the 8th to 20th week, but slows thereafter, and finally ceases at birth. In the third phase (maturation), the cells enter the prophase of the first meiotic division, acquire a ring of granulosa cells, and become definitive oocytes within the primary follicles.

It is well to remember that all oocytes are derived from the primitive germ cells. Blandau and co-workers (1963) have recorded, cinematographically, in the mouse, the ameboidlike migration of primitive germ cells from the yolk sac to the germinal ridges. The primitive oogonia, furthermore, continue movements locally within the developing ovary even after the pachytene stage of meiosis is reached.

There is no evidence of *neogenesis* of human ova. Of the total number of primary oocytes at birth, estimated to be about 2,000,000, and at puberty to be 400,000 to 500,000 (Baker, 1963), only 400 to 500 will actually be ovulated; the majority degenerate in situ (see Chapter 3, p. 33). After puberty, several oocytes may begin to enlarge during each cycle, but ordinarily only one reaches full maturity.

The primary oocytes increase in size and cuboidal follicular cells proliferate to form increasingly thick coverings around them (Fig. 5-2). The follicular cells, furthermore, deposit on the surface of the oocyte an *acellular* glycoprotein mantle that thickens gradually to form the *zona pellucida* (Figs. 5-2, 5-3). Irregular fluid-filled spaces between the follicular cells then coalesce to form an antrum. The radially elongated follicular cells that surround the zona pellucida form the *corona radiata* (Fig. 5-2). A solid mass of follicular cells, the *cumulus oophorus* (*discus proligerus*), surrounds the ovum in a developing vesicular ovarian follicle (Figs. 5-2, 5-3). As the follicle nears maturity, the cumulus projects further into the antrum and, as a consequence, the oocyte appears to be supported by this column of follicular cells. At this stage, the follicle may vary from 6 to 12 mm in diameter and lies immediately beneath the surface of the ovary.

The formation of the oocyte completes the first meiotic division, which was begun before birth, during the final stage of transformation of the primordial follicle into the mature graafian follicle. The important result is

follicular   nucleus of   zona   cumulus
cells   primary oocyte   pellucida   oophorus

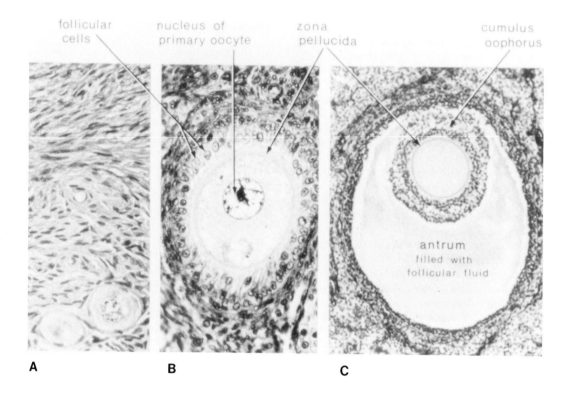

antrum
filled with
follicular fluid

A   B   C

Figure 5-2. Photomicrographs of sections from ovaries of adult women. **A.** Ovarian cortex showing two primordial follicles that contain primary oocytes that have completed the prophase of the first meiotic division and have entered the dictyotene stage, a "resting" stage between prophase and metaphase (×250). **B.** Growing follicle that contains a primary oocyte, surrounded by the zona pellucida and a stratified layer of follicular cells (×250). **C.** An almost mature follicle with a large antrum. The oocyte, embedded in the cumulus oophorus, does not show a nucleus because it has been sectioned tangentially (×100). (*From Moore: The Developing Human, 3rd ed. Philadelphia, Saunders, 1982.*)

the formation of two daughter cells, each with 23 chromosomes but of greatly unequal size. One receives almost all of the cytoplasm of the mother cell and becomes a secondary oocyte; the other, the first polar body, receives very little cytoplasm. The polar body lies between the zona pellucida and the vitelline membrane of the secondary oocyte.

Not only is there a chosen (or dominant) follicle—there is a dominant oocyte since it is the only oocyte in the preovulatory follicle that matures; all others do not develop beyond the immature dictyate state (Channing and associates, 1982). It is believed that a cybernin (Chapter 3, p. 60) called *oocyte maturation inhibitor* may serve an important role in oocyte maturation. Oocyte maturation inhibitor appears to be present in all follicles except preovulatory ones. From the results of a variety of experiments beginning with those of Chang (1955), it seems reasonably clear that a substance in follicular fluid that arises from granulosa cells inhibits oocyte maturation.

As summarized by Channing and Pomerantz (1981), there is in human (and other mammalian) follicular fluid an inhibitor of oocyte maturation—of molecular weight of less than 2000—which is probably a polypeptide that is secreted by granulosa cells. The action of oocyte maturation inhibitor is probably mediated by cells of the cumulus. LH, in all likelihood, acts on the chosen follicle to block the action of the oocyte maturation inhibitor.

In studies of tubal ova, Hertig and Rock (1944) found that the first polar body is cast off while still in the ovary. A second division is consummated in the formation of the second polar body at about the moment that the sperm penetrates the egg.

A most interesting, and unsolved, riddle in this field is the mechanism(s) that prevents all follicles but one from undergoing simultaneous maturation and ovulation during the first, or any given, cycle. The factors that normally are believed to be responsible for allowing only one ovum to reach maturity each month are considered subsequently and in Chapter 3 (p. 60).

In ova of women, the second maturation division is completed only if the ovum is fertilized. If penetration by a spermatozoan does not occur within a few hours of ovulation, the ovum begins to degenerate; it is believed, however, that the ovum is capable of being fertilized successfully for 15 to 18 hours after ovulation (Blandau,

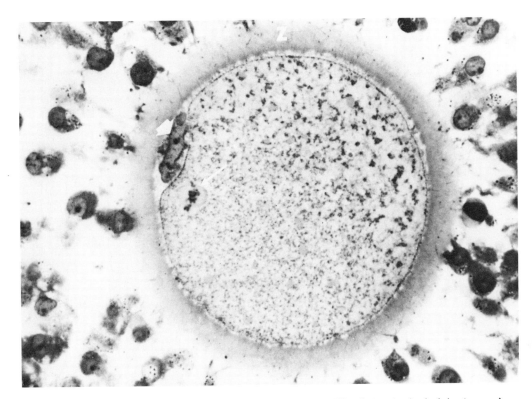

Figure 5-3. Light micrograph of a human follicular oocyte. The first polar body (*short arrow*) has been liberated and lies in the perivitelline space, which separates the oocyte from the zona pellucida (Z). The oocyte chromosomes are aligned on the equator of the meiotic spindle (*long arrow*). They will remain in this position until penetration of the fertilizing spermatozoan, when the second meiotic division will resume. The cells of the cumulus oophorus are more dispersed than in the previous stages. Some of them are undergoing regression, as shown by the presence of numerous fat droplets in the cytoplasm and pyknosis of nuclei. These features represent the onset of the denudation of the oocyte, a process that will be completed in the oviduct (×1500). (*From Ferenczy and Richart (eds): The Female Reproductive System. Dynamics of Scan and Electron Microscopy. New York, Wiley, 1974.*)

1975). Although it is not certain that the first polar body always undergoes subsequent division, fertilized ova have been found that were accompanied by three polar bodies. During maturation, the diameter of the human ovum increases from 19 μm in the original oocyte to 135 μm in the fully mature ovum, a sevenfold increase in size.

Spermatogenesis

In the male embryo, as previously described in the female, the primordial germ cells enter the developing gonad during the fifth week but locate in the medulla of the fetal testis, rather than in the cortex, as do the germ cells in the ovary. There, the germ cells are incorporated into irregularly shaped primitive sex cords that are composed of cells that are derived from the surface epithelium.

At birth, the sex cords are solid and only later do lumens form, which become the seminiferous tubules. Two kinds of cells are found in the sex cords. One cell type is larger than the other, is located along the base-

ment membrane, and in these cells there is a pale-staining nucleus with one or more nucleoli; it is this cell type that probably represents the primordial germ cell. The other cell type is also found along the basement membrane, but is much smaller, and in these cells there are coarsely granulated nuclei; these cells cease to proliferate at birth and become sustentacular (Sertoli) cells.

The nuclear changes that ensue during spermatogenesis are analogous to those in oogenesis. Each primary spermatocyte enters the long prophase of the first meiotic division. Upon completion of the first reduction division, secondary spermatocytes are formed, in each of which there is the haploid number of chromosomes; unlike the products of the first meiotic division of the ovum, however, the secondary spermatocytes receive equal shares of cytoplasm from the parent cell. Almost immediately after formation, the secondary spermatocytes begin the second meiotic division, which results in the production of four spermatids. Theoretically, each primary spermatocyte, after two meiotic divisions, gives rise to four spermatids, which are analogous (chromosomally) to the mature ovum and the second polar body,

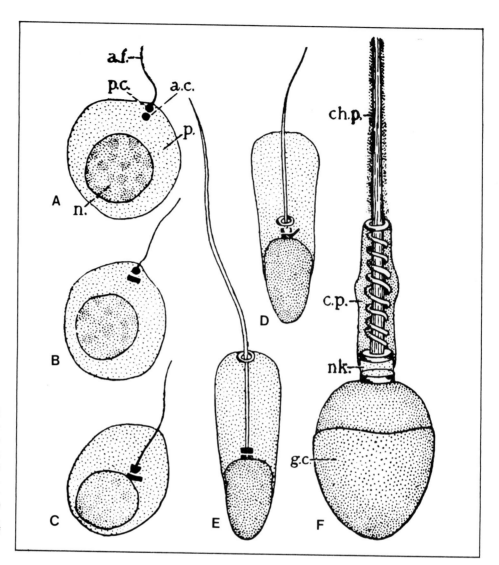

Figure 5-4A–F. The development of spermatozoa (Meves): a.c. = anterior centrosome; a.f. = axial filament; c.p. = connecting pieces; ch.p = chief piece; glc. = galea capitis; n. = nucleus; nk. = neck; p. = protoplasm; p.c. = posterior centrosome. (*From Greep (ed): Histology. McGraw Hill, New York, 1954.*) (*Courtesy of Blakiston.*)

but which develop, subsequently, into spermatozoa (Fig. 5-1).

Immediately after spermatids are formed, these cells undergo extensive changes in shape to become spermatozoa (Fig. 5-4). In the newly formed spermatid, there are a spherical nucleus, prominent Golgi, and many mitochondria. An initial change in the Golgi is the appearance of the dense *acrosomic granule*, which later forms a thin membrane over the surface of the nucleus, that is, the head cap. The centrioles migrate to the pole of the nucleus opposite the head cap and form the flagellum, while the nucleus becomes condensed and slightly flattened and elongated. At the same time, mitochondria move toward the flagellum to form a collar around the axial filament. Distally, the mitrochondrial collar is limited by an annular structure, and together with the centriole, the collar and ring form the middle portion of the spermatozoan. The cytoplasm and the Golgi material that are not incorporated into the spermatozoan are cast off. Though only slightly motile when first entering the

seminiferous tubules, the spermatozoa become fully motile in the epididymis (Figs. 5-4, 5-5).

TRANSPORT OF OVA AND SPERMATOZOA

Tubal Transport

Eddy and Pauerstein (1980) have presented an excellent review of the anatomy and physiology of the fallopian tube. In women, the ovaries normally lie free in the peritoneal cavity except for the supporting mesovarium and ovarian ligament. About the time of ovulation, however, the fimbriae of the oviduct, possibly as the consequence of appropriate hormonal and neural (doubtful) regulation, are believed to cover completely the ovary at the site of ovulation. Ovulation is not an explosive phenomenon; instead, as the stigma is digested by proteolytic enzymes, there is a gentle outpouring of the contents of the follicle, including the egg, which is surrounded by

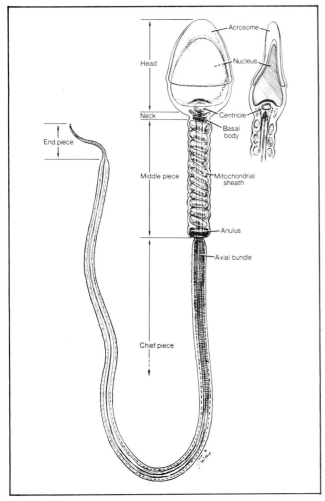

Figure 5-5. Ultramicroscopic structure of human spermatozoan.

or else, theoretically, the ovum may cross inside the uterus and migrate up to the opposite tube (*internal migration*). Presumptive clinical evidence of migration of the ovum includes a successful intrauterine pregnancy in women who have only one tube and only the contralateral ovary. It is likely that the entire subject of migration of the ovum in women has received more attention than it deserves. In consideration of known normal anatomic relationships, as observed at laparotomy, both tubes usually are freely mobile, and the fimbriated extremities lie posterior to the uterus and in rather close approximation. In view of the recognized motility of the fallopian tubes, it is reasonable to presume that the ovum may be taken up directly by the opposite tube, without recourse to complicated explanations that involve mechanisms of internal or external migration.

Transport of Spermatozoa

During human coitus, in each ejaculate, on average, there is a volume of 2 to 5 ml in which there are approximately 70 million sperm per milliliter that are deposited in the vagina. Between 80 and 90 percent of these more than 100 million spermatozoa are presumed to be normal forms, but perhaps fewer than 200 actually reach the site of fertilization, namely, the ampulla of the tube. For successful fertilization, Eddy and Pauerstein (1980) asked the important question as to why ". . . so many sperm are required in the ejaculate when so few arrive at the site of fertilization?" Only one spermatozoan must meet, in the upper portion of the fallopian tube, the single mature ovum that is released during each ovulatory cycle.

Sperm reach the site of fertilization in the ampulla of the oviduct shortly (often only 5 minutes) after ejaculation, a time that is much faster than can be explained by the flagellar action of spermatozoa. Eddy and Pauerstein are of the view that there are reservoirs (i.e., the ejaculate and the uterus may be considered as reservoirs for spermatozoa) whereas "the cervix, uterotubal junctions, and possibly the oviductal isthmus may be considered as barriers to the passage of sperm." An unbelievably sharp decrement occurs in the number of sperm between those deposited in the vagina and those that reach the ampulla of the fallopain tube (cf. Eddy and Pauerstein, 1980).

It still remains a biologic curiosity that spermatozoa can reach the ampulla of the fallopian tube with such rapidity from the time of insemination. Indeed, it has been reported that this transit time may be no more than 5 minutes, but, on average, a time of 4 to 6 hours seems more reasonable. The loss of sperm in the ejaculate, however, is remarkable. In one study, it was estimated that for every 14 million sperm deposited in the vagina, only one could be recovered from the fallopian tubes within 15 to 45 minutes of insemination. From these data, it is clear that there are mechanisms that are operative in the genital tract of women that provide for accelerated transport of sperm—at rates that are considerably greater than can be accounted for by sperm

the zona pellucida and the cumulus oophorus. The cumulus cells appear to be important for uptake and transport of the ovum by the oviduct. In the oviduct of the monkey, ciliary action is believed to be the prominent force in the movement of the ovum in the tube, whereas peristalsis appears to be so in the rabbit (Blandau, 1975). The relative contribution of each of these mechanisms in sperm and ovum transport in women is not known. Since, in mammals, fertilization usually occurs in the ampulla, whatever the roles of the tubal cilia and peristalsis may be, an adequate theory must be one whereby movement of ova and spermatozoa in opposite directions can be explained.

Migration of Fertilized Ovum

In most mammals, the fertilized ovum migrates through the oviduct and reaches the cavity of the uterus about 3 to 4 days after ovulation. In women, the ovum is believed to be able to wander across the pelvis and then to be taken up by the opposite tube (*external migration*)

migration by flagellation. It is believed that movement of spermatozoa that is caused by flagellar action is necessary for maintenance of the sperm in suspension and in the facilitation of transport; moreover, such movement is believed to be necessary for transit of the spermatozoan through the cumulus oophorus and zona pellucida of the ovum.

Blandau (1975) believes that the spermatozoa must make their own way through the mucus that fills the cervical canal. The first spermatozoa appear to burrow through the mucus by chemical as well as mechanical means; the leaders among the spermatozoa very likely depolymerize the cervical mucus by releasing proteases that are contained in the acrosome, and thereby render the mucus more easily penetrable by the spermatozoa that follow and successfully enter the uterine cavity. The uterine cavity in vivo may well be nearly obliterated except for canals that extend from the internal os of the cervix to the uterotubal junctions; as the consequences of such canals, sperm are directed to the oviduct.

FERTILIZATION

As soon as the sperm penetrates the zona pellucida and comes in contact with the vitelline membrane, a second polar body is formed and the female pronucleus, as well as the male pronucleus, are evident in the ovum. Ordinarily, the penetration of the zona pellucida and vitelline membrane by one sperm acts in a manner to inhibit entry by other sperm; but, at times, more than one sperm does enter. The mechanism by which the sperm penetrates the zona pellucida is not defined clearly, but probably involves enzymatic action. Materials other than genetic material that are contained in the sperm degenerate within the ovum.

Zona Pellucida

Dickman and Noyes (1961) found that the zona pellucida in the rat is shed from the blastocyst during the fifth day after fertilization. The shedding, moreover, appears unrelated to a specific uterine environment, but rather is an intrinsic manifestation of growth and maturation of the blastocyst. The zona clearly is not necessary for implantation; on the contrary, its removal is a prerequisite for implantation, at least in the laboratory rodents studied thus far.

Presently, and even more so heretofore, the cause of involuntary infertility in as many as 20 to 35 percent of couples is unknown. By conventional testing, both partners appeared to be normal and, yet, pregnancy was not achieved. These findings were obviously suggestive that a variety of undefined and, at that time, undetectable factors were important in the processes that lead to gametogenesis, gamete maturation, fertilization, transport of fertilized ova, implantation, and embryogenesis. For a variety of reasons, it was suspected that there was a "male" factor involved in a large proportion of in-

stances of unexplained infertility. At that time, in the evaluation of male fertility, we were restricted to evaluation by history and by physical examination and by evaluation of seminal ejaculates for volume, sperm concentration, morphology, and motility. Even then, it was reasonable to assume that these data gave us little insight into sperm survival, cervical penetration, migration, or capacity for oocyte penetration and fertilization. And this is to say nothing of the potential—and perhaps the likelihood—that antibodies of either male or female origin can act to inhibit—in one manner or another—the capacity of sperm to reach and thence to fertilize a receptive ovum.

Possibly, the most obvious cause of unexplained infertility is that based upon an immunologic disorder. The difficulty, to date, with this proposition is the development of immunologic tests with sufficient specificity to permit conclusions to be drawn from the results obtained. Many reports appear to be anecdotal and others are replete with what appear to be the findings of false positives, that is, antisperm antibodies in biologic fluid(s) of women known to be fertile or even to be pregnant. As stated by Warren R. Jones (1980), "human semen is an antigenic nightmare."

A novel test was introduced in 1976 by Yanagimachi and colleagues to assess the capacity of human spermatozoa to fertilize. This test is dependent upon the capacity of the sperm of one species, man, to penetrate the ovum of another species, provided that the acellular, sperm-resistant (possibly specific antigen-containing) zona pellucida of such ova are removed. These investigators demonstrated that capacitated human spermatozoa could penetrate zona-free hamster eggs. Thereafter, there was decondensation of the sperm chromatin and pronucleus formation—events analogous to those of fertilization. In some clinics, this test is proving to be correlated reasonably well with male fertility. It also is of particular potential importance that there appear to be zona pellucida-specific antigens. Antizonal antibodies appear to react with eggs in such a manner that binding receptors for sperm are masked; thus, fertilization cannot take place. Indeed, there are reports of infertility due to the presence of circulating antizonal antibodies, but the status of this entity is as yet not clear. Nonetheless, the possibility is real of an antizonal antibody to produce passive and even temporary infertility in this day of monoclonal antibody technology.

Aging of Gametes

The increased incidence of the trisomy 21 variety of Down syndrome late in reproductive life is well established. It may be related to an increased tendency toward nondysjunction in ova that have remained dormant in the ovary for 40 years or more. Although the incidence of this syndrome in the population as a whole is only 3 per 2000 live births, the incidence rises to about 1 in 100 in women by age 40.

Tesh and Glover (1969) noted that gametes of aging males also exerted deleterious effects on the embryo and fetus. They reported that aging of rabbit sperm in the male reproductive tract led to a decrease in the capacity for fertilization. Moreover, if eggs were fertilized by such sperm, an increase in embryonic anomalies resulted. Friedman (1981) found that the risk of new autosomal dominant mutations in children is increased many times among the offspring of fathers who are 40 years of age or older. Indeed, he found that such risk was similar to that of Down syndrome in infants of 35- to 40-year-old mothers.

Vickers (1969) observed that delayed fertilization also led to an increase in chromosomal anomalies of the embryo. In mice, in which fertilization was delayed (7 to 13 hours), triploidy, for example, was increased ninefold. Vickers postulated that the chromosomal aberrations may have resulted from errors in meiosis, fertilization, or cleavage.

IN VITRO FERTILIZATION

In most infertility clinics—and in particular in those that are charged with primary care—the most perplexing problem may be that related to infertility as a consequence of tubal occlusion from infectious, surgical, or other cause. In many such cases, surgical repair of the fallopian tube to effect patency, even by use of the most modern microsurgical techniques, was not possible or in the immediate future a reasonable alternative. This seemed a tragic conclusion in couples where regular, ovulatory cycles were occurring in the woman and sperm normal in quality and quantity were present in the man. The only viable therapeutic alternative, of many tested, was that of in vitro fertilization, that is, the removal of a mature ovum from the ovary of a woman whose fallopian tubes were occluded, followed by in vitro fertilization with sperm, and reimplantation of the fertilized egg into the uterine cavity. Indeed, more than 1200 embryos fertilized in vitro have been placed in utero with a recent success rate in terms of pregnancy and delivery of a healthy infant of 20 percent (Edwards and Steptoe 1983).

The grave problems of in vitro fertilization that were envisioned by some are not yet apparent. There are technical advances to be made: the means of optimizing the likelihood of retrieval of mature ova; endocrine and sonographic monitoring of follicular development; evaluation of oocyte maturation by measurement of follicular fluid hormones; evaluation of success and optimization of in vitro fertilization; and idealization of choice of embryo(s) for reimplantation and, means of reimplantation. Barring unforeseen long-range problems that we cannot ignore, those of us who originally were counted among the skeptics must now salute the pioneers of this field for their conviction, courage, perseverance, and humanitarianism.

DEVELOPMENT OF FERTILIZED OVUM

Cleavage of the Ovum

The mature ovum, after fertilization, becomes a zygote that then undergoes segmentation, or cleavage, into blastomeres. With the accumulation of fluid between the blastomeres, the blastocyst is formed. Although it is not strictly correct to refer to segmenting zygotes as ova, the earliest stages of human development have traditionally been so designated. The blastocyst, or fertilized "ovum," then implants in the endometrium, and thence the fetal membranes and germ layers of the embryo are formed. Although the distinction between embryo and fetus is essentially arbitrary, it is customary to refer to the human conceptus, from fertilization through the first 8 weeks of development, as an *embryo,* and from 8 weeks after ovulation until term, as a *fetus.* During the embryonic period, the major organ systems are formed, and, during fetal life, histogenesis, or differentiation and maturation of the tissues, proceeds.

The first typical mitotic division of the segmentation nucleus of the zygote results in the formation of two blastomeres. In a photomicrograph of a living segmenting ovum of the monkey (Fig. 5-6), the suspension of blastomeres and polar bodies in the perivitelline fluid that is surrounded by the zona pellucida is shown. In the fertilized human ovum (Fig. 5-7), there are similar changes.

Within the fallopian tube, the fertilized ovum undergoes slow cleavage for 3 days: indeed, fertilized human ova that are recovered from the uterine cavity may be comprised of only 12 blastomeres. As the blastomeres continue to divide, a solid mulberrylike ball of cells, the *morula,* is produced. The gradual accumulation of fluid within the morula results in formation of the blastocyst, at one pole of which there is a compact mass of cells, the *inner cell mass,* which is destined to produce the embryo (Fig. 5-8) and the outer layer of cells, the *trophoblast,* which provides nourishment to the ovum.

The Early Human Ovum

In the presumably normal two-celled egg that was flushed from the oviduct (Fig. 5-7A), Hertig and co-workers (1954) found that the blastomeres and a polar body that was free in the perivitelline fluid were surrounded by a thick zona pellucida (cf., see fertilized ovum of monkey, Fig. 5-6A). They provisionally considered as abnormal the four cleavage stages with 5, 8, 9, and 11 to 12 blastomeres that they found in the uterine cavity, but they recovered morphologically normal stages that were comprised of 12 and 58 cells. The normal, fertilized ovum, still surrounded by zona pellucida, measured 0.150 mm in the fresh state. In the 58-cell morula (Fig. 5-7B), the outer cells can be distinguished (presumably, those that are destined to produce the trophoblast; and from the inner cells, those that form the embryo). The

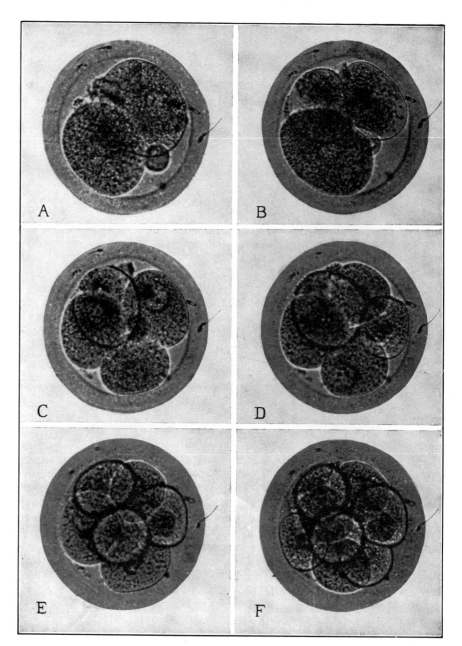

Figure 5-6. Photomicrographs (×300) of living monkey fertilized ovum showing its cleavage divisions. The fertilized ovum was washed out of the tube and cultivated in plasma; its growth changes were recorded cinematographically. The illustations are enlargements from single frames of the film. **A.** Two-cell stage, 29 hours and 30 minutes after ovulation. **B.** Three-cell stage, 36 hours and 4 minutes after ovulation. **C.** Four-cell stage, 37 hours and 35 minutes after ovulation. **D.** Five-cell stage, 48 hours and 39 minutes after ovulation. **E.** Six-cell stage, 49 hours exactly after ovulation. **F.** Eight-cell stage, 48 hours and 48 minutes after ovulation. These cleavages normally occur as the ovum passes down the fallopian tube. Note the spermatozoan in the zona pellucida. (*After Lewis and Hartman: Contrib Embryol 24:187, 1933.*)

next stage that was obtained was a 107-cell blastocyst (blastodermic vesicle) that was no larger than the earlier cleavage stages, despite the accumulated fluid (Fig. 5-7C). It measured 0.153 × 0.155 mm in diameter before fixation and after the disappearance of the zona pellucida. The eight formative (embryo-producing) cells were surrounded by 99 trophoblastic cells. The fertilized "ovum," now a blastocyst, was ready for implantation.

Implantation

Before implantation, the zona pellucida disappears and the blastocyst adheres to the endometrial surface. After erosion of the epithelium, the blastocyst sinks into the endometrium. From the findings of Hertig and Rock (1945), it is apparent that, in women, the pole of the blastocyst at which the inner cell mass is located enters first.

One of the earliest implantation sites discovered by Hertig and Rock (1944, 1945) is shown in Figure 5-9. It measured only 0.36 × 0.31 mm; its discovery was truly a remarkable achievement. The blastocyst that is shown in Figure 5-9 was believed to be in the process of entering the endometrium, with its thin, outer wall still within the uterine cavity. An implanting ovum at a similar stage of development, 7½ days after fertilization, is shown in Figure 5-10. It appears to have been flattened in the process of penetrating the uterine epithelium; the en-

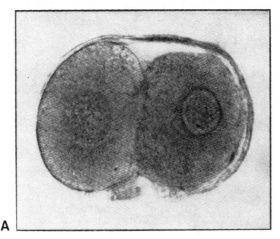

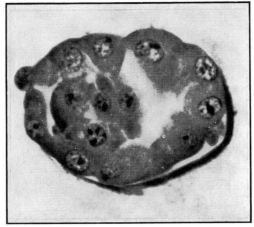

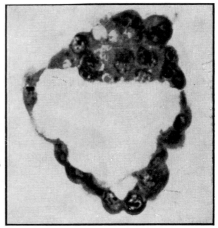

Figure 5-7. Human preimplantation stages. **A.** Two-celled stage. Intact fertilized ovum surrounded by zona pellucida, photographed after fixation. Washed from fallopian tube about 1½ days after conception. Nuclei shimmer through granular cytoplasm. Polar body in perivitelline space (*Carnegie Collection No. 8698.* (×500). **B.** 58-celled blastula with intact zona pellucida found in uterine cavity 3 to 4 days after conception. Thin section showing outer (probably trophoblastic) and inner (embryo-forming) cells and beginning segmentation cavity (*Carnegie Collection No. 8794* (×600). **C.** 107-celled blastocyst found free in uterine cavity about 5 days after conception. A shell of trophoblastic cells enveloping fluid-filled blastocele and inner mass consisting of embryo-forming cells (*Carnegie Collection No. 8663* (×600). (*From Hertig and associates: Contrib Embryol 35:199, 1954.*)

largement and multiplication of the trophoblastic cells in contact with the endometrium alone are responsible for the increase in size of the implanted blastocyst as compared with the free one. The hole in the uterine epithelium that is created by the fertilized ovum 9½ days after fertilization (Fig. 5-11) as it implants is indicative of the size of the zygote at the time of erosion of the surface. The defect is bounded by a zone of maternal epithelium that became shriveled as the trophoblast spread out beneath it. When correction was made for the additional artifactual shrinkage, which results from preparation of the histologic sections, the diameter of the fertilized ovum at the moment of implantation was estimated to be 0.23 mm. According

to Hertig and Rock (1945), implantation of the smallest human zygote takes place 6 days after fertilization.

Mechanism of Implantation

Although little is known of the fundamental nature of implantation in women, some information (based primarily on findings of studies of lower species) is available. As the blastocyst contacts the endometrium, syncytiotrophoblast is differentiated from cytotrophoblast. Development of syncytiotrophoblast undoubtedly is a major factor in the successful invasion of the endometrium. In women, a full decidual response is not elicited

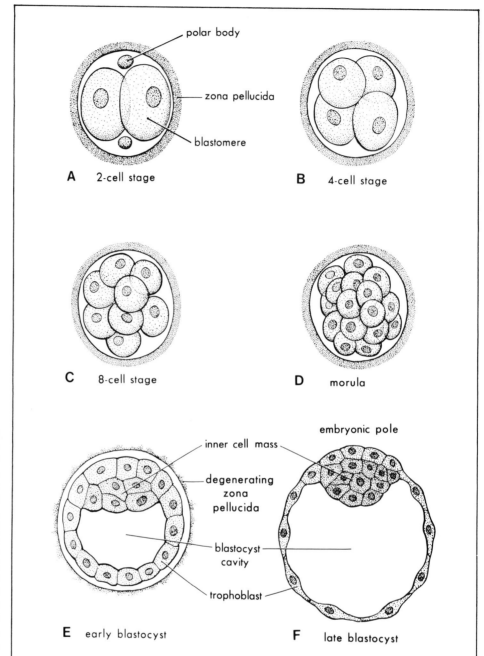

Figure 5-8. Drawings illustrating cleavage of the zygote and formation of the blastocyst. **A** to **D** show various stages of cleavage. The period of the morula begins at the 12- to 16-cell stage and ends when the blastocyst forms, which occurs when there are 50 to 60 blastomeres present. **E** and **F** are sections of blastocysts. The zona pellucida has disappeared by the late blastocyst stage (5 days). The polar bodies shown in **A** are small, nonfunctional cells that soon degenerate. (*From Moore: The Developing Human, 3rd ed. Philadelphia, Saunders, 1982.*)

until the trophoblast has eroded the superficial uterine epithelium.

Whereas, in women, the free blastocystic period is 4 to 6 days, in some species, there is a "developmental diapause," or delayed implantation, during which time the blastocysts may remain unattached for much longer intervals (6 months or more in the pine marten).

Free blastocysts that were recovered from the uterus of the cow and the sheep and kept frozen in liquid nitrogen for up to 3 weeks have been implanted successfully in recipient animals to produce normal offspring. Human ova have been fertilized in vitro and many suc-

cessful pregnancies have been reported since the original one by Steptoe and Edwards (1978).

Development of Fertilized Ovum After Implantation

At 7½ days of development, the stage shown in Figure 5-10, the wall of the blastocyst that faces the uterine lumen consists of a single layer of flattened cells, whereas the thicker opposite wall is comprised of two zones—the trophoblast and the embryo-forming inner cell mass. Signs of injury are apparent in maternal tis-

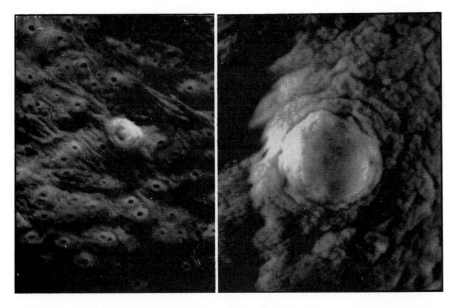

Figure 5-9. Low- and high-power photographs of surface view of an early human implantation obtained on day 22 of cycle, less than 8 days after conception. Site was slightly elevated and measured 0.36 by 0.31 mm. Mouths of uterine glands appear as dark spots surrounded by halos. (*Carnegie Collection No. 8225.*) (*From Hertig and Rock: Am J Obstet Gynecol 47:149, 1944.*)

sues that are in contact with trophoblast; the decidua, immediately adjacent, appears to be condensed, perhaps as a result of withdrawal of water by the invading trophoblast. Within the trophoblast, two subdivisions are distinguishable, the *cytotrophoblast,* which consists of individual cells with relatively pale-staining cytoplasm, and the *syncytiotrophoblast,* in which dark-staining nuclei are distributed irregularly within a common basophilic cytoplasm. In the trophoblast, mitotic figures are confined to the cellular elements. As early as 7½ days after fertilization, the inner cell mass, now called the *embryonic disc,* is already differentiated into a thick plate of primitive ectoderm and an underlying layer of endoderm. Between the embryonic disc and the trophoblast appear some small cells that soon enclose a space that will become the amnionic cavity.

To illustrate the next stage of development, a thin section of the 9½-day fertilized ovum (Fig. 5-11) is

shown; the increase in size is principally the result of development of the syncytium, which comprises a complex network of protoplasmic strands that enclose irregular fluid-filled spaces, the *lacunae,* that later become confluent. The embryonic disc now consists of a "dorsal" ectoderm that is composed of tall columnar cells and a "ventral" endoderm, which is formed of somewhat irregular cells. The remainder of the blastocyst is occupied by a proteinaceous coagulum, which is limited externally by a layer of flattened cells (the *exocoelomic* or *Heuser membrane*), the origin of which is uncertain. The amnionic cavity dorsal to the embryonic disc is now well-defined. With regard to the amnion, it seems reasonable that at least the epithelium is delaminated from the trophoblast. There is no convincing evidence that the inner-cell mass produces any of the extraembryonic mesoderm.

As the embryo enlarges, more maternal tissue is de-

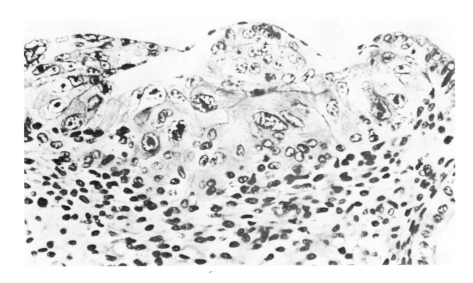

Figure 5-10. An implanting human blastocyst 7½ days after fertilization. (*From Potter and Craig: Pathology of the Fetus and the Infant. Chicago, Year Book, 1975.*)

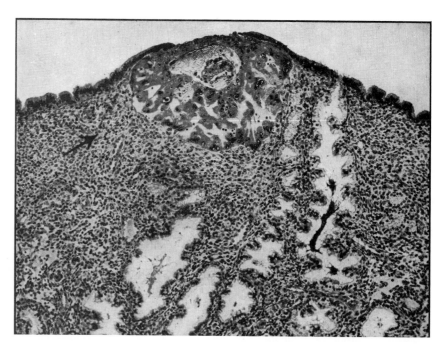

Figure 5-11. A thin section of fertilized ovum obtained on 25th day of cycle, 9½ days or less after fertilization. Area still exposed to uterine lumen as in Figure 5-14. Syncytiotrophoblast, a complex network fills enlarged implantation site. Within cytotrophoblastic shell, two-layered embryo and amnion-forming cells. Arrow is pointed to zone of enlarged stromal cells. (*Carnegie Collection No. 8004.*) Photomicrograph ×100. (*From Hertig and Rock: Contrib Embryol 31:65, 1945.*)

stroyed and the walls of the capillaries thereof are eroded; the result is that maternal blood enters the lacunae. With deeper burrowing of the blastocyst into the decidua, the trophoblastic strands branch to form the solid primitive villi that traverse the lucunae. Originally located over the entire surface of the fertilized ovum, the villi disappear later except over the most deeply implanted portion, that is, the site destined to be that of the placenta. The mesenchyme first appears as isolated cells within the cavity of the fertilized ovum. When the cavity is lined completely with mesoderm, it is termed the *chorionic vesicle,* and its membrane, now called the *chorion,* is composed of trophoblasts and mesenchyme.

In the 12-day embryo, as shown in Figure 5-12, the diameter is almost 1 mm. The mesenchymal cells within the cavity are most numerous about the embryo, where they eventually condense to form the *body stalk* that serves to join the embryo to the nutrient chorion and, later, develop into the umbilical cord. Thereafter, the site of entry of the blastocyst into the endometrium is covered by regenerated epithelium. The defect per se is plugged by fibrin and cellular debris. The syncytiotrophoblast of the chorionic shell is permeated by a system of intercommunicating channels or trophoblastic lucunae that contain maternal blood. At the same time, in the surrounding endometrial stroma, there develops a decidual reaction that is characterized by enlargement of the connective tissue cells and storage therein of glycogen. The amnionic cavity is then lined by ectoderm, which apparently is contiguous with that of the embryonic disc. At this stage, the endoderm probably delaminates from the inferior surface of the embryonic disc and soon spreads peripherally beyond the disc to line the blastocoele; this process results in the formation of the yolk sac. The remainder of the blastocyst is filled with primary mesoderm, which consists of sparse mesenchymal cells in a loose matrix. It is believed that the mesoderm arises from the trophoblast, but its precise mode of origin in man remains to be elucidated.

The Germ Layers

In Figures 5-13 and 5-14, the amnion and yolk sacs with both epithelial and mesenchymal components are illustrated. The body stalk, from which the caudal end of the embryo arises, also can be recognized at this stage. Cellular proliferation in the embryonic disc marks the beginning of a thickening in the midline that clearly is indicative of the embryonic axis and is called the *primitive streak.* Cells spread out laterally from the primitive streak between ectoderm and endoderm to form the mesoderm. These three germ layers give rise to the various organs of the developing embryo. From the *ectoderm* are derived the entire nervous system, central and peripheral, and the epidermis, with such derivatives as the crystalline lens and the hair. The *endoderm* develops into the lining of the gastrointestinal tract, from pharynx to rectum, and such derivative organs as the liver, pancreas, and thyroid. The dermis, the skeleton, the connective tissues, the vascular and urogenital systems, and most skeletal and smooth muscle arise from the *mesoderm.* The cavity that later divides the somatic and visceral sheets of intraembryonic mesoderm is the *coelom.*

Formation of the Somites

During the third week after fertilization (fifth week of gestation), the primitive streak becomes a prominent structure and the cephalic and caudal ends of the embryo become distinguishable. As cells proliferate rapidly

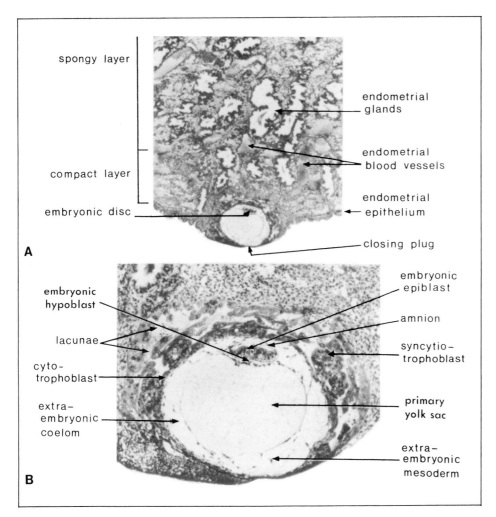

Figure 5-12. A. Section through the implantation site of a human embryo 12 days after fertilization. The embryo is embedded in the compact layer of endometrium (×30). B. Higher magnification of the conceptus and surrounding endometrium (×100). (*From Hertig and Rock: Contrib Embryol 29:127, 1941. Courtesy of Carnegie Institution of Washington, as modified by Moore: The Developing Human, 2nd ed. Philadelphia, Saunders, 1977.*)

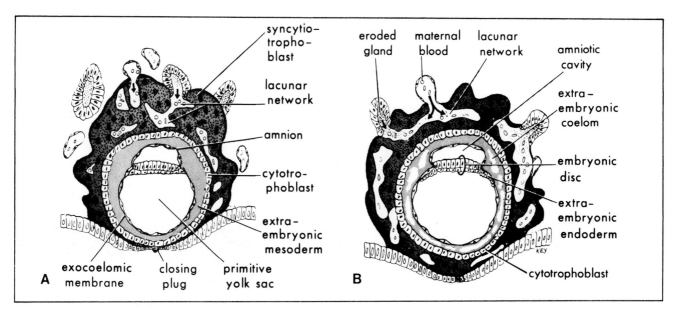

Figure 5-13. Drawings of sections through implanted blastocysts. A. 10 days; B. 12 days after fertilization. This stage of development is characterized by the intercommunication of the lacunae filled with maternal blood. Note in B that large cavities have appeared in the extraembryonic mesoderm, forming the beginning of the extraembryonic coelom. Also, note that extraembryonic endodermal cells have begun to form on the inside of the primary yolk sac. (*From Moore: The Developing Human, 2nd ed. Philadelphia, Saunders, 1977.*)

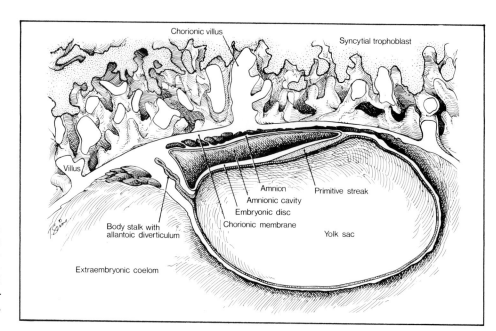

Figure 5-14. Median view of a drawing of a wax reconstruction of Mateer fertilized ovum, showing the amnionic cavity and its relations to chorionic membrane and yolk sac (×50). (*After Streeter: Contrib Embryol 9:389, 1920.*)

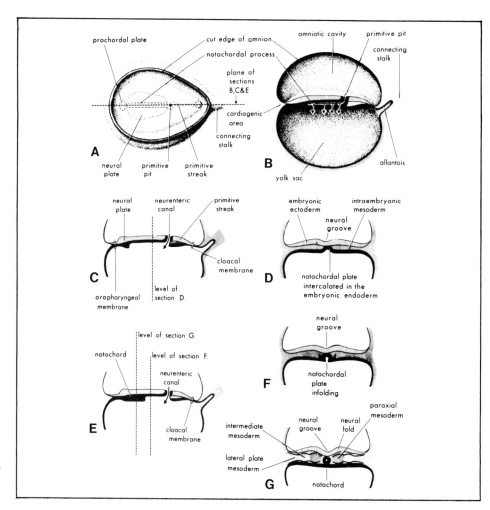

Figure 5-15. Drawings illustrating final stages of notochord development. **A.** Dorsal view of the embryonic disc at about 18 days, exposed by removing the amnion. **B.** Three-dimensional sagittal section of the embryo. **C.** and **E.** Sagittal sections of embryos of about 18 to 19 days. **D., F.,** and **G.** Transverse sections of the embryonic disc. (*From Moore: The Developing Human, 3rd ed. Philadelphia, Saunders, 1982.*)

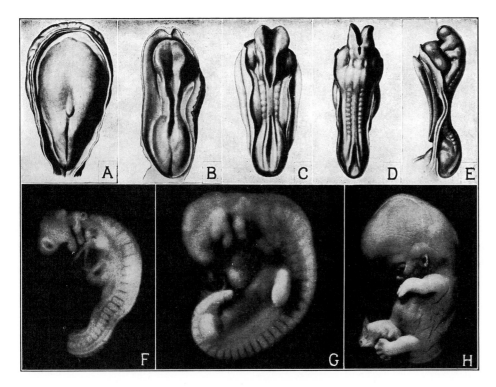

Figure 5-16. Human embryogenesis. (*Carnegie Collection*). **A.** Heuser, ×30, 19 days. **B.** Ingalls, ×28. **C.** Payne, ×23. **D.** Corner, ×23. **E.** Atwell, ×15.5, 21 to 22 days. **F.** ×12, fourth week. **G.** ×8.5, fifth week. **H.** ×2.5, eighth week. (*From Streeter: Sci Monthly 32:495, 1931.*)

and spread laterally from the primitive streak, a midline *primitive groove* develops. Simultaneously, the yolk sac enlarges, and, hence, the embryonic disc is spread out upon it. In Figure 5-14, there is shown a well-defined body stalk into which a narrow endodermal diverticulum, the allantois, has extended. In many mammals, the allantois develops into a large sac that vascularizes the chorion. A forward extension of the primitive streak, the *notochord* (Fig. 5-15), constitutes the primordial supporting structure of vertebrates and remains as a continuous column of cells throughout embryonic life. Remnants of the notochord persist in the adult as the nucleus pulposus of the intervertebral discs.

Since differentiation of structures proceeds from cephalic to caudal ends in a sequence characteristic of all vertebrate embryos, most of the substance of the early embryo will enter into formation of the head; the subsequent development of the primitive streak provides material for the rest of the body. Soon, there develops a *neural groove* as neural folds arise on either side. The cavity of the future neural tube is connected with the future lumen of the gut by the *neurenteric canal*. As the neural folds develop, the underlying lateral mesoderm is divided into discrete blocks—the *somites* that give rise to the skeletal and connective tissues, the muscles, and the dermis. The first three or four somites enter into formation of the occipital region of the head. The primordium of the heart already has appeared beneath the pharynx and is separated from the yolk sac by a fold that also lifts the cephalic end of the embryo above the level of the yolk sac. In Figure 5-16A–E, the elevation of the neural folds is shown, as is the closure of these folds to form a tube, which is wider from the outset in the re-

gion of the fourth pair of somites. Although the head remains relatively enormous during the embryonic period, the rest of the body takes form after the fourth week, and the head becomes smaller in proportion. By the seventh week after fertilization, the neck can be recognized, the tail filament has disappeared, and the embryo can be identified as human. From the eighth week after fertilization, changes in the shape of the human fetus are less striking. Some of the principal features are outlined in Chapter 8.

REFERENCES

Baker TG: A quantitative and cytological study of germ cells in human ovaries. Proc R Soc (Biol) 158:417, 1963

Beer AE, Neaves WB: Antigenic status of semen from the viewpoints of the female and the male. Fertil Steril 29:3, 1978

Blandau R: Personal communication, 1975

Blandau RJ, White BJ, Rumery RE: Observations on the movements of the living primordial germ cells in the mouse. Fertil Steril 14:482, 1963

Brewer JI: A normal human ovum in a stage preceding the primitive streak. Am J Anat 61:429, 1938

Chang MC: The maturation of rabbit oocytes in culture and their maturation, activation, fertilization, and subsequent development in the fallopian tubes. J Exp Zool 128:378, 1955

Channing CP, Pomerantz SH: Studies on an oocyte maturation inhibitor partially purified from porcine and human follicular fluids. In Franchimont P, Channing CP (eds): Intragonadal Regulation of Reproduction. New York, Academic, 1981, pp 81–96

Channing CP, Anderson LD, Hoover DJ, Kolena J, Osteen KG, Pomerantz SH, Tanabe K: The role of nonsteroidal regulators in control of oocyte and follicular maturation. Rec Prog Horm Res 38:331, 1982

Dickman Z, Noyes RW: Zona pellucida at the time of implantation. Fertil Steril 12:310, 1961

Eddy CA, Pauerstein CJ: Anatomy and physiology of the fallopian tube. Clin Obstet Gynecol 23:1177, 1980

Edwards RG, Steptoe PC: Current status of in-vitro fertilisation and implantation of human embryos. Lancet 2:1265, 1983

Friedman JM: Genetic disease in the offspring of older fathers. Obstet Gynecol 57:745, 1981

Hertig AT, Rock J: On the development of the early human ovum with special reference to the trophoblast of the previllous stage: A description of 7 normal and 5 pathologic human ova. Am J Obstet Gynecol 47:149, 1944

Hertig AT, Rock J: Two human ova in the previllous stage, having a developmental age of about 7 and 9 days respectively. Contrib Embryol 31:65, 1945

Hertig AT, Rock J, Adams EC, Mulligan WJ: On the preimplantation stages of the human ovum. Contrib Embryol 35:199, 1954

Heuser C, Hertig AT, Rock J: Two human embryos showing early stages of the definitive yolk sac. Contrib Embryol 31:85, 1945

Jones WR: Immunologic infertility—Fact or fiction? Fertil Steril 33:577, 1980

Pinkerton JHM, McKay DG, Adams EC, Hertig AT: Development of the human ovary: Study using histochemical technics. Obstet Gynecol 18:152, 1961

Steptoe PC, Edwards RG: Birth after the reimplantation of human embryo (letter). Lancet 2:366, 1978

Streeter GL: A human embryo (Mateer) of the presomite period. Contrib Embryol 9:389, 1920

Tesh JM, Glover TD: Aging of rabbit spermatozoa in the male tract and its effect on fertility. J Reprod Fertil 20:287, 1969

Vickers AD: Delayed fertilization and chromosomal anomalies in mouse embryos. J Reprod Fertil 20:69, 1969

Yanagimachi R, Yanagimachi H, Rogers BJ: The use of zona-free animal ova as a test-system for the assessment of the fertilizing capacity of human spermatozoa. Biol Reprod 15:471, 1976

6
The Placenta and Fetal Membranes

Benirschke (1981) states that . . . "The placenta is the most accurate record of the infant's prenatal experiences." Scientific interest in the placenta derives not only from its enormous diversity of form and function but also from the unique metabolic, endocrine, and immunologic properties of trophoblasts. Benirschke goes on to suggest that . . . "Physicians generally are uncomfortable with the task of examining the placenta. Yet, it is a task they should willingly undertake . . . submitting this organ to a reasonably knowledgeable look and touch can provide much insight into prenatal life; the results are often helpful in caring for the neonate; the findings provide a record pediatricians and obstetricians can use to plan the future care for mother and child; and, most important, much of what can be learned cannot be put into the maternal prenatal history if the information is discarded with the organ."

EVOLUTION OF KNOWLEDGE OF THE PLACENTA

The term *placenta* is believed to have been introduced by Realdus Columbus in 1559 when he used the Latin word for a *circular cake*. In 1937, Mossman defined *placenta* as that portion of the fetal membranes that was in apposition with or fused to the uterine mucosa. Historically, however, as pointed out by Boyd and Hamilton (1970), man's knowledge of the "afterbirth" can be traced far into human history. In the Old Testament, the placenta was considered as the External Soul and was sometimes described as being tied up in the so-called "Bundle of Life" that probably included the umbilical cord. It is believed that Aristotle (384-322 B.C.) was the first to use the word *chorion*. It was not, however, until the early 16th century, a time of renaissance of anatomy, that opinions concerning the function of the placenta were given. But even then, as pointed out by Boyd and Hamilton, Leonardo da Vinci (1452-1515) and Vesalius (1514-1564) illustrated the human placenta incorrectly. To his credit, however, Vesalius, in 1555, corrected his error in the second edition of his outstanding book (Boyd and Hamilton, 1970).

The concept of circulation of blood in the placenta apparently was introduced by Harvey in 1628, but it was John Mayow who more adequately described the nature of the fetal circulation. It can be appreciated that the endocrine function of the placenta was not recognized until much later because the function of hormones in general must necessarily have preceded such an elucidation. It was not until 1564 that Arantius, by way of careful placental dissections, discounted the concept that there was continuity between the maternal and fetal vascular systems. Harvey, in 1651, set forth clearly that there was a fetal arterial and venous circulation to the placenta, but it was Malpighi, in 1660, who set forth the concept of a capillary network as the anatomic basis for the regional circulation. By way of the findings of many celebrated anatomists, there was, by the end of the 17th century, a remarkably accurate concept of the structure and functional significance of the human placenta. The basic idea that there was a "placental barrier" clearly already was formulated in the late 17th or early 18th century.

William Hunter, in 1774, is credited with the first accurate description of the decidua and, even then, he distinguished a parietal lining (decidua vera) from a capsular one. Later, John Hunter (1821) described the decidua basalis. It was probably William and John Hunter, although each claimed credit separately, who accurately described what we now know as the intervillous spaces. It was not until the middle of the 19th century that the true nature of the chorionic villi were appreciated; by 1880, however, the basic knowledge of the nature of blood circulation in the intervillous space was established. In 1882, a notable contribution was made by Langhans, who demonstrated clearly that the villi were covered by two layers of cells. Indeed, it is the inner layer of cells, the cytotrophoblasts, that are referred to as the Langhans cells. It was in 1889 that the term "trophoblast" was introduced by Hubrecht to distinguish the portion of blastocyst that does not contribute to the cellular portion of the embryo. The superficial layer of the chorionic villi was eventually demonstrated to be syncytial in nature and is now generally referred to as the syncytiotrophoblast.

DEVELOPMENT OF THE HUMAN PLACENTA

Early Trophoblasts

In the discussion of the earliest stages of placentation in the human (see Chapter 5), the wall of the primitive blastodermic vesicle is described as consisting of a single layer of ectoderm. Hertig (1962) observed that as early as 72 hours after fertilization, the 58-cell blastula had differentiated into 5 embryo-producing cells and 53 cells that were destined to form trophoblasts. Although trophoblasts have not been identified before nidation of the ovum, both cellular and syncytial trophoblasts are apparent in the earliest implanted blastocyst of the monkey. Indeed, some evidence has been presented that suggests that the secretion of human chorionic gonadotropin (hCG) by the blastocyst may precede implantation. Soon after implantation, the trophoblasts proliferate rapidly and invade the surrounding decidua. In cytolytic and invasive behavior, in histologic appearance by way of the characteristic cytoplasmic vacuolization, and in ultrastructure, the early trophoblasts resemble choriocarcinoma (see Chapter 23, p. 454). As invasion of the endometrium proceeds, maternal blood vessels are invaded and cytoplasmic vacuoles coalesce to form larger lacunae that soon are filled with maternal blood. As the lacunae join, a complicated labyrinth is formed that is partitioned by solid trophoblastic columns. The trophoblast-lined labyrinthine channels and the solid cellular columns form the intervillous space and primary villous stalks, respectively. Much of our knowledge of the formation of the intervillous space in both the human and the macaque is based on the findings of the classic studies of Wislocki and Streeter (1938).

Chorionic Villi

Villi may be easily distinguished in the human placenta on about the 12th day after fertilization. When the solid trophoblast is invaded by a mesenchymal cord, presumably derived from cytotrophoblast, secondary villi are formed. After angiogenesis occurs in situ from the mesenchymal cores, the villi that are formed are termed tertiary. Maternal venous sinuses are invaded early; but, until the 14th or 15th day after fertilization, maternal arterial blood does not enter the intervillous space. By about the 17th day, both fetal and maternal blood vessels are functional and a placental circulation is established. The fetal circulation is completed when the blood vessels of the embryo are connected with chorionic blood vessels, which are probably formed in situ from cytotrophoblast. In some villi, in which there is absence of an angiogenesis, there results a lack of circulation, and the villi may distend with fluid and form vesicles. A striking exaggeration of this process is present in the development of hydatidiform mole (see Chapter 23, p. 446).

Proliferation of cellular trophoblasts at the tips of the villi produces the cytotrophoblastic cell columns, which are not invaded by mesenchyme but are anchored to the decidua at the basal plate. Thus, the floor of the intervillous space consists of cytotrophoblasts from the cell columns, peripheral syncytium of the trophoblastic shell (trophectoderm), and decidua of the basal plate. The chorionic plate, which consists of the two trophoblasts externally and fibrous mesoderm internally, forms the roof of the intervillous space.

Between the 18th and 19th days of development, the blastocyst (including the chorionic shell) measures 6×2.5 mm in diameter. At this time, the embryo is in the primitive-streak stage and its maximal length is 0.6 to 0.7 mm. The trophoblastic shell is thick, with villi formed of cytotrophoblastic projections, a central core of chorionic mesoderm in which blood vessels are developing, and an external covering of syncytiotrophoblast, or syncytium. The blastocyst is buried in the decidua and is separated from the myometrium by the decidua basalis and from the uterine epithelium by the decidua capsularis. The embryo itself is trilaminar, and the endoderm is continuous with the lining of the yolk sac. An intermediate layer of intraembryonic mesoderm can be traced and is found to be contiguous with the extraembryonic mesoderm, which later forms part of the walls of the amnion and yolk sac and connects the embryonic structures to the chorionic mesoderm by the body stalk, or abdominal pedicle, the forerunner of the umbilical cord. At this stage, the secondary or definitive yolk sac is lined completely by endoderm. External to the yolk sac, the fluid-filled exocoelomic cavity is found, the early formation of which prevents approximation of the yolk sac and trophoblasts in the human and hence precludes formation of a choriovitelline placenta.

By about 3 weeks after fertilization, the relations of chorion to decidua are clearly evident in the human embryo. The chorionic membrane consists of an inner connective tissue layer and an outer epithelium from which rudimentary villi project. The connective tissue consists of spindly cells with protoplasmic processes within a loose intercellular matrix. The trophoblasts differentiate into cuboidal or nearly round cells with clear cytoplasm and light-staining vesicular nuclei (cytotrophoblasts or Langhans cells) and an outer syncytium that contains irregularly scattered, dark-staining nuclei within a coarsely granulated cytoplasm (syncytiotrophoblast).

In early pregnancy, the villi are distributed over the entire periphery of the chorionic membrane; grossly, an ovum dislodged from the endometrium at this stage of development appears shaggy (Fig. 6-1). The villi in contact with the decidua basalis proliferate to form the leafy chorion, or *chorion frondosum,* the fetal component of the placenta, whereas those in contact with the decidua capsularis cease to grow and undergo almost complete degeneration. The greater part of the chorion, thus denuded of villi, is designated as the smooth, or bald chorion, or the *chorion laeve.* It is formed, according to Hertig (1962), as the result of a combination of direct pressure and interference with its vascular supply. Generally, the chorion laeve is more nearly opaque than is

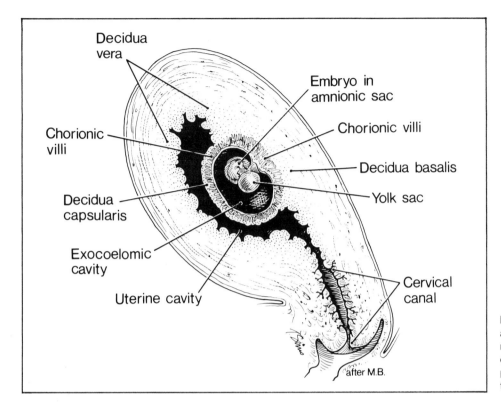

Decidua
vera

Embryo in
amnionic sac

Chorionic villi

Chorionic
villi

Decidua basalis

Decidua
capsularis

Yolk sac

Exocoelomic
cavity

Cervical
canal

Uterine cavity

after M.B.

Figure 6-5. Chorion frondosum and chorion laeve of early pregnancy. Three portions of the decidua (basalis, capsularis, and parietalis, or vera) are also illustrated.

dometrium for implantation and nutrition of the blastocyst. In pregnant women, the decidual reaction is not completed until several days after nidation. It commences first around maternal blood vessels, spreading in waves throughout the mucosa of the uterus. During development of the decidua, the endometrial stromal cells enlarge and form polygonal or round *decidual cells*. The nuclei become round and vesicular, and the cytoplasm becomes clear, slightly basophilic, and surrounded by a translucent membrane.

During pregnancy, the decidua thickens; eventually, a depth of 5 to 10 mm is attained. With a magnifying glass, furrows and numerous small openings, which represent the mouths of uterine glands, can be detected. The portion of the decidua directly beneath the site of implantation forms the *decidua basalis;* that portion that overlies the developing ovum and separates it from the rest of the uterine cavity is the *decidua capsularis* (Figs. 6-5, 6-6). The remainder of the uterus is lined by *decidua vera* or *decidua parietalis*.

During the early months of pregnancy, there is a space between the decidua capsularis and the decidua vera since the gestational sac does not fill the entire uterine cavity. By the fourth month, the enlarging sac fills the uterine cavity; and, with fusion of the decidua capsularis and parietalis, the uterine cavity is obliterated. The decidua capsularis is most prominent at about the second month of pregnancy; at this time, it consists of decidual cells that are covered by a single layer of flattened epithelial cells without traces of glands; internally, it is in contact with the chorion laeve.

The decidua vera and the decidua basalis each are composed of three layers: a surface, or compact zone (*zona compacta*); a middle portion, or spongy zone (*zona spongiosa*) in which there are glands and numerous small blood vessels; and, a basal zone (*zona basalis*). The zona compacta and the zona spongiosa together form the functional zone (*zona functionalis*). The basal zone remains after delivery and gives rise to new endometrium. As pregnancy advances, the glandular epithelium of the decidua vera changes from a cylindrical to a cuboidal or flattened form, and at times, it even resembles endothelium. After the fourth month of pregnancy, because of uterine distension, the decidua vera gradually thins from a maximal height of 1 cm in the first trimester to only 1 or 2 mm at term.

Histology

The compact layer of the decidua consists of large, closely packed, epithelioid, polygonal, lightly staining cells with round, vesicular nuclei (Fig. 6-7). Many stromal cells appear stellate, particularly when the decidua is edematous, with long protoplasmic processes that anastomose with those of adjacent cells. Numerous small round cells that contain very little cytoplasm are scattered among typical decidual cells, especially early in pregnancy. Formerly, these cells were considered to be lymphocytes, but are now regarded as precursors of new decidual elements. In the early months of pregnancy, ducts of uterine glands are found in the decidua compacta, but these become less obvious in late pregnancy.

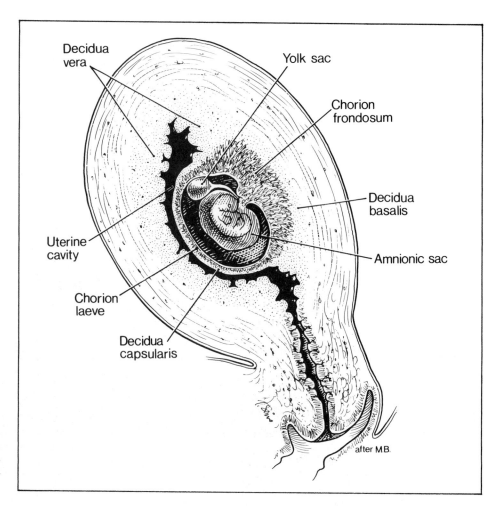

Figure 6-6. More advance stage of pregnancy, showing atrophic chorion laeve and chorion frondosum (chorionic villi) proliferating into decidua basalis.

The spongy layer of the decidua consists of large distended glands, which often are markedly hyperplastic but are separated by minimal stroma. At first, the glands are lined by typical cylindrical uterine epithelium, in the cells of which there is abundant secretory activity. Presumably, the glandular secretion contributes to the nourishment of the ovum during its histrotrophic phase, before the establishment of a placental circulation. The epithelium gradually becomes cuboidal or even flattened; later, it degenerates and is sloughed to a greater extent into the lumens of the glands. The interglandular stroma of the spongy zone undergoes little change during pregnancy.

From the basal zone of the decidua vera (not to be confused with decidua basalis) some of the endometrium regenerates during the puerperium (see Chapter 19, p. 367). In comparing the decidua vera at 4 months gestation with the early proliferative endometrium it is clear that, during decidual transformation of the endometrial stroma, there is marked hypertrophy but only slight hyperplasia.

The decidua basalis enters into the formation of the *basal plate* of the placenta and differs, histologically, from the decidua vera in two respects (Fig. 6-8). First, the spongy zone of the decidua basalis consists mainly of arteries and widely dilated veins; by term, the glands

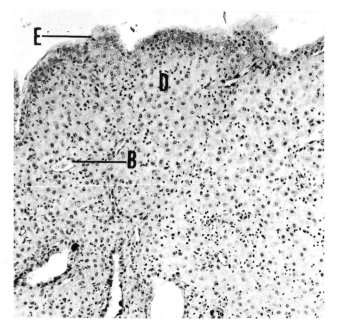

Figure 6-7. Photomicrograph of decidua vera (parietalis) in which epithelium (E), decidualized stromal cells (D), and blood vessels (B) are shown. (*Courtesy of Dr. Ralph M. Wynn.*)

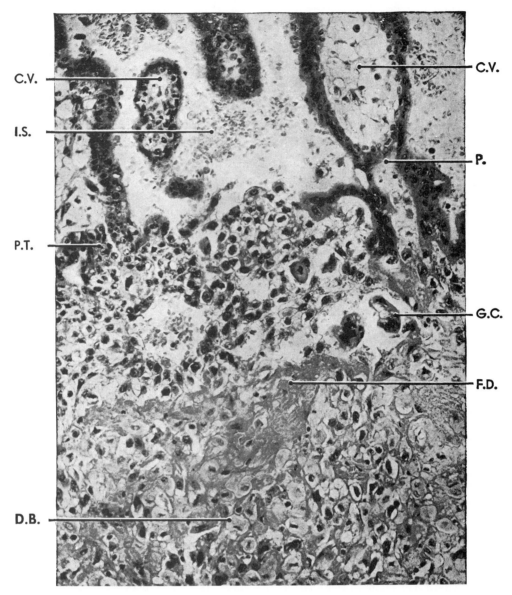

Figure 6-8. Section through junction of chorion and decidua basalis. Fourth month of gestation. C.V. = chorionic villi; D.B. = decidua basalis; F.D. = fibrinoid degeneration; G.C. = giant cell; I.S. = intervillous space containing maternal blood; P. = fastening villus; P.T. = proliferating trophoblast.

have virtually disappeared. Second, the decidua basalis is invaded extensively by trophoblastic giant cells that appear as early as the time of implantation. The number and depth of penetration of the giant cells vary greatly. Although generally confined to the decidua, these cells may penetrate the myometrium. In such circumstances, the number and invasiveness of such cells may be so extensive as to be suggestive of choriocarcinoma to the inexperienced observer.

Aging of the Decidua. Where invading trophoblasts meet the decidua, there is a zone of fibrinoid degeneration, namely, the *Nitabuch layer.* Whenever the decidua is defective, as in placenta accreta (see Chapter 34, p.

712), the Nitabuch layer usually is absent. There also is an inconstant deposition of fibrin, that is, the *Rohr stria,* at the bottom of the intervillous space and surrounding the fastening villi. McCombs and Craig (1964) found that decidual necrosis is a normal phenomenon in the first and probably the second trimesters. The presence of necrotic decidua (obtained through curettage after spontaneous abortion in the first trimester) should not, therefore, be interpreted necessarily as either a cause of, or an effect of, the abortion.

Histochemistry and Ultrastructure. In their elegant studies of placental histochemistry, Wislocki and Dempsey (1948, 1955) found that there is difficulty in distinguishing, with conventional stains, trophoblast from decidua in the basal plate. They observed differences, however, in the distribution of RNA and mitochondria and characteristic "capsules" that surround individual decidual cells. Wynn's electron microscopic findings (1967) of the human basal plate were demonstrative that this complex region of the placenta is composed of intimately related fetal and maternal cells. Well-preserved trophoblastic and endometrial cells are rarely in direct contact, however, but rather remain separated by degenerating tissue and fibrinoid. The giant cells in the region are derived from the syncytium or else arise from differentiation of cytotrophoblasts in situ. These syncytial masses may be hormonally active late in pregnancy. Moe (1969) confirmed these findings by showing that there is no intimate contact between apparently viable cytotrophoblasts and decidua. The immunologic implications of these cellular relations are discussed subsequently.

Bioactive Substances in Decidua. As described in Chapter 4, the concentration of prolactin in amniotic fluid is extraordinarily high compared with the levels of prolactin in fetal or maternal plasma. It now is reasonably clear that this prolactin arises in the decidua (Riddick and co-workers, 1983). There are a number of lines of evidence in favor of this conclusion: Prolactin concentrations in decidua are extraordinarily high; the synthesis of prolactin persists in decidual tissue maintained in organ culture; prolactin has been isolated from culture medium of dispersed decidual cells in monolayer culture; pituitary and decidual prolactin are immunologically indistinguishable, as are the biologic activities of pituitary and decidual prolactin; cyclohexamide treatment of decidual tissue in culture inhibits prolactin secretion; radiolabeled leucine is incorporated into prolactin by decidual tissue; and, bromocryptine treatment of pregnant women, while causing a striking reduction in the concentration of prolactin in fetal and maternal plasma, does not affect the concentration of prolactin in amniotic fluid. The factor(s) that regulates prolactin secretion in decidua is not clearly defined. For example, those factors known to affect, either negatively or positively, the rate of secretion of prolactin by the anterior pituitary, for example, dopamine and dopamine agonists and thyrotropin-releasing hormone, do not act either in vivo or in vitro to alter the rate of decidual prolactin secretion. It has been reported that arachidonic acid, but not prostaglandins E_2 and $F_{2\alpha}$, will attenuate the rate of decidual prolactin secretion. The physiologic role of prolactin produced in decidua is not known. Since all or most all of prolactin produced in decidua enters amnionic fluid, it has been speculated that there may be a role for this hormone in solute and water transport across the chorioamnion and, thus, in the maintenance of amnionic fluid volume homeostasis. Various other roles for decidual prolactin have been suggested but, presently, these must be considered as speculative. Excellent reviews of the synthesis of prolactin in decidua have been presented by Tyson and McCoshen (1983) and by Bigazzi (1983).

It now also seems likely that relaxin and 1,25-dihydroxyvitamin D_3 are produced in decidua of women.

Polyamine Synthesis and Metabolism in Decidua. Many investigators have established the probability that the accelerated production of the polyamines, viz., putrescine, spermidine, and spermine, is essential in processes that involve both hypertrophy and hyperplasia. Human pregnancy would seem to be a physiologic process in which extraordinary rates of polyamine production exist. Not only is there a rapidly growing fetus and placenta but there is extensive hypertrophy of the uterus and other tissues as well. Yet, as discussed in Chapter 9, increased levels of polyamines are demonstrable in the urine of pregnant women only briefly during pregnancy at about 12 to 14 weeks gestation. The enzyme that catalyzes the first and rate-limiting step in polyamine formation, ornithine decarboxylase, is present in and has been characterized in decidua of women (Garza and co-workers, 1983). Thus, it seems enigmatic and, in view of the growth of the fetus, disappointing that the levels of polyamines in maternal blood and urine are not reflective of the rate of growth of fetus, decidua, and uterine hypertrophy; if this were the case, it could be that the measurement of polyamines would be useful as an index of fetal growth. An explanation, however, may be offered for this apparent paradox. The activity of the enzyme diamine oxidase, formerly known as histaminase, rises dramatically in blood of pregnant women early in pregnancy at about the time that the levels of polyamines begin to decline, namely, at about 14 weeks gestation. The importance of this observation is that diamine oxidase is the enzyme that catalyzes the metabolism of putrescine. Thus, it may be that the rate of polyamine synthesis is strikingly accelerated and increases throughout pregnancy but the rate of catabolism of these compounds is greater than the rate of synthesis. This is easily envisioned when one considers that diamine oxidase activity in plasma of pregnant women may increase a thousandfold by 20 weeks gestation (Ahlmark, 1944). It is believed that this increased amount of diamine oxidase is principally of decidual origin (Swanberg, 1948). For this reason and others, many investigators have determined the activity of diamine oxidase in plasma of pregnant women in the hope of using such values as an index of fetal well-being. Although some correlates appear to exist, it now is generally accepted that such measurements are not of specific usefulness in alterations in clinical management plans (Resnik and Levine, 1969).

BIOLOGY OF THE TROPHOBLAST

Origin of the Syncytiotrophoblast

Of all placental components, the trophoblast is the most variable in structure, function, and development. Its invasiveness provides for attachment of the blastocyst to the uterus; its role in nutrition of the conceptus is reflected in its name; and, its function as an endocrine organ is required for the maintenance of pregnancy. Morphologically, the trophoblast may be cellular or syncytial and it may appear as uninuclear cells or multinuclear giant cells. The true syncytial character of the human syncytiotrophoblast (syncytium) has been confirmed by electron microscopy. The mechanism of growth of the syncytium, however, has remained a mystery in view of the discrepancy between the increase in the number of nuclei in the syncytiotrophoblast and only equivocal evidence of intrinsic nuclear replication. Mitotic figures are completely absent from the syncytium, being confined to the cytotrophoblasts. To distinguish amitotic nuclear proliferation within the syncytium from cytotrophoblastic origin of the syncytiotrophoblast, Galton (1962) employed microspectrophotometry, based on the Feulgen method for measuring DNA. He noted a diploid, unimodal distribution of DNA in the syncytium at a time of rapid placental growth, whereas a high proportion of cytotrophoblastic nuclei contained DNA in excess of the dipoid amount, reflecting synthesis of DNA in interphase nuclei preparatory to division (see Chapter 5). Galton concluded that the rapid accumulation of nuclei in the syncytiotrophoblast is explained by cellular proliferation within the cytotrophoblast, followed by a coalescence of daughter cells in the syncytium.

Further evidence was provided by Richart (1961), who found early incorporation of tritium-labeled thymidine in cytotrophoblasts but not in the syncytium. Midgley and co-workers (1963) subsequently extended the idea and found that although tritium-labeled thymidine appeared at first only in the nuclei of the cytotrophoblasts, the radiolabel could be detected 22 hours later in the syncytiotrophoblast; this finding is indicative that the syncytium is derived from cytotrophoblasts and is a mitotic end stage.

Ultrastructure

From the electron microscopic studies of Wislocki and Dempsey (1955), the basic data upon which the functional interpretation of placental fine structure is based were provided. The prominent microvilli of the syncytial surface, which corresponds to the so-called brush border observed by light microscopy, and associated pinocytotic vacuoles and vesicles are related to the absorptive and secretory functions of the placenta. In the Langhans cells, which persist to term although often compressed against the trophoblastic basal lamina, the ultrastructural simplicity is retained. In these cells, there are a few specialized organelles, abundant free ribosomes, but scant ergastoplasm. Desmosomes connect individual Langhans cells with one another and with the syncytium, from which complete plasma membranes are absent. Ultrastructurally, the syncytium is relatively complex and contains abundant endoplasmic reticulum, Golgi bodies, and mitochondria, as well as numerous secretory granules, lipid droplets, and highly convoluted plasma membranes; the syncytial nuclei are electron dense, and the abundant ribosomes and granular endo-

plasmic reticulum of the syncytial cytoplasm are correlated with a high content of the ribonucleoprotein and deep basophilia. As the syncytium matures, the fine structural changes are reflective of functional maturation. In early syncytiotrophoblast, there often is a microvesicular endoplasmic reticulum; later, at the height of active synthesis of proteins, flattened ergastoplasmic channels assume prominence; and, still later, associated with storage and transport of proteins, dilated cisternae of endoplasmic reticulum appear, the largest of which are visible with the light microscope. Secretory granules, at least those believed to contain glycoproteins, and osmiophilic lipid granules correspond to PAS-positive and sudanophilic droplets, respectively (Figs. 6-9–6-11).

As the placenta matures, the collagen-rich stromal connective tissue decreases, as do the numbers of fibroblasts and Hofbauer cells. The human placental membrane may be reduced, anatomically, to a thin covering of trophoblast, capillary endothelium, and trophoblastic and endothelial basement membranes that are separated

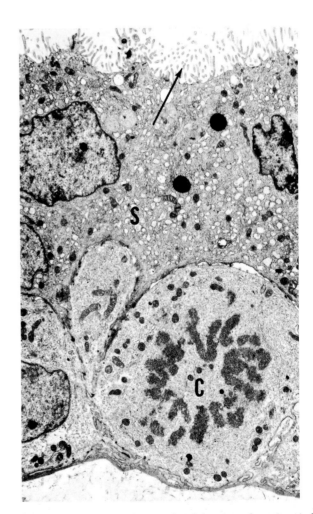

Figure 6-9. Electron micrograph of human placenta at 6 weeks gestation. Note prominent border of microvilli (*arrow*), syncytium (S), and mitotic figure in cytotrophoblast (C). (*Courtesy of Dr. Ralph M. Wynn.*)

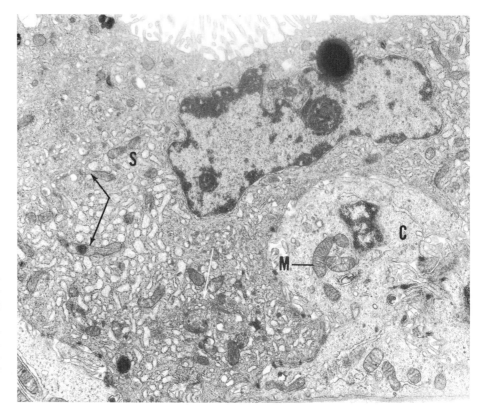

Figure 6-10. First-trimester human placenta, showing well-differentiated synytiotrophoblast (S) with numerous mitochondria (*black arrows*) and Golgi complexes (*white arrow*). Cytotrophoblast (C) has large mitochondria (M) but few other organelles. (*Courtesy of Dr. Ralph M. Wynn.*)

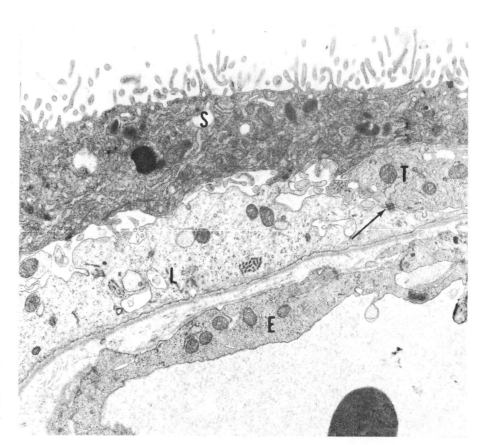

Figure 6-11. Term human placenta showing electron-dense syncytium (S), Langhans cells (L), transitional cytotrophoblast (T), and capillary endothelium (E). Arrow points to desmosome. (*Courtesy of Dr.Ralph M. Wynn.*)

106

by mere wisps of connective tissue. Although at term there is focal villous degeneration, morphologic evidence of activity in all layers persists. Since not only in the trophoblast but also in the endothelium and even the basal laminas there may be evidence of pinocytosis and other metabolic activity, it is not necessarily reasonable to equate the number of layers in the histologic "barrier" with functional efficiency of the placenta. Reduction of the number of layers may result in more rapid transplacental passage of substances to which the laws governing simple diffusion apply, but metabolites regulated by "carrier systems" are not proportionally affected. As for pinocytosis, a virtually continuous system of vesicles and vacuoles may be found that extend from the syncytial surface to the capillary endothelium. Boyd and co-workers (1968) described a direct connection of some of these vacuoles with the perinuclear space, which receives tubular communications with the endoplasmic reticulum. The term *barrier* as applied to placental physiology should therefore be replaced by the more accurate term, *placental membrane.* The number of layers, furthermore, is a poor index of the true approximation of the circulations, since in the six-layered epitheliochorial placenta of the pig, the indentation of both fetal and maternal epithelium by the respective capillaries results in a rather close vascular relation.

Localization of Placental Hormones. That the syncytium is a source of placental steroids has not been questioned seriously since Wislocki's histochemical localization in the syncytiotrophoblast of sudanophilic droplets, which he associated with estrogen and progesterone. Thiede and Choate (1963) localized chorionic gonadotropin by immunofluorescent techniques to the syncytium. A much smaller amount appeared in the amnion, but no specific fluorescence was detected in the cytotrophoblasts. In combined ultrastructural and immunofluorescent studies, Pierce and Midgley (1963), working with human choriocarcinoma tissue, likewise detected chorionic gonadotropin in the syncytium but not in the cytotrophoblast. Sciarra and co-workers (1963) noted that the protein hormone placental lactogen was in the syncytium but not in the Langhans cells. Wynn and Davies (1965) demonstrated, by electron microscopy, that in the syncytium were there subcellular organelles that are required for synthesis of proteins, particularly abundant endoplasmic reticulum and well-developed Golgi complexes, whereas the cytotrophoblast was, ultrastructurally, simple.

CIRCULATION IN THE MATURE PLACENTA

Since, functionally, the placenta represents a rather intimate presentation of the fetal capillary bed to maternal blood, the gross anatomy is concerned primarily with vascular relations. The human placenta at term is a discoid organ that measures approximately 15 to 20 cm in diameter and 2 to 3 cm in thickness. It weighs approximately 500 g and, generally, is located in the uterus anteriorly or posteriorly near the fundus. The fetal side is covered by transparent amnion beneath which the fetal vessels course, with arteries that pass over veins. Sections through the placenta in situ are presented in Figures 6-12, 6-13, 6-14; amnion, chorion, chorionic villi, and intervillous spaces, decidual plate, and myometrium are shown. The maternal surface of the placenta (Fig. 6-15) is divided into irregular lobes by furrows that are produced by septa, which consist of fibrous tissue in which there are sparse vessels confined mainly to the bases. The broad-based septa ordinarily do not reach the chorionic plate; thus, these provide only incomplete partitions.

Fetal Circulation

Fetal blood flows to the placenta through the two umbilical arteries in which deoxygenated, or "venous," blood is transported. The vessels branch repeatedly beneath the amnion and again within the dividing villi and form capillary networks in the terminal divisions (Figs. 6-16, 6-17). Blood with a significantly higher oxygen content returns to the fetus from the placenta through the single umbilical vein (see Chapter 8, p. 147).

Maternal Circulation

Only relatively recently has the mechanism of the maternal placental circulation been explained in physiologic terms. Insofar as fetal homeostasis is dependent on efficient placental circulation, the extensive efforts of investigators to elucidate the factors that are important in the regulation of the flow of blood into and from the intervillous space have led to important practical applications in obstetrics. An adequate theory must be one in which an explanation is offered for the mechanism by which blood may actually leave the maternal arterial circulation, flow into an amorphous space that is lined by trophoblastic syncytium rather than capillary endothelium, and return through maternal veins without producing arteriovenouslike shunts that would prevent the blood from remaining in contact with the villi for sufficient time to effect adequate exchange.

It was not until the objective studies of Ramsey and her co-workers (1963, 1966) that a "physiologic" mechanism of placental circulation, consistent with both experimental and clinical findings, was available (Fig. 6-17). Discarding the less precise corrosion techniques of her predecessors, Ramsey and colleagues, by careful, slow injections of radiocontrast material under low pressure, so as to avoid disruption of the circulation, proved that the venous exits as well as the arterial entrances are scattered at random over the entire base of the placenta. The maternal blood that enters through the basal plate is driven by the head of maternal arterial pressure high up toward the chorionic plate before lateral dispersion occurs. After bathing the chorionic villi, the blood drains

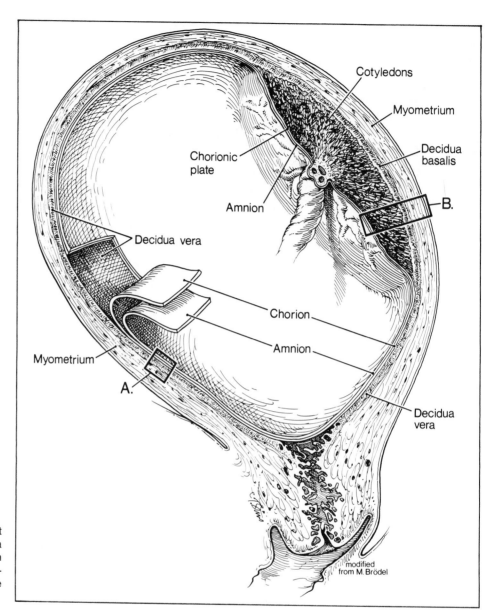

Figure 6-12. Uterus of pregnant woman showing normal placenta in situ. **A.** Location of section shown in Figure 6-13. **B.** Location of section shown in Figure 6-14.

through venous orifices in the basal plate and enters the maternal veins. Thus, the maternal blood traverses the placenta randomly without preformed channels and is propelled by the maternal arterial pressure. The spiral arteries are generally perpendicular and the veins are parallel to the uterine wall; this arrangement facilitates closure of the veins during uterine contractions and prevents squeezing of essential maternal blood from the intervillous space. According to Brosens and Dixon (1963), there are about 120 spiral arterial entries into the intervillous space of the human placenta at term, from which blood is discharged in spurts in a manner that displaces the adjacent villi, as described by Borell and co-workers (1958).

Ramsey and Harris (1966) compared the uteroplacental vasculature and circulation of the rhesus monkey with those of women. The most significant morphologic variation is the greater dilatation of the uteroplacental arteries in women. In women, particularly in early pregnancy, there may be multiple openings from a single arterial stem into the intervillous space. Eventually, the force of the spurts of blood is dissipated with the creation of a small lake of blood approximately 5 mm in diameter about halfway toward the chorionic plate. The closeness of the villi is such that the flow of blood is slowed; thereby, adequate time is provided for exchange.

Ramsey's concept is supported by the findings of numerous arteriographic studies in which it clearly has been shown that the spiral arterial spurts are associated with the "lakes" and by the results of many pressure studies in which it was demonstrated that there was clo-

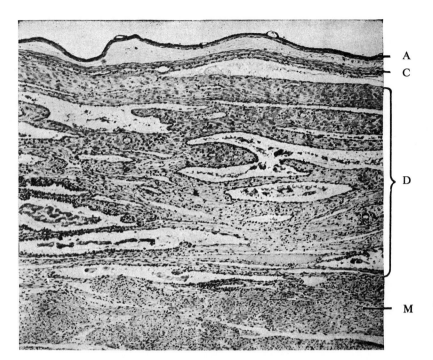

A
C

D

M

Figure 6-13. Section of fetal membranes and uterus opposite placental site at A in Figure 6-12. A, amnion; C, chorion; D, decidua parietalis; M, myometrium.

sure of uteroplacental veins at the beginning of uterine contractions. Corroboration has been provided by the results of cineradioangiography, in which it was shown how, in the macaque, debouching streams from the spiral arteries connect with and develop into the small lakes, which then disperse in a general effusion of blood throughout the intervillous space (Fig. 6-18).

In Ramsey's motion pictures, the effect of myometrial contractions upon placental circulation is shown unequivocally to involve diminution of arterial inflow and cessation of venous drainage. By continued observation of the contrast medium by televised fluoroscopy, the indication was that myometrial contractions cause a slight delay in the appearance of the contrast medium in the veins of the uterine wall when injection was conducted during a strong contraction. The pressure in the intervillous space may be decreased to such an extent that blood cannot be expressed against the prevailing myometrial pressure. Ramsey has provided further evidence of independent activity of the spiral arterioles, as evidenced by the appearance of spurts of blood in different locations even when injections are conducted under conditions of minimal myometrial pressure. Not all endometrial spiral arteries are patent continuously; moreover, blood is not necessarily discharged into the intervillous spaces simultaneously.

In summary, Ramsey's findings are supportive of the proposition that maternal blood enters the intervillous space in spurts that are produced by the maternal blood pressure. The vis a tergo forces blood in discrete streams toward the chorionic plate until the head of pressure is reduced; thereafter, the blood spreads laterally. Continuing influx of arterial blood exerts pressure on the contents of the intervillous space, pushing the blood toward

exits in the basal plate, from which it is drained through uterine and other pelvic veins. During uterine contractions, both inflow and outflow are curtailed, although the volume of blood in the intervillous space is maintained; this situation provides for continual, albeit reduced, exchange.

Freese (1968) provided support for the findings of older anatomic studies in which it was shown that in both the rhesus monkey and women, each placental cotyledon is supplied by one spiral artery, which is located beneath a central empty space. He believed that this relatively hollow central portion of the cotyledon, which he called the intracotyledonary space, is the preferential site of entry of blood. Wigglesworth (1969) suggested that the structure of the fetal cotyledon may determine, in part, the pattern of maternal blood flow through the placenta and that fetal cotyledons develop around the spiral artery. From the variations in structure of the villi in this region, it can be implied that growth occurs around the center of the cotyledon since villi there are less mature. Thus, in the intervillous space, there are arterial, capillary, and venous zones. In this connection, Reynolds and co-workers (1968) demonstrated that the blood pressure was highest around the central cavity of the cotyledon, and that the gradient diminishes radially and toward the subchorial lake. They postulated that Braxton–Hicks contractions (p. 213) are such as to enhance the movement of blood from the center of the cotyledon through the intervillous space.

Bleker and associates (1975), by use of serial sonography in normally laboring women, found that the length, thickness, and surface of the placenta increased during uterine contractions. They attributed these changes to blood distension of the intervillous spaces as

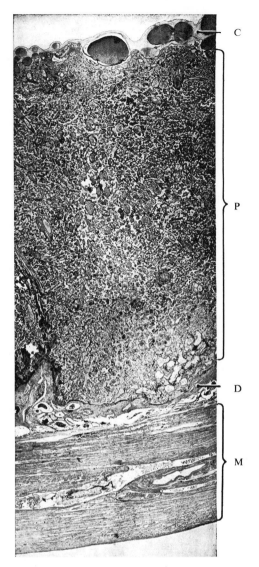

Figure 6-14. Section of placenta and uterus through B in Figure 6-12. C, chorionic plate with fetal blood vessels; P, placental villi; D, decidua basalis; M, myometrium.

the consequence of relatively greater impairment of venous outflow compared with arterial inflow. During contractions, therefore, a somewhat larger volume of blood is available for exchange even though the rate of flow is decreased.

Prostaglandins or prostaglandinlike substances very likely serve an autoregulatory role in placental hemodynamics. Speroff (1975), for example, found a rise in E prostaglandins and an increase in uterine blood flow in response to angiotensin II in pregnant monkeys, whereas treatment with indomethacin caused the opposite effect.

The principal factors that are important in the regulation of the flow of blood in the intervillous space are likely to include arterial blood pressure, intrauterine pressure, the pattern of uterine contraction (including the contour of the individual contraction wave), and other factors that act specifically upon the arteriolar walls. The lack of homogeneity of blood throughout the intervillous space has been emphasized by Fuchs and co-workers (1963), who measured Po_2, Pco_2, pH, and standard bicarbonate in blood samples believed to be from the intervillous space and found considerable variations in the values. The values for some samples were similar to those of arterial blood and yet other values were similar to those of uterine venous blood. They stressed, however, the difficulty of ascertaining with precision the source of blood obtained by transuterine puncture of the placenta.

In studies of the placental circulation in the human, no evidence could be obtained for countercurrent flow, a system by which fetal blood of low oxygen content, as it enters the villous capillaries, would first flow close to maternal blood of low oxygen content and then move in close proximity to progressively more oxygenated maternal blood. In the hemochorial villous placenta of the human, strict countercurrent flow is precluded by the random distribution of villi, in the capillaries of which the direction of fetal-to-maternal flow can bear no fixed relationship.

Harris and Ramsey (1966) published a summary of the findings of their anatomic studies of the uteroplacental vasculature. They found that cytotrophoblastic elements are confined initially to the terminal portions of the uteroplacental arteries but later extend proximally. By the 16th week of gestation, cytotrophoblasts are found in many of the arteries of the inner layer of myometrium. Intraarterial accumulation of trophoblasts ultimately may interfere with the circulation through some of these vessels. The number of arterial openings into the intervillous space is reduced gradually by cytotrophoblasts and by breaching of the walls of the more proximal parts of the arteries by deeply penetrating trophoblasts. Brosens and co-workers (1967) found that the cytotrophoblasts not only breach the maternal spiral vessels but also serve a major role in the progressive conversion to large tortuous channels by replacement of the normal muscular and elastic tissue of the wall by fibrous tissue and fibrinoid. After the 30th week of gestation, a prominent venous plexus separates the decidua basalis from the myometrium; thus, a plane of cleavage for separation of the placenta after delivery of the fetus is provided.

PLACENTAL IMMUNOLOGY

The placenta and fetus appear to defy the laws of transplantation immunology. Today, it is still a mystery how the pregnant woman tolerates the fetal allograft; this obtains in light of the now well-established antigenic competency of both the trophoblast and the fetus. Indeed, the distinguished scientist and Nobel laureate, Medawar (1953), was led to ask, "How does the pregnant mother

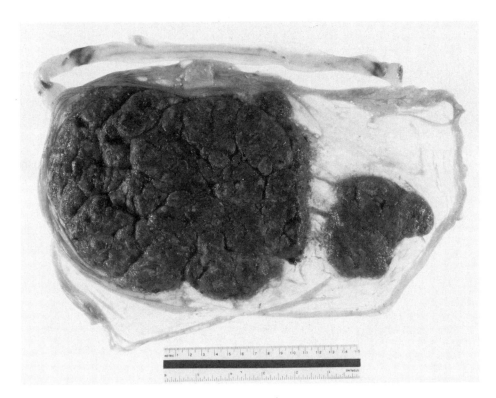

Figure 6-15. Maternal surface of term placenta. Variably discrete, irregularly shaped adjacent lobes are evident plus a large separate (succenturiate) lobe.

contrive to nourish within itself, for many weeks or months, a fetus which is an antigenically foreign body?" Yet, paradoxically, there is evidence that is supportive of the view that the greater the genetic disparity between mother and fetus, the better the pregnancy, at least in terms of placental and fetal weight.

Breaks in the Placental "Barrier"

The failure of the placenta to maintain absolute integrity of the fetal and maternal circulations is documented by the findings of numerous studies of the passage of cells between mother and fetus in both directions, and best

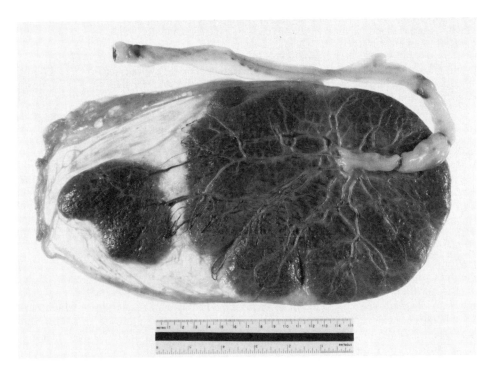

Figure 6-16. Fetal surface of term placenta. Fetal vessels are visible beneath the amnion overlying the placenta. The fetal vessels extend to the adjacent separate (succenturiate) lobe.

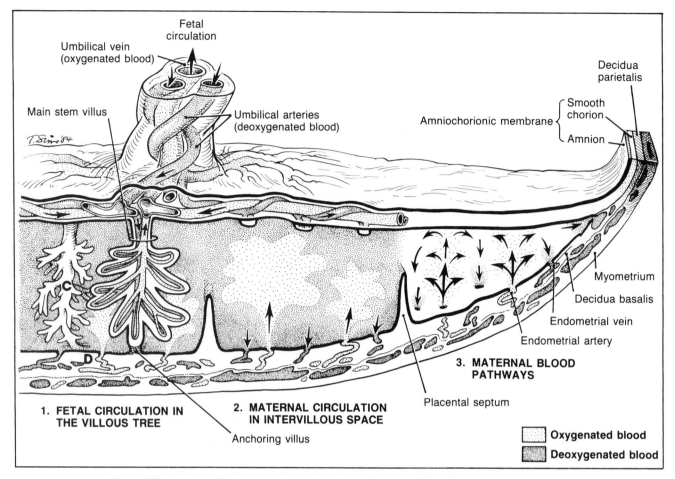

Figure 6-17. Schematic drawing of a section through a full-term placenta: 1. The relation of the villous chorion (C) to the decidua basalis (D) and the fetal placental circulation. 2. The maternal placental circulation. Maternal blood flows into the intervillous spaces in funnel-shaped spurts, and exchanges occur with the fetal blood as the maternal blood flows around the villi. 3. The inflowing arterial blood pushes venous blood into the endometrial veins, which are scattered over the entire surface of the decidua basalis. Note that the umbilical arteries carry deoxygenated fetal blood to the placenta and that the umbilical vein carries oxygenated blood to the fetus. Note that the cotyledons are separated from each other by placental (decidual) septa of the maternal portion of the placenta. Each cotyledon consists of two or more main stem villi and their many branches. (*Based on Moore: The Developing Human. Philadelphia, Saunders, 1982, p 116.*)

exemplified clinically by the occurrence of erythroblastosis fetalis (see Chapter 38, p. 772). Typically, a few fetal blood cells are found in the mother's blood; rarely, the fetus may exsanguinate by way of bleeding into the maternal circulation (see Chapter 28, p. 771). Leukocytes from the fetus may replicate in the mother; leukocytes bearing a Y chromosome have been identified in blood of women for up to 5 years after giving birth to a son (Ciaranfi and colleagues, 1977). Desai and Creger (1963) labeled maternal leukocytes and platelets with atabrine and found that such cells crossed the placenta from mother to fetus. Lymphocytes passing into the fetus create the possibility of *chimerism,* the subject of a review by Benirschke (1970). If the maternal cells then colonize, a "graft-versus-host" reaction, that is, an autoimmune process, may result.

Cells of fetal origin, other than constituents of the blood, also have been identified in the maternal circulation. Cells that are morphologically identical with trophoblasts have been identified in uterine venous blood (Douglas and colleagues, 1959) as well as in cord blood (Salvagio and co-workers, 1960). The immunologic significance of continuous release of fetal elements into the maternal circulation remains to be identified.

Immunologic Considerations

Except in parthenogenesis, or in situations in which both parents are genetically almost identical, the fetus and trophoblast confront the mother with foreign antigens. Furthermore, a fertilized egg that is transplanted to a recipient's uterus may result in a pregnancy with immu-

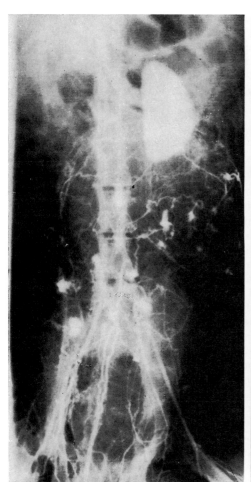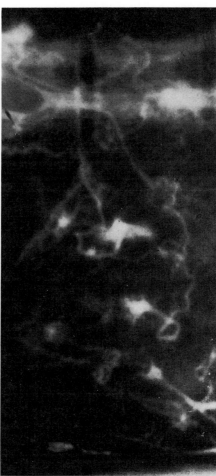

Figure 6-18. Left. Radiogram 6 seconds after injection of a radiopaque contrast medium into the right femoral artery of a monkey on day 111 of pregnancy. The primary placenta is below on the left; the secondary placenta is above on the right. **Right.** High magnification of an artery at the center of the secondary placenta in the same monkey. (*Courtesy of Dr. Elizabeth M. Ramsey.*)

nologic characteristics of a homograft. Interspecific hybrids, analogous to heterografts, represent even more flagrant violations of the laws of immunology. Attempts to explain the survival of the "homograft" have occupied the attention of several of the world's outstanding biologists. An explanation based on antigenic immaturity of the fetus must be discarded in light of Billingham's demonstration (1964) that transplantation antigens appear very early in life. A second explanation, based on diminished immunologic reactivity of the mother during pregnancy, provides only an ancillary factor in the prevention of the development of maternal isoimmunization during pregnancy in a few species. If the uterus were an immunologically privileged site, as in a third explanation, advanced ectopic pregnancies could never occur. Clearly, however, the trophoblast is immunologically privileged since transplantation immunity can be evoked and expressed in the uterus as elsewhere; the survival of the homograft must be related to a peculiarity of the fetus and placenta rather than of the uterus. A fourth explanation is one that involves a physiologic barrier between fetus and mother. Lanman and colleagues (1962) provided evidence in indirect support for this hypothesis in their experiments in which fertilized rabbit's ova were transferred to a recipient's uterus. Neither prior exposure of the foster mother to skin grafts

from the parents nor reexposure to homografts of these donors at the time of egg transfer or at midpregnancy adversely affected the pregnancy. Kobayashi and coworkers (1979) have reported a dose-dependent suppression of the bidirectional mixed lymphocyte reaction by progesterone in concentrations comparable to those in the placenta. Therefore, they suggest a role for progesterone at its site of production in immunoregulation during pregnancy. Siiteri and co-workers (1977) previously demonstrated that the rejection of grafted hamster skin is delayed by the presence of progesterone implants.

One reasonable explanation for the survival of the homograft appears to be a fairly complete anatomic separation of maternal and fetal circulations. Examinations of the placenta under comparative electron microscopy have been supportive of the concept of a prime role of the trophoblast in maintaining the "immunologic barrier." In all placentas examined with the electron microscope, at least one layer of trophoblast has been shown to persist essentially throughout gestation.

The suggestion by Kirby and co-workers (1964) that deposition of fibrinoid was a general phenomenon of mammalian placentation was one that rekindled interest in these amorphous deposits. (We have used the term *fibrinoid* in the restricted conventional sense of the histopathologist to refer to a group of substances recognized with the light microscope.) Although fibrinoids are not demonstrable in all mammalian placentas, a submicroscopic glycocalyx that coats most trophoblastic plasma membranes may be found with the electron microscope. Still, it is not clear whether these polysaccharide barriers serve as mechanical barriers to the passage of transplantation antigens from fetus to mother, or else to provide for local shields from maternal lymphocytes.

Maternal lymphocyte function is altered during pregnancy, as reflected by a reduction in phytohemagglutinin-induced transformation (Finn and associates, 1972; Purtilo and colleagues, 1972). It was suggested by Finn (1975) that lymphocytes possess individual-specific surface repellent molecules and that these can cross the placenta and coat maternal lymphocytes, thus preventing an attack on fetal cells. It also has been suggested that various secretory products of the trophoblast, for example, hCG and progesterone, and a host of newly discovered pregnancy-specific proteins (Chapter 7), may act to confer immunologic privilege.

Finn and associates (1977) posed an attractive explanation for the tolerance of the fetus and placenta by the mother. They demonstrated that maternal and fetal lymphocytes were tolerant of each other in the bidirectional mixed lymphocyte reaction. They believed that the tolerance between maternal and fetal cells was due largely to a genetic mechanism since the bidirectional mixed lymphocyte reaction between parents and older children also was reduced when compared with that between randomly selected control subjects. Tolerance between maternal and fetal cells was not demonstrated in a unidirectional mixed lymphocyte reaction, suggesting that, for tolerance, viability of both cell populations is required. They postulated that the mother has two al-

lelic surface markers, one of which must pass to the cells of the fetus, so that there is a common marker on maternal and fetal cells. These markers are mutually repellent and act to keep the cell surfaces sufficiently separated to prevent contact between major HLA antigens, thereby preventing an immunologic reaction.

THE AMNION

The human amnion develops either by delamination from the cytotrophoblast about the seventh or eighth day of development of the normal ovum or else it develops essentially as an extension of the fetal ectoderm. Initially, a minute vesicle (see Fig. 5-13), the amnion develops into a small sac that covers the dorsal surface of the embryo. As the amnion enlarges, the growing embryo is gradually engulfed and prolapses into the amnionic cavity. Distension of the amnionic sac eventually brings it into contact with the interior of the chorion; apposition of the mesoblasts of chorion and amnion near the end of the first trimester results in the obliteration of the extraembryonic coelom. The amnion and chorion, although adherent, are never connected intimately and usually can be separated easily, even at term.

The normal amnion is 0.02 to 0.5 mm in thickness. Normally, the epithelium consists of a single layer of nonciliated, cuboidal cells. According to Bourne (1962), there are five layers, comprising, from within outward, epithelium, basement membrane, the compact layer, the fibroblastic layer, and the spongy layer. In electron microscopic studies of amnion by Wynn and French (1968) and by Hoyes (1968), however, such sharply defined layers were not defined (Fig. 6-19).

Bourne (1962) was unable to find blood vessels or

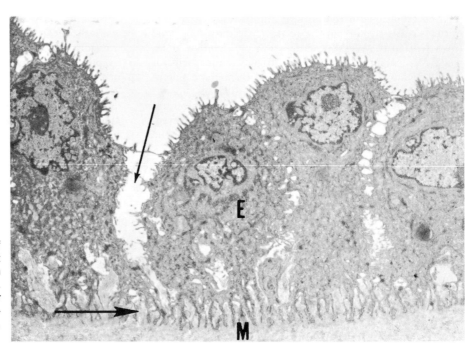

Figure 6-19. Electron micrograph of human amnion at term obtained at time of cesarean section. Epithelium (E) and mesenchyme (M) are shown. Thin arrow indicates intercellular space. Thick arrow points to specializations of basal plasma membranes. (*Courtesy of Dr. Ralph M. Wynn.*)

nerves in the amnion at any stage of development and, despite the occurrence of suggestive spaces in the fibroblastic and spongy layers, he could not identify distinct lymphatic channels.

At term, small rounded plaques often are found on the amnion, particularly near the attachment of the umbilical cord. These *amnionic caruncles* consist of stratified squamous epithelium that histologically resembles skin (see Chapter 23, p. 461).

Fetal Membranes and Steroid Hormone Metabolism

Studies directed toward a definition of the role of the fetal membranes in the initiation of parturition were undertaken by MacDonald and co-workers (1974). Among the early findings was the clear demonstration that in both the amnion and chorion laeve there are extensive enzymatic capabilities for steroid hormone metabolism, including 5α-reductase, 3β-hydroxysteroid dehydrogenase, $\Delta^{5\text{-}4}$-isomerase, 20α-hydroxysteroid oxidoreductase, 17β-hydroxysteroid oxidoreductase, and other enzyme activities.

The fetal membranes contain glycerophospholipids that are enriched in arachidonic acid, the obligate precursor of prostaglandins E_2 and $F_{2\alpha}$. In the fetal membranes, there also is a phospholipase A_2 as well as other enzymes that catalyze the release of arachidonic acid, likely the rate-limiting step in prostaglandin biosynthesis (see Chapter 15, p. 301).

AMNIONIC FLUID

The normally clear fluid that collects within the amnionic cavity increases in quantity as pregnancy advances until near term, when, normally, the volume decreases somewhat. An average volume of slightly less than 1000 ml is found at term, although the volume may vary widely, that is, from a few milliliters to many liters in abnormal conditions (oligohydramnios and polyhydramnios, or hydramnios). The origin, composition, and function of the amnionic fluid are discussed further in Chapter 8 (p. 169).

UMBILICAL CORD AND RELATED STRUCTURES

Development of the Cord and Related Structures

The yolk sac and the umbilical vesicle into which it develops are quite prominent at the beginning of pregnancy. At first, the embryo is a flattened disc that is interposed between amnion and yolk sac. Since the dorsal surface grows faster than the ventral surface, in association with the elongation of the neural tube, the embryo bulges into the amnionic sac and the dorsal part of the yolk sac is incorporated into the body of the em-

bryo to form the gut. The allantois projects into the base of the body stalk from the caudal wall of the yolk sac or, later, from the anterior wall of the hindgut. As pregnancy progresses, the yolk sac becomes smaller and its pedicle relatively longer. By about the middle of the third month of gestation, the expanding amnion obliterates the exocoelom, fuses with the chorion laeve, and thereafter covers the bulging placental disc and the lateral surface of the body stalk, which is then called the umbilical cord, or funis. Remnants of the exocoelom in the anterior portion of the cord may contain loops of intestine, which continue to develop outside the embryo. Although the loops are withdrawn, the apex of the midgut loop retains its connection with an attenuated vitelline duct that terminates in a crumpled, highly vascular sac that is 3 to 5 cm in diameter and lies on the surface of the placenta between amnion and chorion or in the membranes just beyond the placental margin, where occasionally it may be identified at term.

In an electron microscopic study, Hoyes (1969) confirmed that the endoderm of the yolk sac is the origin of fetal blood cells. The ultrastructural features of the epithelium of the yolk sac are those usually associated with a tissue that serves as a site of transfer of metabolites.

The three vessels in the cord at term normally are two arteries and one vein. The right umbilical vein usually disappears early during fetal development, leaving only the original left vein. By section of any portion of the cord near the center, the small duct of the umbilical vesicle, lined by a single layer of flattened or cuboidal epithelial cells, is found. In sections just beyond the umbilicus, but never at the maternal end of the cord, another duct that represents the allantoic remnant occasionally is found. The intraabdominal portion of the duct of the umbilical vesicle, which extends from umbilicus to intestine, usually atrophies and disappears, but occasionally it remains patent, forming the Meckel diverticulum. The most common vascular anomaly in man is the absence of one umbilical artery. This subject is discussed further in Chapter 23 (p. 459).

Structure and Function of the Cord

The umbilical cord, or funis, extends from the fetal umbilicus to the fetal surface of the placenta. Its exterior is dull white, moist, and covered by amnion, through which the three umbilical vessels may be seen. Its diameter is 1 to 2.5 cm, with an average length of 55 cm but a range of 30 to 100 cm. Folding and tortuosity of the vessels, which are longer than the cord itself, frequently create nodulations on the surface, or *false knots*, which, essentially, are varices. The matrix of the cord consists of Wharton Jelly (Figs. 6-20, 6-21). After fixation, the umbilical vessels appear empty, but the presentation in Figure 6-21 is more accurately representative of the situation in vivo, when the vessels are not emptied of blood. The two arteries are smaller in diameter than the vein. When fixed in its normally distended state, the umbilical artery exhibits transverse intimal *folds of Hobo-*

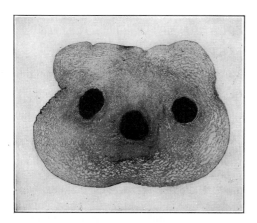

Figure 6-20. Cross section of umbilical cord fixed after blood vessels had been emptied. The umbilical vein, carrying oxygenated blood to the fetus, is in the center; on either side are the two umbilical arteries carrying deoxygenated blood from the fetus to the placenta. (*From Reynolds: Am J Obstet Gynecol 68:69, 1954.*)

ken across part of its lumen (Chacko and Reynolds, 1954). The mesoderm of the cord, which is of allantoic origin, fuses with the amnion.

The egress of blood from the umbilical vein is by way of two routes—the ductus venosus, which empties directly into the inferior vena cava, and, by way of numerous smaller openings, into the fetal hepatic circulation and thence into the inferior vena cava by way of the hepatic vein. The blood takes the path of least resistance through these alternate routes. Resistance in the ductus venosus is controlled by a sphincter, which is situated at the origin of the ductus at the umbilical recess and innervated by a branch of the vagus nerve.

Ellison and co-workers (1970) studied the innervation of the umbilical cord of the rat by means of locali-

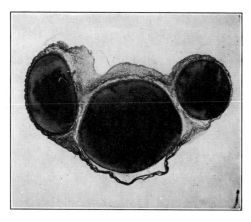

Figure 6-21. Cross section of same umbilical cord shown in Figure 6-20, but through a segment from which the blood vessels had not been emptied. This photograph probably represents more accurately the conditions in utero. (*From Reynolds: Am J Obstet Gynecol 68:69, 1954.*)

zation of acetylcholinesterase and catecholamines. Cholinesterase-positive nerves were confined to the periarterial plexus whereas adrenergic nerves were not found in the cord. By these techniques, certain nerves could be traced to the placenta but not into it. Although several recent investigators, relying on histochemical methods, have reported the finding of nerves in placenta and amnion, confirmation of these findings by use of ultrastructural techniques is lacking. The innervation of the placenta and membranes thus remains an open question.

REFERENCES

Ahlmark A: Studies on the histaminolytic power of plasma with special reference to pregnancy. Acta Physiol Scan (suppl 28) 9:1, 1944

Benirschke K: Spontaneous chimerism in mammals: A critical review. In Current Topics in Pathology. Berlin, Springer-Verlag, 1970, p. 1

Benirschke K: The placenta: How to examine it and what you can learn. Contemp Obstet Gynecol 17:117, 1981

Billingham RE: Transplantation immunity and the maternal–fetal relation. N Engl J Med 270:667, 720, 1964

Bigazzi M: Specific endocrine function of human decidua. Semin Reprod Endocrinol 1:343, 1983

Bleker OP, Kloosterman GJ, Mieras DJ, Oosting J, Salle HJA: Intervillous space during uterine contractions in human subjects: An ultrasonic study. Am J Obstet Gynecol 123:697, 1975

Borell U, Fernstrom I, Westman A: (An arteriographic study of the placental circulation.) Geburtshilfe Frauenheilkd 18:1, 1958

Bourne GL: The Human Amnion and Chorion. Chicago, Year Book, 1962

Boyd JD, Hamilton WJ: The Human Placenta. Cambridge, England, Heffer, 1970

Boyd JD, Boyd CAR, Hamilton WJ: Observations of the vacuolar structure of the human syncytiotrophoblast. Z Zellforsch Mikrosk Anat 88:57, 1968

Brosens I, Dixon HG: The anatomy of the maternal side of the placenta. Br J Obstet Gynaecol 73:357, 1963

Brosens I, Robertson WB, Dixon HB: The physiological response of the vessels of the placental bed to normal pregnancy. J Pathol Bact 98:569, 1967

Chacko AW, Reynolds SRM: Architecture of distended and nondistended human umbilical cord tissues, with special references to the arteries and veins. Contrib Embryol 35:135, 1954

Ciaranfi A, Curchod A, Odartchenko N: Survie de lymphocytes foetaux dans de sang maternel post-partum. Schweiz Med Wschr 107:134, 1977

Crawford JM: A study of human placental growth with observations on the placenta in erythroblastosis foetalis. Br J Obstet Gynaecol 66:885, 1959

Desai RG, Creger WP: Maternofetal passage of leukocytes and platelets in man. Blood 21:665, 1963

Douglas GW, Thomas L, Carr M. Cullen NM, Morris R: Trophoblast in the circulating blood during pregnancy. Am J Obstet Gynecol 78:960, 1959

Ellison JP, Hibbs RG, Ferguson MA, Mahan M, Blasini EJ: The innervation of the umbilical cord. Anat Rec 166:302, 1970

Finn R: Survival of the genetically incompatible fetal allograft. Lancet 1:835, 1975

Finn R, St. Hill CA, Govan AJ, Ralfs IG, Gurney FJ, Denye V: Immunological responses in pregnancy and survival of fetal homograft. Br Med J 3:150, 1972

Finn R, Davis JC, St. Hill CA, Hipkin LJ: Fetomaternal bidirectional mixed lymphocyte reaction and survival of fetal allograft. Lancet 1:200, 1977

Freese UE: The uteroplacental vascular relationship in the human. Am J Obstet Gynecol 101:8, 1968

Fuchs F, Spackman T, Assali NS: Complexity and nonhomogenicity of the intervillous space. Am J Obstet Gynecol 86:226, 1963

Galton M: DNA content of placental nuclei. J Cell Biol 13:183, 1962

Garza JR, MacDonald PC, Johnston JM, Casey ML: Characterization of ornithine decarboxylase activity in human uterine decidua vera. Am J Obstet Gynecol 145:509, 1983

Harris JWS, Ramsey EM: The morphology of human uteroplacental vasculature. Contrib Embryol 38:43, 1966

Hertig AT: The placenta: Some new knowledge about an old organ. Obstet Gynecol 20:859, 1962

Hoyes AD: Fine structure of human amniotic epithelium in early pregnancy. Br J Obstet Gynecol 75:949, 1968

Hoyes AD: The human foetal yolk sac: An ultrastructural study of four specimens. Z Zellforsch 99:469, 1969

Kirby DRS, Billington WD, Bradbury S, Goldstein DJ: Antigen barrier of the mouse placenta. Nature (London) 204: 548, 1964

Kobayashi H, Mori T, Suzuki A, Nishimura T, Nishimoto H, Harada M: Suppression of mixed lymphocyte reaction by progesterone and estradiol-17β. Am J Obstet Gynecol 134:255, 1979

Lanman JT, Dinerstein J, Fikrig S: Homograft immunity in pregnancy: Lack of harm to fetus from sensitization of mother. Ann NY Acad Sci 99:706, 1962

MacDonald PC, Schultz FM, Duenhoelter JH, Gant NF, Jimenez JM, Pritchard JA, Porter JC, Johnston JM: Initiation of human parturition: I. Mechanism of action of arachidonic acid. Obstet Gynecol 44:629, 1974

McCombs HL, Craig MJ: Decidual necrosis in normal pregnancy. Obstet Gynecol 24:436, 1964

Medawar PB: Some immunological and endocrinological problems raised by the evolution of viviparity in vertebrates. Symp Soc Exp Biol 11:320, 1953

Midgley AR Jr, Pierce GB Jr, Deneau GA, Gosling JRS: Morphogenesis of syncytiotrophoblast in vivo: An autoradiographic demonstration. Science 141:349, 1963

Moe N: The deposits of fibrin and fibrin-like materials in the basal plate of the normal human placenta. Acta Pathol Microbiol Scand 75:1, 1969

Pierce GB Jr, Midgley AR Jr: The origin and function of human syncytiotrophoblastic giant cells. Am J Pathol 43:153, 1963

Purtilo DT, Hallgren H, Yunis EJ: Depressed maternal lymphocyte response to phytohaemagglutinin in human pregnancy. Lancet 1:769, 1972

Ramsey EM, Davis RW: A composite drawing of the placenta to show its structure and circulation. Anat Rec 145:366, 1963

Ramsey EN, Harris JWS: Comparison of uteroplacental vasculature and circulation in the rhesus monkey and man. Contrib Embryol 38:59, 1966

Resnik R, Levine RJ: Plasma diamine oxidase activity in pregnancy: A reappraisal. Am J Obstet Gynecol 104:1061, 1969

Reynolds SRM, Freese UE, Bieniarz J, Caldeyro-Barcia R, Mendez-Bauer C, Escarcena L: Multiple simultaneous intervillous space pressures recorded in several regions of the hemochorial placenta in relation to functional anatomy of the fetal cotyledon. Am J Obstet Gynecol 102:1128, 1968

Richart RM: Studies of placental morphogenesis: I. Radioautographic studies of human placenta utilizing tritiated thymidine. Proc Soc Exp Biol Med 106:829, 1961

Riddick DH, Daly DC, Walters CA: The uterus as an endocrine compartment. Clin Perinatol 10:627, 1983

Salvaggio AT, Nigogosyan G, Mack HC: Detection of trophoblasts in cord blood and fetal circulation. Am J Obstet Gynecol 80:1013, 1960

Sciarra JJ, Kaplan SL, Grumbach MM: Localization of antihuman growth hormone serum within the human placenta: Evidence for a human chorionic-growth-hormone-prolactin. Nature (London) 199:1005, 1963

Siiteri PK, Febres F, Clemens LE, Jeffry Chang R, Gondos B, Sites D: Progesterone and maintenance of pregnancy: Is progesterone nature's immunosuppressant? Ann NY Acad Sci 286:384, 1977

Speroff L: An autoregulatory role for prostaglandins in placental hemodynamics: Their possible influence on blood pressure in pregnancy. J Reprod Med 15:181, 1975

Swanberg H: Source of histaminolytic enzyme in blood of pregnant women. Acta Physiol Scand 16:83, 1948

Thiede HA, Choate JW: Chorionic gonadotropin localization in the human placenta by immunofluorescent staining: II. Demonstration of hCG in the trophoblast and amnion epithelium of immature and mature placentas. Obstet Gynecol 22:433, 1963

Thomson AM, Billewicz WZ, Hytten FE: The weight of the placenta in relation to birthweight. Br J Obstet Gynaecol 76:865, 1969

Tyson JE, McCoshen JA: Decidual prolactin: An enigmatic cybernin in human reproduction. Semin Reprod Endocrinol 1:197, 1983

Wigglesworth JS: Vascular anatomy of the human placenta and its significance for placental pathology. J Obstet Gynaec Brit Comm 76:979, 1969

Wislocki GB, Dempsey EW: The chemical histology of human placenta and decidua with reference to mucoproteins, glycogen, lipids and acid phosphatase. Am J Anat 83:1, 1948

Wislocki GB, Dempsey EW: Electron microscopy of the human placenta. Anat Rec 123:133, 1955

Wislocki GB, Streeter GL: On the placentation of the macaque (Macaca mulatta), from the time of implantation until the formation of the definitive placenta. Contrib Embryol 27:1, 1938

Wynn RM: Comparative electron microscopy of the placental junctional zone. Obstet Gynecol 29:644, 1967

Wynn RM: Fetomaternal cellular relations in the human basal plate: An ultrastructural study of the placenta. Am J Obstet Gynecol 97:832, 1967

Wynn RM, Davies J: Comparative electron microscopy of the hemochorial villous placenta. Am J Obstet Gynecol 91:533, 1965

Wynn RM, French GL: Comparative ultrastructure of the mammalian amnion. Obstet Gynecol 31:759, 1968

7

The Placental Hormones

The endocrine alterations that accompany pregnancy in women are perhaps the most remarkable that are recorded in mammalian physiology or pathophysiology. Consider the following: each day, in a pregnant woman at or near term, there is the production of 15 to 20 mg of estradiol-17β, 50 to 100 mg of estriol, 250 to 600 mg of progesterone, 1 to 2 mg of aldosterone, and 3 to 12 mg of deoxycorticosterone; furthermore, there are striking increases in the levels of plasma renin, angiotensinogen, and angiotensin II, together with the daily production of 1 g of human placental lactogen (hPL), massive quantities of human chorionic gonadotropin (hCG), and, likely human chorionic thyrotropin (hCT), chorionic ACTH, and other products of pro-opiomelanocortin and possibly the hypothalamiclike releasing and inhibiting hormones TRH, LHRH, corticotropin releasing factor (CRF), and somatostatin, as well as a variety of proteins (pregnancy-specific) that are unique to pregnancy or neoplastic processes. Thus, one of the most remarkable physiologic events of pregnancy may be the establishment of mechanisms whereby the gravid woman and her fetus are able to adapt to this unusual endocrine milieu. These latter issues will be considered in more detail in Chapter 9.

CHORIONIC GONADOTROPIN

History

The evolution of our understanding of the biologic, physiologic, and chemical nature of human chorionic gonadotropin (hCG) occupies an important niche in the history of obstetrics. It is interesting to recall that the first species in which a chorionic gonadotropin was discovered was the human. Hirose (1919) is credited with the first demonstration of a trophic effect of human placental tissue fragments on the ovaries and uteri of the rabbit. Indeed, it was the demonstration of the "pregnancy hormone" in urine of pregnant women by Ascheim and Zondek (1927) that formed the basis for the original consideration of the placenta as an endocrine organ and subsequently the basis of a test for pregnancy. Hertz (1980) relates the story of an interesting conversation that he had with Dr. Bernhard Zondek. In that conversation, Hertz says, Zondek recounted with good humor that he once chastized his technician for the reporting of a positive pregnancy test that was obtained with the urine of a man. Hertz recounts that the matter was complicated further since the man's last name was the same as that of one of the pregnant women whose urine was tested in the same assay. Ultimately, it was found that the man in question was one in whom there was a testicular tumor that was producing hCG. Zondek, says Hertz, made amends and never doubted that technician's findings again.

The discovery of the "pregnancy hormone" led to the development of the first pregnancy test and even the laity were familiar with the "A-Z" test and the "Friedman" test because, as Hertz points out, these became household terms (Chapter 10, and Table 10-1). Indeed, the "A-Z" test, or variations on the theme, namely stimulation of the follicles of the ovaries of experimental animals, including the induction of ovulation in induced ovulators (rabbits) by urine of pregnant women was the standard test for pregnancy in women for more than 40 years.

Zondek believed that there were two pregnancy-related gonadotropin activities because he observed that concentrates of urine of pregnant women evoked both follicular development and ovulation and corpus luteum formation. For these reasons, he believed that there were two separate agents and he referred to these putative agents as prolan A and prolan B.

Soon there was considerable controversy as to the relationship between the gonadotropin(s) in urine of pregnant women and those extracted from pituitary tissue. Hertz recounts the history and the resolution of this controversy as follows: In 1931, Zondek and others emphasized that, by use of the bioassay procedures employed, there was, in the urine of postmenopausal women, follicle stimulating activity. It also was demonstrated that whereas the avian gonad and the ovary of the immature rhesus monkey are responsive to extracts of the pituitary, there was no such response to concentrates of urine of pregnant women. Convincing evidence that the two preparations (namely, pituitary extracts and concentrates of urine of pregnant women) were different in gonadotropin properties was obtained by Reichert and co-workers (1932), who demonstrated that the hypophysectomized rat was virtually unresponsive to extracts of urine of pregnant women but readily responsive to extracts of pituitary tissue.

In 1938, the placental source of hCG was established further and verified by Gey, Jones, and Hellman, who demonstrated the production of the hormone by trophoblastic cells maintained in tissue culture. Finally, in 1948, the hormone was crystallized by Claesson and co-workers.

From the work of these pioneering investigators, we have come to know (a) the nature of as well as the structure of hCG, (b) in large measure, the molecular events involved in its mechanism of action, (c) the nature of its biosynthesis and processing, (d) the utility of this protein hormone in the evaluation of certain neoplastic processes, and (e) trials have even been conducted in women to ascertain if the hormone could be used as an antigen for the development of antibodies to hCG as a means of immunization against pregnancy.

We now know that hCG is a glycoprotein (molecular weight ~37,000 to 38,000) with a high carbohydrate content. The molecule is comprised of two dissimilar subunits, designated α and β, that are noncovalently linked. These subunits have been separated, isolated in pure form, and the primary structure of each has been characterized. The carbohydrate content of the native molecule is about 30 percent, the highest carbohydrate content of any human hormone. The carbohydrate content, and especially the terminal sialic acid, may protect the molecule from catabolism; in fact, the enzymatic removal of the terminal sialic acid by use of specific enzymes greatly accelerates the rate of clearance of hCG from the circulation.

The α- and β-subunits of hCG are held together by electrostatic and hydrophobic forces that can be separated by treatment with acidified urea. The nature of the purified subunits is of considerable interest to both investigators and clinicians. There is no intrinsic biologic activity in either separated subunit; if the subunits are recombined, however, nearly 100 percent of bioactivity is restored. The primary structures of all human glycoprotein hormone α-subunits are nearly, if not completely, identical; in contrast, while sharing certain similarities, it has been shown that there are distinctive differences among the amino acid sequences of the β-subunits of hFSH, hTSH, as well as those of hCG and hLH. The β-subunits of hCG and LH, however, are more similar one to the other; 80 percent of the first 115 amino acid residues of LH and hCG are identical, but in the hCG β-subunit, there are 30 additional amino acid residues at the COOH-terminal that are distinctive. Recombination of α- and β-subunits of the various glycoproteins gives rise to a molecule with biologic activity characteristic of the hormone from which the β-subunit was derived.

It now is apparent that the synthesis of the α- and β-chains of hCG also are regulated separately. The two subunits are translated from separate messenger RNAs (mRNAs) rather than in tandem from a single mRNA.

The rate of synthesis of the β-subunit is limiting with respect to the synthesis of the complete hCG molecule. Trophoblasts of normal placenta and of hydatidiform mole and choriocarcinoma secrete the α- and β-subunits as well as hCG; however, there is a large excess of α-subunits in placenta and in plasma of pregnant women whereas the β-subunit is present in small or undetectable quantities. Interestingly, the same obtains with respect to the synthesis and secretion of the α- and β-subunits of LH by the pituitary. The subunits of hCG are synthesized as pre-subunits, which are somewhat larger than the native proteins of the two units of hCG. The pre-subunit is processed to its native form prior to hCG assembly.

The rate of secretion of hCG may be subject to trophic regulation. By way of example, it has been demonstrated that a number of agents act to increase hCG secretion by trophoblasts in vitro. Among these are butyrated derivatives of cyclic AMP, LHRH, and epidermal growth factor; on the other hand, dibutyryl cyclic GMP, AMP, insulin, progesterone, epinephrine, or prostaglandin do not cause an augmentation of hCG secretion.

Cellular Site of Origin and Biological Aspects of hCG Action

Human chorionic gonadotropin is believed to be produced principally by syncytiotrophoblast rather than cytotrophoblast, as pointed out in Chapter 6 (p. 107).

It is perhaps paradoxical, however, that the greatest concentration of hCG in plasma of pregnant women is found when there are the greatest number of cytotrophoblasts, viz., in early pregnancy, at 8 to 10 weeks gestation, and in complicated pregnancies in which there is a reappearance of cytotrophoblasts, for example, with Rh isoimmunization and an affected fetus and in pregnancies complicated by maternal diabetes mellitus. It is possible, as is addressed subsequently, that LHRH, of cytotrophoblastic origin, stimulates, in a paracrine fashion, the secretion of hCG by the syncytiotrophoblast in a manner analogous to the stimulation of pituitary LH release by LHRH of hypothalamic origin.

The most apparent function of hCG in women is to maintain the function of the corpus luteum during early pregnancy. Until recently, however, this action of hCG, while accepted without question from the findings of Bradbury and co-workers (1950), seemed to offer an incomplete explanation for the physiologic role of hCG. Bradbury and colleagues demonstrated that the life-span of the corpus luteum in nonpregnant women could be prolonged by the administration of hCG to such women. Yet, the maximum concentrations of hCG in plasma of pregnant women are attained at a time in gestation when the function of the corpus luteum, with respect to progesterone formation, has declined, viz., at 8 to 10 weeks gestation (Fig. 7-1). Although not rigorously proven, a tentative explanation for these several obser-

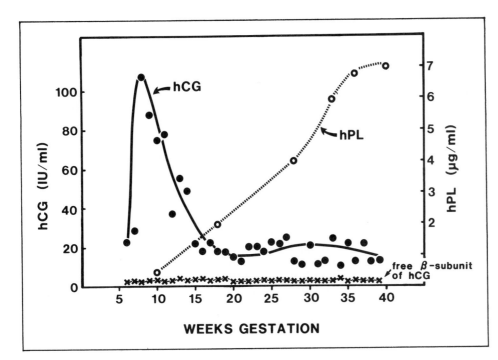

Figure 7-1. Mean concentration of chorionic gonadotropin (hCG) and placental lactogen (hPL) in serum of women throughout normal pregnancy. Free β-subunit of hCG is in low concentration or else is undetectable throughout pregnancy. The concentration of free α-subunit of hCG in serum increases gradually during pregnancy in a manner similar to that of hPL, albeit in much smaller amounts than hPL. (*Data from Ashitaka et al., 1980, and Selenkow et al., as reviewed by Goebelsman, 1970; Courtesy of Dr. L. Casey.*)

vations may be that hCG, in high concentrations at 8 to 10 weeks gestation, may serve to "down-regulate" the hCG/LH receptors in corpus luteum; the consequence could be a decrease in the rate of cholesterol side-chain cleavage and, thereby, a reduction in the rate of corpus luteum progesterone secretion at a time in gestation when trophoblasts are capable of producing sufficient progesterone for the maintenance of pregnancy.

Moreover, fetal testicular testosterone secretion is maximum at the same time that the rate of secretion of hCG also is maximum. Thus, at a time in fetal development prior to vascularization of the fetal pituitary, by way of the hypophysial portal vessels, hCG can serve to act on fetal testes as an LH surrogate to promote testosterone synthesis and secretion and thereby male sexual differentiation at a critical time in fetal development.

In the human ovary, appropriately primed by follicle-stimulating hormone (FSH), hCG induces ovulation and is sometimes so used as a luteinizing hormone (LH) surrogate in the treatment of infertility due to anovulation and hypogonadotropic hypogonadism. In this context, it is important to note that the half-life of hCG is quite long (24 to 37 hours) compared with that of LH (2 hours), which may account for the longer life-span of the corpus luteum after ovulation induction with hCG than with that induced by LH (Chapter 3).

A role in the maintenance of cholesterol side-chain cleavage for hCG in the placenta and in the stimulation of aromatization must be considered; moreover, a role for hCG in the provision of immunologic privilege to the trophoblast has been suggested.

The methods for assaying hCG are of considerable importance, since these assays form the basis for the ma-

jority of tests for pregnancy in women. Until recently, neither the immunoassays nor bioassays commonly employed for pregnancy testing were absolutely specific for hCG. The similarity of the immunologic determinants in the α-chains, but not β-chains, of the various glycoprotein hormones accounts for the cross-reactivity when immunoassay procedures are employed by use of antibodies directed against native LH or hCG. The apparent hCG activity in biologic fluids at times was found to differ appreciably, depending upon whether immunoassay or bioassay was employed. Wide and Hobson (1967), and also Bridson and associates (1970), demonstrated that hCG synthesized in vitro by cloned choriocarcinoma cells yielded values twice as great by immunoassay as by bioassay. They suggested that the reduction in biologically active material compared with that found employing urinary hCG was the result of alterations in the hormone molecule after it was secreted by the trophoblast. We now know, however, that such cells secrete the α-chain, the β-chain, and hCG; the separate chains are biologically inactive but are recognized by antibodies in varying reactivities. Some of the techniques in current clinical use for detecting chorionic gonadotropin in biologic fluids are considered further in Chapter 10 (p. 214).

With the recognition that LH and hCG were composed of an α- and β-subunit, that the two subunits of each molecular species could be separated and purified, and that the β-subunits of each were structurally distinct, at least at the COOH-terminus, Vaitukaitis and colleagues (1972) set out to develop antibodies that would recognize, specifically, the β-subunit of hCG. Thereby, an antibody would be available that could discriminate between LH and hCG. The development of such an antibody has become an incredibly useful tool for elucidation of physiologic processes, early detection of pregnancy in cases of infertility, and for monitoring hCG production in persons with neoplastic trophoblastic disease, both before and during treatment.

The rate of excretion of chorionic gonadotropin into the urine of pregnant women increases rapidly between the 30th and 60th day of pregnancy, with peak levels attained between the 60th and 70th days of gestation. Thereafter, the levels of hCG decrease slowly, and a nadir is reached between the 100th and 130th days at a low level that is maintained throughout the remainder of gestation. The levels of hCG in the serum are closely parallel to those in the urine, rising rapidly from approximately 1 IU/ml by 6 weeks after the commencement of the last menstrual period to an average value of about 100 IU/ml between the 60th and 80th days after the last menses (Fig. 7-1). Although most curves constructed from mean values for hCG in serum or urine are quite similar, such curves are not such as to emphasize the considerable variations in the levels of this hormone in blood or urine among individual women at the same time of gestation.

Whereas the pattern of hCG secretion in pregnancy is well-defined, as cited, the levels of the α- and β-subunit in plasma of pregnant women are appreciably different from those of the intact molecule. As cited, the levels of the β-subunit are low or undetectable throughout human pregnancy (Fig. 7-1). On the other hand, the levels of the α-subunit increase gradually and steadily until about 30 weeks gestation when a plateau is attained that is maintained for the remainder of pregnancy, similar to the pattern of human placental lactogen (Fig. 7-1), as is discussed subsequently (Ashitaka and co-workers, 1980).

Significantly higher levels of hCG are likely to be found in pregnancies with multiple fetuses, in pregnancies with a single erythroblastic fetus resulting from maternal isoimmunization, and especially in women with hydatidiform mole and choriocarcinoma. Interestingly, many nontrophoblastic tumors produce hCG, and Yoshimoto and co-workers (1979) have demonstrated that many normal tissues also secrete hCG, in small amounts. Recently, it was shown that the β-subunit of hCG is produced in fetal kidney (McGregor and co-workers, 1981). Borkowski and Muquardt (1979) found that hCG could be detected, albeit in very small amounts, in the blood of 12 of 16 blood donors who were believed to be normal men.

Metabolic Disposition of hCG

The metabolic clearance rate (MCR) of hCG is about 3 ml per minute, that is, about 4 liters of plasma are cleared of hCG each day. The renal clearance of hCG as the native molecule accounts for 30 percent of the total MCR, the remainder being metabolized by pathways other than renal excretion, probably in liver and kidney

(Nisula and Wehmann, 1980). The MCR of the β-subunit and of the α-subunit are about 10-fold and 30-fold, respectively, greater than that of native hCG. On the other hand, the renal clearance rate of the subunits are considerably less than that of hCG. Thus, renal clearance is not the means by which the subunits in plasma are cleared so rapidly, according to Nisula and Wehmann.

HUMAN PLACENTAL LACTOGEN

Human placental lactogen (hPL) is detectable in the trophoblast as early as the third week after ovulation. This hormone was described first by Ito and Higashi in 1961. In 1962, Josimovich and MacLaren isolated the hormone and characterized it as a polypeptide that was found in extracts of human placenta and retroplacental blood. Since in hPL there is both potent lactogenic and growth hormone–like activity and an immunochemical resemblance to human growth hormone, it first was called *human placental lactogen,* or chorionic growth hormone. Later, it was referred to as chorionic somatomammotropin. Recently, most authors returned to the original terminology, namely, human placental lactogen. Grumbach and Kaplan (1964) found, by immunofluorescence studies, that this hormone, like hCG, was concentrated in the syncytiotrophoblast.

This protein consists of a single polypeptide chain with a molecular weight of about 22,000 (Li and co-workers, 1968). Placental lactogen contains 191 amino acid residues, compared with 188 in human growth hormone; the amino acid sequence in each hormone also is quite similar. The gene for hPL has been cloned, and the nucleotide sequence for DNA complementary to the mRNA encoding for hPL has been determined (Shine and colleagues, 1977).

The genes for both hPL and human growth hormone are known to be located in close linkage on chromosome 17 (Fiddes and co-workers, 1980; Owerbach and colleagues, 1980). On the other hand, the gene for prolactin is located on chromosome 6 (Owerbach and co-workers, 1981). It is speculated, therefore, that the gene encoding for hPL may have risen by duplication of the hGH gene (for review, see Kaplan and Grumbach, 1981). Incredibly, at term, hPL represents 7 to 10 percent of the peptides synthesized by placental ribosomes. The synthesis of hPL is stimulated by insulin and cAMP. PGE_2 and $PGF_{2\alpha}$ seem to inhibit the secretion of hPL. The MCR of hPL, 175 liters per day, is considerably greater than that of hCG, and the production rate near term, 1 g or more per day, is the greatest of any known hormone in the human.

Placental lactogen can be detected in the serum of pregnant women as early as the sixth week of gestation (or 4 weeks after fertilization). The concentration of hPL rises steadily until about the 36th week of pregnancy and the concentration in maternal blood is approximately proportional to placental mass. The concentration of hPL in maternal serum, as measured by radioimmunoassay, reaches levels in late pregnancy higher than that of any other known protein hormone (Fig. 7-1). These high levels, coupled with a very short half-life in the circulation, attest to a rate of production of hPL by the placenta of considerable magnitude. Very little hPL is found in the circulation of the human fetus or in the urine of the mother or newborn; the concentration of the hormone in amnionic fluid is somewhat lower than that in maternal plasma. Since hPL is secreted primarily into the maternal circulation, with only very small amounts found in cord blood, it appears that the role of the hormone in pregnancy, if any, is mediated through action in maternal rather than in fetal tissues.

It has been postulated that hPL participates, directly or indirectly, in a number of profound metabolic actions. These putative actions include lipolysis and an increase in the levels of circulating free fatty acids, thereby providing a source of energy for maternal metabolism and fetal nutrition, and the inhibition of both the uptake of glucose and of gluconeogenesis in the mother, thereby sparing both glucose and protein (see Chapter 9, p. 189). The alleged antiinsulin action of hPL is believed to lead to an increase in maternal levels of insulin, which favors protein synthesis; this, in turn, ensures a mobilizable source of amino acids for transport to the fetus. The presence of the hormone, however, does not appear to be required for a successful pregnancy outcome. Nielsen and associates (1979) described a pregnancy in which hPL could not be identified in either maternal serum or in the placenta when analyzed by several techniques in a number of laboratories. Since the account of Nielson and co-workers, other cases of very low or undetectable levels of hPL in otherwise normal pregnancies have been described. It has been estimated that deficiency in hPL production may occur in about 1 of 12,000 pregnancies. Hubert and associates (1983) found that the level of mRNA encoding for hPL in placental tissue of a pregnancy in which hPL in maternal plasma was undetectable was very low compared with that in a normal placenta.

Spellacy and Buhi (1969) could not detect hPL in the early postpartum period and also noted a deficient output of pituitary growth hormone at this time. They suggested that this relative lack of insulin antagonists is associated with low fasting levels of blood glucose during this period.

HPL production is not restricted to the trophoblast. The hormone has been detected by direct radioimmunoassay in sera from men and women with various malignancies, other than those originating in trophoblast or gonad, including bronchogenic carcinoma, hepatoma, lymphoma, and pheochromocytoma (Weintraub and Rosen, 1970).

Possible indications in clinical obstetrics for assaying hPL are considered in Chapter 14 (p. 280). A clear utility for the measurement of hPL in high-risk pregnancy has not been established.

CHORIONIC THYROTROPIN AND ADRENOCORTICOTROPIN

There is evidence, albeit somewhat controversial, that the placenta produces a human chorionic thyrotropin (hCT), but there is little or no evidence that there is a significant biologic role for this substance in normal human pregnancy. The neoplastic trophoblast of hydatidiform mole and choriocarcinoma may produce a family of chorionic thyrotropins, but the increased thyroid-stimulating activity in pregnant women and especially in those with neoplastic trophoblastic disease can be attributed chiefly to the thyroid-stimulating properties of hCG.

The placenta may be a tissue that contributes to the ACTH that is present in maternal plasma in pregnancy. In pregnant women, the plasma levels of ACTH increase throughout pregnancy; nonetheless, the levels of ACTH at all times in pregnancy (before labor) are lower than those found in men and nonpregnant women. (There is convincing evidence that ACTH does not cross the placenta.) The administration of dexamethasone to pregnant women does not cause suppression of the levels of free cortisol in urine as it does in men and nonpregnant women.

An ACTH-like protein has been isolated from placental tissue and considerable evidence has accrued to support the proposition that this compound is of placental origin, but perhaps chemically distinct from pituitary ACTH. There are several lines of evidence that are supportive of the likelihood that ACTH is produced in chorionic tissue. Odagiri and colleagues (1979) found that ACTH, lipotropin, and β-endorphin are all found in placental extracts and presumably are derived from the same or a similar 31K precursor molecule, pro-opiome-

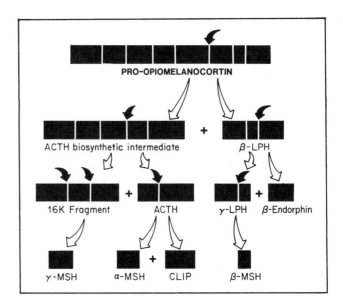

Figure 7-2. Processing of pituitary pro-opiomelanocortin (31K protein). (*Courtesy of Dr. A. Barnes.*)

lanocortin (Fig. 7-2), as are the pituitary peptides, and Liotta and colleagues (1979) found that ACTH is produced by dispersed placental cells.

Dexamethasone treatment does not alter the levels of ACTH in placental tissue whether the ACTH is measured by bioassay or immunoassay. By use of experiments to evaluate the formation of ACTH and ACTH-like compounds, the incorporation of [^{35}S]methionine and [^{3}H]leucine into ACTH and related peptides by dispersed trophoblastic cells was demonstrated. By use of pulse-chase studies, the radiolabel was first incorporated into a high-molecular-weight ($\sim$34,000) peptide similar to that of the ACTH, β-LPH precursor of the pituitary and hypothalamus. With longer incubations, the radiolabel disappeared progressively from the high-molecular-weight form and began to appear, in increasing amounts, in smaller peptides that corresponded to peptides with antigenic determinants of ACTH and α-MSH, as well as β-lipotropin and β-endorphin.

Nonetheless, the physiologic significance of placental ACTH and related compounds is unclear. For a review of the placental processing of pro-opiomelanocortin, see Simpson and MacDonald (1981) and Krieger (1982).

HYPOTHALAMIC-LIKE RELEASING HORMONES OF THE PLACENTA

In placenta, there is an appreciable amount of immunoreactive *luteinizing hormone–releasing hormone* (LHRH) (Siler-Khodr and Khodr, 1978). Interestingly, these investigators also demonstrated that immunoreactive LHRH was present in the cytotrophoblast, but not in the syncytiotrophoblast. More recently, Siler-Khodr (1983) has referred to this substance as hCG-releasing hormone. Gibbons and co-workers (1975) and Khodr and Siler-Khodr (1980) have demonstrated that the human placenta can synthesize both LHRH and *thyrotropin-releasing hormone* (TRH) in vitro.

Indeed, for each known hypothalamic-releasing hormone or inhibiting hormone described, namely LHRH, TRH, corticotropin-releasing hormone (CRF), and somatostatin, there are reports of analogous hormones produced in human placenta (cf. Siler-Khodr, 1983). The role of these hypothalamic-like releasing or inhibiting hormones in chorionic tissue, however, cannot be resolved presently. It is interesting to speculate that the finding of these substances in placental tissue is indicative that there may be a hierarchy of control of formation of chorionic trophic agents such as hCG, chorionic thyrotropin, and pro-opiomelanocortin-derived peptides of the placenta.

PREGNANCY-"SPECIFIC" PROTEINS

In the past 10 to 15 years, a host of proteins have been discovered that many investigators refer to as "pregnancy-specific" or "pregnancy-related." For the most part, these "newly-discovered" proteins were identified by use of antibodies developed in animals against the serum of pregnant women. The resulting antibodies in animal serum were treated with serum of men or nonpregnant women to remove antibodies not specific for proteins of human pregnancy; remaining antibodies were directed toward antigens specific in, or in far greater concentration in, serum of pregnant women. The residual antiserum was then used to isolate proteins peculiar to the serum of pregnant women. Many investigators have employed this approach, and, in consequence, it is estimated that 20 or more such proteins have been isolated recently (Klopper, 1981). This estimate, however, is difficult to make with certainty because there is no consistent nomenclature or precise standards for identification of these pregnancy-related proteins. Thus, at the time of this writing, it is highly likely that a number of investigators are studying the same protein but are reporting their findings with their own nomenclature for that given protein. By way of example, Klopper points out that pregnancy-associated globulin is also known as pregnancy zone protein and by six other names as well. Presently, the lines of investigation of the physiologic or pathophysiologic relevance of these proteins is one that follows a familiar path; early pregnancy diagnosis, relation to fetal well-being, immunosuppression, tumor marker, implantation, etc. The field is confusing and, as yet, lacks clarity of direction. Nonetheless, it is one to be mindful of, and hopeful for.

ESTROGENS

Mechanism of Estrogen Formation in Pregnancy

Near term, normal pregnancy in women constitutes a hyperestrogenic state of near unbelievable magnitude. In many normally pregnant women, the amount of estrogen produced daily is equivalent to that produced, on average, by no fewer than 1000 premenopausal women in 1 day. By way of another analogy, during the course of normal pregnancy, the gravid woman produces more estrogen than an ovulatory woman could produce in 150 years. The mechanism of estrogen formation in normal pregnant women, however, differs strikingly from that in nonpregnant premenopausal women. In summary:

1. The placenta is the site of origin of estrogens during pregnancy in women.
2. The placenta synthesizes estrogens from externally supplied prehormones that are transported to trophoblasts by way of maternal and fetal plasma.
3. The disproportionately elevated levels of estriol in blood and urine of pregnant women result from the synthesis of estriol in the placenta, principally from the conversion, by aromatization, of 16α-hydroxydehydroisoandrosterone sulfate, most of which arises in the fetus.

Thus, during normal human pregnancy, there is a hyperestrogenic state of continually increasing proportion that terminates abruptly after delivery of the fetus and placenta. There is no doubt that the site of origin of the increased amounts of estrogens in pregnant women is the placenta. As early as the seventh week of gestation, more than 50 percent of estrogens entering the maternal circulation is of placental origin (Siiteri and MacDonald, 1966). Indeed, Diczfalusy and Borell (1961) demonstrated that the levels of urinary estrogens do not decrease after bilateral oophorectomy performed as early as the 78th day of pregnancy. Similar results were obtained in several studies of urinary estrogen excretion by pregnant women after surgical removal of the corpus luteum. Thus, it is evident that the ovary is not a quantitatively important source of estrogens after the first few weeks of pregnancy in women.

As pointed out in Chapter 3, the principal estrogen secreted by the ovary in nonpregnant women is estradiol-17β, while that of extraglandular origin is estrone, and from these two estrogens the multiple estrogenic metabolites in urine of nonpregnant women are derived. In nonpregnant women, the ratio of the concentration of urinary estriol to that of estrone plus estradiol-17β is approximately 1:1. During pregnancy, however, this ratio increases to 10:1 or more near term (Brown, 1956). This disproportionate increase in estriol formation during human pregnancy results from the placental formation of estriol from 16α-hydroxylated C_{19}-steroids, principally 16α-hydroxydehydroisoandrosterone sulfate, rather than from an alteration in the fractional conversion of estrone and estradiol-17β to estriol in mother or fetus or from 16α-hydroxylation in placenta.

The biosynthetic pathways of estrogen formation in the placenta differ considerably from those in other endocrine organs. From the results of in vitro studies, it is clear that estrogens of ovarian origin arise de novo, that is, from acetate or cholesterol (Fig. 3-12). It has not been possible, however, to demonstrate that acetate or cholesterol, or even progesterone, can serve as a precursor for estrogen biosynthesis in the placenta. The placenta appears to lack steroid 17α-hydroxylase activity, and, consequently, the conversion of C_{21}-steroids to C_{19}-steroids, the precursors of estrogen, is not possible.

Ryan (1959), in classic experiments, demonstrated that there is an exceptionally high capacity to convert certain C_{19}-steroids to estrone and estradiol-17β in placental tissue. He found that dehydroisoandrosterone, androstenedione, and testosterone were converted efficiently to estrone, estradiol-17β, or both, by placental preparations in vitro. These findings ultimately led to an investigation of the role of C_{19}-steroids in maternal or fetal blood or both as precursors for the biosynthesis of estrogen in placenta.

Amoroso (1960) deduced that the placenta, might, through its abundant enzymatic activity, bring about the formation of active agents by way of the conversion of inactive materials derived from elsewhere in the body. Support for this deduction was provided by Frandsen and Stakeman (1961), who found that in the urine of women pregnant with an anencephalic fetus there was approximately one tenth the amount of estrogens than is present in women pregnant with a normal fetus at the same stage of gestation. Pointing to the characteristic absence of the fetal zone of the adrenal cortex in anencephalic fetuses, Frandsen and Stakeman postulated that the fetal adrenal was the site of origin of a substance(s) that serves as the precursor of placental estrogen.

Plasma-Borne Precursors

The first proof that the placenta utilizes plasma-borne precursors was provided by the demonstration that radiolabeled dehydroisoandrosterone sulfate, introduced into maternal blood, was converted extensively to estrogens by the placenta (Baulieu and Dray, 1963; Siiteri and MacDonald, 1963). It also was shown that other C_{19}-steroids, namely, dehydroisoandrosterone, androstenedione, and testosterone, when introduced into the maternal circulation, also were converted to estrogens. The abundance of dehydroisoandrosterone sulfate in the plasma, however, and its much longer half-life uniquely qualified it as the principal circulating precursor of placental estrone and estradiol-17β. The arrival of dehydroisoandrosterone at the site of conversion as the sulfate ester does not preclude its utilization in the synthesis of estrogen; this obtains because the placenta normally is a rich source of sulfatase activity (Pulkkinen, 1961; Warren and Timberlake, 1962). By infusing radiolabeled dehydroisoandrosterone sulfate into pregnant women, it was shown that as early as the seventh week of gestation there is readily demonstrable conversion of circulating maternal dehydroisoandrosterone sulfate to estradiol-17β. By the 30th week of pregnancy, 25 percent or more of dehydroisoandrosterone sulfate in the maternal plasma is converted to estradiol-17β by the placenta. Additionally, maternal dehydroisoandrosterone sulfate is converted to estriol by way of an estrone–estradiol-17β independent pathway (MacDonald and Siiteri, 1965a) to be described below. The rapid utilization of circulating maternal dehydroisoandrosterone sulfate for placental estrogen biosynthesis undoubtedly accounts, in part, for the progressive decrease in the concentration of dehydroisoandrosterone sulfate in the plasma of pregnant women as pregnancy progresses (Migeon et al., 1955), as well as the decrease of the 11-deoxy-17-ketosteroids excreted in the urine of pregnant women.

In extensive studies of the metabolism of maternal plasma dehydroisoandrosterone sulfate during the course of human gestation, Gant and co-workers (1971) found that there was a striking increase in the rate of clearance of dehydroisoandrosterone sulfate from plasma of normally pregnant women at term compared with its clearance in men and nonpregnant women. Whereas the metabolic clearance rate of dehydroisoandrosterone sulfate in men and nonpregnant women is 6 to 8 liters per 24 hours, the rate of clearance of this substance from plasma of pregnant women at term is increased by 10- to

20-fold. Since the maternal adrenal production rate of dehydroisoandrosterone sulfate is not significantly changed during the course of human pregnancy, the concentration in plasma must decrease with increasing rates of clearance.

The increase in clearance of dehydroisoandrosterone sulfate from the plasma of pregnant women appears to be attributable principally to two processes: (1) its removal through conversion to estradiol-17β by the trophoblasts and (2) an increased rate of metabolism that is attributable to increased 16α-hydroxylation of dehydroisoandrosterone sulfate in the maternal compartment. Approximately 30 percent of dehydroisoandrosterone sulfate in the plasma of pregnant women is converted to 16α-hydroxydehydroisoandrosterone sulfate. Although the extent of these conversions is high, the maternal adrenal does not produce significantly increased quantities of dehydroisoandrosterone sulfate during pregnancy; therefore, the fetal adrenal constitutes the principal source of placental estriol precursor.

By use of the principle of determining the total rate of clearance of dehydroisoandrosterone sulfate and simultaneously the fraction of that clearance that is attributable uniquely to the trophoblastic utilization of dehydroisoandrosterone sulfate for the formation of estradiol-17β, Gant and co-workers (1971) developed a method for determining the placental clearance of dehydroisoandrosterone sulfate through estradiol-17β formation. In normally pregnant, ambulatory women near term, the placental clearance of maternal plasma dehydroisoandrosterone sulfate to estradiol-17β is approximately 25 ml per minute. On the other hand, in women whose pregnancies are complicated by pregnancy-induced hypertension, the placental clearance is markedly reduced. By use of this technique to monitor placental function, Gant and associates (1976) demonstrated that there was a consistent decrease in placental clearance in both normal and hypertensive women after sodium depletion induced by the ingestion of low salt diets or else the administration of diuretics. Moreover, the metabolic clearance rates of dehydroisoandrosterone sulfate in young primigravid women who ostensibly were normal, but identified as being at risk for the development of pregnancy-induced hypertension (i.e., the loss of angiotensin II pressor refractoriness early in pregnancy), were found to be higher than those in young primigravid women who remained normotensive at similar stages of gestation (see Chapter 27, p. 539). The results of these studies, together with those of others who found increased plasma renin levels early in pregnancy, as well as increased concentrations of estriol early in pregnancy in women who later developed pregnancy-induced hypertension compared with those found in women who remained normotensive, suggest that preeclampsia is preceded by a state of hyperplacentosis (Robertson and co-workers, 1971).

As pregnancy advances, however, the utilization of maternal plasma dehydroisoandrosterone sulfate accounts for only a small fraction of the estrogens produced by the placenta. The observation by Frandsen and Stakemann (1961) of lower excretion of estrogens in women pregnant with an anencephalic fetus, in whom the fetal zone of the adrenal cortex characteristically is absent, together with the finding of high levels of dehydroisoandrosterone sulfate in the cord blood of normal infants (Colas and co-workers, 1964), suggested that precursors secreted by the fetal adrenal contributed appreciably to the synthesis of placental estrogens. Confirmation of this hypothesis was provided by the experiments of Bolté and co-workers (1964), who demonstrated that dehydroisoandrosterone sulfate, introduced into the umbilical artery and perfused through the placenta in situ, was converted to estrone and estradiol-17β.

Although dehydroisoandrosterone sulfate, circulating in both fetal and maternal plasma, is utilized in the production of estrone and estradiol-17β by the placenta, an explanation was still required for the inordinately large amount of estriol that is present in the urine of pregnant women. The estriol in the urine of pregnant women cannot be accounted for on the basis of metabolism of estrone and estradiol-17β. In this regard, it is important to recall that Brown (1956) and Fishman and associates (1961) demonstrated that the metabolism of estradiol-17β in pregnant women was not significantly different from that found in nonpregnant women. Moreover, it has not been possible to demonstrate the conversion of more than trace amounts of estradiol-17β to estriol in the placenta, indicating that the critical step of 16α-hydroxylation necessary for the conversion of estrone or estradiol-17β to estriol is not efficiently performed by placental tissue. Consequently, several other explanations were offered to account for the formation of estriol in pregnancy.

One of the several hypotheses held that placental estrone and estradiol-17β are circulated to the fetus and therein converted to estriol, which thereafter reenters the maternal circulation (Fishman et al., 1961; Gurpide et al., 1962). Another explanation, advanced by Bolté and co-workers (1964), held that the fetus converts placental estrone to 16α-hydroxyestrone, which then circulates back to the placenta, where reduction to estriol occurs. A third explanation requires the production of a 16α-hydroxy-C$_{19}$-steroid in the fetus or mother as a circulating precursor for placental biosynthesis of estriol. Although all three explanations are supported by data, quantitatively, the third mechanism is the most important.

Ryan (1959) also had demonstrated the 16α-hydroxylated C$_{19}$-steroids such as 16α-hydroxydehydroisoandroxterone, 16α-hydroxy-Δ^4-androstenedione, and 16α-hydroxytestosterone were converted efficiently to estriol by preparations of human placental tissue. In addition, large amounts of 16α-hydroxydehydroisoandrosterone sulfate are found in umbilical cord blood (Colas et al., 1964). Finally, the conversion of radiolabeled 16α-hydroxydehydroisoandrosterone and 16α-hydroxydehydroisoandrosterone sulfate, introduced into the maternal circulation, to radiolabeled estriol was

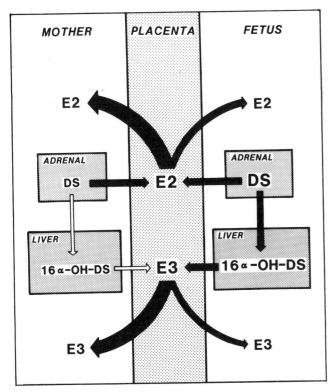

Figure 7-3. Schematic presentation of the biosynthesis of estrogen in human placenta. Near term, 50 percent of estradiol-17β is derived from fetal adrenal dehydroisoandrosterone sulfate (DS) and 50 percent from maternal DS. On the other hand, 90 percent of estriol in placenta arises from fetal 16α-OH-dehydroisoandrosterone sulfate (16α-OH-DS) and only 10 percent from all other sources. Most (80 to 90 percent) of steroids produced in placenta are secreted into the maternal blood. (*Courtesy of Dr. L. Casey.*)

demonstrated (Siiteri and MacDonald, 1965b; Madden and associates, 1978).

Thus, the adrenal cortices of both mother and fetus are the sites of origin of precursors of placental estrogens. In the absence of the fetal zone of the adrenal cortex, as in anencephaly, the rate of formation of placental estrogens (especially estriol) is limited severely due to the lack of precursor formation in the fetus. Verification of the diminished levels of precursors in anencephalic fetuses was provided by the finding of low levels of dehydroisoandrosterone sulfate in cord blood of such newborns (Nichols, 1958). In addition, it was shown that almost the total production of estrogens in women pregnant with an anencephalic fetus at 33 to 40 weeks of gestation can be accounted for by the placental utilization of maternal plasma dehydroisoandrosterone sulfate (MacDonald and Siiteri, 1965b). Furthermore, in such pregnancies, the production of estrogens can be increased by the administration of ACTH, which stimulates the rate of dehydroisoandrosterone sulfate secretion by the maternal adrenal. Finally, placental pro-

duction of estrogens can be decreased in women pregnant with an anencephalic fetus by the administration of a potent glucocorticosteroid, which suppresses ACTH secretion and thus decreases the rate of secretion of dehydroisoandrosterone sulfate from the maternal adrenal cortex (MacDonald and Siiteri, 1965b).

In women with Addison disease, there is decreased excretion of estrogens in urine during pregnancy (Baulieu and co-workers, 1956), although the decrease is principally in the urinary estrone and estradiol-17β fractions, since the fetal contribution to the synthesis of estriol, particularly in the latter part of pregnancy, is of paramount importance. A schematic representation of the pathways of estrogen formation in the placenta is presented in Figure 7-3.

The extraordinary efficiency of the placenta in the aromatization of C_{19}-steroids may be exemplified by two considerations. First, Edman and associates (1981) found that the placental clearance of maternal plasma androstenedione to estradiol-17β was very similar (when corrected for total blood cleared) to the estimated blood flow to the placenta. Second, it is very rare that a female fetus is virilized in a pregnant woman who is known to have an androgen-secreting ovarian tumor. This finding is indicative that the placenta efficiently converts aromatizable androgens to estrogens, thereby precluding transplacental passage of the androgen from the mother to the fetus. Indeed, it may be that the female fetuses who are virilized in women with an androgen-producing tumor are those in whom a nonaromatizable C_{19}-steroid androgenic steroid is produced by the tumor, for example, 5α-dihydrotestosterone.

The Human Fetal Adrenal

Thus, there is a major role for the fetal adrenal cortex in the biosynthesis of estrogen by the human placenta. Indeed, the human fetal adrenal is a unique organ; comparatively, the fetal adrenal is the largest organ of the fetus. Moreover, it is a unique structure in other ways. More than 85 percent of the fetal adrenal gland is normally composed of a fetal zone that is not present in the adrenals of adults. At term, the weight of the fetal adrenals approximates the weight of the adrenals of the adult.

Although direct measurements of fetal adrenal secretory activity have not been possible, it can be estimated that in some fetuses the adrenals must produce 100 to 200 mg of steroids per day. If one considers that the normal production of steroids by the adrenals of the nonstressed, resting adult rarely exceeds 20 to 30 mg per day, it is apparent that the fetal adrenal is a truly remarkable endocrine organ.

Immediately after birth, the fetal adrenal cortex undergoes rapid involution and the weight of the adrenals decreases strikingly during the first few weeks of life. The size attained by the adrenals of the human fetus just prior to birth is not achieved again until late in adolescent life (Fig. 7-4). Based on the importance of the fetal adrenal in the biogenesis of placental estrogen pre-

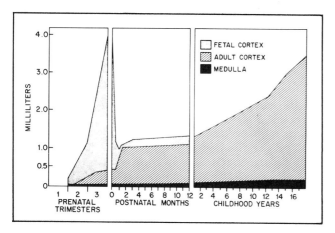

Figure 7-4. Size of the adrenal gland and its component parts in utero, during infancy, and during childhood. (*Adapted from Bethune: The Adrenal Cortex, A Scope Monograph. Kalamazoo, MI, Upjohn, 1974.*)

cursors, and the potential importance of the fetal adrenal secretions in the initiation of labor (Chapter 15), and in fetal lung maturation (Chapter 8), considerable interest and investigative efforts have been directed toward an elucidation of the factors that act to regulate the steroidogenic activity and growth of the fetal adrenals.

Early Fetal Adrenal Development

Early in embryonic life, the fetal adrenal is composed of cells that resemble those of the fetal zone of the fetal adrenal cortex; these cells rapidly appear and proliferate prior to the time that vascularization of the pituitary by the hypothalamus is complete. This suggests that the early development of the fetal adrenal is under trophic influences that do not conform to those of the adult. Either ACTH is secreted by the fetal pituitary in the absence of hypothalamic-corticotropin-releasing factor, or else ACTH arises from source(s) other than the fetal pituitary, for example, from chorionic ACTH that is synthesized by trophoblast. ACTH does not cross the placenta. Even in the anencephalic fetus, the fetal adrenal sometimes grows normally until approximately 20 weeks gestation. At this time, in the anencephalic fetus, a progressive decrease in fetal adrenal size usually occurs. In the normal fetus, however, the adrenal continues to grow, and during the last 5 to 6 weeks of gestation, there is a sharp increase in the rate of growth of the fetal adrenal. The results of a variety of studies suggest that the rate of fetal adrenal growth and steroid secretion are not controlled by a single trophic stimulus but rather by a multiplicity of influences, which, acting in concert, result in the peculiar development, growth rate, and steroid synthetic pattern that are characteristic of the fetal adrenal. First, there is a relative deficit in the expression of the enzyme complex 3β-hydroxysteroid dehydrogenase, $\Delta^{5,4}$-isomerase in the fetal adrenal. The absence of effective expression of this enzyme attenuates the conversion of pregnenolone to progesterone, an

obligatory step in cortisol biosynthesis, and also precludes the conversion of dehydroisoandrosterone to androstenedione. Serra and associates (1971) demonstrated, however, that the lack of expression of the activity of this enzyme is not because of an absence of the enzyme but rather because its expression is inhibited by the high levels of progesterone, and possibly estrogen, as described by Bongiovanni and associates (1967). In any event, the failure of expression of 3β-hydroxysteroid dehydrogenase enzyme activity will result in a decrease in the capacity for cortisol biosynthesis from cholesterol and pregnenolone. This set of events sets the stage for the potential of a cycle that can be envisioned to act to control the activity and growth of the fetal adrenal.

The early growth of the fetal adrenal, prior to the development of hypothalamic control of the pituitary by way of the hypophysial portal blood, may be, in part, the consequence of the elaboration of chorionic ACTH (p. 123). Several investigators suggest that in early pregnancy an ACTH-like substance is elaborated from the placenta. If this were true, the production of chorionic ACTH would reach a nadir at about 120 to 140 days of gestation. At this time, vascularization of the pituitary by way of the long hypophysial–portal vessels has been completed, and theoretically, at least, corticotropin-releasing factor from the fetal brain could now influence the release of ACTH by the fetal anterior pituitary. In the absence of adequate pituitary production of ACTH (e.g., in the anencephalic fetus), it is conceivable that the adrenal would begin to undergo involution at about 20 weeks of gestation. It appears, however, that ACTH alone does not produce the total physiologic response observed in fetal adrenal growth and steroid secretion, as it has been demonstrated that there is a continual decrease in the concentration of ACTH in human fetal plasma as pregnancy progresses (Winters and associates, 1974).

For the reasons just cited, a second trophic agent is envisioned that could act cooperatively with ACTH to stimulate the fetal adrenal cortex in its rate of growth and steroid secretion. Many investigators have sought to identify the "second trophic stimulus" of the fetal adrenal. Every compound known to be secreted by the pituitary (Fig. 7-2) and each of the peptide hormones of the placenta have been considered to be candidates for this role. The results of recent investigations, however, are consistent with the view that an alternative explanation(s) may be more appropriate to account for stimulation of the growth and high rate of steroid excretion by the fetal adrenal.

The Source of Cholesterol Used as Steroid Precursor by the Fetal Adrenal.
As cited, the output of steroids from the fetal adrenal is enormous. Indeed, fetal adrenal steroid hormone production alone requires the utilization of an amount of cholesterol equivalent to one fourth to one fifth of the total daily LDL-cholesterol turnover in the adult. If the relative size of the fetus is taken into account, it can be computed that the rate of turnover of the cholesterol pool in the fetus must be six times that

of the total cholesterol turnover in the adult simply to accommodate the needs of the fetal adrenal for steroidogenesis. From this analysis, we believe that the more cogent question to ask first is, "What is the source of fetal adrenal steroid precursor?" rather than, "What is the alternate adrenocorticotrophic agent?" Others have proposed that progesterone and pregnenolone produced by the placenta may serve as precursors for fetal adrenal cortisol and dehydroisoandrosterone sulfate biosynthesis, respectively. A role for fetal plasma progesterone as precursor in the biosynthesis of adrenal cortisol, however, is unlikely, for suppression of fetal pituitary ACTH by the administration of glucocorticosteroids to the mother results in a striking reduction of cortisol in fetal plasma without a concomitant reduction in progesterone levels. Recall that ACTH acts to increase cholesterol side-chain cleavage activity, the enzyme that catalyzes the conversion of cholesterol to pregnenolone, an enzymatic reaction that precedes those that effect the conversion of progesterone to cortisol. Thus, the conversion of progesterone to cortisol proceeds by way of enzymatic reactions largely independent of acute ACTH control. The conversion of radiolabeled progesterone, introduced into the fetal circulation, to radiolabeled cortisol has been demonstrated. The relative importance, however, of this pathway of cortisol formation compared with that of the de novo synthesis of fetal cortisol from cholesterol is probably small. It is clear, however, that the utilization of pregnenolone in the fetal circulation cannot account for more than a tiny fraction of the enormous quantity of dehydroisoandrosterone sulfate secreted by the fetal adrenals near term.

We come then to what we now consider to be a most important issue with respect to the regulation of fetal adrenal steroidogenesis; namely, what is the source of cholesterol that is used for fetal adrenal steroidogenesis? Several investigators have demonstrated that fetal adrenal tissue, in vitro, can synthesize steroid hormones. From these findings, it is clear that the fetal adrenal also can synthesize cholesterol from two-carbon fragments, viz., acetate. The rate of cholesterol synthesis by fetal adrenal tissue, however, is such that this source of cholesterol can account for only a fraction of the steroids produced by the fetal adrenals at term. Thus, the fetal adrenal must assimilate cholesterol from the circulation in order to meet the demands for optimal steroidogenesis. In plasma, cholesterol and cholesterol esters are present principally in the form of lipoproteins. Lipoproteins are designated according to density as determined by ultracentrifugation, for example, very low-density lipoprotein (VLDL), low-density lipoprotein (LDL), and high-density lipoprotein (HDL). In studies of human fibroblasts in culture, Goldstein and Brown (1974) demonstrated the presence of specific plasma membrane receptors with high affinity for LDL. After binding of LDL to the plasma membrane receptor, LDL is internalized by an adsorptive endocytotic process. The internalized endocytotic vesicles fuse with lysosomes and the hydrolytic enzymes of the lysosomes catalyze the hydrolysis of the protein component of LDL, which gives rise to amino acids, and the hydrolysis of the cholesterol esters of LDL, which gives rise to cholesterol and fatty acids.

In elegantly designed studies, Goldstein and Brown (1974), Anderson and associates (1976), and Faust and colleagues (1977), have shown that in most human tissues there are plasma membrane receptors for LDL. Simpson and co-workers (1979) conducted experiments designed to ascertain whether human fetal adrenals utilize circulating lipoproteins as a source of cholesterol for steroidogenesis. Employing explants of human fetal adrenal tissue maintained in organ culture, they found that when LDL was present in the culture medium, there was a marked stimulation of steroidogenesis by ACTH-treated fetal adrenal tissue. HDL was much less effective than LDL, and VLDL was devoid of stimulatory activity. Carr and associates (for review, see Carr and Simpson, 1981) also evaluated the relative contributions of cholesterol synthesized de novo and cholesterol derived from the uptake of LDL for fetal adrenal steroidogenesis. First, they found that the activity of the rate-limiting enzyme in de novo cholesterol synthesis in the fetal adrenal, 3-hydroxy-3-methylglutaryl coenzyme A (HMG CoA) reductase, was sufficient to account for only a fraction of the cholesterol required for fetal adrenal steroidogenesis. Second, they demonstrated that if LDL were removed from the medium of fetal adrenal explants in organ culture, the rate of steroidogenesis decreased, even in the presence of ACTH. Thus, the fetal adrenal is highly dependent upon circulating LDL as a source of cholesterol for steroidogenesis. Indeed, alterations in LDL-cholesterol levels in cord plasma appear to be highly dependent, inversely, upon the rate of fetal adrenal steroid biosynthesis before birth (Parker and associates, 1980, 1983a, 1983b).

Therefore, an important question to be addressed is the source of circulating cholesterol in the human fetus. Pitkin and co-workers (1972), from the results obtained in studies of subhuman primates, and in the study of one human pregnancy, concluded that no more than 20 percent of cholesterol in fetal plasma could be attributed to transfer from the mother. A model of cholesterol metabolism in the fetal adrenal proposed by Carr and Simpson (1981) is presented in Figure 7-5. The low level of LDL-cholesterol in the plasma of the fetus is probably due to the rapid utilization of LDL by the fetal adrenal for steroidogenesis. The levels of LDL-cholesterol are high in umbilical cord plasma of the anencephalic newborn in whom the adrenal is atrophic. Moreover, there is a higher level of LDL in infants of women with hypertension in whom estriol levels are low; thus, there is an inverse correlation between the cord plasma levels of LDL and dehydroisoandrosterone sulfate.

Fetal Growth Factors as Trophic Stimuli for the Fetal Adrenal. In addition to ACTH, the cholesterol contained in plasma lipoprotein, especially that in LDL, appears to occupy a crucial role in fetal adrenal steroidogenesis. Nonetheless, the likelihood that there is yet another trophic stimulus for the fetal adrenal is still

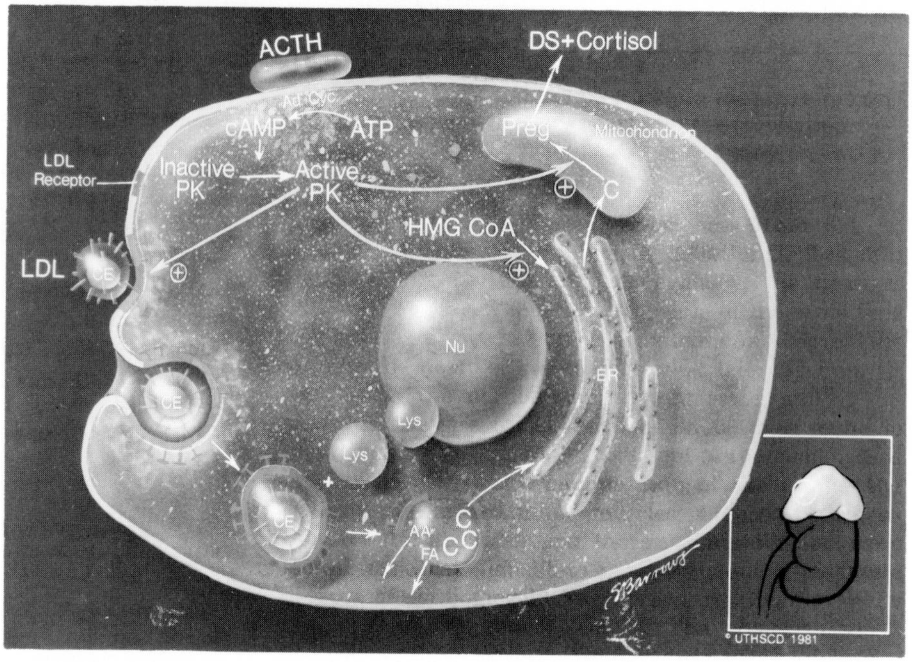

Figure 7-5. A model proposed for the regulation of fetal adrenal steroidogenesis, lipoprotein utilization, and cholesterol metabolism in the human fetal gland. Lys = lysosome; Nu = nucleus; ER = endoplasmic reticulum; Ad. Cyc. = adenylate cyclase; Preg = pregnenolone; CE = cholesterol esters; AA = amino acids; C = cholesterol; FA = fatty acids; PK = protein kinase; + = stimulation. (*From Carr and Simpson, 1981, with permission.*)

attractive. The unique pattern of fetal adrenal secretion, that is, the secretion of large amounts of dehydroisoandrosterone sulfate and small amounts of cortisol, is reminiscent of the adrenal steroid secretory patterns observed in women with virilizing adrenal adenomas.

In yet another pathophysiologic state, namely, hyperprolactinemia due to pituitary microadenomas, high plasma levels of dehydroisoandrosterone sulfate and normal levels of cortisol are observed commonly. Importantly, when such women were treated with bromocriptine, dehydroisoandrosterone sulfate levels in plasma decreased appreciably. Thus, a second hormone that may serve a role in fetal adrenal steroidogenesis is fetal pituitary prolactin. In support of this view, it has been demonstrated that while ACTH levels in fetal plasma decline throughout the course of gestation, increasing concentrations of prolactin are observed. Indeed, the concentrations of prolactin during the last 5 weeks of pregnancy increase and are maintained at a high level during the time of maximum fetal adrenal growth (Winters et al., 1975).

Prolactin will cause cholesterol storage in some endocrine glands. ACTH, on the other hand, promotes the cleavage of the cholesterol side chain to give rise to pregnenolone. These two events working in concert in the face of a relative deficit in the expression of the enzyme 3β-hydroxysteroid dehydrogenase would favor the production of dehydroisoandrosterone or its sulfate by the fetal adrenal. As discussed previously, dehydroisoandrosterone sulfate of fetal adrenal origin serves, ultimately, as the principal precursor for placental estrogen production. The estrogen thus produced could serve to perpetuate the cyclicity of the dualistic trophic stimulus of the fetal adrenal. The increasing production of estrogen favors the release of prolactin by the pituitary.

Most investigators, including ourselves, have been unable, however, to show a direct stimulatory effect of prolactin on fetal adrenal tissue. Therefore, it appears that if there is a role for prolactin in fetal adrenal growth and steroidogenesis, it must be indirect, for example, by way of acting to effect the growth of the fetal adrenal without necessarily affecting steroid synthesis directly or else by increasing the availability of LDL. Indeed, it now seems likely that the third trophic agent (ACTH and LDL being the first two discovered) will be one or several substances that act as growth-promoting factors.

Postnatal Adrenal Changes. After birth, there is a precipitous decrease in the concentration of prolactin in the plasma of newborns and a concomitant decrease in the size and the rate of secretion of steroids by the adrenals of the newborn child.

MEASUREMENT OF URINARY OR PLASMA ESTRIOL DURING PREGNANCY AS A TEST OF FETAL WELL-BEING

Rationale

With the discovery that the urine of pregnant women contains large amounts of estrogens that originate in the placenta, measurements of the urinary metabolites of these hormones have been conducted in an attempt to provide an index of "placental function" or "fetal well-being." Because the principal estrogen in the urine of pregnant women is estriol, many investigators concentrated on developing reliable methods for the measurement of this metabolite. The discovery that the fetus serves an important role in contributing precursors for the synthesis of estriol strengthened the possibility that abnormalities in pregnancy may be recognized by abnormal rates of excretion of estriol in urine of pregnant women.

Urinary Estriol

It has long been known that fetal death is accompanied by a striking reduction in the levels of urinary estrogens. Moreover, Cassmer (1959) demonstrated that ligation of the umbilical cord with the fetus and placenta left in situ was followed by an abrupt and striking decrease in the production of placental estrogens. These findings were subject to at least two interpretations.

The first holds that maintenance of the fetal circulation is essential to the functional endocrine integrity of the placenta. This explanation is unlikely to be correct, however, because in Cassmer's preparation the placental production of progesterone was maintained at "preligation" levels after ligation of the umbilical cord.

A second explanation of the marked decrease in urinary estrogens after fetal death is that after umbilical cord ligation there is an elimination of an important source of precursors of placental estrogen biosynthesis, namely, the fetus. The quantitative importance of fetal precursors of placental estriol in normal pregnancy is amply demonstrated by the low levels of urinary estriol in pregnancies with an anencephalic or dead fetus.

The principal influence upon levels of estriol in the urine of pregnant women, therefore, is not the biosynthetic integrity of the placenta (except in rare instances) but rather the availability of precursors of placental estrogens, principally of fetal adrenal origin. The clinical usefulness of the measurements of estriol as corroborative evidence of fetal death is well established, but whether a clinically useful index of placental function or evaluation of the condition of the living fetus is provided by measurement of urinary or plasma estriol is still not proven. *The clinical value of these tests can be established only by proof of increased infant salvage resulting directly from therapeutic regimens predicated upon the results of estriol measurements.* The development of this aspect of obstetric endocrinology was discussed extensively by Frandsen and Stakemann (1963), who reviewed the development of methods for measuring urinary estriol and described reliable procedures that they developed for the estimation of urinary estriol throughout normal human pregnancy. The range of variation in the amount of urinary estriol excreted among different normal pregnant women is great, as illustrated in Figure 7-6. With reliable urine collections and accurate chemical methods, however, Frandsen found that the day-to-day variation of estriol excretion by the same woman was relatively small; in four fifths of the women in his study, there was less than 20 percent day-to-day variation in estriol levels during the last 30 weeks of pregnancy.

The interpretation of "abnormal" levels of urinary or plasma estriol associated with possibly or definitely abnormal pregnancies must be made with caution and with appreciation of several factors:

1. The wide range of normal values for estriol in plasma or urine severely restricts the significance of a single measurement that falls in the "normal range" (Fig. 7-6).
2. In view of the difficulties of accurately ascertaining both duration of gestation and completeness of urine collection, and of eliminating technical errors, a *single measurement that falls considerably outside the "normal range" must be verified.*
3. Restriction of the supply of placental precursors of estriol—as in anencephaly, isolated fetal pituitary ACTH deficiency, or during the administration of potent glucocorticosteroids to the mother—will result in decreased production of placental estriol, independent of placental function.
4. Factors apparently unrelated to the fetoplacental unit may be associated with decreased urinary estriol levels. For example, Taylor and colleagues (1963) found low levels of urinary estriol in women with acute pyelonephritis who subsequently recovered and delivered a healthy infant. Moreover, low levels of estriol are found during the ingestion of certain drugs, including certain antibiotics, phenobarbital, and even aspirin (Castellanos and associates, 1975).
5. Low levels of urinary and plasma estriol have been observed that resulted from a placental deficiency of sulfatase activity (France and Liggins, 1969), a situation that precludes the utilization of the sulfurylated precursors, dehydroisoandrosterone sulfate or 16α-hydroxydehydroisoandrosterone sulfate, for placental estrogen biosynthesis. The infants (all males who later develop the skin disorder ichthyosis) of these pregnancies are apparently normal at birth, but labor may not occur at term and is seemingly difficult to induce in some affected cases.

For these reasons, there is general agreement that a single measurement of the level of urinary estriol may not reliably or accurately reflect the status of the fetoplacental unit. Repeated measurements to confirm the results or to identify a pattern are, therefore, essential.

High rates of excretion of estriol may occur in women with multiple fetuses and in some sensitized Rh-negative women who are pregnant with an erythroblastic fetus (Greene and Touchstone, 1963; Taylor and associates, 1963). It also is theoretically possible that women pregnant with a fetus affected by congenital adrenal hyperplasia will have elevated levels of urinary estriol as a result of the increased production of C_{19}-steroids by the affected fetal adrenal cortex.

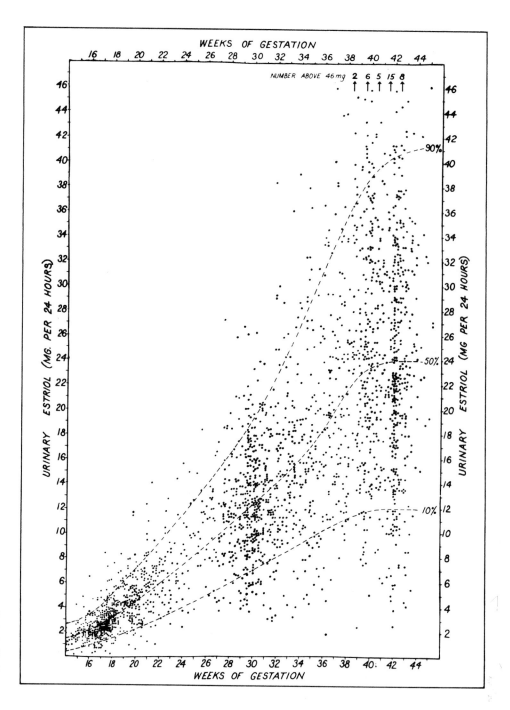

Figure 7-6. Urinary estriol values from 14 weeks of gestation showing 10th, 50th, and 90th percentiles. (*From Beischer et al: Am J Obstet Gynecol 103:483, 1969.*)

Plasma Estriol

In addition to the utilization of urinary estriol levels to monitor high-risk pregnancies, plasma estriol has been similarly employed for the same purpose. Generally, the results of plasma estriol measurements by a variety of techniques, as well as total plasma estrogens, have correlated well with the results of urinary estrogen determinations. Advantages of the utilization of plasma estriol include ease of collection of blood compared with 24-hour urine collections and avoidance of technical difficulties both in the collection and in the processing of urine.

Estetrol

Some interest was directed towards the possible merits of measuring plasma or urinary estetrol to monitor fetal well-being. Estetrol is 15α-hydroxyestriol; two features of this metabolite make it uniquely representative of fetal metabolic function. First, it is derived principally from estriol, the production of which is attributable primarily to the utilization of fetal precursors; and, second, estetrol is produced almost exclusively in the fetus. The 15α-hydroxylation capability of the fetus and requisite for the formation of estetrol is not demonstrable in the maternal compartment. Thus, estetrol represents a compound, the production of which is dependent principally upon fetal precursors and upon fetal metabolism for its finite and final formation. To date, however, the results reported are not supportive of the view that the measurement of estetrol is advantageous over that of estriol determinations in the monitoring of pregnancies in which the fetus may be at high risk.

Clinical Utility

One of the greatest problems in obstetric management today is the proper timing of delivery when complications of a given pregnancy threaten the life or well-being of the fetus. The difficult, but common, problem is to choose between prematurity, on the one hand, and a high risk for the fetus if intrauterine existence in a deteriorating environment is continued, on the other hand. In such situations, notably diabetes mellitus, pregnancy-induced or chronic hypertension, poor previous obstetric history, fetal growth retardation, suspected postmaturity, and others, the need for an accurate index of fetal well-being is urgent. The results of future studies may substantiate the value of measurements of urinary or plasma estriol (or estetrol) as the free, conjugated, or total estriol pool as a guide to obstetric management in these difficult situations. This prospect seems unlikely, however, after so many years of poor experiences. Barnes (1965) emphasized that there is little evidence that therapy based on levels of urinary estriol increase the rate of infant salvage beyond that accomplished by sound clinical judgment alone. Moreover, the results of the only prospective, controlled study reported to date suggest that the measurement of estriol has little or no clinical utility in reducing perinatal mortality or morbidity (Duenhoelter and associates, 1976). Specifically, the results of this study were supportive of the proposition that expert clinical management offers the greatest potential to date for the reduction of perinatal mortality and morbidity and that the measurement of hormones produced by the placenta offers no unique insight into a complicated pregnancy in which the fetus is at high risk.

For these reasons, we do not employ estriol measurements in the management of pregnancies in which the fetus is considered to be at risk. In a study of pregnancies complicated by mild chronic hypertension, Arias and Zamora (1979) also found that estriol measurements were of no utility in the management of such complicated pregnancies. Similarly, Schneider and associates (1978) concluded that 24-hour urinary estriol excretion measured three times per week was of no value in management of postterm pregnancies.

Other investigators who do employ estriol measurements in obstetric management generally agree that the levels of estriol do not always accurately reflect the well-being of the fetus. Hagerman (1979), for example, has written, "It seems likely that the greatest value of the test (plasma estriol) resides in the predictive value of a negative result, which can provide a modest degree of reassurance that the status of the infant is satisfactory. No laboratory test is perfect, and this one is less informative than some. Nevertheless, it is probably as good as, or better than, many other tests used in this area of clinical medicine. The overall classification of correct results with an efficiency of 59 percent is satisfactory. The false-negative rate is disappointingly high." His comments support the need for better tests rather than the perpetuation of some of those that have been used commonly for years even though they are, in fact, of little predictive value.

PROGESTERONE

Site of Production

Progesterone production is accomplished by the placental utilization of maternal lipoprotein-cholesterol in syncytiotrophoblast. Although much more progesterone than estrogen is produced during normal human pregnancy, correspondingly much less was known about its biosynthesis until recently. The placenta produces large amounts of progesterone during pregnancy, and as documented in the review of Diczfalusy and Troen (1961), little production of progesterone takes place in the ovary after the first few weeks of gestation. Surgical removal of the corpus luteum or even bilateral oophorectomy conducted during the seventh to tenth weeks of pregnancy does not result in a decrease in the rate of urinary excretion of pregnanediol, the principal metabolite of progesterone. During normal human pregnancy, there is a gradual increase in the levels of plasma progesterone as well as those of estradiol-17β and estriol, as shown in Figure 7-7.

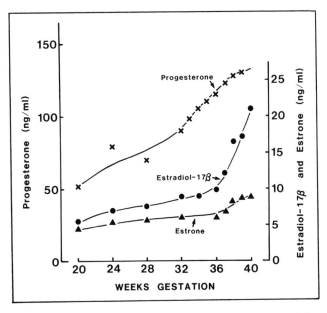

Figure 7-7. Mean plasma levels (± standard error mean) for progesterone, unconjugated estradiol-17β, and unconjugated estriol in 33 normal women during the last 9 weeks before delivery. (*Adapted from Tungsubutra and France, Aust NZ J Obstet Gynaecol, 18:97, 1978. Courtesy Dr. L. Casey.*)

Production Rate

Isotope dilution techniques for the measurement of endogenous rates of hormone production were first applied to the study of progesterone production in pregnancy. The results of these studies, conducted by Pearlman in 1957, indicated that the daily production of progesterone in late pregnancy is about 250 mg. The results of studies in which other methods have been employed are in agreement with that value.

Source of Cholesterol Precursor for Progesterone Biosynthesis

The biosynthetic origin of placental progesterone was an enigma until recently. Solomon and colleagues (1954) demonstrated that in vitro perfusion of the placenta with radiolabeled cholesterol resulted in the formation of radiolabeled progesterone. In addition, incubation of Δ^5-pregnenolone with placental tissue preparations also resulted in the formation of progesterone, and an exceedingly great capacity of the placenta to convert Δ^5-pregnenolone to progesterone has been demonstrated by the in situ placental perfusion studies conducted in Diczfalusy's laboratories.

Although the placenta produces a prodigious amount of progesterone, there is a very limited capacity for the biosynthesis of cholesterol in this organ. The rate of incorporation of radiolabeled acetate into cholesterol by placental tissue proceeds very slowly and the activity of the rate-limiting enzyme in cholesterol biosynthesis, viz., 3-hydroxy-3 methylglutaryl coenzyme A (HMG-CoA) reductase, in placental tissue microsomes is limited.

By in vivo studies, Bloch (1945) and Werbin and co-workers (1957) demonstrated that after the intravenous administration of radiolabeled cholesterol to pregnant women, the specific activity of urinary pregnanediol was similar to that of plasma cholesterol. Hellig and associates (1970) also demonstrated that maternal plasma cholesterol was the principal precursor (up to 90 percent) of progesterone biosynthesis in human pregnancy.

Role of Lipoprotein Cholesterol

In studies similar to those described by use of fetal adrenal tissue, Simpson and associates (for review, see Simpson and MacDonald, 1981) have shown that the placenta preferentially utilizes lipoprotein cholesterol for progesterone biosynthesis. Thus, the formation of placental progesterone, like that of placental estrogens, occurs through the utilization of circulating precursors; unlike estriol, however, which is formed principally from the utilization of fetal adrenal precursors, placental progesterone biosynthesis proceeds by way of the utilization of a maternal precursor, which is taken up in the form of LDL-cholesterol.

These findings not only provide new insights into the biochemical mechanisms of placental progesterone formation, but also may provide insights into other aspects of maternal–placental–fetal physiology. The rate of progesterone secretion may be largely dependent on the number of LDL receptors on the plasma membrane of the trophoblasts and, thereby, primarily independent of uteroplacental blood flow. This holds for several reasons:

1. Cholesterol side-chain cleavage by placental mitochondria is continually in a highly activated state. Some investigators have taken this to mean that the placenta is under constant trophic stimulation and that hCG may be the trophic substance. Indeed, a hierarchy of control of placental hormone production was suggested from the finding of immunoreactive LHRH in placental tissue (Siler-Khodr and Khodr, 1978).
2. De novo cholesterol synthesis by the placenta is very limited.
3. The fetus contributes little or no precursors for placenta progesterone biosynthesis.
4. Maternal levels of LDL-cholesterol should never be rate limiting in the placental assimilation of cholesterol from the maternal circulation.

Importantly, perhaps, the metabolism of LDL by the trophoblasts will result in the hydrolysis of LDL-protein and cholesterol esters. This is an important consideration because such a prodigous amount of LDL is processed each day by the near-term placenta. In fact, it can be computed that the placenta alone may process an amount of LDL-cholesterol equal to the total daily LDL turnover in nonpregnant women. The hydrolysis of the protein component of LDL gives rise to amino acids, many of which are essential amino acids. The hydrolysis of the cholesterol esters of LDL gives rise to cholesterol, which is utilized for progesterone biosynthesis, and to fatty acids. The principal fatty acid of LDL-cholesterol esters is linoleic acid, an essential fatty acid. It seems reasonable to speculate, therefore, that the metabolism of LDL by the trophoblasts constitutes a means of obtaining cholesterol for placental progesterone biosynthesis and a mechanism for sequestering essential fatty acids and amino acids for transport to the fetus. Interestingly, Simpson and Burkhart (1979) also found that progesterone, in concentrations similar to those found in placental tissue, inhibits the activity of the enzyme that catalyzes the esterification of cholesterol. It can be envisioned that this physiologic event will serve to ensure a supply of cholesterol for progesterone biosynthesis by preventing the sequestration of cholesterol into an inappropriate storage form, viz., cholesterol esters, and to protect essential fatty acids from reesterification with cholesterol.

The intimate relationships that exist between the fetus and placenta in the production of estrogen cannot be demonstrated in the case of progesterone. Fetal death, ligation of the umbilical cord in situ, and anencephaly all are conditions associated with very low maternal plasma levels and urinary excretion of estrogens, but a concomitant decrease in plasma levels of progesterone excretion of pregnanediol to anywhere near the same extent does not occur in these situations until some indeterminate time after fetal death.

Secretion of Placental Steroids into the Maternal and Fetal Compartments

The estrogens that are synthesized in trophoblast enter the maternal circulation preferentially. In fact, Gurpide and co-workers (1966) have shown that more than 90 percent of the estradiol-17β and estriol that are formed in the trophoblast are secreted into the maternal compartment. The same is true of progesterone that is formed in the trophoblast. Specifically, Gurpide and co-workers (1972) found that 85 percent or more of the progesterone that is formed in trophoblast enters the maternal compartment, and that very little of the progesterone in the maternal circulation enters the fetus.

Surprisingly, estradiol-17β, and not estrone, preferentially enters the maternal compartment whereas the reverse appears to be true for the fetus (Walsh and McCarthy, 1981; Gurpide and co-workers, 1982). This finding, however, as Gurpide and colleagues point out, may be due to extratrophoblastic conversion of estradiol-17β to estrone in fetal tissues or erythrocytes. Recently, we have discovered an interesting phenomenon with respect to the distribution of trophoblastically formed steroids to the maternal and fetal compartments in pregnancies in which decreased uteroplacental blood flow was suspected. In newborn infants of women with pregnancy-induced hypertension, chronic hypertension, and the more severe forms of diabetes mellitus, the umbilical cord plasma levels of estrogens and progesterone are significantly greater than in newborn infants of normal women. We interpret these findings as follows: By virtue of the nature of the hemochorioendothelial placentation in the human, the vast majority (90 percent or more) of steroids produced in trophoblast enter the maternal intervillous space because maternal blood is directly bathing the syncytiotrophoblast. Nevertheless, with a reduction in blood flow to the intervillous spaces, there may be a relative redistribution of trophoblastic steroid in favor of the fetal compartment and thereby an increase in the concentration of trophoblastically formed steroids in the umbilical vein, even in the face of a decrease in total placental estrogen formation, which, in turn, decreases estrogen levels in the maternal compartment. The validity of this concept may become important in consideration of the role of estrogen in fetal lung maturation, which we know may be accelerated in fetuses of women in whom uteroplacental blood flow is presumed to be reduced (Chapter 8).

REFERENCES

Amoroso EC: Comparative aspects of the hormonal functions. In Villee CA (ed): The Placenta and Fetal Membranes. Baltimore, Williams and Wilkins, 1960, p 3

Anderson RGN, Goldstein JL, Brown MS: Localization of low-density lipoprotein receptors on plasma membranes of normal human fibroblasts and their absence in cells from a familial hypercholesterolemia homozygote. Proc Natl Acad Sci USA 73:2434, 1976

Arias F, Zamora J: Antihypertensive treatment and pregnancy outcome in patients with mild chronic hypertension. Obstet Gynecol 53:489, 1978

Ascheim S, Zondek B: (Anterior pituitary hormone and ovarian hormone in the urine of pregnant women.) Klin Wochensehr 6:248, 1927

Ashitaka Y, Nishimura R, Takemori M, Tojo S: Production and secretion of hCG and hCG subunits by trophoblastic tissue. In Segal S (ed): Chorionic Gonadotropins. New York, Plenum, 1980, p 151

Barnes AC: Discussion of paper by JW Greene. Am J. Obstet Gynecol 91:688, 1965

Baulieu EE, Bricaire H, Jayle MF: Lack of secretion of 17-hydroxycorticosteriods in a pregnant woman with Addison's disease. J Clin Endocrinol 16:690, 1956

Baulieu EE, Dray F: Conversion of H^3-dehydroisoandrosterone (3β-hydroxy-Δ^5-androsten-17-one) sulfate to H^3-estrogens in normal pregnant women. J Clin Endocrinol 23:1298, 1963

Beischer NA, Brown JB, Smith MA, Townsend L: Studies in prolonged pregnancy. II. Clinical results and urinary excretion in prolonged pregnancy. Am J Obstet Gynecol 103:483, 1969

Bloch K: The biological conversion of cholesterol to pregnanediol. J Biol Chem 157:661, 1945

Bolté E, Mancuso S, Eriksson G, Wiqvist N, Diczfalusy E: Studies on the aromatisation of neutral steroids in pregnant women: 1. Aromatisation of C-19 steriods by placenta perfused in situ. Acta Endocrinol 35:535, 1964a

Bolté E, Mancuso S. Eriksson G, Wiqvist N, Diczfalusy E: Studies on the aromatisation of neutral steroids in pregnant women: 2. Aromatisation of dehydroisoandrosterone and of its sulphate administered simultaneously into a uterine artery. Acta Endocrinol 45:560, 1964b

Bolté E, Mancuso S, Eriksson G, Wiqvist N, Diczfalusy E: Studies on the aromatization of neutral steroids in pregnant women: 3. Over-all aromatization of dehydroisoandrosterone sulfate circulating in the foetal and maternal compartments. Acta Endocrinol 45:576, 1964c

Bongiovanni AM, Eberlein WR, Goldman AS, New M: Disorders of adrenal steroid biogenesis. Rec Prog Horm Res 23:375, 1967

Borkowski A, Maquardt C: Human chorionic gonadotropin in the plasma of normal, nonpregnant subjects. N Engl J Med 301:298, 1979

Bradbury JT, Brown WE, Guay LA: Maintenance of the corpus luteum and physiologic action of progesterone. Rec Prog Horm Res 5:151, 1950

Bridson WE, Ross GT, Kohler PO: Immunologic and biologic activity of chorionic gonadotropin synthesized by cloned choriocarcinoma cells in tissue culture. Clin Res 18:356, 1970

Brown JB: Urinary excretion of oestrogens during pregnancy, lactation, and the reestablishment of menstruation. Lancet 1:704, 1956

Carr BR, Simpson ER: Lipoprotein utilization and cholesterol synthesis by the human fetal adrenal gland. Endocrine Reviews 2:306, 1981

Cassmer O: Hormone production of the isolated human placenta. Acta Endocrinol 32(Suppl):45, 1959

Castellanos JM, Aranda M, Cararach J, Cararach V: Effect of aspirin on oestriol excretion in pregnancy. Lancet 1:859, 1975

Claesson L, Hogberg B, Rosenberg T, Westman A: Crystalline human chorionic gonadotropin and its biological action. Acta Endocrinol 1:1, 1948

Colas A, Heinrichs WL, Tatum HJ: Pettenkofer chromogens in the maternal and fetal circulations: Detection of 3β, 16α-dihydroxyandrost-5-en-17-one in umbilical cord blood. Steroids 3:417, 1964

Diczfalusy E, Borell U: Influence of oophorectomy on steroid excretion in early pregnancy. J Clin Endocrinol 21:1119, 1961

Diczfalusy E, Troen P: Endocrine functions of the human placenta. Vit Horm 19:229, 1961

Duenhoelter JH, Whalley PJ, MacDonald PC: An analysis of the utility of plasma immunoreactive estrogen measurements in determining delivery time of gravidas with a fetus considered at high risk. Am J. Obstet Gynecol 125:889, 1976

Edman CD, Toofanian A, MacDonald PC, Gant NF: Placental clearance rate of maternal plasma androstenedione through placental estradiol formation: An indirect method of assessing uteroplacental blood flow. Am J Obstet Gynecol 141:1029, 1981

Faust JR, Goldstein JL, Brown MS: Receptor-mediated uptake of low density lipoprotein and utilization of its cholesterol for steroid synthesis in cultured mouse adrenal cells. J Biol Chem 252:4861, 1977

Fiddes JC, Seeburg PH, DeNoto FM, Hallewell RA, Baxter JD, Goodman HM: Structure of genes for human growth hormone and chorionic somatomammotropin. Proc Natl Acad Sci USA 76:4294, 1979

Fishman J, Brown JB, Hellman L, Zumoff B, Gallagher TF: Estrogen metabolism in normal and pregnant women. J Biol Chem 237:1489, 1961

France JT, Liggins GC: Placental sulfatase deficiency. J Clin Endocrinol 29:138, 1969

Frandsen VA, Stakemann G: The site of production of oestrogenic hormones in human pregnancy: Hormone excretion in pregnancy with anencephalic foetus. Acta Endocrinol 38:383, 1961

Frandsen VA, Stakemann G: The urinary excretion of oestriol during the early months of pregnancy. Acta Endocrinol 44:196, 1963

Gant NF, Hutchinson HT, Siiteri PK, MacDonald PC: Study of the metabolic clearance rate of dehydroisoandrosterone sulfate in pregnancy. Am J. Obstet Gynecol 111:4:555, 1971

Gant NF, Madden JD, Siiteri PK, MacDonald PC: The metabolic clearance rate of dehydroisoandrosterone sulfate. IV. Acute effects of induced hypertension, hypotension, and natriuresis in normal and hypertensive pregnancies. Am J Obstet Gynecol 124:143, 1976

Gey GO, Jones GES, Hellman LM: The production of a gonadotrophic substance (prolan) by placental cells in tissue culture. Science 88:306, 1938

Gibbons JM, Mitnick M, Chieffo V: In vitro biosynthesis of TSH- and LH-releasing factors by human placenta. Am J Obstet Gynecol 121:127, 1975

Goebelsmann U: Middle and late gestation. In Mishell DR, Davajan V (eds): Reproductive Endocrinology, Infertility and Contraception. Philadelphia, Davis, 1979, p 132

Goldstein JL, Brown MS: Binding and degradation of low density lipoproteins by cultured human fibroblasts. J Biol Chem 249:5153, 1974

Greene JW, Touchstone JC: Urinary estriol as an index of placental function. Am J Obstet Gynecol 85:1, 1963

Grumbach MM, Kaplan SL: On placental origin and purification of chorionic growth hormone-prolactin and its immunoassay in pregnancy. Trans NY Acad Sci 27:167, 1964

Gurpide E, Angers M, VandeWiele R, Lieberman S: Determination of secretory rates of estrogens in pregnant and nonpregnant women from the specific activities of urinary metabolites. J Clin Endocrinol 22:935, 1962

Gurpide E, Schwers J, Welch MT, VandeWiele RL, Lieberman S: Fetal and maternal metabolism of estradiol during pregnancy. J Clin Endocrinol Metab 26:1355, 1966

Gurpide E, Tseng J, Escarcena L, Fahning M, Gibson C, Fehr P: Feto-maternal production and transfer of progesterone and uridine in sheep. Am J Obstet Gynecol 113:21, 1971

Hagerman DD: Clinical use of plasma total estriol measurements late in pregnancy. J Reprod Med 23:179, 1979

Hellig HD, Gattereau D, Lefevre Y, Bolté E: Steroid production from plasma cholesterol: I. Conversion of plasma cholesterol to placental progesterone in humans. J Clin Endocrinol Metab 30:624, 1970

Hertz R: Early studies of chorionic gonadotropin and antihormones. In Segal SJ (ed): Chorionic Gonadotropin. New York, Plenum, 1980, p 1

Hirose T: Experimentalle histologische studie fur genese corpus luteum. Mitt ad med Fakultd t Univ Z U Tokyo 23:63, 1919

Hubert C, Descombey D, Mondon F, Daffos F: Plasma human chorionic somatomammotropin deficiency in a normal pregnancy is the consequence of low concentration of messenger RNA coding for human chorionic somatomammotropin. Am J Obstet Gynecol 147:676, 1983

Ito Y, Higashi K: Studies on prolactin-like substance in human placenta. II. Endocrinol Jpn 8:279, 1961

Josimovich JB, MacLaren JA: Presence in human placenta and term serum of highly lactogenic substance immunologically related to pituitary growth hormone. Endocrinology 71:209, 1962

Kaplan SN, Grumbach MM: Chorionic somatomammotropin in primates. In Novy MD, Resko JA (eds): Fetal Endocrinology. New York, Academic, 1983, p 127

Khodr GS, Siler-Khodr TM: Placental luteinizing hormone-releasing factor and its synthesis. Science 207:315, 1980

Klopper A: The new placental proteins: Their role in pregnancy. In Givens JR (ed): Endocrinology of Pregnancy. Chicago, Year Book, 1981, p 203

Krieger DT: Placenta as a source of "brain" and "pituitary hormones". Biol Reprod 26:55, 1982

Li CH, Grumbach MM, Kaplan SL, Josimovich JB, Friesen H, Cati KG: Human chorionic somatomammotropin (HCS), proposed terminology for designation of a placental hormone. Experientia 24:1288, 1968

Liotta A, Osathanondh R, Ryan KJ, Krieger DT: Presence of corticotropin in human placenta: Demonstration of in vitro synthesis. Endocrinology 101:1552, 1977

MacDonald PC, Siiteri PK: The conversion of isotope-labeled dehydroisoandrosterone and dehydroisoandrosterone sulfate to estrogen in normal and abnormal pregnancy. In Paulsen CA (ed): Estrogen Assays in Clinical Medicine. Seattle, University of Washington Press, 1965a, p 251

MacDonald PC, Siiteri PK: Origin of estrogen in women pregnant with an anencephalic fetus. J Clin Invest 44:465, 1965b

Madden JD, Gant NF, MacDonald PC: Studies of the kinetics of conversion of maternal plasma dehydroisoandrosterone sulfate to 16α-hydroxydehydroisoandrosterone sulfate, estradiol and estriol. Am J Obstet Gynecol 132:392, 1976

McGregor WG, Raymoure WJ, Kuhn RW, Jaffe RB: Fetal tissue can synthesize a placental hormone: Evidence for chorionic gonadotropin β-subunit synthesis by human fetal kidney. J Clin Invest 68:306, 1981

Migeon CJ, Keller AT, Holmstrom EG: Dehydroisoandrosterone, androsterone and 17-hydroxycorticosteroid levels in maternal and cord plasma in cases of vaginal delivery. Bull Johns Hopkins Hosp 97:415, 1955

Nichols J, Lescure OL, Migeon CJ: Levels of 17-hydroxycorticosteroids and 17-ketosteroids in maternal and cord plasma in term anencephaly. J Clin Endocrinol 18:444, 1958

Nielsen PV, Pedersen J, Kampmann E-M: Absence of human placental lactogen in an otherwise uneventful pregnancy. Am J Obstet Gynecol 135:322, 1979

Nishula BC, Wehmann R: Distribution, metabolism, and excretion of human chorionic gonadotropin and its subunits in man. In Segal S (ed): Chorionic Gonadotropin. New York, Plenum, 1980, p 199

Odagiri E, Sherrill BJ, Mount CD, Nicholson WE, Orth DN: Human placental immunoreactive corticotropin, lipotropin, and β-endorphin. Evidence for a common precursor. Proc Natl Acad Sci USA 16:2027, 1979

Owerbach D, Martial JA, Baxter JD, Rutler WJ, Shows TB: Genes for growth hormone, chorionic somatomammotropin, and growth hormone-like gene on chromosome 17 in humans. Science 209:289, 1980

Owerbach D, Rutter WJ, Cooke NE, Martial JA, Shows TB: The prolactin gene is located on chromosome 6 in humans. Science 212:815, 1981

Parker CR Jr, Simpson ER, Bilheimer DW, Leveno KJ, Carr BR, MacDonald PC: Inverse relation between low-density lipoprotein-cholesterol and dehydroisoandrosterone sulfate in human fetal plasma. Science 208:512, 1980

Parker CR Jr, Carr BR, Winkel CA, Casey ML, Simpson ER, MacDonald PC: Hypercholesterolemia due to elevated low-density lipoprotein-cholesterol in newborns with anencephaly and adrenal atrophy. J Clin Endocrinol Metab 57:37, 1983a

Parker CR Jr, Carr BR, Simpson ER, MacDonald PC: Decline in the concentration of low-density lipoprotein-cholesterol in human fetal plasma near term. Metabolism 32:919, 1983b

Pearlman WH: (16-³H)Progesterone metabolism in advanced pregnancy and in oophorectomized-hysterectomized women. Biochem J 67:1, 1957

Pitkin RM, Connor WE, Lin DS: Cholesterol metabolism and placental transfer in the pregnant rhesus monkey. J Clin Invest 51:2584, 1972

Pulkkinen MO: Arylsulphatase and the hydrolysis of some steroid sulphates in developing organism and placenta. Acta Physiol Scand 52, Suppl 180, 1961

Reichert FL, Pencharz FI, Simpson ME, Meyer K, Evans HM: Relative ineffectiveness of prolan in hypophysectomized animals. Am J Physiol 100:157, 1932

Robertson JIS, Weir RJ, Dusterdieck GO, Fraser R, Tree M: Renin, angiotensin, and aldosterone in human pregnancy and the menstrual cycle. Scot Med J 16:183, 1971

Ryan KJ: Metabolism of C-16-oxygenated steroids by human placenta: The formation of estriol. J Biol Chem 234:2006, 1959

Schneider JM, Olson RW, Curet LB: Screening for fetal and neonatal risk in the postdate pregnancy. Am J Obstet Gynecol 131:473, 1978

Serra GB, Perez-Palacios G, Jaffe RB: Enhancement of 3β-hydroxysteroid dehydrogenase-isomerase in the human fetal adrenal by removal of the soluble cell fraction. Biochem Biophys Acta 244:186, 1971

Shine J, Seeburg PH, Marial JA, Baxter JD, Goodman HM: Construction and analysis of recombinant DNA for human chorionic somatomammotropin. Nature 270:494, 1977

Siiteri PK, MacDonald PC: The utilization of circulating dehydroisoandrosterone sulfate for estrogen synthesis during human pregnancy. Steroids 2:713, 1963

Siler-Khodr TM, Khodr GS: Content of luteinizing hormone-releasing factor in the human placenta. Am J Obstet Gynecol 130:216, 1978

Siler-Khodr TM: Hypothalamic-like peptides of the placenta. Semin Reprod Endocrinol 1:321, 1983

Simpson ER, MacDonald PC: Endocrine physiology of the placenta. Ann Rev Physiol 43:163, 1981

Simpson ER, Burkhart M: Acyl CoA:cholesterol acyl transferase activity in human placental microsomes: Inhibition by progesterone. Arch Biochem Biophy 200:79, 1980

Simpson ER, Carr BR, Parker CR, Milewich L, Porter JC, MacDonald PC: The role of serum lipoproteins in steriodogenesis by the human fetal adrenal cortex. J Clin Endocrinol Metab 49:164, 1979

Solomon S, Lentz AL, VandeWiele RL, Lieberman S: Pregnenolone as intermediate in the biogenesis of progesterone and the adrenal hormones. Proc Am Chem Soc abstract 29C, 1954

Spellacy WN, Buhi WC: Pituitary growth hormone and placental lactogen levels measured in normal term pregnancy and at the early and late postpartum periods. Am J Obstet Gynecol 105:888, 1969

Taylor ES, Hassner A, Bruns PD, Drose VE: Urinary estriol excretion of pregnant patients with pyelonephritis and Rh isoimmunization. Am J Obstet Gynecol 85:10, 1963

Vaitukaitis JL, Braunstein GD, Ross GT: A radioimmunoassay with specifically measured chorionic gonadotropin in the presence of human luteinizing hormone. Am J Obstet Gynecol 113:751, 1972

Warren JC, Timberlake CE: Steroid sulfatase in the human placenta. J Clin Endocrinol 22:1148, 1962

Weintrab D, Rosen SW: Ectopic production of human chorionic somatomammotropin (HCS) in patients with cancer. Clin Res 18:375, 1970

Werbin H, Plotz EJ, LeRoy GV, David ME: Cholesterol: A precursor of estrone in vivo. J Am Chem Soc 79:1012, 1957

Wide L, Hobson B: Immunological and biological activity of human chorionic gonadotropin in urine and serum of pregnant women and women with a hydatidiform mole. Acta Endocrinol 54:105, 1967

Winters AJ, Colston C, MacDonald PC, Porter JC: Fetal plasma prolactin levels. J Clin Endocrinol Metab 41:626, 1975

Winters AJ, Oliver C, Colston C, MacDonald PC, Porter JC: Plasma ACTH levels in the human fetus and neonate as related to age and parturition. J Clin Endocrinol Metab 39:269, 1974

Worley RJ, Everett RB, Madden JD, MacDonald PC, Gant NF: Fetal considerations. Metabolic clearance rate of maternal plasma dehydroisoandrosterone sulfate. Semin Perinatol 2:15, 1978

Yoshimoto Y, Wolfsen AR, Hirose F, Odell WD: Human chorionic gonadotropin-like material: Presence in normal human tissues. Am J Obstet Gynecol 134:729, 1979

Zondek B: Die hormone des ovariums und des hypophysenvordelappens. Berlin, Springer, 1931

8
The Morphologic and Functional Development of the Fetus

Since World War II, and especially during the last two decades, our knowledge of fetal development, function, and environment has increased remarkably. As an important consequence, the status of the fetus has been elevated to that of a patient who should be given the same meticulous care by the physician that we long have given the pregnant woman. Investigations of the nature of human life in utero have been and will continue to be among the most rewarding in all of biology, and these are of great clinical importance as well. In this chapter, we consider the development of the normal fetus; techniques for identifying fetal well-being, or fetal health, are considered in greater detail in Chapter 14, and anomalies, injuries, and diseases that affect the fetus and newborn infant are addressed in Chapters 37, 38, and 39.

The Embryo and Fetus at Various Times in Pregnancy

The different terms that commonly are used to indicate the duration of pregnancy and, thus, fetal age are somewhat confusing. *Menstrual age* or *gestational age* is estimated from the first day of the last menstrual period, or about 2 weeks before ovulation and fertilization, or nearly 3 weeks before implantation of the fertilized ovum. About 280 days, or 40 weeks, elapse, on average, between the first day of the last menstrual period and delivery of the infant; 280 days correspond to 9⅓ calendar months, or 10 units of 28 days each. The unit of 28 days has been referred to commonly, but imprecisely, as a lunar month of pregnancy; actually, the time from one new moon to the next is 29½ days.

The usual practice for obstetricians is to calculate the gestational age on the basis of menstrual age of a given pregnancy. Embryologists, however, cite events in days or weeks from the time of ovulation (*ovulation age*) or fertilization (*fertilization age*), the latter two being nearly identical. Occasionally, it is of some value to divide the period of gestation into three units of three calendar months each, or *trimesters,* since some important obstetric milestones may be designated conveniently by trimesters. The possibility of spontaneous abortion, for example, is limited principally to the first

trimester of pregnancy, whereas the likelihood of survival of the prematurely born infant is confined, with some exceptions, to pregnancies that reach the third trimester.

A short description of various periods of development of the ovum and embryo is presented. For a more detailed description, based on Streeter's (1920) timetables of human development ("Horizons"), the reader is referred to the text by Hamilton and Mossman (1972).

The Ovum. During the first 2 weeks from the time of ovulation, there are several successive phases of development that are identified as follow: (1) ovulation, (2) fertilization of the ovum, (3) formation of free blastocyst (the events of the first week after ovulation are illustrated diagrammatically in Figure 8-1), and (4) implantation of the blastocyst, a process that begins at the end of the first week after ovulation. Primitive chorionic villi begin to form after implantation. It is conventional to refer to the products of conception after the development of chorionic villi not as a fertilized ovum but as an embryo. The early stages of preplacental development are discussed in Chapter 5 and the formation of the placenta in Chapter 6.

The Embryo. The beginning of the embryonic period is taken as the beginning of the third week after ovulation, or the fifth week after the onset of the last menstrual period, and coincides in time with the expected time of menstruation. Most pregnancy tests in clinical use usually are positive by this time (see Chapter 10, p. 213). The embryonic disc is well defined and the body stalk is differentiated. At this stage, the chorionic sac measures approximately 1 cm in diameter (Figs. 8-2, 8-3). The chorionic villi at this time are distributed equally around the circumference of the chorionic sac. There is a true intervillous space that contains maternal blood and villous cores in which there is angioblastic chorionic mesoderm.

By the end of the fourth week *after ovulation,* the chorionic sac measures 2 to 3 cm in diameter, and the embryo about 4 to 5 mm in length (Fig. 8-4). The heart and pericardium are very prominent because of the dila-

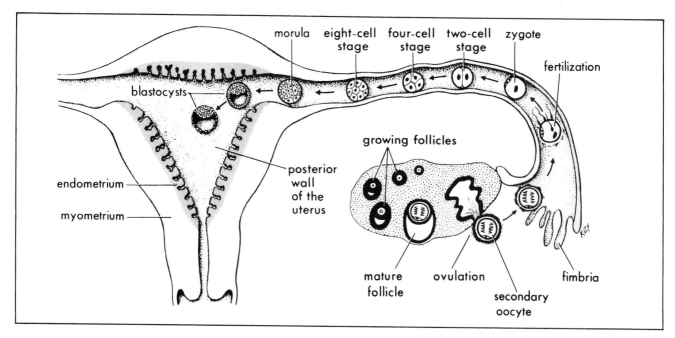

Figure 8-1. Diagrammatic summary of the ovarian cycle, fertilization, and human development during the first week. Developmental stage 1 begins with fertilization and ends when the zygote forms. Stage 2 (days 2 to 3) comprises the early stages of cleavage (from 2 to about 16 cells, or the morula). Stage 3 (days 4 to 5) consists of the free unattached blastocyst. Stage 4 (days 5 to 6) is represented by the blastocyst attaching to the center of the posterior wall of the uterus, the usual site of implantation. (*From Moore: The Developing Human, 3rd ed. Philadelphia, Saunders, 1982.*)

tation of the chambers of the heart. Arm and leg buds are present, and the amnion is beginning to ensheath the body stalk, which thereafter becomes the umbilical cord.

At the end of the sixth week from the time of ovulation, or about 8 weeks after the onset of the last menstrual period, the embryo is 22 to 24 mm in length, and the head is quite large compared with the trunk. Fingers and toes are present, and the external ears form definitive elevations on either side of the head.

The end of the embryonic period and the beginning of the fetal period are arbitrarily considered by most em-

bryologists to occur 8 weeks after ovulation, or 10 weeks after the onset of the last menstrual period. At this time, the embryo is nearly 4 cm long. Few, if any, new major structures are formed thereafter; development during the fetal period of gestation consists of growth and maturation of structures that were formed during the embryonic period.

Three Lunar Months. By the end of the 12th week of pregnancy by menstrual age, or 10 weeks since ovulation, the crown–rump length of the fetus is 6 to 7 cm (Figs.

Figure 8-2. Early human embryos. Only the chorion adjacent to the body stalk is shown. Small outline to right of each embryo gives its actual size. Ovulation ages: **A.** Carnegie collection (presomite), 19 days. **B.** (7 somites), 21 days. **C.** (17 somites), 22 days. (*After drawings and models in the Carnegie Institution.*)

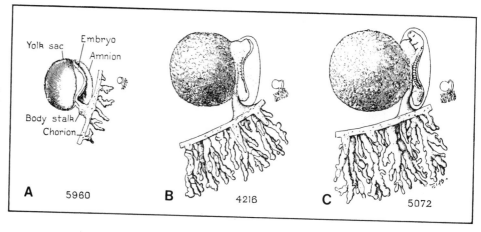

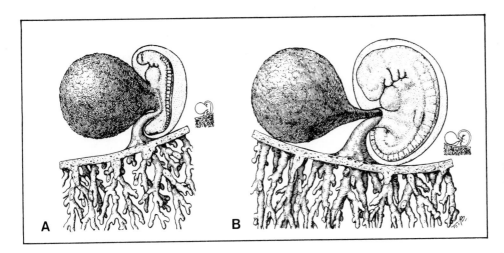

Figure 8-3. Early human embryos. Small outline to right of each embryo gives its actual size. Ovulation ages: **A.** 22 days. **B.** 23 days. (*After drawings and models in the Carnegie Institution.*)

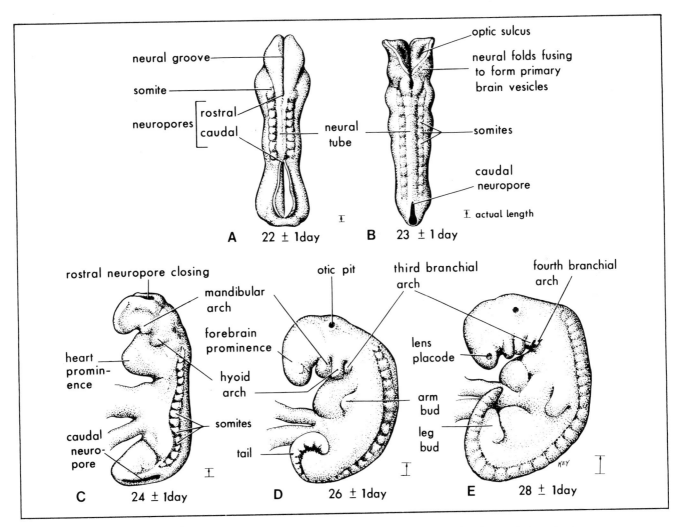

Figure 8-4. Three- to four-week-old embryos. **A, B.** dorsal views of embryos during stage 10 of development (about 22 to 23 days) showing 8 and 12 somites, respectively. **C, D, E.** lateral views of embryos during stages 11, 12, and 13 of development (24 to 28 days), showing 16, 27, and 33 somites, respectively. (*From Moore: The Developing Human, 3rd ed. Philadelphia, Saunders, 1982.*)

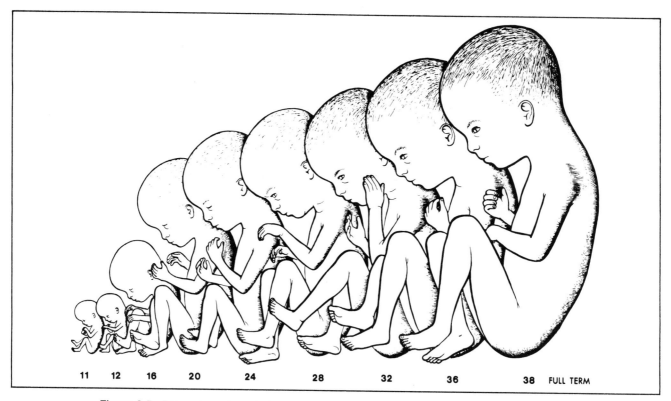

11   12   16   20   24   28   32   36   38   FULL TERM

Figure 8-5. The embryonic period ends at the point of the eighth week after fertilization; by this time, the beginnings of all essential structures are present. The fetal period, extending from the ninth week until birth, is characterized by growth and elaboration of structures. Sex is clearly distinguishable by 12 weeks. (*From Moore: The Developing Human, 3rd ed. Philadelphia, Saunders, 1982.*)

8-5, 8-6), and by this time the uterus usually is palpable just above the symphysis pubis. Centers of ossification have appeared in most bones, the fingers and toes have become differentiated and are provided with nails, scattered rudiments of hair appear, and the external genitalia are beginning to show definite signs of male or female sex. A fetus born at this time may make spontaneous movements if still within the amnionic sac or if immersed in warm saline.

Four Lunar Months. By the end of the 16th week, by menstrual age, the crown–rump length of the fetus is 12 cm, and it weighs about 110 g. By careful examination of the external genital organs, the sex of the fetus can be identified.

Five Lunar Months. The end of the fifth lunar month, or 20 weeks, is the midpoint of pregnancy or gestation, as estimated from the onset of the last normal menstrual

Figure 8-6. Sketches showing methods of measuring the length of embryos. **A.** Greatest length. **B, C.** Crown–rump length. **D.** Crown–heel length. (*From Moore: The Developing Human, 3rd ed. Philadelphia, Saunders, 1982.*)

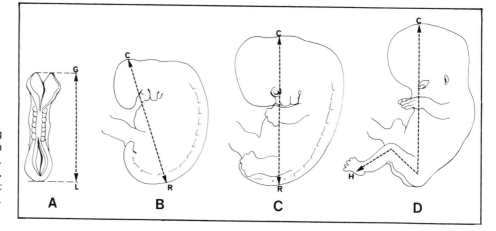

A   B   C   D

period. The fetus now weighs somewhat more than 300 g. The skin has become less transparent, a downy lanugo covers its entire body, and some scalp hair is visible.

Six Lunar Months. By the end of the 24th week, the fetus weighs about 650 g. The skin is characteristically wrinkled, and fat is deposited beneath it. The head is comparatively still quite large; eyebrows and eyelashes usually are recognizable. A fetus born at this period will attempt to breathe, but almost always dies shortly after birth.

Seven Lunar Months. By the end of the 28th week after the onset of the last menstrual period, a crown–rump length of about 25 cm is attained and the fetus weighs about 1100 g. The thin skin is red and covered with vernix caseosa. The pupillary membrane has just disappeared from the eyes. An infant born at this time in gestation moves his limbs quite energetically and cries weakly. The infant, with expert care, may survive.

Eight Lunar Months. At the end of the eighth lunar month, or 32 weeks, the fetus has attained a crown–rump length of about 28 cm and a weight of about 1800 g. The surface of the skin is still red and wrinkled. Infants born at this period, with proper care, usually survive.

Nine Lunar Months. At the end of 36 weeks gestation, the average crown–rump length of the fetus is about 32 cm and the weight is about 2600 g. Because of the deposition of subcutaneous fat, the body has become more rotund and the previous wrinkled appearance of the face is lost. Infants born at this time have an excellent chance of survival with proper care.

Ten Lunar Months. Term is reached at 10 lunar months, or 40 weeks after the onset of the last menstrual period. At this time the fetus is fully developed, with the characteristic features of the newborn infant to be described here. The average crown–rump length of the fetus at term is about 36 cm, and the weight is approximately 3400 g, with variations to be discussed subsequently and plotted in Figure 37-1.

Length of Fetus

Because of the variability in the length of the legs and the difficulty of maintaining them in extension, measurement of the sitting height (crown to rump) is more accurate than that of the standing height (Fig. 8-5). The average sitting height and weight of the fetus at the end of each lunar month were ascertained by Streeter (1920) from 704 specimens and still are similar to those found more recently, as shown in Table 8-1. Such values are approximate; generally, however, the length is a more

TABLE 8-1. CRITERIA FOR ESTIMATING AGE DURING THE FETAL PERIOD

Age (Weeks)		CR Length (mm)*	Foot Length (mm)*	Fetal Weight (g)†	Main External Characteristics
Menstrual	Fertilization				
11	9	50	7	8	Eyes closing or closed. Head more rounded. External genitalia still not distinguishable as male or female. Intestines are in the umbilical cord.
12	10	61	9	14	Intestine in abdomen. Early fingernail development.
14	12	87	14	45	Sex distinguishable externally. Well-defined neck.
16	14	120	20	110	Head erect. Lower limbs well developed.
18	16	140	27	200	Ears stand out from head.
20	18	160	33	320	Vernix caseosa present. Early toenail development.
22	20	190	39	460	Head and body (lanugo) hair visible.
24	22	210	45	630	Skin wrinkled and red.
26	24	230	50	820	Fingernails present. Lean body.
28	26	250	55	1000	Eyes partially open. Eyelashes present.
30	28	270	59	1300	Eyes open. Good head of hair. Skin slightly wrinkled.
32	30	280	63	1700	Toenails present. Body filling out. Testes descending.
34	32	300	68	2100	Fingernails reach finger tips. Skin pink and smooth.
38	36	340	79	2900	Body usually plump. Lanugo hairs almost absent. Toenails reach toe tips.
40	38	360	83	3400	Prominent chest; breasts protrude. Testes in scrotum or palpable in inguinal canals. Fingernails extend beyond finger tips.

* These measurements are averages and so may not apply to specific cases; dimensional variations increase with age. The method for taking CR (crown–rump) measurements is illustrated in Figure 8-5.B.

† These weights refer to fetuses that have been fixed for about two weeks in 10 percent formalin. Fresh specimens usually weigh about 5 percent less.

(*From Moore: The Developing Human, 2nd ed. Philadelphia, Saunders, 1977.*)

accurate criterion of the age of a fetus than is the weight.

Haase (1875) suggested that, for clinical purposes, the length in centimeters of the fetus measured from crown to heel may be approximated during the first 5 months by squaring the number of the lunar month to which the pregnancy has advanced and, in the second half of pregnancy, by multiplying the month by 5.

Weight of the Newborn

The average term infant at birth weighs about 3000 to 3600 g, depending upon race, parental economic status, size of the parents, and parity of the mother, with boys about 100 g (3 ounces) heavier than girls (Fig. 37-1). From the observations of Gruenwald (1967) and other investigators, it is established that during the second half of pregnancy the fetal weight increases in a linear manner with time until about the 37th week of gestation, and then it slows in rate variably. Gruenwald emphasized that the principal determinants of the extent to which fetal growth late in pregnancy departs from the previously linear pattern are related in large part to the socioeconomic status of the mother. In general, the greater the socioeconomic deprivation, the slower the rate of fetal growth late in pregnancy.

Birth weights over 5000 g occur occasionally, but most tales of huge babies vastly exceeding this figure are based on hearsay and inaccurate measurements at best. Presumably, the largest baby recorded in the medical literature is that described by Belcher (1916), a stillborn female weighing 11,340 g (25 pounds). In spite of these exceptional cases of macrosomia, extreme skepticism is justified in accepting reports concerning phenomenally heavy newborns. Term infants, however, frequently weigh less than 3200 g and sometimes as little as 2250 g (5 pounds) or even less. In the past, it was customary, when the birth weight was 2500 g or less, to classify the infant as premature even though in some instances the low birth weight was not the consequence of prematurity but rather was due to growth retardation.

The many factors intimately involved in fetal growth are considered further in this chapter in the sections on placental transfer and fetal nutrition (pp. 145, 167), as well as in Chapters 13 and 37.

Fetal Head

Obstetrically, the head of the fetus is a most important part, since an essential feature of labor is the adaptation between the fetal head and the maternal bony pelvis. Only a comparatively small part of the head of the fetus at term is represented by the face; the rest is composed of the firm skull, which is made up of two frontal, two parietal, and two temporal bones, along with the upper portion of the occipital bone and the wings of the sphenoid. These bones are not united rigidly, but rather are separated by membranous spaces, the *sutures* (Fig. 8-7). The most important sutures are the *frontal,* between the two frontal bones, the *sagittal,* between the two parietal bones, the two *coronals,* between the frontal and parietal bones, and the two *lambdoids,* between the posterior margins of the parietal bones and upper margin of the occipital bone. With vertex presentation, all the sutures are palpable during labor, except the *temporal* sutures, which are situated on either side between the inferior margin of the parietal and upper margin of the temporal bones, are covered by soft parts and cannot be felt in the living fetus.

Where several sutures meet, an irregular space forms, which is enclosed by a membrane and designated a *fontanel* (Fig. 8-7). Three such structures usually are distinguished, namely, the greater, the lesser, and the temporal fontanels. The *greater,* or *anterior, fontanel* is a lozenge-shaped space situated at the junction of the sagittal and the coronal sutures. The *lesser,* or *posterior, fontanel* is represented by a small triangular area at the intersection of the sagittal and lambdoid sutures. Both may be felt readily during labor, and the localization of these fontanels gives important information concerning the presentation and position of the fetus. The *temporal,* or *casserian,* fontanels, situated at the junction of the lambdoid and temporal sutures, have no diagnostic significance.

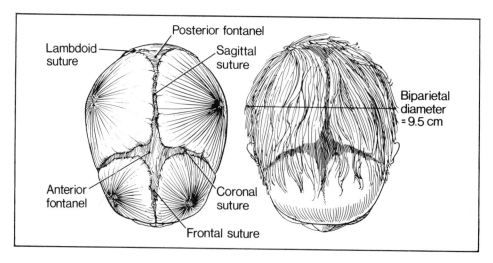

Figure 8-7. Fetal head at term showing various fontanels, sutures, and diameter.

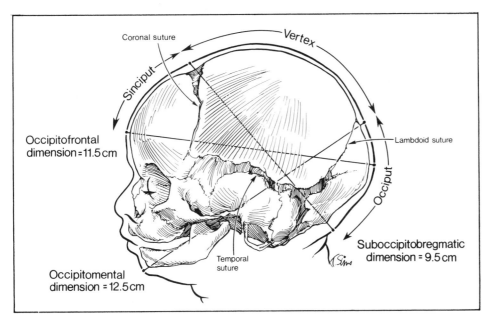

Figure 8-8. Diameters of the fetal head at term.

It is customary to measure certain critical *diameters* (Fig. 8-8) and *circumferences* of the infant's head. The diameters most frequently used and the average lengths thereof are:

1. The *occipitofrontal* (11.5 cm), which follows a line extending from a point just above the root of the nose to the most prominent portion of the occipital bone.
2. The *biparietal* (9.5 cm), the greatest transverse diameter of the head, which extends from one parietal boss to the other.
3. The *bitemporal* (8.0 cm), the greatest distance between the two temporal sutures.
4. The *occipitomental* (12.5 cm), from the chin to the most prominent portion of the occiput.
5. The *suboccipitobregmatic* (9.5 cm), which follows a line drawn from the middle of the large fontanel to the undersurface of the occipital bone just where it joins the neck (Figs. 8-7, 8-8).

The greatest circumference of the head, which corresponds to the plane of the occipitofrontal diameter, averages 34.5 cm, and the smallest circumference, corresponding to the plane of the suboccipitobregmatic diameter, is 32 cm. As a rule, white infants have larger heads than do nonwhite infants, boys somewhat larger than girls, and the infants of multiparas larger heads than those of nulliparas.

Because of the widely varying mobility between the bones of the skull at the sutures, fetal heads differ appreciably in adaptation to the maternal pelvis by *molding.* The bones of the calvarium of one fetus may be soft and readily molded, whereas those of another are firmly ossified, only slightly mobile, and therefore incapable of allowing a significant reduction in the dimensions of the fetal head.

Fetal Brain

As pregnancy advances, the fetal brain changes remarkably in appearance, as well as in function (Fig. 8-9). Therefore, it is possible to identify fetal age rather precisely from the external appearance of the brain (Dolman, 1977).

PLACENTAL TRANSFER

General Concepts

A major function of the placenta is to transfer oxygen and a great variety of nutrients from the mother to the fetus and, conversely, convey carbon dioxide and other metabolic wastes from fetus to mother. To appreciate the complexity of the placenta as an organ of transfer, it is necessary only to consider that the placenta, and to a limited extent the attached membranes, supply all material for fetal growth and energy production while removing all products of fetal catabolism.

There are no continuous direct communications between the fetal blood in the vessels of the chorionic villi and the maternal blood in the intervillous space. Throughout most of pregnancy, nearly all the erythrocytes in the fetal circulation can be shown to be rich in fetal hemoglobin, whereas only rarely does an erythrocyte in the maternal circulation contain fetal hemoglobin. The one exception to this generalization regarding the independence of the circulations is the development of occasional breaks in the chorionic villi, permitting the escape of varying numbers of fetal erythrocytes into the maternal circulation (see Chapter 6, p. 111). This leakage is the clinically significant mechanism by which some Rh negative women become sensitized by the erythrocytes of their Rh positive fetus (see Chapter 38, p. 774). These occasional leaks, however, do not controvert the

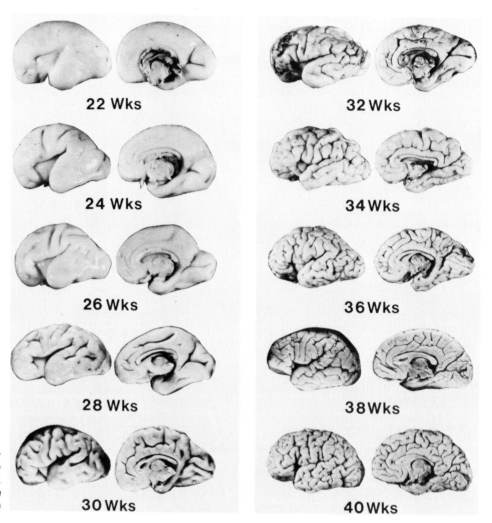

Figure 8-9. Characteristic configuration of fetal brains from 22 to 40 weeks of gestation at 2-week intervals. (*From Dolman: Arch Pathol Lab Med 101:193, 1977.*)

basic principle that no *gross* intermingling of the macromolecular constituents of the two circulations occurs. The transfer of substances from mother to fetus and from fetus to mother, therefore, depends primarily on the mechanisms that permit the transport of such substances through the intact chorionic villus.

At least nine variables determine the effectiveness of the human placenta as an organ of transfer:

1. The concentration in the maternal plasma of the substance under consideration and in some instances the extent to which it is bound to another compound.
2. The rate of maternal blood flow through the intervillous space.
3. The area available for exchange across the villous epithelium.
4. In case the substance is transferred by diffusion, the physical properties of the tissue barrier, interposed between blood in the intervillous space and blood in the fetal capillaries.
5. For any substance actively transported, the capacity of the biochemical machinery of the placenta for effecting active transfer.

6. The amount of the substance metabolized by the placenta during transfer.
7. The area for exchange across the fetal capillaries in the placenta.
8. The concentration in the fetal blood of the substance, exclusive of any that is bound.
9. The rate of fetal blood flow through the villous capillaries.

Unfortunately, in human pregnancy many of these processes cannot be measured accurately in either the mother or the fetus. In recent years, however, techniques have been developed for doing so in experimental animals.

The Intervillous Space

The intervillous space functions as the depot from which materials are transferred, either passively or actively, through the chorionic epithelium to the fetal vessels, and where substances from the fetus enter the maternal circulation. Since this process of transfer supplies the fetus with oxygen as well as nutriment and provides for elimination of metabolic waste products in addition, the chorionic villi and the intervillous space, together, function for the fetus as a lung, gastrointestinal tract, and kidney.

The circulation of maternal blood within the intervillous space has been considered in detail in Chapter 6. The residual volume of the intervillous space of the delivered term placenta measures about 140 ml; however, the normal volume of the intervillous space before delivery is probably twice this value (Aherne and Dunnill, 1966). Uteroplacental blood flow near term has been estimated to be about 600 ml per minute, with most of the blood apparently going through the intervillous space. Although much remains to be learned about the hemodynamics of the intervillous space even in normal pregnancy, on the basis of a variety of animal studies, as well as clinical observations made in women, the following conclusions can be drawn: Uterine contractions reduce blood flow through the intervillous space, the degree of reduction depending in large part upon the intensity of the contraction. Blood pressure within the intervillous space is significantly less than uterine arterial pressure but somewhat greater than uterine venous pressure. Uterine venous pressure, in turn, varies depending upon several factors, including posture. When the mother is supine, for example, pressure in the lower part of the inferior vena cava is elevated; consequently, in this circumstance, pressure in the uterine and ovarian veins and, in turn, the intervillous space, is elevated. An even greater increase in intervillous pressure is likely when the mother stands.

The hydrostatic pressure in the capillaries of the chorionic villi is probably not appreciably different from that in the intervillous space. During normal labor, the rise in fetal blood pressure must parallel the pressure in the amnionic fluid and the intervillous space. Otherwise, the capillaries in the chorionic villi would collapse and fetal blood flow through the placenta would cease.

Chorionic Villus

Substances that pass from the maternal blood to the fetal blood must traverse trophoblast, stroma, and fetal capillary wall. These layers would have a minimal aggregate thickness of 3 to 6 μm, according to Wislocki (1955). Although the histologic "barrier" separates the maternal and fetal circulations, it does not behave uniformly like a simple physical barrier, because throughout pregnancy it either actively or passively permits, facilitates, and adjusts the amount and rate of transfer of a wide range of substances to the fetus. Certain histologic alterations in the villus with advancing pregnancy appear to enhance placental permeability. As the duration of pregnancy increases, the prominence of Langhans cells, or cytotrophoblast, decreases and the villous epithelium consists predominantly of syncytiotrophoblast. The walls of the villous capillaries likewise become thinner, and the relative number of fetal vessels increases in relation to the villous connective tissue.

Several attempts have been made to estimate the total surface area of chorionic villi in the human pla-

centa at term. The planimetric measurements made by Aherne and Dunnill (1966) of the villous surface area of the placenta closely correlated with fetal weight. They calculated that the total surface area at term was approximately 10 square meters.

Transfer by Diffusion

Most substances with a molecular weight less than 500 can diffuse readily through the placental tissue interposed between the maternal and fetal circulations. Molecular weight clearly has a bearing on the rate of transfer by diffusion; all other things being equal, the smaller the molecule, the more rapid is the rate. Diffusion, however, is by no means the only mechanism of transfer of compounds with a low molecular weight. The placenta actually facilitates the transfer of a variety of such compounds, especially those that are in low concentration in maternal plasma but are essential for the rapid growth of the fetus.

Simple diffusion appears to be the mechanism involved in the transfer of oxygen, carbon dioxide, and water, and most but not all electrolytes. Anesthetic gases also pass through the placenta rapidly and do so apparently by simple diffusion.

Insulin, steroid hormones from the adrenal, and hormones from the thyroid may cross the placenta but do so at very slow rates. The hormones synthesized by the placenta enter both the maternal and fetal circulations but not necessarily to the same degree. For example, the concentrations of chorionic gonadotropin and placental lactogen are appreciably lower in fetal plasma than in maternal plasma. Substances of very high molecular weight do not usually traverse the placenta, but there are pronounced exceptions, such as immune γ-globulin G (IgG) with a molecular weight of about 160,000.

Transfer of Oxygen and Carbon Dioxide. Normal values for oxygen, carbon dioxide, and pH in maternal and fetal blood, as calculated by Longo (1972), are presented in Table 8-2. Because of the continuous passage of oxygen from the maternal blood in the intervillous

TABLE 8-2. NORMAL VALUES FOR OXYGEN, CARBON DIOXIDE, AND pH IN HUMAN MATERNAL AND FETAL BLOOD

	Uterine		Umbilical	
	Artery	Vein	Vein	Artery
Po_2 (mm Hg)	95	40	27	15
O$_2$Hb (percent saturation)	98	76	68	30
O$_2$ content (ml/dl)	15.8	12.2	14.5	6.4
Hemoglobin (g/dl)	12.0	12.0	16.0	16.0
O$_2$ capacity (ml O$_2$/dl)	16.1	16.1	21.4	21.4
Pco_2 (mm Hg)	32	40	43	48
CO$_2$ content (mM/L)	19.6	21.8	25.2	26.3
HCO$_3$ (mM/L)	18.8	20.7	24.0	25.0
pH	7.40	7.34	7.38	7.35

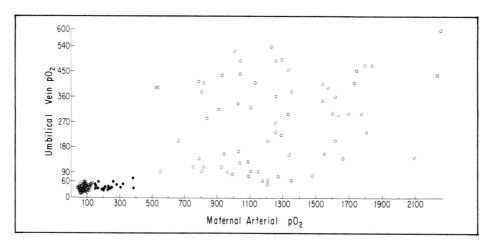

Figure 8-10. Changes in umbilical vein blood Po_2 during progressively increasing maternal blood Po_2. Note that when the maternal blood Po_2 was raised to about 300 mm Hg by ventilating the maternal lungs with 100 percent oxygen (*black dots*), umbilical vein blood Po_2 remained below 60 mm Hg. This illustrates the boundary imposed on fetal oxygenation. Only when maternal blood Po_2 was increased by hyperbaric oxygenation (*open circles*) did the fetal blood Po_2 increase to high levels. (*From Assali: In Gluck (ed): Modern Perinatal Medicine. Chicago, Year Book, 1974.*)

space to the fetus, the oxygen saturation of this blood resembles that in the maternal capillaries and is less than that of the mother's arterial blood. The average oxygen saturation of intervillous space blood is estimated to be 65 to 75 percent, with a partial pressure (Po_2) of about 30 to 35 mm Hg. The oxygen saturation of umbilical vein blood is similar, but with an oxygen partial pressure somewhat lower. In the estimations reported for the Po_2 of blood from the intervillous space, inconsistently high or low figures are often encountered, suggesting that if the needle is actually in the intervillous space, the blood is not thoroughly mixed. If the needle or electrode were placed at a point where it is bathed by a jet of arterial blood into the intervillous space, the estimate of oxygen saturation becomes falsely high, whereas the reverse holds if the needle or electrode is placed at a location where the circulation is relatively sluggish. The collection of umbilical venous or arterial blood at delivery that is truly representative of the oxygenation in utero is also fraught with errors.

Despite the relatively low Po_2, the fetus does not normally suffer from lack of oxygen. The human fetus probably behaves like the lamb fetus, which has a cardiac output considerably greater per unit of body weight than does the adult. The high cardiac output and, late in pregnancy, the increased oxygen-carrying capacity of fetal blood as the consequence of fetal hemoglobin and a higher hemoglobin concentration compensate effectively for the low oxygen tension. Both of these mechanisms are considered further in this chapter in the sections on Fetal Circulation and Fetal Blood. Additional evidence that the fetus does not normally experience lack of oxygen is supplied by measurement of the lactic acid content of fetal blood, which is only slightly higher than that of the mother.

Assali and co-workers (1968b, 1974) were able to raise the Po_2 in the umbilical vein of the lamb fetus by 10 mm Hg when the mother breathed 100 percent oxygen at atmospheric pressure. They detected no fall in uteroplacental or umbilical blood flow in response to 100 percent oxygen. When the ewe breathed hyperbaric oxygen that raised the maternal arterial Po_2 to 1300 mm Hg, uteroplacental blood flow did not change and umbilical flow decreased only slightly, although the Po_2 in umbilical blood rose to nearly 600 mm Hg (Fig. 8-10). With normally functioning maternal and fetal circulations, therefore, oxygen can be delivered across the placenta, at least to the fetus of the sheep, under increased tension and without remarkably restricting umbilical blood flow. Employing the usual clinical equipment for providing oxygen to the mother, the increase is modest, however.

There are no precise measurements of the ability of the human fetus to withstand severe hypoxia. Myers (1970) measured the tolerance of the brain of the monkey fetus to hypoxia induced by cord compression with complete cessation of flow. The rates at which bradycardia, hypotension, and acidosis developed varied with gestational age—the more mature the fetus, the more rapid the rate of deterioration.

In general, the transfer of carbon dioxide from the fetus to the mother obeys the same laws as those described for oxygen, although carbon dioxide traverses the chorionic villus more rapidly than does oxygen. Near term, the partial pressure of carbon dioxide in the umbilical arteries is estimated to average about 48 mm Hg, or about 5 mm or so more than in the maternal blood in the intervillous space. Fetal blood has somewhat less affinity for carbon dioxide than does the blood of the mother, thereby favoring the transfer of carbon dioxide from the fetus to the mother. Also, mild hyperventilation by the pregnant woman results in a fall in P_{CO_2}, favoring a transfer of CO_2 from the fetal compartment into the blood of the gravida.

Selective Transfer

Although diffusion is an important method of placental transfer, the chorionic villus exhibits enormous selectivity in transfer, maintaining different concentrations of a variety of metabolites on the two sides of the villus. One example of this selectivity is in the transfer of the two isomers of histidine, as demonstrated by Page (1957). D-Histidine, the unnatural isomer, traverses the placenta more slowly, coming to equilibrium with the fetal blood within 3 or 4 hours. If only passive transfer by simple diffusion were involved, L-histidine, the natural isomer, would be expected to behave similarly, but in the case of this isomer, equilibrium is attained within a few minutes. The concentrations of a number of substances that are not synthesized by the fetus are several times higher in fetal than in maternal blood. Ascorbic acid is a good example of this phenomenon. This crystalline substance of relatively low molecular weight chemically resembles the pentose and hexose sugars and might be expected to traverse the placenta by simple diffusion. The concentration of ascorbic acid, however, is two to four times higher in fetal plasma than in maternal plasma (Braestrup, 1937; Manahan and Eastman, 1938). The unidirectional transfer of iron across the placenta provides another example of the unique capabilities of the human placenta for transport. Typically, iron is present in the plasma at a lower concentration in the gravida than in the fetus, and, at the same time, the iron-binding capacity of the plasma is much greater in the pregnant woman than in the fetus. Nonetheless, iron is transported actively from maternal to fetal plasma, and in the human fetus the amount transferred appears to be independent of maternal iron status (Pritchard, unpublished).

Intrauterine infections caused by viruses, bacteria, and protozoa are occasionally encountered. Many viruses, including those responsible for rubella, chickenpox, measles, mumps, smallpox, vaccinia, poliomyelitis, cytomegalic inclusion disease, coxsackie virus disease, and western equine encephalitis, may cross the placenta and infect the fetus. *Treponema pallidum, Toxoplasma,* and *Plasmodium* species, and *Mycobaterium tuberculosis* may similarly produce intrauterine infection. With protozoal and bacterial, but not necessarily viral, infections, there is almost always histologic evidence of involvement of the placenta.

Rarely, malignancies in the pregnant woman can be transferred to the placenta and to the fetus. Approximately 50 percent of these are malignant melanomas or hematopoietic in origin (Read and Platzer, 1981).

PHYSIOLOGY OF THE FETUS

Fetal Circulation

Since practically all materials needed for growth and maintenance are brought to the fetus from the placenta by the umbilical vein, the fetal circulation must differ fundamentally from that of the adult (Fig. 8-11). The single umbilical vein in the umbilical cord carries oxygenated, nutriment-bearing blood from the placenta to the fetus. The *umbilical vein* enters the fetus through the umbilical ring and ascends along the anterior abdominal wall to the liver. The vein then divides into the portal sinus and the ductus venosus, the former carrying blood to the hepatic veins primarily of the left side of the liver and the latter or major "branch" of the umbilical vein traversing the liver to enter directly the *inferior vena cava*. The blood flowing to the fetal heart from the inferior vena cava, therefore, consists of an admixture of oxygenated blood that passes through the ductus venosus and less well oxygenated blood that collects from most of the veins below the level of the diaphragm. As a consequence, the oxygen content of blood delivered to the heart from the inferior vena cava is decreased with respect to that leaving the placenta, but it is greater than that from the superior vena cava.

As emphasized by Dawes (1962), the *foramen ovale* opens directly off the inferior vena cava so that blood from the inferior vena cava is, for the most part, immediately deflected by the crista dividens through the foramen ovale into the left atrium. Little or none of the less well oxygenated blood from the *superior vena cava* normally passes through the foramen ovale. The preferential flow of blood from the inferior vena cava through the foramen ovale to the left atrium bypasses the right ventricle and pulmonary circulation and permits delivery of more highly oxygenated blood to the left ventricle than if complete admixture had occurred in the right atrium. The more highly oxygenated blood that passes through the foramen ovale and is ejected from the left ventricle perfuses two vital organs, the heart and the brain. The blood that is typically venous in character, coming from the superior vena cava and ejected from the right ventricle into the pulmonary trunk, is, for the most part, shunted through the *ductus arteriosus* into the descending aorta. Only about one third of the blood goes through the lungs.

The lamb fetus has been studied intensively by several groups of investigators who believe that the circulatory function of the mature lamb fetus is similar in many respects to that of the mature human fetus. Before birth, in man and in sheep, both ventricles of the fetal heart, as the consequence of the shunts just described, work in parallel rather than in series. Attempts to measure cardiac output in the lamb fetus have yielded somewhat variable results. Assali (1974) and associates (1968a) have ascertained a mean value of about 225 ml/kg per minute but with considerable individual variation; Paton

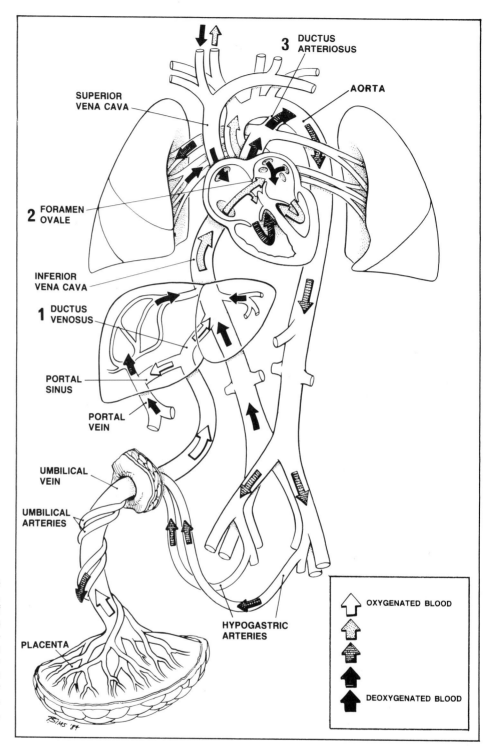

Figure 8-11. The intricate nature of the fetal circulation is evident. The degree of oxygenation of blood in various vessels differs appreciably from that in the postnatal state as the consequences of oxygenation being provided by the placenta rather than the lungs and the presence of three major vascular shunts: **1.** Ductus venosus. **2.** Foramen ovale. **3.** Ductus arteriosus.

and co-workers (1973) found very similar values in baboon fetuses. Such a high fetal cardiac output, which per unit of weight is about three times that of an adult at rest, would help to compensate for the low oxygen content of fetal blood. The high cardiac output is accomplished in part by the fast heart rate of the fetus and a low systemic (peripheral) resistance.

Before birth and expansion of the lungs, the high pulmonary vascular resistance accounts for the high pressure and the low blood flow in the fetal pulmonary circuit. At the same time, resistance to flow through the ductus arteriosus and the umbilicoplacental circulation is low, probably accounting for the overall low fetal systemic vascular resistance. It is estimated that in the fetal lamb about one half the combined output of the two ventricles goes to the placenta. Rudolph and Heymann (1968), by injecting isotopically labeled plastic microspheres into the fetal lamb circulation at various sites, determined the distribution of cardiac output during the last third of gestation to be roughly as follows: placenta, 41 percent; carcass, 35 percent; brain, 5 percent; heart, 5 percent; gastrointestinal tract, 5 percent; lungs, 4 percent; kidneys, 2 percent; spleen, 2 percent; liver (hepatic artery only), 2 percent.

Blood is returned to the placenta through the two *hypogastric arteries, which become the umbilical arteries* distally.

After birth, the umbilical vessels, the ductus arteriosus, the foramen ovale, and the ductus venosus normally constrict or collapse, and consequently the hemodynamics of the fetal circulation undergo pronounced changes. According to Assali (1974) and associates (1968), clamping of the umbilical cord and expansion of the fetal lungs, either through spontaneous breathing or artificial respiration, promptly induce a variety of hemodynamic changes in sheep. The systemic arterial pressure initially falls slightly, apparently the result of the reversal in the direction of blood flow in the ductus arteriosus, but it soon recovers and then rises above the control value. They concluded that several factors played a role in regulating the flow of blood through the ductus arteriosus, including the difference in pressure between the pulmonary artery and aorta and especially the oxygen tension of the blood passing through the ductus arteriosus. They were able to influence flow through the ductus arteriosus by altering the Po_2 of the blood. When the lungs were ventilated with oxygen and the Po_2 rose above 55 mm Hg, ductus flow dropped, but ventilation with nitrogen, initially at least, returned the ductus flow to the original pattern.

The effects from variations in oxygen tension of blood flowing through the ductus arteriosus are thought to be mediated through the actions of prostaglandins on the ductus. Prostaglandins E_1 and E_2 dilate the constricted ductus arteriosus and are intimately involved in maintaining normal patency in utero. Inhibitors of prostaglandin synthetase, when given to the mother, may lead to premature closure of the ductus arteriosus (see Chapter 37, p. 753) but can be used postnatally to induce closure of a patent ductus arteriosus (Brash and associates, 1981).

With expansion of the lungs, pressures in the right ventricle and pulmonary arteries fall because of the marked decrease in pulmonary vascular resistance. Theoretically, at least, an increase in the left arterial pressure above that of the right atrium would close the foramen ovale. There is some disagreement, however, as to when closure actually occurs. The experiments of Barclay and co-workers (1939) are consistent with the view that functional closure of the foramen ovale occurs within several minutes of birth. Arey (1946), however, stated that anatomic fusion of the two septa of the foramen ovale is not completed until about 1 year after

birth, and that in 25 percent of cases perfect closure is never attained. When the foramen ovale remains functionally patent, circulatory disturbances of variable gravity result.

The more distal portions of the hypogastric arteries, which course from the level of the bladder along the abdominal wall to the umbilical ring and into the cord as umbilical arteries, undergo atrophy and obliteration within 3 to 4 days after birth, to become the *umbilical ligaments;* intraabdominal remnants of the umbilical vein form the *ligamentum teres.* The ductus venosus constricts and its lumen closes, resulting in the formation of the *ligamentum venosum.*

Using a pulsed doppler technique and B-mode ultrasonic imaging of the human umbilical cord, Gill and co-workers (1981) calculated that umbilical blood flow increased from 22 to 100 ml per minute at 22 weeks of gestation to 300 ml per minute at 37 to 38 weeks, after which there was a modest reduction until delivery.

Fetal Blood

Hematopoiesis is demonstrable first in the yolk sac of the very early embryo. The next major site of erythropoiesis is the liver and finally the bone marrow. The contributions made by each site throughout the growth and development of the embryo and fetus are demonstrated graphically in Figure 8-12. The first erythrocytes formed are nucleated, but as fetal development progresses, more and more of the circulating erythrocytes are nonnucleated. As the fetus grows, not only does the volume of blood in the common circulation of the fetus and placenta increase but the hemoglobin concentration rises as well. As shown by the studies of Walker and Turnbull (1953), the hemoglobin of fetal blood rises to the adult male level of about 15.0 g/dl at midpregnancy,

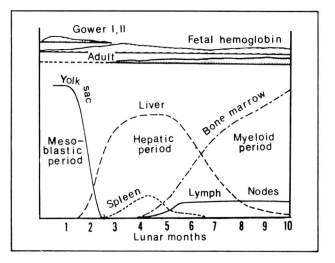

Figure 8-12. Sites of hematopoiesis and kinds of hemoglobin synthesized at various stages of fetus development. (*From Brown: Biology of Gestation, Vol. II. The Fetus and Neonate. New York, Academic, 1968, p 361.*)

and at term it is somewhat higher. Fetal blood at or near term is characterized, therefore, by a high hemoglobin concentration that is high by maternal standards. The reticulocyte count falls from a very high level in the very young fetus to about 5 percent at term. Pearson (1966), using a variety of techniques, found the life-span of erythrocytes from more mature fetuses to be approximately two thirds that of erythrocytes of normal adults; erythrocytes of less mature fetuses have even shorter life-spans. These data are supportive of the concept that fetal erythrocytes are "stress erythrocytes." The erythrocytes of the fetus differ structurally and metabolically from those of the adult. Fetal erythrocytes are more deformable, which helps to offset their higher viscosity (Smith and co-workers, 1981). The fetus is capable of making erythropoietin in increased amounts when severely anemic and of excreting it into the amnionic fluid (Finne, 1966; Živný and co-workers, 1982).

Precise measurements of the volume of blood contained in the human fetoplacental circulation are lacking. Usher, Shepard, and Lind (1963), however, have measured the volume of blood of term normal infants very soon after birth and noted an average of 78 ml/kg when immediate cord-clamping was carried out. Gruenwald (1967) found the volume of blood of fetal origin contained in the placenta after prompt cord-clamping to average 45 ml/kg of fetus. Thus, fetoplacental blood volume at term is approximately 125 ml/kg of fetus. Pritchard and co-workers (unpublished observations) measured the volumes of blood in infants with erythroblastosis fetalis as well as in their placenta and cord immediately after delivery. The "fetoplacental" blood volume in these circumstances was very close to 120 ml/kg of infant weight.

In the embryo and fetus, the globin moiety of much of the hemoglobin differs from that of the normal adult. In the embryo, three major forms of hemoglobin may be found (Pearson, 1966). The most primitive forms are Gower-1 and Gower-2. The globin moiety of Gower-1 consists of four ε-peptide chains per molecule of protein, whereas in Gower-2 there are two α- and two ε-chains. All normal hemoglobins elaborated after Gower-1 contain a pair of α-chains, but the other pair of peptide chains differs for each kind of hemoglobin. Hemoglobin F (so-called fetal hemoglobin, or alkaline-resistant hemoglobin) contains a pair of α-peptide chains and a pair of γ-chains per molecule of hemoglobin. Actually, two varieties of γ-chains have been identified in hemoglobin F, their ratios changing steadily as the fetus and infant mature (Huisman and colleagues, 1970; Fadel and Abraham, 1981). As shown in Figure 8-13, hemoglobin A, the fourth hemoglobin to be formed by the fetus and the major hemoglobin formed after birth in normal persons, is present after the 11th week of gestation in progressively greater amounts as the fetus matures (Pataryas and Stammatoyannopoulos, 1972). The globin of hemoglobin A is made up of a pair of α-chains and a pair of β-chains. Hemoglobin A₂, the globin of which contains a pair of α-chains and a pair of δ-chains, is present in very

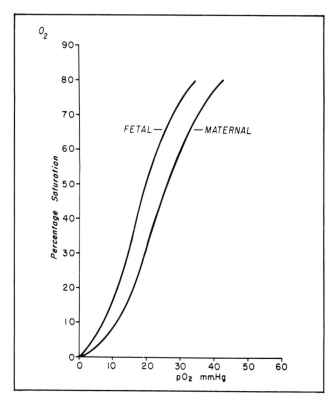

Figure 8-13. Oxygen dissociation curves of fetal and maternal human bloods prepared at pH 7.40. (*Courtesy of Dr. André Hellergers.*)

small concentrations in the mature fetus but increases after birth. Thus, as growth proceeds, there is a shift not only in the amounts but also in the kinds of globin synthesized by the embryo and fetus.

As demonstrated in Figure 8-13, at any given oxygen tension and at identical pH, fetal erythrocytes that contain mostly hemoglobin F bind more oxygen than do erythrocytes containing nearly all hemoglobin A. The major reason for this difference is that hemoglobin A binds 2,3-diphosphoglycerate more avidly than does hemoglobin F (De Verdier and Garby, 1969) and 2,3-diphosphoglycerate so bound lowers the affinity of the hemoglobin molecule for oxygen. The increased oxygen affinity of the fetal erythrocyte results from a lower concentration of 2,3-diphosphoglycerate than is present in the maternal erythrocyte, in which the 2,3-diphosphoglycerate level is increased compared to the nonpregnant state (see Chapter 9, p. 191). Gilbert, Lis, and Longo (1983) noted that at higher temperatures the affinity of fetal blood for oxygen decreases. They concluded that increases in fetal temperature as a consequence of maternal hyperthermia could intensify fetal hypoxia.

Since fetal erythrocytes formed late in pregnancy contain less hemoglobin F and more hemoglobin A than do the cells formed earlier, the content of hemoglobin F of the fetal erythrocytes falls somewhat during the latter weeks of pregnancy. At term, about three fourths of the total hemoglobin normally is hemoglobin F. During the first 6 to 12 months after delivery, the proportion of hemoglobin F continues to fall, eventually to reach the low level found in erythrocytes of normal adults (Schulman and Smith, 1953).

Evidence of a physiologic role for erythropoietin in fetal erythropoiesis has been provided by Zanjani and co-workers (1974). The injection of antierythropoietin into the sheep fetoplacental circulation was followed by a fall in reticulocytes and incorporation of radioiron into erythrocytes; moreover, induction of anemia in the fetus resulted in elevated levels of erythropoietin–like material. In utero the fetal liver, rather than the kidney, appears to be an important source of erythropoietin.

The kinds and numbers of leukocytes in the fetus are highly variable, depending upon the degree of maturity and the impact of labor.

The concentrations of several coagulation factors at birth are appreciably below the levels that develop within a few weeks after birth. (Sell and Corrigan, 1973). The factors that are low in cord blood are II, VII, IX, X, XI, XII, XIII, and fibrinogen. Without prophylactic vitamin K, vitamin K–dependent coagulation factors usually decrease even further during the first few days after birth, especially in breast-fed infants, and may lead to hemorrhage in the newborn infant (Shearer and co-workers, 1982) (see Chapter 38, p. 782). Platelet counts in cord blood are in the normal range for nonpregnant adults, while fibrinogen levels are somewhat less than in nonpregnant adults. For reasons unknown, the time for conversion of fibrinogen in plasma to fibrin clot when thrombin is added (thrombin time) is somewhat prolonged compared with that of older children and adults. The measurement of factor VIII coagulant activity in the cord is of value in accurately making or excluding the diagnosis of hemophilia in male infants (Kasper and colleagues, 1964). Functional factor XIII (fibrin-stabilizing factor) levels in plasma are significantly reduced compared to those in normal adults (Henriksson and co-workers, 1974), but the clinical diagnosis of factor XIII deficiency is usually made by observing a continuous "ooze" from the umbilical stump. Nielsen (1969) described the finding of low levels of plasminogen and somewhat increased fibrinolytic activity in cord plasma compared to that in maternal plasma. This may be due to a structurally and functionally different fetal plasminogen (Estelles and co-workers, 1980).

The mean total plasma protein and plasma albumin concentrations in maternal and cord blood are similar. For example, Foley and associates (1978) identified maternal and cord total plasma proteins to average 6.5 and 5.9 g/dl, respectively, with maternal and cord plasma albumin levels of 3.6 and 3.7 g/dl, respectively.

Near term, the immunoglobulin IgG is present in approximately the same concentrations in cord and maternal sera but IgA and IgM are considerably lower in cord serum. Although IgA and IgM of maternal origin are effectively excluded from the fetus, IgG crosses the placenta with considerable efficiency (Gitlin and colleagues, 1972). All four major subclasses of IgG appear to cross the placenta from mother to fetus but whether by the same or different transport systems is not clear (Gitlin, 1974). *Increased amounts of IgM are found in the fetus only after the immune mechanism has been provoked into antibody response by an infection in the fetus.*

The viscosities of maternal and cord bloods are similar (Foley and associates, 1978). The increase in viscosity imposed by the higher hematocrit of cord blood is offset by the lower levels of fibrinogen and IgM in the cord plasma and by the more deformable fetal erythrocyte (Smith and co-workers, 1981).

Urinary System

Two primitive urinary systems, the pronephros and the mesonephros, precede the development of the metanephros. Embryologic failure of either of the first two may result in anomalous development of the definitive urinary system.

By the end of the first trimester, the nephrons have some capacity for excretion through glomerular filtration, although the kidneys are functionally immature throughout fetal life. The ability to concentrate and modify the pH of urine is quite limited even in the mature fetus. Fetal urine is hypotonic with respect to fetal plasma because of low concentrations of electrolytes. In the lamb fetus, and most likely in the human fetus, the fraction of the cardiac output perfusing the kidneys is low and renal vascular resistance is high, compared with these values later in life (Assali and colleagues, 1968a; Rudolph and Heymann, 1968). In the lamb fetus, urine flow varies considerably in response to stress. Transient marked fetal polyuria post-operatively that apparently dissipates with recovery of fetal well-being has been noted by Gresham and co-workers (1972).

Urine is usually found in the bladder even in small fetuses. Wladimiroff and Campbell (1974) estimated urine production by human fetuses using an ultrasonic method to determine bladder volumes. They report a mean production of 10 ml per hour at 30 weeks, with an increase at term to 27 ml per hour, or 650 ml per day. A maternally administered diuretic (furosemide) increases fetal urine formation. Kurjak and associates (1981) confirmed Wladimiroff and Campbell's work and measured fetal glomerular filtration rates and fetal tubular water reabsorption. All three measurements were decreased in 33 percent of growth-retarded infants and in 17 percent of infants of diabetic mothers. All values were normal in anencephalic fetuses and in cases of polyhydramnios.

After obstruction of the urethra, the bladder, ureters, and renal pelves may become quite dilated; the bladder may become sufficiently distended that dystocia results. The kidneys in these circumstances seem capable of excreting urine until back pressure ultimately destroys the renal parenchyma. Kidneys are not essential for survival in utero but are important in the control of the composition and volume of amnionic fluid (see Chapter 23, p. 463). Abnormalities that cause chronic anuria most often are accompanied by oligohydramnios and by hypoplasia of the lungs.

RESPIRATORY SYSTEM

Maturation of Fetal Lung

The timetable and identification of the biochemical maturation of the fetal lung is of considerable importance and concern to the obstetrician because functional immaturity of the lung at birth leads to the development of the respiratory distress syndrome. Kiedel and Gluck (1975), as well as Farrell and Avery (1975), have succinctly related the history of the clinical identification of the respiratory distress syndrome. The signs and symptoms of this disorder were described first in 1903 by Hocheim, who observed a nebulous lining in the lungs of two infants who died shortly after birth. His observation led to the use of the descriptive phrase, "hyaline membrane disease," to describe the pathologic features of the respiratory distress syndrome. In 1929, von Neergard compared the pressure–volume curves of lungs distended with air with those of lungs distended with a gum arabic solution; from the results of these studies he concluded that the forces that promote deflation or collapse of the air-containing lung result principally from surface tension at the air–tissue interface of the alveolus. Clements (1957) found that a surface tension–lowering material was present in saline extracts of lung lavage material. Subsequently, it was demonstrated that the surface-active components of the alveoli are attributable to the properties of a complex lipoprotein, viz., *surfactant.* Klaus and associates (1961) demonstrated that the principal surface-active component of surfactant was attributable to a specific lecithin, namely, dipalmitoyl-phosphatidylcholine, a unique phosphatidylcholine moiety in which palmitate is present in both the *sn*-1 and *sn*-2 positions of the glycerophospholipid. This is a peculiar species of phosphatidylcholine; it is rare to find a saturated fatty acid in both the *sn*-1 and -2 positions of a glycerophospholipid. Avery and Mead (1959) were the first to point out that the respiratory distress syndrome is caused by a deficiency in surfactant biosynthesis in fetal and neonatal lung. Subsequently, several investigators have shown that augmented surfactant synthesis normally appers in fetal lungs according to a developmental timetable; moreover, it is known that of the 40 cell types of the lung, surfactant is formed specifically in the type II pneumonocytes that line the alveoli.

The recognition of the importance of the role of surfactant in the prevention of respiratory distress syndrome led many investigators to study the composition of surfactant (Fig. 8-14). There are several unique features that are characteristic of the glycerophospholipid composition of this complex lipoprotein. Ninety percent of surfactant (dry weight) is lipid, and approximately 80 percent of the glycerophospholipids are comprised of phosphatidylcholines (lecithins); importantly, however, a

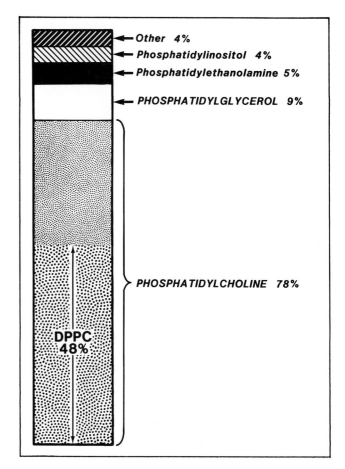

Figure 8-14. Glycerophospholipid composition of "mature" surfactant. Surfactant is especially enriched in lecithin (phosphatidylcholine) and, in particular, the surface-active dipalmitoylphosphatidylcholine (DPPC, 48 percent). The phosphatidylglycerol content of surfactant (8 to 15 percent) is also very high. (*Courtesy Dr. L. Casey.*)

single phosphatidylcholine, namely, dipalmitoylphosphatidylcholine (disaturated phosphatidylcholine or disaturated lecithin), accounts for nearly 50 percent of the glycerophospholipids of surfactant. There is also an unusually high content of phosphatidylglycerol in surfactant, viz., 9 to 15 percent, an amount that is much greater than what is found in any other mammalian tissue (White, 1973). Phosphatidylglycerol is the second most surface-active component of surfactant, but, more importantly, phosphatidylglycerol appears to confer a certain unique feature to the surfactant moiety, a surface-active property that is over and above what can be attributed to its surface tension–lowering properties alone. This, as yet ill-defined, action of phosphatidylglycerol is believed to be important in the prevention of the respiratory distress syndrome because infants born before the appearance of phosphatidylglycerol in surfactant are at increased risk of development of the respiratory distress syndrome even when the dipalmitoylphosphatidylcholine content of the surfactant is normal for mature lungs.

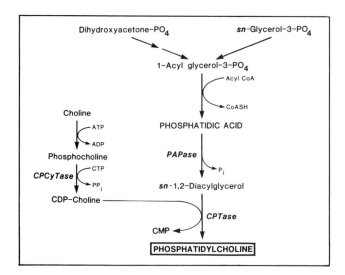

Figure 8-15. Biosynthetic pathway for phosphatidylcholine (lecithin) synthesis in type II pneumonocytes. PAPase = phosphatidate phosphohydrolase; CPTase = choline phosphotransferase; CPCyTase = choline phosphate cytidylyltransferase; CDP = choline diphosphate; CMP = cytidine monophosphate. (*Courtesy Dr. L. Casey.*)

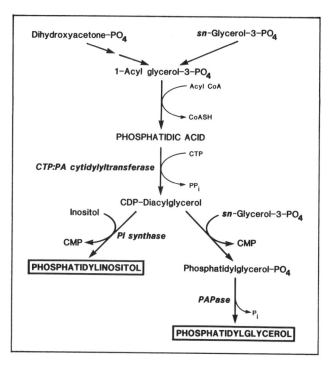

Figure 8-16. Biosynthetic pathway for the synthesis of phosphatidylinositol and phosphatidylglycerol in type II pneumonocytes. CTP:PA = cytidine triphosphate: phosphatidic acid. For other abbreviations, see Figure 8-15. (*Courtesy Dr. L. Casey.*)

In an elegant series of studies, Gluck and associates (1967, 1970, 1971, 1972, 1974) demonstrated that an increasing concentration of dipalmitoylphosphatidylcholine (lecithin) in amnionic fluid, relative to that of sphingomyelin (the lecithin to sphingomyelin, or L/S, ratio), constitutes an index of fetal lung maturation. These studies were successful because of the ingenious idea of determining the concentration of sphingomyelin as a reference for glycerophospholipid synthesis by the lung in general, whereas the measurement of acetone-precipitable dipalmitoylphosphatidylcholine (disaturated lecithin) is a specific index of surfactant synthesis in type II pneumonocytes. More recently, Hallman, Gluck, and coworkers (1976) demonstrated that the identification of phosphatidylglycerol in amnionic fluid is also an indicator of lung maturation. From these diverse observations, it is apparent that augmented synthesis of surfactant, and specifically that which is enriched with dipalmitoylphosphatidylcholine and phosphatidylglycerol, is essential in the successful preparation of the fetal lung for the transition from a water–alveolar interface to an air–alveolar interface, events that must take place if alveolar collapse on expiration is to be prevented after birth. Thus, the regulation of the rate of synthesis of dipalmitoylphosphatidylcholine and phosphatidylglycerol in fetal lung is of signal importance. The biosynthetic pathways involved in the formation of the glycerophospholipids of surfactant are illustrated in Figures 8-15, 8-16, and 8-17.

Biosynthetic Regulation of Surfactant Formation
In the biosynthesis of phosphatidylcholine and phosphatidylglycerol, several common reactions are involved. The glycerol backbone for phosphatidylcholine, phosphatidylinositol, and phosphatidylglycerol synthesis (phosphatidic

acid) is provided from either glycerol-3-phosphate or dihydroxyacetone phosphate, or both (Figs. 8-15, 8-16). It is noteworthy that glycerol-3-phosphate originates from glycerol in tissues in which there is glycerolkinase activity and from glucose through glycolysis. Glycerol-3-phosphate is acylated in a stepwise fashion in a process that gives rise to phosphatidic acid in which there are two of a variety of fatty acids. The acyl donor to the glycerol backbone is fatty acid–coenzyme A (CoA). Generally, there is a saturated fatty acid in the *sn*-1 position and an unsaturated fatty acid in the *sn*-2 position of phosphatidic acid. In lung tissue, however, there is considerable capacity for the de novo synthesis of palmitic acid and thus a greater likelihood of finding palmitate in the *sn*-2 position in lung tissue than in other tissues. In the biosynthesis of phosphatidic acid by lung tissue, however, there is no evidence for preferential incorporation of palmitoyl-CoA in the *sn*-2 position.

It also is important to note that phosphatidic acid is a substrate common to the formation of the two principal surface-active glycerophospholipids, namely, dipalmitoylphosphatidylcholine and phosphatidylglycerol (Figs. 8-15, 8-16, 8-17). Thus, the metabolism of phosphatidic acid constitutes a critical branch point in the regulation of the biosynthesis of the principal surface-active glycerophospholipids of surfactant.

Lecithin (Dipalmitoylphosphatidylcholine) of Surfactant
Let us consider first the biosynthesis of dipalmitoylphosphatidylcholine. Phosphatidic acid is hydrolyzed, through the action of the enzyme phosphatidate phosphohydrolase

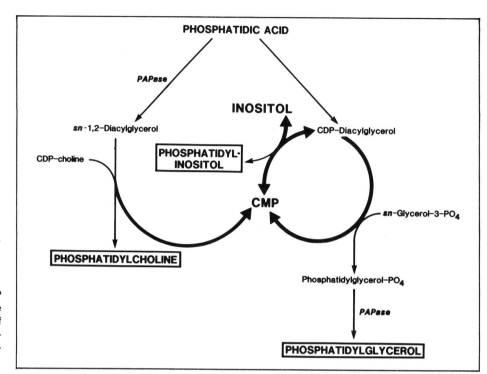

Figure 8-17. The proposed CMP cycle for the regulation of the relative rates of synthesis of phosphatidylcholine, phosphatidylinositol, and phosphatidylglycerol. (*Courtesy Dr. L. Casey.*)

(PAPase), to give sn-1,2-diacylglycerols (Fig. 8-15). The sn-1,2-diacylglycerols serve as a co-substrate with cytidine diphosphate (CDP)-choline in the formation of phosphatidylcholines. This latter reaction is catalyzed by the enzyme choline phosphotransferase (CPTase). The co-substrate, CDP–choline, is formed in a sequence of reactions; through the action of choline kinase, phosphorylcholine is formed. Phosphorylcholine, in turn, is converted to CDP–choline in a reaction that is catalyzed by cytidine triphoshate (CTP)–phosphocholine cytidylyltransferase (CTP-CyT) (Fig. 8-15). In the resultant phosphatidylcholines, there may be a saturated fatty acid, commonly palmitic acid, in the sn-1 position, whereas an unsaturated fatty acid may be present in the sn-2 position. Obviously, some molecular rearrangement of such phosphatidylcholines must occur to produce dipalmitoylphosphatidylcholine, the surface-active lecithin. Two separate mechanisms have been proposed to account for the enrichment of phosphatidylcholines with palmitic acid in the sn-2 position. In both mechanisms, the action of the enzyme, phospholipase A_2, is required. The action of phospholipase A_2 results in the deacylation of glycerophospholipids at the sn-2 position. One product of this reaction is sn-1-palmitoyllysophosphatidylcholine. This lysophosphatidylcholine product may be acylated with palmitoyl–CoA through the action of acyltransferase, resulting in the product, dipalmitoylphosphatidylcholine (Lands, 1958). It is interesting that this pathway was demonstrated first in lung tissue. Alternatively, the remodeling of phosphatidylcholine can come about as the result of the transfer of the acyl moiety from the sn-1 position of an sn-1-palmitoyllysophosphatidylcholine to the sn-2 position of a second sn-1-palmitoyllysophosphatidylcholine. Dipalmitoylphosphatidylcholine can also be formed by way of this pathway. This latter mechanism for remodeling phosphatidylcholine was demonstrated originally in liver tissue (Marinetti, 1958), but it also has been demonstrated in lung tissue (van den Bosch and colleagues, 1965).

Much effort has been directed toward defining the regulatory mechanisms that act to bring about accelerated surfactant biosynthesis as the fetal lungs mature. A number of investigators, working in the laboratories of Dr. John M. Johnston, have accumulated considerable evidence in support of the view that the enzyme PAPase occupies a central regulatory role in the biosynthesis of the glycerophospholipids of surfactant (Delahunty and colleagues, 1979; Herbert and associates, 1978; Jimenez and colleagues, 1974, 1975, 1976; Johnston and co-workers, 1978a and b; Rosenfeld and associates, 1979; Schultz and colleagues, 1974; Spitzer and associates, 1975; Douglas and co-workers, 1983). The specific activity of PAPase in fetal rabbit lung tissue increases dramatically just prior to the time that dipalmitoylphosphatidylcholine begins to accumulate in fetal lung. In view of this striking increase in the specific activity in PAPase in fetal rabbit lung tissue just prior to the lecithin "surge," Johnston, Jimenez and colleagues evaluated the activity of PAPase in human amnionic fluid as a function of gestational age. They found that PAPase was present in amnionic fluid and that the specific activity of this enzyme began to increase at about 29 to 32 weeks of gestation (Fig. 8-18). Moreover, the increase in PAPase activity in amniotic fluid preceded, or was concomitant with, the increase in the L/S ratio.

These investigators also demonstrated that the specific activity of PAPase in the nasopharyngeal fluid of the newborn infant was greater than that in amnionic fluid, suggesting that PAPase in amnionic fluid arises by secretion from fetal lung tissue. Thus, PAPase is translocated from the type II pneumonocytes into the alveolar space and thence into the bronchi and is swept into the amnionic fluid by fetal thoracic movements. It appears the PAPase and surfactant are secreted by the type II pneumonocytes as a closely associated unit, viz., the lamellar body, by a process that likely involves the microtubular system (Figs. 8-19, 8-20, 8-21).

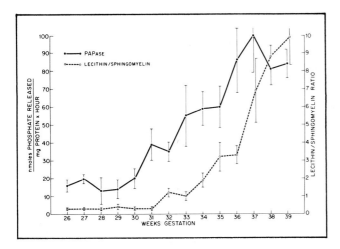

Figure 8-18. Specific activity of PAPase in human amnionic fluid as a function of fetal gestational age, and the relationship of PAPase specific activity to the L/S ratio. (*From Jimenez and Johnston: Pediatr Res 10:767, 1976.*)

Johnston and associates (1978a and b) also found that the hydrolysis of phosphatidylglycerol phosphate to give rise to phosphatidylglycerol was catalyzed by PAPase, and that the enzyme previously presumed to be phosphatidylglycerol phosphate hydrolase (PGPase) (Fig. 8-16) was, in fact, PAPase. Thus, the increase in activity of PAPase in fetal lung may bring about a series of events that serve to regulate the rate and nature of surfactant formation in developing lungs.

1. PAPase catalyzes the hydrolysis of phosphatidic acid to give rise to diacylglycerol, the co-substrate for phosphatidylcholine formation.

2. Diacylglycerol, in increased concentrations, brings about an activation of the enzyme CTP-phosphocholine cytidylyltransferase, which catalyzes the reaction, giving rise to CDP-choline, the other co-substrate for phosphatidylcholine biosynthesis.

3. PAPase also is the enzyme that catalyzes the hydrolysis of phosphatidylglycerol phosphate to give rise to phosphatidylglycerol.

The regulation of phosphatidylglycerol synthesis warrants careful investigation since Hallman, Gluck, and co-workers have shown that increased concentrations of phosphatidylglycerol, together with decreased concentrations of phosphatidylinositol, in surfactant also herald lung maturation. Furthermore, it has been shown that phosphatidylglycerol also acts to increase the activity of the lung tissue enzyme, CTP-phosphocholine cytidylyltransferase, an enzyme necessary for phosphatidylcholine biosynthesis. Moreover, some infants who are born of diabetic mothers develop the respiratory distress syndrome despite high concentrations of dipalmitoylphosphatidylcholine in their amnionic fluid. The surfactant in lung and amniotic fluid of affected fetuses and neonates is characterized by low levels of phosphatidylglycerol and high levels of phosphatidylinositol. Thus, an understanding of the regulation of formation of phosphatidylglycerol becomes of crucial importance in a consideration of the final biochemical events in fetal lung maturation.

Phosphatidylglycerol and Phosphatidylinositol of Surfactant

Presently, the control of phosphatidylinositol and phosphatidylglycerol biosynthesis is incompletely understood. It seems likely that the decrease in concentration of phosphatidylinositol that is associated with a concomitant increase in phosphatidylglycerol in surfactant with lung maturation is brought about by a change in the flux of

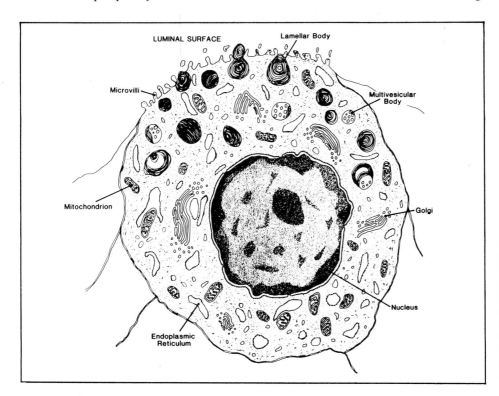

Figure 8-19. Type II pneumonocyte. There are prominent microvilli on the apical surface identifiable. Many multivesicular bodies, the precursor of lamellar bodies, and many lamellar bodies (rich in surfactant) that are migrating toward the luminal surface prior to extrusion into the alveolar space are illustrated. (*Courtesy Dr. L. Casey.*)

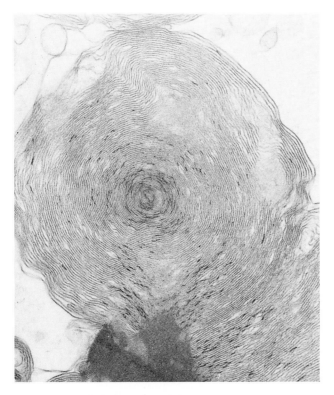

Figure 8-20. Transmission electron micrograph of fused human fetal lung lamellar bodies. (*Courtesy of Dr. J. Snyder and Dr. John M. Johnston.*)

CDP–diacylglycerol through the pathways involved in the synthesis of these acidic glycerophospholipids (Bleasdale and colleagues, 1979) (Figs. 8-16, 8-17). In any event, it is known that with fetal lung maturation there is first a "surge" in phosphatidylcholine synthesis, followed, in time, by an increase in phosophatidylglycerol and a concomitant decrease in phosphatidylinositol in surfactant (Fig. 8-22).

From an evaluation of the metabolic pathways involved in the biosynthesis of phosphatidylglycerol and phosphatidylinositol, it was difficult to envision a mechanism that could account for (1) the increase in phosphatidylcholine synthesis for surfactant formation with lung maturation, which thereafter is followed in time by an (2) increase in phosphatidylglycerol content and (3) a concomitant decrease in phosphatidylinositol concentration in surfactant. The difficulty in resolving the mechanisms involved was related to the proposition that each of these glycerophospholipids is derived ultimately from a common precursor, viz., phosphatidic acid; moreover, phosphatidylinositol and phosphatidylglycerol are both derived from a common precursor that is a product of phosphatidic acid, namely CDP–diaclyglycerol. How, then, can there be a reciprocal relationship between the rates of formation of phosphatidylglycerol and phosphatidylinositol when both are biosynthesized from common precursors?

A potential solution to this apparent paradox is provided by the findings of elegant studies conducted by Johnston, Bleasdale, and associates (Bleasdale and associates, 1979; Quirk and co-workers, 1980; Bleasdale and Johnston, 1982). First, they demonstrated that the phosphatidylinositol synthetase reaction is *reversible* (Fig. 8-16, 8-17). Hereto-

fore, this was not generally believed to be physiologically important. Nonetheless, the reaction that catalyzes the conversion of CDP–diacylglycerol and *myo*-inositol to phosphatidylinositol and cytidine monophosphate (CMP) is reversible in the presence of CMP in optimum concentrations—the latter issue is of great importance when we consider the temporal relationships that exist between increased phosphatidylcholine formation and the subsequent decline in phosphatidylinositol synthesis in favor of phosphatidylglycerol in the formation of "mature" surfactant. For the moment, suffice it to say that the reversibility of the reaction(s) catalyzed by phosphatidylinositol synthetase is such as to permit the possibility of a flux of the common precursor, CDP–diacylglycerol, to phosphatidylglycerol at the expense of phosphatidylinositol.

The first indication of maturation of the fetal lung with respect to accelerated surfactant formation is the increased synthesis and secretion of dipalmitoylphosphatidylcholine. At this time, phosphatidylinositol levels in surfactant are high and those of phosphatidylglycerol are low (Fig. 8-22). Moreover, it is only later in maturation, after a considerable increase in the rate of lecithin synthesis, that there is, simultaneously, an increase in phosphatidylglycerol and a decrease in phosphatidylinositol in surfactant. These several observations (together with the demonstration of the reversibility of the reaction catalyzed by phosphatidylinositol synthetase) led to the concept of a CMP cycle, a concept first fostered by Johnston, Bleasdale, and colleagues (for review, see Bleasdale and Johnston, 1984).

The first evidence of accelerated surfactant synthesis, that is, increased synthesis of dipalmitoylphosphatidylcholine, may come about as a consequence of a maturational increase in PAPase activity and a resultant increase in diacylglycerol synthesis en route to the formation of phosphatidylcholine. As a by-product of this reaction, there is an increase in the rate of formation of CMP (Fig. 8-15).

Based on the proposition that CMP is a co-substrate for the reverse reaction that is catalyzed by phosphatidylinositol synthetase, namely, PI + CMP ⇌ CDP–diacylglycerol + *myo*-inositol, it seemed reasonable that accelerated phosphatidylcholine synthesis would promote the flux of phosphatidylinositol through CDP–diacylglycerol and thence to phosphatidylglycerol phosphate and on to phosphatidylglycerol. The latter reaction should not be rate limiting because, as stated, PAPase catalyzes the hydrolysis of phosphatidylglycerophosphate to phosphatidylglycerol; moreover, for practical purposes, the hydrolysis of phosphatidylglycerol phosphate is irreversible. Let us then take stock of the role of CMP in these reactions: (1) increased phosphatidylcholine biosynthesis gives rise to increased CMP, (2) the forward reaction of the phosphatidylinositol synthetase enzyme gives rise to CMP, and (3) in the formation of phosphatidylglycerol phosphate from CDP–diacylglycerol, CMP is a product. Thus, a CMP cycle is established with respect to the relative rates of formation of the glycerophospholipids of surfactant (Fig. 8-17). It has been suggested that the activation of this CMP cycle is initiated first by way of an increase in phosphatidylcholine formation. In consequence, CMP levels rise, phosphatidylinositol conversion to CDP–diacylglycerol is favored, and the resultant CDP–diacylglycerol can be re-routed toward phosphatidylglycerol. Thus, the concentration of phosphatidylcholine in surfactant rises first; thereafter, the levels of phosphatidylinositol decrease while the concentration of phosphatidylglycerol increases—features characteristic of "mature" surfactant.

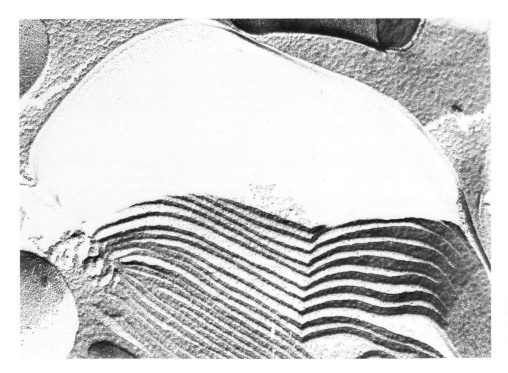

Figure 8-21. Freeze-fracture scanning electron micrograph of a lamellar body. (*Courtesy of Dr. R. C. Reynolds and Dr. John M. Johnston.*)

Alterations in the Timetable of "Mature" Surfactant Formation

If this were a correct formulation of the means by which the relative amounts of glycerophospholipids in surfactant are regulated, it can be envisioned that certain physiologic or pathophysiologic events may cause a delay in the time-table of lung maturation. By way of example, if the levels of plasma *myo*-inositol were elevated, phosphatidylinositol

formation, at the expense of phosphatidylglycerol, would be favored (Fig. 8-17). This pattern of surfactant formation, that is, one rich in phosphatidylcholine and phosphatidyl-inositol and deficient in phosphatidylglycerol, is character-istic of that found in some newborn infants of diabetic mothers. Such infants are at greater risk of respiratory dis-tress syndrome, in spite of high levels of lecithin in amni-onic fluid. Inositolemia and inositol intolerance are common

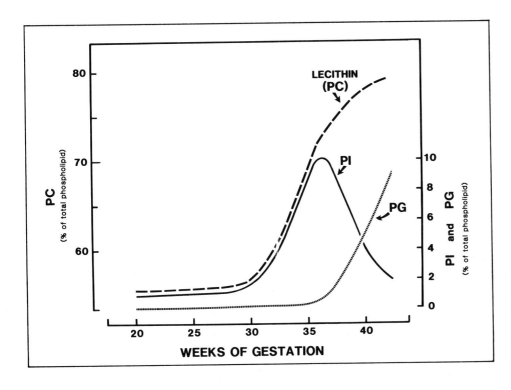

Figure 8-22. Relation between the levels of lecithin [dipalmitoyl-phosphatidylcholine (PC)], phos-phatidylinositol (PI), and phos-phatidylglycerol (PG) in amnionic fluid as a function of gestational age. (*Courtesy Dr. L. Casey.*)

in persons with diabetes mellitus. Quirk and Bleasdale (1984) have presented an in-depth review of the maturation of the fetal lung in pregnancies complicated by maternal diabetes mellitus.

In this regard, it is known that early in gestation, the concentration of *myo*-inositol in fetal plasma is much greater than that in maternal plasma. As pregnancy progresses, however, the concentration of *myo*-inositol in fetal plasma declines. This is believed to be an important maturational event because only a limited amount of lung tissue *myo*-inositol arises by de novo synthesis; the remainder is obtained by lung tissue in an energy-dependent uptake of *myo*-inositol from blood. It has been suggested, therefore, that the developmental decline in *myo*-inositol concentrations in blood may favor a decrease in phosphatidylinositol synthesis in favor of phosphatidylglycerol by way of an alteration in flux of CDP–diacylglycerol. Hyperinositolemia in the fetus of a woman with diabetes mellitus could lead to a delay in the developmental change in surfactant composition from one that is rich in phosphatidylinositol to one that is rich in phosphatidylglycerol.

Hormonal Regulation of Surfactant Formation in Human Fetal Lung

Although it is of signal importance to elucidate the biochemical events involved in the synthesis and release of surfactant, it is equally important to define the mechanisms involved in the control of the synthesis and release of surfactant. Many substances have been proposed as potentially important in these processes. The interest of most investigators who have directed their attention to this question, however, has been centered on only a few agents. Of these, the most intensively investigated compounds are hormones, in particular, cortisol and other glucocorticosteroids.

Cortisol and Fetal Lung Maturation

The basis for suspecting that glucocorticosteroids stimulate surfactant secretion was provided first by Liggins (1969). He observed that there appeared to be accelerated lung maturation in prematurely delivered lambs that had received glucocorticosteroids prior to birth. Since that time, many investigators have suggested that fetal cortisol is the natural trigger for augmented surfactant synthesis. It has been observed that the administration of glucocorticosteroids to the fetus causes an increase in the rate of incorporation of radiolabeled choline into phosphatidylcholine in fetal rabbit lungs (Barrett and colleagues, 1975; Farrell and Zachman, 1973) and fetal rat lungs (Russell and associates, 1974). The inclusion of glucocorticosteroids in the medium of human fetal lung tissue explants (Ekelund and co-workers, 1975) and mixed lung cells (rabbit) grown in tissue culture (Smith and Torday, 1974) resulted in increased incorporation of radiolabeled choline into phosphatidylcholine. The administration of glucocorticosteroids to rabbit fetuses causes an increase in the specific activity of lung CPTase (Farrell and Zachman, 1973), lipoprotein lipase (Hamosh and associates, 1977), and PAPase (Brehier and co-workers, 1978). On the other hand, Rooney and co-workers (1975) and Brehier and colleagues (1977) could not demonstrate an increase in the specific activity of CPTase or glycerolphosphate phosphatidyltransferase after glucocorticosteroid administration in the rabbit. Glucocorticosteroid receptors have been demonstrated in cytosolic and nuclear fractions prepared from fetal lung tissues (Ballard and Ballard, 1972; Giannopoulus, 1973).

There is evidence in support of the view that glucocorticosteroids, when administered in large amounts to the mother at certain critical times during gestation, effect an increase in the rate of maturation of the human fetal lung, as indicated by a reduced incidence of respiratory distress syndrome in newborn infants of such glucocorticosteroid-treated mothers compared with that in those of mothers who were not so treated (Liggins and Howie, 1972). The precise role of glucocorticosteroids in fetal lung maturation has not been fully defined, however, and, from the evidence available it cannot be concluded that cortisol is the single physiologic regulator of the activities of enzymes involved in surfactant formation in most species, including man. There is little doubt that the administration of glucocorticosteroids to pregnant women during the 29th to 33rd week of gestation is associated with a reduced incidence of respiratory distress in their prematurely born infants, but various conclusions have been reached regarding the mechanism(s) by which such treatment is effective. Some investigators have found that the lecithin (phosphatidylcholine)-to-sphingomyelin ratio in amnionic fluid increases after glucocorticosteroid treatment of the mother (Spellacy and colleagues, 1973; Zuspan and associates, 1977); Liggins and Howie, however, found no consistent increase. Some investigators have found a temporal relationship between the levels of cortisol in amnionic fluid and increasing lecithin-to-sphingomyelin ratios (Fencl and colleagues, 1975; Tan and co-workers, 1976); yet we (Milewich and associates, 1978) and others (Sivakumaran and associates, 1975) have found no such relationship. Murphy (1975) found a significant correlation between the level of cortisol in umbilical cord plasma and the lecithin-to-sphingomyelin ratio in amnionic fluid; Sybulski and Manghan (1976) did not. Murphy found a relationship between the levels of cortisol in cord plasma and the subsequent development of respiratory distress syndrome in newborn infants; Hauth and associates (1978) did not.

It should be emphasized, however, that the failure to find a correlation between the levels of cortisol in umbilical cord plasma and in amnionic fluid with alterations in the L/S ratio in the amnionic fluid and with the subsequent development of respiratory distress syndrome should be viewed with caution. This obtains since it is likely that the metabolic clearance rate of plasma cortisol in the fetus increases as a function of the size of the fetus and its vascular volume. Thus, the levels of fetal plasma cortisol may remain relatively constant during the latter few weeks of gestation, at a time when the rate of cortisol secretion by the fetal adrenal may be rising appreciably. If this were the case, then static measurements of fetal plasma cortisol at one point in time, namely, the time of birth, would not be reflective of the rate of secretion of cortisol by the fetal adrenal cortex. At the same time, the level of cortisol in amnionic fluid may not necessarily be reflective of the rate of cortisol secretion by the fetal adrenal. This results from the fact that cortisone, arising in the maternal compartment, can be converted to cortisol by the human fetal membranes (Murphy, 1977). Moreover, alterations in the rate of excretion of cortisol sulfate by the developing fetal kidneys, together with increasing clearance of substances in amnionic fluid through increased fetal "breathing" and fetal swallowing as gestation advances, as well as transport from the amnionic fluid to the maternal compartment, are factors likely to give rise to significant alterations in the levels of cortisol in amnionic fluid that are independent of the rate of secretion of cortisol by the fetal adrenal cortex. Nonetheless, Johnson and colleagues (1978) found that the administration of glucocorticosteroids to pregnant subhuman primates was not associated with an increase in surfactant content in the fetal lungs. Rather, they found that the principal alteration in the fetal lungs of corticosteroid-treated pregnant monkeys was a decrease in the content of collagenous tissue.

Thus, in view of the failure to find a consistent relationship between glucocorticosteroid administration and an increase in activity of an enzyme involved in surfactant synthesis, the failure to find consistently a response in phosphatidylcholine formation (as indicated by an increased L/S ratio) after the administration of glucocorticosteroids to pregnant women, and the failure to demonstrate consistently a temporal relationship between increased cortisol (as indicated by cortisol levels in amnionic fluid or in umbilical cord plasma) and increased surfactant formation, some investigators have concluded that cortisol may not be the only trigger for augmented surfactant formation in the maturing human fetal lung (Hauth and co-workers, 1978). This conclusion is strengthened by the well-known clinical observation that the respiratory distress syndrome is not necessarily observed in many human neonates in whom the capacity to secrete cortisol is limited. Such infants include those with anencephaly, adrenal hypoplasia, and congenital adrenal hyperplasia. It may be that cortisol is one of several hormones that act cooperatively to effect fetal lung maturation. For example, cortisol is believed to stabilize the ribosomal–endoplasmic reticulum complex of mammary tissue such that this organ can respond to prolactin and insulin and thereby secrete milk (Oka and Topper, 1971).

Prolactin and Fetal Lung Maturation

Winters and colleagues (1975) found that the levels of prolactin in fetal plasma increased strikingly during the last few weeks of human pregnancy. Hauth and co-workers (1978) found that the rise in fetal prolactin levels was temporally related to the increase in the L/S ratio in amnionic fluid (Fig. 8-23). They also suggested that a role for prolactin in fetal lung maturation can be envisioned by recalling that prolactin has a profound effect on the gills of fish, the phylogenetic homologue of lung (Lam, 1969), and that there are certain metabolic similarities between the maturing human lung and the prolactin-stimulated mammary gland. For example, these two tissues share a common and almost unique lipid biosynthetic capability, namely, an extraordinary capacity to incorporate palmitic acid into the sn-2 position of the glycerophospholipids of surfactant and into the sn-2 position of triacylglycerols of milk (Breckenridge and associates, 1969). Prolactin acts to increase the capacity of mammary tissue that is maintained in culture to synthesize fatty acids (Hollowes and colleagues, 1973) and other milk constituents such as casein and lactose (Turkington and co-workers, 1973). In type II cell tumors of the lung, and presumably nontumorous type II pneumonocytes, there is a greater capacity for synthesizing palmitic acid than there is in the other cells of the lung (Voelker and associates, 1976). It has been shown that prolactin administration to fetal rabbits results in an increase in the phosphatidylcholine concentration of the fetal lung (Hamosh and Hamosh, 1977). (Interestingly, the action of

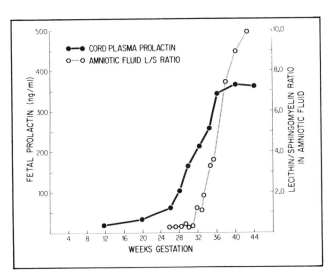

Figure 8-23. Temporal relationship between fetal plasma prolactin concentrations and the amnionic fluid L/S ratio. (*From Hauth et al.: Obstet Gynecol 51:81, 1978.*)

prolactin in mammary tissue is dependent upon pretreatment of such tissue with glucocorticosteroids and insulin.)

On the other hand, it should be pointed out that Ballard and colleagues (1978) were unable to induce increased phosphatidylcholine content in the lung tissue of rabbit fetuses by prolactin treatment. Specifically, after the injection of prolactin into fetal rabbits, they did not find an increase in phosphatidylcholine concentration of similar magnitude to that found by Hamosh and Hamosh. Moreover, Ballard and associates administered prolactin to sheep fetuses and again were unable to find an increase in the phosphatidylcholine content of the tracheal fluid of such treated sheep fetuses. It should be noted, however, that the lecithin content of tracheal fluid in the sheep fetus does not rise during glucocorticosteroid treatment. It has been reported that the newborn infant of a woman treated with bromocriptine did not suffer from respiratory distress syndrome (Bigazzi and colleagues, 1979) even though such treatment caused low levels of prolactin in fetal blood. This finding is important because the levels of prolactin in the mother and in the newborn infant of this bromocriptine-treated woman were quite low. On the other hand, the level of prolactin in amnionic fluid of this subject was not reduced. [Amnionic fluid prolactin is believed to arise in decidua and is not subject to dopaminergic regulation (Chapters 6 and 7).] Johnson and associates (1979) have proposed that prolactin in amnionic fluid, inspired into the fetal alveoli during fetal thoracic movements, may serve an important role in the maturation of fetal lungs. Thus, as in the case of cortisol, one cannot conclude that prolactin, either of fetal pituitary or amnionic fluid origin, is the sole stimulant for the biochemical maturation of the fetal lung.

Nonetheless, it has been found that the concentration of prolactin in umbilical cord plasma and the incidence of respiratory distress syndrome are inversely correlated (Table 8-3). In the study by Hauth and co-workers it was found that in those infants in whom the prolactin concentration in cord plasma was equal to or greater than 200 ng/ml, respiratory distress occurred uncommonly—0 percent in infants delivered from 29.5 to 33 weeks of gestation and 5

TABLE 8-3. THE INCIDENCE OF RESPIRATORY DISTRESS AND CORD PLASMA PROLACTIN LEVELS IN VARIOUS GESTATIONAL AGE GROUPS

Gestational Age At Delivery (Wks)	Incidence of Respiratory Distress Syndrome				
	Newborn Cord Plasma Prolactin				
	(<200 ng/ml)		(≧200 ng/ml)		
	Incidence	Percent	Incidence	Percent	P*
∠26	4/4	100	0/0		—
26.5–29	12/14	86	0/0		—
29.5–33	20/26	80	0/10	0	<0.001
33.5–36	7/25	28	2/43	5	<0.01
≧36.5	1/20	5	2/50	4	0.64

* Computed from the exact probability test of Fisher.
(From Hauth et al: Obstet Gynecol 51:81, 1978.)

percent in infants delivered from 33.5 to 36 weeks of gestation. When the prolactin level in cord plasma was less than 200 ng/ml, respiratory distress occurred often—80 percent in infants delivered from 29.5 to 33 weeks, and 28 percent in those delivered from 33.5 to 36 weeks. All infants delivered from 25 to 29 weeks of gestation had prolactin levels less than 200 ng/ml; among these infants, the incidence of respiratory distress was 89 percent. Smith and co-workers (1978) also measured cord plasma prolactin levels in 58 newborns ranging from 27 weeks of gestation to term. They found that the incidence of respiratory distress was markedly increased in those infants in whom the cord plasma prolactin levels were less than 140 ng/ml, as compared to those in whom the prolactin levels were greater than 140 ng/ml. Gluckman and associates (1978) also found that infants who develop respiratory distress had lower prolactin plasma concentrations at the time of birth than did those infants who did not develop respiratory distress. Similar findings were reported by Grosso and colleagues (1980).

It can be argued that augmented surfactant biosynthesis and increased prolactin secretion are independent milestones in fetal lung maturation. The presence of prolactin receptors in fetal lung tissue (Josimovich and co-workers, 1977), however, and the demonstrated participation of prolactin in lipid biosynthesis by the fetal lung and by mammary tissue are supportive of the view that there is a role for prolactin in the process of augmented surfactant formation. Additional support for this proposed action of prolactin in the biochemical maturation of the fetal lung is provided by the finding that the incidence of respiratory distress syndrome in premature infants born of heroin addicts is markedly decreased (Glass and associates, 1971). Opiates, for example, morphine, are potent stimuli for prolactin secretion (Tolis and colleagues, 1975). These several lines of evidence taken together have led some investigators to the conclusion that increased prolactin secretion and augmented synthesis of surfactant by the human fetus during the last trimester of gestation may be causally related, and that prolactin and cortisol may act in concert to bring about augmented surfactant synthesis.

Snyder and colleagues (1981) have developed an elegant system for the study of human fetal lung maturation in vitro. They find that there is a striking morphologic and biochemical maturation in explants of fetal lung tissue (16 to 20 weeks of gestational age abortuses) that are maintained in organ culture. In such tissues, there is a remarkable increase in phosphatidylcholine formation and a rapid (4 to 5 days of culture) appearance of multivesicular bodies and lamellar bodies in type II pneumonocytes in these tissues. In such preparations, Mendelson and co-workers (1981) found that cortisol plus prolactin (but neither hormone alone) caused a profound acceleration in the rate of increase in phosphatidylcholine synthesis by human fetal lung tissue in organ culture. Thus, cortisol and prolactin, acting in concert, may be the lead hormones in the orchestration of a multihormonal stimulation of surfactant biosynthesis in fetal lung.

If the account presented were an accurate evaluation of the events that transpire in vivo, it could easily be envisioned that other hormones might serve a supportive role in this orchestration of fetal lung maturation. Estrogens affect phospholipid turnover in many tissues, act to promote prolactin release from the anterior pituitary, and, in many tissues, may be involved in the synthesis of prolactin receptors. (For a review of the role of prolactin in fetal lung maturation, see Quirk and colleagues, 1982.)

Estrogens and Fetal Lung Maturation

It is interesting that in many of the tissues in which there are prolactin receptors, there also are receptors for estrogens. In fact, it appears that estrogens, directly or indirectly, act to regulate the number of prolactin receptors in the liver and mammary gland (Gelato and co-workers, 1975; Kelly and associates, 1975; Posner and colleagues, 1975). Many of the actions of prolactin and estrogens appear to be interrelated, especially with regard to lipid metabolism and growth. Estrogens are anabolic steroids that are known to regulate lipoprotein synthesis in the liver (Luskey and co-workers, 1974) and lipid metabolism in the rat uterus (Chan and colleagues, 1976). Increased lipid synthesis is one of the earliest and most dramatic responses of the rat uterus to estrogenic hormones (Aizawa and Mueller, 1961). Spooner and Gorski (1972) showed that estrogens caused enhanced fatty acid synthesis and an increase in rate of the incorporation of choline into glycerophospholipids of the rat uterus. Dickey and Robertson (1969) found that maternal and neonatal urinary estrogens in infants in whom respiratory distress subsequently developed were decreased. Pasqualini and associates (1976), studying guinea pig fetuses, demonstrated a high concentration of estradiol-17β receptors in lung tissue cytosol as well as nuclear binding of the steriod. Moreover, the number of estrogen receptors in the lung of the guinea pig fetus increased with gestational age (Sumida and colleagues, 1977). Mendleson and associates (1980) have demonstrated high-affinity estrogen binding in cytosolic fractions prepared from rat and human fetal lung tissues. Moreover, Khosla and Rooney (1979) found that when pregnant rabbits were injected with estradiol-17β, fetal lung surfactant content was increased. Rooney and Brehier (1982) suggested that the estrogen-induced increase in the incorporation of choline into phosphatidylcholine is mediated by changes in CTP–phosphocholine cytidylyltransferase activity.

Thyroxine and Fetal Lung Maturation

A role for thyroxine in the rate of surfactant synthesis has been proposed by a number of investigators. Thyroxine administration to rabbit fetuses at 24 to 25 days of gestation is associated with accelerated maturation of the fetal lung and an early appearance of osmophilic lamellar inclusions within the type II pneumonocytes (Rooney and colleagues, 1974; Wu and associates, 1971, 1973). Smith and Torday (1974) found that thyroxine treatment was associated with an increased incorporation of choline into phosphatidylcholine in cultured cells prepared from rabbit fetuses of 28 days of gestation. On the other hand, Rooney and co-workers found no effect of thyroxine treatment on the activities of lysophosphatidic acid acyltransferase, CPTase, CDP-diglyceride–inositol phosphatidyltransferase, glycerolphosphate phosphatidyltransferase, acyltransferase, or fatty acid biosynthesis. Mason (1973), in a study of the effect of thyroxine treatment on the concentration of dipalmitoylphosphatidylcholine in lungs of hyperthyroid and in euthyroid rats, found that thyroxine had little effect on the concentration of dipalmitoylphosphatidylcholine. Thus, the role of thyroxine, if any, in the biochemical maturation of the fetal lung type II pneumonocyte is unclear.

Conclusion. Presently, it seems reasonable to conclude that the hormonal stimulation of surfactant synthesis in the type II pneumonocytes of developing fetal lung is brought about by a complex interaction of several hormones. It is well established that pretreatment of breast tissue with estrogens, followed by cortisol, prolactin, and insulin treatment, is essential for lactation. Perhaps a similar sequence of events leads to accelerated surfactant formation in maturing fetal lungs.

Respiration

Within a very few minutes after birth, the respiratory system must be able to provide oxygen as well as eliminate carbon dioxide if the neonate is to survive. Development of air ducts and alveoli, pulmonary vasculature, and muscles of respiration, and coordination of their activities through the central nervous system to a degree that allows fetal survival, at least for a time, can be demonstrated by the end of the second trimester of pregnancy. The majority of fetuses born before this time succumb immediately or during the next few days from respiratory insufficiency, as pointed out in Chapter 38 (p. 769).

Movements of the fetal chest wall have been detected by sophisticated ultrasonic techniques as early as 11 weeks of gestation (Boddy and colleagues, 1975). From the beginning of the fourth month, the fetus is capable of respiratory movement sufficiently intense to move amnionic fluid in and out of the respiratory tract. In the roentgenogram in Figure 8-24, obtained 26 hours after injection of Thorotrast into the amnionic sac, the contrast medium is present in fetal lung. Davis and Potter (1946) reported that the longer the exposure in utero after a single injection of Thorotrast, the greater the apparent concentration in the lungs.

Duenhoelter and Pritchard (1976, 1977) demonstrated in both the human and the rhesus monkey fetus that chromium-labeled erythrocytes and other labeled particles injected into the amnionic sac accumulated in the lungs as well as the gastrointestinal tract (Fig. 8-25).

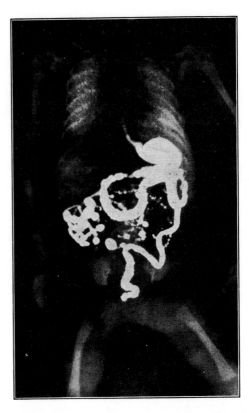

Figure 8-24. X-ray of 115-g fetus in which Thorotrast is present in the lungs, esophagus, stomach, and entire intestinal tract following injection of Thorotrast into the amnionic cavity 26 hours before delivery. This demonstrates not only intrauterine respiration of the fetus but also active swallowing of amnionic fluid by the fetus. (*From Davis and Potter: JAMA 131:1194, 1946.*)

They concluded that throughout the last two trimesters progressively larger volumes of amnionic fluid are normally inspired and presumably expired by the fetus. The pressure changes with some inspirations are sufficient to account for such movement in the rhesus fetus (Martin and co-workers, 1974).

Boddy and Dawes (1975) identified fetal breathing movements in the normal human fetus that are episodic and irregular, their frequency typically ranging from 30 to 70 per minute. Asphyxia was followed by cessation of normal breathing movements and the initiation of gasping respiratory efforts. Such cessation of normal respiratory movements may be the consequence of increased levels of fetal β-endorphin (Browning and co-workers, 1983) (see Chapter 9, p. 202). For an extensive overview of the physiology of fetal breathing and state of the art of the clinical usefulness of analysis of fetal breathing movements, the reader is urged to consult the review by Patrick (1980).

Vagitus Uteri. Crying in utero is a rare phenomenon. Following rupture of the membranes, air may gain access to the amnionic cavity and be inspired by the fetus.

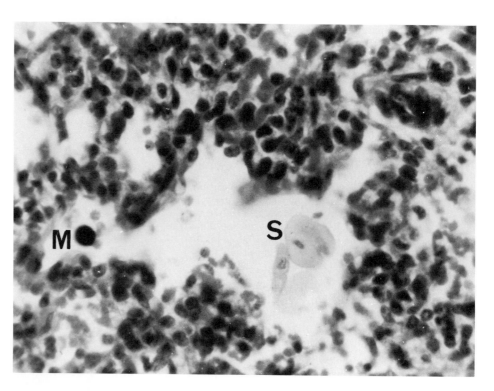

Figure 8-25. Photomicrograph of lung of a near-term rhesus fetus delivered 24 hours after labeling the amnionic fluid with radio-strontium-labeled microspheres as well as chromium-labeled erythrocytes. Contained in the alveolus immediately adjacent to the dense microsphere (M) are labeled erythrocytes that were also inhaled, as were fetal squamous cells, or squames (S). From the amount of chromium within the lungs, it was calculated that at least 62 ml of amnionic fluid was inhaled in 24 hours by a fetus that weighed 281 g. (*From Duenhoelter and Pritchard: Am J Obstet Gynecol 125:306, 1976.*)

Thiery and associates (1973) described three cases in which fetal crying was heard during vaginal examination, amnioscopy, or application of a clip electrode to the fetus. Fetal hiccuping is a more common phenomenon and frequently is appreciated by the mother.

DIGESTIVE SYSTEM

By the 11th week of gestation, the small intestine undergoes peristalsis and is capable of transporting glucose actively (Koldovsky and colleagues, 1965). Gastrointestinal function is sufficiently developed at 4 months to allow the fetus to swallow amnionic fluid, absorb much of the water from it, and propel unabsorbed matter as far as the lower colon (Fig. 8-24). Hydrochloric acid and some adult digestive enzymes are present in very small amounts in the early fetus. In the premature infant, transient deficiencies of these enzymes are often present, depending upon the gestational age of the infant when born (Lebenthal and colleagues, 1983).

Fetal swallowing at various stages of pregnancy has been measured by introducing a small volume of maternal erythrocytes labeled with isotopic chromium into the amnionic sac and subsequently measuring the chromium that accumulated in the gastrointestinal tract either directly in fetuses that succumbed from immaturity after delivery or in the meconium and feces passed after birth by more mature fetuses (Pritchard, 1965, 1966). Term-size fetuses were thought to swallow relatively large volumes of amnionic fluid; in one study, the amount appeared to average nearly 450 ml of amnionic fluid per 24 hours. Gitlin and associates (1972) found that the rate of clearing of radiolabeled albumin from amnionic fluid, presumably by swallowing, was very similar to this value. It is likely, however, that the volumes of amnionic fluid swallowed directly by the fetus are somewhat less than what has been reported. Probably part of the label in the amnionic fluid was removed by inhalation and the inspired label, in turn, was either absorbed across the lung or was propelled from the lung by ciliary movement into the pharynx from which it was swallowed (Duenhoelter and Pritchard, unpublished).

Fetal swallowing appears to have little effect on the amnionic fluid volume early in pregnancy, because the volume swallowed is small in comparison with the total volume of amnionic fluid present. Late in pregnancy, however, the volume of amnionic fluid appears to be regulated to some degree by fetal swallowing, for when swallowing is inhibited, hydramnios is common (see Chapter 23, p. 463).

The act of swallowing may enhance growth and development of the alimentary canal and condition the fetus for alimentation after birth, although anencephalic fetuses, which usually swallow little amnionic fluid, have gastrointestinal tracts that appear normal. In late pregnancy, swallowing serves to remove some of the insoluble debris that is normally shed into the amnionic sac and sometimes abnormally excreted into it. The undigested portions of the swallowed debris can be identified in meconium collected at birth. The amnionic fluid swallowed probably contributes little to the caloric requirements of the fetus but may contribute essential nutrients. Gitlin (1974) demonstrated that late in pregnancy about 0.8 g of soluble protein, approximately one-half albumin, appears to be ingested by the fetus each day.

Meconium consists not only of undigested debris from swallowed amnionic fluid but, to a larger degree, of various products of secretion, excretion, and desquamation by the gastrointestinal tract. The dark greenish-black appearance is caused by pigments, especially biliverdin. Hypoxia has been implicated in the evacuation of meconium from the large bowel into the amnionic fluid. This mechanism may result from the release of arginine vasopressin from the fetal pituitary in response to hypoxia. The arginine vasopressin so released stimulates the smooth muscle of the colon to contract, resulting in intraamnionic defecation (DeVane and co-workers, 1982). Small-bowel obstruction may lead to vomiting in utero (Shrand, 1972). Indeed, fetuses who suffer from congenital chloride diarrhea may have diarrhea in utero, which leads to hydramnios and premature delivery (Holmberg and associates, 1977).

LIVER AND PANCREAS

Hepatic function in the fetus differs in several ways from that of the adult. Many enzymes of the fetal liver are present in considerably reduced amounts compared to later life. The liver has a very limited capacity for converting free *bilirubin* to bilirubin diglucuronoside (see Chapter 38 p. 779). The more immature the fetus, the more deficient is the system for conjugating bilirubin.

Because the life-span of the fetal erythrocyte is shorter than that of the normal adult, relatively more bilirubin is produced. Only a small fraction of the bilirubin is conjugated by the fetal liver and excreted through the biliary tract into the intestine and ultimately oxidized to biliverdin. Bashore and associates (1969) and Bernstein and co-workers (1969) demonstrated that radiolabeled unconjugated bilirubin is cleared promptly from monkey and dog fetal circulation by the placenta to the maternal liver where it is conjugated and excreted through maternal bile. The transfer of the unconjugated bilirubin across the placenta, however, is bidirectional. This observation is supported by the rarely encountered case of high levels of unconjugated bilirubin in maternal plasma. Conjugated bilirubin is not exchanged to any significant degree between mother and fetus.

Glycogen appears in low concentration in fetal liver during the second trimester of pregnancy, but near term there is a rapid and marked increase in normal fetuses to levels two to three times those in adult liver. After delivery, the glycogen content falls precipitously.

The exocrine function of the fetal pancreas appears to be limited but not necessarily absent. For example, radioiodine-labeled human albumin injected into the amnionic sac and swallowed by the fetus is absorbed from the fetal intestine. It is not absorbed as undigested protein, however, because the iodine is excreted promptly in the maternal urine when pretreatment with iodide has been provided to enhance the clearance of the digested radiolabeled iodine (Pritchard, 1965).

Insulin-containing granules can be identified in the fetal pancreas by 9 weeks of gestation, and plasma *insulin* is detectable at 12 weeks (Adam, 1969). The fetal pancreas responds to hyperglycemia by increasing plasma insulin (Obenshain and colleagues, 1970). Although the precise role played by insulin of fetal origin is not clear, fetal growth must be determined to a considerable extent by the amounts of basic nutrients from the mother and, through the action of insulin, the anabolism of these materials by the fetus. Insulin levels are high in serum from infants of diabetic mothers and in other large-for-gestational-age infants, but insulin levels are low in infants who are small for gestational age (Brinsmead, Liggins, 1979). Proof that insulin of fetal origin helps meet the needs of the diabetic mother is lacking.

Glucagon has been identified in the pancreas at 8 weeks of gestation. Induced hypoglycemia and infused alanine increase glucagon levels in the rhesus monkey mother, but similar stimuli to the fetus do not. Within 12 hours of birth, however, the infant is capable of responding (Chez and co-workers, 1975). Moreover, fetal α-cells of the pancreas are capable of responding to L-dopa (Epstein and associates, 1977). Therefore, α-cell nonresponsiveness to hypoglycemia and infused alanine likely is the consequence of failure of glucagon release rather than inadequate production of the hormone.

OTHER ENDOCRINE GLANDS

Before the end of the first trimester, the fetal pituitary is able to synthesize and store pituitary hormones. Growth hormone, corticotropin (ACTH), prolactin, luteinizing hormone, and follicle-stimulating hormone have been identified in the pituitary of the human fetus by 10 weeks of gestation. Moreover, the fetal pituitary is responsive to hypophysiotropic hormones and is capable of secreting these hormones from early in gestation (Grumbach and Kaplan, 1974).

Winters and co-workers (1974) have shown that by the 12th week ACTH levels are high in fetal plasma and remain so until late in pregnancy, when they decrease significantly. As gestation advances, however, *prolactin* in fetal plasma rises remarkably, to levels on the average six times greater at 35 to 42 weeks gestation than at 16 to 19 weeks. Fetal prolactin is considered further in Chapter 7 (p. 130.

The levels of pituitary *growth hormone* are rather high in cord blood, although the role for the hormone in fetal growth and development is not clear. Decapitation in utero does not appreciably impair the growth of the rest of the animal fetus, as shown by Bearn (1967) as well as others. Furthermore, human anencephalic fetuses with little pituitary tissue are not remarkably different in weight from normal fetuses.

The fetal pituitary produces and releases β-endorphin in a manner irrespective of maternal plasma levels.

TABLE 8-4. PHASES OF THYROID MATURATION IN THE HUMAN FETUS AND NEWBORN INFANT

Phase	Events	Gestational Age
I	Embryogenesis of pituitary–thyroid axis	2–12 weeks
II	Hypothalamic maturation	10–35 weeks
III	Development of neuroendocrine control	20 weeks to 4 weeks after birth
IV	Maturation of peripheral monodeiodination systems	30 weeks to 4 weeks after birth

(*From Fisher: Ross Conference on Obstetrical Decisions and Neonatal Outcome, San Diego, May, 1979.*)

Furthermore, cord blood levels of β-endorphin and β-lipotrophin have been reported to decrease with declining fetal pH but correlate in a positive manner with fetal Pco_2 (Browning and co-workers, 1983) (see p. 163, and Chapter 9, p. 202). The pituitary–thyroid system is capable of function by the end of the first trimester (Table 8-4). Until midpregnancy, however, secretion of thyroid-stimulating hormone and thyroid hormones is low. There is a considerable increase after this time (Fisher, 1975; Fisher and Klein, 1981). Probably very little *thyrotropin* crosses the placenta from mother to fetus, whereas the long-acting thyroid stimulators (LATS) and LATS Protector do so when present in high concentrations in the mother (see Chapter 28, p. 605). Also, maternal IgG antibodies against thyroid-stimulating hormone (TSH) may cross the placenta (Lazarus and associates, 1983).

The human placenta actively concentrates iodide on the fetal side, and throughout the second and third trimesters of pregnancy the fetal thyroid concentrates iodide more avidly than does the maternal thyroid. Therefore, the hazard to the fetus of administering to the mother either radioiodide or appreciable amounts of ordinary iodide is obvious.

Thyroid hormones of maternal origin cross the placenta to a very *limited* degree, with triiodothyronine crossing more readily than thyroxin. The fetus is dependent upon hormone produced by the fetal thyroid gland. From the fact that athyreotic cretins generally have euthyroid mothers it can be inferred that a normal rate of maternal thyroid secretion cannot compensate for inadequate fetal glandular synthesis.

Immediately after birth there are major changes in thyroid function and metabolism. Atmospheric cooling evokes sudden and marked increase in thyrotropin secretion that, in turn, causes a progressive increase in serum thyroxine levels, maximal 24 to 36 hours after birth. There are nearly simultaneous elevations of serum triiodothyronine levels.

There is good evidence that the fetal parathyroids elaborate *parathormone* by the end of the first trimester, and the glands appear to respond in utero to regulatory stimuli. Newborn infants of mothers with hyperparathyroidism, for example, may suffer hypocalcemic tetany.

It has been suggested that lack of *antidiuretic hormone* production by the fetus accounts for the lack of urine-concentrating ability in the newborn infant. Several investigators have found that the levels of arginine vasopressin in umbilical cord plasma are strikingly increased compared with the levels found in maternal plasma (Chard and associates, 1971; Polin and co-workers, 1977). Additionally, arginine vasopressin in cord and fetal blood appears to be elevated by fetal stress (DeVane and Porter, 1980; DeVane and co-workers, 1982).

The *adrenal* of the human fetus is very much larger in relation to total body size than is that of the adult; the bulk of the enlargement is made up of the central or so-called fetal zone of the adrenal cortex. The normally hypertrophied fetal zone involutes rapidly after birth. The fetal zone is scant to absent in rare instances where the fetal pituitary is missing. The function of the fetal adrenal and the control of fetal adrenal steroidogenesis are discussed in detail in Chapter 7 (p. 127).

The fetal adrenal synthesizes *aldosterone*. In one study, aldosterone levels in cord plasma near term exceeded those in maternal plasma, as did renin and renin substrate (Katz and colleagues, 1974). The renal tubules of the newborn, and presumably the fetus, appear relatively insensitive to aldosterone (Kaplan, 1972).

Siiteri and Wilson (1974) demonstrated synthesis of *testosterone* by the fetal testis from progesterone and pregnenolone by 10 weeks of gestation. Before the development of primary and graafian follicles in the second half of gestation the capacity for steroidogenesis by the ovary is limited (Grumbach and Kaplan, 1974).

Components of the fetoplacental endocrine system very likely play a prominent role in the initiation of spontaneous labor, as discussed in Chapter 15.

NERVOUS SYSTEM AND SENSORY ORGANS

Synaptic function is developed sufficiently by the eighth week of gestation to demonstrate flexion of the neck and trunk (Temiras and co-workers, 1968). If the fetus is removed from the uterus during the tenth week, spontaneous movements may be observed, although movements in utero are usually not felt by the mother until several weeks later. At 10 weeks, local stimuli may evoke squinting, opening the mouth, incomplete finger closure, and plantar flexion of the toes. Complete finger closure is achieved during the fourth lunar month. Swallowing and respiration are also evident during the fourth lunar month (Figs. 8-24, 8-25) but the ability to suck is not present until the sixth month or even later (Lebenthal and associates, 1983). During the third trimester of pregnancy, integration of nervous and muscular function proceeds rapidly.

By the seventh lunar month, the eye is sensitive to light, but perception of form and color is not complete until long after birth.

The internal, middle, and external components of the ear are well developed by mid-pregnancy. The fetus apparently hears some sounds in utero as early as the 24th to 26th week of gestation (Westin, 1968).

Taste buds are histologically evident in the third lunar month; by the seventh month of gestation, the fetus is responsive to variations in the taste of ingested substances.

IMMUNOLOGY

Infections in utero have provided an opportunity to examine some of the mechanisms for immune response by the human fetus. The opinion that the fetus is immunologically incompetent is no longer tenable. Indeed, morphologic evidence of immunologic competence in the human fetus has been reported as early as 13 weeks of gestational age by Altshuler (1974), who described infection of the placenta and fetus by cytomegalovirus with characteristic severe inflammatory cell proliferation as well as virus inclusions. Moreover, synthesis by fetal organs of components of complement late in the first trimester has been demonstrated by Kohler (1973). All components of human complement are produced at an early stage of fetal development. In cord blood at or near term, the average level for most components of complement are about one half the values for adults (Adinolfi, 1977).

In the absence of a direct antigenic stimulus in the fetus, such as infection, the immunoglobulins in the fetus consist almost totally of species of immune globulin G (IgG) synthesized by the mother and subsequently transferred across the placenta by both diffusion and active transport, as described on page 147 of this chapter. Therefore, the antibodies in the fetus and the newborn infant most often reflect the immunologic experiences of the mother.

Differing from many animals, the human newborn infant does not acquire much in the way of passive immunity from the absorption of humoral antibodies ingested in the colostrum. Nonetheless, immune globulin A (IgA) ingested in colostrum may provide protection against enteric infections, because the antibody resists digestion and is effective on mucosal surfaces. The same is possibly true for IgA ingested with amnionic fluid before delivery.

In the adult, production of immune globulin M (IgM) in response to antigen is superseded in a week or so predominantly by production of IgG. In contrast, the IgM response remains the dominant one for weeks to months in the fetus and newborn. IgM serum levels in umbilical cord blood and identification of specific antibodies may be of aid in the diagnosis of intrauterine infection.

The transfer of some IgG antibodies from mother to fetus is harmful rather than protective to the fetus. The classic clinical example of antibodies of maternal origin that are dangerous to the fetus is hemolytic disease of the fetus and newborn resulting from Rh isoimmunization. In this disease, maternal antibody to fetal erythrocyte antigen crosses the placenta to destroy the fetal erythrocytes (see Chapter 38, p. 772).

NUTRITION OF THE FETUS

During the first 2 months of pregnancy, the embryo consists almost entirely of water; in later months, relatively more solids are added. The amounts of water, fat, nitrogen, and certain minerals in the fetus at successive weeks of pregnancy are shown in Table 8-5, adapted from Widdowson (1968). Because of the small amount of yolk in the human ovum, growth of the fetus from the very early stage of development depends on nutrition obtained from the mother. During the first few days after implantation, the nutrition of the fertilized ovum is derived directly from the interstitial fluid of the endometrium and from the surrounding maternal tissue, which has undergone proteolysis due to trophoblastic invasion. Within the next week, the forerunners of the

TABLE 8-5. TOTAL AMOUNTS OF FAT, NITROGEN, AND MINERALS IN THE BODY OF THE DEVELOPING FETUS

Body Weight (g)	Approximate Fetal Age (weeks)	Water (g)	Fat (g)	N (g)	Ca (g)	P (g)	Mg (g)	Na (mEq)	K (mEq)	Cl (mEq)	Fe (mg)	Cu (mg)	Zn (mg)
30	13	27	0.2	0.4	0.09	0.09	0.003	3.6	1.4	2.4	—	—	—
100	15	89	0.5	1.0	0.3	0.2	0.01	9	2.6	7	5.1	—	—
200	17	177	1.0	2.8	0.7	0.6	0.03	20	7.9	14	10	0.7	2.6
500	23	440	3.0	7.0	2.2	1.5	0.10	49	22	33	28	2.4	9.4
1000	26	860	10	14	6.0	3.4	0.22	90	41	66	64	3.5	16
1500	31	1270	35	25	10	5.6	0.35	125	60	96	100	5.6	25
2000	33	1620	100	37	15	8.2	0.46	160	84	120	160	8.0	35
2500	35	1940	185	49	20	11	0.58	200	110	130	220	10	43
3000	38	2180	360	55	25	14	0.70	240	130	150	260	12	50
3500	40	2400	560	62	30	17	0.78	280	150	160	280	14	53

(From Widdowson: In Assali (ed): Biology of Gestation, Vol. II, The Fetus and Neonate. New York, Academic, 1968.)

intervillous space arise, comprising at first simply lacunae filled with maternal blood. During the third week after ovulation, blood vessels appear in the chorionic villi. During the fourth week after ovulation, a cardiovascular system, and thereby a true circulation, has formed both within the embryo and between the embryo and the chorionic villi.

Ultimately, the maternal diet is the source of the nutrients supplied to the fetus. The mother eats varying amounts and kinds of food several times a day. In turn, the food is digested, its constituents are absorbed, and, for the most part, they are immediately stored. The storage forms are then made available continuously in an orderly way to meet the demands for energy, tissue, repair, and new growth, including pregnancy. Three major storage depots, namely, the liver, muscle, and adipose tissue, and the storage hormone, insulin, are involved intimately in the metabolism of the nutrients absorbed from the maternal gut. Insulin is released from the maternal islands of Langerhans in response to various materials liberated from food during digestion and absorption. The secretion of insulin is sustained by rising levels of blood glucose and amino acids. The net effect is to store glucose as glycogen primarily in the liver and muscle, to retain some amino acids as protein, and to store the excess as fat. This storage of maternal fat peaks in the second trimester and then declines as fetal demands increase in late pregnancy (Pipe and colleagues, 1979).

During the fasting state, glucose is released from glycogen, but glycogen stores are not large in the mother and cannot in themselves provide an adequate amount of glucose to meet the requirements of the mother and fetus for energy and growth. The cleavage of stored triglycerides in adipose tissue, however, provides the mother with energy in the form of free fatty acids. The process of lipoylsis is activated directly or indirectly by a number of hormones, including glucagon, norepinephrine, placental lactogen, glucocorticoids, and thyroxine. Neutral fat does not cross the placenta but glycerol does. The extent of transport of free fatty acids is not known, although Szabo and associates (1969) noted active transfer of palmitic acid from the maternal to the fetal side of the human placenta perfused in vitro. Portman and coworkers (1969), furthermore, demonstrated rapid transfer of palmitic and linoleic acids from mother to fetus in subhuman primates. Glucose and the naturally occurring forms of amino acids, of course, readily cross the placenta to the fetus. It appears that glucose transfer across the placenta is carrier-mediated, or "facilitated," although this is not an established fact (Hay, 1979). The placenta and, in turn, the fetus are not exposed to a constant supply of glucose because even in normal pregnant women the plasma levels may vary by up to 75 percent. Although the fetus is quite dependent on his mother for nutrition, he is not a passive parasite. He can actively participate through appropriate humoral and metabolic interaction in providing for his own nutrition.

The placenta is known to concentrate a large number of amino acids intracellularly from maternal plasma (Lemons, 1979). The actual uptake of amino acids by the placenta occurs by diffusion and by active transport. Presumably, fetal uptake of amino acids is dependent to an appreciable extent upon this concentrating capacity of the placenta. Essential amino acids for the fetus include methionine, cystine, histidine, isoleucine, leucine, lysine, phenylalanine, threonine, tryptophan, and valine (Lemons, 1979).

Because glucose is a major nutrient for growth and energy in the fetus, it would seem advantageous during pregnancy, as emphasized by Freinkel (1979), for the operational mechanisms to be those that minimize glucose utilization by the mother and thereby make the limited maternal supply available to the fetus. One metabolic action of placental lactogen, a hormone normally present in abundance in the mother but not the fetus, is to block the peripheral uptake and utilization of glucose by the mother while promoting the mobilization and utilization of free fatty acids. Placental lactogen does not appear to be absolutely required for a normal pregnancy outcome, however. Nielsen and co-workers (1979), and subsequently others, have described otherwise normal pregnancies in which *no* placental lactogen could be identified by any of the techniques applied in several laboratories.

For obvious reasons, a great deal of investigative effort continues to be focused on maternal nutrition and its effect on the growth and development of the fetus. Fetal size is not just a function of fetal age. For example, in maternal diabetes mellitus without significant maternal vascular disease, the fetus is much larger typically than normal; if severe maternal vascular disease further complicates the diabetes, however, the fetus may be appreciably smaller than normal (see Chapter 28, p. 601). Page (1970), in an interesting theoretical discussion of fetal growth, analyzed the factors known to control the delivery of a primary nutrient, glucose, to the fetus. Because maternal hyperglycemia leads to increased transfer of glucose across the placenta, he suggested that hyperglycemia and hyperinsulinemia in the fetus together accelerate fetal growth. Brinsmead and Liggins (1979) have observed insulin levels to be higher in cord plasma from large-for-gestational-age infants and lower when infants were small for gestational age.

Factors leading to growth retardation in the human fetus are complex. Growth retardation might result from insufficient concentration of a nutrient in the maternal arterial plasma, inadequate uterine blood flow and placental perfusion, reduced functional surface area of the chorionic villi, impairment of placental transport mechanisms, inadequate vascularity of the chorionic villi, or insufficient umbilical blood flow to transfer the nutrient in appropriate amounts from the placenta to the fetus (see Chapter 37). Maternal dietary deficiencies among species in which the weight of the fetus is relatively large compared with the mother's weight, and in which the duration of gestation is short, commonly cause fetal growth retardation. However, in instances where fetal size is slight compared with that of the mother and the duration of gestation is long, it has been difficult to demonstrate a clear-cut correlation between maternal nutritional deficiency and fetal growth retardation (see Chapter 13, p. 250). It is possible that subtle but nonetheless deleterious changes in the human fetus may be induced by faulty maternal nutrition, be it either undernutrition or the ingestion of excessive amounts of nutrients, including protein (Stein and colleagues, 1978).

AMNIONIC FLUID

The fluid filling the amnionic sac serves several important functions. It provides a medium in which the fetus can readily move, cushions him against possible injury, helps him maintain an even temperature, and provides, when appropriately tested, useful information concerning the health and maturity of the fetus (see Chapter 14). If the presenting part of the fetus is not closely applied to the lower uterine segment during labor, the hydrostatic action of the amnionic fluid may also be important in dilating the cervical canal.

By the 12th day after fertilization of the ovum, a cleft enclosed by primitive amnion has formed adjacent to the embryonic plate. Rapid enlargement of the cleft and fusion of the surrounding amnion first with the body stalk, and later with the chorion, create the amnionic sac, which fills with an essentially colorless fluid. The amnionic fluid increases rapidly to an average volume of 50 ml at 12 weeks of gestation and 400 ml at midpregnancy; it reaches a maximum of about 1 liter at 36 to 38 weeks of gestation. The volume then decreases as term approaches, and, if the pregnancy is prolonged, amnionic fluid may become relatively scant (see Chapter 37, p. 761). There are rather marked individual differences in amnionic fluid volume, however, as reported by Fuchs (1966). Similar data reported by Gillibrand (1969) are shown in Figure 8-26. The physician performing amniocentesis for diagnostic purposes soon appreciates the considerable variability in the volume of amnionic fluid present at the same time in different pregnancies as well as at different times in the same pregnancy.

The composition and volume of amnionic fluid change as pregnancy advances. In the first half of pregnancy, the fluid has essentially the same composition as maternal plasma except for a much lower protein concentration, and it is nearly devoid of particulate matter. As gestation advances, phospholipids, primarily from the lung, accumulate in the fluid and variable amounts of particulate matter, in the form of desquamated fetal cells, lanugo and scalp hair, and vernix caseosa, are shed into the fluid. The concentrations of various solutes also change significantly and, as a consequence, the osmolality decreases on the average about 20 to 30 mOsm, or about 10 percent, as shown in Figure 8-26.

Ions and small molecules move rapidly into and out of amnionic fluid but at rates that are specific for each substance. In contrast to bulk movement of amnionic fluid, as with swallowing, this process involves simply

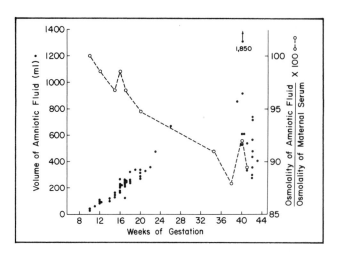

Figure 8-26. Amnionic fluid volume (*black dots*) and osmolality (*open circles*). The first and second trimesters are characterized by a rather orderly increase in volume, but at term the volume is quite variable. The osmolality decreases in approximately linear fashion as pregnancy advances. (*From Gillibrand: Br J Obstet Gynaecol 76:893, 1969.*)

molecular or ionic trade across a membrane without necessarily inducing changes in volume or concentration (Plentl, 1968).

There is no single mechanism that will account for all the variations in composition and volume of amnionic fluid that have been observed during the course of a normal pregnancy. One relatively simple explanation is that amnionic fluid in early pregnancy is a product primarily of the amnionic membrane covering the placenta and cord. It is likely that fluid also passes across the fetal skin at this time (Lind and colleagues, 1972). As the pregnancy advances, the surface of the amnion expands and the volume of fluid increases, but from about the fourth month the fetus is capable of modifying amnionic fluid composition and volume by urinating and swallowing progressively larger amounts of fluid. At the same time, movement of fluid into and out of the respiratory tract is likely to modify further the volume and composition of amnionic fluid.

As gestation advances, fetal urine makes an increasingly important contribution to the amnionic fluid. Fetal urine is quite hypotonic compared with maternal or fetal plasma, because of the lower electrolyte concentration in the urine, but it contains more urea, creatinine, and uric acid than does plasma. The net effect is that the osmolality of fluid decreases with increasing length of gestation. These observations have been shown to exist in utero as early as the 24th week of pregnancy. Mandelbaum and Evans (1969) examined urine obtained inadvertently from the fetal bladder at the time of attempted transfusion and compared the concentrations of several of the constituents of the urine with those of amnionic fluid. Even at 24 weeks of gestation, the urea and creatinine concentrations were two to three times higher in the urine, whereas the concentrations of sodium, potassium, and chloride were only about one third to one fifth as great as those in the amnionic fluid. The admixture of sizable volumes of fetal urine with the amnionic fluid, therefore, would logically be expected to lower the osmolality, as shown in Figure 8-26, and, at the same time, raise the concentration of urea, creatinine, and uric acid. Indeed, late in pregnancy, amnionic fluid normally differs from plasma in precisely these ways.

The fetus swallows amnionic fluid during much of pregnancy. Often, but not always, a great excess of amnionic fluid (hydramnios) develops whenever fetal swallowing is greatly impaired (see Chapter 23, p. 463). A classic example of a lesion in which fetal swallowing cannot take place and thereby leads to hydramnios is fetal esophageal atresia. Conversely, when urination in utero cannot take place, as in instances of renal agenesis or atresia of the urethra, the volume of amnionic fluid typically surrounding the fetus is extremely limited (oligohydramnios).

Although lack of fetal swallowing with continuous production of normal amounts of fluid by the amnion and by the fetal kidneys may lead to hydramnios, this mechanism is certainly not the sole cause of hydramnios. Progressive hydramnios has been observed in instances in which a normal fetus was known to ingest relatively large amounts of amnionic fluid, and in which maternal diseases known to predispose to hydramnios, such as diabetes, were not identified (Pritchard, 1966). Presumably, in these instances, increased production by the amnion, or unlikely, intense fetal polyuria, or even both, cause the increase in amnionic fluid volume. Whether the respiratory tract is involved at times in the development of hydramnios is not clear. What is clear, however, is that if the volume of amnionic fluid is reduced to abnormal levels, as may occur in anephric fetuses or in instances of early and prolonged rupture of the fetal membranes, fetal pulmonary hypoplasia may result to such a severe degree that extrauterine life is impossible (Fliegner and co-workers, 1981; Wigglesworth and Desai, 1982).

SEX OF THE FETUS

Sex Ratio

The accepted secondary sex ratio, that is, the sex ratio of human fetuses that reach viability, is approximately 106 males to 100 females. This figure has been obtained by the examination of term and premature infants. Many attempts have been made to establish a sex ratio for fetuses of earlier gestational age. In general, such studies have been misleading, for, as Wilson (1926) showed, the appearance of external genitals are an unreliable index of sex before the 50-mm stage.

Since, theoretically, there should be as many Y-bearing as X-bearing sperm, the primary sex ratio, or the ratio at the time of fertilization, should be 1:1. If so, the secondary sex ratio of 106:100 is suggestive that more fe-

males than males are lost during the early months of pregnancy. Establishment of the primary sex ratio in man is at present impracticable, for it requires the recovery and assignment of zygotes that fail to cleave and blastocysts that fail to implant. The results of Carr's studies (1963), nevertheless, suggest that the primary sex ratio in the human is unity.

Sexual Differentiation

One of the greatest responsibilities of the obstetrician is the assignment of sex to the newborn. An incorrect assignment of sex portends grave psychologic and social problems for the baby and family. Yet, we are of the view that sex assignment can be made correctly even in newborns with ambiguity of the external genitalia. To address this issue, and to address the issue of establishing a definitive diagnosis as to the cause of development of ambiguous external genitalia, the mechanisms of normal and abnormal sexual differentiation must be considered. It is clear that male phenotypic sexual differentiation is directed by the testis. *In the absence of the testis, female differentiation ensues irrespective of the genetic sex.*

Genetic sex, XX or XY, is established at the time of fertilization of the ovum. Thereafter, however, the initial development of male and female embryos is identical. It is the differentiation of the primordial gonad into testis or ovary that heralds the establishment of gonadal sex (Fig. 8-27). In the development of gonadal differentiation, it is known that the Y chromosome is of paramount importance in the direction of gonadal differentiation into testes. Nonetheless, it still is not clear how the Y chromosome directs testicular differentiation. It is known that there are male-specific, cell-surface proteins, for example, the H-Y antigen(s), that are correlated with testicular development in many species. Indeed, evidence has been presented that the H-Y antigen(s) actually induces testicular differentiation (Ohono and associates, 1978). It may be, however, that the structural gene that specifies the H-Y antigen is located on an autosome with positive regulation caused by a loci on the Y chromosome and a negative regulatory control caused by a loci on the X chromosome (Wolf, 1981). As pointed out by Silvers and colleagues (1982), however, there likely are a number of male-specific antigens; presently, no invariable relation can be defined between the presence of a given antigen and the development of a testis. Nonetheless, with establishment of the gonadal sex, there is the very rapid development of the phenotypic sex.

For example, Jost (1973) found that when castration of the rabbit fetus was conducted before differentiation of the genital anlagen, all newborns were phenotypic females with female external genitalia and the müllerian ducts had developed into uterus, fallopian tubes, and upper vagina. On the other hand, if castration of the fetus was conducted before differentiation of the genital anlagen and this was followed by implantation of a testis on one side, the phenotype of all fetuses was male; the

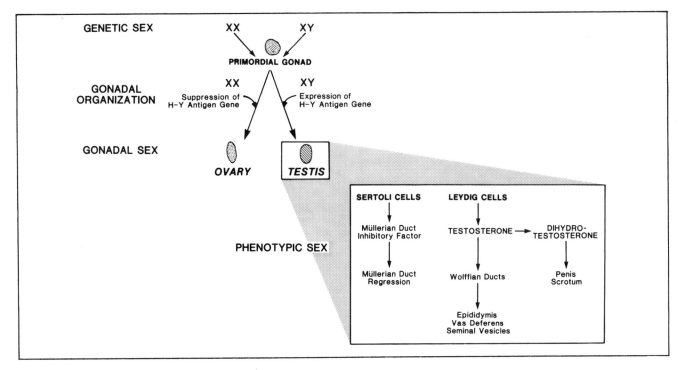

Figure 8-27. Sexual differentiation. Genetic sex is established at the time of fertilization of the ovum. At a time thereafter, the primordial gonad is acted upon by male-specific substances [e.g., H-Y antigen(s)] that effect the organization of the gonad as a testis, the secretions of which effect male phenotypic sex differentiation. (*Courtesy Dr. L. Casey.*)

external genitalia of such fetuses were masculinized; and, on the side of the testicular implant there was wolffian duct development in that a vas deferens, epididymis, and seminal vesicle were formed. On the side of the testicular implant, müllerian structures, namely, uterine horn and fallopian tube, were not present. On the other hand, the müllerian duct did develop on the side of castration in which there was no testis graft. Jost also found that if after castration of the fetus at the sexually indifferent stage a testosterone pellet was implanted on one side (in the site of a removed gonad), the external genitalia masculinized, as did the wolffian duct; the müllerian duct did not regress, however, that is, the uterine horn and fallopian tubes did develop in spite of the "androgen" implant.

These fundamental observations, together with those of Wilson and collaborators (Wilson and Gloyna, 1970; Wilson and Lasnitzki, 1971), form the basic framework of our understanding of the mechanisms of sexual differentiation. Wilson and Gloyna convincingly demonstrated that in most androgen responsive tissues, the androgen, testosterone, is converted to 5α-dihydrotestosterone in a reaction catalyzed by the enzyme, 5α-reductase. In these tissues, androgen action is expressed by way of this 5α-reduced metabolite. The 5α-dihydrostestosterone is bound to a cytosolic binding protein and the steroid-receptor protein complex is translocated to the nucleus, where it becomes associated with chromatin. Thus, in the genital tubercle and urogenital sinus,

testosterone acts only after conversion to 5α-dihydrotestosterone. There is a notable and important exception to this generalization for testosterone action in genital tissues, however. Wilson and Lasnitzki also demonstrated that testosterone, as testosterone, acts on the wolffian duct of the embryo to cause development of the male ductal system; indeed, this action of testosterone is expressed before 5α-reductase activity is detectable in this tissue.

Based on these observations, the biochemical basis of sexual differentiation can be formulated, as illustrated diagrammatically in Figure 8-27 and summarized below:

1. Genetic sex is established at the time of fertilization of the ovum.
2. Gonadal sex is determined by organizing factor(s) that may arise on autosomes, but by way of genic action that is affected positively by factors encoded on loci on the Y chromosome or negatively by factors encoded on loci on the X chromosome. By way of these coordinated processes, differentiation of the primitive gonad as a testis is accomplished.
3. The fetal testis (Sertoli cells) elaborates a proteinaceous substance called müllerian duct regression (or inhibitory) factor (a protein, ca. 35,000 daltons) that acts to cause regression of the müllerian duct, that is, it causes failure of development of uterus, fallopian tube, and upper

vagina. Müllerian duct regression factor is produced by the Sertoli cells of the seminiferous tubules; importantly, recall that the seminiferous tubules appear in fetal gonads before the Leydig cells, the cellular site of origin of testosterone. Therefore, regression of the müllerian ducts is initiated at a time in fetal development before testosterone secretion commences. Müllerian duct regression factor acts locally, that is, near its site of formation; therefore, if a testis were absent on one side, the müllerian duct on that side would persist and the uterus and fallopian tubes would develop therefrom.

4. The fetal testis, under the influence of the action of chorionic gonadotropin initially and thence fetal pituitary LH, secretes testosterone that acts directly on the wolffian duct to effect the development of the vas deferens, epididymides, and seminal vesicles. Testosterone, of fetal testicular origin, enters the blood, reaches the genital tubercle and urogenital sinus, and, in these tissues, is converted to 5α-dihydrotestosterone, the active androgen that brings about the virilization of the external genitalia.

The development of ambigious genitalia is brought about, invariably, by abnormal androgenic representation in utero. This means, simply, too much androgen for an embryo that was destined to be female, or too little androgenic representation for an embryo or a fetus that was destined to be male. In the case of the fetus destined to be male, inadequate androgenic representation may be caused by deficient fetal testicular secretion of testosterone or else by a deficiency in responsiveness to testosterone or 5α-dihydrotestosterone in tissues that nominally respond to androgen.

Based on these premises, we believe that all abnormalities of sexual differentiation can be identified in one of three general categories:

- Category 1. Female pseudohermaphroditism.
- Category 2. Male pseudohermaphroditism.
- Category 3. Dysgenetic gonads and true hermaphroditism.

Category 1. Female Pseudohermaphroditism. In this category, we find abnormalities that conform to several guidelines: (1) müllerian duct regression factor is *not* produced; (2) androgen exposure of the embryo and fetus is variable; (3) karyotype is 46,XX; and (4) ovaries are present. Therefore, all subjects in this category were destined to be female by virtue of genetic and gonadal sex. Thus, the only abnormality that can occur is androgenic excess. Because müllerian duct regression factor was not produced, there will be a uterus, fallopian tubes, and upper vagina in each subject in this category. If such embryos were exposed to a small androgenic excess reasonably late in embryonic (early fetal) development, the only abnormality would be slight clitoral hypertrophy, with an otherwise normal female phenotype. With some-

what greater androgenic excess, clitoral hypertrophy and posterior labial fusion may develop. With progressively increasing androgenic excess, somewhat earlier in embryonic development, there is greater virilization. This process of virilization can proceed through the formation of labioscrotal folds, the development of a urogenital sinus (in which the vagina empties into the posterior urethra), and even to the development of a penile urethra with scrotal formation, the "empty scrotum" syndrome. The cause of female pseudohermaphroditism is excessive androgen for a fetus that is destined to be female. The androgenic excess most commonly arises from the fetal adrenal by virtue of excess secretion of androgen or androgen prehormones in instances of enzymatic defects in the pathway to cortisol formation in the adrenal cortex, that is, congenital adrenal hyperplasia. With inadequate cortisol synthesis, it is presumed that ACTH secretion is elevated. Excessive stimulation of the adrenals leads to excessive secretion of cortisol precursors and metabolites thereof, including androgens and prehormones that can be converted to true androgens, principally androstenedione, which is converted to testosterone in extraglandular tissues. The enzyme deficiency may involve any of the five enzymatic reactions in the pathway to cortisol biosynthesis, namely, cholesterol side-chain cleavage, 3β-hydroxysteroid dehydrogenase, 17β-hydroxylase, 21-hydroxylase, or 11β-hydroxylase.

Another cause of female pseudohermaphroditism is fetal androgenic excess that is due to excessive androgen arising in the maternal compartment. Excess androgen in the mother may arise as a result of secretion from maternal ovaries, that is, hyperreactio lutealis, or from tumors of the maternal ovary, for example, luteomas, arrhenoblastomas, hilar cell tumors, and so on. Commonly, however, the female fetus of a pregnant woman with an androgen-secreting tumor is not virilized. During most, and perhaps all, of pregnancy, the female fetus is protected from androgen excess in the mother because of the extraordinary capacity of the trophoblast to convert aromatizable C_{19}-steroids (androgens) to estrogens (see Chapter 7).

In addition, if certain drugs are given to pregnant women, virilization of their female fetuses may occur. Most commonly, such drugs are synthetic progestins. It is not altogether clear how progestins cause virilization of the female fetus. On one hand, some of these compounds, especially those of the 19-nortestosterone configuration, may act on fetal tissues as androgens. On the other hand, these agents may act to inhibit aromatization in the placenta and thus allow the transfer to the fetus of androgens that escape aromatization. In summary, all subjects of Category 1 can become normal, fertile women if the proper diagnosis is made and appropriate therapy is initiated.

Category 2. Male Pseudohermaphroditism. In this category, we find abnormalities that conform to several guidelines: (1) müllerian duct regression factor is produced; (2) androgenic representation is variable; (3) karyotype is 46,XY; and, (4) testes, or else no gonads, are

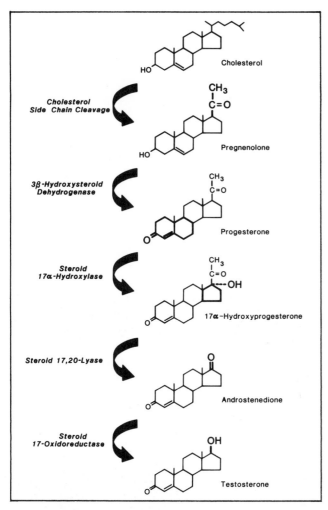

Figure 8-28. Biosynthetic pathway of testosterone formation in the testis. There are five enzymatic reactions involved in the conversion of cholesterol to testosterone. A defect in each of these enzymes has been identified as the cause of inadequate fetal testicular testosterone production. (*Courtesy of Dr. L. Casey.*)

present. All subjects in this category were destined to be male by virtue of genetic sex. Thus, the abnormalities in sexual differentiation are the result of incomplete virilization.

Diminished masculinization can be caused by inadequate production of testosterone by the fetal testis or else by diminished responsiveness of the genital anlagen to normal quantities of androgen. Since müllerian duct regression factor is produced during embryonic life in these subjects, there is no uterus, fallopian tubes, or upper vagina. Deficient testosterone production may occur if there is an enzymatic defect in the testis that involves any one of the five enzymes in the biosynthetic pathway to testosterone formation (Fig. 8-28). Defects in each of these enzymatic reactions, as a cause of abnormal sex differentiation, have been described.

If the testes regress during embryonic or fetal life, there will, thereafter, be deficient testosterone produc-

tion. Such an occurrence has been referred to as embryonic testicular regression (Edman and associates, 1977).

Deficiencies in androgen responsiveness may be due to inadequate or abnormal androgen receptor macromolecules or both in the cytosol of androgen responsive tissues or else may be due to failure of conversion of testosterone to 5α-dihydrotestosterone in such tissues due to deficient 5α-reductase enzyme activity.

The most extreme form of the disorders of androgen resistance is that of testicular feminization. In this entity, there appears to be little or no tissue responsiveness to androgen. In affected subjects, there is a female phenotype and a short, blind-ending vagina, no uterus or fallopian tubes, and no wolffian duct structures. At the expected time of puberty, testosterone levels in such women rise to values similar to or greater than those found in normal adult men. Nonetheless, virilization does not occur and even sexual hair, that is, pubic and axillary hair, does not develop, presumably because of resistance to androgen action. Presumably, because of androgen resistance at the level of the brain and pituitary, LH levels are elevated in these women. In response to LH, in high concentrations, there also is increased testicular secretion of estrogen compared with that found in normal men (MacDonald and colleagues, 1979). The increased estrogen, together with the absence of androgen responsiveness, may act in concert to cause feminization, that is, breast development. In the disorder referred to as incomplete testicular feminization, there appears to be slight androgen responsiveness. In such subjects, there ordinarily is modest clitoral hypertrophy at birth; at the expected time of puberty, however, virilization does not occur, although pubic and axillary hair do develop. These women also develop feminine breasts, presumably through the same endocrine mechanisms as in women with the complete form of testicular feminization (Madden and co-workers, 1975).

A third syndrome of androgen resistance has been referred to as familial male pseudohermaphroditism, Type I (Wilson and colleagues, 1974). This entity is commonly referred to as Reifenstein syndrome but constitutes a spectrum of abnormalities of genital virilization varying from a phenotype similar to that of women with incomplete testicular feminization to that of a male phenotype with only a bifid scrotum, infertility, and gynecomastia. In these subjects, androgen resistance was also established by the demonstration of diminished 5α-dihydrotestosterone binding capacity in fibroblasts grown in culture from genital skin biopsies.

A fourth form of androgen resistance is caused by a deficiency, in androgen-responsive tissues, of the enzyme activity, 5α-reductase. Since androgen action in the genital tubercle and urogenital sinus is mediated by the action of 5α-dihydrotestosterone, in persons with 5α-reductase deficiency there are female external genitalia (modest clitoral hypertrophy). Since androgen action in the wolffian duct of the embryo is mediated by testosterone per se, however, in such persons there are well-developed epididymides, seminal vesicles, vas deferens;

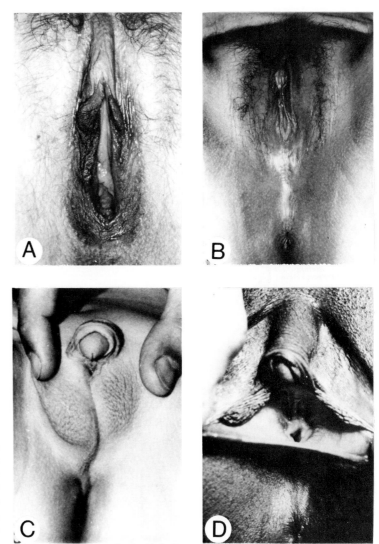

Figure 8-29. External genitalia of representative patients with male pseudohermaphroditism due to androgen resistance. **A.** Testicular feminization. **B.** Incomplete testicular feminization. **C.** Familial male pseudohermaphroditism, Type I (Reinfenstein syndrome). **D.** 5-Reductase deficiency. (*From Wilson and MacDonald, In Metabolic Basis of Inherited Disease. New York, McGraw-Hill, 1978.*)

the male ejaculatory ducts empty into the vagina (Walsh and associates, 1974).

A composite photograph of the genitalia of subjects with each of the four types of androgen resistance is shown in Figure 8-29.

Enzymatic defects in testicular testosterone biosynthesis give rise to decreased rates of fetal testosterone secretion; incomplete masculinization of the external genitalia is the consequence. The phenotype of such newborns is variable in the degree of ambiguity because the degree of enzyme deficiency varies.

The phenotype of subjects with embryologic testicular regression is dependent upon the time in embryonic life that the fetal testes regressed. The time course of gonadal development and sexual differentiation is illustrated in Figure 8-30.

Edman and associates (1977) analyzed the phenotypes of reported cases of agonadism in 46,XY persons, and in three of their own cases. They compared these findings with those that would be expected to occur if the testes regressed at various stages of development according to embryologic findings of the time course of sexual differentiation in man (Jirasek, 1967, 1970, 1971). They found that a spectrum of phenotypes (cases a–i, Fig. 8-30) had been described; among affected persons, the phenotypes varied from normal female with absent uterus, fallopian tubes, and upper vagina, to that of a normal male, but with anorchia. Since müllerian regression commences before virilization is initiated in embryonic life, such a spectrum of phenotypes was to be expected if testicular regression were to occur at various times during the process of sexual differentiation.

Category 3. In this category of our classification, we find subjects with abnormalities of sexual differentiation that conform to several guidelines: (1) müllerian duct regression factor was not produced; (2) fetal androgen production among subjects was variable; (3) karyotype varies among subjects and commonly is abnormal; and, (4) gonads are not present, neither ovaries nor testes. In all of the subjects of this category, there is a uterus, fallopian tubes, and upper vagina. In the majority of sub-

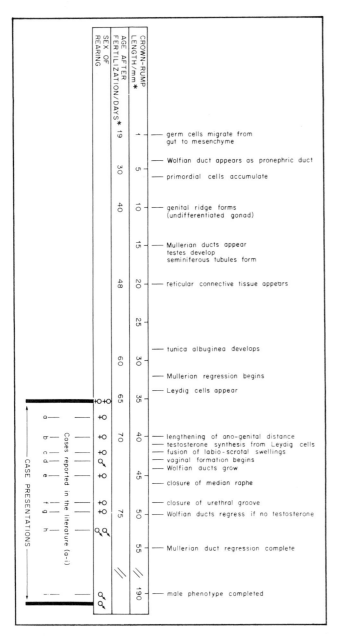

Figure 8-30. The temporal relations of the sequence or morphologic changes that occur during male embryogenesis, and a comparison of this sequence to the phenotypes reported in subjects with embryologic testicular regression.

jects in Category 3, dysgenetic gonads are found. With the typical case of gonadal dysgenesis (e.g., those with Turner syndrome) there is a female phenotype; at the time of expected puberty, however, sexual infantilism persists. In some persons with gonadal dysgenesis, there are ambiguous genitalia, a finding that is indicative that an abnormal gonad produced androgen, albeit in small amounts, during embryonic development. Generally, in such subjects, we find mixed gonadal dysgenesis, that is, a dysgenetic gonad on one side and an abnormal testis or

dysontogenetic tumor on the other side. In most subjects with true hermaphroditism, the guidelines for Category 3 are met. True hermaphrodites are those persons in whom both ovarian and testicular tissues are present; and, in particular, the germ cells, namely, ova and sperm, of both sexes are formed.

Preliminary Diagnosis

A preliminary diagnosis of the etiology and pathogenesis of genital ambiguity can be made at the time of birth of an affected child. By rectal examination of the newborn, the experienced examiner can ascertain whether the child has a uterus. If the uterus is present, the diagnosis must be female pseudohermaphroditism, testicular or gonadal dysgenesis, or true hermaphroditism. A family history of congenital adrenal hyperplasia is helpful. If the uterus is not present, the diagnosis is male pseudohermaphroditism. Androgen resistance and enzymatic defects in testicular testosterone biosynthesis are familial.

Sex Assignment

The critical decision of sex assignment by the obstetrician, in our view, is an easy, although sometimes painful, decision to make. In our judgment, any newborn with ambiguity of the genitalia so severe that the urethral opening is onto the perineum should be designated as female. This conclusion is reached on the basis of several considerations: (1) All persons in Category 1 of our classification (i.e., female pseudohermaphroditism) can be normal, fertile women. (2) The subjects of Category 2 of this classification either cannot produce testosterone or else are refractory to its action. Moreover, all of the subjects of Category 2 are infertile. (3) Presently, reconstruction of the penis in persons with androgen resistance in such a manner that a sexually functional organ is produced is difficult, if not impossible.

REFERENCES

Adam PAJ, Teramo K, Raiha N, Gitlin D, Schwartz R: Human fetal insulin metabolism early in gestation: Response to acute elevation of the fetal glucose concentration and placental transfer of human insulin-I-131. Diabetes 18:409, 1969

Adinolfi M: Human complement: Onset and site of synthesis during fetal life. Am J Dis Child 131:1015, 1977

Aherne W, Dunnill MS: Morphometry of the human placenta. Br Med Bull 22:1, 1966

Aizawa Y, Mueller GC: The effect in vivo and in vitro of estrogens on lipid synthesis in the rat uterus. J Biol Chem 236:381, 1961

Altshuler G: Immunologic competence of the immature human fetus. Obstet Gynecol 43:811, 1974

Arey LB: Developmental Anatomy: A Textbook and Laboratory Manual of Embryology, 5th ed. Philadelphia, Saunders, 1946

Assali NS: In Gluck L (ed): Modern Perinatal Medicine. Chicago, Year Book, 1974

Assali NS, Morris JA: Maternal and fetal circulations and their interrelationships. Obstet Gynecol Survey 19:923, 1964

Assali NS, Bekey GA, Morrison LW: Fetal and neonatal circulation. In Assali NS (ed): Biology of Gestation, Vol II. The Fetus and Neonate. New York, Academic, 1968a

Assali NS, Kirschbaum TH, Dilts PV: Effects of hyperbaric oxygen on uteroplacental and fetal circulation. Circ Res 22:573, 1968b

Avery ME, Mead J: Surface properties in relation to atelectasis and hyaline membrane disease. Am J Dis Child 97:517, 1959

Ballard PL, Ballard RA: Glucocorticoid receptors and the role of glucocorticoids in fetal lung development. Proc Natl Acad Sci USA 69:2668, 1972

Ballard PL, Gluckman PD, Brehier A, Kitterman JA, Kaplan SL, Rudolph AM, Grumbach MM: Failure to detect an effect of prolactin on pulmonary surfactant and adrenal steroids in fetal sheep and rabbits. J Clin Invest 62:879, 1978

Barclay AE, Barcroft J, Barron DH, Franklin KJ: Radiographic demonstration of circulation through heart in adult and in foetus, and identification of ductus arteriosus. Br J Radiol 12:505, 1939

Barrett CT, Sevanian A, Kaplan SA: Cyclic AMP (cAMP) and surfactant production: New means for enhancing lung maturation in the fetus. Pediatr Res 9:394, 1975

Bashore RA, Smith F, Schenker S: Placental transfer and disposition of bilirubin in the pregnant monkey. Am J Obstet Gynecol 103:950, 1969

Bearn JG: Role of fetal pituitary and adrenal glands in the development of the fetal thymus of the rabbit. Endocrinology 80:979, 1967

Belcher DP: A child weighing 25 pounds at birth. JAMA 67:950, 1916

Bernstein RB, Novy MJ, Piasecki GJ, Lester R, Jackson BT: Bilirubin metabolism in the fetus. J Clin Invest 48:1678, 1969

Bigazzi M, Ronga R, Lancranjan I, Ferraro S, Branconi F, Buzzoni P, Martorana G, Scarselli GF, Del Pozo E: A pregnancy in an acromegalic woman during bromocriptine treatment: Effects on growth hormone and prolactin in maternal, fetal, and amniotic compartments. J Clin Endocrinol Metab 48:9, 1979

Bleasdale JE, Johnston JM: CMP-dependent incorporation of [^{14}C] glycerol 3-phosphate into phosphatidylglycerol and phosphatidylglycerol phosphate by rabbit lung microsomes. J Biochim Biophys Acta, 710:377, 1982

Bleasdale JE, Johnston JM: Development Biochemistry of Lung Surfactant. In Nelson GH (ed): Pulmonary Development and Transition to Extrauterine Life. New York, Marcell Dekker, 1984, in press

Bleasdale JE, MacDonald PC, Johnston JM: Fetal lung maturation: The biochemistry of surfactant production: In DiRenzo GC, Hawkins PF (eds): Perinatal Medicine: Update and Controversies. London, Wiley, 1984, in press

Bleasdale JE, Wallis P, MacDonald PC, Johnston JM: Characterization of the forward and reverse reactions catalyzed by CDP-diacylglycerol: Inositol transferase in rabbit lung tissue. Biochim Biophys Acta 575:135, 1979

Boddy K, Dawes GS: Fetal breathing. Br Med Bull 31:3, 1975

Braestrup PW: Studies of latent scurvy in infants: II. Content of ascorbic (cevitamic) acid in the blood serum of women in labor and in children at birth. Acta Paediat 19 (Suppl 1):328, 1937

Brash AR, Hickey DE, Graham TP, Stahlman MT, Oates JA, Cotton RB: Pharmacokinetics of indomethacin in the neonate. Relation of plasma indomethacin levels to response of the ductus arteriosus. N Engl J Med 305:67, 1981

Breckenridge WC, Makai L, Kuksis A: Triglyceride structure of human milk fat. Can J Biochem 47:761, 1969

Brehier A, Benson BJ, Williams MC, Mason RJ, Ballard PL: Corticosteroid induction of phosphatidic acid phosphatase in fetal rabbit lung. Biochem Biophys Res Commun 77:886, 1977

Brinsmead MW, Liggins GC: Somatomedin-like activity, prolactin, growth hormone and insulin in human cord blood. Aust N Z Obstet Gynaec 19:129, 1979

Brown A: Biology of Gestation, Vol II. The Fetus and Neonate. New York, Academic, 1968

Browning AJF, Butt WR, Lynch SS, Shakespear RA: Maternal plasma concentrations of β-endorphin and γ-lipotrophin throughout pregnancy. Br J Obstet Gynaecol 90:1147, 1983

Carr D: Chromosome studies in abortuses and stillborn infants. Lancet 2:603, 1963

Chan L, Jackson RL, O'Malley BW: Synthesis of very low density lipoproteins in the cockerel. Effects of estrogen. J Clin Invest 58:368, 1976

Chard T, Hudson CN, Edwards CRW, Boyd NRH: Release of oxytocin and vasopressin by the human foetus during labour. Nature 234:352, 1971

Chez RA, Mintz DH, Reynolds WA, Hutchinson DL: Maternal–fetal plasma glucose relationships in late monkey pregnancy. Am J Obstet Gynecol 121:938, 1975

Clements JA: Surface tension of lung extracts. Proc Soc Exp Biol Med 95:170, 1957

Davis ME, Potter EL: Intrauterine respiration of the human fetus. JAMA 131:1194, 1946

Dawes GS: The umbilical circulation. Am J Obstet Gynecol 84:1634, 1962

Delahunty TJ, Spitzer HL, Jimenez JM, Johnston JM: Phosphatidate phosphohydrolase activity in porcine pulmonary surfactant. Am Rev Resp Dis 119:75, 1979

DeVane GW, Porter JC: An apparent stress-induced release of arginine vasopression by human neonates. J Clin Endocrinol Metab 51:1412, 1980

DeVane GW, Naden RP, Porter JC, Rosenfeld CR: Mechanism of arginine vasopressin release in the sheep fetus. Pediatr Res 16:504, 1982

De Verdier CH, Garby L: Low binding of 2,3-diphosphoglycerate to hemoglobin F. Scand J Clin Lab Invest 23:149, 1969

Dickey RP, Robertson AF: Newborn estrogen excretion. Am J Obstet Gynecol 104:551, 1969

Dolman CL: Characteristic configuration of fetal brains from 22 to 40 weeks gestation at two week intervals. Arch Pathol Lab Med 101:193, 1977

Douglas WHJ, Sommers-Smith SK, Johnston JM: Phosphatidic acid phosphohydrolase (PAPase) activity as a marker for surfactant synthesis in organotypic cultures of type II alveolar pneumonocytes. J Cell Sci 60:199, 1983

Duenhoelter JH, Pritchard JA: Unpublished observations

Duenhoelter JH, Pritchard JA: Fetal respiration: Quantitative measurements of amnionic fluid inspired near term by human and rhesus fetuses. Am J Obstet Gynecol 125:306, 1976

Duenhoelter JH, Pritchard JA: Fetal respiration. A review. Am J Obstet Gynecol 129:326, 1977

Edman CD, Winters AJ, Porter JC, Wilson J, MacDonald PC: Embryonic testicular regression. A clinical spectrum of XY agonadal individual. Obstet Gynecol 49:208, 1977

Ekelund L, Arvidson G, Åstedt B: Cortisol induced accumulation of phospholipids in organ culture of human fetal lung. Scand J Clin Lab Invest 35:419, 1975

Epstein M, Chez RA, Oakes GK, Mintz DH: Fetal pancreatic glucagon responses in glucose-intolerant nonhuman primate pregnancy. Am J Obstet Gynecol 127:268, 1977

Estelles A, Aznar J, Gilabert J, Parrilla JJ: Dysfunctional plasminogen in full-term newborn. Pediatr Res 14:1180, 1980

Fadel HE, Abraham EC: Minor fetal hemoglobins in relation to gestational age. Am J Obstet Gynecol 141:704, 1981

Farrell PM, Zachman RD: Induction of choline phosphotransferase and lecithin synthesis in the fetal lung by corticosteroids. Science 179:297, 1973

Farrell PM, Avery ME: Hyaline membrane disease. Am Rev Resp Dis 111:657, 1975

Fencl M, Tulchinsky D: Total cortisol in amniotic fluid and fetal lung maturation. N Engl J Med 292:133, 1975

Finne PH: Antenatal diagnosis of the anemia in erythroblastosis. Acta Paediatr Scand 55:609, 1966

Fisher DA: Fetal thyroid hormone metabolism. Contemporary Ob/Gyn 3:47, 1975

Fisher DA, Klein AH: Thyroid development and disorders of thyroid function in the newborn. N Engl J Med 304:702, 1981

Fliegner JR, Fortune DW, Eggers TR: Premature rupture of the membranes, oligohydramnios and pulmonary hypoplasia. Aust N Z J Obstet Gynaecol 21:77, 1981

Foley ME, Isherwood DM, McNicol GP: Viscosity, haematocrit, fibrinogen and plasma proteins in maternal and cord blood. Br J Obstet Gynaecol 85:500, 1978

Freinkel N: Homeostatic factors in fetal carbohydrate metabolism. In Wynn RM (ed): Fetal Homeostasis. New York, Appleton, 1969, vol IV

Fuchs F: Volume of amniotic fluid at various states of pregnancy. Clin Obstet Gynecol 9:449, 1966

Gelato M, Marshall S, Boudreau M, Bruni J, Campbell GA, Meit J: Effects of thyroid and ovaries on prolactin binding activity in rat liver. Endocrinology 96:1292, 1975

Giannopoulus G: Glucocorticoid receptors in lung. I. Specific binding of glucocorticoids to cytoplasmic components of rabbit fetal lung. J Biol Chem 248:3876, 1973

Gilbert RD, Lis L, Longo LD: Temperature effects on O_2 affinity of fetal blood. Presented at the 30th Annual Meeting of the Society for Gynecologic Investigation, Washington, DC, March 17–20, 1983

Gill RW, Trudinger BJ, Garrett WJ, Kossoff G, Warren PS: Fetal umbilical venous flow measured in utero by pulsed Doppler and B-mode ultrasound. I. Normal pregnancies. Am J Obstet Gynecol 139:720, 1981

Gillibrand PN: Changes in amniotic fluid volume with advancing pregnancy. J Obstet Gynaecol Br Commonw 76:527, 1969

Gitlin D: Protein transport across the placenta and protein turnover between amnionic fluid, maternal and fetal circulation. In Moghissi and Hafez (eds): The Placenta. Springfield, IL, Thomas, 1974

Gitlin D, Kumate J, Morales C, Noriega L, Arevalo N: The turnover of amniotic fluid protein in the human conceptus. Am J Obstet Gynecol 113:632, 1972

Glass L, Rajegowda BK, Evans HE: Absence of respiratory distress syndrome in premature infants of heroin-addicted mothers. Lancet 2:685, 1971

Gluck L, Motoyama EK, Smits HL, Kulovich MV: The biochemical development of surface activity in mammalian lung. I. The surface-active phospholipids; the separation and distribution of surface-active lecithin in the lung of the developing rabbit fetus. Pediatr Res 1:237, 1967

Gluck L, Landowne RA, Kulovich MV: Biochemical development of surface activity in mammalian lung: III. Structural changes in lung lecithin during development of the rabbit fetus and newborn. Pediatr Res 4:352, 1970

Gluck L, Kulovich MV, Borer RC, Brenner PH, Anderson GG,

Spellacy WN: Diagnosis of the respiratory distress syndrome by amniocentesis. Am J Obstet Gynecol 109:440, 1971

Gluck L, Kulovich MV, Eidelman AI, Cordero L, Khazin AF: Biochemical development of surface activity in mammalian lung: IV. Pulmonary lecithin synthesis in the human fetus and newborn and etiology of the respiratory distress syndrome. Pediatr Res 6:81, 1972

Gluck L, Kulovich MV, Borer RC: The interpretation and significance of the lecithin-sphingomyelin ratio in amniotic fluid. Am J Obstet Gynecol 120:142, 1974

Gluckman PD, Ballard PL, Kaplan SL, Liggins GC, Grumbach MM: Prolactin in umbilical cord blood and the respiratory distress syndrome. J Pediatr 93:1011, 1978

Gresham EL, Rankin JHG, Makowski EL, Meschia G, Battagia FC: Fetal renal function in unstressed pregnancies. J Clin Invest 51:149, 1972

Grosso DS, MacDonald CP, Thomasson JE, Christian CD: Relationship of newborn serum prolactin to the respiratory distress syndrome and maternal hypertension. Am J Obstet Gynecol 137:569, 1980

Gruenwald P: Growth of the human foetus. In McLaren A (ed): Advances in Reproductive Physiology. New York, Academic, 1967

Grumbach MM, Kaplan SL: Fetal pituitary hormones and the maturation of central nervous system regulation of anterior pituitary function. In Gluck L (ed): Modern Perinatal Medicine. Chicago, Year Book, 1974

Haase W: Maternity annual report for 1875. Charite Annalen 2:669, 1875

Hallman M, Kulovich MV, Kirkpatrick E, Sugarman RG, Gluck L: Phosphatidylinositol and phosphatidylglycerol in amniotic fluid: Indices of lung maturity. Am J Obstet Gynecol 125:613, 1976

Hamilton WJ, Mossman HW: Human Embryology, 4th ed. Baltimore, Williams & Wilkins, 1972

Hamosh M, Hamosh P: The effect of prolactin on the lecithin content of fetal rabbit lung. J Clin Invest 59:1002, 1977

Hauth JC, Parker CR, MacDonald PC, Porter JC, Johnston JM: Role of fetal prolactin in lung maturation. Obstet Gynecol 51:81, 1978

Hay WW Jr: Fetal glucose metabolism. Semin Perinatol 3:157, 1979

Henriksson P, Hedner V, Nilsson IM, Boehm J, Robertson B, Lorand L: Fibrin-stabilization factor XIII in the fetus and the newborn infant. Pediatr Res 8:789, 1974

Herbert WNP, Johnston JM, MacDonald PC, Jimenez JM: Fetal lung maturation: Human amniotic fluid phosphatidate phosphohydrolase activity through normal gestation and its relation to the lecithin/sphingomyelin ratio. Am J Obstet Gynecol 132:373, 1978

Hocheim H: Cited by Kiedel W, Gluck L, in Scarpelli (ed): Pulmonary Physiology of the Fetus, Newborn, and Child. Philadelphia, Lea and Febiger, 1975

Hollowes RC, Wang DY, Lewis DJ: The stimulation by prolactin and growth hormone of fatty acid synthesis in explants from rat mammary glands. J Endocrinol 57:265, 1973

Holmberg C, Perheentupa J, Launiala K, Hallman N: Congenital chloride diarrhea. Arch Dis Childhood 52:255, 1977

Huisman THJ, Schroder WA, Brown AK: Changes in the nature of human fetal hemoglobin during the first year of life. Presented before Society for Pediatric Research, Atlantic City, NJ, May 1, 1970

Jimenez JM, Johnston JM: Fetal lung maturation: IV. The release of phosphatidic acid phosphohydrolase and phospholipids into the human amniotic fluid. Pediatr Res 10:767, 1976

Jimenez JM, Schultz FM, MacDonald PC, Johnston JM: Fetal lung maturation: II. Phosphatidic acid phosphohydrolase in human amniotic fluid. Gynecol Invest 5:245, 1974

Jimenez JM, Schultz FM, Johnston JM: Fetal lung maturation. III. Amniotic fluid phosphatidic acid phosphohydrolase (PAPase) and its relation to the lecithin/sphingomyelin ratio. Am J Obstet Gynecol 46:588, 1975

Jirasek JE: The relationship between the structure of the testis and differentiation of the external genitalia and phenotype in man. In Wolstenholm, O'Connor (eds): Ciba Foundation Colloquia on Endocrinology. Endocrinology of the Testis. Boston, Little, Brown, 1967

Jirasek JE: The relationship between differentiation of the testicle, genital ducts and external genitalia in fetal and postnatal life. In Rosenberg, Paulsen (eds): The Human Testis: Advances in Experimental Medicine and Biology. New York, Plenum Press, 1970, vol 10.

Jirasek JE: Development of the genital system in human embryos and fetuses. Development of the Genital System and Male Pseudohermaphroditism. Baltimore, Johns Hopkins Press, 1971

Johnson JWC, Mitzner W, Lindon WJ, Palmer AE, Scott R, Kearney K: Glucocorticoids and the rhesus fetal lung. Am J Obstet Gynecol 130:905, 1978

Johnson JWC, Tyson JE, Mitzner W, London W, Palmer A, Andreassen B, Beck J: Prolactin and rhesus fetal lung characteristics. Presented before Society for Gynecologic Investigation, San Diego, Calif, March 21, 1979

Johnston JM, Porter, JC, MacDonald PC: The biosynthesis and hormonal regulation of surfactant formation. In Gatt S, Freysz L, Mandel P (eds): Enzymes of Lipid Metabolism. New York, Plenum, 1978a, p 327

Johnston JM, Reynolds G, Wylie MB, MacDonald PC: The phosphohydrolase activity in lamellar bodies and its relationship to phosphatidylglycerol and lung surfactant formation. Biochim Biophys Acta 531:65, 1978b

Josimovich JB, Merisko K, Boccella L: Binding of prolactin by fetal rhesus cell membrane fractions. Endocrinology 100:557, 1977

Jost A, Vigier B, Prepin J: Studies on sex differentiation in mammals. Rec Prog Horm Res 29:1, 1973

Kaplan S: Disorders of the endocrine system. In Assali NS (ed): Pathophysiology of Gestation: III. Fetal and Neonatal Disorders. New York, Academic, 1972

Kasper CK, Hoag MS, Aggeler PM, Stone S: Blood clotting factors in pregnancy: Factor VIII concentrations in normal and AHF-deficient women. Obstet Gynecol 24:242, 1964

Katz FH, Beck P, Makowski EL: The renin-aldosterone system in mother and fetus at term. Am J Obstet Gynecol 118:51, 1974

Kelly PA, Posner BI, Friesen HG: Effects of hypophysectomy, ovariectomy, and cycloheximide on specific binding sites for lactogenic hormones in rat liver. Endocrinology 97:1408, 1975

Khosla SS, Rooney SA: Stimulation of fetal lung surfactant production by administration of 17β-estradiol to the maternal rabbit. Am J Obstet Gynecol 133:213, 1979

Kiedel W, Gluck L: In Scarpelli E (ed): Pulmonary Physiology of the Fetus, Newborn, and Child. Philadelphia, Lea and Febiger, 1975, p 96

Klaus MH, Clements JA, Havel RJ: Composition of surface-active material isolated from beef lung. Proc Natl Acad Sci USA 47:185, 1961

Kohler PF: Maturation of the human complement system. J Clin Invest 52:671, 1973

Koldovsky O, Heringova A, Jirsova U, Jirasek JE, Uher J: Transport of glucose against a concentration gradient in everted sacs of jejunum and ileum of human fetuses. Gastroenterology 48:185, 1965

Kurjak A, Kirkinen P, Latin V, Ivankovic D: Ultrasonic assessment of fetal kidney function in normal and complicated pregnancies. Am J Obstet Gynecol 141:266, 1981

Lam TJ: Effect of prolactin on loss of solutes via the head region of the early-winter marine threespine stickelback (Gasterosteus aculeatus L., form tacherus) in fresh water. Can J Zool 47:865, 1969

Lands WE: Metabolism of glycerolipids: A comparison of lecithin and triglyceride synthesis. J Biol Chem 231:883, 1958

Lazarus JH, John R, Ginsberg J, Hughes IA, Shewring G, Smith BR, Woodhead JS, Hall R: Transient neonatal hyperthyrotrophinaemia: A serum abnormality due to transplacentally acquired antibody to thyroid stimulating hormone. Br Med J 286:592, 1983

Lebenthal E, Wynn RJ, Lebenthal H: Digestive disorders in neonates. Part 1. Gastrointestinal ontogeny. Perinatol Neonatol, March, 1983

Lemons JA: Fetal placental nitrogen metabolism. Semin Perinatol 3:177, 1979

Liggins GC: Premature delivery of foetal lambs infused with glucocorticoids. J Endocrinol 45:515, 1969

Liggins GC, Howie MB: A controlled trial of antepartum glucocorticoid treatment of prevention of the respiratory distress syndrome in premature infants. Pediatrics 50:515, 1972

Lind R, Kendall A, Hytten FE: The role of the foetus in the formation of amniotic fluid. J Obstet Gynaecol Br Commonw 79:289, 1972

Longo L: Disorders of placental transfer. In Assali NS (ed): Pathophysiology of Gestation. New York, Academic, 1972, vol II

Luskey KL, Brown MS, Goldstein JL: Stimulation of the synthesis of very low density lipoproteins in rooster liver by estradiol. J Biol Chem 249:5939, 1974

MacDonald PC, Madden JD, Brenner PF, Wilson JD, Siiteri PK: Origin of estrogen in normal men and in women with testicular feminization. J Clin Endocrinol Metab 49:905, 1979

Madden JD, Walsh PC, MacDonald PC, Wilson JD: Clinical and endocrinological characterization of a patient with syndrome of incomplete testicular feminization. J Clin Endocrinol 41:751, 1975

Manahan CP, Eastman NJ: The cevitamic acid content of fetal blood. Bull Johns Hopkins Hosp 62:478, 1938

Mandelbaum B, Evans TN: Life in the amniotic fluid. Am J Obstet Gynecol 104:365, 1969

Marinetti GV, Erbland J, Witter RF, Petix J, Stotz E: Metabolic pathways of lipolecithin in a soluble rat-liver system. Biochim Biophys Acta 30:223, 1958

Martin CB, Murata Y, Petrie RH: Respiratory movements in fetal rhesus monkeys. Am J Obstet Gynecol 119:934, 1974

Mason RJ: Disaturated lecithin concentration of rabbit tissues. Am Rev Resp Dis 107:678, 1973

Mendelson CR, Johnston JM, MacDonald PC, Snyder JM: Multihormonal regulation of surfactant synthesis by human fetal lung in vitro. J Clin Endocrinol Metab 53:307, 1981

Mendelson CR, MacDonald PC, Johnston JM: Estrogen binding in human fetal lung cytosol. Endocrinology 106:368, 1980

Milewich L, Johnston JM, Bradfield DJ, Herbert WNP, MacDonald PC, Jimenez JM: The relationship of amniotic fluid dehydroisoandrosterone sulfate (DS) and cortisol (F) concentrations with lecithin to sphingomyelin (L/S) ratios during human gestation. Pediatr Res 12:397, 1978 (abstr)

Moore KL: The Developing Human, 3rd ed. Philadelphia, Saunders, 1982

Murphy BEP: Coritsol and cortisone levels in the cord blood at delivery of infants with and without the respiratory distress syndrome. Am J Obstet Gynecol 119:1112, 1975

Murphy BEP: Chorionic membrane as an extra-adrenal source of foetal cortisol in human amniotic fluid. Nature 266:179, 1977

Myers RE: Fetal brain tolerance to umbilical cord compression according to gestational age. Presented at the 17th Annual Meeting of the Society for Gynecologic Investigation, New Orleans, April 2, 1970

Nielsen NC: Coagulation and fibrinolysin in normal women immediately postpartum and in newborn infants. Acta Obstet Gynecol Scand 48:371, 1969

Nielsen PV, Pedersen J, Kampmann E-M: Absence of human placental lactogen in an otherwise uneventful pregnancy. Am J Obstet Gynecol 135:322, 1979

Obenshain SS, Adam PAJ, King KC, Teramo K, Raivio KO, Räihä N, Schwartz R: Human fetal insulin response to sustained maternal hyperglycemia. N Engl J Med 283:566, 1970

Ohno S, Najai Y, Cicares S: Testicular cells lyso-stripped of H-Y antigen organize ovarian follicle-like aggregates. Cytogenet Cell Genet 20:351, 1978

Oka T, Topper YJ: Hormone-dependent accumulation of rough endoplasmic reticulum in mouse mammary epithelial cells in vitro. J Biol Chem 246:7701, 1971

Page EW: Transfer of materials across the human placenta. Am J Obstet Gynecol 74:705, 1957

Page EW: Problems of nutrition in the perinatal period. Report of the 60th Ross Conference on Pediatric Research, Columbus, Ohio, 1970

Page EW, Glendening MB, Margolis A, Harper HA: Transfer of D- and L-histidine across the human placenta. Am J Obstet Gynecol 73:589, 1957

Pasqualini JR, Sumida C, Gelly C: Cytosol and nuclear [^{3}H]oestradiol binding in the foetal tissues of guinea pig. Acta Endocrinol 83:811, 1976

Pataryas HA, Stammatoyannopoulos G: Hemoglobins in human fetuses: Evidence for adult hemoglobin production after the 11th gestational week. Blood 39:688, 1972

Paton JB, Fisher DE, DeLannoy CW, Behrman RE: Umbilical blood flow, cardiac output, and organ blood flow in the immature baboon fetus. Am J Obstet Gynecol 117:560, 1973

Patrick J (ed): Fetal Breathing Movements. Semin Perinatol 4:249, 1980

Pearson HA: Recent advances in hematology. J Pediatr 69:466, 1966

Pipe NGJ, Smith T, Halliday D, Edmonds CJ, Williams C, Coltart TM: Changes in fat, fat-free mass and body water in human normal pregnancy. Br J Obstet Gynaecol 86:929, 1979

Plentl AA: Physiology of the placenta: III. Dynamics of amniotic fluid. In Assali NS (ed): Biology of Gestation, Vol I, The Maternal Organism. New York Academic, 1968

Polin RA, Husain MK, James LS, Frantz AG: High vasopressin concentrations in human umbilical cord blood—lack of correlation with stress. J Perinat Med 5:114, 1977

Portman OW, Behrman RE, Soltys P: Transfer of free fatty acids across the primate placenta. Am J Physiol 216:143, 1969

Posner BI, Kelly PA: Prolactin receptors in rat liver: Possible induction by prolactin. Science 188:57, 1975

Pritchard JA: Deglutition by normal and anencephalic fetuses. Obstet Gynecol 25:289, 1965

Pritchard JA: Fetal swallowing and amniotic fluid volume. Obstet Gynecol 28:606, 1966

Pritchard JA: Unpublished observations

Quirk JG, Bleasdale, JE: Fetal lung maturation in the pregnancy complicated by diabetes mellitus. In DiRenzo GC, Hawkins PF (eds): Perinatal Medicine: Updates and Controversies. London, Wiley, 1984, in press

Quirk JG, Bleasdale JE: Myo-inositol homeostasis in the human fetus. Obstet Gynecol 62:41, 1983

Quirk JG, Bleasdale JE, MacDonald PC, Johnston JM: A role for cytidine monophosphate in the regulation of the glycerophospholipid composition of surfactant in developing lung. Biochem Biophys Res Commun 95:985, 1980

Quirk JG, MacDonald PC, Johnston JM: Role of fetal pituitary prolactin in fetal lung maturation. Semin Perinatol 6:328, 1982

Read EJ Jr, Platzer PB: Placental metastasis from maternal carcinoma of the lung. Obstet Gynecol 58:387, 1981

Rooney SA, Brehier A: The CDP-choline pathway: cholinephosphate cytidylyl-transferase. In Farrell PM (ed): Lung Development: Biological and Clinical Perspectives. New York, Academic, 1982, vol 1, p 317

Rooney SA, Gross I, Motoyama EK, Warshaw JB: Effects of cortisol and thyroxine on fatty acid and phospholipid biosynthesis in fetal rabbit lung. Physiologist 17:323, 1974

Rooney SA, Gross J, Gassenheimer LN, Motoyama EK: Stimulation of glycerolphosphate phosphatidyltransferase activity in fetal rabbit lung by cortisol administration. Biochim Biophys Acta 398:433, 1975

Rosenfeld CR, Andujo O, Johnston JM, Jimenez JM: Phosphatidate phosphohydrolase (PAPase) and phospholipids (PL) in tracheal (TF) and amniotic (AF) fluid during ovine gestation. Pediatr Res 13:363, 1979

Rudolph AM, Heymann MA: The fetal circulation. Ann Rev Med 19:195, 1968

Russell BJ, Nugent L, Chernick V: Effects of steroids on the enzymatic pathways of lecithin production in fetal rabbits. Biol Neonat 24:306, 1974

Schulman I, Smith CH: Fetal and adult hemoglobins in premature infants. Am J Dis Child 86:354, 1953

Schultz FM, Jimenez JM, MacDonald PC, Johnston JM: Fetal lung maturation. I. Phosphatidic acid phosphohydrolase in rabbit lung. Gynecol Invest 5:222, 1974

Sell EJ, Corrigan JJ Jr: Platelet counts, fibrinogen concentrations, and factor V and factor VIII levels in healthy infants according to gestational age. J Pediatr 82:1028, 1973

Shearer MJ, Rahim S, Barkhan P, Stimmler L: Plasma vitamin K$_1$ in mothers and their newborn babies. Lancet 2:460, 1982

Shrand II: Vomiting in utero with intestinal atresia. Pediatrics 49:767, 1972

Siiteri PK, Wilson JD: Testosterone formation and metabolism during male sex differentiation in human embryo. J Clin Endocrinol 38:113, 1974

Silvers WK, Glasser DL, Eicher EM: H-Y antigen, serologically detectable male antigen and sex determination. Cell 28:439, 1982

Sivakumaran T, Duncan ML, Effer SB, Younglai EV: Relationship between cortisol and lecithin/sphingomyelin ratios in human amniotic fluid. Am J Obstet Gynecol 122:291, 1975

Smith BT, Torday JS: Factors affecting lecithin synthesis by fetal lung cells in culture. Pediatr Res 8:848, 1974

Smith II CM, Tukey DP, Krivit W, White JG: Fetal red cells (FC) differ in elasticity, viscosity, and adhesion from adult red cells (AC). Pediatr Res 15:588, 1981

Smith YF, Mullan DK, Hamosh M, Scanlon JW, Hamosh P: Prolactin and human lung maturation. Pediatr Res 12:569, 1978

Snyder JM, Johnston JM, Mendelson CR: Differentiation of type II cells of human fetal lung in vitro. Cell Tissue Res 220:17, 1981

Spellacy WN, Buhi WC, Riggall FC, Holsinger KL: Human amniotic fluid lecithin/sphingomyelin ratio changes with estrogen or glucocorticoid treatment. Am J Obstet Gynecol 115:216, 1973

Spitzer HL, Johnston JM: Characterization of phosphatidate phosphohydrolase activity associated with isolated lamellar bodies. Biochim Biophys Acta 531:275, 1978

Spitzer HL, Rice JM, MacDonald PC, Johnston JM: Phospholipid biosynthesis in lung lamellar bodies. Biochem Biophys Res Commun 66:17, 1975

Spooner PM, Gorski J: Early estrogen effects on lipid metabolism in the rat uterus. Endocrinology 91:1273, 1972

Stein Z, Susser M, Rush D: Prenatal nutrition and birth weight: Experiments and quasi-experiments in the past decade. J Reprod Med 21:287, 1978

Streeter GL: Weight, sitting height, head size, foot length, and menstrual age of the human embryo. Contrib Embryol 11:143, 1920

Sumida C, Gelly C, Nugyen BL, Pasqualini JR: Cytosol and nuclear ^{3}H-estradiol receptors in fetal guinea pig kidney, lung, and uterus during fetal development. Acta Endocrinol (Suppl 212)85:36, 1977

Sybulski S, Manghan GB: Relationship between cortisol levels in umbilical cord plasma and development of the respiratory distress syndrome in premature newborn infants. Am J Obstet Gynecol 125:239, 1976

Szabo AJ, Grimaldi RCD, Jung WF: Palmitate transport across perfused human placenta. Metabolism 18:406, 1969

Tan SY, Gewolb IH, Hobbins JC: Unconjugated cortisol in human amniotic fluid: Relationship to lecithin/sphingomyelin ratio. J Clin Endocrinol Metab 43:412, 1976

Temiras PS, Vernadakis A, Sherwood NM: Development and plasticity of the nervous system. In Assali NS (ed): Biology of Gestation, VII. The Fetus and Neonate. New York, Academic, 1968

Thiery M, Yo Le Sian A, Vrijens M, Janssens D: Vagitus uterinus. J Obstet Gynaecol Brit Commonw 80:183, 1973

Tolis G, Hickey J, Guyda H: Effect of morphine on serum growth hormone, cortisol, prolactin, and thyroid stimulating hormone in man. J Clin Endocrinol Metab 41:797, 1975

Turkington RW, Majumderi GC, Kadohama N: Hormone regulation of gene expression in mammary cells. Rec Prog Horm Res 29:417, 1973

Usher R, Shephard M, Lind J: The blood volume of the newborn infant and placental transfusion. Acta Paediatr 52:497, 1963

Van Den Bosch J, Bonte HA, vanDeenen LLM: On the anabolism of lipolecithin. Biochim Biophys Acta 98:648, 1965

Voelker DR, Ten-Ching L, Snyder F: Fatty acid biosynthesis and dietary regulation in pulmonary adenomas. Arch Biochem Biophys 176:753, 1976

Von Neergaad K: Neue auffassungen uber einen grundbegriff de Atemmechanik Die Retrakionskraft der Lunge Abhängig von der Oberfläch enspannung in den Alveolen. Z Ges Expt Med 66:373, 1929

Walker J, Turnbull EPN: Haemoglobin and red cells in the human foetus and their relation to the oxygen content of the blood in the vessels of the umbilical cord. Lancet 2:312, 1953

White DA: In Ansell GB, Dawson RMC, Hawthorne JN (eds): Form and Function of Phospholipids. Amsterdam, Elsevier, 1973, p 441

Widdowson EM: Growth and composition of the fetus and newborn. In Assali NS (ed): Biology of Gestation, Vol II. The Fetus and Neonate. New York, Academic, 1968

Wigglesworth JS, Desai R: Is fetal respiratory function a major determinant of perinatal survival? Lancet 1:264, 1982

Wilson JD, Gloyna RE: The intranuclear metabolism of testosterone in the accessory organs of reproduction. Rec Prog Horm Res 26:309, 1970

Wilson JD, Harrod MJ, Goldstein JL, Hemsell DL, MacDonald PC: Familial incomplete male pseudohermaphroditism, Type I. Evidence for androgen resistance and variable clinical manifestation in a family with Reifenstein syndrome. N Engl J Med 290:1097, 1974

Wilson JD, Lasnitzki I: Dihydrotestosterone formation in fetal tissues of the rabbit and rat. Endocrinology 89:659, 1971

Wilson JD, MacDonald PC; Male pseudohermaphroditism due to androgen resistance: Testicular feminization and related syndromes. In Stanbury JB, Wyngaarden JD, Frederickson DS (eds): The Metabolic Basis of Inherited Disease. New York, McGraw-Hill, 1978

Wilson KM: Correlation of external genitalia and sex-glands in the human embryo. Contrib Embryol 18:23, 1926

Winters AJ, Colston C, MacDonald PC, Porter JC: Fetal plasma prolactin levels. J Clin Endocrinol Metab 41:626, 1975

Winters AJ, Oliver C, Colston C, MacDonald PC, Porter JC: Plasma ACTH levels in the human fetus and neonate as related to age and parturition. J Clin Endocrinol Metab 39:269, 1974

Wislocki GB: In Villee CA (ed): Gestation. Transactions of the First Conference. New York, The Josiah Macy Jr Foundation, 1955

Wladimiroff JW, Campbell S: Fetal urine-production rates in normal and complicated pregnancy. Lancet 1:151, 1974

Wolf U: Genetic aspects of H-Y antigen. Hum Genet 58:25, 1981

Wu B, Kikkawa Y, Orzalesi MM, Motoyama EK, Kaibara M, Zigas CJ, Cook CD: Accelerated maturation of fetal rabbit lungs by thyroxine. Physiologist 14:253, 1971

Wu B, Kikkawa Y, Orzalesi MM, Motoyama EK, Kaibara M, Zigas CJ, Cook CD: The effect of thyroxine on the maturation of fetal rabbit lungs. Biol Neonat 22:161, 1973

Zanjani ED, Peterson EN, Gordon AS, Wasserman LR: Erythropoietin production in the fetus: Role of the kidney and maternal anemia. J Lab Clin Med 83:281, 1974

Živný J, Kobilková J, Neuwirt J, Andrasová V: Regulation of erythropoiesis in fetus and mother during normal pregnancy. Obstet Gynecol 60:77, 1982

Zuspan FR, Cordero L, Semchyshyn S: Effects of hydrocortisone on lecithin-sphingomyelin ratio. Am J Obstet Gynecol 128:571, 1977

9
Maternal Adaptation to Pregnancy

The biochemical, physiologic, and anatomic adaptations that occur during the short span of human pregnancy are profound. Many of these changes begin soon after fertilization and continue throughout gestation. An equally astounding fact is that the pregnant woman returns almost completely to her prepregnancy state following delivery and lactation. The understanding of these adaptations to pregnancy remains a major goal of obstetrics, for without such knowledge it is difficult to impossible to understand the disease processes—pregnancy-induced or coincidental—that can threaten women during pregnancy and the puerperium.

UTERUS

Hypertrophy and Dilatation

The uterus has a remarkable capacity to increase rapidly in size during pregnancy and then to return essentially to its original state within a few weeks. In the nonpregnant woman, the uterus is an almost solid structure with a cavity of 10 ml or less; during pregnancy, it is transformed into a relatively thin-walled muscular container of sufficient capacity to accommodate the fetus, placenta, and amnionic fluid. The total volume of the contents of the uterus at term averages about 5 liters but may be as much as 10 liters or more, so that by the end of pregnancy the uterus has achieved a capacity that is 500 to 1000 times greater than in the nonpregnant state. A corresponding increase in weight occurs. The body of the uterus at term weighs approximately 1100 g, compared to about 70 g or so in the nonpregnant woman. During pregnancy, uterine enlargement involves stretching and marked hypertrophy of existing muscle cells, whereas the appearance of new muscle cells is limited. At the time of parturition, a single myometrial cell is about 500 μm in length and the nucleus is eccentrically placed in the thickest part of the cell. The cell is surrounded by an irregular array of collagen fibrils. The force of contraction is transmitted from the contractile proteins of the muscle cell to the surrounding connective tissue through the reticulum of collagen (Carsten, 1968).

Accompanying the increase in size of the uterine muscle cells during pregnancy is an accumulation of fibrous tissue, particularly in the external muscular layer, together with a considerable increase in elastic tissue. The network thus formed adds materially to the strength of the uterine wall. There is, concomitantly, a great increase in the size and number of blood vessels and lymphatics in the uterus. The veins that drain the placental site are transformed into large uterine sinuses. Hypertrophy of the nerve supply of the uterus also takes place, exemplified by the increase in size of Frankenhäuser cervical ganglion.

During the first few months of pregnancy, hypertrophy of the uterine wall is probably stimulated chiefly by the action of estrogen and perhaps that of progesterone. It is apparent that the early hypertrophy of the uterus is not entirely the result of mechanical distension by the products of conception because similar uterine changes occur when the embryo is implanted in the fallopian tube or ovary. After the third month, the increase in uterine size is, in large part, due to the effect of pressure exerted by the expanding products of conception.

Rapid growth of tissues is correlated with increased synthesis of *polyamines*. The polyamines—spermidine and spermine and their immediate precursor, putrescine—are believed to play crucial roles in tissue growth and cell hypertrophy. (For review see Russell and Durie, 1978.) Russell and colleagues (1978) reported that polyamine levels in the urine of normally pregnant women are strikingly elevated and that the highest levels are attained at 13 to 14 weeks of gestation (Fig. 9-1). It is interesting to speculate that the increased rate of synthesis of polyamines at this time in gestation is related to the hypertrophy of the myometrium that occurs during this stage of pregnancy.

During the first few months of pregnancy, the uterine walls become considerably thicker than in the nonpregnant state, but as gestation advances the walls gradually thin. At term, the walls of the uterine corpus are for the most part 1.5 cm or less in thickness. Early in pregnancy, the uterus loses the firmness and resistance characteristic of the nonpregnant organ. In the later months, the uterus is changed into a muscular sac with thin, soft, readily indentable walls, demonstrable by the ease with which the fetus can usually be palpated through the abdominal wall and by the readiness with which the uterine walls yield to the movements of the fetal extremities.

The enlargement of the uterus is not symmetric;

181

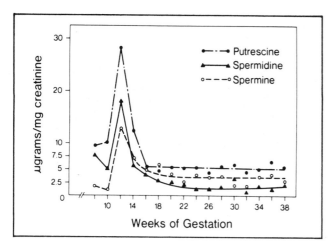

Figure 9-1. Polyamines in the urine of women with normal pregnancies are plotted as a function of weeks of gestation. Each point is the mean value of results obtained in the urine of at least five separate women. (*From Russell and colleagues, 1978.*)

rather it is most marked in the fundus. The differential growth is readily apparent by observing the relative positions of the attachments of the fallopian tubes and ovarian ligaments. In the early months of pregnancy, these structures insert only slightly below the apex of the fundus, whereas in the later months, they are inserted slightly above the middle of the uterus. The position of the placenta also influences the extent of uterine hypertrophy, since the portion of the uterus surrounding the placental site enlarges more rapidly than does the myometrium distal to the site of placental implantation.

Arrangement of the Muscle Cells

The musculature of the pregnant uterus is arranged in three strata: an external hoodlike layer, which arches over the fundus and extends into the various ligaments; an internal layer, consisting of sphincterlike fibers around the orifices of the tubes and the internal os; and, lying between these two layers, a dense network of muscle fibers perforated in all directions by blood vessels. The main portion of the uterine wall is formed by the middle layer, which consists of an interlacing network of muscle fibers between which extend the blood vessels. Each cell in this layer has a double curve, so that the interlacing of any two gives approximately the form of a Figure 8. As a result of this arrangement, when the cells contract after delivery they constrict the penetrating blood vessels and thus act as ligatures.

The muscle cells composing the uterine wall in pregnancy, especially in its lower portion, overlap one another like shingles on a roof. One end of each fiber arises beneath the serosa of the uterus and extends obliquely downward and inward toward the decidua, forming a large number of muscular lamellae that are interconnected by short muscular processes. When the tissue is slightly spread apart, it appears sieve–like and, on closer examination, is found to comprise innumerable rhomboidal spaces.

Changes in Uterine Size, Shape, and Position

As the uterus increases in size, it also undergoes important modifications in shape. For the first few weeks, its original pear shape is maintained, but as pregnancy advances the corpus and fundus soon assume a more globular form, becoming almost spherical by the third lunar month. Subsequently, the organ increases more rapidly in length than in width and assumes an ovoid shape (Fig. 6-14).

By the end of 12 weeks, the uterus has become too large to remain wholly within the pelvis. Thereafter, as the uterus continues to enlarge, it contacts the anterior abdominal wall, displaces the intestines laterally and superiorly, and continues to rise, ultimately reaching almost to the liver. As the uterus rises, tension is exerted upon the broad ligaments, which partly unfold their median and lower portions, and upon the round ligaments.

During pregnancy, the uterus is movable. With the pregnant woman standing, the longitudinal axis of the uterus corresponds to an extension of the axis of the pelvic inlet. The abdominal wall supports the uterus and, unless it is quite relaxed, maintains this relation between the long axis of the uterus and the axis of the pelvic inlet. When the pregnant woman is supine, the uterus falls back to rest upon the vertebral column and the adjacent great vessels, especially the inferior vena cava and the aorta.

With ascent of the uterus from the pelvis, it usually undergoes rotation to the right, resulting in the left margin facing anteriorly. This *dextrorotation* probably results in large measure from the presence of the rectosigmoid on the left side of the pelvis. However, *levorotation* occurs occasionally, especially if there is a pelvic or low abdominal mass on the right side, for example, a transplanted kidney.

Changes in Contractility

From the first trimester of pregnancy onward, the uterus undergoes irregular contractions, which normally are painless. In the second trimester such contractions may be detected by bimanual examination. The relaxed uterus transiently becomes firm and then returns to its original relaxed state. Since attention was first called to this phenomenon by Braxton Hicks, the contractions have been known by his name. Such contractions appear unpredictably and sporadically, are usually non-rhythmic, and their intensity, according to Alvarez and Caldeyro-Barcia (1950), is somewhat more than 8 cm of water. Until the last month of gestation, *Braxton Hicks contractions* are infrequent but increase in frequency during the last week or two. At this time, the contractions may occur as often as every 10 to 20 minutes and also may assume some degree of rhythmicity. Late in pregnancy these contractions may cause some discomfort and account for so-called false labor.

Uteroplacental Blood Flow

The delivery of most substances essential for the growth and metabolism of the fetus and placenta, as well as the removal of most metabolic wastes, is dependent upon adequate perfusion of the placental intervillous space. Placental perfusion by maternal blood depends, in turn, upon blood flow to the uterus through the uterine and ovarian arteries. There is no question that there is a progressive increase in uteroplacental blood flow during pregnancy. The reported values, which average roughly 500 ml per minute late in pregnancy, must be viewed as approximations because of inherent errors in the methods of measurement as well as the undoubtedly appreciable changes in uterine blood flow that likely are induced by various body positions (Kauppila and associates, 1980).

Assali and co-workers (1953, 1960), Metcalfe and colleagues (1955), and Blechner and associates (1975), employing the nitrous oxide method to estimate uteroplacental blood flow in human pregnancy, found that the total flow averages about 500 ml per minute at term. Browne and Veall (1953) arrived at approximately the same values, using the rate of disappearance of ^{24}Na.

Rekonen and co-workers (1976) attempted measurement of intervillous and myometrial blood flow in pregnant women in the supine position using intravenously injected ^{133}Xe. They obtained mean values for intervillous flow of 135 ml per minute per deciliter and myometrial flow of 7.7 ml per minute per 100 g. Thus for a placenta of 500 g and a uterus of 1000 g, uteroplacental blood flow estimated by this technique averaged 750 ml per minute. There was appreciable variation among individuals, although reproducibility in the same individual was good.

Edman and colleagues (1979) calculated minimal placental intervillous blood flow from the placental clearance rate of maternal plasma Δ^4-androstenedione through placental estradiol-17β formation. They reported values of approximately 450 ml of blood per minute for placental intervillous flow at or near term.

Campbell and co-workers (1983) reported on the use of pulsed doppler techniques to study wave forms in uterine wall arteries in normal and complicated pregnancies. In cases of fetal hypoxia, fetal growth retardation, and in hypertensive pregnancies, the systolic pulsatile pattern was high and the diastolic flow of blood was low. This method may prove to be a means of assessing uterine perfusion in normal and compromised pregnancies.

Assali and co-workers (1968), and others, using electromagnetic flow meters, studied the effects of spontaneous and oxytocin-induced labor on uteroplacental blood flow in sheep and dogs at term. They noted that uterine contractions, either spontaneous or induced, caused a decrease in uterine blood flow that was roughly proportional to the intensity of the contraction; a tetanic contraction caused a precipitous fall in uterine blood flow. Harbert and associates (1969) made similar observations in gravid monkeys, and the same pattern of change undoubtedly occurs during the myometrial contractions of human parturition.

Control of Uteroplacental Blood Flow

The factors that control uteroplacental perfusion remain largely unknown. However, through the use of animal models and indirect methods of assessing uteroplacental perfusion in the human, a partial understanding is evolving.

Increases in total uterine blood flow occur progressively throughout gestation in both the human and sheep. However, there is a definite redistribution of blood flow within the gravid ovine (sheep) uterus (Makowski and co-workers, 1968). Prior to pregnancy, uterine blood flow is equally divided between myometrium, endometrium, and future placental implantation sites (caruncles). By the end of the first third of ovine pregnancy, endometrial blood flow is 50 percent of the total. By term, the blood flow to the placental cotyledons accounts for approximately 90 percent of total uterine blood flow (Rosenfeld and associates, 1974).

There appear to be at least two distinct stages of placental development associated with the changes in distribution of ovine uterine blood flow just noted. The first is associated with implantation and is completed near the end of the middle third of pregnancy when placental weight is maximal and total uterine blood flow temporarily plateaus at 400 to 500 ml per minute. The second stage occurs during the last third of pregnancy. At this time, there is no further placental growth. Despite this, vessel diameters increase without an increase in the number of endothelial cells (Teasdale, 1976) and placental blood flow doubles to values of approximately 900 to 1000 ml per minute. These observations imply, at least, that vasodilation is occurring at this time.

What actually induces the increase in uterine blood flow during the first two thirds of ovine pregnancy is not clearly understood. There is, however, no doubt that it is in part the consequence of increasing placental size and number of blood vessels (Teasdale, 1976). An additional factor may be the localized production of Wharton jelly, a major component of which is glucosamine. Greiss and Wagner (1983) have shown that glucosamine can induce significant increases in uteroplacental blood flow and may function locally to redistribute blood flow early in pregnancy from the endometrium and myometrium to the uterine caruncles and placental cotyledons. The role, if any, of prostaglandins at this stage or later in pregnancy remains to be defined.

During the last third of ovine pregnancy, the increase in maternal–placental blood flow occurs principally by means of vasodilation whereas fetal–placental blood flow is increased by a continuing increase in placental vessels (Teasdale, 1976). This appears to result in an optimal match of maternal and fetal placental blood flows such that maternal–fetal transfer is maximal. It appears likely that this late pregnancy vasodilation is at least in part the consequence of estrogen stimulation (Rosenfeld and co-workers, 1976). The administration of estradiol-17β to late pregnant sheep can increase placental blood flow by as much as 25 percent without a change in perfusion pressure, further evidence of placental vasodilation (Rosenfeld and co-workers, 1976).

The observation that the estrogen-induced increase in uterine blood flow (vasodilation) could be partially blocked

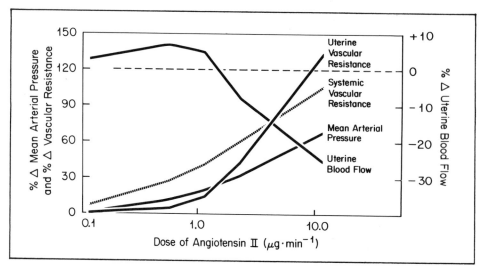

Figure 9-2. The relative changes in uterine blood flow, mean arterial pressure, systemic vascular resistance, and uterine vascular resistance during the systemic infusion of angiotensin II in term pregnant ewes. Responses were recorded after 4 to 5 minutes of stabilization at each dose of angiotensin II. (*From Rosenfeld, 1984.*)

by surgical and/or anesthetic stress (Rosenfeld and associates, 1973; Killam and colleagues, 1973) is consistent with the hypothesis that these particular uterine vascular systems are likely responsive to a number of vasoactive compounds such as catecholamines and angiotensin II. This hypothesis has been confirmed.

Catecholamines

Both epinephrine and norepinephrine have been shown to result in significant decreases in placental perfusion in sheep even in the absence of any change in arterial blood pressure (Rosenfeld and co-workers, 1976; Rosenfeld and West, 1977). Such a response is probably the consequence of a greater sensitivity to catecholamine by the uteroplacental vascular beds when compared to the systematic vasculature. It is worrisome to speculate that any stressful situation (pain, anesthesia, and/or surgery) that results in an elevation of catecholamines may decrease uteroplacental perfusion even in the absence of an elevation in blood pressure.

Angiotensin II

Refractoriness to angiotensin II pressor effects appears to be a normal characteristic of both human (Chesley and associates, 1965; Gant and co-workers, 1973) and ovine pregnancy (Rosenfeld and Gant, 1981; Naden and Rosenfeld, 1981). Despite this marked refractoriness of the systemic vasculature to angiotensin II, the uterine vasculature in sheep is even more refractory (Rosenfeld and Gant, 1981; Naden and Rosenfeld, 1981). This is clearly illustrated in Figure 9-2, where greater changes in mean arterial blood pressure and systemic vascular resistance are seen at lower doses of infused angiotensin II when compared to changes in uterine vascular resistance. This observation has been confirmed and expanded by Matsuura and co-workers (1984).

The clinical implications of uterine vascular refractoriness to angiotensin II are not readily apparent but may be of significance. This physiologic response may result in a potential advantage to the fetus in cases where there is a decreased refractoriness of the systemic vasculature to pressor agents (increased sensitivity to pressor agents), as occurs in women destined to develop pregnancy-induced hypertension (Gant and associates, 1973) and where uterine

vascular refractoriness to pressor agents is maintained at least initially. This would be expected to result in an increased uteroplacental perfusion in such patients prior to the development of actual hypertension. Such a situation has been reported to occur (Gant and associates, 1972; Gant and co-workers, 1976). As increasing vasoconstriction occurs, for example, in women destined to develop pregnancy-induced hypertension, uterine vascular resistance eventually increases and a progressive fall in uteroplacental perfusion follows (Fig. 9-3). This is analogous to the effect observed on the uteroplacental vasculature that occurs at higher doses of infused angiotensin II (Fig. 9-2), when uterine vascular resistance exceeds mean arterial pressure, resulting in a decrease in uterine blood flow.

The above observations have additional clinical significance as to whether mild to moderate increases in blood pressure as occurs in women with chronic hypertension should be treated with antihypertensive drugs during pregnancy. Antihypertensive drugs may cause a greater decrease in systemic blood pressure than in uterine vascular resistance, thereby resulting in a greater fall in uterine perfusion. Gant and colleagues (1976) reported that uteroplacental perfusion appeared to be higher in pregnancies complicated by moderate essential hypertension than in normotensive patients. This also may be the consequence of an increased arterial blood pressure (less refractoriness of the systemic vascular tree to pressor agents) and a greater refractoriness of the uterine vasculature to pressor agents, resulting in an increased blood flow, as described above in studies of women destined to develop pregnancy-induced hypertension and in the angiotensin II studies conducted during ovine pregnancy.

Although many of the above studies have been conducted in pregnant sheep, thus far these studies are consistent with less extensive and certainly less invasive studies conducted during human pregnancy. The interested reader is referred to the review by Rosenfeld (1984).

Changes in the Cervix

During pregnancy, pronounced softening and cyanosis of the cervix occurs, often demonstrable as early as a month after conception. These changes comprise two of

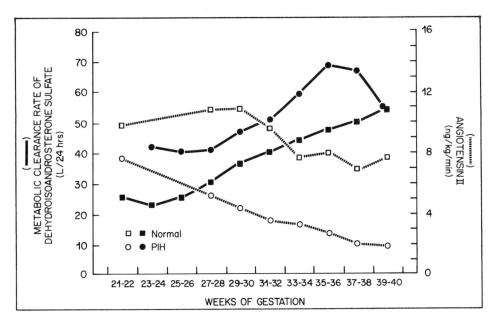

Figure 9-3. Comparison of the metabolic clearance rate of dehydroisoandrosterone sulfate and the amount of angiotensin II required to evoke a standard pressor response in primigravidas who remained normotensive (*squares*) and in primigravidas who subsequently developed pregnancy-induced hypertension (*circles*).

the very earliest physical signs of pregnancy. The factors responsible for these changes are increased vascularity and edema of the entire cervix, together with hypertrophy and hyperplasia of the cervical glands.

As shown in Figures 9-4 and 9-5, the glands of the cervical mucosa undergo such marked proliferation that by the end of pregnancy, they occupy approximately one half of the entire mass of the cervix, rather than a small fraction, as in the nonpregnant state. Moreover, the septa separating the glandular spaces become progressively thinner, resulting in the formation of a structure resembling a honeycomb, the meshes of which are filled

with tenacious mucus. Soon after conception a clot of very thick mucus obstructs the cervical canal. At the onset of labor, if not before, this so-called *mucus plug* is expelled, resulting in a "bloody show." The glands near the external os proliferate beneath the stratified squamous epithelium of the portio vaginalis, giving the cervix the velvety consistency characteristic of pregnancy.

So-called *erosions of the cervix* are common during pregnancy. These lesions are customarily red and velvety in appearance and are covered by columnar epithelium, spreading from the external os to involve the

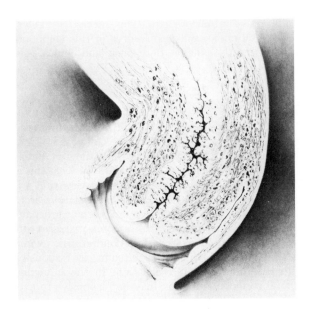

Figure 9-4. Cervix in the nonpregnant woman.

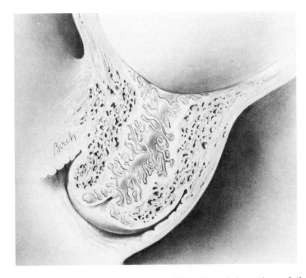

Figure 9-5. Cervix in pregnancy. Note the elaboration of the mucosa into a honeycomblike structure, the meshes of which are filled with a tenacious mucus—the so-called mucus plug.

portio vaginalis of the cervix to various degrees. The high frequency of cervical "erosions" in pregnancy is best explained on the basis that they are not abnormal, but instead represent an extension, or *eversion*, of the proliferating endocervical glands and the columnar endocervical epithelium. Although the term erosion implies an "eating out" or ulceration of the covering epithelium, the cause in pregnancy is rarely inflammatory.

During pregnancy, there is a change in the consistency of the cervical mucus. In the great majority of pregnant women, cervical mucus, spread and dried on a glass slide, is characterized by fragmentary crystallization, or "beading," typical of the effect of progesterone (see Chapter 4, p. 75). Arborization of the crystals, or "ferning," however, is not necessarily associated with a poor outcome of pregnancy (Salvatore, 1968). Chrétien (1978), employing scanning electron microscopy, studied the structural variations in cervical mucus during normal pregnancy.

During pregnancy, basal cells near the squamocolumnar junction of the cervix, histologically, are likely to be prominent in size, shape, and staining qualities. These changes are considered by most authorities to be estrogen-induced (Hellman and colleagues, 1954).

Although the cervix contains a small amount of smooth muscle, its major component is connective tissue. The cervix undergoes profound changes during pregnancy, especially during labor, and these must involve its collagen-rich connective tissue (see Chapter 15, p. 306).

OVARIES AND OVIDUCTS

Ovarian Function

Ovulation ceases during pregnancy and the maturation of new follicles is suspended. As a rule, only a single corpus luteum of pregnancy can be found in the ovaries of pregnant women. In gonadotropin-induced pregnancies, Yoshima and associates (1969) found that the level of plasma progesterone reached a nadir by the eighth week of pregnancy (sixth week postovulation) and then rose again. Such a nadir was not observed by Tulchinsky and Hobel (1973) in spontaneous ovulatory cycles but instead a less rapid increase or plateau in plasma progesterone levels was seen. By contrast, maternal plasma 17α-hydroxyprogesterone levels continued to decline to a level only somewhat higher than those found during the luteal phase. Thus, the corpus luteum of pregnancy most likely functions maximally during the first 6 to 7 weeks of pregnancy (4 to 5 weeks postovulation) but thereafter contributes relatively little to progesterone production during the remainder of human pregnancy. This has been confirmed in vivo by the surgical removal of the corpus luteum before 7 weeks of gestation (5 weeks postovulation), which results in a rapid fall in maternal serum progesterone and abortion (Csapo and co-workers, 1973).

Relaxin

Relaxin is a protein hormone secreted by the corpus luteum during human pregnancy (see Chapter 3, p. 56). It is detectable in serum by the time of the first missed menses and is believed to be secreted in a pattern similar to that of human chorionic gonadotropin. Thus the secretion of this corpus luteum hormone differs from that of the steroids of the corpus luteum. Whereas 17α-hydroxyprogesterone and presumably progesterone secretion by the corpus luteum has declined to neglible rates by the seventh to eighth week of pregnancy (5 to 6 weeks postovulation), relaxin secretion continues throughout pregnancy.

The decidua has been reported to be a source of relaxin but significant amounts of human relaxin have not as yet been obtained from these tissues. The amounts of relaxin present are very low in comparison with the amounts produced by the corpus luteum of pregnancy (Bryant-Greenwood, 1982).

The role of relaxin, if any, during human pregnancy remains to be defined. Although relaxin is a major myometrial inhibitory substance in guinea pig gestation (Porter, 1972), the compound does not appear to be essential to the maintenance of human pregnancy (Bryant-Greenwood, 1982). It may be that relaxin is involved in "ripening" the human cervix prior to the initiation of parturition (Steinetz and co-workers, 1980; and Porter, 1980). It has been used for this purpose in a small double-blind randomized clinical trial (Evans and co-workers, 1983).

Although a great deal remains to be learned about relaxin, a significant advance was made in this direction by Hudson and co-workers (1983), who reported the successful identification of a genomic clone from which the structure of the entire coding region of a human pre-prorelaxin gene was defined. This advance allowed these investigators to *synthesize* an apparently authentic biologically active human relaxin. This success is likely to ensure a continuous and pure source of this compound, which will greatly enhance both basic and clinical studies.

Pregnancy Luteoma

In 1963, Sternberg described a solid ovarian tumor that developed during pregnancy that was composed of large acidophilic luteinized cells. The observations of Krause and Stembridge (1966), Garcia-Bunuel and co-workers (1975) and others, are consistent with the view that a luteoma of pregnancy represents an exaggeration of the luteinization reaction of the ovary of normal pregnancy and is not a true neoplasm. The luteoma regresses after delivery, and normal ovarian function returns, even in those instances in which the luteoma is responsible, transiently, for maternal virilization. In the immediate puerperal state, the luteoma may be responsive to exogenously administered hCG (Cohen and associates, 1982).

Even though maternal virilization may be prominent, the fetus is not always affected, presumably because of the protective role of the placenta through its high capacity to convert androgens to estrogens (Edman and co-workers, 1979). However, there is no question that a fetus can in some cases be virilized (Verkauf and co-workers, 1977; Hensleigh and Woodruff, 1978; Cohen and associates, 1982).

> Why one fetus will be virilized and another not remains incompletely understood. Edman and associates (1979) presented good evidence that the androgens produced in at least two cases of luteoma of pregnancy are rapidly and extensively converted into estrogens, thus acting to protect the fetus. Cohen and associates (1982) speculated that, in some cases, the high androgen levels might in fact suppress testosterone-binding globulin, resulting in more free testosterone. Another possibility is that 5α-reductase activity is increased (or not suppressed), resulting in higher concentrations of 5α-dihydrotestosterone. Even more critical is the time at which androgen levels are presented to the fetal compartment. That is, if excessive androgen levels are present early enough in pregnancy, their concentration may exceed the enzymatic capacity of a small placenta to clear the androgens into estrogens.

Other Changes

A *decidual reaction* on and beneath the surface of the ovaries, similar to that found in the endometrial stroma, is usual in pregnancy and is commonly observed at cesarean section. These elevated patches of tissue bleed easily and may, on first glance, resemble freshly torn adhesions. Similar decidual reactions are occasionally seen on the posterior uterine serosa and upon or within other pelvic or even extrapelvic abdominal organs.

The enormous caliber of ovarian veins inspected at cesarean section is startling. Through actual measurement, Hodgkinson (1953) found that the diameter of the ovarian vascular pedicle increased during pregnancy from 0.9 cm to approximately 2.6 cm at term.

Oviducts

The musculature of the fallopian tubes undergoes little hypertrophy during pregnancy. The epithelium of the tubal mucosa is flattened during gestation, compared to that of the nonpregnant state. Decidual cells may develop in the stroma of the endosalpinx, but a continuous decidual membrane is not formed.

VAGINA AND OUTLET

During pregnancy, increased vascularity and hyperemia develop in the skin and muscles of the perineum and vulva and there is softening of the normally abundant connective tissue of these structures.

Increased vascularity prominently affects the vagina. The copious secretion and the characteristic violet color of the vagina during pregnancy (Chadwick sign), similar to the changes that occur in the cervix during pregnancy,

probably result chiefly from hyperemia. The vaginal walls undergo striking changes, seemingly in preparation for the distension that occurs during labor, with a considerable increase in thickness of the mucosa, loosening of the connective tissue, and hypertrophy of the smooth-muscle cells to nearly the same extent as in the uterus. These changes effect such an increase in length of the vaginal walls that sometimes, in parous women, the lower portion of the anterior vaginal wall protrudes slightly through the vulvar opening. The papillae of the vaginal mucosa also undergo considerable hypertrophy, creating a fine hobnailed appearance.

Vaginal Secretion

The considerably increased cervical and vaginal secretion during pregnancy consists of a somewhat thick, white discharge. Its pH is acidic, varying from 3.5 to 6, the result of increased production of lactic acid from glycogen in the vaginal epithelium by the action of *Lactobacillus acidophilus*. The acidic pH probably serves to control the rate of multiplication of pathogenic bacteria in the vagina.

Vaginal Cytology

Early in pregnancy the vaginal epithelial cells are similar to those found during the luteal phase of the menstrual cycle (see Chapter 4, p. 74), but as pregnancy advances two patterns of response are seen:

1. Small intermediate cells, called navicular cells by Papanicolaou, are found in abundance in small, dense clusters. The ovoid navicular cell contains a vesicular, somewhat elongated nucleus.
2. Vesicular nuclei without cytoplasm, or so-called naked nuclei, are evident, along with an abundance of *Lactobacillus,* a normal organism in the vagina.

ABDOMINAL WALL AND SKIN

Striae Gravidarum

In the later months of pregnancy, reddish, slightly depressed streaks commonly develop in the skin of the abdomen and sometimes in the skin over the breasts and thighs. These striae gravidarum occur in about one half of all pregnant women. In multiparous women, in addition to the reddish striae of the present pregnancy, glistening, silvery lines that represent the cicatrices of previous striae are seen frequently.

Diastasis Recti

Occasionally, the muscles of the abdominal walls do not withstand the tension to which they are subjected, and the rectus muscles separate in the midline, creating a diastasis recti of varying extent. If severe, a considerable portion of the anterior uterine wall is covered by only a layer of skin, attenuated fascia, and peritoneum. In extreme instances, herniation of the gravid uterus through the diastasis may be so great that the fundus of the uterus drops below the level of the pelvic inlet when the woman is standing.

Pigmentation

In many women, the midline of the abdominal skin becomes markedly pigmented, assuming a brownish-black color to form the *linea nigra.* Occasionally, irregular brownish patches of varying size appear on the face and neck, giving rise to *chloasma* or *melasma gravidarum* (*"mask of pregnancy"*), which, fortunately, usually disappears, or at least regresses considerably, after delivery. Oral contraceptives may cause similar pigmentation in these same women. There is very little known of the nature of these pigmentary changes, although melanocyte-stimulating hormone, a polypeptide similar to ACTH, has been shown to be remarkably elevated from the end of the second month of pregnancy until term. Estrogen and progesterone have been reported to exert a melanocyte-stimulating effect (Diczfalusy and Troen, 1961).

Cutaneous Vascular Changes

Angiomas, called *vascular spiders,* develop in about two thirds of white women and approximately 10 percent of black women during pregnancy (Bean and colleagues, 1949). These are minute, red elevations on the skin, particularly common on the face, neck, upper chest, and arms, with radicles branching out from a central body. The condition is often designated as nevus, angioma, or telangiectasis. *Palmar erythema* is also frequently encountered in pregnancy, having been observed by Bean and associates in about two thirds of white women and one third of black women. The two conditions frequently occur together but are of no clinical significance and disappear in most women shortly after the termination of pregnancy. The high incidence of vascular spiders and palmar erythema in pregnancy is most probably the consequence of the hyperestrogenemia of pregnancy.

BREASTS

During pregnancy, striking changes occur in the breasts. In the early weeks, the pregnant woman often experiences tenderness and tingling of the breasts. After the second month, the breasts increase in size and become nodular as a result of hypertrophy of the mammary alveoli. As the breasts increase in size, delicate veins become visible just beneath the skin. The changes in the nipples and areolae are even more characteristic. The nipples become considerably larger, more deeply pigmented, and more erectile. After the first few months, a thick, yellowish fluid, *colostrum,* often can be expressed from the nipples by gentle massage. At that time, the areolae be-

comes broader and more deeply pigmented. The depth of pigmentation varies with the woman's complexion. Scattered through the areolae are a number of small elevations, the so-called glands (follicles) of Montgomery, which are hypertrophic sebaceous glands. If the increase in size of the breasts is very extensive, striations similar to those observed in the abdomen may develop. Histologic and functional changes of the breasts induced by pregnancy and lactation are discussed further in Chapter 19 (p. 369).

METABOLIC CHANGES

In response to the rapidly growing fetus and placenta and their increasing demands, the pregnant woman undergoes metabolic changes that are numerous and intense. Certainly no other physiologic event in postnatal life induces such profound metabolic alterations.

Weight Gain

Most of the increase in weight that occurs during pregnancy is attributable to the uterus and its contents, the breasts, and increases in blood volume and extravascular extracellular fluid. A smaller fraction of the increased weight is the result of metabolic alterations that result in an increase in cellular water and deposition of new fat and protein, so-called maternal reserves. Chesley (1944) reported that the average total weight gain in pregnancy was 24 pounds (11 kg). During the first trimester, the average gain was 2 pounds (1 kg), compared to about 11 pounds (5 kg) during each of the last two trimesters. Much more recently, Hytten (1981) reported similar, but somewhat higher, average weight gains for English women (Table 9-1).

Water Metabolism

Increased retention of water is a normal physiologic alteration of pregnancy. Marked retention of water, however, with the development of edema, is commonly present with pregnancy-induced hypertension.

At term, the water content of the fetus, placenta, and amnionic fluid amounts to about 3.5 liters. Approximately 3.0 liters more water accumulates as a result of increases in the maternal blood volume and in the size of the uterus and the breasts. Thus, the minimum amount of extra water that the average woman could be expected to retain during normal pregnancy is about 6.5 liters. Clearly demonstrable pitting edema of the ankles and legs occurs in a substantial proportion of pregnant women, especially at the end of the day, before retiring. This accumulation of fluid, which may amount to a liter or so, is caused by an increase in venous pressure below the level of the uterus because of the increased venous pressure that occurs in all body positions except the lateral recumbent.

The amount of water to be mobilized and excreted

TABLE 9-1. DISTRIBUTION OF WEIGHT GAIN DURING PREGNANCY

Tissue/Fluid	Increase in Weight in Grams (and Pounds)* up to:			
	10 weeks	*20 weeks*	*30 weeks*	*40 weeks*
Fetus	5 (0.01)	300 (0.7)	1500 (3.3)	3400 (7.5)
Placenta	20 (0.04)	170 (0.4)	430 (0.9)	650 (1.4)
Amnionic Fluid	30 (0.07)	350 (0.8)	750 (1.7)	800 (1.8)
Uterus	140 (0.3)	320 (0.7)	600 (1.3)	970 (2.1)
Breasts	45 (0.1)	180 (0.4)	360 (0.8)	405 (0.9)
Blood	100 (0.2)	600 (1.3)	1300 (2.9)	1250 (2.8)
Extracellular Extravascular Fluid (no edema present)	0 (0)	30 (0.06)	80 (0.2)	1680 (3.7)
Subtotal	340 (0.7)	1950 (4.3)	5020 (11.1)	9155 (20.2)
Maternal Reserves	310 (0.7)	2050 (4.5)	3480 (7.7)	3345 (7.4)
Total Weight Gain	650 (1.4)	4000 (8.8)	8500 (18.7)	12,500 (27.5)

* Where possible, numbers were rounded to the nearest one-tenth pound.
(*Modified from Hytten and Chamberlain, 1981, p 221, Table 7.8.*)

by the mother after delivery will depend upon the amount retained during pregnancy, the degree of hydration or dehydration during labor, and the amount of blood lost at delivery. In normal primiparas without demonstrable edema before vaginal delivery, weight loss during the first 10 days after delivery averaged nearly 5 pounds (2 kg) (Dennis and Bytheway, 1965).

Protein Metabolism

The products of conception, as well as the uterus and maternal blood, are relatively rich in protein rather than fat or carbohydrate. Nonetheless, their protein content is rather small compared with the total body protein of the mother. At term, the fetus and placenta together weigh about 4 kg and contain approximately 500 g of protein, or about one half of the total increase normally induced by pregnancy (Hytten and Leitch, 1971; Widdowson, 1968). The remaining 500 g of protein is added to the uterus as contractile protein, to the breasts primarily in the glands, and to the maternal blood in the form of hemoglobin and plasma proteins. At the same time, the concentrations of several plasma proteins are altered by pregnancy. The albumin concentration decreases significantly (p. 201) while fibrinogen rises (p. 193). The concentrations of IgG, IgA, and IgM fall somewhat (Amino and colleagues, 1978).

Dietary protein requirements during pregnancy and lactation are discussed in Chapter 13 (p. 252).

Carbohydrate Metabolism

Pregnancy is potentially diabetogenic. Diabetes mellitus may be aggravated by pregnancy and clinical diabetes may appear in some women only during pregnancy. Consequently, considerable attention has been focused on the metabolism of carbohydrates and insulin in preg-

nant women. In healthy women, the fasting plasma glucose concentration falls somewhat during pregnancy (Fig 9-6). The effect of normal pregnancy on *insulin* levels is disputed. Increased fasting levels of insulin have been reported by some investigators (Bleicher and colleagues, 1964; Spellacy and associates, 1963) while others have found them to be unchanged (Taylor and co-workers, 1978) or even lower during prenancy (Tyson and associates, 1976).

Bleicher and associates (1964) presented the concept that the lower fasting glucose levels and the higher concentration of plasma free fatty acids found normally in pregnant women result from a state of "accelerated starvation" brought about by the "host–parasite" relation between mother and conceptus. During pregnancy, there are safeguards that spare utilization of glucose by maternal tissues while allowing "parasitization" of glucose and gluconeogenic precursors by the fetus to continue. The placenta is known to synthesize and secrete a growth-hormone-like substance, placental lactogen (p. 201). This hormone promotes lipolysis, bringing about an increase in plasma free fatty acids, and thereby provides alternative fuel substrates for the mother. The ability of placental lactogen to oppose the action of insulin results in increased maternal requirements for insulin during pregnancy. However, it should be pointed out that otherwise quite normal pregnancy outcomes have been achieved in the absence of detectable amounts of this potent hormone.

Estrogens, progesterone, and cortisol may also contribute to the diabetogenic predisposition apparent in pregnancy. Progesterone given to monkeys was shown by Beck (1969) to produce a marked increase in the plasma insulin response to intravenous glucose similar to that noted in human pregnancy. Moreover, Beck and Wells (1969) found that the potent synthetic estrogen, mestranol (ethinyl estradiol-3-methyl ether), caused not

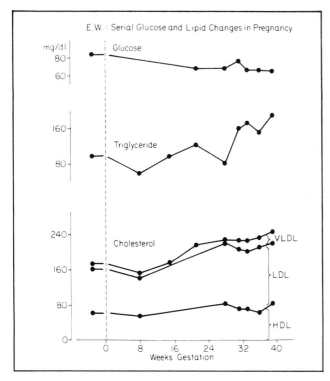

Figure 9-6. Serial changes in concentrations of glucose and lipids during normal pregnancy. VLDL = very low-density lipoproteins; LDL = low-density lipoproteins; HDL = high-density lipoproteins. (*From Knopp RH: Contemporary Ob/Gyn 12:83, 1978.*)

only an increased plasma insulin response to intravenous glucose but also a decreased sensitivity to the hypoglycemic action of exogenous insulin. Only the subjects with limited ability to increase insulin production demonstrated decreased glucose tolerance after mestranol treatment, presumably became of failure to compensate for insulin resistance induced by mestranol. Plasma cortisol levels are increased appreciably during pregnancy, but much of the increase represents hormone bound to transcortin.

Insulinase activity has been found in the human placenta. It seems unlikely, however, that accelerated degradation of insulin by placental insulinase contributes appreciably to the diabetogenic state induced by pregnancy, since the rate of degradation of radiolabeled insulin in vivo does not appear to differ among pregnant and nonpregnant women (Burt and Davidson, 1974).

The role of glucagon during pregnancy is not totally defined. Hornnes and Kuhl (1980) measured glucagon and insulin responses to a standard glucose stimulus in the same women late in normal pregnancy and again postpartum. The insulin response to glucose infusion was increased 3.8 times in late pregnancy. The glucagon suppression was similar in late pregnancy and the puerperium. These results are consistent with the view that β-cell sensitivity to a glucose challenge is significantly increased in normal pregnant women, but the α-cell sen-

sitivity to a glucose stimulus is unaltered during pregnancy.

By means of intravenous glucose tolerance tests distinct differences in the magnitude and duration of the induced hyperglycemia between normal pregnant and nonpregnant women have not been demonstrated. Employing oral glucose tolerance tests, the hyperglycemia induced may persist somewhat longer than in normal nonpregnant women, probably because of slower and therefore more prolonged absorption of glucose. This explanation may be an oversimplification of the problem. The hypoglycemic effect of tolbutamide is not nearly so great in normal pregnant women as it is in nonpregnant women, even though insulin release appeared to be appreciably greater (Spellacy and associates, 1965). The decreased hypoglycemic effect of tolbutamide in pregnancy results mainly from the increased peripheral resistance to insulin action that is induced by pregnancy.

The frequent occurrence of *glucosuria* in healthy women during pregnancy results from increased glomerular filtration and less effective renal tubular absorption than in the nonpregnant state (Davison and Hytten, 1975).

Fat Metabolism

Plasma lipids increase appreciably during the latter half of pregnancy. This increase involves total lipids, esterified and nonesterified cholesterol, phospholipids, neutral fat, lipoproteins, and free fatty acids. The magnitude of some of the changes is illustrated in Table 9-2 and Figure 9-6. Cholesterol, triglyceride, and lipoprotein levels decrease at different rates after delivery (Potter and Nestel, 1979) and the rate of this decrease can be increased significantly by breast-feeding (Darmady and Postle, 1982).

In pregnant women, starvation induces much more intense ketonemia and ketonuria than it does in nonpregnant women. Women at midpregnancy who before abortion were starved experimentally for upward of 4 days demonstrated remarkably increased levels of

TABLE 9-2. CHANGES IN SERUM LIPIDS (FASTING) INDUCED BY PREGNANCY

	Nonpregnant	37–40 Weeks	Percent Change
Serum Total Lipids (mg/dl)	711	1039	+46
Serum Total Cholesterol (mg/dl)	178	249	+40
Esterified Cholesterol (%)	74	77	—
Serum Phospholipids (mg/dl)	256	350	+37
Free Fatty Acids (μEq/L)	768	1226	+60

(*Data from deAlvarez and associates: Am J Obstet Gynecol 82:1096, 1961; and Burt: Obstet Gynecol 15:460, 1960.*)

plasma free fatty acids, glycerol, and ketones as glucose fell more than one third. Similar changes occurred in amnionic fluid (Kim and Felig, 1972).

Hytten and Thomson (1968) and Pipe and co-workers (1979) concluded that storage of fat occurs primarily during midpregnancy, the fat being deposited mostly in central rather than peripheral sites. Later in pregnancy, as the nutritional demands of the fetus increase remarkably, storage of fat decreases. Hytten and Thompson cited some evidence that progesterone may act to reset a "lipostat" in the hypothalamus; at the end of pregnancy the lipostat returns to its previous nonpregnant level and the added fat is lost. Such a mechanism for energy storage, theoretically at least, might protect the mother and fetus during times of prolonged starvation or hard physical exertion.

Mineral Metabolism

The requirements for iron during pregnancy are considerable, and often exceed the amounts available (p. 192). With respect to most other minerals, pregnancy induces little change in their metabolism other than their retention in amounts equivalent to those utilized for growth of fetal and, to a lesser extent, maternal tissues (see Chapter 8, p. 167, Chapter 13, p. 252).

Copper and ceruloplasmin in the plasma increase considerably early in pregnancy, because of the increases in estrogens, which will produce the same changes when administered to nonpregnant subjects (Russ and Raymunt, 1956). Vir and co-workers (1981) reported that copper levels in hair were similar in nonpregnant and pregnant women, but values in pregnancy decreased from the first through the third trimester. They added that there was a significant positive correlation between third-trimester maternal hair and serum copper levels and neonatal weight but a significant negative correlation with respect to maternal serum copper and neonatal head circumference.

During pregnancy, calcium and magnesium levels are reduced very slightly, the reduction probably reflecting for the most part the lowered plasma protein concentration and, in turn, the consequent decrease in the amount of each electrolyte that is bound to protein. However, Fogh-Anderson and Schultz-Larsen (1981) have calculated a small but significant increase in free calcium ion concentration in late pregnancy by correcting for blood pH changes. Serum phosphorus levels are within the nonpregnant range. The status of zinc metabolism in pregnancy, as discussed in Chapter 13 (p. 253), is not clearly understood.

Acid–Base Equilibrium and Blood Electrolytes

Normally, the pregnant woman hyperventilates, compared with the nonpregnant subject, and this causes a respiratory alkalosis by lowering the P_{CO_2} of the blood. A moderate reduction in plasma bicarbonate from about 26 mmol to about 22 mmol/L *partially* compensates for the respiratory alkalosis. As a result, there is only a minimal increase in blood pH (Sjöstedt, 1962). The increase in blood pH shifts the oxygen dissociation curve to the left and increases the affinity of maternal hemoglobin for oxygen (Bohr effect), thereby decreasing the oxygen-releasing capacity of maternal blood. Thus, the hyperventilation, which results in a reduced maternal P_{CO_2}, facilitates transport of carbon dioxide from the fetus to the mother but *appears to impair* release of oxygen from the mother's blood to the fetus. The increase in blood pH, however, while minimal, stimulates an increase in 2,3-diphosphoglycerate in maternal erythrocytes (Tsai and co-workers, 1982) that counteracts the Bohr effect by shifting the oxygen dissociation curve back to the right, facilitating oxygen release to the fetus. These subtle but important changes ensure that the fetus has every advantage in blood gas exchange.

Total protein in plasma is decreased slightly during pregnancy. The serum osmolality and the concentration of potassium and sodium are reduced about 3 percent.

HEMATOLOGIC CHANGES ASSOCIATED WITH NORMAL PREGNANCY

Blood Volume and Iron Metabolism

The maternal blood volume increases markedly during pregnancy. In a study of 50 normal women, the blood volumes at or very near term averaged about 45 percent above their nonpregnant levels (Pritchard, 1965). This increase is similar to that described by Caton and associates (1949), Dahlström and Ihrman (1960), and Ueland (1976).

The degree of expansion varies considerably; in some women there is only a modest increase and in others their blood volume nearly doubles. A fetus is not essential for the development of hypervolemia during pregnancy, for increases in blood volume identical with those found during normal pregnancy have been demonstrated in some women with hydatidiform mole (Pritchard, 1965).

The pregnancy-induced hypervolemia serves to meet the demands of the enlarged uterus, with its greatly hypertrophied vascular system, to protect the mother and, in turn, the fetus against the deleterious effects of impaired venous return in the supine and erect positions, and, very importantly, to safeguard the mother against the adverse effects of blood loss associated with parturition.

The maternal blood volume starts to increase during the first trimester, expands most rapidly during the second trimester, and then rises at a much slower rate during the third trimester to attain a plateau during the last several weeks of pregnancy.

The increase in blood volume results from an increase in both plasma and erythrocytes. The usual pattern is that of an initial rise in the plasma volume, followed by an increase in the volume of circulating erythrocytes. Although more plasma than erythrocytes is usually added to the maternal circulation, the increase in the volume of circulating erythrocytes is considerable, averaging, in the 50 women previously mentioned, about 450 ml of erythrocytes, or an increase of about 33 percent. The importance of this increase in creating a demand for iron is discussed below. The increase in the volume of circulating erythrocytes in pregnancy is accomplished by acccelerated production rather than by prolongation of the life-span of the erythrocyte (Pritchard and Adams, 1960).

The mean age of circulating maternal red cells is lower during the latter half of pregnancy because the rate of red cell production exceeds that of destruction. The *mean cell volume* is increased, with the red blood cell becoming more spherical due to a decreased diameter and an increased thickness (Bolton and Street, 1982).

Moderate erythroid hyperplasia is present in the bone marrow, and the reticulocyte count is elevated slightly during normal pregnancy. This is almost certainly due to the increased levels of erythropoietin that have been noted in maternal plasma and urine during pregnancy (Jepson, 1969; Živný and associates, 1982; Cotes and Canning, 1983).

Jepson and Friesen (1968) reported that administration of placental lactogen, purified from human placenta, to polycythemic mice accelerated the incorporation of iron into their erythrocytes, an effect that was abolished by its incubation with antibody to placental lactogen but not with antisheep erythropoietin. Cotes and Canning (1983) reported that serum erythropoietin levels and placental lactogen were significantly related. Again, it is pointed out that apparently quite normal pregnancies have been observed with no detectable levels of placental lactogen.

Changes in Hematocrit

In spite of the augmented erythropoiesis, the concentrations of hemoglobin and erythrocytes, as well as the hematocrit, commonly decrease slightly during normal pregnancy. In Sturgeon's careful study (1959), in which iron was readily available to the mother for erythropoiesis, he found that the hemoglobin concentration at term averaged 12.1 g, as compared with a level of 13.3 g/dl for nonpregnant women. In a similar study, the hemoglobin concentration at term averaged 12.5 g, with a level below 11.0 g/dl present in only 6 percent of the pregnant subjects (Pritchard and Hunt, 1958). In many more recent studies these results have been confirmed. A hemoglobin concentration below 11.0 g/dl, especially late in pregnancy, probably should be considered as abnormal and usually due to iron deficiency, rather than to the physiologic hypervolemia of pregnancy (see Chapters 13 and 28, pp. 252 and 563).

Iron Stores

It has been stated commonly that the total body iron content averages about 4 g, or slightly more, in the adult. This value, however, applies to normal men. In

TABLE 9-3. MEASUREMENT OF HEMOGLOBIN IRON AND IRON STORES IN HEALTHY YOUNG WOMEN (NEVER PREGNANT AND NEVER EXPERIENCED ABNORMAL BLOOD LOSS)

	Average	Range
Age	23	21 to 26
Weight (kg)	60	49 to 72
Height (in)	65	60 to 68
HGB Concentration (g/dl)	14.1	13.0 to 15.6
Serum Iron Concentration (μg/dl)	105	76 to 132
HGB Mass (g)	443	358 to 492
HGB Iron (mg)	1505	1210 to 1670
Iron Stores* (mg)	347	150 to 629

* Iron converted to hemoglobin in response to repeated phlebotomy. (*From Pritchard and Mason, 1964.*)

healthy young women of average size, the body iron content is probably not much more than half that amount (Table 9-3). Commonly, iron stores of normal young women are only about 0.3 g (Pritchard and Mason, 1964; Scott and Pritchard, 1967). As in men, heme iron in myoglobin and enzymes and tranferrin-bound circulating iron together total only a few hundred milligrams. The total iron content of normal adult women, therefore, is probably in the range of 2.0 to 2.5 g.

Iron Requirements

The iron requirements of normal pregnancy total about 1 g (Fig. 9-7). About 300 mg are actively transferred to the fetus and placenta (Widdowson and Spray, 1951) and about 200 mg are lost through various normal routes of excretion. These are obligatory losses and occur even

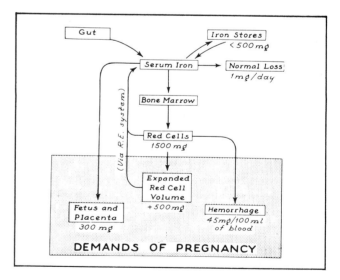

Figure 9-7. The iron requirements of normal pregnancy. The 300 mg of iron transferred to the fetus are permanently lost from the mother. The 500 mg incorporated into maternal hemoglobin usually are not all lost; the amount recovered for storage depends upon the amount of blood lost at and after delivery.

when the mother is iron deficient. The average increase in the total volume of circulating erythrocytes of about 450 ml during pregnancy, when iron is available, utilizes another 500 mg of iron because 1 ml of normal erythrocytes contains 1.1 mg of iron. Practically all the iron for these purposes is utilized during the latter half of pregnancy. Therefore, the iron requirement becomes quite large during the second half of pregnancy, averaging 6 to 7 mg per day (Pritchard and Scott, 1970). Since this amount of iron is not available from body stores in most women, the desired increase in maternal erythrocyte volume and hemoglobin mass will not develop unless exogenous iron is made available in adequate amounts. In the absence of added exogenous iron, the hemoglobin concentration and hematocrit fall appreciably as the maternal blood volume increases. Hemoglobin production in the fetus, however, will not be impaired, because the placenta obtains iron from the mother in amounts sufficient for the fetus to establish normal hemoglobin levels even when the mother has severe iron-deficiency anemia.

The amounts of iron absorbed from diet, together with that mobilized from stores, is usually insufficient to meet the demands imposed by pregnancy, even though iron absorption from the gastrointestinal tract appears to be moderately increased during pregnancy (Hahn and associates, 1951). Supplemental iron, therefore, is valuable during the latter half of pregnancy, and for several weeks after delivery if the infant is to be breast-fed (see Chapter 13, p. 252).

Without supplemental iron, the maternal *plasma iron concentration* often decreases during pregnancy. Undoubtedly, in most instances, iron deficiency contributes significantly to the fall. The *plasma iron-binding capacity* (transferrin) increases during pregnancy even when iron deficiency has been eliminated by appropriate treatment (Sturgeon, 1959). When administered to nonpregnant women, estrogen has been shown to produce an increase in plasma transferrin levels comparable to those of pregnancy.

Blood Loss

Not all the iron added to the maternal circulation in the form of hemoglobin is necessarily lost from the mother. During normal vaginal delivery and through the next few days, only about one half of the erythrocytes added to the maternal circulation during pregnancy are lost from the majority of women by way of the placental implantation site, the placenta itself, the episiotomy wound and lacerations, and in the lochia. On the average, an amount of maternal erythrocytes corresponding to about 600 ml of predelivery blood is lost during and after vaginal delivery of a single fetus (Newton, 1966; Pritchard, 1965; Ueland, 1976). The average blood loss associated with cesarean section or with the vaginal delivery of twins is about 1 liter, or nearly twice that lost with the delivery of a single fetus (Pritchard, 1965; Ueland, 1976; Wilcox and co-workers, 1959). Unfortunately, it is not rare for the quantity of erythrocytes lost to equal or exceed the added volume accumulated during pregnancy.

Generally, the pattern of change in maternal blood volume during labor, vaginal delivery, and puerperium is as follows: (1) there is some hemoconcentration during labor, which varies with the degree of muscular activity and dehydration; (2) during and soon after delivery there is a further reduction in volume that closely parallels the amount of blood lost; (3) during the first few days of the puerperium there is little change or a slight increase in blood volume, especially if hemoconcentration during labor or blood loss at delivery was sizable; (4) by 1 week after delivery there is a further reduction in plasma volume to the extent that the maternal blood volume is only slightly greater than several months later (McLennan and co-workers, 1959; Pritchard, 1965).

Following delivery, any excess circulating hemoglobin above the amount normally present in the nonpregnant state ultimately yields iron for storage. The mechanism by which this occurs is most likely not accelerated erythrocyte destruction during the late puerperium, but rather normal destruction with reduced production of new erythrocytes. A similar process occurs after a normal nonanemic person receives transfused cells, or when a normal person with polycythemia, induced by high altitude, returns to sea level.

Leukocytes

The blood leukocyte count varies considerably during normal pregnancy (Efrati and co-workers, 1964). Usually it ranges from 5000 to 12,000 per mm³. During labor and the early puerperium it may become markedly elevated, attaining levels of 25,000 or even more; however, the increase averages 14,000 to 16,000 per mm³ (Taylor and co-workers, 1981). The cause for the marked increase is not known, but the same response occurs during and after strenuous exercise. It probably represents the reappearance in the circulation of leukocytes previously shunted out of the active circulation.

Beginning quite early in pregnancy, the activity of alkaline phosphatase in the leukocytes is increased. Elevated leukocyte alkaline phosphatase activity is not peculiar to pregnancy but occurs in a wide variety of conditions, including most inflammatory states. During pregnancy there is a neutrophilia that consists predominantly of mature forms; however, by close examination of smears of the peripheral blood of pregnant women, one can find an occasional myelocyte.

Blood Coagulation

The levels of several blood coagulation factors are increased during pregnancy. Plasma fibrinogen (factor I) measured as thrombin-clottable protein in normal pregnant women, averages very close to 300 mg and ranges from about 200 to 400 mg/dl. During normal pregnancy the concentration of fibrinogen increases about 50 percent, to average about 450 mg late in pregnancy, with a range from approximately 300 to 600 mg/dl. The increase in the concentration of fibrinogen undoubtedly contributes greatly to the striking increase in the blood *sedimentation rate* in normal pregnancy (Ozanne and co-workers, 1983). The increased sedimentation rate in pregnancy, therefore, has no diagnostic or prognostic value when employed for the usual clinical purpose, such as the assessment of the activity of lupus erythematosus.

Other clotting factors, the activities of which are inceased appreciably during normal pregnancy, are factor VII (proconvertin), factor VIII (antihemophiliac globulin), factor IX (plasma thromboplastin component or Christmas factor), and factor X (Stuart factor). Usually the level of factor II (prothrombin) is increased only slightly, whereas those of factors XI (plasma thromboplastin antecedent) and XIII (fibrin-stabilizing factor) are decreased somewhat during pregnancy (Coopland and associates, 1969; Kasper and colleagues, 1964; Talbert and Langdell, 1964). The Quick one-stage prothrombin time and the partial thromboplastin time are both shortened slightly as pregnancy progresses.

Some investigators have described a moderate decrease in the number of platelets per unit volume (Pitkin and Witte, 1979). This may be the consequence of increased platelet consumption throughout normal pregnancy (Fay and co-workers, 1983). The clotting times of whole blood in either plain glass tubes (wettable surface) or silicone-coated or plastic tubes (nonwettable surface) do not differ significantly in normal pregnant and nonpregnant women. Some, but not all, of the pregnancy-induced changes in the levels of coagulation factors can be duplicated by the administration of one of several of the commonly used estrogen plus progestin contraceptive tablets (Fletcher and Alkajaersig, 1969).

High-molecular-weight soluble fibrin–fibrinogen complexes circulate in normal pregnancy. Also, an increased capacity for neutralizing heparin has been described, as well as a lower level of antithrombin III. Some of these alterations in coagulation factors during normal pregnancy may be equated with a continuing low-grade process of intravascular coagulation (Fletcher and co-workers, 1979). Bonnar (1978) employing electron microscopy, identified fibrin deposited in the intervillous space of the placenta and in the walls of the spiral arteries that supply blood to the intervillous space.

During normal pregnancy, the level of maternal plasminogen (profibrinolysin) in plasma increases considerably, a phenomenon that can be induced by estrogen treatment. Even so, fibrinolytic, or plasmin, activity, measured either as the time for clotted plasma to dissolve or as the time for the clotted euglobulin fraction from plasma to undergo lysis, is distinctly prolonged compared with that of the normal nonpregnant state. Åstedt (1972) implicated the placenta in the reduced fibrinolytic activity that characterizes normal pregnancy, since normally delivery is promptly followed by an increase in plasma fibrinolytic activity (Ratnoff and co-workers, 1954). At the same time, fibrin degradation products usually rise slightly after delivery (Woodfield and associates, 1968).

CARDIOVASCULAR SYSTEM

During pregnancy and the puerperium there are remarkable changes involving the heart and the circulation.

Heart

Typically, the resting pulse rate increases about 10 to 15 beats per minute during pregnancy. As the diaphragm is elevated progressively during pregnancy, the heart is displaced to the left and upward, while at the same time it is rotated somewhat on its long axis. As a result, the apex of the heart is moved somewhat laterally from its position in the normal nonpregnant state, and an increase in the size of the cardiac silhouette is found in roentgenograms (Fig. 9-8). The extent of these changes is influenced by the size and position of the uterus, the strength of the abdominal muscles, and the configurations of the abdomen and thorax. Variability of these factors makes it difficult to precisely identify moderate degrees of cardiomegaly by physical examination or by simple roentgenographic studies. The physician must, therefore, be cautious in making a diagnosis of pathologic cardiomegaly during pregnancy.

In several studies using frontal and sagittal roentgenograms, the cardiac volume was found to increase normally by about 75 ml, or a little more than 10 percent, between early and late pregnancy (Ihrman, 1960). Such an increase in cardiac volume might involve slight hypertrophy, dilatation, or, more likely, both. Katz and co-workers (1978) studied left ventricular performance during pregnancy and the puerperium using echocardiography. Both left ventricular wall mass and end-diastolic dimensions were observed to increase during pregnancy, as did heart rate, calculated stroke volume, and cardiac output. The changes in stroke volume were directly pro-

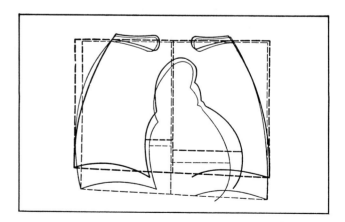

Figure 9-8. Change in cardiac outline that occurs in pregnancy. The light lines represent the relations between the heart and thorax in the nonpregnant woman, and the heavy lines represent the conditions existing in pregnancy. These findings are based on teleoroentgenograms and represent the average findings in 33 women. (*From Klafen and Palugyay: Arch Gynaekol 131:347, 1927.*)

portional to end-diastolic volume, implying, at least, that there is little change in the inotropic state of the myocardium during normal pregnancy and the puerperium.

During pregnancy some of the cardiac sounds may be altered to the extent that they would be considered abnormal in the absence of pregnancy. Cutforth and MacDonald (1966) obtained phonocardiograms at varying stages of pregnancy in 50 normal women and documented the following changes:

- *Heart sounds:* An exaggerated splitting of the first heart sound with increased loudness of both components; no definite changes in the aortic and pulmonary elements of the second sound; a loud, easily heard third sound.
- *Heart murmurs:* A systolic murmur in 90 percent of pregnant women, intensified during inspiration in some or expiration in others, and disappearing very shortly after delivery; a soft diastolic murmur transiently in 19 percent; continuous murmurs arising apparently in breast vasculature in 10 percent.

The physician must be cautious when interpreting the significance of murmurs during pregnancy, especially systolic murmurs.

Normal pregnancy induces no characteristic changes in the *electrocardiogram* other than slight deviation of the electrical axis to the left as a result of the altered position of the heart.

Cardiac Output

During normal pregnancy, the arterial blood pressure and vascular resistance decrease while the blood volume, maternal weight, and basal metabolic rate increase. Each of these events would be expected to affect cardiac output, with some leading to decreased output but others causing an increase. It is now evident that cardiac output *at rest,* when measured in the lateral recumbent position, increases appreciably during the first trimester and remains elevated during the second and third trimesters. Typically, cardiac output in late pregnancy is appreciably higher when the woman is in the lateral recumbent position than when she is supine, since in the supine position the large uterus and its contents often impede venous return to the heart (Kerr, 1965; Lees and co-workers, 1968). Ueland and Hansen (1969), for example, found that cardiac output increased 1100 ml (22 percent) when the pregnant woman was moved from her back onto her side. According to Milsom and Forssman (1984), in normal pregnant women during the third trimester, cardiac output and stroke volume are greatest when the women are in the left lateral recumbent position.

Cardiac output in response to physical activity by the ambulatory woman must be greater late in pregnancy than it would be if she were not pregnant. Increase in mass alone demands such a response.

During the first stage of labor, maternal cardiac output increases moderately, and during the second stage of labor, with vigorous expulsive efforts, the cardiac output is appreciably greater. Most of the increase in cardiac output induced by pregnancy is lost very soon after delivery (Ueland and Metcalfe, 1975).

Reviews of cardiac function and cardiovascular physiology have been provided more recently by Metcalfe and co-workers (1981) and by Hankins and associates (1983).

Circulation

The posture of the pregnant woman affects *arterial blood pressure.* Typically, blood pressure in the brachial artery is highest when the gravida is sitting, lowest when lying in the left lateral recumbent position, and intermediate when supine, except for some women who become quite hypotensive in the supine position. Usually, arterial blood pressure decreases to a nadir during the second trimester or early third trimester, and rises thereafter. Any sustained rise of 30 mm systolic or 15 mm diastolic under basal conditions is indicative of an abnormality, most likely pregnancy-induced hypertension (see Chapter 27, p. 525).

The antecubital *venous pressure* remains unchanged during pregnancy, but in the supine position the femoral venous pressure rises steadily from 8 cm of water pressure early in pregnancy to 24 cm at term (Fig. 9-9). Employing radiolabeled tracers, Wright and co-workers (1950) and many others have demonstrated that blood flow in the legs is retarded during pregnancy except when the subjects are in the lateral recumbent position. This tendency toward stagnation of blood in the lower extremities during the latter part of pregnancy is attributable to the occlusion of the pelvic veins and inferior

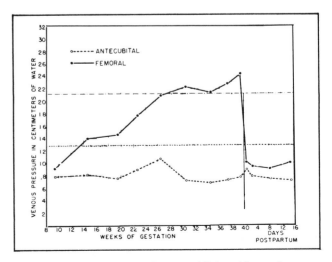

Figure 9-9. Serial changes in antecubital and femoral venous blood pressure throughout normal pregnancy and early puerperium. These measurements were made on women in the supine position. (*From McLennan, 1943.*)

vena cava by pressure of the enlarged uterus. The elevated venous pressure returns to normal if the pregnant woman lies on her side and immediately after delivery of the infant by cesarean section (McLennan, 1943). From a clinical viewpoint, the retarded blood flow and increased venous pressure in the legs, which are demonstrable in the latter months of pregnancy, are of great importance. These alterations contribute to the dependent edema frequently experienced by women as they approach term and to the development of varicose veins in the legs and vulva, as well as hemorrhoids.

Other Circulatory Effects from Supine Position

In the supine position, the large uterus of pregnancy rather consistently compresses the venous system that returns blood from the lower half of the body to the extent that cardiac filling may be reduced and cardiac output decreased. Infrequently, this causes significant arterial hypotension, sometimes referred to as the supine hypotensive syndrome (Howard and colleagues, 1953). Moreover, Bieniarz and associates (1968) observed that in the supine position the large pregnant uterus may compress the aorta sufficiently to lower arterial blood pressure below the level of compression. They demonstrated that the usual sphygmomanometric measurement of blood pressures in the brachial artery does not provide a reliable estimate of the pressure in the uterine or other arteries that lie distal to the compression exerted on the aorta by the gravid uterus and its contents. When the pregnant woman is supine, uterine arterial pressure is significantly lower than that in the brachial artery. In the presence of systemic hypotension, as occurs with spinal anesthesia, the decrease in uterine arterial pressure is even more marked than in arteries above the level of compression of the aorta. Gant and associates (1974) reported that an appreciable number of women destined to develop pregnancy-induced hypertension exhibited a more than 20 mm Hg increase in diastolic blood pressure when they were turned from the lateral to the supine position. These investigators called this a supine pressor test. The exact mechanism responsible for this response remains to be defined.

Blood Flow to Skin

Increased cutaneous blood flow in pregnancy serves to dissipate excess heat generated by the increased metabolism imposed by pregnancy (Burt, 1950; Spetz, 1964).

RESPIRATORY TRACT

Anatomic Changes

The level of the diaphragm rises about 4 cm during pregnancy. The subcostal angle widens appreciably as the transverse diameter of the thoracic cage increases about 2 cm. The thoracic circumference increases about 6 cm

but not sufficiently to prevent a reduction in the residual volume of air in the lungs created by the elevated diaphragm. The idea that the elevated diaphragm was "splinted" during normal pregnancy has been disproven using fluoroscopic studies (Möbius, 1961). Diaphragmatic excursion is actually greater during pregnancy than in the nonpregnant woman. As a result, the tidal volume increases.

Pulmonary Function

At any stage of normal pregnancy, the amount of oxygen delivered by the increase in tidal volume clearly exceeds the oxygen need imposed by the pregnancy. Moreover, the amount of hemoglobin in the circulation and, in turn, the total oxygen-carrying capacity increase appreciably during normal pregnancy, as does cardiac output. As the consequence, *maternal arteriovenous oxygen difference* is decreased during pregnancy.

The respiratory rate is changed little during pregnancy but the *tidal volume, minute ventilatory volume, and minute oxygen uptake* increase appreciably as pregnancy advances (Table 9-4). The *maximum breathing capacity* and *forced or timed vital capacity* are not altered appreciably. The *functional residual capacity* and the *residual volume* of air are decreased as the consequence of elevation of the diaphragm. *Lung compliance* is unaffected by pregnancy whereas *airway conductance* is increased and *total pulmonary resistance* is reduced. Gee and associates (1967) speculated that increased airway conductance from decreased bronchomotor tone may be effected by progesterone action.

The *closing volume,* that is, the lung volume at which airways in the dependent parts of the lung begin to close during expiration, has been considered to be higher in pregnancy by some investigators but not by others (Baldwin and associates, 1977).

An increased awareness of a desire to breathe is common even early in pregnancy (Milne and colleagues, 1978) and may be interpreted as dyspnea, which, in turn, suggests pulmonary or cardiac abnormalities even though most often none exists. The increased tidal volume normally lowers slightly the blood P_{CO_2}, causing

TABLE 9-4. RESTING RESPIRATORY FUNCTION

Function	Not Pregnant	Pregnant	Change (%)
Respiratory Rate	15	16	—
Tidal Volume (ml)	487	678	+39*
Minute Ventilation (ml)	7270	10,340	+42*
Minute O_2 Uptake	201	266	+32*
Vital Capacity (ml)	3260	3310	+ 1
Maximum Breathing Capacity (% of predicted)	102	97	− 5
Inspiratory Capacity (ml)	2625	2745	+ 5
Residual Volume (ml)	965	770	−20*

* Highly significant differences.
(*From Cugell and associates: Am Rev Tuberc 67:568, 1953.*)

mild respiratory alkalosis, which is partially compensated for by a lowering of the bicarbonate concentration.

The increased respiratory effort and, in turn, the reduction in P_{CO_2} during pregnancy are most likely induced in large part by progesterone and to a lesser degree estrogen. Oral medroxyprogesterone has been administered to stimulate an increased respiratory drive in obese nonpregnant subjects who hypoventilate (Sutton and co-workers 1975). The site of action of the hormones appears to be central, that is, the stimulatory effect acts directly on the respiratory center.

Although pulmonary function is not impaired by pregnancy, disease of the respiratory tract may be more serious during gestation. Important factors are undoubtedly the increased oxygen requirements imposed by pregnancy and perhaps an increase in closing volume, especially when supine.

URINARY SYSTEM

Remarkable changes in both structure and function take place in the urinary tract during normal pregnancy.

Kidney

The kidney increases slightly in size during pregnancy. Bailey and Rolleston (1971), for example, found that the kidney was 1.5 cm longer during the early puerperium than when measured 6 months later.

Glomerular filtration rate (GFR) and renal plasma flow (RPF) increase early in pregnancy, the former as much as 50 percent by the beginning of the second trimester, and the latter not quite so much (Chesley, 1963; Sims, 1963; and Dunlop, 1981). The precise mechanism by which RPF and GFR are increased in pregnancy has not been identified. The elevated GFR has been found by most investigators to persist to term (Fig. 9-10), whereas the RPF decreases during the third trimester.

Most studies of renal function conducted during pregnancy have been performed while the subjects were supine, a position that late in pregnancy may produce marked systemic hemodynamic changes (see p. 196) that lead to alterations in several aspects of renal function. Late in pregnancy, for instance, urinary flow and sodium excretion are affected significantly by posture, averaging less than half the rate of excretion in the supine position, compared to the lateral recumbent position.

Whereas posture clearly affects sodium and water excretion in late pregnancy, its impact on GFR and RPF seems to be much more variable. Chesley and Sloan (1964), for example, found GFR and RPF to be commonly reduced when the pregnant woman was in the supine position, whereas Dunlop (1976) identified little or no reduction. Pritchard and associates (1955) detected decreases in GFR and RPF while supine compared to lateral recumbent in some, but not most, of the late pregnant women studied. Ezimokhai and associates

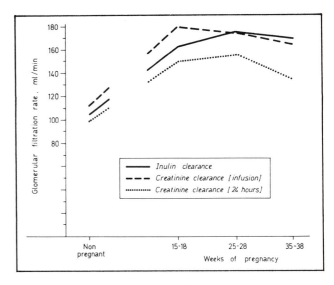

Figure 9-10. Mean glomerular filtration rate in healthy women over a short period with infused inulin (*solid line*), simultaneously as creatinine clearance during the inulin infusion (*broken line*), and over 24 hours as endogenous creatinine clearance (*dotted line*). (*From Davison and Hytten, 1974.*)

(1981) have presented good evidence that the late-pregnancy decrease in RPF is not due simply to a positional effect. Davison and Hytten (1974) have rightfully pointed out that an estimate of glomerular filtration rate is only valid for the conditions under which it is measured and that changes with posture represent the real-life situation rather than artifact.

A possible cause of the changes in renal function in the supine position compared to the lateral recumbent is reduced venous return to the heart, which results from obstruction of the inferior vena cava and iliac veins by the large pregnant uterus, which could lead to reduction in cardiac output and, in turn, lowering of RPF and GFR. The sequence of events, however, does not appear to be essential to the mechanism that triggers sodium and water retention when supine. In a woman at term with a renal transplant in the right iliac fossa, a change to the supine from the lateral recumbent position had no obvious effect on water and sodium excretion or on GFR (Pritchard, unpublished).

Another possible mechanism to account for decreased sodium and water excretion in supine pregnant women is elevated ureteral pressure. Fulop and Brazeau (1970) induced increased tubular reabsorption of sodium and water in dogs by elevating ureteral pressure moderately. Pritchard and associates (1955) were not able to prevent such decreases in the supine position following the insertion of ureteral catheters well above the pelvic brim; however, increased intraureteric pressure may not have been completely prevented by this maneuver.

It has been suggested by some that the release of antidiuretic hormone (ADH) plays a role, but ADH is probably not essential, as postural changes have produced similar reductions in a pregnant woman with severe diabetes insipidus (Whalley and co-workers, 1961).

Loss of Nutrients

One unusual feature of the pregnancy-induced changes in renal excretion is the remarkably increased amounts of various nutrients in the urine. Amino acids and water-soluble vitamins are lost in the urine of pregnant women in much greater amounts than in the urine of nonpregnant women (Hytten and Leitch, 1971).

Tests of Renal Function

The results of several of the tests of renal function in general clinical use may be altered during normal pregnancy and therefore be quite misleading. During pregnancy the concentrations in plasma of creatinine and urea normally decrease as a consequence of the increased GFR. At times, the urea concentration may be so low as to suggest impaired hepatic synthesis, which sometimes occurs with severe liver disease.

Creatinine clearance is a useful test of renal function in pregnancy provided that complete urine collection is made over an accurately timed period, preferably several hours at least. *Urine concentration tests* may give results that are misleading (Davison and colleagues, 1981). During the day, pregnant women tend to accumulate water in the form of dependent edema (see p. 188), and at night, while recumbent, they mobilize this fluid and excrete it via the kidneys. This reversal of the usual nonpregnant diurnal pattern of urinary flow causes nocturia and the nighttime excretion of urine more dilute than in the nonpregnant state. The failure of a pregnant woman to excrete a concentrated urine after withholding fluids for approximately 18 hours does not necessarily mean renal damage. The kidney, in fact, in these circumstances functions perfectly normally by excreting mobilized extracellular fluid of relatively low osmolality. *Dye excretion tests,* such as the timed measurement of the amount of injected phenolsulfonphthalein (PSP) excreted in the urine, may also be misleading during pregnancy. The dye may very well be excreted by the kidney, but at low rates of urinary flow it is not collected and measured because of stagnation of urine in the considerably dilated renal pelves and ureters (see below).

Urinalysis

Glucosuria during pregnancy is not necessarily abnormal. The appreciable increase in glomerular filtration, together with impaired tubular reabsorptive capacity for filtered glucose, accounts in most cases for the glucosuria. Chesley (1963) calculated that for these reasons alone about one sixth of all pregnant women should spill glucose in the urine. Even though glucosuria is common during pregnancy, the possibility of diabetes mellitus cannot be ignored. *Proteinuria* does not occur normally during pregnancy except occasionally in slight amounts during or soon after vigorous labor. If not the result of contamination during collection, blood cells in the urine during pregnancy are compatible with a diagnosis of uri-

nary tract disease. Difficult labor and delivery, of course, can cause hematuria because of trauma to the lower urinary tract.

Hydronephrosis and Hydroureter

In pregnant women, after the uterus rises completely out of the pelvis, it rests upon the ureters, compressing them at the pelvic brim. Increased intraureteral tonus above the level of the pelvic brim compared with that of the pelvic portion of the ureter has been identified (Rubi and Sala, 1968). No such differences were demonstrable in nonpregnant women.

Typically, ureteral dilatation above the pelvic brim is more marked on the right side. Schulman and Herlinger (1975) found ureteral dilatation to be greater on the right side in 86 percent of pregnant women studied (Fig. 9-11). A similar result has been reported by Peake and co-workers (1983) using ultrasonographic techniques rather than intravenous pyelograms. The unequal degrees of dilatation may result from a cushioning provided the left ureter by the sigmoid colon and perhaps from greater compression of the right ureter as the consequence of dextrorotation of the uterus. Bellina and co-

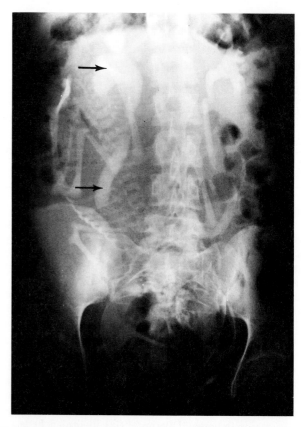

Figure 9-11. Normal intravenous pyelogram at 36 weeks gestation. Pregnancy-induced hydronephrosis (*upper arrow*) and hydroureter (*lower arrow*) are more marked on the mother's right side. Elongation, dilatation, and peristalsis of the ureter create the appearance of discontinuity of the ureter.

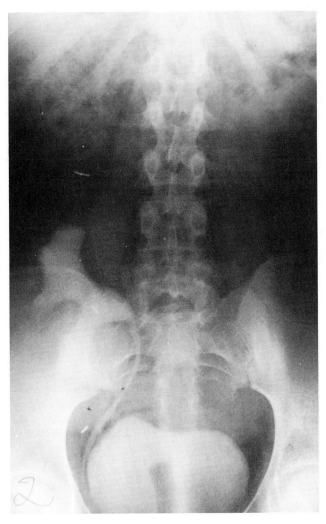

Figure 9-12. A. Intravenous pyelogram of renal transplant: Before pregnancy.

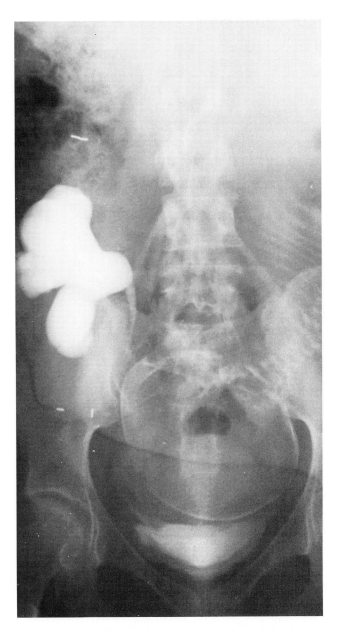

Figure 9-12. B. Intravenous pyelogram of renal transplant: Late in pregnancy. Marked levorotation of the uterus was identified at cesarean section.

workers (1970) emphasized that the right ovarian vein complex, which is remarkably dilated during pregnancy, lies obliquely over the right ureter and may contribute significantly to right ureteral dilatation.

Another possible mechanism causing hydronephrosis and hydroureter is hormonal, presumably an effect of progesterone. Major support for this concept was provided by Van Wagenen (1939), who described in the monkey further dilatation of the ureters after removal of the fetus if the placenta remained in situ. The relatively abrupt onset of dilatation in women at midpregnancy, described by Schulman and Herlinger (1975), is more consistent with ureteral compression from a translocated enlarging uterus than a humoral effect.

Elongation accompanies distension of the ureter, which is frequently thrown into curves of varying size, the smaller of which may be sharply angulated, producing, at least theoretically, partial or complete obstruction. These so-called kinks are poorly labeled, as the term connotes obstruction. They are, usually, merely single or double curves, which, when viewed in the roentgenogram taken in the same plane as the curve, appear as more or less acute angulations of the ureter (Fig. 9-11). Another exposure at right angles nearly always identifies them to be more gentle curves than kinks. The ureter, in both its abdominal and pelvic portions, undergoes not only elongation but frequently lateral displacement by the pressure of the enlarged uterus.

Remarkable pregnancy-induced hydronephrosis with some degree of hydroureter has been demonstrated after transplant of a donor kidney to the iliac fossa (Fig. 9-12A,B). In this particular subject, the creatinine clearance increased from 75 ml per minute very early in preg-

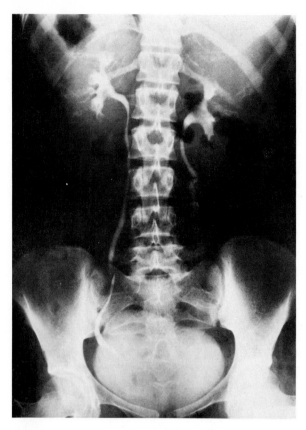

Figure 9-13. Intravenous pyelogram 1-week postpartum on the same woman as in Figure 9-11. There has been rapid resolution of much of the pregnancy-induced hydronephrosis and hydroureter evident in Figure 9-11.

nancy to 120 ml per minute during the third trimester, a normal response for pregnancy.

After delivery, there is resolution so that by 6 to 8 weeks the urinary tract has returned to prepregnancy dimensions (Fig. 9-13). The stretching and dilatation do not continue sufficiently long to impair permanently the elasticity of the ureter unless infection supervenes. These changes induced by pregnancy have been reviewed by Fainstat (1963) and by Schulman and Herlinger (1975).

Urinary Bladder

There are few significant anatomic changes in the bladder before the fourth month of pregnancy. From that time onward, however, the increased size of the uterus, together with the hyperemia that affects all pelvic organs and the hyperplasia of the muscle and connective tissues, elevates the bladder trigone and causes thickening of its posterior, or intraureteric, margin. Continuation of this process to the end of pregnancy produces marked deepening and widening of the trigone. The bladder mucosa undergoes no change other than an increase in the size and tortuosity of its blood vessels.

Toward the end of pregnancy, particularly in nullip-

aras in whom the presenting part often engages before the onset of labor, the entire base of the bladder is pushed forward and upward, converting the normal convex surface into a concavity. As a result, difficulties in diagnostic and therapeutic procedures are increased greatly. In addition, the pressure of the presenting part impairs the drainage of blood and lymph from the base of the bladder, often rendering the area edematous, easily traumatized, and probably more susceptible to infection. Both urethral pressure and length have been shown to be decreased in women following vaginal but not abdominal delivery (van Geelen and co-workers, 1982). These investigators suggested that a weakness of the urethral sphincter mechanism due to pregnancy and/or delivery may play a role in the pathogenesis of urinary stress incontinence.

Normally there is little residual urine in nulliparas, but occasionally it develops in multiparas with relaxed vaginal walls and cystoceles. Incompetence of the ureterovesical valve may supervene, with the consequent probability of vesicoureteral reflux of urine.

GASTROINTESTINAL TRACT

As pregnancy progresses, the stomach and intestines are displaced by the enlarging uterus. As the result of the positional changes in these viscera, the physical findings in certain diseases are altered. The appendix, for instance, is usually displaced upward and somewhat laterally as the uterus enlarges, and at times it may reach the right flank (Chapter 28, p. 616).

The tone and motility of the gastrointestinal tract are usually decreased, which prolongs the times of gastric emptying and intestinal transit. This may result from the large amounts of progesterone that are present during pregnancy, decreased levels of *motalin,* a hormonal peptide known to have smooth muscle stimulating effects (Christofidis and associates, 1982), or both. During labor, especially after administration of analgesic agents, *gastric-emptying time* is typically appreciably prolonged. A major danger of general anesthesia for delivery is regurgitation and aspiration of either food-laden or highly acidic gastric contents (see Chapter 18, p. 356).

Pyrosis (*heartburn*), common during pregnancy, is most probably caused by reflux of acidic secretions into the lower esophagus, the altered position of the stomach probably contributing to its frequent occurrence. Esophageal and gastric tone are altered by pregnancy, with intraesophageal pressures being lower and intragastric pressures higher in pregnant women. At the same time, esophageal peristalsis has lower wave speed and lower amplitude (Ulmsten and Sundström, 1978). These changes favor gastroesophageal reflux.

The gums may become hyperemic and softened during pregnancy and may bleed when mildly traumatized, as with a toothbrush. A focal, highly vascular swelling of the gums, the so-called *epulis* of pregnancy, develops occasionally but typically regresses spontaneously after delivery. There is no good evidence that pregnancy per se incites tooth decay.

Hemorrhoids are fairly common during pregnancy. They are caused in large measure by constipation and the elevated pressure in veins below the level of the enlarged uterus.

LIVER AND GALLBLADDER

Liver

Although the liver in some animals increases remarkably in size during pregnancy, there is no evidence of such an increase in human pregnancy (Combes and Adams, 1971). Moreover, by histologic evaluation of liver obtained by biopsy, including examination with the electron microscope, it has been demonstrated that no distinct changes in liver morphology occur in response to normal pregnancy (Adams and Ashworth, unpublished; Ingerslev and Teilum, 1946). The results of the very few measurements of hepatic blood flow during pregnancy are conflicting; there is perhaps a slight increase.

Some of the laboratory tests commonly used to evaluate hepatic function yield appreciably different results during normal pregnancy. Moreover, the changes induced by pregnancy often occur in the same direction as those found in patients with hepatic disease. Total *alkaline phosphatase* activity in serum almost doubles during normal pregnancy and commonly reaches levels that would be considered abnormal in the nonpregnant woman. Much of the increase can be attributed to alkaline phosphatase isozymes from the placenta, which are heat-stable up to 65°C. Whether all of the increase is caused by enzymes of placental origin is not clear, since nonpregnant women given estrogen in amounts comparable with those found in pregnancy frequently have increased serum alkaline phosphatase activity in their blood (Song and Kappas, 1968). Mendenhall (1970), as part of a study of the effects of pregnancy on several serum proteins, reconfirmed the presence of a decrease in *plasma albumin* concentration, showing it to average 3.0 g/dl late in pregnancy compared with 4.3 g/dl in nonpregnant women. The reduction in serum albumin, combined with a slight increase in globulins in plasma that occur normally during pregnancy, results in a decrease in the albumin to globulin ratio similar to that seen in certain hepatic diseases. Plasma *cholinesterase* activity is reduced during normal pregnancy, as it is in certain liver diseases. The magnitude of the decrease is about the same as the decrease in the concentration of albumin (Pritchard, 1955).

Leucine aminopeptidase activity is markedly elevated in serum from pregnant women; at term it reaches a level approximately three times the nonpregnant value. The increase in total serum leucine aminopeptidase activity during pregnancy results from the appearance of a pregnancy-specific enzyme (or enzymes) with distinct substrate specificities (Song and Kappas, 1968). This pregnancy-induced aminopeptidase has oxytocinase activity.

Combes and associates (1963) demonstrated that the capacity of the liver for excreting sulfobromophthalein into bile is somewhat decreased during normal pregnancy, while, at the same time, the ability of the liver to extract and store sulfobromophthalein is increased. The administration of estrogens to nonpregnant women induces comparable changes (Mueller and Kappas, 1964). *Spider nevi and palmer erythema,* both of which occur in patients with liver disease, are commonly found in normal pregnant women, most likely as a result of the increased circulating estrogens during pregnancy, but they disappear soon after delivery.

Gallbladder

Gallbladder function is altered during pregnancy. Potter (1936) noted that at the time of cesarean section the gallbladder is quite often distended but hypotonic; moreover, aspirated bile is quite thick. It is commonly accepted that pregnancy predisposes to formation of gallstones (see Chapter 28, p. 615).

ENDOCRINE GLANDS

Some of the most important endocrine changes of pregnancy have been discussed elsewhere, especially in Chapter 7.

Pituitary

The pituitary enlarges somewhat during pregnancy. Although there have been suggestions that it may increase in size sufficiently to compress the optic chiasma and reduce the visual fields, such visual changes during normal pregnancy are either absent or minimal. Striking enlargement of microadenomas of the pituitary can occur, however, during pregnancy.

The maternal pituitary gland is not essential for the maintenance of pregnancy. There now are a number of women who have undergone hypophysectomy, completed pregnancy successfully, and undergone spontaneous labor while receiving glucocorticosteroids along with thyroid hormone and vasopressin. Extensive destruction of both the maternal and the fetal pituitary glands in monkeys during the second trimester does not interrupt gestation (Hutchinson and co-workers, 1962). In these hypophysectomized primates, marked adrenal atrophy did not occur; thus the placenta may be a source of an adrenal corticotropin in this species.

Pituitary Growth Hormone

Although human placental lactogen (hPL) is abundant in the pregnant woman's blood, the level of pituitary growth hormone is decreased. After delivery, hPL rapidly disappears, but pituitary growth hormone remains quite low for some time (Spellacy and Buhi, 1969). The relative lack of these hormones, with the loss of their diabetogenic effect, may account in part for the usually abrupt and rather marked reduction in insulin requirements of women with diabetes mellitus during the early puerperium.

Prolactin

During the course of human gestation, there is a marked increase in the levels of prolactin in the maternal plasma. In fact, the levels increase to such an extent that mean concentrations of 150 ng/ml, values ten times greater than those in normal nonpregnant women, are observed at term (Friesen and co-workers, 1972; Riggs and colleagues, 1977). Paradoxically, following delivery, there is a decrease in plasma prolactin concentration even in the lactating mother. During early lactation, there are pulsatile bursts of secretion of prolactin, apparently in response to suckling. The physiologic cause of the marked increase in prolactin prior to parturition is unknown. Given the marked increase in secretion that occurs in the experimental animal under estrogen influence, however, it is tempting to relate the increase in prolactin secretion during pregnancy to the increase in estrogens in the gravid woman. Moreover, it is likely that the action of prolactin in mediating lactalbumin synthesis is inhibited during the course of pregnancy by the steroid hormone progesterone. Thus, following delivery, with the removal of the inhibitory influence of progesterone, lactation may proceed.

Prolactin is also found, throughout the course of gestation, in high concentration in the fetal plasma, attaining highest concentrations during the last 5 weeks of pregnancy (Winters and associates, 1975). Considerable evidence has accrued that is supportive of the view that prolactin in fetal plasma is of fetal pituitary origin and not of maternal pituitary origin.

For reasons not yet clearly understood, the concentrations of prolactin in the amnionic fluid are highest early in gestation and, in fact, levels of 10,000 ng/ml can be observed in the amnionic fluid at 20 weeks of gestation. Several groups of investigators have presented convincing evidence that the uterine decidua is one site of synthesis of at least a part of the prolactin in amnionic fluid. The levels of prolactin in amnionic fluid decrease after about 24 weeks of gestation such that by term the concentrations are one tenth those observed in early pregnancy (Friesen and colleagues, 1972).

β-Lipotrophin

The major precursor for a number of pituitary and probably chorionic peptide hormones is pro-opiomelanocortin, a large peptide chain that is split at a variety of sites by specific proteolytic enzymes (see Chapter 7, p. 123, and Fig. 7-2). One of the major fragments from this process is a 91-amino acid chain, β-lipotrophin. This compound may then be broken again to yield two additional

fragments, one a 51-amino acid peptide called γ-lipotrophin and the other a 31-amino acid chain called β-endorphin. β-Endorphin is a potent endogenous opioid that is elevated in a variety of stressful situations, in parallel with pituitary ACTH and in maternal plasma at delivery (Csontas and co-workers, 1979; Fletcher and associates, 1980; Genazzani and colleagues, 1981; Goland and associates, 1981).

Maternal plasma concentrations of β-lipotrophin, β-endorphin, and γ-lipotrophin are increased steadily throughout pregnancy (Browning and co-workers, 1983a, 1983b; Newnham and associates, 1983). The levels of the three compounds are lower in women delivering vaginally who have epidural anesthesia than in women receiving either a narcotic or no analgesics. The specific physiologic function for these opioid agents in maternal plasma during pregnancy and labor has not been established. However, such agents obviously could serve to blunt the pain of childbirth.

Browning and co-workers (1983b) have speculated that a flaccid baby with depressed respiratory drive may be the consequence of fetal acidosis increasing the opioid agent, β-endorphin, to very high levels that, in turn, depress respiratory drive and result in a depressed neonate.

Thyroid

During pregnancy there is slight enlargement of the thyroid caused by hyperplasia of the glandular tissue and increased vascularity. Normal pregnancy does not cause goiter, and any goiter in pregnancy should be considered as pathologic (Levy and co-workers, 1980). The basal metabolic rate increases progressively during normal pregnancy by as much as 25 percent. Most of this increase in oxygen consumption, however, is the result of the metabolic activity of the products of conception. If the body surface of the fetus is considered along with that of the mother, the predicted and the measured basal metabolic rates are quite similar.

Thyroxine. Beginning as early as the second month of pregnancy, the concentration of *thyroxine* rises sharply in the mother's plasma to a plateau, which is maintained until after delivery. The plateau is reached at levels of from 9 to 16 μg/dl of thyroxine as compared with 5 to 12 μg/dl in nonpregnant euthyroid women.

Such an elevation of circulating thyroid hormone should not be indicative of hyperthyroidism. During pregnancy, the *thyroxine-binding proteins* of plasma, principally an α-globulin, are considerably increased. Mulaisho and Utiger (1977) provide the following mean values for thyroid-binding globulin levels in plasma: 7.1 mg/dl in the first trimester, 9.0 mg/dl in the second, and 8.9 mg/dl in the third trimester, compared to a value of 3.6 mg/dl for normal nonpregnant women. Even though the total concentrations of thyroxine and triiodothyronine are elevated, the amounts of unbound, or effective, hormone are not appreciably higher (Osathanondh and colleagues, 1976). The increase in circulating estrogens

TABLE 9-5. COMPARISON OF EFFECTS OF PREGNANCY AND OF ESTROGEN ADMINISTRATION ON TESTS USED TO EVALUATE THYROID FUNCTION

Tests	Normal Pregnancy	Estrogen Administration	Hyper-thyroidism
Basal Metabolic Rate	Increased	Not Increased	Increased
Total Thyroxine	Increased	Increased	Increased
Thyroxine-Binding Globulin	Increased	Increased	Not increased
Free Thyroxine	Not increased	Not increased	Increased
Total Triiodothyronine	Increased	Increased	Increased
Free Triiodothyronine	Not increased	Not increased	Increased
Radioiodine Uptake (percent)	Increased	Not increased	Increased
Absolute Iodine Uptake	Not increased	Not increased	Increased
Triiodothyronine Resin Uptake	Decreased	Decreased	Increased
Serum Cholesterol Level	Increased	Variable	Decreased

during pregnancy is presumably the major cause of these changes in circulating hormones and binding capacity, for they can be reproduced by administering estrogen, including most oral contraceptives, to nonpregnant women. Although the normal early increase in thyroxine and thyroid-binding globulin and the decrease in triiodothyronine resin uptake are sometimes absent in women destined to abort, the abortion almost certainly does not result from failure of hormones and binding protein to increase, but rather is due to an abnormal conceptus.

During pregnancy, there is increased uptake of ingested radioiodide by the maternal thyroid gland, again suggesting a hyperthyroid state. Aboul-Khair and associates (1964), however, claimed that although the clearance of inorganic iodine is increased by the thyroid gland during pregnancy, the absolute uptake is not increased. They concluded that the thyroid enlargement of pregnancy simply compensates for the lower concentration of circulating iodide available for synthesis of thyroxine.

Hershman and Starnes (1969), as well as others, identified a thyrotropic substance obtained from human placenta, but the role of chorionic thyrotropin, if any, in stimulating the thyroid is unclear. In women with hydatidiform moles, increased thyroid activity is probably due primarily to the action of chorionic gonadotropin, which is known to have intrinsic thyroid-stimulating activity.

Resin Uptake of Triiodothyronine. In 1957, Hamolsky and associates reported that the in vitro uptake of radioactive triiodothyronine by erythrocytes was increased during incubation with serum from hyperthyroid subjects but decreased with serum from hypothyroid subjects or pregnant women. Furthermore, the administration of estrogen lowered the uptake of triiodothyronine. The decreased uptake by erythrocytes, or by resin, both in pregnancy and following administration of estrogen, is clearly the result of increased binding of the triiodothyronine to thyroid-binding proteins, especially α-globulin. The change in uptake is similar in time of appearance to that of thyroxine, but in the opposite direction. *Therefore, an elevated plasma thyroxine level*

and simultaneously a lowered uptake of triiodothyronine by resin are indicative of hyperestrogenemia, including that induced by pregnancy or by estrogen-containing oral contraceptives. In Table 9-5, the pregnancy-induced changes, those found in hyperthyroidism, and those induced by administration of estrogen, are compared.

Thyroxine, thyroxine-binding capacity, and triiodothyronine resin uptake values in cord serum are less than those in maternal serum but greater than levels in nonpregnant adults (Russell and colleagues, 1964).

Parathyroid

Both increased and decreased plasma levels of parathyroid hormone have been reported in pregnancy. Reitz and co-workers (1977) and Pitkin and Gebhardt (1977) reported that the level of hormone during the third trimester was about twice that of normal nonpregnant controls whereas Whitehead and associates (1981) reported normal nonpregnant levels or even slightly decreased values. In general, the level of ionized calcium in plasma is of major importance in the operation of a feedback mechanism regulating the secretion of parathyroid hormone, but it has been reported that the level of ionized calcium does not increase during normal pregnancy (Pitkin and Gebhardt, 1977) or only increases slightly (Fogh-Anderson and Schultz-Larsen, 1981). Reitz and co-workers suggest that during pregnancy a new "set point" exists between the levels of parathyroid hormone and ionized calcium.

Calcitonin, which originates in the parafollicular, or C cells, of the thyroid, may protect the skeleton during calcium stress by opposing the tendency of 1,25-dihydroxyvitamin D and parathyroid hormone to resorb bone. During pregnancy and lactation, calcitonin levels in plasma are appreciably higher than in nonpregnant women and are comparable to those seen in men and in women who are using estrogen–progestin contraceptives (Hillyard and colleagues, 1978; Stevenson and co-workers, 1979; Whitehead and associates, 1981).

Plasma 1,25-dihydroxyvitamin D (1,25-$(OH)_2$D) levels are increased in normal pregnancy (Kumar and co-workers,

1980; Whitehead and associates, 1981). The action of 1,-25(OH)$_2$D is to increase intestinal absorption of calcium during pregnancy. The stimulus responsible for this increase is unknown but human placental lactogen and estrogen have been suggested as possible agents (Kumar and co-workers, 1980).

Adrenal

In normal pregnancy, there is probably very little morphologic change in the maternal adrenal.

Cortisol. There is a considerable increase in the concentration of circulating cortisol, but much of it is bound by the cortisol-binding globulin, *transcortin*. The rate of secretion of cortisol by the maternal adrenal is not increased; it is probably decreased compared to the nonpregnant state. The metabolic clearance rate of cortisol, however, is lower during pregnancy, as indicated by the fact that in a pregnant woman, the half-life of intravenously injected radiolabeled cortisol is nearly twice as long as it is in nonpregnant women (Migeon and associates, 1957). Administration of estrogen, including those in most oral contraceptives, causes changes in levels of cortisol and transcortin similar to those of pregnancy.

In early pregnancy, the levels of circulating corticotropin (ACTH) are strikingly reduced. As pregnancy progresses, the levels of ACTH and free cortisol rise. This apparent paradox is not completely understood. Nolten and Rueckert (1981) have presented evidence that the higher free cortisol levels observed in pregnancy are the result of a "resetting" of the maternal feedback mechanisms to higher levels. They further propose that the "resetting" might result from *tissue refractoriness* to cortisol. Thus an elevated free cortisol would be needed during pregnancy to maintain homeostasis.

Aldosterone. As early as the 15th week of normal pregnancy, the maternal adrenal secretes considerably increased amounts of aldosterone. By the third trimester, about 1 mg per day is secreted. If sodium intake is restricted, aldosterone secretion is even further elevated (Watanabe and co-workers, 1963). At the same time, levels of renin and angiotensin substrate are normally increased, especially during the latter half of pregnancy (Geelhoed and Vander, 1968; Massani and associates, 1967). This gives rise to increased angiotensin II plasma levels that appear to account for the markedly elevated secretion of aldosterone. It has been suggested that the elevated secretion of aldosterone during normal pregnancy affords protection against the natriuretic effect of progesterone (Landau and Lugibihl, 1961). Progesterone administered to nonpregnant women is associated with a prompt and marked increase in aldosterone excretion (Laidlaw and colleagues, 1962).

Deoxycorticosterone. There is a striking increase in the maternal plasma levels of deoxycorticosterone (DOC) during the last trimester of pregnancy. Brown

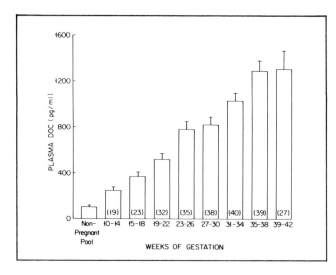

Figure 9-14. Plasma deoxycorticosterone (DOC) in primigravid women. (*From Parker and co-workers, 1980.*)

and co-workers (1972) and Nolten and associates (1978) found that in nonpregnant women and during the first two trimesters of pregnancy the levels of plasma DOC are less than 10 ng/dl. During the last few weeks of pregnancy, DOC levels rise to 150 ng/dl or more (Fig. 9-14). The origin of these increased amounts of DOC is not clear. Interestingly, Nolten and associates found that the administration of a potent glucocorticosteroid, dexamethasone, to pregnant women to reduce ACTH secretion is not accompanied by a reduction in plasma DOC levels. Moreover, ACTH administration to pregnant women is not accompanied by an increase in plasma DOC concentration.

These findings, together with the finding of significant quantities of DOC in the fetal circulation and of DOC sulfate in the amnionic fluid, led these investigators to suggest that the increased levels of DOC in maternal plasma arise in the fetus. This may be true. Alternatively, it has been suggested (Winkel and colleagues, 1980) that maternal plasma progesterone may serve as a precursor for DOC biosynthesis in the maternal compartment. These investigators demonstrated that [^{3}H]progesterone administered to pregnant and nonpregnant persons is converted to [^{3}H]DOC because [^{3}H]tetrahydro DOC is found in the urine of such subjects. The extent of conversion of plasma progesterone to DOC (based on the ^{3}H:^{14}C ratio of urinary tetrahydro DOC following the intravenous infusion of [^{3}H]progesterone and [^{14}C]DOC) is approximately 1 percent. It is not yet clear, however, whether the DOC derived from the conversion of plasma progesterone ever enters the circulation as DOC. It seems likely that this conversion occurs in the maternal liver. If this is true, it is possible that the DOC derived by conversion of progesterone in the hepatocyte is reduced to tetrahydro DOC before it leaves the liver cell. The fractional conversion of plasma progesterone to urinary tetrahydro DOC is similar in nonpregnant and pregnant humans. There may be a threshold level of plasma progesterone that is reached before DOC, derived from progesterone conversion, has access to maternal plasma. Such an occurrence could have profound physiologic and pathophysiologic consequences, in instances of large placental mass and high plasma progesterone levels, for example, multiple pregnancy, hydatidiform mole, and with hydrops fetalis or possibly in cases of pregnancy-induced hypertension (see Chapter 27, p. 526).

Other Steroids

As discussed in Chapter 7 (p. 125), the levels of *dehydroisoandrosterone sulfate* circulating in maternal blood and excreted in the urine are not increased during normal pregnancy, but rather decreased as a consequence of an increased rate of removal, through extensive 16α-hydroxylation in the maternal liver and estrogen formation in the placenta.

The maternal plasma levels of *androstenedione* and *testosterone* are increased during pregnancy. This finding is not totally explained by alterations in the metabolic clearance rates of these androgens. On the one hand, maternal plasma androstenedione and testosterone are converted to estradiol in the placenta, which increases the rate of clearance, but, on the other hand, there is an increased amount of testosterone–estradiol-binding globulin in plasma of pregnant women that retards the rate of testosterone clearance. Thus, there is an increased plasma production rate of maternal testosterone and androstenedione during human pregnancy. The source of this increased androgen production is unknown but it probably originates in the ovary. Interestingly, little or no testosterone in maternal plasma enters the fetal circulation as testosterone. Even when massive testosterone levels are found in the circulation of pregnant women with androgen-secreting tumors, the testosterone level in umbilical cord venous plasma is likely to be too low to be detected. This finding is the result of the almost complete conversion of testosterone to 17β-estradiol by the trophoblast (Edman and associates, 1979).

MUSCULOSKELETAL SYSTEM

Progressive *lordosis* is a characteristic feature of normal pregnancy. Compensating for the anterior position of the enlarging uterus, the lordosis shifts the center of gravity back over the lower extremities. There is increased mobility of the sacroiliac, sacrococcygeal, and the pubic joints during pregnancy, presumably as a result of hormonal changes. Their mobility may contribute to the alteration of maternal posture and, in turn, cause discomfort in the lower portion of the back, especially late in pregnancy. During the last trimester of pregnancy, aching, numbness, and weakness are occasionally experienced in the upper extremities, possibly as a result of the marked lordosis, with anterior flexion of the neck and slumping of the shoulder girdle, which, in turn, produces traction on the ulnar and median nerves (Crisp and DeFrancesco, 1964).

PRECOCIOUS AND LATE PREGNANCY

The youngest mother whose history is authenticated is Lina Medina, who was delivered by cesarean section in Lima, Peru, on May 15, 1939. It was claimed that she was 4 years and 8 months old, but a careful review of her birth records indicates that she may have been 5 years and 8 months of age. In either event, it is a record.

Ms. Medina related to a reporter (The National Enquirer, September 30, 1980) that she always knew that the child who had been reared as her brother had come from her own body, but she did not completely comprehend the significance of this until she was about 11. Her son, Gerardo (named for the doctor who performed the cesarean section), was 10 years old before he knew that Lina was his mother.

Ms. Medina went on to marry Raul Gonzalez and has had one child in this marriage. Gerardo married at age 18 and had two daughters. He died on September 8, 1979, of an apparent heart attack at the age of 40.

Although true precocious puberty, as suffered by Lina Medina, is still very uncommon, the average age of menarche and ovulation is appreciably lower than it was several decades ago (see Chapter 4, p. 76). The mean age of menarche in the United States is now estimated to be 12.3 years.

As a consequence of earlier menarche, and perhaps of greater sexual freedom, most obstetric services have witnessed a marked increase in the number of extremely young pregnant women.

Although it was predicted by some that long-term suppression of ovulation by oral contraceptives might result in continued ovulation for years after the usual time of menopause, there is no evidence to support the occurrence of such a phenomenon. Pregnancy after the age of 47 years is uncommon. In a careful review of the literature from 1860 to 1964 on this subject, Wharton (1964) cited 26 women over the age of 50 with normal pregnancy; the oldest was said to be 63. The paucity of reports of pregnancy in women of advanced age is probably an underestimate of the prevalence, but it nevertheless indicates the rarity of pregnancy in the sixth decade of life.

Horger and Smythe (1977) have reviewed the pregnancy experiences of 440 women whose ages ranged from 40 to 54 years. Pregnancy terminated in abortion in 22 percent, one half of which were electively induced. The perinatal mortality rate was 101 per 1000 (10.1 percent) and neonatal morbidity, including low birth weight, was increased. Hypertensive disorders were common. Abruptio placentae complicated 16 pregnancies (4.6 percent) and in 5 instances the infants were stillborn. One woman died in the postpartum period from carcinoma of the pancreas. Similar outcomes have been reported by Naeye (1983).

REFERENCES

Aboul-Khair SA, Crooks J, Turnbull AC, Hytten FE: The physiological changes in thyroid function during pregnancy. Clin Sci 27:195, 1964

Adams RH, Ashworth CT: unpublished observation

Alvarez H, Caldeyro-Barcia R: Contractility of the human uterus recorded by new methods. Surg Gynecol Obstet 91:1, 1950

Amino N, Tanizawa O, Miyai K, Tanaka F, Hayashi C, Kawashima M, Ichihara K: Changes in serum immunoglobulins IgG, IgA, IgM, and IgE during pregnancy. Obstet Gynecol 52:415, 1978

Assali NS, Dilts PV, Plentl AA, Kirschbaum TH, Gross SJ: Physiology of the placenta. In Assali NS (ed); Biology of Gestation: The Maternal Organism. New York, Academic, 1968, vol I

Assali NS, Douglass RA, Baird WW, Nicholson DB, Suyemoto R: Measurement of uterine blood flow and uterine metabolism: IV. Results in normal pregnancy. Am J Obstet Gynecol 66:248, 1953

Assali NS, Rauramo L, Peltonen T: Measurement of uterine blood flow and uterine metabolism: VIII. Uterine and fetal blood flow and oxygen consumption in early pregnancy. Am J Obstet Gynecol 79:86, 1960

Åstedt B: Significance of placenta in depression of fibrinolytic activity during pregnancy. J Obstet Gynaecol Br Commonw 79:205, 1972

Bailey RR, Rolleston GL: Kidney length and ureteric dilatation in the puerperium. J Obstet Gynaecol Br Commonw 78:55, 1971

Baldwin GR, Moorthi DS, MacDonnell KF: New lung functions and pregnancy. Am J Obstet Gynecol 127:235, 1977

Barron WM, Lindheimer MD: Renal function during pregnancy. Contemporary Ob/Gyn, 21:179, 1983

Bean WB, Cogswell R, Dexter M, Embick JF: Vascular changes of the skin in pregnancy-vascular spiders and palmar erythema. Surg Gynecol Obstet 88:739, 1949

Beck P: Effects of gonadal hormones and contraceptive steroids on glucose and insulin metabolism. In Salhanick HA, Kipnis DM, Vande Wiele RL (eds): Metabolic Effects of Gonadal Hormones and Contraceptive Steroids. New York, Plenum, 1969

Beck P, Wells C: Comparison of mechanisms underlying carbohydrate intolerance in subclinical diabetic women during pregnancy and during postpartum oral contraceptive steroid treatment. J Clin Endocrinol 29:807, 1969

Bellina JH, Dougherty CM, Mickal A: Pyeloureteral dilation and pregnancy. Am J Obstet Gynecol 108:356, 1970

Bieniarz J, Branda LA, Maqueda E, Morozovsky J, Caldeyro-Barcia R: Aortocaval compression by the uterus in late pregnancy: III. Unreliability of the sphygmomanometric method in estimating uterine artery pressure. Am J Obstet Gynecol 102:1106, 1968

Blechner JN, Stenger VG, Prystowsky H: Blood flow to the human uterus during maternal metabolic acidosis. Am J Obstet Gynecol 121:789, 1975

Bleicher SJ, O'Sullivan JB, Freinkel N: Carbohydrate metabolism in pregnancy: V. The interrelations of glucose, insulin, and free fatty acids in late pregnancy and postpartum. N Engl J Med 271:866, 1964

Bolton FG, Street MJ, Pace AJ: Changes in erythrocyte volume and shape in pregnancy. Br J Obstet Gynecol 89:1018, 1982

Bonnar J: Hemostatic function and coagulopathy during pregnancy. In Wynn R (ed): Obstetrics and Gynecology Annual: 1978. New York, Appleton, p. 195

Brown RD, Strott CA, Liddle GW: Plasma desoxycorticosterone in normal and abnormal human pregnancy. J Clin Endocrinol Metab 35:736, 1972

Browne JCM, Veall N: The maternal placental blood flow in normotensive and hypertensive women. J Obstet Gynaecol Br Emp 60:142, 1953

Browning AJF, Butt WR, Lynch SS, Shakespear RA, Crawford JS: Maternal and cord plasma concentrations of β-lipotrophin, β-endorphin, and γ-lipotrophin at delivery; effect of analgesia, Br J Obstet Gynaecol 90:1152, 1983a

Browning, AJF, Butt WR, Lynch SS, Shakespear RA: Maternal plasma concentrations of β-endorphin and γ-lipotrophin throughout pregnancy. Br J Obstet Gynaecol 90:1147, 1983b

Bryant-Greenwood GD: Relaxin as a new hormone. Endo Rev 3:62, 1982

Burt CC: Forearm and hand blood flow in pregnancy. In: Toxaemias of Pregnancy. Ciba Foundation Symposium. Philadelphia, Blakiston, 1950, p 151

Burt RL, Davidson IWF: Insulin half-life and utilization in normal pregnancy. Obstet Gynecol 43:161, 1974

Campbell S, Griffin DF, Pearce JM, Diaz-Recasens J, Cohen-Overbeek TE, Willson K, Teague MJ: New doppler technique for assessing uteroplacental blood flow. Lancet 1:675, 1983

Carsten ME, Regulation of myometrial composition, growth, and activity. In Assali NS (ed): Biology of Gestation: The Maternal Organism. New York, Academic, 1968, vol I

Caton WL, Roby CC, Reid DE, Gibson JG: Plasma volume and extravascular fluid volume during pregnancy and the puerperium. Am J Obstet Gynecol 57:471, 1949

Chesley LC: Weight changes and water balance in normal and toxic pregnancy. Am J Obstet Gynecol 48:565, 1944

Chesley LC: Renal function during pregnancy. In Carey HM (ed): Modern Trends in Human Reproductive Physiology. London, Butterworths, 1963

Chesley LC, Sloan DM: The effect of posture on renal function in late pregnancy. Am J Obstet Gynecol 89:754, 1964

Chesley LC, Talledo OE, Bohler CS, Zuspan FP: Vascular reactivity to angiotensin II and norepinephrine in pregnant and nonpregnant women. Am J Obstet Gynecol 91:837, 1965

Chrétien FC: Ultrastructure and variations of human cervical mucus during pregnancy and the menopause. Acta Obstet Gynecol Scand 57:337, 1978

Christofides ND, Ghatei MA, Bloom SR, Borberg C, Gillmer MDG: Decreased plasma motilin concentrations in pregnancy. Br Med J 285:1453, 1982

Cohen DA, Daughaday WH, Weldon VV: Fetal and maternal virilization associated with pregnancy. Am J Dis Child 136:353, 1982

Combes B, Adams RH: Pathophysiology of the liver in pregnancy. In Assali NS (ed): Pathophysiology of Gestation. New York, Academic, 1971, vol I

Combes B, Shibata H, Adams R, Mitchell BD, Trammell V: Alterations in sulfobromophthalein sodium-removal mechanisms from blood during normal pregnancy. J Clin Invest 42:1431, 1963

Coopland A, Alkjaersig N, Fletcher AP: Reduction in plasma factor XIII (fibrin stabilization factor) concentration during pregnancy. J Lab Clin Med 73:144, 1969

Cotes PM, Canning CE, Lind T: Changes in serum immunoreactive erythropoietin during the menstrual cycle and normal pregnancy. Br J Obstet Gynecol 90:304, 1983

Crisp WE, DeFrancesco A: The hand syndrome of pregnancy. Obstet Gynecol 23:433, 1964

Csapo AI, Pulkkinen MO, Wiest WG: Effects of hysterectomy and progesterone replacement in early pregnant patients. Am J Obstet Gynecol 115:759, 1973

Csontos K, Rust M, Hollt V, Mahr W, Kromer W, Teschemacher HJ: Elevated plasma β-endorphin levels in pregnant women and their neonates. Life Sci 25:835, 1979

Cutforth R, MacDonald CB: Heart sounds and murmurs in pregnancy. Am Heart J 71:741, 1966

Dahlström H, Ihrman K: A clinical and physiological study of pregnancy in a material from Northern Sweden. IV. Observations on the blood volume during and after pregnancy. Acta Soc Med Upsal 65:295, 1960

Darmady JM, Postle AD: Lipid metabolism in pregnancy. Br J Obstet Gynaecol 89:211, 1982

Davison JM, Hytten FE: Glomerular filtration during and after pregnancy. J Obstet Gynaecol Br Commonw 81:588, 1974

Davison JM, Hytten FE: The effect of pregnancy on the renal handling of glucose. Br J Obstet Gynaecol 82:374, 1975

Davison JM, Vallotton MB, Lindheimer MD: Plasma osmolality and urinary concentration and dilution during and after pregnancy. Evidence that lateral recumbency inhibits maximal urinary concentrating ability. Br J Obstet Gynaecol 88:472, 1981

Dennis KJ, Bytheway WR: Changes in the body weight after delivery. J Obstet Gynaecol Br Commonw 72:94, 1965

Diczfalusy E, Troen P: Endocrine functions of the human placenta. Vitam Horm 19:229, 1961

Dunlop W: Investigations into influence of posture on renal plasma flow and glomerular filtration rate during late pregnancy. Br J Obstet Gynaecol 83:17, 1976

Dunlop W: Serial changes in renal haemodynamics during normal human pregnancy. Br J Obstet Gynaecol 88:1, 1981

Edman CD, Devereux WP, Parker CR, MacDonald PC: Placental clearance of maternal androgens: A protective mechanism against fetal virilization. Proc Soc Gynecol Invest 67, 1979 (abstr)

Efrati P, Presentey B, Margalith M, Rozenszajn L: Leukocytes of normal pregnant women. Obstet Gynecol 23:429, 1964

Evans MI, Dougan MB, Moawad AH, Evans WJ, Bryant-Greenwood GD, Greenwood FC: Ripening of the human cervix with porcine ovarian relaxin. Am J Obstet Gynecol 147:410, 1983

Ezimokhai M, Davison JM, Philips PR, Dunlop W: Non-postural serial changes in renal function during the third trimester of normal human pregnancy. Br J Obstet Gynaecol 88:465, 1981

Fainstat T: Ureteral dilation in pregnancy: A review. Obstet Gynecol Survey 18:845, 1963

Fay RA, Hughes AO, Farron NT: Platelets in pregnancy: Hyperdestruction in pregnancy. Obstet Gynecol 61:238, 1983

Fletcher AP, Alkjaersig N: Thromboembolism and contraceptive medications: Incidence and mechanism. In Salhanick HA, Kipnis DM, Vande Wiele RL (eds): Metabolic Effects of Gonadal Hormones and Contraceptive Steroids. New York, Plenum, 1969

Fletcher AP, Akljaersig NK, Burstein R: The influence of pregnancy upon blood coagulation and plasma fibrinolytic enzyme function. Am J Obstet Gynecol 134:743, 1979

Fletcher JE, Thomas TA, Hill RG: β-Endorphin and parturition. Lancet 1:310, 1980

Fogh-Andersen N, Schultz-Larsen P: Free calcium ion concentration in pregnancy. Acta Obstet Gynecol Scand 60:309, 1981

Friesen H, Hwang P, Guyda H, Tolis G, Tyson J, Myers R: A radioimmunoassay for human prolactin. In Prolactin and Carcinogenesis. Proceedings of the Fourth Tenovus Workshop, Cardiff, March 1972. Cardiff, Wales, Alpha Omega Alpha, August 1972

Fulop M, Brazeau P: Increased ureteral back pressure enhances renal tubular sodium reabsorption. J Clin Invest 49:2315, 1970

Gant NF, Chand S, Worley RJ, Whalley PJ, Crosby UD, MacDonald PC: A clinical test for predicting the development of acute hypertension in pregnancy. Am J Obstet Gynecol 120:1, 1974

Gant NF, Daley GL, Chand S, Whalley PJ, MacDonald PC: A study of angiotensin II pressor response throughout primigravid pregnancy. J Clin Invest 52:2682, 1973

Gant NF, Madden JD, Siiteri PK, MacDonald PC: A sequential study of the metabolism of dehydroisoandrosterone sulfate in primigravid pregnancy. Excerpta Medica Int Congr Series 273:1026, 1972

Gant NF, Madden JD, Chand S, Worley RJ, Strong JS, MacDonald PC: Metabolic clearance rate of dehydroisoandrosterone sulfate. V. Studies of essential hypertension complicating pregnancy. Obstet Gynecol 47:319, 1976

Garcia-Bunuel R, Berek JS, Woodruff JD: Luteomas of pregnancy. Obstet Gynecol 45:407, 1975

Gee JBL, Packer BS, Millen JE, Robin ED: Pulmonary mechanics during pregnancy. J Clin Invest 46:945, 1967

Geelhoed GW, Vander AJ: Plasma renin activities during pregnancy and parturition. J Clin Endocrinol 28:412, 1968

Genazzani AR, Facchinetti F, Parrini D: β-Lipotrophin and β-endorphin plasma levels during pregnancy. Clin Endocrinol 141:409, 1981

Goland RS, Wardlaw SL, Stark RI, Frantz AG: Human plasma β-endorphin during pregnancy, labor and delivery. J Clin Endocrinol Metab 52:74, 1981

Greiss Jr FC, Wagner WD: Glycosaminoglycans: Their distribution and potential vasoactive action in the nonpregnant and pregnant ovine uterus. Am J Obstet Gynecol 145:1041, 1983

Hahn PF, Carothers EL, Darby WJ, Martin M, Sheppard CW, Cannon RO, Beam AS, Densen PM, Peterson JC, McClellan GS: Iron metabolism in human pregnancy as studied with the radioactive isotope ^{59}Fe. Am J Obstet Gynecol 61:477, 1951

Hamolsky MW, Stein M, Freedberg AS: The thyroid hormone-plasma protein complex in man: II. A new in vitro method for study of "uptake" of labelled hormonal components by human erythrocytes. J Clin Endocrinol 17:33, 1957

Hankins, GDV, Wendel GD, Whalley PJ, Quirk Jr JG: Cardiovascular monitoring in high-risk pregnancy. Perinatol Neonatol 7:29, 1983

Harbert GM, Cornell GW, Littlefield JB, Kayan JB, Thornton WN: Maternal hemodynamics associated with uterine contraction in gravid monkeys. Am J Obstet Gynecol 104:24, 1969

Hellman LM, Rosenthal AH, Kistner RW, Gordon R: Some factors influencing the proliferation of the reserve cells in the human cervix. Am J Obstet Gynecol 67:899, 1954

Hensleigh PA, Woodruff JD: Differential maternal-fetal response to androgenizing luteoma or hyperreactio luteinalis. Obstet Gynecol 33:262, 1978

Hershman JM, Starnes WR: Extraction and characterization of a thyrotropic material from the human placenta. J Clin Invest 48:923, 1969

Hillyard CJ, Stevenson JC, MacIntyre I: Relative deficiency of plasma-calcitonin in normal women. Lancet 2:961, 1978

Hodgkinson CP: Physiology of the ovarian veins in pregnancy. Obstet Gynecol 1:26, 1953

Horger EO III, Smythe AR II: Pregnancy in women over forty. Obstet Gynecol 49:257, 1977

Hornnes PJ, Kuhl C: Plasma insulin and glucagon responses to isoglycemic stimulation in normal pregnancy and post partum. Obstet Gynecol 55:425, 1980

Howard BK, Goodson JH, Mengert WR: Supine hypotensive syndrome in late pregnancy. Obstet Gynecol 1:371, 1953

Hudson P, Haley J, John M, Cronk M, Crawford R, Haralambidis J, Gregear G, Shine J, Niall H: Structure of a genomic clone encoding biologically active human relaxin. Nature 301:628, 1983

Hutchinson DL, Westoner JL, Well DW: The destruction of the maternal and fetal pituitary glands in subhuman primates. Am J Obstet Gynecol 83:857, 1962

Hytten FE, Chamberlain G: Clinical Physiology in Obstetrics. Oxford, Blackwell, 1981

Hytten FE, Leitch I: The Physiology of Human Pregnancy, 2nd ed. Philadelphia, Davis, 1971

Hytten FE, Thomson AM: Maternal physiological adjustments. In Assali NS (ed): Biology of Gestation: The Maternal Organism. New York, Academic, 1968, vol I

Ihrman K: A clinical and physiological study of pregnancy in material from northern Sweden. VII. The heart volume during and after pregnancy. Acta Soc Med Uppsala 65:326, 1960

Ingerslev M, Teilum G: Biopsy studies on the liver in pregnancy: II. Liver biopsy on normal pregnant women. Acta Obstet Gynecol Scand 25:352, 1946

Jepson JH, Friesen HG: The mechanism of action of human placental lactogen on erythropoiesis. Br J Haematol 15:465, 1968

Kasper CK, Hoag MS, Aggelar PM, Stone S: Blood clotting factors in pregnancy: Factor VIII concentrations in normal and AHF-deficient women. Obstet Gynecol 24:242, 1964

Katz R, Karliner JS, Resnik R: Effects of a natural volume overload state (pregnancy) on left ventricular performance in normal human subjects. Circulation 58:434, 1978

Kauppila A, Koskinen M, Puolakka J, Tuimala R, Kuikka J: Decreased intervillous and unchanged myometrial blood flow in supine recumbency. Obstet Gynecol 55:203, 1980

Kerr MG: The mechanical effects of the gravid uterus in late pregnancy. J Obstet Gynaecol Br Commonw 72:513, 1965

Killam AP, Rosenfeld CR, Battaglia FC, Makowshi EL, Meschia G: Effect of estrogens on the uterine blood flow of oophorectomized ewes. Am J Obstet Gynecol 115:1045, 1973

Kim YJ, Felig P: Maternal and amniotic fluid substrate levels during caloric deprivation in human pregnancy. Metabolism 21:507, 1972

Klafen, Palugyay: Arch Gynaekol 131:347, 1927

Krause DE, Stembridge VA: Luteomas of pregnancy. Am J Obstet Gynecol 95:192, 1966

Kumar R, Cohen WR, Epstein FH: Vitamin D and calcium hormones in pregnancy. N Engl J Med 302:1143, 1980

Laidlaw JC, Ruse JL, Gornall AG: The influence of estrogen and progesterone on aldosterone excretion. J Clin Endocrinol 22:161, 1962

Landau RL, Lugibihl K: The catabolic and natriuretic effects of progesterone in man. Recent Prog Horm Res 17:249, 1961

Lees MM, Scott DB, Slawson KB, Kerr MG: Haemodynamic changes during caesarean section. J Obstet Gynaecol Br Commonw 75:546, 1968

Levy RP, Newman DM, Rejali LS, Barford DAG: The myth of goiter in pregnancy. Am J Obstet Gynecol 137:701, 1980

MacLennan, AH, Green RC, Bryant-Greenwood GD, Green-

wood FC, Seamark RF: Cervical ripening with combinations of vaginal prostaglandin $F2_{\alpha}$, estradiol, and relaxin. Obstet Gynecol 58:601, 1981

McLennan CE: Antecubital and femoral venous pressure in normal and toxemic pregnancy. Am J Obstet Gynecol 45:568, 1943

McLennan CE, Lowenstein JM, Sayler CB, Richards EM: Blood volume changes immediately after delivery. Stanford Med Bull 17:152, 1959

Makowski EL, Meschia G, Droegemueller W, Battaglia FC: Distribution of uterine blood flow in the pregnant sheep. Am J Obstet Gynecol 101:409, 1968

Manasc B, Jepson J: Erythropoietin in plasma and urine during human pregnancy. Can Med Assoc J 100:687, 1969

Massani ZM, Sanguinetti R, Gallegos R, Raimondi D: Angiotensin blood levels in normal and toxemic pregnancies. Am J Obstet Gynecol 99:313, 1967

Matsuura S, Naden RP, Gant NF Jr, Parker CR, Rosenfeld CR: Effect of hypertonic saline on vascular responses to angiotensin II in pregnancy. Am J Obstet Gynecol 147:231, 1983

Mendenhall HW: Serum protein concentrations in pregnancy: I. Concentrations in maternal serum. Am J Obstet Gynecol 106:388, 1970

Metcalfe J, McAnulty JH, Ueland K: Cardiovascular physiology. Clin Obstet Gynecol 24:693, 1981

Metcalfe J, Romney SL, Ramsey LH, Reid DE, Burwell CS: Estimation of uterine blood flow in normal human pregnancy at term. J Clin Invest 34:1632, 1955

Migeon CJ, Bertrand J, Wall PE: Physiological disposition of $4\text{-}^{14}C$ cortisol during late pregnancy. J Clin Invest 36:1350, 1957

Milne JS, Howie AD, Pack AI: Dyspnoea during normal pregnancy. Br J Obstet Gynaecol 85:260, 1978

Milsom I, Forssman L: Factors influencing aortocaval compression in late pregnancy. Am J Obstet Gynecol 148:764, 1984

Möbius Wvon: Atmung und Schwangerschaft. Munch Med Wochenschr 103:1389, 1961

Mueller MN, Kappas A: Estrogen pharmacology: I. The influence of estradiol and estriol on hepatic disposal of sulfobromophthalein (BSP) in man. J Clin Invest 43:1905, 1964

Mulaisho C, Utiger RD: Serum thyroxine-binding globulin: Determination by competitive ligand-binding assay in thyroid disease and pregnancy. Acta Endocrinol 85:314, 1977

Naden RP, Rosenfeld CR: Effect of angiotensin II on uterine and systemic vasculature in pregnant sheep. J Clin Invest 68:468, 1981

Naeye RL: Maternal age, obstetric complications and the outcome of pregnancy. Obstet Gynecol 61:210, 1983

Newnham JP, Tomlin S, Ratter SJ, Bourne GL, Rees LH: Endogenous opiod peptides in pregnancy. Br J Obstet Gynaecol 90:535, 1983

Newton M: Postpartum hemorrhage. Am J Obstet Gynecol 94:711, 1966

Nolten WE, Lindheimer MD, Oparil S, Ehrlich EN: Desoxycorticosterone in pregnancy. I. Sequential studies of the secretory patterns of desoxycorticosterone, aldosterone and cortisol. Am J Obstet Gynecol 132:414, 1978

Nolten WE, Rueckert PA: Elevated free cortisol index in pregnancy: Possible regulatory mechanisms. Am J Obstet Gynecol 139, 1981

Osathanondh R, Tulchinsky D, Chopra IJ: Total and free thyroxine and triiodothyronine in normal and complicated pregnancy. J Clin Endocrinol Metab 42:98, 1976

Ozanne P, Linderkamp O, Miller FC, Meiselman HJ: Erythrocyte aggregation during normal pregnancy. Am J Obstet Gynecol 147:576, 1983

Parker CR, Everett RB, Whalley PJ, Quirk JG, Gant NF, MacDonald PC: Hormone production during pregnancy in the primigravid patient. II. Plasma levels of deoxycorticosterone throughout pregnancy of normal women and women who developed pregnancy-induced hypertension. Am J Obstet Gynecol 138:626, 1980

Peake SL, Roxburgh HB, Langlois SLP: Ultrasonic assessment of hydronephrosis of pregnancy. Radiology 146:167, 1983

Pipe NGJ, Smith T, Halliday D, Edmonds CJ, Williams C, Coltart TM: Changes in fat, fat free mass and body water in human normal pregnancy. Br J Obstet Gynaecol 86:929, 1979

Pitkin RM, Gebhardt MP: Serum calcium concentrations in human pregnancy. Am J Obstet Gynecol 127:775, 1977

Pitkin RM, Witte DL: Platelet and leukocyte counts in pregnancy. JAMA 242:2696, 1980

Porter DG: Relaxin and cervical softening. In Anderson AM, Ellwood DA (eds): The Cervix in Pregnancy and Labour. Edinburgh, Churchill Livingston, 1980

Porter DG: Myometrium of the pregnant guinea pig: The probable importance of relaxin. Biol Reprod 7:458, 1972

Potter JM, Nestel PJ: The hyperlipidemia of pregnancy in normal and complicated pregnancies. Am J Obstet Gynecol 133:165, 1979

Potter MG: Observations of the gallbladder and bile during pregnancy at term. JAMA 106:1070, 1936

Pritchard JA: Plasma cholinesterase activity in normal pregnancy and in eclamptogenic toxemias. Am J Obstet Gynecol 70: 1083, 1955

Pritchard JA: Changes in the blood volume during pregnancy and delivery. Anesthesiology 26:393, 1965

Pritchard JA: Personal observations

Pritchard JA, Adams RH: Erythrocyte production and destruction during pregnancy. Am J Obstet Gynecol 79:750, 1960

Pritchard JA, Hunt CF: A comparison of the hematologic responses following the routine prenatal administration of intramuscular and oral iron. Surg Gynecol Obstet 106:516, 1958

Pritchard JA, Mason RA: Iron stores of normal adults and their replenishment with oral iron therapy. JAMA 190:897, 1964

Pritchard JA, Scott DE: Iron demands during pregnancy. In Hallberg, Hariverth, Vannotti (eds): Iron Deficiency-Pathogenesis: Clinical Aspects and Therapy. London, Academic, 1970, p 173

Pritchard JA, Barnes AC, Bright RH: The effect of the supine position on renal function in the near-term pregnant woman. J Clin Invest 34:777, 1955

Ratnoff OD, Colopy JE, Pritchard JA: The blood-clotting mechanism during normal parturition. J Lab Clin Med 44:408, 1954

Reitz RE, Thomas AD, Woods JR, Weinstein RL: Calcium, magnesium, phosphorus, and parathyroid hormone interrelationships in pregnancy and newborn infants. Obstet Gynecol 50:701, 1977

Rekonen A, Luotola H, Pitkänen M, Kuikka J, Pyörälä M: Measurement of intervillous and myometrial blood flow by an intravenous ^{133}Xe method. Br J Obstet Gynaecol 83:723, 1976

Riggs LA, Lein A, Yen SSC: Pattern of increase in circulating prolactin levels during human gestation. Am J Obstet Gynecol 129:454, 1977

Rosenfeld CR: Consideration of the uteroplacental circulation in intrauterine growth. Semin Perinatol 8:42, 1984

Rosenfeld CR, Barton MD, Meschia G: Effects of epinephrine on distribution of blood flow in the pregnant ewe. Am J Obstet Gynecol 124:156, 1976

Rosenfeld CR, Gant NF Jr: The chronically instrumented ewe. A model for studying vascular reactivity to angiotensin II in pregnancy. J Clin Invest 67:486, 1981

Rosenfeld CR, Killam AP, Battaglia FC, Makowski EL, Meschia G: Effect of estradiol-17,β on the magnitude and distribution of uterine blood flow in nonpregnant, oophorectomized ewes. Pediatr Res 7:139, 1973

Rosenfeld CR, Morriss FH Jr, Makowski EL, Meschia G, Battaglia FC: Circulatory changes in the reproductive tissues of ewes during pregnancy. Gynecol Invest 5:252, 1974

Rosenfeld CR, West J: Circulatory response to systemic infusion of norepinephrine in the pregnant ewe. Am J Obstet Gynecol 127:376, 1977

Rubi RA, Sala NL: Ureteral function in pregnant women: III. Effect of different positions and of fetal delivery upon ureteral tonus. Am J Obstet Gynecol 101:230, 1968

Russ EM, Raymunt J: Influence of estrogens on total serum copper and caeruloplasmin. Proc Soc Exp Biol Med 92:465, 1956

Russell DH, Durie BGM: Polyamines and Biochemical Markers of Normal and Malignant Growth. In: Progress in Cancer Research and Therapy. New York, Raven, 1978, vol 8

Russell DH, Giles HR, Christian CD, Campbell JL: Polyamines in amniotic fluid, plasma, and urine during normal pregnancy. Am J Obstet Gynecol 132:649, 1978

Russell KP, Rose H, Starr P: Further observations on thyroxine interactions in the newborn at delivery and in the immediate neonatal period. Am J Obstet Gynecol 90:682, 1964

Salvatore CA: Cervical mucus crystallization in pregnancy. Obstet Gynecol 32:226, 1968

Schulman A, Herlinger H: Urinary tract dilatation in pregnancy. Br J Radiol 48:638, 1975

Scott DE, Pritchard JA: Iron deficiency in healthy young college women. JAMA 199:897, 1967

Sims EAH: The kidney in pregnancy. In Strauss MG, Welt LG (eds): Diseases of the Kidney. Boston, Little, Brown, 1963

Sjöstedt S: Acid–base balance of arterial blood during pregnancy, at delivery, and in the puerperium. Am J Obstet Gynecol 84:775, 1962

Song CS, Kappas A: The influence of estrogens, progestins and pregnancy on the liver. Vitam Horm 26:147, 1968

Spellacy WN, Buhi WC: Pituitary growth hormone and placental lactogen levels measured in normal term pregnancy and at the early and late postpartum periods. Am J Obstet Gynecol 105:888, 1969

Spellacy WN, Goetz FC: Plasma insulin in normal late pregnancy. N Engl J Med 268:988, 1963

Spellacy WN, Goetz FC, Greenberg BZ, Schoeller KL: Tolbutamide response in normal pregnancy. J Clin Endocrinol 25:1251, 1965

Spetz S: Peripheral circulation during normal pregnancy. Acta Obstet Gynecol Scand 43:309, 1964

Steinetz BG, O'Byrne EM, Kroc RL: The role of relaxin in cervical softening during pregnancy in mammals. In Naftolin F, Stubblefield PG (eds): Dilatation of the Uterine Cervix, Connective Tissue Biology and Clinical Management. New York, Raven, 1980

Sternberg WH: Non-functioning ovarian neoplasms. In Grady HG, Smith DE (eds): International Academy of Pathology Monograph. No 3, The Ovary. Baltimore, Williams & Wilkins, 1963

Stevenson JC, Hillyard CJ, MacIntyre I, Cooper H, Whitehead MI: A physiological role for calcitonin: Protection of the maternal skeleton. Lancet 2:769, 1979

Sturgeon P: Studies of iron requirements in infants: III. Influence of supplemental iron during normal pregnancy on mother and infant. A. The mother. Br J Haematol 5:31, 1959

Sutton FD, Zwillich CW, Creagh E, Pierson DJ, Weil JV: Progesterone for outpatient treatment of Pickwickian Syndrome. Ann Intern Med 83:476, 1975

Talbert LM, Langdell RD: Normal values of certain factors in the blood clotting mechanism in pregnancy. Am J Obstet Gynecol 90:44, 1964

Taylor DJ, Phillips P, Lind T: Puerperal haematological indices. Br J Obstet Gynaecol 88:601, 1981

Taylor GO, Modie JA, Agbedana EO: Serum free fatty acids, insulin and blood glucose in pregnancy. Br J Obstet Gynaecol 85:592, 1978

Teasdale F: Numerical density of nuclei in the sheep placenta. Anat Rec 185:186, 1976

Tsai CH, deLeeuw NKM: Changes in 2,3-diphosphoglycerate during pregnancy and puerperium in normal women and in β-thalassemia heterozygous women. Am J Obstet Gynecol 142:520, 1982

Tulchinsky D, Hobel CJ: Plasma human chorionic gonadotropin, estrone, estradiol, estriol, progesterone, and 17α-hydroxyprogesterone in human pregnancy. III. Early normal pregnancy. Am J Obstet Gynecol 117:884, 1973

Tyson JE, Austin K, Farinholt J, Fiedler J: Endocrine-metabolic response to acute starvation in human gestation. Am J Obstet Gynecol 125:1073, 1976

Ueland K: Maternal cardiovascular dynamics. VII. Intrapartum blood volume changes. Am J Obstet Gynecol 126:671, 1976

Ueland K, Hansen JM: Maternal cardiovascular dynamics: II. Posture and uterine contractions. Am J Obstet Gynecol 103:1, 1969

Ueland K, Metcalfe J: Circulatory changes in pregnancy. Clin Obstet Gynecol 18:41, 1975

Ulmsten U, Sundström G: Esophageal manometry in pregnant and nonpregnant women. Am J Obstet Gynecol 132:260, 1978

van Geelen JM, Lemmens WAJG, Eskes TKAB, Martin Jr CB: The urethral pressure profile in pregnancy and after delivery in healthy nulliparous women. Am J Obstet Gynecol 144:636, 1982

Van Wagenen G, Jenkins RH: An experimental examination of factors causing ureteral dilatation of pregnancy. J Urol 42:1010, 1939

Verkauf BS, Reiter EO, Hernandez L, Burns SA: Virilization of mother and fetus associated with luteoma of pregnancy: A case report with endocrinologic studies. Am J Obstet Gynecol 129:274, 1977

Vir SC, Love AHG, Thompson W: Serum and hair concentrations of copper during pregnancy. Am J Clin Nutr 34:2382, 1981

Watanabe M, Meeker CI, Gray MJ, Sims EAH, Solomon S: Secretion rate of aldosterone in normal pregnancy. J Clin Invest 42:1619, 1963

Whalley PJ, Roberts AD, Pritchard JA: The effects of posture on renal function during pregnancy in a patient with diabetes insipidus. J Lab Clin Med 58:867, 1961

Wharton LR: Normal pregnancy with living children in women past the age of fifty. Am J Obstet Gynecol 90:672, 1964

Whitehead M, Lane G, Young O, Campbell S, Abeyasekera G, Hillyard CJ, MacIntyre I, Phang KG, Stevenson JC: Interrelations of calcium-regulating hormones during normal pregnancy. Br Med J 283:10, 1981

Widdowson EM: Growth and composition of the fetus and newborn. In Assali NS (ed): Biology of Gestation: The Fetus and Neonate, Vol II. New York, Academic, 1968

Widdowson EM, Spray CM: Chemical development in utero. Arch Dis Child 26:205, 1951

Wilcox CF, Hunt AB, Owen CA: The measurement of blood lost during cesarean section. Am J Obstet Gynecol 77:772, 1959

Winkel CA, Parker CR Jr, Milewich L, Simpson ER, Gant NF, MacDonald PC: The conversion of plasma progesterone to deoxycorticosterone (DOC) in men, nonpregnant and pregnant women, and adrenalectomized subjects: Evidence for steroid 21-hydroxylase activity in non-adrenal tissues. J Clin Invest 66:803, 1980

Winters AJ, Colston C, MacDonald PC, Porter JC: Fetal plasma prolactin levels. J Clin Endocrinol Metab 41:626, 1975

Woodfield DG, Cole SK, Allan AGE, Cash JD: Serum fibrin degradation products throughout normal pregnancy. Br Med J 4:665, 1968

Wright HP, Osborn SB, Edmonds DG: Changes in rate of flow of venous blood in the leg during pregnancy, measured with radioactive sodium. Surg Gynecol Obstet 90:481, 1950

Yoshima T, Strott CA, Marshall JR, Lipsett MD: Corpus luteum function early in pregnancy. J Clin Endocrinol Metab 29:225, 1969

Živný J, Kobilková J, Neuwirt J, Andrasová V: Regulation of erythropoiesis in fetus and mother during normal pregnancy. Obstet Gynecol 60:77, 1982

10
Diagnosis of Pregnancy

Every physician who assumes the responsibility for the medical care of any woman under the age of 50, irrespective of the nature of the physician's practice or special interest, must always consider the question, "Is she pregnant?" Failure to do so often leads to incorrect diagnoses, inappropriate therapy, and, at times, to medicolegal embroilment. Ordinarily, the diagnosis of pregnancy should offer little difficulty. Most often, the woman is aware of the likelihood of pregnancy when she consults a physician, although she may not volunteer this information unless asked specifically. At times, however, the diagnosis of pregnancy is not easy to make, but rarely is it impossible if appropriate clinical and laboratory tests are conducted.

Mistakes in diagnosis are made most frequently in the first several weeks of pregnancy while the uterus is still a pelvic organ. Although it is possible to mistake the uterus of pregnancy, even at term, for a tumor of some nature, such errors usually are the result of hasty or careless examination.

The diagnosis of pregnancy is based upon certain symptoms and signs that are found by careful physical examination and upon results of laboratory tests. The signs and symptoms of pregnancy are classified into three groups: positive signs, probable signs, and presumptive evidence.

POSITIVE SIGNS OF PREGNANCY

The three positive signs of pregnancy are (1) identification of the fetal heart action separately and distinctly from that of the woman, (2) perception of active fetal movements by the examiner, and (3) recognition of the embryo and fetus most any time in pregnancy by sonographic techniques or the more mature fetus roentgenographically in the latter half of pregnancy.

Identification of Fetal Heart Action

Hearing or observing the pulsations of the fetal heart assures the diagnosis of pregnancy. Contractions of the fetal heart can be identified by auscultation with a special fetoscope (Fig. 17-2A,B), by use of the doppler principle with ultrasound, and by use of sonography (Chapter 14, p. 279). The heart beat of the fetus can be detected by auscultation with a stethoscope by 17 weeks gestation, on average, and by 19 weeks in nearly all pregnancies (Jimenez and co-workers, 1979). Normally, the fetal heart rate ranges from 120 to 160 beats a minute and is heard as a double sound resembling the tick of a watch under a pillow. It is not sufficient for establishing the diagnosis of pregnancy merely to "hear" the "fetal" heart; it must be proved to be distinctly different from that of the maternal pulse. During much of pregnancy, the fetus moves freely in the amnionic fluid; consequently, the site on the maternal abdomen where the fetal heart sounds can be heard best will vary as the position of the fetus varies.

Several instruments are available that make use of the *doppler principle* to detect the action of the fetal heart. By use of these instruments, ultrasound is directed toward the moving blood of the fetus. The sound reflected by the moving blood undergoes a shift in frequency, the echo of which is detected by a receiving crystal immediately adjacent to the transmitting crystal. Because of the difference in heart rates, pulsatile flow in the fetus is differentiated easily from that of the mother unless there is severe fetal bradycardia or significant maternal tachycardia. Fetal cardiac action can be detected with appropriate equipment in which the doppler principle is employed almost always by the 10th to 12th week of gestation.

Echocardiography can be used to detect fetal heart action as early as 48 days after the first day of the last normal menses (Robinson, 1972).

Real time sonography can be used to detect fetal heart action and fetal movement after the second month of pregnancy.

Upon auscultation of the abdomen in the later months of pregnancy, the examiner may often hear sounds other than those produced by fetal heart action, the most common of which are (1) the funic (umbilical cord) souffle, (2) the uterine souffle, (3) sounds resulting from movement of the fetus, (4) the maternal pulse, and (5) the gurgling of gas in the intestines of the woman.

The funic, or umbilical cord, souffle is caused by the rush of blood through the umbilical arteries. It is a sharp, whistling sound that is synchronous with the fetal pulse and can be heard in perhaps 15 percent of pregnancies. It is inconstant, sometimes being distinctly rec-

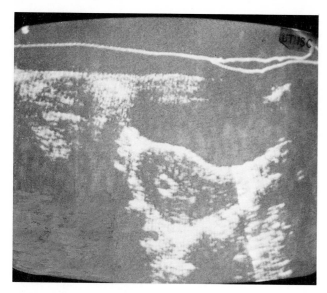

Figure 10-1. Longitudinal sonogram in which a gestation sac at 5 to 6 weeks of gestational (menstrual) age is demonstrated. (*Courtesy of Dr. R. Santos.*)

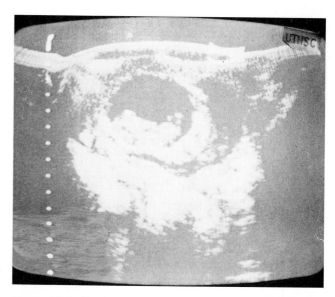

Figure 10-2. Transverse sonographic view of amnionic sac in which there is a fetus of 10 to 12 weeks of gestational age. (*Courtesy of Dr. R. Santos.*)

ognizable at the time of one examination but not found on other occasions.

The uterine souffle is heard as a soft, blowing sound that is synchronous with the maternal pulse, and usually is heard most distinctly during auscultation of the lower portion of the uterus. This sound is produced by the passage of blood through the dilated uterine vessels and is characteristic not only of pregnancy but of any condition in which the blood flow to the uterus is greatly increased. Accordingly, a uterine souffle may be heard in nonpregnant women with large uterine myomas or large tumors of the ovaries.

Frequently, the maternal pulse can be heard distinctly by auscultation of the abdomen; in some women, the pulsation of the aorta is unusually loud. Occasionally during examination, the pulse of the mother may become so rapid as to simulate the fetal heart sounds. In addition to the sounds described, it is not unusual to hear certain other sounds that are produced by the passage of gases or liquids through the intestines of the pregnant woman.

Perception of Fetal Movements

The second positive sign of pregnancy is the detection, by the examiner, of movements by the fetus. After about 20 weeks gestation, active fetal movements can be felt, at indeterminate intervals, by placing the examining hand on the woman's abdomen. These fetal movements vary in intensity, from a faint flutter early in pregnancy to brisk motions at a later period; the latter are sometimes visible as well as palpable. Occasionally, somewhat similar sensations may be produced by contractions of the intestines or the muscles of the abdominal wall of the pregnant woman, although these should not deceive an experienced examiner.

Sonographic Recognition of the Fetus

A normal intrauterine pregnancy may be demonstrated by pulse-echo sonography after only 4 to 5 weeks of amenorrhea (Fig. 10-1). After 6 weeks of amenorrhea, the small white gestational ring is so characteristic that failure to identify such raises doubts about pregnancy. Thus, there may be sonographic confirmation of pregnancy by the time that some of the common tests for human chorionic gonadotropin (hCG) in urine become positive. By careful scanning, distinct echoes from the embryo can be demonstrated within the gestational ring by 8 weeks after commencement of the last normal menstrual period. Moreover, from the length of the embryo, the gestational age can be estimated quite accurately (Fig. 10-2).

In addition to the early identification of normal pregnancy, the findings of sonography also may allow for the identification of those gestations in which there is a blighted ovum, that is, the embryo is dead and an abortion will occur ultimately. The characteristic features of a blighted ovum are (1) loss of definition of the gestational sac, (2) an unusually small gestational sac, and (3) the absence of echoes emanating from the fetus after 8 weeks gestation (Chapter 24).

By 11 weeks of amenorrhea, normally the pregnancy ring is no longer distinctly identifiable in the uterine cavity by sonography. By this time, however, fetal heart action usually can be detected with equipment that utilizes the doppler effect or by real time sonography. By the 14th week, the fetal head and thorax can be identified; soon thereafter, the placental site can be visualized by ultrasound techniques.

Subsequently, ultrasonography can be used successfully to identify the number of fetuses, the presenting part(s), various fetal anomalies, hydramnios, and to assess the rate of fetal growth by measuring, serially, the biparietal diameter of the fetal head and the circumference of the fetal abdomen.

Sonography usually provides as much information (and often much more) as does radiography without the potential, albeit undefined, risks of irradiation. To date, no adverse effects on the human embryo or fetus have been identified from exposure to energies comparable to those used in clinical sonographic examinations.

Radiographic Recognition of the Fetus

Whenever the fetal skeleton can be distinguished radiologically, the diagnosis of pregnancy is certain. This method of positive identification of pregnancy is usually not valid until after 16 weeks of gestation. By x-ray examination, Bartholomew and co-workers (1921) were able to make a positive diagnosis of pregnancy by 20 weeks gestation in only one third of the women examined who were pregnant, and only in one half by 24 weeks. Just how early the fetal skeleton is visible in the roentgenogram depends, in part, upon the thickness of the abdominal wall of the mother and the radiologic technique employed. Foci of ossification in the fetus have been demonstrated as early as 14 weeks, although ordinarily the gestation must reach 16 weeks or more before the fetal skeleton can be visualized. Roentgenography may be of value in differentiating the uterus of pregnant women from abdominal tumors, especially when the fetus is more mature but dead.

PROBABLE EVIDENCE OF PREGNANCY

The probable signs of pregnancy include (1) enlargement of the abdomen, (2) changes in the shape, size, and consistency of the uterus, (3) changes in the cervix, (4) Braxton Hicks contractions, (5) ballottement, (6) outlining the fetus, and (7) results of endocrine tests.

Enlargement of the Abdomen

By 12 weeks of gestation, the uterus can usually be felt through the abdominal wall just above the symphysis as a tumor; thereafter, the uterus increases in size gradually up to the end of pregnancy. In general, any enlargement of the abdomen during the childbearing period of women is strongly suggestive of pregnancy.

The abdominal enlargement is usually less pronounced in nulliparous than in multiparous women in whom some of the abdominal musculature tone has been lost; indeed, in some multiparous women, the abdominal wall is so flaccid that the uterus sags forward and downward, producing a pendulous abdomen. This difference in abdominal tone between first and subsequent pregnancies is so obvious that it is not rare for women in the latter part of a second pregnancy to suspect a twin pregnancy because of the increased size of their abdomen, as compared with that in the corresponding month of their previous pregnancy. The abdomen of the pregnant woman also undergoes significant changes in shape depending on her body position. The uterus is, of course, much less prominent when the woman is in the supine position.

Changes in Size, Shape, and Consistency of the Uterus

During the first few weeks of pregnancy, the increase in size of the uterus is limited principally to the anteroposterior diameter, but at a little later period of gestation, the body of the uterus is almost globular; an average diameter of 8 cm is attained by 12 weeks of pregnancy. On bimanual examination, the uterine body of pregnancy feels doughy or elastic and sometimes becomes exceedingly soft.

At about 6 to 8 weeks after the onset of the last period, the sign of Hegar becomes manifest. With one hand on the abdomen and two fingers of the other hand in the vagina, the still-firm cervix is felt, with the elastic body of the uterus above the compressible soft isthmus, which is between the two. Occasionally, the softening at the isthmus is so marked that the cervix and the body of the uterus seem to be separate organs. The inexperienced examiner may mistake the cervix for a small uterus, and the softened body of the fundus for a tumor of the ovaries or oviducts. The sign of Hegar is not, however, positively diagnostic of pregnancy, since occasionally it may be present when the walls of the nonpregnant uterus are excessively soft for reasons other than pregnancy.

Changes in the Cervix

By 6 to 8 weeks gestation, the cervix often becomes considerably softened. In primigravidas, the consistency of the cervix surrounding the external os is more similar to that of the lips of the mouth than to that of the nasal cartilage, as in nonpregnant women. Other conditions, however, may bring about softening of the cervix. Estrogen–progestin contraceptives, for example, commonly act to cause some softening and congestion of the uterine cervix.

As pregnancy advances, the cervical canal may become sufficiently patulous as to admit the tip of the examiner's finger. In certain inflammatory conditions, as well as with carcinoma, the cervix may remain firm during pregnancy, yielding only with the onset of labor, if at all.

Braxton Hicks Contractions

The uterus during pregnancy undergoes palpable but ordinarily painless contractions at irregular intervals from early stages of gestation. These may be enhanced in number and amplitude by massaging the uterus. These Braxton Hicks contractions, however, are not positive signs of pregnancy, since similar contractions sometimes are observed in uteri of women with hematometra and occasionally in uteri in which there are soft myomas, especially those of the pedunculated, submucous variety. The detection of Braxton Hicks contractions, however, may be helpful in excluding the existence of an ectopic abdominal pregnancy.

Ballottement

Near midpregnancy, the volume of the fetus is small compared with that of the volume of amnionic fluid; consequently, sudden pressure exerted on the uterus may cause the fetus to sink in the amnionic fluid and then rebound to its original position, with the tap felt by the examining finger.

Outlining the Fetus

In the second half of pregnancy, the outlines of the fetal body may be palpated through the maternal abdominal wall, and the outlining of the fetus becomes easier the nearer to term. Occasionally, subserous myomas may be of such a size and shape as to simulate the fetal head or small parts, or both, thus causing serious diagnostic errors. A positive diagnosis of pregnancy cannot be made, therefore, on this sign alone.

Endocrine Tests

The presence of hCG in maternal plasma and its excretion in urine provides the basis for the endocrine tests for pregnancy. HCG may be identified in body fluids by any one of a variety of immunoassay or bioassay techniques. *Hormonal tests that are commonly performed in the physician's office or clinic or in clinical laboratories do not absolutely identify the presence or absence of pregnancy.*

In this time of wide utilization of the principles of radioimmunoassay for the measurement of thousands of compounds, at a time when radioreceptor assays are common, as are radioenzymatic assays and the use of monoclonal antibodies, it seems strange that we were obliged to use bioassays for the evaluation of hCG in biologic fluids for nearly 4 decades. On the other hand, it obviously was necessary to establish the general principles of immunoassay before these could be applied to the measurement of hCG as a means of sensitive and accurate testing for pregnancy. Also, in retrospect, it is reasonably impressive to recall that several of the bioassays for hCG, especially that employing the development of ovarian hyperemia in the immature rat as the endpoint, were, while insensitive, remarkably accurate within 4 to 5 weeks after ovulation or at least by the time of the second missed menses.

Today, almost 60 years later, we are faced with the enviable decision of using a test for hCG that is so sensitive and specific that hCG production in some nonpregnant persons in whom there are no tumors can be detected. As cited in Chapter 7, it has been shown that a variety of normal tissues may produce hCG. Yet, as usually is the case, we pay for what we get. The more sensitive and precise the test, the more time, equipment,

and expense is involved. Fortunately, for the vast majority of pregnancy testing conducted, there are inexpensive test kits available that can be used for tests to be conducted quickly, that is, in 1 to 2 minutes, with high accuracy and—with certain precautions—high precision.

Almost without exception, chemical detection of pregnancy involves the demonstration of hCG in blood or urine of the test subject. Many different test systems are available in "kit" form commercially. Each, however, is dependent upon one of two principles: (1) recognition of hCG by an antibody to the hCG molecule; or (2) recognition of hCG by a receptor for hCG and LH (luteinizing hormone).

In the case of antibody recognition, antibodies have been raised against hCG (which also recognize LH) and these are the most commonly employed; antibodies with high specificity for the β-subunit of hCG with little cross reactivity against LH (see Chapter 7), and antibodies raised against the α-subunit of hCG and LH (which are identical) are also used.

The radioreceptor assay is one in which plasma membranes of bovine corpora lutea are employed. In such preparations, there are receptor sites with high affinity for hCG and LH. Thus, although such an assay is sensitive, by use of such preparations, one cannot distinguish between hCG and LH.

In immunoassay procedures, the principle of hemagglutination inhibition of erythrocytes is employed or the prevention of flocculation of hCG-coated particles, for example, latex particles to which hCG is covalently bound.

In radioassays, [^{125}I]iodohCG is used as the radiolabeled ligand for antibodies raised against hCG and is dependent upon displacement of (or competition with) the radioligand by nonradiolabeled hCG in the biologic sample to be tested. In radioimmunoassays, "free" and "bound" [^{125}I]iodohCG are separated and radioactivity that is unbound is assayed. From a construction of standard curves, hCG is quantified with great accuracy and sensitivity by this method of radioimmunoassay. If the test employed is so sensitive that it detects very small amounts of hCG (with an antibody that also recognizes LH), the results may give rise to a positive test for pregnancy in nonpregnant women, especially in problem cases, because of the cross reactivity of circulating or excreted LH. At the time of menopause, for example, amenorrhea not infrequently causes considerable fear of a possible pregnancy. At the same time, the levels of pituitary gonadotropins in plasma and urine are usually elevated in the postmenopausal woman and may be the cause of a false positive pregnancy test. If, however, the sensitivity of the pregnancy test is reduced in order to exclude a false positive result from LH, some early pregnancies will not be identified because the levels of hCG are too low to be detected. The false negative test is most likely to be encountered during the first few days of pregnancy or after the fourth month, although with abnormal pregnancies, such as a tubal pregnancy, hCG may be present only in small amounts and therefore not identified by the less sensitive methods of testing.

The production of hCG begins very early in the course of pregnancy and indeed may even precede the time of nidation. Thereafter, the levels of hCG rise very rapidly in early pregnancy, with an estimated doubling time of hCG concentrations in plasma of 1.4 to 2.0 days (Chartier and colleagues, 1979). Certainly with a sensitive test, for example, the radioimmunoassay employing antibodies directed against the β-subunit of hCG (which is specific for hCG and does not cross react significantly with LH), the pregnancy hormone can be demonstrated by 8 to 9 days after ovulation.

The concentration of hCG in urine rises rapidly, as pointed out in Chapter 7 (p. 122). A good rule of thumb is that the concentration of hCG contained in 1 liter of maternal plasma is equivalent to that contained in 24 hours of urine. Thus, if the urine excreted per 24 hours were 1 liter, the concentration of hCG in serum and in urine would be similar. Most of the commonly used immunologic tests for pregnancy in which latex fixation of hCG is used are able to detect 1.5 to 3 IU/ml. With some of the hemagglutination inhibition tube tests, 0.25 to 1 IU/ml can be detected. If the rate of urine excretion during the time of collection were 1 liter per 24 hours, the detectable hCG concentration among the various tests would be equivalent to the concentration of 0.25 to 3 IU of hCG per milliliter of serum. Rarely do concentrations of LH reach this level, even in postmenopausal women. Ordinarily, concentrations of LH at the time of the midcycle LH surge reach levels on the order of 40 to 60 mIU/ml of plasma. We have observed that non-hCG protein, nonspecific substances in urine, or even in tap water, are more likely to give rise to false positive pregnancy tests employing the latex fixation immunoassay procedures than is increased LH excretion either at midcycle or in the postmenopausal woman. Moreover, many investigators have cautioned against freezing urine prior to testing. Freezing of urine commonly gives rise to false positive tests whereas storage of urine in the refrigerator at 4°C does not.

Specific tests for hCG, namely, those utilizing the antibody directed against recognition sites on the β-subunit of hCG, are currently available commercially. These tests are conducted with serum by radioimmunoassay and are exquisitely sensitive. Theoretically, these tests should provide greater specificity, since the β-subunit of hCG differs antigenetically from the β-subunit of LH. The various antibodies developed to the β-subunit cross react variably with those of the β-subunit of LH or with the total LH moiety. Thus, greater accuracy and great sensitivity is possible. Special equipment, however, is required to conduct radioimmunoassay, viz., gamma counter, centrifuges, and, in some cases, incubators.

"Do It Yourself" Test Kits. Today there are several over-the-counter pregnancy test kits for use at home that range in price from $8.99 to $17.98 (Dallas, 1984). In each of the tests, the principle of hemagglutination inhibition using sheep erythrocytes with antibodies to hCG is employed with the subject's urine. The experience to date has been that women who used the test at home experienced a relatively low ($\cong$ 5 percent) false positive rate, but a high false negative ($\cong$ 20 percent) result. Valanis and Perlman (1982) evaluated the prevalence of use of home pregnancy testing kits among a wide distribution of subjects according to age, race, and socioeconomic status. These investigators also investigated test results. They found that among the women interviewed, namely, 144 women in the settings of a private physician's office, a Planned Parenthood clinic, and a public obstetrics–gynecology clinic, almost one third of the subjects had used a home pregnancy testing kit. They also found that the false negative test result incidence was almost 25 percent, and that only one third of the subjects complied with test-kit instructions. They also found a greater use frequency among white women compared with black women and greater use among middle-class income women and private physician patients. These investigators voiced concern about the high false negative test results even among women who did ultimately seek medical advice. In this study, only women who did initiate medical care were evaluated. Physician opinion is divided concerning the wisdom of making pregnancy testing available to nonprofessionals. Some argue that such tests will give results that will prompt women to see physicians earlier. We are of the view that the reverse may be more likely in those complicated situations in which early physician consultation is urgently needed.

The kits commercially available to offices and laboratories that employ failure of agglutination of latex particles to detect hCG in urine contain two reagents. One is a suspension of latex particles coated with or covalently bound to hCG and the other contains a solution of hCG antibody. To test for hCG, one drop of urine is mixed with one drop of the antibody-containing solution on a black glass slide. If no hCG is present in the urine, antibody will remain available to agglutinate the hCG-coated latex particles, which are added subsequently. Agglutination of the latex particles can be observed easily when a bright light source is illuminated against the dark background of the glass slide. If hCG is present in the urine, it binds to the antibody and thus prevents antibody-induced agglutination of the hCG-coated latex particles. Therefore, the pregnancy test is positive if no agglutination occurs; the pregnancy test is negative when agglutination occurs.

Radioreceptor Assay

Saxena and Landesman (1978) have reviewed the development and utilization of a radioreceptor assay for hCG. This assay makes use of the high-affinity receptors on plasma membrane preparations of responsive tissues, for example, bovine corpora lutea. The radioreceptor assay does not distinguish between LH and hCG. It requires the utilization of radiolabeled hCG and approximately 2 hours to conduct. The test does offer the advantages of good accuracy and applicability to serum testing (Boyko and Russell, 1979.)

TABLE 10-1. BIOLOGIC TESTS FOR PREGNANCY

Name	Test Animal	End Point	Time of Test
Aschheim-Zondek	Mice or Rats	Corpus Luteum Formation	5 days
Friedman	Rabbits	Corpus Luteum Formation	48 hr
Ovarian Hyperemia (Beck and Co-workers)	Rats	Hyperemia	12–18 hr
Frog Test (Wiltberger, Miller)	Female	Extrusion of Eggs	24 hr
Toad Test (Galli Mainini, Shapiro)	Male	Extrusion of Sperm	2–5 hr

Bioassay

Few, if any, of the bioassay techniques that have been employed in the past to detect hCG are still in use. Of these, the rat ovarian hyperemia test was probably the most satisfactory for general pregnancy testing. Several of the previously employed bioassay methods are of some historical interest and are listed in Table 10-1.

Progesterone-induced and synthetic progestin-induced withdrawal uterine bleeding was used in the past in attempts to differentiate pregnancy from other causes of amenorrhea. In the absence of pregnancy, withdrawal bleeding usually occurs 3 to 5 days after the last dose of the progestin in estrogen-producing anovulatory women. This response, of course, requires an estrogen-primed endometrium. Withdrawal of the progestin results in uterine bleeding if there is little or no endogenous progesterone production. If there is sufficient production of endogenous progesterone or if the endometrium is not estrogen-primed, no bleeding occurs: the latter is a false positive test. In general, this method offers little that cannot be accomplished by carefully evaluating the woman's history and by ascertaining, at the time of pelvic examination, whether there is any cervical mucus, and, if so, whether the spread and dried mucus crystallizes to form a fern or a cellular pattern (see Chapter 4, pp. 74, 75). If copious thin mucus is present, and if a fern pattern develops on drying, early pregnancy is very unlikely and the woman almost certainly will sustain uterine bleeding after treatment with and withdrawal from progestin. If little cervical mucus is present, and a highly cellular pattern forms, she may or may not be pregnant. If not pregnant, she may or may not develop uterine bleeding after receiving progestin, depending upon her own supply of endogenous progesterone. Moreover, currently there is the fear that progestins are potential teratogens (see Chapter 40, p. 818). Therefore, progestins should not be used in women who are believed to be pregnant except in unusual circumstances, for example, removal of the corpus luteum prior to the eighth week of pregnancy (see Chapter 3).

Summary

None of the chemical tests for pregnancy is sufficiently accurate to provide positive proof of pregnancy. Unfortunately, the same or even greater error rate in tests conducted by women at home may give rise to false security or unnecessary alarm if the likely validity of the results of such tests cannot be evaluated in light of other signs or symptoms.

Measurement of hCG in Gynecic Emergencies and Other Trophoblastic Disorders

Ectopic pregnancy (Chapter 22) is a common gynecologic disorder that may present a variety of difficulties in diagnosis and management. Commonly, the routinely used clinical tests for pregnancy, when the embryo is implanted outside the endometrial cavity (ectopic pregnancies) are negative for hCG. This may be due to a variety of reasons, probably the most common being reduction in placentation for the stage of gestation because of the ectopic site of implantation, disruption of trophoblasts by hemorrhage, embryonic death, and so forth. Nonetheless, hCG is present in plasma and urine of most women with ectopic pregnancies, albeit in lower concentrations, generally, than in women with normal intrauterine pregnancies at comparable stages of gestation. In many instances of unruptured ectopic pregnancy, the diagnosis may be difficult (Chapter 22). For this reason, the detection of hCG in biologic fluids of such women or the demonstration of a declining concentration of the levels of hCG may be of considerable assistance in reaching a definitive diagnosis. By use of radioimmunoassay procedures with antibodies directed toward the β-subunit of the molecule, this goal ordinarily is achieved. The same is true of the use of radioreceptor assays; these, however, as pointed out, do not distinguish between LH and hCG. If the case in point is not an emergency situation, the demonstration of a decline in hCG levels early in pregnancy or else a failure of the levels to increase with time is indicative of impending spontaneous abortion or else ectopic pregnancy. Unfortunately, the reverse does not obtain. Namely, normal levels of hCG may be found in women in whom there is an ectopic pregnancy. Recall that early in pregnancy the levels of hCG in plasma double every 2 days, on average. If this doubling time can be demonstrated, a successful pregnancy outcome will be expected in 90 percent of cases (cf. Pelosi and associates, 1983). This same doubling time in the increase in plasma levels of hCG is found in only 20 percent of women with an ectopic pregnancy. By way of example, Kadar and colleagues (1981) found that the level of hCG in plasma increased by at least 66 percent in 48 hours early in normal pregnancy but by less than this amount in women with an ectopic pregnancy.

By use of sensitive assays for hCG, positive results have been obtained in 80 to 99 percent of proven cases of ectopic pregnancy by various investigators. It is important to remember, however, that low or falling levels of hCG are not such as to distinguish between ectopic pregnancy and impending spontaneous abortion.

Lagrew and colleagues (1983) found that the concentration of hCG in plasma of pregnant women increased in an exponential fashion between 30 and 60 days of pregnancy (dated from last menses). By use of a regression line constructed from measurement of hCG in a large population of pregnant women, these investigators found that the level of hCG at this time in pregnancy was an accurate reflection of gestation duration. Thus, in women with infertility and ovulation induction or in other instances in which the last normal menses may not be appropriate for pregnancy dating, the levels of hCG in early pregnancy may be useful.

Sensitive tests for hCG in biologic fluids are also of specific utility in the management of persons with neoplastic trophoblastic disease, especially in the evaluation of the results of and effectiveness of treatment.

In some cases of elective abortion, postabortion evaluation of persistence of hCG may be useful in evaluating the possibility of persistent trophoblastic function, which could be indicative of the possibilities that abortion was not accomplished (e.g., very early in pregnancy—menstrual extraction), that abortion was incomplete, or that the pregnancy was (and is) ectopically implanted. Yet another explanation could be that a twin pregnancy existed, but only one fetus (placenta) was removed. Given the long half-life of hCG, early postabortal testing for hCG, however, is of little utility. Postabortion follow-up testing for hCG, if indicated, is best conducted 2 to 3 weeks after the procedure (Derman, moderator; Corson, Horwitz, Lau, Solderstrom, panelists, 1981).

PRESUMPTIVE EVIDENCE OF PREGNANCY

The presumptive evidence of pregnancy comprises largely subjective symptoms and signs that are appreciated by the woman. These signs include (1) cessation of menses, (2) changes in the breasts, (3) discoloration of the vaginal mucosa, (4) increased skin pigmentation and the appearance of abdominal striae, and (5) especially important, whether the woman perceives herself as being pregnant. The symptoms include (1) nausea with or without vomiting, (2) disturbances in urination, (3) fatigue, and (4) the perception of fetal movement.

Cessation of Menses

In a healthy woman who previously has had spontaneous, cyclic, and predictable menstruation, the abrupt cessation of menstruation is strongly suggestive of pregnancy. Not until 10 days or more after the time of expected onset of the menstrual period, however, is the absence of menses a reliable indication of pregnancy. When the second period is missed, the probability of pregnancy is very much greater.

Although cessation of menstruation is an early and very important indication of pregnancy, gestation may begin without prior menstruation, and uterine bleeding that is suggestive of menstruation to the woman is occasionally noted after conception. In certain Oriental countries where girls marry at a very early age, and in sexually promiscuous groups, pregnancy sometimes occurs before menarche. Indeed, we have managed the pregnancies of a girl who had four children without ever having a menstrual period. She delivered her fourth child at age 16, and conceived her first child at age 13, before menarche. Nursing mothers, who usually do not menstruate during lactation, sometimes conceive at that time, and, more rarely, women who believe they have passed the menopause may become pregnant. Conversely, during the first half of pregnancy, one or two episodes of bloody discharge, reminiscent of menstruation, are not uncommon, but almost without exception such bleeding is brief and scant. In a series of 225 consecutive gravidas who did not abort, Speert and Guttmacher (1954) observed that macroscopic vaginal bleeding, which occurred between the time of conception and the 196th day of pregnancy, was reported by 22 percent of these women. In the absence of any cervical lesion, the bleeding began on or before the 40th day in 8 percent. Speert and Guttmacher interpreted such bleeding to be physiologic, the consequence of implantation. Bleeding during pregnancy was three times more frequent among multiparas than among primigravidas. Of 83 multiparas, 25 percent experienced bleeding. Instances in which women are said to have "menstruated" every month throughout pregnancy are of questionable authenticity, and true uterine bleeding during pregnancy is undoubtedly the result of some abnormality of the reproductive organs. Bleeding per vagina at any time during pregnancy must be regarded as abnormal.

Absence of menstruation may result from a number of conditions other than pregnancy. Probably the most common cause of a delay in the onset of the menstrual period is anovulation, which in turn may be the consequence of a number of factors that include emotional disorders, for example, the fear of pregnancy. Environmental changes as well as a variety of chronic disease processes also may suppress ovulation by inducing anestrogenic or estrogenic anovulation.

Changes in the Breasts

Generally, the breast changes that accompany pregnancy (see Chapter 9) are quite characteristic in primiparas but are less obvious in multiparas, whose breasts may contain a small amount of milk or colostrum for months or even years after the birth of their last child. Occasionally, changes in the breasts similar to those produced by pregnancy are found in women with prolactin-secreting pituitary tumors and in women taking certain tranquilizers that induce hyperprolactinemia. Instances also have been reported of such breast changes occurring in women with spurious or imaginary pregnancy (pseudocyesis) or after repeated stimulation of the breasts.

Discoloration of the Vaginal Mucosa

During pregnancy, the vaginal mucosa frequently appears dark bluish or purplish-red and congested (the sign of Chadwick).

This appearance of the vagina is taken as presumptive evidence of pregnancy but is not conclusive, since such vaginal changes may be observed in any condition that causes intense congestion of the pelvic organs.

Increased Skin Pigmentation and the Appearance of Abdominal Striae

These cutaneous manifestations are common to, but not diagnostic of, pregnancy. These signs may be absent during gestation and, conversely, may be associated with the use of estrogen–progestin contraceptives.

SYMPTOMS OF PREGNANCY

Nausea With or Without Vomiting

Commonly, pregnancy is characterized by disturbances of the digestive system, manifested particularly by nausea and vomiting. The so-called morning sickness of pregnancy usually commences during the early part of the day but passes off in a few hours, although occasionally it persists longer and may occur at other times. This disturbing symptom usually appears about 6 weeks after the commencement of the last menstrual period and disappears spontaneously 6 to 12 weeks later.

Disturbances in Urination

During the first trimester of pregnancy, the enlarging uterus, by exerting pressure on the urinary bladder, may cause frequent micturition. The frequency of urination diminishes gradually during pregnancy as the uterus rises up into the abdomen. This symptom reappears near the end of pregnancy, however, when the fetal head descends into the maternal pelvis.

Fatigue

Easy fatigability is such a frequent characteristic of early pregnancy that it affords a noteworthy diagnostic clue.

The Sensation of Fetal Movement

Sometime between 16 and 20 weeks after the onset of the last menstrual period, the pregnant woman usually becomes conscious of slight fluttering movements in the abdomen, with these movements gradually increasing in intensity. These are caused by fetal activity, and the time that these are first appreciated by the mother is designated as "quickening," or the perception of life. This sign provides only corroborative evidence of pregnancy and in itself is of little diagnostic value. It is, however, a milestone of pregnancy progression that, if accurate, can be corrobative evidence of the duration of gestation.

DIFFERENTIAL DIAGNOSIS OF PREGNANCY

Often the uterus of pregnancy is mistaken for other tumors occupying the pelvis or abdomen; less frequently, the opposite error is made. The uterine changes of the early weeks of pregnancy may be simulated by enlargement of the uterus due to myomas, hematometra, adenomyosis, or by apparent enlargement that is actually due to a contiguous extrauterine mass or masses. As a rule, the enlarged uterus in these circumstances is firmer than it is in pregnancy and is less elastic and boggy. Except in hematometra, moreover, such conditions are usually not attended by cessation of the menses. If uncertainty remains, however, reexamination in a few weeks will usually allow for the correct diagnosis to be established.

SPURIOUS PREGNANCY

Imaginary pregnancy, or *pseudocyesis,* usually occurs in women nearing the menopause or in women who intensely desire to be pregnant. Such women may present all the subjective symptoms of pregnancy in association with a considerable increase in the size of their abdomen, caused either by deposition of fat, by gas in the intestinal tract, or by abdominal fluid. In such women, the menses do not as a rule disappear, but may become unpredictable in time of onset and in amount and duration of bleeding. Changes in the breasts, including enlargement, the appearance of galactorrhea, and increased areolar pigmentation sometimes occur. In a majority of these women, there is morning sickness, probably of psychogenic origin.

The ingestion of a variety of phenothiazines can lead to amenorrhea, breast enlargement, hyperprolactinemia and galactorrhea, and even false positive pregnancy tests. Obviously, the underlying emotional problem may be compounded by these changes.

The supposed fetal movements that are perceived by women with pseudocyesis can be ascribed to contractions of the intestines of the woman or the muscles of her abdominal wall, but occasionally these are so marked as even to deceive physicians. Careful examination of such women usually leads to a correct diagnosis without great difficulty since the small uterus can be palpated on bimanual examination. The greatest difficulty encountered in the care of such women may be that of convincing them of the correct diagnosis. Psychotic women may persist for years in the delusion that they are pregnant.

DISTINCTION BETWEEN FIRST AND SUBSEQUENT PREGNANCIES

Occasionally, it is of practical importance to ascertain whether a woman is pregnant for the first time or has previously borne children. Ordinarily, but not always, there are indelible traces of a former term pregnancy.

In a nullipara, the abdomen is usually tense and firm, and the uterus is felt through it with difficulty. The characteristic old abdominal striae and the distinctive changes in the breasts are absent. The labia majora are usually in close apposition and the frenulum is intact. The vagina is usually narrow and characterized by well developed rugae. The cervix is softened but usually does not admit the tip of the examiner's finger until the very end of pregnancy.

In multiparas, the abdominal wall is usually lax and, at times, pendulous, and through it the uterus is palpated readily. In addition to the pink abdominal striae associated with the present pregnancy, the silvery cicatrices of past pregnancies also may be present. Usually the breasts are not as firm as in women during their first pregnancy and frequently in the skin over the breast tissue there are striae similar to those on the abdomen. The vulva of women who previously have delivered vaginally usually gapes open to some extent, the frenulum has disappeared, and the hymen is transformed into the myrtiform caruncles. In multiparas who previously have delivered vaginally, the external os, even in the early months of pregnancy, may admit the tip of the examiner's finger, which can be carried up to the internal os. Moreover, the sites of healed lacerations of the cervix can usually be identified.

IDENTIFICATION OF FETAL LIFE OR DEATH

In the early months of pregnancy, the diagnosis of fetal death may present difficulty. Unless special ultrasonic techniques are employed, the diagnosis of fetal death can be made with certainty only after it can be shown by repeated examinations that the uterus has remained constant in size or there actually has been a decrease in size of the uterus over a number of weeks. Since the placenta may continue to produce hCG for several weeks after death of the embryo or fetus, a positive endocrine test for pregnancy does not necessarily prove that the fetus is alive.

In the latter half of pregnancy, the cessation of fetal movements usually alerts the woman to the possibility of fetal death, but if fetal cardiac action can still be identified distinct from that of the mother, the fetus is certainly alive. If, by careful auscultation, the fetal heart tones are not heard, however, the fetus probably is dead. There is a possibility of error, of course, especially in

pregnancies in which the fetal heart is remote from the examiner, for example, if the woman is obese or if hydramnios exists.

Ultrasonic instruments in which the doppler shift principle is employed, as described on page 211, are of considerable value in the evaluation of pregnancies in which the fetal heart cannot be heard by auscultation with a stethoscope. The use of doppler ultrasound is especially valuable when fetal death is suspected but fetal heart action can be identified. If fetal heart action is not demonstrated after careful examination, it can be stated that very likely, but not absolutely, the fetus is dead. Real-time ultrasonographic examination when carefully performed will serve to identify accurately the presence or absence of fetal heart motion.

If the fetus has been dead for some time, it can usually be shown by careful examination that the uterus does not correspond in size to the estimated duration of pregnancy or actually that the uterus has become smaller than previously observed. With the death of the fetus, maternal weight gain usually ceases; not infrequently there is even a slight decrease in her weight. At the same time, retrogressive changes usually have occurred in the breasts. Ordinarily, the diagnosis of fetal death cannot be made from the findings of a single examination, but fetal death certainly must be considered when the signs just mentioned are identified and fetal cardiac action cannot be detected.

Occasionally, a positive diagnosis of fetal death can be established by palpating the collapsed fetal skull through the partially dilated cervix; in that event, the loose bones of the fetal head feel as though these are contained in a flabby bag.

There are three principal radiologic signs of fetal death:

1. Significant overlap of the skull bones (the sign of Spalding), caused by liquefaction of the brain, a process that requires several days to develop. A similar sign may develop occasionally with a living fetus, for example, when the fetal head is compressed in the maternal pelvis.
2. Exaggerated curvature of the fetal spine. Since the development of this sign depends on maceration of the spinous ligaments, its development also requires several days; moreover, mild degrees of curvature of the spine in living fetuses may be misleading.
3. Demonstration of gas in the fetus is an uncommon but reliable sign of fetal death (Fig. 10-3).

In instances in which the fetus has been dead for several days to weeks, the amnionic fluid is red to brown and usually turbid rather than nearly colorless and clear. The finding of such anmionic fluid is not absolutely diagnostic of fetal death, however, since prior hemorrhage into the amnionic sac, as sometimes occurs during amniocentesis, may lead to similar discoloration of the amnionic fluid even though the fetus is alive.

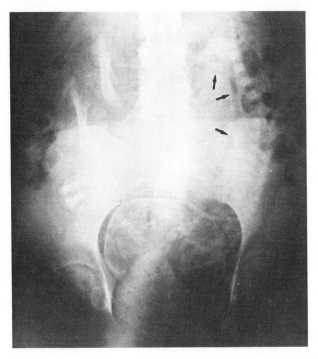

Figure 10-3. Fetal death is established by the presence of gas in a major vessel. The close proximity to the fetal spine implies that the vessel is the aorta.

REFERENCES

Bartholomew RA, Sale BE, Calloway JT: Diagnosis of pregnancy by the roentgen ray. JAMA 76:912, 1921

Boyko WL, Russell HT: Evaluation and clinical application of the quantitative radioreceptor assay for serum hCG. Obstet Gynecol 54:737, 1979

Chadwick JR: Value of the bluish coloration of the vaginal entrance as a sign of pregnancy. Trans Am Gynecol Soc 11:399, 1886

Chartier M, Roger M, Barrat J, Michelon B: Measurement of plasma chorionic gonadotropin (hCG) and β-hCG activities in the late luteal phase: Evidence of the occurrence of spontaneous menstrual abortions in infertile women. Fertil Steril 31:134, 1979

Derman R, Corson LS, Horwitz CA, Lau HD, Solderstrom R: Early diagnosis of pregnancy: A symposium. J Reprod Med 26:149, 1981

Jimenez JM, Tyson JE, Santos-Ramos R, Duenhoelter JH: Comparison of obstetric and pediatric evaluation of gestational age. Pediatr Res 13:498, 1979

Kadar N, Caldwell BV, Romero R: A method of screening for ectopic pregnancy and its indications. Obstet Gynecol 58:162, 1981

Lagrew DC, Wilson EA, Jawad MJ: Determination of gestational age by serum concentrations of human chorionic gonadotropin. Obstet Gynecol 61:37, 1981

Pelosi MC, Apuzzi J, Dwyer JW: Early diagnosis of pregnancy. Part I: Workup and laboratory tests. The Female Patient 8:38, 1983

Robinson HP: Detection of fetal heart movement in first trimester of pregnancy using pulsed ultrasound. Br Med J 4:66, 1972

Santos R: Personal communication, 1979

Saxena BB, Landesman R: Diagnosis and management of pregnancy by the radioreceptor assay of human chorionic gonadotropin. Am J Obstet Gynecol 131:97, 1978

Speert H, Guttmacher AF: Frequency and significance of bleeding in early pregnancy. JAMA 155:172, 1974

Valanis BG, Perlman CS: Home pregnancy testing kits: Prevalence of use, false-negative rates, and compliance with instructions. Am J Public Health 72:1034, 1982

11

The Normal Pelvis

The mechanisms of labor are essentially processes of accommodation of the fetus to the bony passage through which it must pass. Accordingly, the size and shape of the pelvis are of extreme importance in obstetrics. In both women and men, the pelvis forms the bony ring through which the body weight is transmitted to the lower extremities, but in women it assumes a special form that adapts it to childbearing (Fig. 11-1).

The adult pelvis is composed of four bones: the sacrum, the coccyx, and the two innominate bones. Each innominate bone is formed by the fusion of the ilium, the ischium, and the pubis. The innominate bones are joined firmly to the sacrum at the sacroiliac synchondroses, and to one another at the symphysis pubis. Consideration of the pelvis will be limited to those peculiarities of importance in childbearing.

PELVIC ANATOMY FROM THE OBSTETRIC POINT OF VIEW

The linea terminalis demarcates the *false pelvis* from the *true pelvis* (Fig. 11-2). The false pelvis lies above the linea terminalis and the true pelvis below this anatomic boundary. The false pelvis is bounded posteriorly by the lumbar vertebrae and laterally by the iliac fossae; in front the boundary is formed by the lower portion of the anterior abdominal wall. The false pelvis varies considerably in size among women according to the flare of the iliac bones, but is of no particular obstetric significance.

The true pelvis lies beneath the linea terminalis and is the portion important in childbearing. The true pelvis is bounded above by the promontory and alae of the sacrum, the linea terminalis, and the upper margins of the pubic bones, and below by the pelvic outlet. The cavity of the true pelvis can be compared with an obliquely truncated, bent cylinder with its greatest height posteriorly, since its anterior wall at the symphysis pubis measures about 5 cm and its posterior wall about 10 cm (Figs. 11-3, 11-4). With the woman upright, the upper portion of the pelvic canal is directed downward and backward, and its lower course curves and becomes directed downward and forward.

The walls of the true pelvis are partly bony and partly ligamentous. The posterior boundary is the anterior surface of the sacrum, and the lateral limits are

formed by the inner surface of the ischial bones and the sacrosciatic notches and sacrosciatic ligaments. In front, the true pelvis is bounded by the pubic bones, the ascending superior rami of the ischial bones, and the obturator foramina that they partially enclose.

The side walls of the true pelvis of the normal adult woman converge somewhat; therefore, if the planes of the ischial bones of the pelvis of a normal adult woman were extended downward, they would meet near the knee. Extending from the middle of the posterior margin of each ischium are the ischial spines, which are of great obstetric importance, because a line drawn between them usually represents the shortest diameter of the pelvic cavity. Moreover, since the ischial spines can be felt readily by vaginal or rectal examination, they serve as valuable landmarks in determining the level to which the presenting part of the fetus has descended into the true pelvis.

The sacrum forms the posterior wall of the pelvic cavity. Its upper anterior margin, corresponding to the body of the first sacral vertebra and designated as the promontory, may be felt on vaginal examination and can provide a landmark for clinical pelvimetry. Normally, the sacrum possesses a marked vertical and a less pronounced horizontal concavity, which, in abnormal pelves, may undergo important variations. A straight line drawn from the promontory to the tip of the sacrum usually measures 10 cm, whereas the distance along the concavity averages 12 cm.

In women the appearance of the pubic arch is characteristic. The descending inferior rami of the pubic bones unite at an angle of 90 to 100 degrees to form a rounded arch under which the fetal head may readily pass (Fig. 11-1).

PLANES AND DIAMETERS OF THE PELVIS

Because of the peculiar shape of the pelvis, it is difficult to describe the exact location of an object therein. For convenience, the pelvis has long been described as having four imaginary planes: (1) the plane of the pelvic inlet (superior strait), (2) the plane of the pelvic outlet (inferior strait), (3) the plane of greatest pelvic dimensions, and (4) the plane of the midpelvis (least pelvic dimensions).

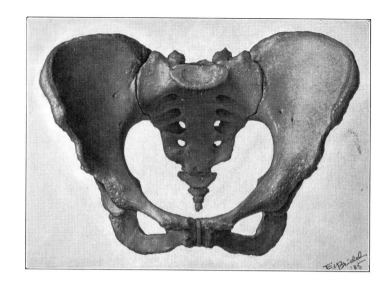

Figure 11-1. Normal female pelvis.

Pelvic Inlet

The pelvic inlet (superior strait) is bounded posteriorly by the promontory and alae of the sacrum, laterally by the linea terminalis, and anteriorly by the horizontal rami of the pubic bones and symphysis pubis (Figs. 11-1, 11-4). The configuration of the inlet of the pelvis of women typically is more nearly round than ovoid. Caldwell and co-workers (1934) identified roentgenographically a nearly round or "gynecoid" pelvic inlet in 50 percent of the pelves of white women.

Four diameters of the pelvic inlet are usually described: the anteroposterior, the transverse, and two obliques. The obstetrically important anteroposterior diameter is the shortest distance between the promontory of the sacrum and the symphysis pubis and is designated the *obstetric conjugate* (Figs. 11-3, 11-4). Normally, the obstetric conjugate measures 10 cm or more, but it may be considerably shortened in abnormal pelves.

The transverse diameter is constructed at right angles to the obstetric conjugate and represents the greatest distance between the linea terminalis on either side. It usually intersects the obstetric conjugate at a point about 4 cm in front of the promontory (Fig. 11-4).

Each of the oblique diameters extends from one of the sacroiliac synchondroses to the iliopectineal eminence on the opposite side of the pelvis. They average just under 13 cm and are designated right and left, re-

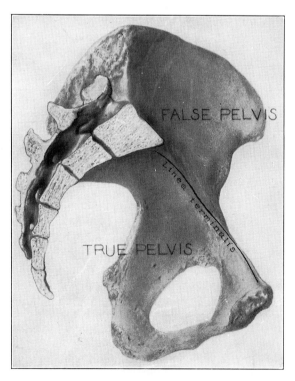

Figure 11-2. Sagittal section of pelvis showing false and true pelvis.

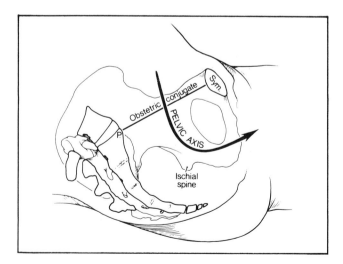

Figure 11-3. The cavity of the true pelvis is comparable to an obliquely truncated, bent cylinder with its greatest height posteriorly. Note the curvature of the pelvic axis.

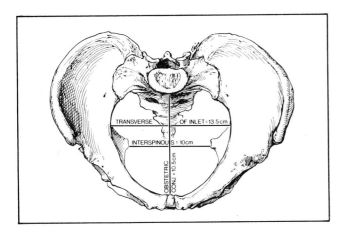

Figure 11-4. Adult female pelvis demonstrating anteroposterior and transverse diameters of the pelvic inlet and transverse (interspinous) diameter of the midpelvis; the obstetric conjugate normally is greater than 10 cm.

spectively, according to whether they originate at the right or left sacroiliac synchondrosis.

The anteroposterior diameter of the pelvic inlet that has been identified as the *true conjugate* does not represent the shortest distance between the promontory of the sacrum and symphysis pubis (Fig. 11-5). The shortest distance is the *obstetric conjugate,* which is the shortest anteroposterior diameter through which the head must pass in descending through the pelvic inlet (Figs. 11-3, 11-4, 11-5).

The obstetric conjugate cannot be measured directly with the examining fingers; therefore, various instruments have been designed in an effort to obtain such a measurement, but no instrument has proven to be reliable. For clinical purposes, it is sufficient to estimate the length of the obstetric conjugate indirectly by measuring the distance from the lower margin of the symphysis to the promontory of the sacrum, that is, the *diagonal conjugate,* and subtracting 1.5 to 2 cm from the result, according to the height and inclination of the symphysis pubis (see Pelvic Size and Its Estimation, p. 226).

Pelvic Outlet

The outlet of the pelvis consists of two approximately triangular areas not in the same plane but having a common base, which is a line drawn between the two ischial tuberosities. The apex of the posterior triangle is at the tip of the sacrum; the lateral boundaries are the sacrosciatic ligaments and the ischial tuberosities. The anterior triangle is formed by the area under the pubic arch. Three diameters of the pelvic outlet are usually described: the anteroposterior, the transverse, and the posterior sagittal. The anteroposterior diameter extends from the lower margin of the symphysis pubis to the tip of the sacrum (11.5 cm). The transverse diameter is the distance between the inner edges of the ischial tuberosities (10.0 cm). The posterior sagittal diameter extends from the tip of the sacrum to a right-angled intersection

with a line between the ischial tuberosities (7.5 cm) (Fig. 11-6).

Midpelvis

The midpelvis at the level of the ischial spines (midplane, or plane of least pelvic dimensions) is of particular importance following engagement of the fetal head in obstructed labor. The interspinous diameter of 10.0 cm, or somewhat more, is usually the smallest diameter of the pelvis (Fig. 11-4). The shortest anteroposterior diameter, at the level of the ischial spines, normally measures at least 11.5 cm (Fig. 11-5). The posterior component (posterior sagittal diameter) between the sacrum and the intersection with the interspinous diameter is usually at least 4.5 cm.

> The *plane of greatest pelvic dimensions* has no obstetric significance. As the name implies, this plane represents the roomiest portion of the pelvic cavity. It extends from the middle of the posterior surface of the symphysis pubis to the junction of the second and third sacral vertebrae and passes laterally through the ischial bones over the middle of the acetabulum. Its anteroposterior and transverse diameters average about 12.5 cm. Since its oblique diameters terminate in the obturator foramina and the sacrosciatic notches, their length cannot be determined.

Pelvic Inclination. The normal position of the pelvis, in the erect woman, can be reproduced by holding a skeletal specimen with the incisures of the acetabula pointing directly downward. The same result is achieved when the anterior superior spines of the ilium and the pubic tubercles are placed in the same vertical plane (Fig. 11-2).

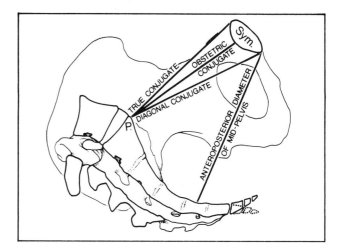

Figure 11-5. Three anteroposterior diameters of the pelvic inlet are illustrated: the true conjugate, the obstetrically important obstetric conjugate, and the clinically measurable diagonal conjugate. The anteroposterior diameter of the midpelvis is shown (P = sacral promontory; Sym = symphysis pubis).

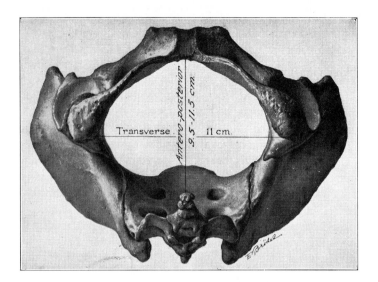

Figure 11-6. Pelvic outlet.

Pelvic Joints. Anteriorly, the pelvic bones are joined together by the symphysis pubis, which consists of fibrocartilage, and by the superior and inferior pubic ligaments; the latter is frequently designated the arcuate ligament of the pubis (Fig. 11-7). The symphysis has a certain degree of mobility, which increases during pregnancy, particularly in multiparas. This fact was demonstrated by Budin (1897), who reported that if a finger was inserted into the vagina of a pregnant woman and she then walked, the ends of the pubic bones could be felt moving up and down with each step. The articulations between the sacrum and innominate bones (*sacroiliac joints*) also have a certain degree of mobility (Fig. 11-8).

Relaxation of the pelvic joints during pregnancy is probably the result of hormonal changes. Abramson and co-workers (1934) observed that relaxation of the symphysis pubis commenced in women in the first half of pregnancy and increased during the last 3 months. These investigators observed that regression of relaxation began immediately after parturition and was completed within 3 to 5 months. The symphysis pubis also increases in width during pregnancy (more in multiparas than in primigravidas) and returns to normal soon after delivery. By careful roentgenographic studies, Borell and Fernstrom (1957) demonstrated that the rather marked mobility of the pelvis of women at term was caused by an upward gliding movement of the sacroiliac joint. The displacement, which is greatest in the dorsal lithotomy position, may cause an increase in the diameter of the outlet of 1.5 to 2 cm.

Because of the elasticity of the pelvic joints in pregnancy, it was formerly thought that positioning the woman in extreme hyperextension increased the obstetric conjugate. To obtain this objective, the woman was placed on her back with her buttocks extending slightly over the edge of the delivery table and with her legs hanging down by their own weight, the so-called

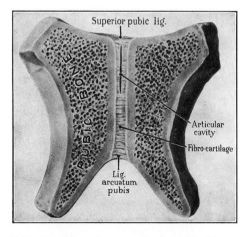

Figure 11-7. Frontal section symphysis pubis. Lig. arcuatum pubis = arcuate pubic ligament. (*From Spalteholz: Hand Atlas of Human Anatomy. Philadelphia, Lippincott, 1933, Vol 1.*)

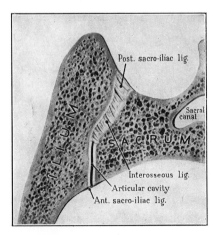

Figure 11-8. Sacroiliac synchondrosis. (*From Spalteholz: Hand Atlas of Human Anatomy. Philadelphia, Lippincott, 1933, Vol 1.*)

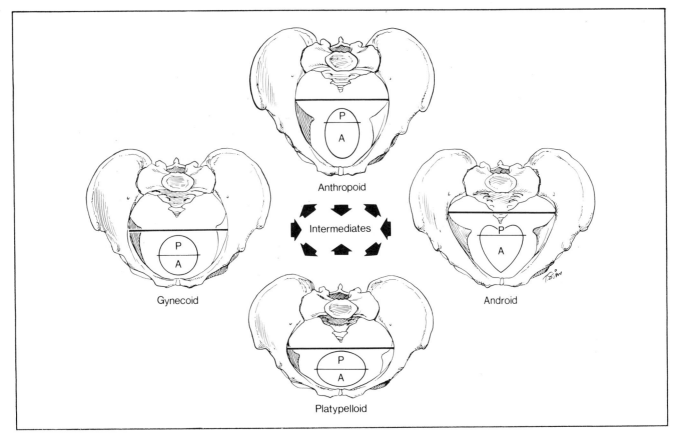

Figure 11-9. The four parent pelvic types. A line passing through the widest transverse diameter divides the inlet into posterior (P) and anterior (A) segments.

Walcher position. From results of roentgenologic studies, Young (1940) and Brill and Danielius (1941) showed clearly that no appreciable increase in pelvic size results from the Walcher position. The position is both useless and very uncomfortable for the mother.

The conversion of the pelvis of the fetus into the adult form, including sexual differences, is considered at the end of this chapter.

PELVIC SHAPES

In years past, when the *potential* hazards of diagnostic x-rays were not fully appreciated but the *real* and immediate risks of cesarean section were known, before antibiotics, x-ray pelvimetry was used with greater frequency in cases of suspected cephalopelvic disproportion or fetal malpresentation. During this same time period, pelvic roentgenography was used as an aid for understanding the general architecture or configuration of the pelvis, apart from its size. Caldwell and Moloy (1933) developed a classification of the pelvis according to shape that is now widely used. Familiarity with such a classification helps the physician to understand the mechanism of labor and to manage labor in pregnancies more intelligently with various types of pelvic contraction.

Caldwell–Moloy Classification

The shapes of posterior and anterior segments of the pelvic inlet are important determinants in this method of classification (Fig. 11-9). A line drawn through the greatest transverse diameter of the inlet divides the inlet into anterior and posterior segments. The character of the posterior segment determines the type of pelvis, and the character of the anterior segment determines the tendency. Many pelves are not pure but mixed types, as, for example, a gynecoid pelvis with android "tendency," meaning that the hindpelvis is gynecoid and the forepelvis is android.

Gynecoid Pelvis. This pelvis displays the anatomic characteristics ordinarily associated with the female pelvis. The posterior sagittal diameter of the inlet is only slightly shorter than the anterior sagittal. The sides of the posterior segment are well rounded, and the forepelvis is also well rounded and wide. Since the transverse diameter of the inlet is either slightly greater than or about the same as the anteroposterior diameter, the inlet in toto is either slightly oval or round. The side walls of the pelvis are straight, the spines are not prominent; the pubic arch is wide, with a transverse diameter at the ischial spines of 10 cm or more. The sacrum is inclined neither anteriorly nor posteriorly. The sacrosciatic notch is well rounded and never narrow. Caldwell and co-workers (1939) ascertained the frequency of the four parent types by study of Todd's collection of pelves. They found the gynecoid pelvis was the most common type, occurring in almost one-half.

Android Type. The posterior sagittal diameter at the inlet is much shorter than the anterior sagittal, limiting the use of the posterior space by the fetal head. The sides of the posterior segment are not rounded but tend to form, with the corresponding sides of the anterior segment, a wedge at their point of junction. The forepelvis is narrow and triangular. The side walls are usually convergent; the ischial spines are prominent; and the subpubic arch is narrowed. The bones are characteristically heavy. The sacrosciatic notch is narrow and high-arched. The sacrum is set forward in the pelvis and is usually straight, with little or no curvature, and the posterior sagittal diameter is decreased from inlet to outlet by the forward inclination. Not infrequently there is considerable forward inclination of the tip.

The extreme android pelvis presages a very poor prognosis for delivery through the vagina. The frequency of difficult forceps operations and stillbirths increases substantially when there is a small android pelvis. The android type makes up one third of pure-type pelves encountered in white women and one sixth in nonwhite women in the Todd collection.

Anthropoid Type. This pelvis is characterized by an anteroposterior diameter of the inlet greater than the transverse, forming more or less an oval anteroposteriorly, with the anterior segment somewhat narrow and pointed. The sacrosciatic notch is large. The side walls are often somewhat convergent, and the sacrum usually has six segments and is straight, making the anthropoid pelvis deeper than the other types.

The ischial spines are likely to be prominent. The subpubic arch is frequently somewhat narrow but well shaped. The anthropoid pelvis is said to be more common in nonwhite women, whereas the android form is more frequent in white women. Anthropoid types make up one fourth of pure-type pelves in white women, in comparison with nearly one half of nonwhite women.

Platypelloid Type. This pelvis is a flattened gynecoid pelvis, with a short anteroposterior and a wide transverse diameter. The latter is set well in front of the sacrum, as in the typical gynecoid form. The angle of the forepelvis is very wide, and the anterior puboiliac and posterior iliac portions of the iliopectineal lines are well curved. The sacrum is usually well curved and rotated backward. Thus, the sacrum is short and the pelvis shallow, creating a wide sacrosciatic notch. The platypelloid pelvis is the rarest of the pure varieties, occurring in less than 3 percent of women.

Intermediate Types. Intermediate or mixed types of pelves are much more frequent than pure types.

PELVIC SIZE AND ITS ESTIMATION

Diagonal Conjugate

In many abnormal pelves, the anteroposterior diameter of the pelvic inlet (the obstetric conjugate) is considerably shortened. It is therefore important to determine its length, but this measurement can be obtained only by roentgenographic techniques. However, the distance from the sacral promontory to the lower margin of the symphysis pubis (the diagonal conjugate) can be measured clinically (Figs. 11-10, 11-11, 11-12). *The diagonal conjugate measurement is most important, and every practitioner of obstetrics should be thoroughly familiar with the technique of its measurement and interpretation.*

For this purpose, the woman should be placed upon an examining table with her knees drawn up and her feet supported by suitable stirrups. If such an examination cannot be arranged conveniently, she should be brought to the edge of the bed, where a firm pillow should be placed beneath her buttocks. The examiner introduces two fingers into the vagina; before measuring the diagonal conjugate, the mobility of the coccyx is evaluated and the anterior surface of the sacrum is palpated. The mobility of the coccyx is tested by palpating it with the fingers in the vagina and attempting to move it to and fro. The anterior surface of the sacrum is then palpated methodically from below upward and its vertical and lateral curvatures are noted. In normal pelves, only the last three sacral vertebrae can be felt without indenting the perineum, whereas in markedly contracted varieties the entire anterior surface of the sacrum is usually readily accessible. Frequently, the mobility of the coccyx and the anatomic features of the lower sacrum may be defined more easily by rectal examination.

Except in extreme degrees of pelvic contraction, in order to reach the promontory of the sacrum, the elbow must be depressed and, unless the examiner's fingers are unusually long, the perineum forcibly indented by the knuckles of the examiner's third and fourth fingers. The index and the second fingers, held firmly together, are carried up and over the anterior surface of the sacrum, where, by sharply depressing the wrist, the promontory is felt by the tip of the second finger as a projecting bony margin at the base of the sacrum. With the finger closely applied to the most prominent portion of the upper sacrum, the vaginal hand is elevated until it contacts the pubic arch, and the immediately adjacent point on the index finger is marked, as shown in Figure 11-10. The hand is withdrawn and the distance between the mark and the tip of the second finger is measured. Because measurement using a pelvimeter often introduces an error of 0.5 to 1 cm, it is better to employ a rigid measuring scale attached to the wall, as shown in Figure 11-11. The diagonal conjugate is thus determined and the obstetric conjugate is computed by deducting 1.5 to 2.0 cm, depending upon the height and inclination of the symphysis pubis, as illustrated in Figure 11-12. If the diagonal conjugate is greater than 11.5 cm, it is justifiable to

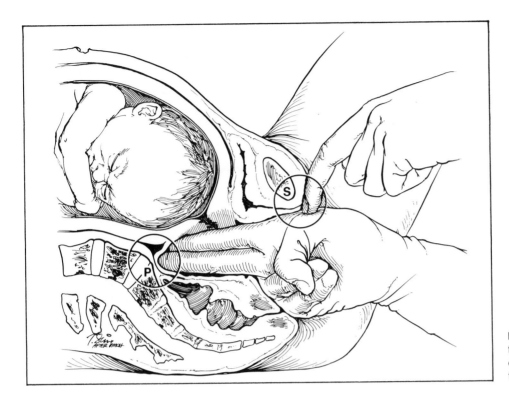

Figure 11-10. Vaginal examination to determine the diagonal conjugate (P = sacral promontory; S = symphysis pubis).

assume that the pelvic inlet is of adequate size for childbirth.

Objection to measurement of the diagonal conjugate is sometimes raised on the basis that it is painful to the patient. It probably causes mild momentary discomfort, but, if properly performed and deferred until the latter half of pregnancy when the distensibility of the vagina and perineum is greater, women object to it no more than to venipuncture.

Transverse contraction of the inlet can be measured only by x-ray pelvimetry. Transverse contractions may exist even in the presence of an adequate anteroposterior diameter.

Engagement. Engagement is the descent of the biparietal plane of the fetal head to a level below that of the pelvic inlet (Figs. 11-13, 11-14). In other words, when the biparietal or largest diameter of the normally flexed head has passed through the inlet, the head is engaged. Although engagement of the fetal head is usually regarded as a phenomenon of labor (and is discussed later in that connection), in nulliparas it commonly occurs during the last few weeks of pregnancy. When it does so, it is confirmatory evidence that the pelvic inlet is adequate for that particular fetal head. With engagement, the fetal head serves as an internal pelvimeter to demonstrate that the pelvic inlet is ample for that particular fetus.

Whether the head is engaged may be ascertained either by rectal or vaginal examination or by abdominal palpation. After gaining experience with vaginal examination, it becomes relatively easy to locate the station of the lowermost part of the fetal head in relation to the level of the ischial spines. If the lowest part of the occiput is at or below the level of the spines, the head is usually, but not always, engaged, since the distance from the plane of the pelvic inlet to the level of the ischial spines approximates 5 cm in most pelves, whereas the distance from the biparietal plane of the unmolded fetal head to the vertex is only about 3 to 4 cm. In these circumstances, the vertex cannot possibly reach the level of the spines unless the biparietal diameter has passed the inlet or unless there has been considerable elongation of the fetal head because of molding and formation of a caput succedaneum (see Chapter 16, p. 329).

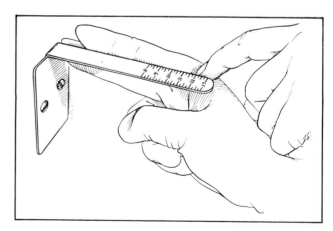

Figure 11-11. Metal scale fastened to wall for measuring the diagonal conjugate diameter as ascertained manually.

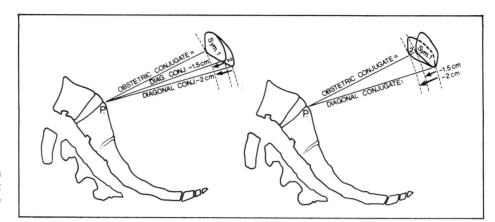

Figure 11-12. Variations in length of diagonal conjugate dependent on height and inclination of the symphysis pubis.

Engagement may be ascertained less satisfactorily by abdominal examination. If, in a mature infant the biparietal plane has descended through the inlet, that plane so completely fills the inlet that the examining fingers cannot reach the lowermost part of the head. Hence, when pushed downward over the lower abdomen, the examining fingers will slide over that portion of the head proximal to the biparietal plane (nape of the neck) and diverge. Conversely, if the head is not engaged, the examining fingers can easily palpate the lower part of the head and will hence converge (Chapter 12, p. 242).

Fixation of the fetal head is descent of the head through the pelvic inlet to a depth that prevents its free movement in any direction when pushed by both hands placed over the lower abdomen; it is not necessarily synonymous with engagement. Although a head that is freely movable on abdominal examination cannot be engaged, fixation of the head is sometimes seen when the biparietal plane is still a centimeter or more above the

pelvic inlet, especially if the head is molded appreciably.

Although engagement is conclusive evidence of an adequate pelvic inlet for the fetus concerned, its absence is by no means always indicative of pelvic contraction. For instance, in Bader's study (1936), labor was entirely normal in 87 percent of the 499 primigravidas with unengaged fetal heads at the onset of labor. Nevertheless, the incidence of contraction of the inlet is higher in this group than in the obstetric population at large.

Outlet Measurements. The other important dimension of the pelvis that is accessible for clinical measurement is the diameter between the ischial tuberosities, variously called the *biischial diameter,* the *intertuberous diameter,* and the *transverse diameter of the outlet.* With the woman in a lithotomy position, the measurement is made from the inner and lowermost aspect of the ischial tuberosities, as shown in Figure 11-15. A measurement of over 8 cm is considered to be normal.

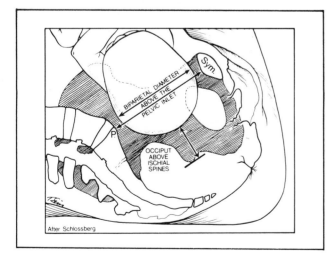

Figure 11-13. When the lowermost portion of the fetal head is above the ischial spines, the biparietal diameter of the head is not likely to have passed through the pelvic inlet and therefore is not engaged (P = sacral promontory; Sym = symphysis pubis).

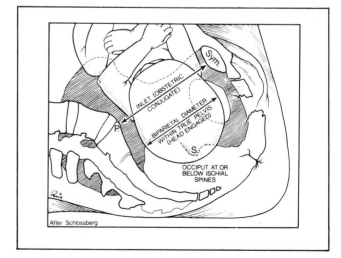

Figure 11-14. When the lowermost portion of the fetal head is at or below the ischial spines, it is usually engaged. Exceptions occur when there is considerable molding or caput formation, or both (P = sacral promontory; Sym = symphysis pubis; S = ischial spine).

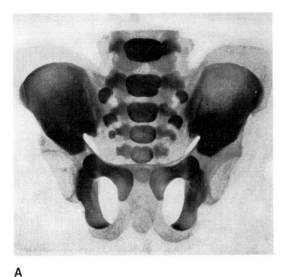

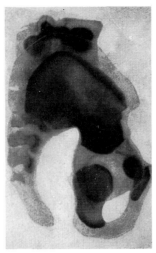

Figure 11-15. Fetal pelvis near term. Frontal (A) and lateral (B) views showing extent of ossification.

A   B

This measurement of the transverse diameter of the outlet can be estimated by placing the closed fist against the perineum between the ischial tuberosities after first measuring the width of the closed fist. Usually the closed fist is wider than 8 cm. The shape of the subpubic arch can be best appreciated if the pubic rami are palpated from the subpubic region to the ischial tuberosities.

Clinical Estimation of Midpelvic Size. Clinical estimation of midpelvic capacity by any direct form of measurement is not possible. If the ischial spines are quite prominent, or if the side walls of the pelvis are felt to converge, or if the concavity of the sacrum is very shallow, suspicion of contraction in this region is aroused, but only by roentgenologic studies can the midpelvis be precisely measured.

X-RAY PELVIMETRY

Status of X-Ray Pelvimetry

The prognosis for successful labor in any given case cannot be established on the basis of x-ray pelvimetry alone, since the pelvic capacity is but one of several factors that determine the outcome. As enumerated by Mengert (1948), there are at least five factors concerned: (1) size and shape of the bony pelvis, (2) size of the fetal head, (3) force of the uterine contractions, (4) moldability of the head, and (5) presentation and position of the fetus. Only the first of these factors is amenable to reasonably precise roentgenologic measurement, and it is the object of x-ray pelvimetry simply to eliminate this one factor from the category of the unknown. X-ray pelvimetry must therefore be regarded merely as an adjunct in the management of a pregnancy with a cephalic fetal presentation in which the mother is suspected of having a contracted pelvis. However, if a vaginal delivery is anticipated for a breech presentation (Chapter 30, p. 658), x-

ray pelvimetry still remains an accepted standard of care in many communities and medical centers (Collea and co-workers, 1980) as well as our own obstetric service.

X-ray pelvimetry has the following advantages over manual estimation of pelvic size:

1. It can provide precision to a degree of mensuration otherwise unobtainable. The clinical importance of such precision becomes evident when the shortcomings of the diagonal conjugate measurement are considered. When the diagonal conjugate exceeds 11.5 cm, the anteroposterior dimension of the inlet (the obstetric conjugate) is very rarely contracted. When the diagonal conjugate is under 11.5, however, it is not always a reliable index of the obstetric conjugate, since the difference between these two diameters, usually about 1.5 cm, may range from less than 1 to more than 2 cm. For example, two primigravidas may have diagonal conjugates of 10.5 cm, but in one the obstetric conjugates may be 10.2 cm and easy vaginal delivery follows, whereas in the other it may be 8.2 cm, in which case cesarean section is obligatory. Such information may prove critical during a breech delivery.
2. It can provide exact mensuration of two important diameters not otherwise obtainable, namely, the transverse diameter of the inlet and the interischial spinous diameter (transverse diameter of the midpelvis).

Indications for X-Ray Pelvimetry

Because of the expense involved, as well as potential radiologic hazards (p. 230), radiographic pelvic measurement is not necessary in the great majority of cases (Joyce and co-workers, 1975; Varner and associates, 1980; Radomsky and Radomsky, 1980; Laube and co-workers, 1981; Barton and colleagues, 1982; Anderson,

1983). There are, however, certain clinical circumstances that point to the probability of pelvic contraction or potential dystocia and may, at times, make x-ray pelvimetry a part of good obstetric practice. These include the following circumstances:

1. Previous injury or disease likely to affect the bony pelvis
2. Breech presentations in which vaginal delivery is anticipated

Before obtaining x-ray pelvimetry, it is essential to ask a singularly important question: "Is the information to be obtained likely to affect the subsequent management of labor and delivery?" If cesarean section almost certainly is going to be performed irrespective of the roentgenographic revelations, the use of x-ray pelvimetry is difficult to justify. At a time in the not too distant past, hospital accreditation agencies demonstrated great concern over cesarean section rates and insisted that consultation be obtained before carrying out cesarean section. Such a formal recommendation was almost unique to this surgical procedure. In these circumstances, the presence of an x-ray report perhaps generated the appearance of the obstetrician doing all that was possible before performing a cesarean section to protect the fetus from further deterioration in utero or from some form of birth trauma. Hopefully, there is no longer a need for this particular form of "defensive medicine."

HAZARDS OF DIAGNOSTIC RADIATION

An increasing awareness of the potential hazards of radiation has focused attention on the true value of diagnostic x-rays in obstetrics as compared with the potential damage to the mother, her fetus, and generations yet unborn. The recognized dangers to the fetus from diagnostic radiation are mutations and increased risk of malignancy later in life. Many, but not all, geneticists and radiobiologists believe, on the basis of animal experimentation, that the only entirely safe dose of irradiation is zero (Brent and Gordon, 1972; Gaulden, 1974).

TABLE 11-1. RISK OF LEUKEMIA AFTER RADIATION EXPOSURE IN UTERO FOR PELVIMETRY

	Approximate Risk Per First 10 Years	Relative Risk
U.S. white children (Control)	1:2800	1
In utero during x-ray pelvimetry	1:2000	1.5
Siblings of leukemic children	1:720	4
Identical twin of leukemic child	1:3	1000

TABLE 11-2. CHILDHOOD LEUKEMIA FOLLOWING ANTEPARTUM X-RAYS

Year	Author	Relative Risk	P
1958	Kaplan	1.37	NS*
1958	Stewart et al.	2.00	<0.05
1959	Murray et al	1.00	NS
1959	Ford et al.	1.66	<0.05
1959	Polhemus and Koch	1.34	<0.05
1960	Court Brown et al.	0.86	NS
1960	Lewis	0.42	NS
1961	Wells and Steer	0.72	NS
1962	McMahon	1.52	<0.05
1964	Gunz and Atkinson	1.13	NS
1965	Ager et al.	1.21	NS
1972	Bross and Natarajan	1.40	<0.05
1973	Diamond et al.	2.81	<0.05
1975	Bithell and Stewart	1.41	<0.05
1975	Oppenheim et al.	1.73	NS

* NS, not statistically significant.
(Adapted from Klapholz H: Evaluation of fetopelvic relationships. In Cohen WR, Friedman EA (eds): Management of Labor. Baltimore, University Park Press, 1983.)

The possibility of childhood malignancy was raised by the report of Stewart and associates in 1956, who identified an increase in leukemia in children of women x-rayed during pregnancy. Since then, there have been several more reports that are supportive of the thesis that diagnostic radiation absorbed by the fetus increases the risk of subsequent development of leukemia and other malignant conditions (Stewart and co-workers, 1958; MacMahon, 1962; Bithell and Stewart, 1975; and Kneale and Stewart, 1976). A comparison made by Brent (1974) of the apparent risk of leukemia developing in various groups with specific epidemiologic and pathologic characteristics is presented in Table 11-1. However, Oppenheim and associates (1975) point out that increased morbidity and mortality has not been identified uniformly among children exposed prenatally to diagnostic x-rays. If the mother underwent roentenographic examination because of a medical indication there was increased morbidity and mortality in the offspring compared to that found in offspring of women in whom the irradiation was routine, for example, with pelvimetry. Certainly not all investigators have reported a risk of leukemia developing in children whose mothers received antepartum x-rays (Table 11-2). *However, the slight risk from x-ray pelvimetry seems justifiable only whenever information critical to the welfare of the fetus or mother is likely to be obtained.*

The concept that x-ray pelvimetry should be limited has been endorsed by the American College of Radiology and American College of Obstetrics and Gynecology. Specifically, in 1979, the Bureau of Radiological Health of the Food and Drug Administration (1980) convened a panel composed of both radiologists and obstetricians to examine the available information on x-ray pelvimetry. A statement concerning the uses of such x-rays was developed and unanimously endorsed by the panel. This statement was adopted by the American College of Radiologists as written by the panel and is presented below (American College of Radiology Bulletin, 1979):

> Pelvimetry is not usually necessary or helpful in making the decision to perform a cesarean section. Therefore, pelvimetry should be performed only when the physician caring for the patient feels that pelvimetry will contribute to the decisions concerning diagnosis or treatment. In those few instances, the reason for requesting the pelvimetry should be written on the patient's chart. This statement does not apply to x-ray examinations for purposes other than measurement of the pelvis.

The following statement by the American College of Obstetricians and Gynecologists was published in the ACOG Newsletter (1979).

> X-ray pelvimetry provides limited additional information to physicians involved in the management of labor and delivery. It should not be a prerequisite to clinical decisions concerning obstetrical management. Reasons for requesting x-ray pelvimetry should be individually established.

Not only have recommendations been made to limit x-ray pelvimetry exposure but similar advice has been given to limit x-ray exposure to the pelvis of any woman at any time in the childbearing years.

In 1977, The American College of Obstetricians and Gynecologists, in cooperation with the American College of Radiology, issued a statement of policy in which the "Guidelines for Diagnostic X-ray Examination of Fertile Women" were enunciated. It was agreed that, "Attempts to schedule abdominal x-ray examinations in relation to a woman's menstrual cycle are of little value. The developing ovum is at risk prior to ovulation as well as subsequently. Thus it is erroneous to assume that any time is 'safer' for radiation exposure than another."

The recommended guidelines were as follows:

1. The use of x-ray examination should be considered on an individual basis. Concern over harmful effects should not prevent the proper use of radiation exposure when significant diagnostic information can be obtained. Preexamination consultation with a radiologist may be useful in obtaining optimal information from the x-ray exposure.
2. There is no measurable advantage to scheduling diagnostic x-ray examinations at any particular time during a normal menstrual cycle.
3. The degree of risk involved in an x-ray examination if the person is pregnant, or may become pregnant, should be explained to the patient and documented in her record.

SEXUAL DIFFERENCES IN THE ADULT PELVIS

The pelvis presents marked sexual differences. Generally, the pelvis of men is heavier, higher, and more conical than that of women. In men the muscular attachments are much more strongly marked, and the iliac bones flare less than in women. The pubic arch in men is more angular and presents an aperture of 70 to 75 degrees, as compared with 90 to 100 degrees in women. In men, the pelvic inlet is smaller and more nearly triangular, and the pelvic cavity is deeper and more conical; the sacrosciatic notch is narrower and the distance between the lower border of the sacrum and the ischial spine smaller than in the pelvis of women.

Pelvis of the Newborn Child

The mechanism by which the pelvis of the fetus is converted into the adult form is of interest since it affords important information about the mode of production of certain varieties of deformed pelves.

The pelvis of the child at birth is partly bony and partly cartilaginous (Fig. 11-15). The innominate bone does not exist as such but is represented by the ilium, ischium, and pubis, which are united by a large Y-shaped cartilage, the three bones meeting in the acetabulum. The iliac crests and the acetabula, as well as the greater part of the ischiopubic rami, are entirely cartilaginous.

The cartilaginous portions of the pelvis gradually give place to bone, but complete union in the acetabulum does not occur until about puberty, occasionally even later. The innominate bones may not, in fact, become completely ossified until between 20 and 25 years of age.

TRANSFORMATION OF THE FETAL INTO ADULT PELVIS

The evolution of the pelvic form is generally believed to involve two sets of factors: developmental and inherent tendencies, and mechanical influences. The process is not entirely the result of mechanical forces as manifested by the existence of sexual and racial differences in the adult pelvis. The mechanical influences that come into play after birth are identical in both sexes, but the sexual differences are, nevertheless, established during the pubertal process.

The part played by developmental and hereditary influences are demonstrated clearly by Litzmann (1861), who showed that the sacrum of women is markedly wider than that of men. At birth, in both sexes, the body of the first sacral vertebra is twice as broad as the alae (100 to 50), but in the adult the ratio becomes 100 to 76 in women, and 100 to 56 in men, indicating a much more rapid growth of the alae in women. Early investigators held that all the changes in the developing pelvis are similarly caused and that the influence of mechanical factors is merely accessory. The growth and development of that portion of the ilium forming the upper boundary of the great sacrosciatic notch profoundly affect the shape and size of the pelvic inlet.

Three mechanical forces are important in bringing about the final shape of the pelvis: body weight, the upward and inward pressure that is exerted by the heads of the femurs, and the cohesive force exerted by the symphysis pubis. So long as the child constantly remains in the recumbent position, these forces are not operative, but as soon as she sits up or walks, the body weight is transmitted through the vertebral column to the sacrum. Inasmuch as the center of gravity is anterior to the sacral promontory, the transmitted force is directed downward, and the other forward. Together the two tend to force the promontory of the sacrum downward and forward toward the symphysis pubis, a process that can be accomplished only by the sacrum rotating about its transverse axis. Its tip tends to become displaced both upward and backward. The strong sacrosciatic ligaments, however, resist this displacement and therefore permit only slight extension, with the result that the partly cartilaginous sacrum becomes bent upon itself just in front of its axis, that is, about the middle of its third vertebra, so that its anterior surface becomes markedly concave from above downward, instead of flat, as previously. At the same time, the body weight forces the bodies of the sacral vertebrae forward so that they project slightly beyond the alae, thereby diminishing the transverse concavity of the sacrum.

Since the anterior surface of the sacrum is wider than the posterior, the bone tends to sink into the pelvic cavity under the influence of the body weight and would prolapse into it completely were it not held in place by the strong posterior iliosacral ligaments that suspend it, as it were, from the posterior superior spines of the ilium. As the sacrum is pushed downward into the pelvic cavity, it exerts traction upon these ligaments, which in turn drag the posterior superior spines inward toward the midline and consequently tend to rotate the anterior portions of the innominate bones outward. Excessive outward rotation is prevented, however, partially by the cohesive force exerted at the symphysis but particularly by the upward and inward pressure exerted by the heads of the femurs. Practically, then, the iliac bone becomes converted into a two-armed lever, with the articular surface of the sacrum serving as a fulcrum; consequently, it bends at the point of least resistance, which is just anterior to the articulation, and thus gives the pelvis a greater transverse and a lesser anteroposterior diameter. At the same time, much of the transverse widening is more apparent than real and is caused by the relative shortening of the true conjugate by the downward and forward displacement of the promontory of the sacrum.

It is evident that the forces just mentioned must act in the same manner in the two sexes, so that whereas they may be important in the transformation of the fetal into the adult pelvis, they do not participate directly in the development of sexual differences in the adult pelvis.

The cohesive force exerted at the symphysis pubis cannot act alone, since it is manifested only when the force exerted by the body weight causes a tendency toward gaping of the pubic bones. The effect of the upward and inward force exerted by the femurs cannot act alone, since it comes into play only when it reacts against the body weight, nor has the action of the body weight alone ever been observed, though theoretically it might be noted in an individual presenting a split pelvis (congenital lack of union at the symphysis pubis) who has never walked. The action of the body weight, however, has been studied experimentally by Freund (1885), who suspended a cadaver by the iliac crests after cutting through the symphysis and found that the innominate bones gaped widely.

The effect of the combined action of the body weight and the force exerted by the femurs has been studied by Litzmann (1861) in persons with congenital absence of the symphysis pubis. In such circumstances, there is a marked transverse widening of the posterior portion of the pelvis, while the force exerted by the femurs causes the anterior portions of the innominate bones to become almost parallel.

The action of the body weight and the cohesive force exerted at the symphysis without the upward and inward pressure exerted by the femurs can be studied in individuals whose lower extremities are absent and occasionally in persons with congenital dislocation of the hips. Holst (1869) described a case in which the lower extremities were congenitally absent and the pelvis was characterized by a marked increase in width and a marked decrease in its anteroposterior diameter. Because of the excessive pressure exerted upon the tubera ischii in the absence of the counteracting force exerted by the femurs, the innominate bones are inwardly rotated so as to turn their crests inward and the tubera ischii outward, thus producing a considerable transverse widening of the inferior strait. More or less similar changes may be observed in cases of congenital dislocation of the hip in individuals who have never walked. The effect of the various mechanical influences is exaggerated in the pelves softened by diseases such as rickets and osteomalacia (see Chapter 31).

REFERENCES

Abramson D, Roberts SM, Wilson PD: Relaxation of the pelvic joints in pregnancy. Surg Obstet Gynecol 58:595, 1934

American College of Obstetricians and Gynecologists: Statement of Policy, "Guidelines for Diagnostic X-ray Examination of Fertile Women." Chicago, May, 1977

American College of Obstetricians and Gynecologists: ACOG Bull 23:10, 11:2, Oct/Nov 1979

American College of Radiology: ACR Bull 35(10):2, October 1979

Anderson N: X-ray pelvimetry: Helpful or harmful? J Fam Pract 17:405, 1983

Ager EA, Schuman LM, Wallace HM, Rosenfield AB, Gullen WH: An epidemiological study of childhood leukemia. J Chronic Dis 18:113, 1965

Bader A: The significance of the unengaged head in primiparous labor. Abstracted in Ber ges Gynak u Geburtsh 31:395, 1936

Barton JJ, Garvaciak JA Jr, Ryan GM: The efficacy of x-ray pelvimetry. Am J Obstet Gynecol 143:304, 1982

Bithell J, Stewart A: Prenatal irradiation and childhood malignancy: A review of British data from the Oxford Survey. Br J Cancer 31:271, 1975

Borell U, Fernstrom I: Movements at the sacroiliac joints and their importance to changes in pelvic dimensions during parturition. Acta Obstet Gynecol Scand 36:42, 1957

Brent RL: Comment and Table on Editorial Page 14. J Reprod Med 12:6, 1974

Brent RL, Gordon RO: Radiation exposure in pregnancy. Curr Probl Radiol 2:1, 1972

Brill HM, Danielius G: Roentgen pelvimetric analysis of Walcher's position. Am J Obstet Gynecol 42:821, 1941

Bross IDJ, Natarajan N: Leukemia from low level radiation. N Engl J Med 287:107, 1972

Budin RC: X-radiography of a Naegele pelvis. Obstetrique Par 2:499, 1897

Caldwell WE, Moloy HC: Anatomical variations in the female pelvis and their effect in labor with a suggested classification. Am J Obstet Gynecol 26:479, 1933

Caldwell WE, Moloy HC, D'Esopo DA: A roentgenologic study of the mechanism of engagement of the fetal head. Am J Obstet Gynecol 28:824, 1934

Caldwell WE, Moloy HC, Swenson PC: The use of the roentgen ray in obstetrics: I. Roentgen pelvimetry and cephalometry; technic of pelviroentgenography. Am J Roentgenol 41:305, 1939

Collea JV, Chein C, Quilligan EJ: The randomized management of term frank breech presentation: A study of 208 cases. Am J Obstet Gynecol 137:235, 1980

Court Brown WM, Doll R, Hill AB: Incidence of leukaemia after exposure to diagnostic x-ray in utero. Br Med J 2:1539, 1960

Diamond EL, Schmerler H, Lilienfeld AM: The relationship of intrauterine radiation to subsequent mortality and development of leukemia in children (a prospective study). Am J Epidemiol 97:283, 1973

Ford DD, Paterson JCS, Treuting WL: Fetal exposure to diagnostic x-rays and leukemia and other malignant disease in childhood. J Natl Cancer Inst 22:1903, 1959

Freund WA: On the so-called kyphotic pelvis. Gynaekol Klin Strassb I, 1, 1885

Gaulden ME: Possible effects of diagnostic X-rays on the human embryo and fetus. J Ark Med Soc 70:424, 1974

Gunz FW, Atkinson HR: Medical radiations and leukaemia: A retrospective survey. Br Med J 1:389, 1964

Holst: Description of the pelvis and the delivery of a 40-year-old female amelus. Holst's Beitrage, Hef. 2, pp 145–148, 1869

Joyce DN, Giwa-Sagie F, Stevenson GW: Role of pelvimetry in active management of labor. Br Med J 4:505, 1975

Kaplan HS: An evaluation of the somatic and genetic hazards of the medical uses of radiation. Am J Roentgenol Radium Ther Nucl 80:696, 1958

Klapholz H: Evaluation of fetopelvic relationships. In Cohen WR, Friedman EA (eds). Management of Labor. Baltimore, University Park Press, 1983, p 33

Kneale GW, Stewart AM: Mantel-Haenszel analysis of Oxford data. I. Independent effects of several birth factors including fetal irradiation. J Natl Cancer Inst 56:879, 1976

Laube DW, Varner MW, Cruikshank DP: A prospective evaluation of x-ray pelvimetry. JAMA 246:2187, 1981

Lewis TLT: Leukaemia in childhood after antenatal exposure to x-rays (a survey at Queen Charlotte's Hospital.) Br Med J 2:1551, 1960

Litzmann CCT: Die Formen des Beckens. Berlin, G Reimer, 1861

McMahon B: Prenatal x-ray exposure and childhood cancer. J Natl Cancer Inst 28:1173, 1962

Mengert WF: Estimation of pelvic capacity. JAMA 138:169, 1948

Murray R, Heckel P, Hempelmann LH: Leukemia in children exposed to ionizing radiation. N Engl J Med 261:585, 1959

Oppenheim BE, Griem ML, Meier P: The effects of diagnostic x-ray exposure on the human fetus: An examination of the evidence. Radiology 114:529, 1975

Polhemus DW, Koch R: Leukemia and medical radiation. Pediatrics 23:453, 1959

Radomsky JW, Radomsky NA: Efficacy of pelvimetry. J Can Med Assoc 31:43, 1980

Stewart A, Webb J, Giles D, Hewitt D: Malignant disease in childhood and diagnostic irradiation in utero. Lancet 2:447, 1956

Stewart A, Webb J, Hewitt D: A survey of childhood malignancies. Br Med J 1:1495, 1958

U.S. Department of Health and Human Resources: The selection of patients for x-ray examinations: The pelvimetry examination. HHS Pub (FDA) 80-8128, July, 1980

Varner MW, Cruikshank DP, Laube DW: X-ray pelvimetry in clinical obstetrics. Obstet Gynecol 56:296, 1980

Wells J, Steer CM: Relationship of leukemia in children to abdominal radiation of mothers during pregnancy. Am J Obstet Gynecol 81:1059, 1961

Young J: Relaxation of pelvic joints in pregnancy: Pelvic arthropathy of pregnancy. Br J Obstet Gynaecol 47:493, 1940

12
Presentation, Position, Attitude, and Lie of the Fetus

Fetal Posture

In the later months of pregnancy the fetus assumes a characteristic posture sometimes described as *attitude* or *habitus* (Fig. 12-1). As a rule, the fetus forms an ovoid mass that corresponds roughly to the shape of the uterine cavity. The fetus becomes folded or bent upon itself in such a manner that the back becomes markedly convex; the head is sharply flexed so that the chin is almost in contact with the chest; the thighs are flexed over the abdomen; the legs are bent at the knees; and the arches of the feet rest upon the anterior surfaces of the legs. Usually the arms are crossed over the thorax or become parallel to the sides, and the umbilical cord lies in the space between them and the lower extremities. This characteristic posture results partly from the mode of growth of the fetus and partly from a process of accommodation to the uterine cavity.

Lie of the Fetus

The lie is the relation of the long axis of the fetus to that of the mother and is either *longitudinal* or *transverse*. Occasionally, the fetal and the maternal axes may cross at a 45 degree angle, forming an *oblique* lie, which is unstable and always becomes longitudinal or transverse during the course of labor. Longitudinal lies are present in over 99 percent of labors at term.

Presentation and Presenting Part

The presenting part is that portion of the body of the fetus that is either foremost within the birth canal or in closest proximity to it; that is, the presenting part is that portion of the fetus that is felt through the cervix on vaginal examination. The presenting part determines the presentation. Accordingly, in longitudinal lies, the presenting part is either the fetal head or the breech, creating cephalic and breech presentations, respectively. When the fetus lies with the long axis transversely, the shoulder is the presenting part. Thus, a shoulder presentation is felt through the cervix on vaginal examination.

Cephalic presentations are classified according to the relation of the head to the body of the fetus (Fig. 12-1). Ordinarily, the head is flexed sharply so that the chin is in contact with the thorax. In this circumstance, the occipital fontanel is the presenting part, although such a presentation is usually referred to as a *vertex* or *occiput presentation*. (The vertex actually lies just in front of the occipital fontanel, and the occiput just behind the fontanel, as illustrated in Figure 8-8.) Much less commonly, the fetal neck may be sharply extended so that the occiput and back come in contact and the face is foremost in the birth canal (*face presentation*). The fetal head may assume a position between these extremes, partially flexed in some cases, with the anterior (large) fontanel, or bregma, presenting (*sinciput presentation*), or partially extended in other cases, with the brow presenting (*brow presentation*). Perhaps the latter two should not be classified as distinct presentations, since these are usually transient. As labor progresses, sinciput and brow presentations are almost always converted into vertex or face presentations by flexion or extension, respectively.

When the fetus presents as a breech, the thighs may be flexed and the legs extended over the anterior surfaces of the body (*frank breech presentation*) (Fig. 12-2), or the thighs may be flexed on the abdomen and the legs upon the thighs (*complete breech presentation*) (Fig. 12-3), and one or both feet, or one or both knees, are lowermost (*incomplete* or *footling breech presentation*) (Fig. 12-4).

Position

Position refers to the relation of an arbitrarily chosen portion of the presenting part of the fetus to the right or left side of the maternal birth canal. Accordingly, with each presentation there may be two positions, right or left. The occiput, chin, and sacrum are the determining points in vertex, face and breech presentations, respectively (Figs. 12-5, 12-6, 12-7, 12-8).

Variety. For still more accurate orientation, the relation of a given portion of the presenting part to the anterior, transverse, or posterior portion of the mother's pelvis is considered. Since there are two positions, it follows that there must be six varieties for each presentation (Figs. 12-5, 12-6, 12-7, 12-8).

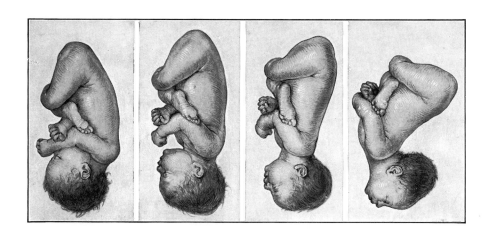

Figure 12-1. Differences in attitude of fetus in vertex, sinciput, brow, and face presentations.

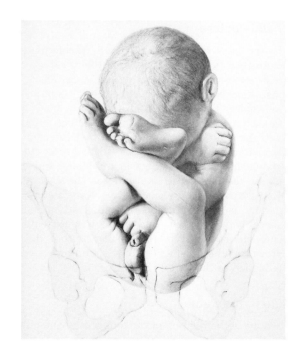

Figure 12-2. Frank breech presentation.

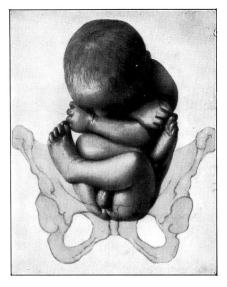

Figure 12-3. Complete breech presentation.

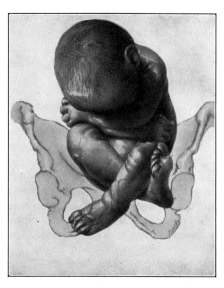

Figure 12-4. Incomplete breech presentation.

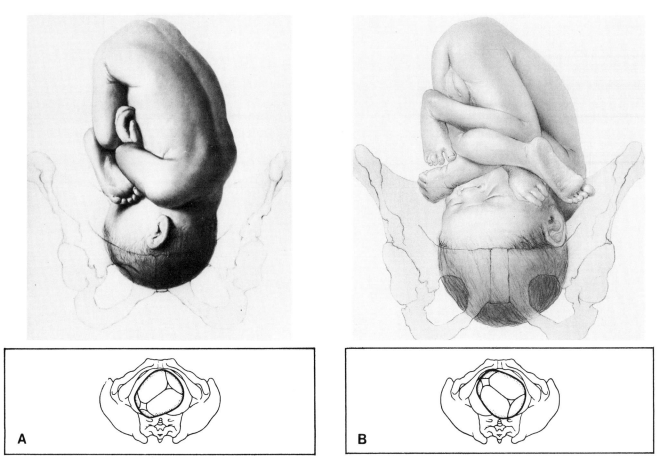

Figure 12-5. Vertex presentation: **A.** Left Occipito-Anterior. **B.** Left Occipito-Posterior.

Nomenclature. Since the presenting part in any presentation may be in either the left or right position, there are left and right occipital, left and right mental, and left and right sacral presentations, which are abbreviated as LO and RO, LM and RM, LS and RS, respectively. Since the presenting part in each of the two positions may be directed anteriorly (A), transversely (T), or posteriorly (P), there are six varieties of each of these three presentations (Figs. 12-5, 12-6, 12-7, 12-8).

In shoulder presentations, the acromion (or the scapula) is the portion of the fetus arbitrarily chosen to orient it with the maternal pelvis. One example of the terminology sometimes employed for the purpose is illustrated in Figure 12-9. The acromion or back of the fetus may be directed either posteriorly or anteriorly and superiorly or inferiorly (see Chapter 30, p. 664). However, since it is impossible to differentiate exactly the several varieties of shoulder presentation by clinical examination and since such differentiation serves no practical purpose, it is customary to refer to all transverse lies of the fetus simply as shoulder presentations.

Frequency of the Various Presentations and Positions. At or near term, the incidence of the various presentations is approximately as follows: vertex, 96 percent; breech, 3.5 percent; face, 0.3 percent; shoulder, 0.4 percent. About two thirds of all vertex presentations are in the left occiput position, and one third in the right.

Although the incidence of breech presentation is only a little over 3 percent at term, it is much greater earlier in pregnancy. White (1956) found the incidence of breech presentation to be 7.2 percent by x-ray examination at the end of the 34th week. A similar frequency was identified sonographically in 1976 by Scheer and Nubar (see Table 30-1). Subsequently, in about one third of nulliparas and two thirds of multiparas, the breech converted to vertex spontaneously before delivery.

Reasons for the Predominance of Cephalic Presentations. Of the several reasons that have been advanced to explain why the fetus at term usually presents by the vertex, the most logical explanation seems to be that this is because the uterus is piriform shaped. Although the fetal head at term is slightly larger than the breech, the entire podalic pole of the fetus, that is, the breech and its flexed extremities, is bulkier than the cephalic pole and more movable. The cephalic pole is comprised of the fetal head only, because the upper extremities are removed some distance, are small, and are less protruding

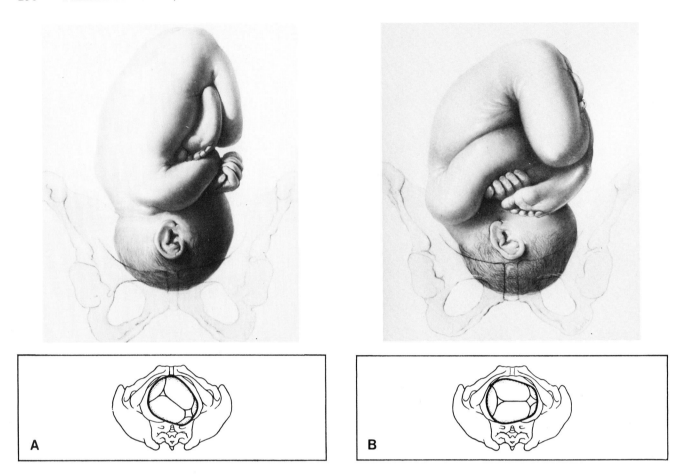

Figure 12-6. Vertex presentation: **A.** Right Occipito-Anterior. **B.** Right Occipito-Transverse.

than the buttocks and lower extremities combined. Until about the 32nd week, the amnionic cavity is large compared to the fetal mass, and there is no crowding of the fetus by the uterine walls. At approximately this time, however, the ratio of amnionic fluid volume to fetal mass becomes altered by relative diminution of amnionic fluid and by increasing fetal size. As a result, the uterine walls are apposed more closely to the fetal parts, and then the fetal lie is more nearly dependent upon the piriform shape of the uterus. The fetus, if presenting by the breech, often changes polarity in order to make use of the roomier fundus for its bulkier and more movable podalic pole. The high incidence of breech presentation in hydrocephalic fetuses is in accord with this theory, since in this circumstance the cephalic pole of the fetus is definitely larger than the podalic pole. However, the fetus need not be alive late in pregnancy for polarity to change (Chapter 30, p. 651).

The cause of breech presentation may be some circumstance that prevents normal version from taking place, for example, a septum that protrudes into the uterine cavity. A peculiarity of fetal attitude, particularly extension of the vertebral column as occurs in frank breeches, also may prevent the fetus from turning.

DIAGNOSIS OF PRESENTATION AND POSITION OF THE FETUS

There are several diagnostic methods that can be used: abdominal palpation, vaginal palpation, combined examination, auscultation, and, in certain doubtful cases, ultrasonography or roentgenography.

Obstetric Palpation

In order to obtain satisfactory results, the examination should be conducted systematically employing the four maneuvers suggested by Leopold and Sporlin (1894). The mother should be on a firm bed or examining table, with her abdomen bared. During the first three maneuvers, the examiner stands at the side of the bed more convenient to him and faces the patient, but he reverses his position and faces her feet for the last maneuver (Fig. 12-10).

First Maneuver. After outlining the contour of the uterus and ascertaining how nearly the fundus approaches the xiphoid cartilage, the examiner gently palpates the fundus with the tips of the fingers of both

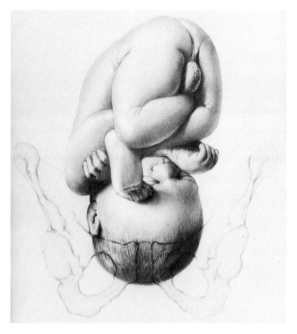

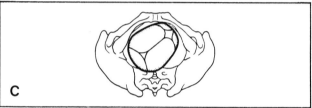

C

Figure 12-6. Vertex presentation: **C.** Right Occipito-Posterior.

hands in order to define which fetal pole is present in the fundus. The fetal breech gives the sensation of a large, nodular body, whereas the head feels hard and round and is more freely movable and ballottable.

Second Maneuver. Having determined which pole of the fetus lies in the fundus, the palms of the examiner's hands are placed on either side of the abdomen and gentle but deep pressure is exerted. On one side, a hard resistant structure is felt, the back, and on the other, numerous nodulations, the small parts. In pregnant women with thin abdominal walls, the fetal extremities can be differentiated readily, but in obese women only irregular nodulations can be felt. In the presence of obesity or considerable amnionic fluid, the back is felt more easily by making deep pressure with one hand while palpating with the other. By next noting whether the back is directed anteriorly, transversely, or posteriorly, a more accurate picture of the orientation of the fetus is obtained.

Third Maneuver. Employing the thumb and fingers of one hand, the examiner grasps the lower portion of the maternal abdomen, just above the symphysis pubis. If the presenting part is not engaged, a movable body will be felt, usually the fetal head. The differentiation between head and breech is made as in the first maneuver. If the presenting part is not engaged, the examination is almost complete; with the location of the fetal head, breech, back, and extremities known, all that remains to be defined is the attitude of the head. If by careful palpation it can be shown that the cephalic prominence is on the same side as the small parts, the head must be

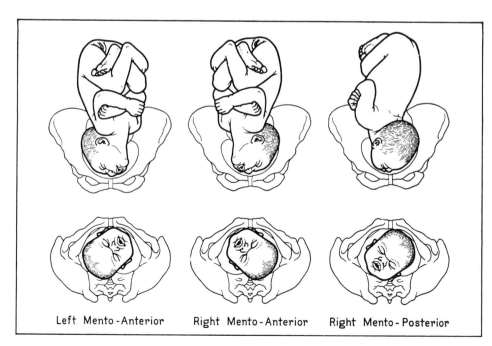

Left Mento-Anterior   Right Mento-Anterior   Right Mento-Posterior

Figure 12-7. Face presentation: Right and left, anterior and posterior positions.

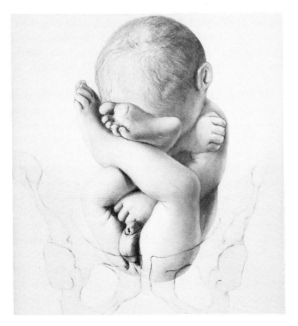

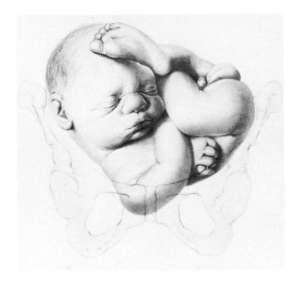

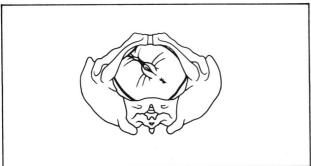

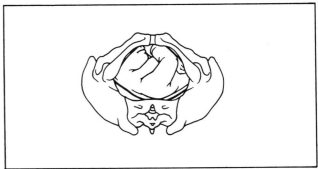

Figure 12-8. Breech presentation: Left sacrum posterior position.

Figure 12-9. Right acromiodorsoposterior (RADP) position. The shoulder of the fetus is to the mother's right, and the back is posterior.

flexed, and therefore the vertex is the presenting part. When the cephalic prominence of the fetus is on the same side as the back, the head must be extended. However, if the presenting part is deeply engaged, the findings from this maneuver are simply indicative of the fact that the lower pole of the fetus is fixed in the pelvis; the details are then defined by the last (fourth) maneuver.

Fourth Maneuver. The examiner faces the mother's feet and, with the tips of the first three fingers of each hand, makes deep pressure in the direction of the axis of the pelvic inlet. If the head presents, one hand is arrested sooner than the other by a rounded body, the cephalic prominence, while the other hand descends more deeply into the pelvis. In vertex presentations, the prominence is on the same side as the small parts, and in face presentations, on the same side as the back. The ease with which the prominence is felt is indicative of the extent to which descent has occurred. In many in-

stances, when the fetal head has descended into the pelvis, the anterior shoulder of the fetus may be differentiated readily by the third maneuver. In breech presentations, the information obtained from this maneuver is less precise.

Abdominal palpation can be performed throughout the latter months of pregnancy and during the intervals between the contractions of labor. The findings provide information about the presentation and position of the fetus and the extent to which the presenting part has descended into the pelvis. For example, so long as the cephalic prominence is readily palpable, the vertex has not descended to the level of the ischial spines. The degree of cephalopelvic disproportion, moreover, can be gauged by evaluating the extent to which the anterior portion of the fetal head overrides the mother's symphysis pubis. With experience, it is possible to estimate the size of the fetus and even to map out the presentation of the second fetus in a twin gestation.

During labor, palpation also may provide informa-

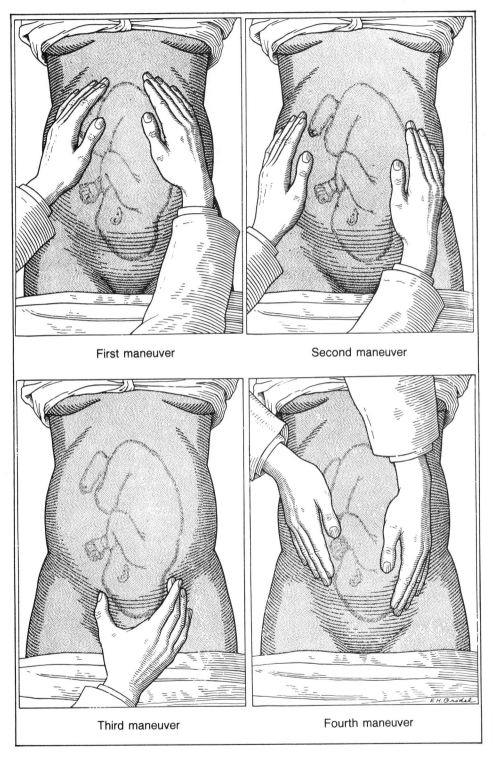

First maneuver

Second maneuver

Third maneuver

Fourth maneuver

E.H.Brödel

Figure 12-10. Palpation in left occiput anterior position (maneuvers of Leopold).

tion about the lower uterine segment. When there is obstruction to the passage of the fetus, a pathologic retraction ring sometimes may be felt as a transverse or oblique ridge extending across the lower portion of the uterus (see Chapter 29, p. 648). Moreover, even in normal cases, the contracting body of the uterus and the passive lower uterine segment may be distinguished by palpation. During a contraction, the upper portion of the uterus is firm or hard, whereas the lower segment feels elastic or almost fluctuant.

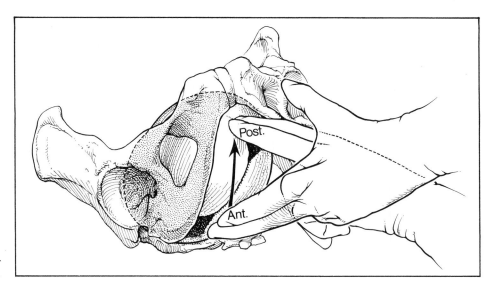

Figure 12-11. Locating the sagittal suture on vaginal examination.

Vaginal Examination

Before labor, the diagnosis of fetal presentation and position by vaginal examination may be somewhat inconclusive, because the presenting part must be palpated through the closed cervix and lower uterine segment. During labor, however, after dilatation of the cervix, important information may be obtained. In vertex presentations, the position and variety are recognized by differentiation of the various sutures and fontanels; in face presentations, by the differentiation of the portions of the face; and in breech presentations, by the palpation of the sacrum and ischial tuberosities.

In attempting to determine presentation and position by vaginal examination, it is advisable to pursue a definite routine, comprised of three maneuvers (Figs. 12-11, 12-12).

1. After the woman is prepared appropriately, as described in Chapter 17, two fingers of either gloved hand of the examiner are introduced into the vagina and carried up to the presenting part. The differentiation of vertex, face, and breech then is accomplished readily.
2. If the vertex is presenting, the examiner's fingers are introduced into the posterior aspect of the vagina. The fingers are then swept forward over the fetal head toward the maternal symphysis (Fig. 12-11). During the performance of this movement, the examiner's fingers necessarily cross the sagittal suture. When it is felt, its course is outlined, with small and large fontanels at the opposite ends.
3. The positions of the two fontanels then are ascertained. The examiner's fingers are passed to the anterior extremity of the sagittal suture, and the fontanel encountered there is examined carefully and identified; then by a circular motion, the fingers are passed around the side of the head

until the other fontanel is felt and differentiated (Fig. 12-12).

Using these three maneuvers, the various sutures and fontanels are located readily, and the possibility of error is lessened considerably. In face and breech presentations, errors are minimized, since the various parts are distinguished more readily.

Auscultation

Auscultation, by itself, does not provide very reliable information concerning the presentation and position of the fetus, but the findings of auscultation sometimes reinforce the results obtained by palpation. Ordinarily, the fetal heart sounds are transmitted through the convex portion of the fetus that lies in intimate contact with the uterine wall. Therefore, fetal heart sounds are heard best through the fetal back in vertex and breech presentations and through the fetal thorax in face presentations. The region of the abdomen in which the fetal heart tones are heard most clearly varies according to the presentation and the extent to which the presenting part has descended. In cephalic presentations, the point of maximal intensity of fetal heart sounds is usually midway between the maternal umbilicus and the anterior superior spine of her ilium, whereas in breech presentations it is usually about level with the umbilicus. In occipitoanterior positions, the heart sounds usually are heard best a short distance from the midline, in the transverse varieties they are heard more laterally, and in the posterior varieties well back in the mother's flank.

Sonography

Improvements in ultrasonographic technique have provided another diagnostic aid of particular value in doubtful cases. In obese women or in women whose abdominal walls are rigid, a sonographic examination may

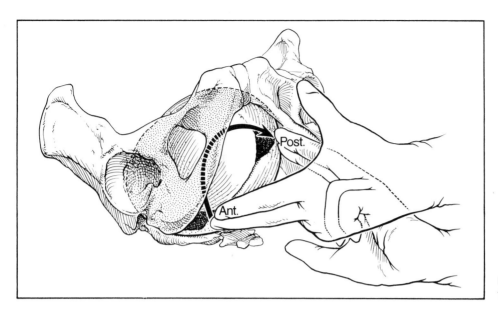

Figure 12-12. Differentiating the fontanels on vaginal examination.

provide information to solve many diagnostic problems and lead to early recognition of a breech or shoulder presentation that might otherwise have escaped detection until late in labor. Employing ultrasonography, the fetal head and body can be located without the potential hazards of radiation (see Chapter 14, p. 278). On some occasions, however, the information obtained roentgenographically far exceeds the minimal risk from a single diagnostic x-ray exposure.

REFERENCES

Leopold, Sporlin: Conduct of normal births through external examination alone. Arch Gynaekol 45:337, 1894

Scheer K, Nubar J: Variation of fetal presentation with gestational age. Am J Obstet Gynecol 125:269, 1976

White AJ: Spontaneous cephalic version in the later weeks of pregnancy and its significance in the management of breech presentation. Br J Obstet Gynaecol 63:706, 1956

13
Prenatal Care

The objective of prenatal care is to assure that every wanted pregnancy culminates in the delivery of a healthy baby without impairing the health of the mother.

Significance

Before the rise of modern obstetrics, the pregnant woman usually had but a single antepartum interview with a physician. At that interview, often not much more was accomplished than an attempt to anticipate the date of delivery. When next seen by the physician, the woman might be in the throes of an eclamptic convulsion, or suffering severe chills and high fever from pyelonephritis, or struggling to expel a very large but dead fetus. Appropriate antepartum care has proven to be of great value in the prevention of such catastrophes.

It hardly needs saying that prenatal care should do no harm. Nonetheless, prenatal care, at times, has been a two-edged sword. Instead of improving pregnancy outcome, on occasion, the exact opposite was brought about in a variety of ways, including inappropriate dietary advice to achieve rigid weight restriction, the unnecessary prescription of potentially dangerous drugs such as powerful diuretics, and the failure to encourage the immediate reporting of an abnormal event, but rather allowing the expectant mother to wait to do so at the next scheduled office or clinic visit.

A priori pregnancy should be considered a normal physiologic state. Unfortunately, the complexity of the functional and anatomic changes that accompany gestation tends in the minds of some to stigmatize normal pregnancy as a disease process. For example, a hemoglobin concentration of 10.5 g/dl is abnormally low for the woman who is not pregnant, but not if she is late in the second trimester of pregnancy; a plasma thyroxine level of 16 μg/dl is normal during pregnancy but is very strongly suggestive of hyperthyroidism in the absence of pregnancy unless the woman is receiving exogenous estrogen. At times, pregnancy imposes other changes that when modest in degree are normal, but when more intense are decidedly abnormal. An example, edema of the feet and ankles after ambulation, is the normal consequence of regional physical forces imposed by the large pregnant uterus and by gravity. Generalized edema obvious in the face, hands, and abdomen, however, is definitely abnormal. It is essential for the physician who assumes responsibility for prenatal care to be very familiar with the changes in normalities as well as abnormalities imposed by pregnancy.

Good prenatal care is vital for the accomplishment of the objective stated at the outset, namely, the delivery of a healthy baby from a healthy mother. An attempt has been made in this chapter to delineate many of the ingredients essential to good prenatal care. **Bad prenatal care may be worse than none.** All too often, inappropriate prenatal care provides the expectant mother with an unwarranted sense of security that allows her to ignore signs and symptoms for which, if left to her own instincts, she would have urgently sought advice.

General Health Care

Systematic health care beginning long before pregnancy undoubtedly proves quite beneficial to the physical and emotional well-being of the mother-to-be and, in turn, her child-to-be. Therefore, prenatal care ideally should be a continuation of a regimen of physician-supervised health care already established for the woman. As the consequence of such a program, acquired diseases and developmental abnormalities, for the most part, will have been recognized before pregnancy and appropriate steps taken to eradicate them or, at least, to minimize their deleterious effects. For example, women with diabetes can and should be advised of the probable benefits for the embryo-fetus to be achieved from near normalization of blood glucose levels before conception (Chapter 28, p. 604). In any event, the mother should be evaluated as early in pregnancy as possible and at appropriate intervals thereafter.

TERMINOLOGY

Definitions

- A *nulligravida* is a woman who is not now and never has been pregnant.
- A *gravida* is a woman who is or has been pregnant irrespective of the pregnancy outcome. With the establishment of the first pregnancy, she be-

comes a primigravida and with successive pregnancies a multigravida.

- A *nullipara* is a woman who has never completed a pregnancy beyond an abortion. She may or may not have aborted previously.
- A *primipara* is a woman who has been delivered once of a fetus or fetuses who reached the stage of viability. Therefore, the completion of any pregnancy beyond the stage of abortion (see Chapter 24, p. 467) bestows parity upon the mother.
- A *multipara* is a woman who has completed two or more pregnancies to the stage of viability. It is the number of pregnancies reaching viability and not the number of fetuses delivered that determines *parity*. Parity is not greater if a single fetus, twins, or quintuplets were delivered, nor fewer if the fetus or fetuses were stillborn.

In certain clinics, it is customary to summarize the past obstetric history of a woman by a series of digits connected by dashes as follows: 6-1-2-6. The first digit refers to the number of term infants, the second to the number of premature infants, the third to the number of abortions, and the fourth to the number of children currently alive. For the example given of 6-1-2-6, the woman has had six term deliveries, one premature delivery, two abortions, and has six children alive at present. This series of digits serves to summarize the obstetric history somewhat better than does the designation *gravida 9, para 7, abortus 2* only when the recipient of the information understands the code.

- A *parturient* is a woman in labor.
- A *puerpera* is a woman who has just given birth.

Normal Duration of Pregnancy

The mean duration of pregnancy calculated from the first day of the last normal menstrual period for a large number of healthy women has been identified to be very close to 280 days, or 40 weeks. Three studies are cited: Kortenoever (1950), in an analysis of 7504 pregnancies, found the average duration to be 282 days. A mean value of 281 days was calculated from the data of the Obstetrical Statistical Cooperative for 77,300 women who underwent spontaneous labor and whose infants weighed at least 2500 g. Nakano (1972) identified for 5596 pregnancies in Osaka, Japan, the mean duration to be 279 days from the first day of the last menstrual period with two standard deviations of ± 17 days. All pregnancies that terminated before 28 weeks gestation were excluded by Nakano, as were breeches and multiple fetuses.

It is customary to estimate the expected date of delivery by adding 7 days to the date of the first day of the last normal menstrual period and counting back 3 months (Naegele's rule). For example, if the woman's last menstrual period began on September 10, the expected date of delivery would be June 17. It is apparent that pregnancy is considered erroneously to have begun about 2 weeks before ovulation if the duration of pregnancy is so calculated from the first day of the last menstrual period. Nonetheless, clinicians persist in using *gestational age* or *menstrual age,* calculated from the first day of the last menstrual period to identify temporal events in pregnancy; embryologists and other reproductive biologists more often employ *ovulatory age,* or *fertilization age,* both of which are typically 2 weeks shorter.

It has become customary to divide pregnancy into three equal parts, or *trimesters,* of slightly more than 13 weeks, or 3 calendar months, each. There are certain major obstetric problems that cluster in each of these time periods. For example, most spontaneous abortions occur during the first trimester, whereas practically all cases of pregnancy-induced hypertension become clinically evident during the third trimester. However, it is no longer true that no infant will survive if born earlier than the third trimester.

The clinical use of trimesters to describe the duration of a specific pregnancy fosters imprecision and should be abandoned. It is inappropriate in case of uterine hemorrhage, as an example, to categorize the problem temporally as "third trimester bleeding." Appropriate management for the mother and her fetus will vary remarkably, depending upon whether the bleeding occurs early or late in the third trimester. *Precise knowledge of the age of the fetus is imperative for ideal obstetric management!* Therefore, expert attention must be given to this important measurement. The clinically appropriate unit of measure is *Weeks of Gestation Completed.*

GENERAL PROCEDURES

Every word and every act by all who come in contact with the pregnant woman should impress upon her both the importance and the availability of prenatal care for her fetus and herself. All too often, especially in public clinics, the strong impression has been propagated that such care is not really available without great expenditure of physical and emotional effort by her, and, too often, of money beyond her ability to pay. It is tragic when women and their fetuses are denied adequate prenatal care simply because of lack of funds. Over and above the humanitarian aspects, the cost for good prenatal care is modest compared to the expense of caring subsequently for serious, but preventable, complications in the mother, her fetus-infant, or both. For example, at Parkland Memorial Hospital not only is the frequency of low-birth-weight infants much higher for pregnancies without prenatal care, but also the cost of caring for the newborn without prenatal care on average is nearly doubled (K. Leveno, personal communication).

It is also unfortunate that, among those who in one way or another come in contact with the pregnant woman who seeks prenatal care, there may be some who display an intolerance for the poor, for the unwed, and for the mother's particular ethnic group. In such circumstances, the best of medical care may go to waste.

Initial Care

Prenatal care should be initiated as soon as there is reasonable likelihood of pregnancy. This may be as early as a few days after a missed menstrual period, especially for the woman who desires an abortion, but it should be no later than the second missed period for anyone.

In order to initiate antepartum care early, a system was developed at Parkland Memorial Hospital that has, in general, proved effective. The woman is seen for initial screening any day of the week without an appointment. At this initial visit nurses with expertness in obstetric care identify the following: (1) the probability of pregnancy (including urine testing for human chorionic gonadotropin when indicated), (2) the woman's desire for the pregnancy to continue, (3) any current health problems, (4) any previous major illnesses, including those in previous pregnancies, (5) the outcomes of previous pregnancies, and (6) all medications being used. The woman is instructed to bring with her at the next visit a few days later all drugs that she has been taking.

Physical evaluation initiated at the initial screening visit by the nurse includes determination of blood pressure, height, and weight.

The following laboratory examinations are initiated at the first visit:

- *Blood:* Hemoglobin, hematocrit, red cell indexes, white blood cell count, platelet count, serologic test for syphilis, identification of blood types and of abnormal antibodies to red cell antigens, and presence of antibody to rubella.
- *Urine:* Glucose, protein, and quantitative culture of clean catch midstream urine to identify significant bacteriuria.

Physicians are continually available in the clinic and are consulted by the nurse whenever a problem is suspected that might require immediate attention. Any woman who is considering abortion is seen by a physician at this time. Moreover, every woman is asked specifically if she wishes to see a physician at this screening visit. Finally, she is given explicit instructions as to how to get help promptly in case a problem develops.

It is difficult to convince the pregnant woman of the importance of prenatal care if, when she seeks it, the physician delays for many weeks her initial care! Even in the absence of identified pregnancy problems, all women are given appointments within 10 days, for completion by a physician of a comprehensive general health evaluation as described below. Previous health records and laboratory data are reviewed at that time.

INITIAL COMPREHENSIVE EVALUATION

Goals

The major goals are (1) to define the health status of the mother and fetus, (2) to determine the gestational age of the fetus, and (3) to initiate a plan for continuing obstetric care. Once the health status of the mother and fetus has been defined, the initial plan for subsequent care may range from relatively infrequent routine visits to

either prompt therapeutic abortion or prolonged hospitalization because of serious maternal or fetal disease.

History. For the most part, the same essentials go into appropriate history taking from the pregnant woman as elsewhere in medicine. The history should be obtained unhurriedly in a reasonably private setting. This is the best time for the physician and for those who assist in providing care for the expectant mother and her fetus to establish the good rapport so necessary for a successful outcome for the pregnancy. Although it is undesirable for the woman to wait for protracted periods of time before interview, it is worse for her to be hurriedly and indifferently interrogated without having her answers appropriately evaluated. **It is mandatory that all data important to the care of the mother and fetus be clearly recorded so that all members of the health care team who use the record can correctly interpret them.**

The *menstrual history* is extremely important. The woman who spontaneously menstruates regularly every 28 days or so is most likely to ovulate at midcycle. Thus, the gestational age (menstrual age) becomes simply the number of weeks since the onset of the last menstrual period. If her menstrual cycles were significantly longer than 28 days to 30 days, ovulation more likely occurred well beyond 14 days or, if the intervals were much longer and irregular, anovulation is likely to have preceded some of the episodes of vaginal bleeding identified as menses. In the latter instance, the menstrual data are unreliable for calculating the duration of the gestation.

It is important to ascertain whether or not *steroidal contraceptives* were used before the pregnancy and, if so, when. It is now common, but not necessarily recommended, for women who sustain regularly recurring withdrawal bleeding while using oral contraceptives cyclically to stop their use and to conceive without any further menstrual-like bleeding. Ovulation, however, may not have resumed 2 weeks after the onset of the last withdrawal bleeding but, instead, at an appreciably later but highly variable date. The difficult problem of predicting the time of ovulation in this circumstance is similar to that in which pregnancy occurs following delivery or abortion prior to the reestablishment of normal menstrual periods.

The possibility of the presence of an *intrauterine device* should be ascertained, since certain pregnancy complications are increased by its presence in utero (see Chapter 40, p. 822). If present, its fate must also be clearly recorded.

Obstetric Examination. The cervix is visualized employing a speculum lightly lubricated but only on the outside of each blade. Next, in order to identify cytologic abnormalities, a gentle swabbing from the lower half of the cervical canal and then a scraping from the squamocolumnar junction are obtained and spread on separate slides and fixed immediately in ether-alcohol or by an appropriate aerosol spray. The outer half of the cervical canal is again swabbed slowly for gonococci and the applicator stick is rolled over Trans-Grow or another suitable transport medium while the container is held vertically to prevent loss of the carbon dioxide–enriched air in the culture bottle. The specimens are labeled immediately and accurately.

Bluish-red passive hyperemia of the cervix is characteristic, but not of itself diagnostic of pregnancy. Dilated, occluded cervical glands bulging beneath the exocervical mucosa, so-called *Nabothian cysts,* may be prominent. If the cervix is dilated appreciably, fetal membranes may be visualized through the cervical canal and implies, at least, that expulsion of the products of conception may be imminent.

The character of vaginal secretions is noted. A moderate amount of white mucoid discharge is normal. The presence of foamy yellow liquid in the vagina is strongly suggestive of *Trichomonas* whereas the presence of a curd-like discharge is consistent with *Candida* infection (p. 263). Material may be swabbed from the vagina for microscopic examination and for culture.

The speculum is removed and the internal pelvic examination is completed by palpation, with special attention given to the consistency, length, and dilatation of the cervix; to the fetal presenting part, especially if late in pregnancy; to the bony architecture of the pelvis; and to any anomalies of the vagina and perineum, including cystocele, rectocele, and relaxed or torn perineum. The vulva and contiguous structures are also carefully inspected. (The pelvic examination is described in more detail in Chapter 17, p. 322.) All cervical, vaginal, and vulvar lesions should be evaluated further by appropriate use of colposcopy, biopsy, culture, or darkfield examination. The perianal region should be visualized and digital rectal examination done to identify hemorrhoids or other lesions.

Between 18 and 32 weeks gestation, there is good correlation between the gestational age of the fetus in weeks and the height of the uterine fundus in centimeters when measured as the distance over the abdominal wall from the top of the symphysis pubis to the top of the fundus. During this time period the height in centimeters equals the gestational age in weeks. Therefore, it is important for the examiner to document carefully the height of fundus, as described below (p. 249).

Physical Examination. The general physical examination includes evaluation of the teeth. Repair of carious teeth should be undertaken promptly. Varicose veins should be looked for and, when identified, frequent postural drainage should be urged and elastic support stockings provided to minimize complications.

Further Instructions. After the history and physical examination have been completed, the expectant mother is instructed about diet, relaxation and sleep, bowel habits, exercise, bathing, clothing, recreation, smoking, drug and alcohol ingestion, and follow-up visits, including steps to take if an appointment is missed. Usually it is possible to assure her that she may anticipate an uneventful preg-

nancy followed by an uncomplicated delivery. **At the same time, she is tactfully instructed about the following danger signals, which must be reported immediately, day or night:**

1. Any vaginal bleeding
2. Swelling of the face or fingers
3. Severe or continuous headache
4. Dimness or blurring of vision
5. Abdominal pain
6. Persistent vomiting
7. Chills or fever
8. Dysuria
9. Escape of fluid from the vagina
10. Marked change in frequency or intensity of fetal movements.

Prognosis. All information obtained should be employed to identify accurately the gestational age of the fetus and to anticipate the kinds and the magnitude of morbidity, both maternal and fetal, that may develop subsequently. Often, when morbidity is anticipated, its intensity can be minimized by appropriate care.

High-Risk Pregnancies. Considerable attention has been directed toward identifying complicated, or "high-risk" pregnancies, and, indeed, risk-assessment programs have been demonstrated to be effective for identifying the majority of pregnancies at increased risk (Hobel and associates, 1979; Sokol and co-workers, 1977). In practice, one problem inherent in such attempts to identify the "high-risk" pregnancy has been a tendency to ignore subsequently the pregnancy that early on had been categorized as "low-risk" yet proved later to be "high-risk." Nonetheless, there are major categories for increased risk that should be identified antepartum and given appropriate consideration in subsequent pregnancy management. These include (1) preexisting medical illness, (2) previous poor pregnancy performance such as perinatal mortality, prematurity, fetal growth retardation, malformations, placental accidents, and maternal hemorrhage, and (3) evidence of maternal undernutrition.

SUBSEQUENT PRENATAL CARE

Return Visits

Traditionally, the timing of subsequent prenatal examinations has been scheduled at intervals of 4 weeks throughout the first 7 months, then every 2 weeks until the last month, and weekly thereafter. Rather often, however, important information can be gained from a more flexible appointment schedule. For example, at midpregnancy, certain clinically discernible events characteristically occur that, when precisely identified, enhance the reliability of the estimate of gestational age of the fetus.

Audible Fetal Heart Sounds. In essentially all pregnancies the fetal heart may be first heard between 16 and 19 weeks of gestation when carefully listened for with a DeLee fetal stethoscope (Fig. 17-2A and B; also, see Chapter 10, p. 211).

Fundal Height. Measurement of the height of the uterine fundus above the symphysis can provide useful information. For example, Jimenez and co-workers (1983) demonstrated that between 20 and 31 weeks of gestation the fundal height in centimeters equaled the gestational age in weeks. Utilizing a tape calibrated in centimeters and applied over the abdominal curvature, they measured the distance from the top of the fundus to the top of the symphysis pubis. The top of the fundus was identified by percussion, as well as by palpation, and the tape was placed there and extended to the top of the symphysis. Quaranta and associates (1981) and Calvert and colleagues (1982) have reported essentially identical observations. *The bladder must be emptied before making the measurement.* Worthen and Bustillo (1980), for example, demonstrated that at 17 to 20 weeks gestation the fundal height was 3 cm higher with a full bladder.

Gestational Age

For the great majority of pregnancies the most important question to be answered through prenatal examination is, "How old is the fetus?" Fortunately, it is possible to identify the gestational age of the fetus with considerable precision through an appropriately timed, carefully performed clinical examination, coupled with knowledge of the time of onset of the last menstrual period. When the date of onset of the last menstrual period and the fundal height are in repeatedly temporal agreement, the duration of gestation can be firmly established. When gestational age cannot be clearly identified, sonography is likely to be of considerable value (see Chapter 14, p. 278).

Later in pregnancy previously acquired precise knowledge of gestational age is of considerable importance since a number of pregnancy complications may develop, for which the optimal treatment will depend on fetal age. For example, with the development of preeclampsia at 38 weeks, very often delivery is the treatment most beneficial to both mother and fetus. However, if the duration of gestation is only 28 weeks when preeclampsia develops, attempts at medical management and delay of delivery may be more beneficial for the quite premature fetus.

Prenatal Surveillance

At each return visit steps are taken to identify the well-being of both the expectant mother and her fetus. Certain information, obtained by interrogation and by examination, is especially important in this regard:

Fetal

1. Fetal heart rate(s)
2. Size of fetus(es), actual and rate of change
3. Amount of amnionic fluid
4. Presenting part and station (late in pregnancy)
5. Fetal activity

Maternal

1. Blood pressure, actual and extent of change
2. Weight, actual and amount of change
3. Symptoms, including headache, altered vision, abdominal pain, nausea and vomiting, bleeding, fluid from vagina, and dysuria
4. Distance to uterine fundus from symphysis
5. A carefully performed vaginal examination late in pregnancy often provides valuable information as follows:
   a. Confirmation of the presenting part
   b. Station (depth in the pelvis) of the presenting part (see Chapter 17, p. 332)
   c. Clinical mensuration of the pelvis and an appreciation of its general configuration (see Chapter 11, p. 226)
   d. The consistency, effacement, and dilatation of the cervix. Digital exploration must be conducted with care lest membranes be ruptured or an undiagnosed low-lying placenta be separated, causing severe hemorrhage.

Subsequent Laboratory Tests. If the initial results were quite normal, most of the procedures need not be repeated. Hematocrit determination and the serologic test for syphilis, if syphilis prevails in the population cared for, should be repeated at about 34 weeks gestation. A cervical culture for gonorrhea may be repeated at the time of the pelvic examination near term, especially if gonorrhea is common.

Routine urine examination at every clinic visit is rarely warranted. Practically all women who develop preeclampsia develop a significant rise in blood pressure, and many have a sudden gain in weight before overt proteinuria develops. Therefore, in general, after the initial examination proteinuria need only be looked for selectively in those women who develop an increase in blood pressure or marked increase in weight. Fasting and postprandial plasma glucose levels are so much more informative than are tests for glucosuria, especially in the case of the woman with a strong family history of diabetes, or previous large infants, or, who during the current pregnancy, has an unusually large fetus. Nonetheless, glucosuria, if detected, should not be ignored.

All pertinent information obtained at each visit must be recorded legibly and be sufficiently descriptive that anyone who uses the pregnancy record at any time can appreciate the significance of the information contained.

NUTRITION DURING PREGNANCY

Throughout most of this century, the diets of pregnant women have been the subject of endless discussions that often resulted in considerable contradiction and confusion. Various enthusiasts have urged pregnant women to adhere to a wide variety of diets, ranging from those that emphasized rigid caloric restriction to those that provided unusually large amounts of protein as well as calories. Faulty reasoning led some obstetricians to advise rigid caloric restriction, a recommendation that stemmed primarily from the observation that a prominent feature of preeclampsia and eclampsia was excessive weight gain. It was not generally appreciated that the abnormal weight gain in preeclampsia and eclampsia resulted from edema rather than excessive caloric intake.

Meaningful studies of nutrition in human pregnancy are exceedingly difficult to design. For ethical reasons, dietary deficiency must not be deliberately produced experimentally in pregnant women. In those instances in which severe nutritional deficiencies have been induced as a consequence of social, economic, or political disaster, coincidental events often have created many variables, the effects of which are not amenable to quantitation. Some past experiences suggest, however, that in otherwise healthy women a state of near starvation is required to establish clear differences in pregnancy outcome, as for example, the acute starvation imposed on pregnant women during the occupation of the Netherlands late in World War II.

During the winter of 1944–45 nutritional deprivation of known intensity prevailed in a well-circumscribed area of the Netherlands. As pointed out by Stein and associates (1972), the type and the degree of nutritional deprivation during the famine was identified with a precision unequaled in any large population before or since. At the lowest point, rations reached 450 kcal per day, with generalized undernutrition rather than selective malnutrition. Shortly after the end of the war, Smith (1947) analyzed the outcomes of pregnancies that were in progress during this 6-month period of famine. The median birth weights of infants were decreased about 8 ounces. The birth weights rose again after food became available in a way that indicated that birth weight can be influenced significantly by starvation during the latter half of pregnancy. The perinatal mortality rate, however, was not altered, nor was the incidence of malformations significantly increased.

Smith also identified the frequency of pregnancy toxemia (preeclampsia–eclampsia), defined by three different sets of criteria, to have declined during the "hunger-winter" of 1944–45. Subsequent analyses of this population by Ribeiro and associates (1982) identified an overall decline in maternal blood pressure near delivery during the famine.

Evidence of impaired brain development has been obtained in some animal fetuses whose mothers during pregnancy had been subjected to intense dietary deprivation. These animal studies, in turn, stimulated interest in the subsequent intellectual development of the young adults in the Netherlands whose mothers had been starved during pregnancy. The comprehensive study by Stein and co-workers (1972) was made possible by the fact that practically all males at age 19 undergo compulsory examination for military service. From the extensive analyses, Stein and associates concluded that the severe dietary deprivation during pregnancy caused no detectable effects on the mental performance of the surviving male offspring.

Caution must be exercised in extrapolating from one species to another. For example, severe protein deprivation of a few days duration in the pregnant rat, in which gestation is only 21 days and in which total fetal weight represents one-fourth of maternal weight, may lead to serious reproductive casualties. In human pregnancy, which lasts 13 times longer and in which fetal weight is only about one-twentieth of that of the mother, failure to ingest protein for the same number of days could hardly be expected to produce an insult of the same intensity.

Weight Gain During Pregnancy

During a normal pregnancy with a single fetus, there is a physiologic basis for a weight gain of at least 20 pounds (9 kg). Typically, there is an increase of 11 pounds of intrauterine contents that include the fetus (7½ pounds), placenta (1½ pounds), and amnionic fluid (2 pounds), in addition to a maternal contribution of 8 pounds from increases in the weights of the uterus (2½ pounds), blood (3½ pounds), and breasts (2 pounds). Also, moderate expansion of interstitial fluid in the pelvis and lower extremities is a normal event attributable to the increased venous pressure created by the large pregnant uterus. In the ambulatory woman, it most likely amounts to at least 3 pounds.

For the woman whose weight is normal before pregnancy, a gain of 20 to 27 pounds appears to be associated with the most favorable outcome of pregnancy (Naeye, 1979). In most pregnant women, this result may be achieved by eating, according to appetite, a diet adequate in calories, protein, essential fatty acids, minerals, and vitamins. Seldom, if ever, should maternal weight gain be restricted deliberately below this level. **Indeed, failure of the pregnant woman to gain weight is an ominous sign.**

Eastman and Jackson (1968) carefully evaluated the relation between maternal weight gain and birth weight in term pregnancies and found that, in general, birth weight paralleled maternal weight gain. The full significance of this relationship is best appreciated when the fate of low-birth-weight infants is considered. The neonatal mortality rate for chronologically mature white newborns weighing 2500 g or less was 45.1 per 1000 live births, in contrast to 6.1 per 1000 live births for those whose weight exceeded 2500 g. Undoubtedly, failure of the mother to gain weight was caused in some instances by associated maternal disease rather than just imposed caloric restriction. Nonetheless, in spite of the reported experiences in the Netherlands, alluded to above, observations such as those of Eastman and Jackson, coupled with those from several well-controlled animal studies demonstrating deleterious effects on the offspring when *severe* maternal caloric restriction was imposed, point out that rigid caloric restriction during pregnancy might prove dangerous to the fetus.

Eastman and Jackson found that the incidence of low birth weight was greatest in pregnant women whose weight was low before pregnancy and whose weight gain was slight during gestation. They recommended that women whose weight before pregnancy is less than 120 pounds be urged to eat according to appetite, at least during the first half of pregnancy, and by 20 weeks, their weight gain reviewed. If less than 10 pounds, someone with nutritional expertise should evaluate the diet and make appropriate corrections so that weight gain approaches a pound a week.

A Task Force on Nutrition of the American College of Obstetricians and Gynecologists (1978) has emphasized that the nutritional status of the expectant mother is more likely to be compromised in any of the following circumstances:

1. She is under 16 years of age.
2. She is economically deprived.
3. She is pregnant for the third time within 2 years.
4. Her past reproductive performance has been poor.
5. She consumes a therapeutic diet in the course of management of some preexisting disease.
6. She is a food faddist.
7. She smokes, drinks, or uses hard drugs.
8. She is appreciably underweight at the outset.
9. The hematocrit drops much below 33 or the hemoglobin concentration falls much below 11 g/dl.
10. Her weight gain for any month during the second and third trimesters is less than 2 pounds.

RECOMMENDED DIETARY ALLOWANCES

Periodically, the Food and Nutrition Board of the National Research Council recommends dietary allowances for women, including those who are pregnant or lactating. Their latest recommendations are summarized in Table 13-1. For certain nutrients, the Board made higher recommendations for the nonpregnant teenager compared to older women of reproductive age. Where there is a difference, the recommended value for 15 to 18 years of age is given for each nutrient unless otherwise stated.

Calories

A daily caloric increase throughout pregnancy of 300 kcal has been recommended by the Food and Nutrition Board. Calories are necessary for energy production. Whenever caloric intake is inadequate, protein may be metabolized as a source of energy, rather than being spared for its vital role in growth and development.

The importance of adequate caloric intake was emphasized by a nutrition intervention study in Guatemala that identified infant birth weights to be larger when the at most marginal diets of the mothers were supplemented (Delgado and associates, 1977). In two of four villages a high protein

TABLE 13-1. RECOMMENDED DAILY DIETARY ALLOWANCES FOR WOMEN 163 CM (64 IN.) TALL AND WEIGHING 55 KG (121 LBS.)

Nutrient	Nonpregnant	Increase	
		Pregnant	Lactating
Kilocalories	2100	300	500
Protein (g)	44*	30	20
Vitamin A (RE)†	800	200	400
Vitamin D (μg)‡	7.5	5	5
Vitamin E (mg T.E.)§	10	2	3
Ascorbic Acid (mg)	60	20	40
Folacin (mg)‖	0.4	0.4	0.1
Niacin (mg)#	14	2	5
Riboflavin (mg)	1.3	0.3	0.5
Thiamin (mg)	1.1	0.4	0.5
Vitamin B$_6$ (mg)	2.0	0.6	0.5
Vitamin B$_{12}$ (μg)	3.0	1.0	1.0
Calcium (mg)	800	400	400
Phosphorus (mg)	800	400	400
Iodine (μg)	150	25	50
Iron (mg)	18	Supplement**	0
Magnesium (mg)	300	150	150
Zinc (mg)	15	5	10

* 46 g if under 19 years of age
† 1 μg retinol = 1 retinol equivalent (R.E.)
‡ As cholecalciferol; 100 International Units = 2.5 μg of cholecalciferol
§ T.E. = tocopherol equivalent
‖ Refers to dietary sources ascertained by Lactobacillus cassei assay; pteroylglutamic acid may be effective in smaller doses
Includes dietary sources of the vitamin plus 1 mg equivalent for each 60 mg of dietary tryptophan
** Increased requirement cannot be met by ordinary diets; therefore supplementation recommended (see text)
(*From Recommended Dietary Allowances, 9th ed., National Academy of Sciences, Washington, D.C., 1980.*)

plus calorie supplement was made available; in the other two villages a drink that provided calories without protein was offered. Birthweights were influenced by the number of calories ingested rather than by the protein content of the supplements. For those pregnancies in which less than 10,000 supplemental kcal were ingested, birth weight averaged 2986 g and 18.3 percent of the infants weighed less than 2500 g. For those pregnancies in which more than 20,000 kcal were consumed in the form of supplements, the mean birth weight was 3120 g, and only 9.4 percent, or one half as many, infants weighed less than 2500 g at birth.

In a more recent investigation of the impact of caloric supplementation on birth weights of infants of Gambian women a threshold effect was apparent (Prentice and coworkers, 1983). Food supplementation that provided throughout much of pregnancy somewhat more than 400 kcal per day on average improved birth weights for infants whose mothers were in marked negative energy balance as the consequence of both food shortage and heavy work load. For example, the frequency of low-birth-weight infants (< 2500 g) decreased sixfold with calorie supplementation of these mothers. However, for women who were in positive energy balance, even though they were consuming only 60 percent of the recommended dietary allowance, supplementation had no demonstrable beneficial effect on birth outcome. These studies serve especially to emphasize the deleterious effect on fetal growth imposed by severe restriction of caloric intake.

Protein. To the basic protein needs of the nonpregnant women for repair of her tissues are added the demands for growth and repair of the fetus, placenta, uterus and breasts, and increased maternal blood volume. During the last 6 months of pregnancy about 1 kg of protein is deposited, amounting to 5 to 6 g per day on average (Hytten and Leitch, 1971). The Food and Nutrition Board has recommended for young nonpregnant women a protein intake of about 0.9 g per day, but an additional 30 g of protein per day is recommended during pregnancy. This is considerably more than the amount recommended by the World Health Organization.

It is desirable that the majority of the protein be supplied from animal sources such as meat, milk, eggs, cheese, poultry, and fish, since they furnish amino acids in optimal combinations. Milk and milk products have long been considered nearly ideal sources of nutrients, especially protein and calcium, for pregnant or lactating women. Nonetheless, milk (lactose) intolerance in the form of gastrointestinal disturbances that include bloating, flatulence, and cramps is a problem in some adults. For example, some degree of lactose intolerance was found in 81 percent of black adults compared to 12 percent of whites in the studies of Bayless and co-workers (1975). As little as 240 ml of milk caused the unpleasant symptoms.

A "high" protein diet has been urged by some enthusiasts who contend that most problems of pregnancy are amenable to manipulation of maternal diet. The desirability of consuming large amounts of protein must be questioned from the standpoint of economics and, perhaps, safety. Analyses of several studies by Stein and associates (1978) have failed to demonstrate improvement in birth weight due specifically to a protein-rich supplement. In fact, they were concerned that the reverse might sometimes be the consequence.

Recently, Zlatnik and Burmeister (1983) used the maternal urinary urea-to-creatinine ratio to evaluate protein intakes and, in turn, the apparent effects of protein intake on anthropometric indices of the newborn. Little difference in birth weights or other anthropometric indices was identified between the lowest decile of protein intake (0.7 g/kg/day) and the highest decile (1.5 g/kg/day).

Minerals. The intakes recommended by the Food and Nutrition Board for a variety of minerals are presented in Table 13-1 and discussed below. There is good evidence that only one mineral, iron, provides any demonstrated benefit when provided as a supplement to pregnant women. Practically all diets that supply sufficient calories for appropriate weight gain will contain enough of the other minerals to prevent a mineral deficiency if iodized salt is used.

Iron. There are increased iron requirements during pregnancy, the reasons for which are discussed in Chapter 9 (p. 192). Of the approximately 300 mg of iron transferred to the fetus and placenta and the 500 mg

incorporated, if available, into the expanding maternal hemoglobin mass, nearly all is utilized during the latter half of pregnancy. During that time, the average iron requirements imposed by the pregnancy itself are about 6 mg a day, and, in addition, there is the need for nearly 1 mg to compensate for maternal excretion, or a total of about 7 mg of iron per day (Pritchard and Scott, 1970). Very few women have sufficient iron stores to supply this amount of iron. Moreover, the diet seldom contains enough iron to meet this demand. The recommendation by the Food and Nutrition Board (Table 13-1) of 18 mg of dietary iron per day for nonpregnant women represents the ceiling imposed by caloric requirements. To ingest any more iron from dietary sources would simultaneously provide an undesirable excess of calories. The Board has acknowledged that because of small iron stores the pregnant woman often will be unable to meet the iron requirements imposed by pregnancy and therefore has recommended supplementation.

Supplementation with medicinal iron is commonly practiced in the United States and elsewhere, although the merits of this practice continue to be questioned by a minority of investigators, as cited below. Scott and co-workers (1970) established that as little as 30 mg of iron supplied in the form of a simple iron salt such as ferrous gluconate, sulfate, or fumarate, and taken regularly once each day throughout the latter half of pregnancy provided sufficient iron to meet the requirements of pregnancy and to protect any preexisting iron stores. Iron, 30 mg daily, as a simple salt, should also provide for the iron requirements of lactation. The pregnant woman may benefit from 60 to 100 mg of iron per day if she is large, has twin fetuses, is late in pregnancy, takes iron irregularly, or her hemoglobin level is somewhat depressed. The woman who is overtly anemic from iron deficiency responds well to 200 mg of iron per day in divided doses (see Chapter 28, p. 564).

The availability for absorption of iron contained in at least some prenatal vitamin–mineral supplements has been questioned (Seligman and associates, 1983). Undoubtedly, calcium and magnesium compounds included in such mixtures can inhibit iron absorption, as they do when taken as antacids. Interestingly, the reaction of at least one provider of such multi-everything preparations has been to reduce markedly the calcium and magnesium content of their "formulation." Why this approach rather than adding more iron is not clear. Presumably, they now consider the previously provided amounts of calcium and magnesium to be superfluous. *A very effective and inexpensive way to avoid impairment of iron absorption by such agents is to prescribe simple iron salts alone!*

Since iron requirements are slight during the first 4 months of pregnancy, it is *not* necessary to provide supplemental iron during this time. Withholding iron supplementation during the first trimester of pregnancy avoids the risk of aggravating nausea and vomiting, which are common at that time. Ingestion of iron at bedtime also appears to minimize the possibility of an

TABLE 13-2. STUDIES OF THE EFFECTS OF IRON SUPPLE-MENTATION DURING PREGNANCY ON HEMOGLOBIN CONCENTRATION, 1958–1982

	Hemoglobin (G/DL)		
	Unsupple-mented	Supple-mented	Differ-ence
Taylor et al (1982)	11.2	12.7	+1.5
Chanarin et al (1977)	11.2	12.8	+1.6
Taylor and Lind (1976)	11.0	12.3	+1.3
Paintin et al (1966)	10.7	12.0	+1.3
De Leeuw et al (1966)	10.9	12.4	+1.5
Chisholm (1966)	11.2	12.4	+1.2
Pritchard and Hunt (1958)	11.3	12.5	+1.2
Average	11.05	12.40	+1.35

adverse gastrointestinal reaction. Moreover, keeping the container of iron tablets in proximity to toothpaste enhances the ability of the expectant mother to remember to ingest the supplement regularly. When she brushes her teeth, she should take an iron tablet! Iron-containing medication must be kept out of the reach of small children lest they ingest a large number of the usually quite attractive tablets or capsules.

Deficiency vs. "Oversufficiency" of Iron

Paintin and co-workers (1966), Taylor and Lind (1976), and a few others at one time or another have insisted that iron supplements stimulate hemoglobin synthesis to an abnormal degree in pregnant women. Moreover, Taylor and Lind questioned whether iron preparations can be given safely to all pregnant women because of a modest increase in mean red cell volume that is likely to follow. A number of studies refute both of these contentions. In brief, evidence has long been available that a higher hemoglobin concentration depends on whether or not iron is available, irrespective of whether or not the iron is derived from oral supplements, from parenteral injection, or simply from stores (Scott and co-workers, 1970). The similarity of the magnitude of the increases observed in several of the studies performed over the past quarter century is apparent in Table 13-2 even though the amounts of iron given varied widely. Importantly, the average increase demonstrated almost universally equals the hemoglobin content of 500 ml of donor blood. The presence or absence of this amount at delivery may determine whether or not a mother is transfused. This is especially true for the 20 percent or so of women who are now delivered by cesarean section!

The moderate increase in maternal mean red cell volume that originally concerned Taylor and Lind (1976) has physiologic bases: (1) recently synthesized red cells of iron-replete individuals are larger than are older red cells and (2) red cells formed by iron-deficient individuals are smaller yet more rigid than are those of iron-replete subjects (Yip and co-workers, 1983). Their rigidity could impair flow in the microcirculation. It should be pointed out that Taylor and co-workers (1982) have now reversed their previous position and state, *"It is concluded that routine oral iron administration should be recommended during pregnancy, certainly after 28 weeks gestation."*

In some circumstances compromised fetal well-being may be associated with an above average maternal hemoglobin concentration (Garn and associates, 1981; Koller, 1982). This has led to the supposition by some that iron ingested prenatally, by stimulating an abnormally high hemoglobin concentration, is actually detrimental and therefore should not be used (Goodlin, 1982). Even vigorous iron administration does not raise the hemoglobin concentration of iron-sufficient women (Taylor and associates, 1982). Almost certainly, reduced blood volume from failure of expansion of plasma volume is the important culprit in the genesis of impaired fetal well-being. Failure of the hemoglobin concentration to fall is but one consequence of inadequate expansion. (If hemoglobin concentration per se were an important factor, phlebotomy or even leeches might come into vogue again!)

Iron supplementation during pregnancy has also been faulted by a few as enhancing the potential for infection based on observations that iron is essential for replication of many kinds of bacteria in vitro and that the risk of infection appears to have been enhanced in some infants by large doses of iron administered parenterally. As pointed out by Stockman (1981), no study has shown any increased risk of infection in infants from iron-fortified formulas and the benefits of iron supplementation far outweigh the possibility of iron excess during a period of life characterized by scant to absent iron stores. We conclude that the same holds true for pregnant women.

Calcium. The expectant mother retains about 30 g of calcium during pregnancy, most of which is deposited in the fetus late in pregnancy (Pitkin, 1975). This amount of calcium represents only about 2.5 percent of the total maternal calcium, most of which is in bone, and which can be readily mobilized for fetal growth. Moreover, Heaney and Skillman (1971) demonstrated increased absorption of calcium by the intestine and progressive retention throughout pregnancy. In a few places in the world *osteomalacia* is still recognized in women who are reproducing but only under the very unusual circumstances of almost total avoidance of sunlight coupled with low vitamin D and calcium intake for very long periods. Bound calcium levels, but probably not ionized calcium, fall slightly in maternal plasma as the concentration of albumin decreases (Chapter 9, p. 191).

Although calcium supplementation during pregnancy has been widely practiced in the United States it is unlikely to be of any benefit. One quart of cow's milk provides approximately 1 g of calcium.

Phosphorous. The ubiquitous distribution of phosphorous assures an adequate intake during pregnancy. Plasma levels of inorganic phosphorus do not differ appreciably from nonpregnant levels.

Zinc. *Severe* zinc deficiency may lead to poor appetite, suboptimal growth, and impaired wound healing. Profound zinc deficiency may cause dwarfism and hypogonadism. It may also lead to a specific skin disorder, acrodermatitis enteropathica.

The concentration of zinc in plasma is only about 1 percent of total body zinc. Moreover, zinc in plasma is almost entirely bound to several plasma proteins and to amino acids. Therefore, most often low plasma concentration of zinc is but the consequence of changes in concentration of the various binders in plasma rather than true zinc depletion (Swanson and King, 1983). Even though the concentration is reduced, the total pool of zinc in plasma of normally pregnant women is actually increased as the consequence of the large increase in plasma volume induced by pregnancy. The rationale for increasing the recommended zinc intake during pregnancy (Table 13-1) is not altogether clear. There is no strong evidence at this time that dietary supplementation with zinc in the United States is of any benefit to the expectant mother or fetus. Meadows and co-workers (1981) have reported the concentration of zinc in leukocytes to be lower in mothers of infants small for gestational age, but whether the low zinc concentration is causally related or merely a marker of fetal growth has not been clarified.

Iodine. The use of iodized salt by all pregnant women is recommended to offset the increased need for fetal requirements and probable increased loss through the maternal kidneys. Severe maternal iodine deficiency in expectant mothers predisposes their offspring to endemic cretinism, characterized by multiple severe neurologic defects. In parts of New Guinea where this condition was endemic, the intramuscular injection of iodized oil into women very early in pregnancy or before successfully prevented cretinism in the offspring (Pharoah and associates, 1971). The ingestion of iodide in large (pharmacologic) amounts during pregnancy may depress thyroid function and induce a sizable goiter in the fetus. The consumption of large amounts of seaweed by food faddists may do the same.

Magnesium. A deficiency in this element as the consequence of pregnancy has not been recognized. Undoubtedly, during prolonged illness with no magnesium intake, the plasma level might become critically low, as it would in the absence of pregnancy. We have observed magnesium deficiency during pregnancy complicated by the consequences of previous intestinal bypass surgery.

Potassium. The concentration of potassium in maternal plasma normally is the same as in nonpregnant plasma or decreases slightly. Potassium deficiency develops in the same circumstances as when the patient is not pregnant. Prolonged nausea and vomiting may lead to hypokalemia and metabolic alkalosis. A previously rather common cause—the use of diuretics—has nearly disappeared.

Sodium. A deficiency of sodium during pregnancy is most unlikely unless diuretics are prescribed or dietary sodium intake is reduced drastically. In general, salting food to taste will provide an abundance of sodium for the pregnant woman. The concentration of sodium in plasma normally decreases a few milliequivalents during pregnancy.

> In the not too distant past much was said about the dangers of inciting preeclampsia–eclampsia through sodium ingestion during pregnancy, and by implication, at least, of the benefits to be achieved from rigid restriction of sodium intake. Next sodium restriction by pregnant women was cited as being detrimental, undoubtedly because rigid sodium restriction in pregnant rats caused abnormalities in the dams' adrenals. About this time it was claimed that extra salt in the maternal diet, especially rock salt, prevented preeclampsia–eclampsia (Robinson, 1958). Nonetheless, the ingestion of exorbitant amounts of sodium may prove harmful. However, there is no good evidence that rigorous sodium restriction is beneficial. Indeed it too may be harmful.

Fluoride. The value of supplemental fluoride during pregnancy has been questioned. Horowitz and Heifetz (1967) investigated the prevalence of caries in temporary and permanent teeth of children with the same postnatal exposure to optimally fluoridated water but different patterns of prenatal exposure. They concluded that there were no meaningful additional benefits from the ingestion of fluoride in water by the expectant mother if the offspring ingested fluoridated water from birth.

Glenn and associates (1982) reported a remarkably lower incidence (99 percent) of caries in children whose mothers ingested 2.2 mg of sodium fluoride daily during pregnancy as compared to those whose mothers used only fluoridated water. They strongly recommended that for structurally superior and caries-free teeth, 2.2 mg of sodium fluoride daily be ingested while fasting, starting during the third month of pregnancy. Obviously, further investigations are needed to confirm the benefits claimed by Glenn and associates and, at the same time, to detect deleterious effects, if any, from the fluoride.

Supplemental fluoride ingested by the lactating woman does not increase the fluoride concentration in her milk, according to Ekstrand (1981).

Vitamins

Most evidence concerning the importance of vitamins for successful reproduction has been obtained from animal experiments. Typically, severe deficiency has been produced in the animal either by withholding the vitamin completely, beginning long before the time of pregnancy, or by giving a very potent vitamin antagonist. The administration of some vitamins in great excess to pregnant animals has been shown to exert deleterious effects on the fetus and newborn.

The practice of supplying vitamin supplements prenatally is a deeply ingrained habit of many obstetricians, even though scientific evidence to show that the usual vitamin supplements are of benefit to either the mother or her fetus is quite meager. The Committee on Maternal Nutrition of the National Research Council pointed out that in the majority of cases routine pharmaceutical supplementation of vitamin and mineral preparations to pregnant women is of doubtful value, except for iron and possibly folic acid. *Such vitamin and mineral preparations should not be regarded as substitutes for food.*

The increased requirements for vitamins during pregnancy (Table 13-1) can in practically all circumstances be supplied by any general diet that provides adequate numbers of calories and amounts of protein, including protein from animal sources. The possible exception is folic acid during times of unusually large requirements, such as pregnancy complicated by protracted vomiting, hemolytic anemia, or multiple fetuses.

Folic Acid. Whereas the advantages to be gained from supplemental iron during pregnancy are quite straightforward, namely, protection against maternal iron deficiency and anemia, the benefits to be derived from folic acid supplementation are not nearly so distinct. In the 1960s several investigators implicated maternal folate deficiency in a variety or reproductive casualties, including placental abruption, pregnancy-induced hypertension (toxemia of pregnancy), and fetal anomalies. For the most part, these reports have not been confirmed (Emery, 1977; Hall, 1977; Whalley and associates, 1969; Pritchard and co-workers, 1969). To date, no one has been able to reduce unequivocally the frequency of these complications simply by administering folic acid during pregnancy.

Smithells and co-workers (1980, 1983) have reported a sevenfold reduction in the anticipated frequency of neural tube defects for pregnancies in which the mothers for at least 28 days before conception, as well as early in pregnancy, received a polyvitamin and mineral supplement that provided 1 mg of folic acid per day.

White and Moffa (1984) have reported an increased incidence of neural tube defects in the fetuses of a species of hamsters especially prone to develop neural tube defects when folic acid was withheld from the maternal diet before and after conception. When folic acid was supplied before and during pregnancy such abnormalities were much less common.

Laurence and associates (1981) reported no recurrence of neural tube defects in a relatively small group of pregnancies among women who ingested folic acid before and during pregnancy. However, some women who entered the study and whose fetuses demonstrated neural tube defects were not included on the basis of suspected noncompliance with the folic acid regime which consisted of 2 mg twice each day. They concluded that folic acid supplementation might be a cheap way of preventing neural tube defects but pointed out that confirmation would require a large, multicenter trial. Unfortunately, subsequent investigations on humans to try to clarify matters have been hampered seriously by questions concerning what studies are now considered ethical.

Evidence is abundant that maternal folate requirements are increased somewhat during pregnancy. In the United States, this increase frequently leads to lowered plasma folate levels, less often to hypersegmentation of neutrophils, infrequently to megaloblastic erythropoiesis, but only rarely to megaloblastic anemia. The amount of folic acid supplement that will prevent these changes varies considerably, depending primarily on the diet consumed by the pregnant woman. Since 1 mg of folic acid orally per day produces a vigorous hematologic response in pregnant women with severe megaloblastic anemia, this amount would almost certainly provide very effective prophylaxis (Pritchard and co-workers, 1969). Chanarin and associates (1968) found that as little as 0.1 mg of folic acid per day raised the blood folate levels to the normal nonpregnant range.

Vitamin B_{12}. The level of vitamin B_{12} in maternal plasma decreases variably in otherwise normal pregnancies (Sauberlich, 1978). The decrease, which is thought to result mostly from a reduction in plasma binders rather than depletion, is prevented only in part by supplementation. However, maternal vitamin B_{12} deficiency can develop in special circumstances. Vitamin B_{12} occurs naturally only in foods of animal origin. It is now established that *strict vegetarians* may give birth to infants whose vitamin B_{12} stores are low. Moreover, since breast milk of a vegetarian mother will most likely contain little vitamin B_{12}, the deficiency may become profound in the breast-fed infant (Higginbottom and associates, 1978).

Excessive ingestion of vitamin C can also lead to a functional deficiency of vitamin B_{12}, as described below under the section on vitamin C.

Vitamin B_6. A variety of biochemical changes induced by vitamin B_6 deficiency, including excessive excretion of xanthurenic acid after the ingestion of a tryptophan load, have been summarized by Sauberlich (1978). Several of the changes also accompany otherwise apparently normal pregnancy and have been identified in women who use estrogen-containing oral contraceptives.

Some investigators have related impaired glucose tolerance during pregnancy to altered metabolic pathways induced by low vitamin B_6 levels and, in turn, a lowering of the biologic activity of endogenous insulin. However, neither the observations of Perkins (1977) nor those of Gillmer and Mazibuko (1979) provide support for this premise. Gillmer and Mazibuko investigated 13 pregnant women who had abnormal glucose tolerance tests and who excreted elevated amounts of xanthurenic acid after a tryptophan load. Treatment with pyridoxine, 100 mg daily for 2 to 3 weeks, restored the urinary excretion of xanthurenic acid to normal levels for nonpregnant individuals but improvement in the glucose tolerance test was observed in only 2 of the 13 pregnant women. There was no change in five and deterioration in six subjects.

As the consequence of some of these observations an appreciable increase in the recommended daily dietary allowance for pyridoxine intake during pregnancy has been urged by some. However, to modify some of the biochemical changes that imply a deficiency of vitamin B_6 during pregnancy requires appreciably more of the vitamin than is now recommended and would be likely to necessitate specific supplementation. For example, Cleary and associates (1975) emphasized that to raise pyridoxal phosphate levels in maternal plasma to those characteristic of normal nonpregnant women required a daily supplement of pyridoxine of more than 2.5 mg. In fact, in some pregnant women daily supplementation with 10 mg did not accomplish this objective. The benefits that might accrue from larger supplements do not appear at this time to warrant so vigorous an undertaking.

> Pyridoxine ingested in large excess can cause dysfunction of the nervous system (Schaumberg and colleagues, 1983). Megadoses of pyridoxine have been implicated in the genesis of a syndrome of progressive sensory ataxia and profound distal limb impairment of position and vibration sense. It is now apparent that a number of vitamins when consumed in large doses can prove toxic. It is unlikely that either the pregnant woman or her fetus is immune to such risks.

The recommendation by the Food and Nutrition Board of the National Research Council calls for 2.0 mg of pyridoxine daily for nonpregnant women and 2.6 mg per day when pregnant or lactating.

Vitamin C. The recommended dietary allowance for vitamin C during pregnancy is 80 mg per day, or about one third more than when nonpregnant (Table 13-1). A reasonable diet should readily provide this amount. The maternal plasma level declines during pregnancy while the cord level is high compared to that of the mother, a phenomenon that is observed with most water-soluble vitamins.

The ingestion of 1 g or more of vitamin C for the prophylaxis of the common cold has become commonplace, even though there is no good evidence that vitamin C when so used is of any benefit. There is evidence that it may prove harmful during pregnancy. Scurvy has been identified in normally fed infants whose mothers had ingested large doses of vitamin C during pregnancy (Cochrane, 1965). Large doses of vitamin C can also interfere with vitamin B_{12} absorption and metabolism. This problem may not be overcome by supplementation with vitamin B_{12} (Herbert, Jacob, 1974).

PRAGMATIC NUTRITIONAL SURVEILLANCE

While the science of nutrition continues in its perpetual struggle to identify the ideal amounts of protein, calories, vitamins, and minerals for the pregnant woman and her fetus, those directly responsible for their care may best discharge their duties as follows:

1. In general, advise the expectant mother to eat what she wants in amounts she desires and salted to taste.

2. Make sure that there is ample food to eat, especially in the case of the socioeconomically deprived woman.
3. Make sure by serially weighing every expectant mother that she is gaining weight, with a goal of at least 20 pounds.
4. At each prenatal visit, explore the food intake by dietary recall to uncover the ingestion of any bizarre diet. In this way the occasional nutritionally absurd diet will be discovered—for example, the ingestion of a peck of grapes per day or a pound of Argo Gloss Starch.
5. Give tablets of simple iron salts that provide 30 to 60 mg of iron daily.

GENERAL HYGIENE

Exercise

In general, it is not necessary for the pregnant woman to limit exercise, provided she does not become excessively fatigued or risk injury to herself or her fetus. The current enthusiasm for jogging has also attracted a number of pregnant women to the endeavor. In fact, several women, even late in pregnancy, have run in marathons of considerable distance without apparent harm to themselves or their fetuses.

Hauth and co-workers (1982) studied fetal heart rate reactivity throughout the third trimester of pregnancy in seven women who jogged at least 1.5 miles three times a week before and during pregnancy. Upon completion of a run the women immediately climbed three flights of stairs to undergo evaluation. Fetal heart reactivity was evident in spite of the vigorous very recent maternal exercise and appreciable fetal tachycardia so induced and which persisted for up to one-half hour.

With some pregnancy complications, the mother and her fetus may benefit significantly from a very sedentary existence; for example, women with pregnancy-induced hypertension appear to do so (see Chapter 27, p. 542), as do women pregnant with two or more fetuses (see Chapter 26, p. 518) and women suspected of having a growth-retarded fetus (see Chapter 37, p. 757).

Employment

It is estimated that more than one third of all women of childbearing age in the United States are now in the labor force and even larger proportions of socioeconomically less fortunate women are working. According to the recent report of Naeye and Peters (1982) working during pregnancy can be deleterious to pregnancy outcome. They identified birth weights of infants whose mothers worked during the third trimester to be 150 to 400 g less than those of newborns whose mothers did not work even though the length of gestation was the same for both groups. Reduction in birth weight was greatest for mothers who were underweight before pregnancy and whose weight gain during pregnancy was low, for mothers who were hypertensive, and for mothers whose work required standing. The data analyzed by them were collected between 1959 and 1966 and therefore these results were possibly influenced by the widespread practice of dietary restrictions and use of drugs then in vogue to try to control weight gain and dependent edema.

Berkowitz and associates (1983) and Murphy and co-workers (1984) did not find physical activity to be detrimental to pregnancy; in fact, they suggested that the opposite is more likely true. It is apparent that the problems associated with attempts to compare pregnancy performance in women who do and do not work during pregnancy are numerous. The financial, sociologic, and medical benefits that have become available recently to more and more working pregnant women are likely to minimize possible adverse effects that might otherwise accrue from working (Saurel and Kaminski, 1983).

Common sense dictates that any occupation that subjects the pregnant woman to severe physical strain should be avoided. Ideally, no work or play should be continued to the extent that undue fatigue develops. Adequate periods of rest should be provided during the working day. Women with previous complications of pregnancy that are likely to be repetitive (for example, low-birth-weight infants) probably should minimize physical work.

Travel. The restriction of travel to short trips had been a rule for obstetric patients until World War II when many women found it necessary to follow their husbands regardless of distance or mode of travel. The data compiled during that era are consistent with the conclusion that travel by the woman without complications has no harmful effect on pregnancy. Travel in properly pressurized aircraft offers no unusual risk. At least every 2 hours, the pregnant woman should walk about. Perhaps the greatest risk with travel, especially international travel, is the development of a pregnancy complication remote from facilities adequate for treatment of the complication.

Bathing. There is no objection to bathing at any time during pregnancy or the puerperium. During the last trimester of pregnancy, the heavy uterus usually upsets the balance of the pregnant woman and increases the likelihood of her slipping and falling in the bathtub. For that reason, tub baths at the end of pregnancy may be inadvisable.

Clothing. The clothing worn during pregnancy should be practical and nonconstricting. Intricate, expensive supporting girdles are no longer used routinely. The increasing mass of the breasts may make them pendulous and painful. In such instances, well-fitting supporting brassieres are indicated. Constricting garters should be avoided during pregnancy because of the interference with venous return and the aggravation of varicosities. Backache and pressure associated with lordotic posture

and a pendulous abdomen may be relieved by a properly fitted maternity girdle. There is no real reason for insisting that the pregnant woman wear only low-heeled shoes, unless she develops backache from the increased lordosis that results from shoes with high heels or if she is unable to maintain good balance.

Bowel Habits. During pregnancy, bowel habits tend to become more irregular, presumably because of generalized relaxation of smooth muscle and compression of the lower bowel by the enlarging uterus early in pregnancy or by the presenting part of the fetus late in pregnancy. In addition to the discomfort caused by the passage of hard fecal material, bleeding and painful fissures in the edematous and hyperemic rectal mucosa may develop. There is also greater frequency of *hemorrhoids* and, much less commonly, of prolapse of the rectal mucosa.

Women whose bowel habits are reasonably normal in the nonpregnant state may prevent constipation during pregnancy by close attention to bowel habits, sufficient quantities of fluid, and reasonable amounts of daily exercise, supplemented when necessary by a mild laxative, such as prune juice, milk of magnesia, bulk-producing substances, or stool-softening agents. The use of nonabsorbable oil preparations has been discouraged because of their possible interference with the absorption of lipid-soluble vitamins. The use of harsh laxatives and enemas is not recommended.

Coitus

Whenever abortion or premature labor threatens, coitus should be avoided. Otherwise it has been generally accepted that in healthy pregnant women sexual intercourse usually does no harm before the last 4 weeks or so of pregnancy. It has long been the custom of many obstetricians to recommend abstinence from intercourse during the last 4 weeks of pregnancy, a recommendation undoubtedly not followed in many instances.

The risks versus possible benefits from intercourse late in pregnancy have not been clearly delineated. Pugh and Fernandez (1953), for example, did not find that intercourse caused premature labor, rupture of the membranes, bleeding, or infection. They concluded that it is not necessary to abstain from coitus during the final weeks of gestation.

Goodlin and associates (1972) were more concerned about possible injurious effects from intercourse late in pregnancy. They identified transient fetal bradycardia with increased uterine tension during maternal orgasms induced by vulval and vaginal manipulation at 39 weeks gestation. The painful uterine contractions ceased within 15 minutes after the last orgasm. Whether such changes commonly accompany orgasm and whether they are harmful to the fetus are not definitely known. They also reported the incidence of orgasm after 32 weeks to have been significantly higher for women who subsequently delivered prematurely. Grudzinkas and co-workers (1979) found no association between gestational age at delivery and the frequency of coitus during the last 4 weeks of pregnancy. However, women who were sexually active in the last 4 weeks showed a higher incidence of fetal distress. Mills and associates (1981) identified no increase in premature rupture of the membranes, low birth weight, or perinatal death among selected women who had sexual intercourse throughout pregnancy. Their study was biased, however, by the exclusion from potential risk of a large number of cases in which intercourse had been interdicted late in pregnancy because of a history of premature birth, spontaneous abortion, bleeding, uterine scar, hypertension, multifetal pregnancy, or stillbirth.

On occasion, the couple's sexual drive in the face of admonishment against intercourse late in pregnancy has led to unusual sexual practices with disastrous consequences. Aronson and Nelson (1967), for instance, describe fatal cases of air embolism late in pregnancy as a result of air blown into the vagina during cunnilingus.

Douches. If douching in pregnancy is desirable because of excessive cervical and vaginal secretions, the following precautions should be observed:

1. Hand bulb syringes must absolutely be forbidden, since several deaths in pregnancy from air embolism have followed their use (Forbes, 1944).
2. The douche bag should be placed not more than 2 feet above the level of the hips to prevent high fluid pressure.
3. The nozzle should not be inserted more than 3 inches through the vulva.

Care of Breasts and Abdomen. Special care of the breasts during pregnancy is often advised to increase the ability to nurse by toughening the nipples and thereby reduce the incidence of cracking and by effecting enlargement and eversion of the nipples. From the available data it is concluded that ointments, massage, and traction on the nipples do not always improve these functions, but such practices are usually harmless. Massages and ointments do not alter significantly the incidence of striae on the breasts or abdomen. In general, the extent of striation is proportional to the size of the uterus and the weight gain of the woman.

Smoking

Mothers who smoke during pregnancy frequently bear smaller infants than do nonsmokers. There is also evidence that smoking mothers have a significantly greater number of unsuccessful pregnancies because of an increase in perinatal deaths. Goldstein (1977) estimated that about 4600 infants die in the United States every year because their mothers smoke. Many of the data to support these statements were presented in the publication, Smoking and Health, Report to the Surgeon General of the Public Health Service (1979).

To explain these adverse effects from smoking various investigators have implicated the following: (1) carbon monoxide and its functional inactivation of fetal and maternal hemoglobin, (2) vasoconstrictor action of nicotine causing reduced perfusion of the placenta, (3) reduced appetite and, in turn, reduced calorie intake by

women who smoke, (4) decreased plasma volume in mothers who smoke, and (5) an unexplained peculiarity in certain women that persists even when they do not smoke.

Astrup and associates (1979), Socol and co-workers (1982), and Bureau and colleagues (1982) implicated carbon monoxide in the genesis of low birth weight on the basis of their studies on women, monkeys, and rabbits. D'Souza and co-workers (1978) identified the hemoglobin level in cord blood to average 17.8 g/dl if the mother smoked during pregnancy compared to 16.3 g/dl if she did not smoke; a plausible explanation to account for these differences in hemoglobin concentrations is bone marrow stimulation from chronic fetal hypoxia. Low birth weight has been described, however, for infants whose mothers did not smoke, but rather had chewed tobacco (Krushna, 1978). Lehtovirta and Forss (1978) reported intervillous blood flow to be acutely reduced during smoking and for 15 minutes afterwards. Monheit and associates (1983) did not alter significantly either uterine or umbilical hemodynamics by infusing nicotine acutely into pregnant sheep in doses that produced blood levels of the alkaloid substantially greater than those reported in humans while smoking. Moreover, Jouppila and co-workers (1983) found no significant change in human fetal blood flow in the thoracic aorta or umbilical vein during and immediately following the mother smoking a cigarette.

Rush (1974) and Davies and co-workers (1976) have contended that lower birth weight of infants whose mothers smoke is primarily the consequence of lower pregnancy weight gain by smoking mothers. However, Haworth and co-workers (1980) identified birth weights to be lower for infants whose mothers smoked than those whose mothers did not, even though maternal weight gain and dietary intake were the same for both groups.

Boomer and Christensen (1982) identified an increased evidence for high maternal hematocrits and low-birth-weight infants in pregnancies of women who smoked. They considered these events to reflect most likely the decrease in plasma volume among pregnant women who smoked described by Pirani and MacGillivray (1978). Yerushalmy (1972) implicated the smoker and not the smoke in the genesis of low birth weight. He reported lower birth weights for infants whose mothers had not yet smoked when the infants were born but who began to smoke subsequently. Most other investigators have not confirmed Yerushalmy's findings. Interestingly, the incidence of preeclampsia has been reported to be somewhat lower in women who smoke (Duffus, MacGillivray, 1968; Underwood and co-workers, 1967).

Hardy and Mellits (1973) could not identify any harmful long-term effects in children of smoking mothers even though they weighed on the average 250 g less and were shorter at birth. Butler and Goldstein (1973), however, based on a sample of several thousand children 7 to 11 years of age, found slight retardation for reading, mathematics, and general ability in children whose mothers smoked during pregnancy.

In the past, a limitation of smoking to no more than 10 cigarettes per day during pregnancy was recommended. In view of the obvious dangers to people who smoke, cigarettes should be avoided completely by women, irrespective of any deleterious effects on pregnancy.

Alcohol

Excessive ingestion of alcohol by the expectant mother is likely to produce abnormalities in the fetus. Chronic alcoholism can lead to fetal maldevelopment, commonly referred to as the *fetal alcohol syndrome.* Jones and associates (1974, 1975) described a common pattern of prenatal and postnatal growth retardation, with characteristic cardiovascular, limb, and craniofacial defects in the offspring of alcoholic mothers. The facial characteristics included short palpebral fissures, short and upturned nose, flattened maxilla, and thinned upper vermillion of the mouth. The children subsequently demonstrated impaired fine and gross motor function and commonly impaired speech. The perinatal mortality rate was 17 percent. At 7 years of age 44 percent of the survivors had an IQ below 80, compared to 9 percent in a control group. Clarren (1981) has provided an excellent summary of the fetal alcohol syndrome.

Women with chronic and severe drinking problems must be discouraged from becoming pregnant until these problems are brought under control. Serious consideration should be given to early pregnancy termination in alcoholic women.

Differences of opinion persist in regard to the possible adverse effects on the fetus from social drinking. For example, Little (1981) has written "the body of research relating moderate alcohol use to adverse fetal development is now too great and too consistent to discount . . . drinking at levels that are generally considered within social norms is not safe for the developing child." Rosett and co-workers (1983), however, found no differences in frequency of abnormalities in offspring born to nondrinkers compared to rare and moderate drinkers. The likelihood of fetal damage from even moderate drinking by the mother appears to be enhanced appreciably by the simultaneous use of a variety of drugs, including analgesics, antidepressants, and anticonvulsants (Poskitt and associates, 1982). From the evidence available the best advice to the woman pregnant or about to become pregnant would seem to be "Don't consume alcohol." Hopefully, the adverse effects of alcohol on pregnancy do not linger after the woman stops drinking.

"Hard" Drugs

Chronic use by the expectant mother of "hard" drugs, including opium derivatives, barbiturates, and amphetamines, in large doses, is harmful to the fetus. Intrauterine distress, low birth weight, and serious compromise as the consequence of drug withdrawal soon after birth have been well documented. Often the mother who uses hard drugs does not seek prenatal care and, even if she does, she may not admit to the use of such substances. Detection of scars from venipunctures may be the first clue. As emphasized elsewhere (see Chapter 38, p. 788),

the management of pregnancy and delivery and successful care of the newborn infant may be extremely difficult. Early abortion should be considered for the addicted pregnant woman who wants to try to "kick the habit."

The effects of maternal marijuana smoking on the human embryo and fetus are not known. Maternal administration of Δ^9tetrahydrocannabol in large amounts is teratogenic in some animals at least.

Care of the Teeth. Examination of the teeth should be included in the prenatal general physical examination. Pregnancy rarely is a contraindication to needed dental treatment. The concept that dental caries are aggravated by pregnancy is unfounded.

Immunization. There has been some concern over the safety of various immunization techniques during pregnancy. The recommendations of the American College of Obstetricians and Gynecologists (1982) with appropriate updating for specific immunizations during pregnancy are summarized below:

1. Cholera	Only to meet international travel requirements
2. Hepatitis A	After exposure; newborns of mothers who are incubating or ill should receive 1 dose after birth (see Chapter 28, p. 613)
3. Hepatitis B	Hepatitis B hyperimmune globulin to infant soon after delivery, followed by vaccination (see Chapter 28, p. 614)
4. Influenza	Evaluate pregnant woman for immunization according to criteria applied to others
5. Measles	Live virus vaccine contraindicated on theoretic grounds during pregnancy; pooled immune globulins for postexposure prophylaxis
6. Mumps	Contraindicated on theoretic grounds during pregnancy
7. Plague	Should be used only if substantial risk of infection

8. Poliomyelitis	Not recommended routinely for adults but mandatory in epidemics or when traveling to endemic area
9. Rabies	Same as nonpregnant
10. Rubella	Contraindicated although teratogenicity of vaccine appears to be negligible (see Chapter 38, p. 786)
11. Tetanus–diphtheria	Give toxoid if no primary series or no booster in 10 years; for postexposure prophylaxis in unvaccinated tetanus immune globulin + toxoid
12. Typhoid	Recommended if traveling in endemic region
13. Varicella	Varicella-zoster immune globulin may be given; indicated for newborns whose mothers developed varicella within 4 days before or 2 after delivery
14. Yellow fever	Immunize before travel to high-risk area but postpone travel if possible

Medications

With rare exception, any drug that exerts a systemic effect in the mother will cross the placenta to reach the embryo and fetus. The effects on the offspring cannot be predicted accurately either from the effects or lack of effects on the mother or from the effects or lack of effects on the offspring of animal species. Widespread use of a medication during pregnancy without recognized adverse effects on the fetus does not guarantee the safety of the medication. Only after many years of use was it established that diphenylhydantoin (Dilantin) and phenobarbital given to women to control epilepsy may both induce fetal malformation and impair synthesis by the fetus and newborn infant of the vitamin K-dependent coagulation factors II, VII, IX, and X (see Chapter 28, p. 608). Not until deliberate, careful, extensive monitoring has failed to identify any adverse effects on the offspring not only in utero or childhood but also in the mature adult, can a drug really be declared to be safe for use in pregnancy. An especially pertinent example of delayed recognition of adverse effects by a drug

that was widely used in obstetrics for a number of years is the induction of several abnormalities of the reproductive organs, including vaginal cancer, in young women whose mothers ingested diethylstilbestrol during pregnancy (see Chapter 25, p. 497).

Even the use of aspirin by the mother has been demonstrated to cause a variety of adverse effects not previously suspected. Maternal ingestion of aspirin induces a degree of platelet dysfunction and diminishes factor XII activity (Bleyer and Breckenridge, 1970; Corby and Schulman, 1971). Shapiro and associates (1976) could find no evidence that the use of aspirin during pregnancy caused perinatal death or reduced birth weight. Moreover, aspirin does not appear to be teratogenic (Slone and co-workers, 1976). However, Australian workers reported that persistent ingestion of analgesic compounds containing salicylates in combination with caffeine or phenacetin or both is associated with an increased incidence of anemia, hemorrhage, prolonged gestation, perinatal mortality, and low birth weight (Collins and Turner, 1975; Turner and Collins, 1974).

Because of aspirin's potentially adverse effects on the hemostatic mechanism and its displacement of bilirubin from protein-binding sites, the use of aspirin should be discouraged, especially late in pregnancy. Acetamenophen has been suggested as a safer alternative; however, we have observed severe maternal hepatic and renal failure and fetal death from acetaminophen toxicity.

The administration of prostaglandin synthease inhibitors, such as indomethacin, will sometimes arrest premature labor but may also cause premature closure of the ductus arteriosus in the fetus.

All physicians should develop the habit early of ascertaining the likelihood of pregnancy before prescribing drugs for any woman, since a number of medications in common use can be injurious to the embryo and the fetus. Package inserts provided by pharmaceutical companies and approved by the Food and Drug Administration should be consulted before drugs are prescribed for pregnant women. **If a drug is administered during pregnancy, the advantages to be gained must clearly outweigh any risks inherent in its use.**

COMMON COMPLAINTS

Nausea and Vomiting

Nausea and vomiting are common complaints during the first half of pregnancy. Typically, nausea and vomiting commence between the first and second missed menstrual period and continue until about the time of the fourth missed period. Nausea and vomiting are usually worse in the morning but may continue throughout the day.

The genesis of pregnancy-induced nausea and vomiting is not clear. Possibly the hormonal changes of pregnancy are responsible. Chorionic gonadotropin, for instance, has been implicated on the basis that its levels are rather high at the same time that nausea and vomiting are most common. Moreover, in women with hydatidiform mole, in which levels of chorionic gonadotropin typically are very much higher than in normal pregnancy, nausea and vomiting are often prominent clinical features. However, Soules and co-workers (1980) found no relationship between the serum levels of chorionic gonadotropin and the incidence and severity of nausea and vomiting in pregnant women, including those with a hydatidiform mole. Emotional factors undoubtedly can contribute to the severity of the nausea and vomiting of pregnancy. Very infrequently, vomiting may be so severe that dehydration, electrolyte and acid–base disturbances, and starvation become serious problems.

Seldom is the treatment of nausea and vomiting of pregnancy so successful that the affected expectant mother is afforded complete relief. However, the unpleasantness and discomfort usually can be minimized. Eating small feedings at more frequent intervals but stopping short of satiation is of value. Since the smell of certain foods often precipitates or aggravates the symptoms, such foods should be avoided as much as possible.

For several years at Parkland Memorial Hospital a combination of doxylamine succinate plus pyridoxine in a specially coated tablet (Bendectin) has been prescribed for pregnancy-induced nausea and vomiting. Usually two tablets taken when retiring and, if necessary, another taken upon arising provided a measure of relief for most women. The preparation is no longer available as the consequence of legal pressures.

> There has been considerable lay publicity which suggested, at least, that the use of Bendectin causes fetal malformations and lawsuits have been initiated based on this assumption. However, data have been published from at least nine series of pregnant women who used Bendectin early in pregnancy and in none was there a significant increase in the frequency of malformations among infants exposed in utero (MacMahon, 1981).

A great variety of other agents has been recommended for treatment. Fairweather (1968), for example, in his comprehensive review of nausea and vomiting in pregnancy, tabulated such bizarre and diverse treatments as hibernotherapy, intravenously administered honey, husband's blood, and the husband's sex hormone (testosterone). These are mentioned only to illustrate the extent to which humankind has gone to try to cope with the aggravation from nausea and vomiting induced somehow by early pregnancy.

Fortunately, effective psychologic support can be offered in the form of reassurance to the pregnant woman that these symptoms nearly always will disappear by the fourth month, and, moreover, that pregnancies in which nausea and vomiting occur are more likely to have a favorable outcome than are those without nausea and vomiting (Yerushalmy and Milkovich, 1965).

The syndrome of nausea and vomiting of great intensity and requiring hospitalization for successful management is referred to as *hyperemesis gravidarum*. Prompt correction of fluid and electrolyte imbalances usually relieves the symptoms (Chapter 28, p. 613). Today therapeutic abortion is rarely required.

Backache

Backache occurs to some extent in some pregnant women. Minor degrees follow excessive strain or fatigue and excessive bending, lifting, or walking. Mild backache usually requires little more than elimination of the strain and occasionally a lightweight maternity girdle.

Severe backaches should not be attributed simply to pregnancy until a thorough orthopedic examination has been conducted. Muscular spasm and tenderness, which are often classified clinically as acute strain or fibrositis, respond well to analgesics, heat, and rest.

In some women, motion of the symphysis pubis and lumbosacral joints, and general relaxation of pelvic ligaments may be demonstrated. In severe cases, the pregnant woman may be unable to walk or even remain comfortable without support furnished by a heavy girdle and prolonged periods of rest. Occasionally, anatomic defects are found, either congenital or traumatic, which may precipitate the complaints. Pain caused by herniation of an intervertebral disc occurs during pregnancy with about the same frequency as at other times.

Varicosities

Varicosities, generally resulting from congenital predisposition, are exaggerated by prolonged standing, pregnancy, and advancing age. Usually varicosities become more prominent as pregnancy advances, as weight increases, and as the length of time spent upright is prolonged.

The symptoms produced by varicosities vary from cosmetic blemishes on the lower extremities and mild discomfort at the end of the day to severe discomfort that requires prolonged rest with the feet elevated.

The treatment of varicosities of the lower extremities is generally limited to periodic rest with elevation of the legs, or elastic stockings, or both. Surgical correction of the condition during pregnancy generally is not advised, although the symptoms rarely may be so severe that injection, ligation, or even stripping of the veins is necessary in order to allow the pregnant woman to remain ambulatory. In general, these operations should be postponed until after delivery. Varicosities of the vulva may be aided by application of a foam rubber pad suspended across the vulva by a belt of the type used with a perineal pad. Rarely, large varicosities may rupture, resulting in profuse hemorrhage.

A severe case of massive varicosities that involved both legs and the vulva of a woman of high parity is demonstrated in Figure 13-1. Treatment during pregnancy consisted of elastic stockings, frequent elevation of the legs throughout the day to provide drainage, and

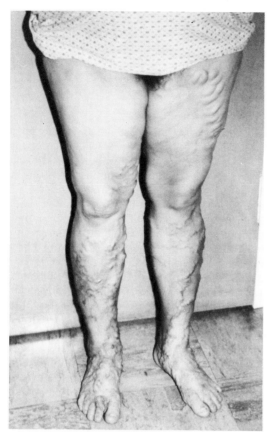

Figure 13-1. Massive varices during pregnancy in a multiparous woman. Well-fitting support hose provided considerable relief until surgical treatment could be applied late in the puerperium.

avoidance of injury to the affected parts. (A leg varix had ruptured with severe hemorrhage, necessitating transfusion shortly before this pregnancy.) Delivery was accomplished spontaneously without laceration. Aggressive ambulation with elastic support stockings was initiated soon after delivery and after tubal sterilization. Surgical intervention with extensive vein stripping was performed late in the puerperium.

Hemorrhoids

Varicosities of hemorrhoidal veins occasionally first appear during pregnancy. More often, pregnancy causes an exacerbation or recurrence of previous symptoms. The development or aggravation of hemorrhoids during pregnancy is related undoubtedly to increased pressure in the hemorrhoidal veins caused by obstruction of venous return by the large pregnant uterus, and to the tendency toward constipation during pregnancy. Usually pain and swelling are relieved by topically applied anesthetics, warm soaks, and agents that soften the stool. Thrombosis of a hemorrhoidal vein can cause considerable pain, but the clot can usually be evacuated by incising

the wall of the involved vein with a scalpel under topical anesthesia.

Bleeding from hemorrhoidal veins occasionally may result in loss of sufficient blood to cause iron deficiency anemia. The loss of only 15 ml of blood results in the loss of 6 to 7 mg of iron, an amount equal to the daily requirements for iron during the latter half of pregnancy. If bleeding is persistent, hemorrhoidectomy may be required. In general, however, hemorrhoidectomy is not desirable during pregnancy, since most often hemorrhoids become asymptomatic soon after delivery.

Heartburn

Heartburn, one of the most common complaints of pregnant women, usually is caused by reflux of gastric or duodenal contents into the lower esophagus (Feeney, 1982). The increased frequency of regurgitation during pregnancy most likely results from the upward displacement and compression of the stomach by the uterus combined with decreased gastrointestinal motility. In some pregnant women, the cardia actually herniates through the diaphragm.

In most pregnant women symptoms are mild and relieved by a regimen of more frequent but smaller meals and avoidance of bending over or lying flat. Antacid preparations may provide considerable relief. Aluminum hydroxide, magnesium trisilicate, or magnesium hydroxide, alone or in combination (for example, Amphojel, Gelusil, Maalox, and milk of magnesia), should be used in preference to sodium bicarbonate. The pregnant woman who tends to retain sodium can become edematous as the result of ingestion of excessive amounts of sodium bicarbonate. Antacids that contain magnesium and aluminum hydroxides impair absorption of iron somewhat but otherwise appear to be quite innocuous (Gant and co-workers, unpublished).

Pica

Occasionally during pregnancy bizarre cravings for strange foods develop and at times for materials hardly considered edible, such as laundry starch, clay, and even dirt. For example, at Parkland Memorial Hospital, interrogation of recently delivered mothers in a single day disclosed that the following items were craved and consumed by them during the current pregnancy: Argo Gloss Starch, flour, baking powder, baking soda, clay, baked dirt, powdered bricks, and frost scraped from the refrigerator (pagophagia).

The ingestion of starch (amylophagia) or clay (geophagia) or related items is practiced more often by socioeconomically less privileged pregnant women. It is unlikely that the craving for these materials is the consequence of hunger but is rather in large part a social custom.

The desire for dry lump starch, clay, chopped ice, or even refrigerator frost has been considered by some to be triggered by severe iron deficiency. Although women with severe iron deficiency sometimes crave these items, and although the craving is usually ameliorated after correction of the iron deficiency, not all pregnant women with pica are necessarily iron-deficient.

Minnich and associates (1968) found that the ingestion of clay, especially Turkish clay and to a lesser extent clays from Georgia and Mississippi, impaired absorption of iron. In Dallas, however, we were unable to demonstrate that either of two Texas clays studied or Argo Gloss Starch reduced absorption of iron significantly (Talkington and associates, 1970).

The consumption of starch in sufficient quantities to provide a significant portion of the calories ingested or to cause ptyalism is not healthful nor is the ingestion of clay to the extent that the intestine is sufficiently filled to cause obstruction of labor or fecal impaction. Nonetheless, it is quite unlikely that either laundry starch or clay free of parasites is distinctly harmful to the pregnancy if consumed in moderation and if the diet is nutritionally adequate.

Ptyalism

Women during pregnancy are occasionally distressed by profuse salivation. The cause of the ptyalism sometimes appears to be stimulation of the salivary glands by the ingestion of starch. This cause should be looked for and eradicated if found.

Fatigue

Early in pregnancy, most women complain of fatigue and desire for excessive periods of sleep. The condition usually remits spontaneously by the fourth month of pregnancy and has no special significance.

Headache

Headache early in pregnancy is a frequent complaint. A few cases may result from sinusitis or ocular strain caused by refractive errors. In the vast majority, however, no cause can be demonstrated. Treatment is largely symptomatic. By the middle of pregnancy, most of these headaches decrease in severity or disappear. The pathologic significance of headaches as the consequence of pregnancy-induced hypertension that develops later in pregnancy is considered in Chapter 27 (p. 541).

Leukorrhea

Pregnant women commonly develop increased vaginal discharge, which in many instances has no pathologic cause. Increased formation of mucus by cervical glands in response to hyperestrogenemia is undoubtedly a contributing factor. If the secretion is troublesome, the woman may be advised to douche with water mildly acidified with vinegar. The precautions for douching listed on page 258 should be stressed.

Occasionally, troublesome leukorrhea is the result of an infection caused by *Trichomonas vaginalis* or *Candida albicans*.

Trichomonas vaginalis. This organism can be identified in as many as 20 percent of women during prenatal examination; however, the infection is symptomatic in a much smaller percentage of pregnant women. Trichomonal vaginitis is characterized by foamy leukorrhea with pruritis and irritation. Trichomonads are readily demonstrated in fresh vaginal secretions as flagellated, pearshaped, motile organisms that are somewhat larger than leukocytes.

It has been suggested that *Trichomonas vaginalis* is a cause of premature labor. However, Mason and Brown (1980) found no difference in birth weights of infants from mothers with or without vaginal infestation with the organism.

Metronidazole (Flagyl) has proved effective in eradicating *Trichomonas vaginalis*. The drug may be administered orally or vaginally. When ingested by the mother, metronidazole crosses the placenta and enters the fetal circulation; the possibility of teratogenicity had been raised if metronidazole were ingested during the first trimester. However, earlier described chromosomal abnormalities following metronidazole therapy for Crohn disease are now thought by the investigators to have been the consequence of sulphasalazine and not metronidazole. In a more recent report they found no increase in frequency of chromosomal abberations after 4 months of therapy (Mitelman and associates, 1980).

Candida albicans. *Candida* (Monilia) can be cultured from the vagina in about 25 percent of women approaching term. Asymptomatic vaginal candidiasis probably requires no treatment. However, it may sometimes cause an extremely profuse irritating discharge. Miconazole nitrate, 2 percent, in a vaginal cream, has been claimed to be highly effective for the treatment of candidiasis during pregnancy (McNellis and co-workers, 1977). Candidiasis is likely to recur, thereby requiring repeated treatment during pregnancy, but usually it subsides at the end of gestation.

Serious fetal infections with *Candida* occur but are rare when compared to the high prevalence of *Candida* in the maternal vagina. Penetration of the fetal membranes, even without gross rupture and invasion of the umbilical cord, can lead to an intense inflammatory response in the fetus with a high mortality rate. The presence of a foreign body such as an intrauterine device in the maternal reproductive tract appears to enhance the risk of fetal infection (Whyte and associates, 1982).

REFERENCES

American College of Obstetricians and Gynecologists: Immunization During Pregnancy. Technical Bulletin, No. 64, May, 1982.

Aronson ME, Nelson PK: Fatal air embolism in pregnancy resulting from an unusual sex act. Obstet Gynecol 30:127, 1967

Astrup P, Olsen HM, Trolle D, Kjeldsen K: Effect of moderate carbon-monoxide-exposure on fetal development. Lancet 2:1220, 1972

Bayless TM, Rothfeld B, Massa C, Wise L, Paige D, Bedine M: Lactose and milk intolerance: Clinical implications. N Engl J Med 292:1156, 1975

Berkowitz GS, Kelsey L, Holford TR, Berkowitz RL: Physical activity and the risk of spontaneous preterm delivery. J Reprod Med 28:581, 1983

Bleyer WA, Breckenridge RT: Studies on the detection of adverse drug reactions in the newborn. JAMA 213:2049, 1970

Boomer AL, Christensen BL: Antepartum hematocrit, maternal smoking and birth weight. J Reprod Med 27:387, 1982

Bureau MA, Monette J, Shapcott D, Paré C, Mathieu J-L, Lippé J, Blovin D, Berthiaume Y, Bégin R: Carboxyhemoglobin concentration in fetal cord blood and in blood of mothers who smoked during labor. Pediatrics 69:371, 1982

Butler NR, Goldstein H: Smoking in pregnancy and subsequent child development. Br Med J 3:573, 1973

Calvert JP, Crean EE, Newcombe RG, Pearson JF: Antenatal screening of measurement of symphysis-fundus height. Br Med J 285:846, 1982

Center for Disease Control: Influenza vaccine: Preliminary statement. Ann Intern Med. 89:373, 1978

Chanarin I, McFayden IR, Kyle R: The physiological macrocytosis of pregnancy. Brit J Obstet Gynaecol 84:504, 1977

Chisholm M: A controlled clinical trial of prophylactic folic acid and iron in pregnancy. J Obstet Gynaecol Brit Comm 73:191, 1966

Clarren SK: Recognition of the fetal alcohol syndrome. JAMA 245:2436, 1981

Cleary RE, Lumeng L, Li Y-K: Maternal and fetal plasma levels of pyridoxal phosphate at term: Adequacy of vitamin B_6 supplementation during pregnancy. Am J Obstet Gynecol 121:25, 1975

Cochrane WA: Overnutrition in prenatal and neonatal life: A problem? Can Med Assoc J 93:893, 1965

Collins E, Turner G: Maternal effects of regular salicylate ingestion in pregnancy. Lancet 2:335, 1975

Corby DG, Schulman I: The effect of antenatal drug administration on aggregation of platelets of newborn infants. J Pediatr 79:307, 1971

Davies DP, Gray OP, Ellwood PC, Abernathy M: Cigarette smoking in pregnancy: Associations with maternal weight gain and fetal growth. Lancet 1:385, 1976

De Leeuw NK, Lowenstein L, Hsieh YS: Iron deficiency and hydremia in normal pregnancy. Medicine 45:201, 1966

Delgado H, Lechug A, Yarbrough C, Martorell R, Klein RE, Irwin M: Maternal nutrition—Its effects on infant growth and development and birthspacing. In Moghissi KS, Evans TN (eds): Nutritional Impacts on Women. Hagerstown, MD, Harper & Row, 1977, p 133

D'Souza SW, Black PM, Williams N, Jennison RF: Effect of smoking during pregnancy upon the haematological values of cord blood. Br J Obstet Gynaecol 85:495, 1978

Duffus G, MacGillivray I: The incidence of preeclamptic toxemia in smokers and non-smokers. Lancet 1:994, 1968

Eastman NJ, Jackson E: Weight relationships in pregnancy: I. The bearing of maternal weight gain and pre-pregnancy weight on birth weight in full term pregnancies. Obstet Gynecol Surv 23:1003, 1968

Ekstrand J: No evidence of transfer of fluoride from plasma to breast milk. Br Med J 283:761, 1981

Emery AEH: Folates and fetal central-nervous-system malformations. Lancet 1:703, 1977

Fairweather DV: Nausea and vomiting in pregnancy. Am J Obstet Gynecol 102:135, 1968

Feeney JG: Heartburn in pregnancy (editorial). Br Med J 284:1138, 1982

Food and Nutrition Board Position Paper on the Relationship of Nutrition to Brain Development and Behavior. Washington, DC, National Academy of Sciences, 1973

Forbes G: Air embolism as complication of vaginal douching in pregnancy. Br Med J 2:529, 1944

Gant NF, Scott DE, Pritchard JA: Unpublished observations

Garn SM, Keating MT, Falkner F: Hematological status and pregnancy outcomes. Am J Clin Nutr 34:115, 1981

Gillmer MDG, Mazibuko D: Pyridoxine treatment of chemical diabetes in pregnancy. Am J Obstet Gynecol 133:499, 1979

Glenn FB, Glenn WD III, Duncan RC: Fluoride tablet supplementation during pregnancy for caries immunity: A study of the offspring produced. Am J Obstet Gynecol 143:560, 1982

Goldstein H: Smoking in pregnancy: Some notes on the statistical controversy. Br J Prevent Soc Med 31:13, 1977

Goodlin RC: Why treat "physiologic" anemias of pregnancy? J Reprod Med 27:639, 1982

Goodlin RC, Keller DW, Raffin M: Orgasm during late pregnancy: Possible deleterious effects. Obstet Gynecol 38:916, 1971

Goodlin RC, Schmidt W, Creevy DC: Uterine tension and fetal heart rate during maternal orgasm. Obstet Gynecol 39:125, 1972

Grudzinkas JG, Watson C, Chard T: Does sexual intercourse cause fetal distress? Lancet 2:692, 1979

Hall MH: Folates and the fetus. Lancet 1:648, 1977

Hardy JB, Mellits ED: Does maternal smoking during pregnancy have a long-term effect on the child? Lancet 2:1332, 1973

Hauth JC, Gilstrap LC III, Widmer K: Fetal heart rate reactivity before and after maternal jogging during the third trimester. Am J Obstet Gynecol 142:545, 1982

Haworth JC, Ellestad-Sayed JJ, King J, Dilling LA: Fetal growth retardation in cigarette-smoking mothers is not due to decreased maternal food intake. Am J Obstet Gynecol 137:719, 1980

Heaney RP, Skillman TG: Calcium metabolism in normal human pregnancy. J Clin Endocrinol 33:661, 1971

Herbert V, Jacob E: Destruction of vitamin B_{12} by ascorbic acid. JAMA 230:241, 1974

Higginbottom MC, Sweetman L, Nyhan WL: A syndrome of methylmalonic aciduria, homocystinuria, megaloblastic anemia and neurologic abnormalities in a vitamin B_{12}-deficient breast-fed infant of a strict vegetarian. N Engl J Med 299:317, 1978

Hobel CJ, Youkeles L, Forsythe A: Prenatal and intrapartum high-risk screening. II. Risk factors reassessed. Am J Obstet Gynecol 135:1051, 1979

Horowitz HS, Heifetz SB: Effects of prenatal exposure to fluoridation on dental caries. Pub Health Rep 82:297, 1967

Hytten FE, Leitch I: The Physiology of Human Pregnancy, 2d ed. Oxford, Blackwell, 1971

Jimenez JM, Tyson JE, Reisch JS: Clinical measures of gestational age in normal pregnancies. Obstet Gynecol 61:438, 1983

Jones KL, Smith DW: The fetal alcohol syndrome. Teratology 12:1, 1975

Jones KL, Smith DW, Streissguth AP, Myrianthopoulos NC: Incidence of fetal alcohol syndrome in offspring of chronically alcoholic women. Pediatr Res 8:440, 1974

Jones KL, Smith DW, Ulleland CN, Streissguth AP: Pattern of malformation in offspring of chronic alcoholic mothers. Lancet 1:7815, 1974

Jouppila P, Kirkinen P, Eik-Nes S: Acute effect of maternal smoking on the human fetal blood flow. Br J Obstet Gynaecol 90:7, 1983

Koller O: The clinical significance of hemodilution during pregnancy. Obstet Gynecol Surv 37:649, 1982

Kortenoever ME: Pathology of pregnancy: Pregnancy of long duration and postmature infant. Obstet Gynecol Surv 5:812, 1950

Krushna K: Tobacco chewing in pregnancy. Br J Obstet Gynaecol 85:726, 1978

Laurence KM, James N, Miller MH, Tennant GB, Campbell H: Double-blind randomised controlled trial of folate treatment before conception to prevent recurrence of neural-tube defects. Br Med J 282:1509, 1981

Lehtovirta P, Forss M: The acute effect of smoking on intervillous blood flow of the placenta. Br J Obstet Gynaecol 85:729, 1978

Little RE: Epidemiologic and experimental studies in drinking and pregnancy: The state of the art. Neurobehav Toxicol Teratol 3:163, 1981

MacMahon B: More on Bendectin. JAMA 246:37, 1981

Mason PR, Brown I McL: Trichomonas in pregnancy. Lancet 2:1025, 1980

McNellis D, McLeod M, Lawson J, Pasquale SA: Treatment of vulvovaginal candidiasis in pregnancy. Obstet Gynecol 50:674, 1977

Mills JL, Harlap S, Harley EE: Should coitus late in pregnancy be discouraged? Lancet 2:136, 1981

Minnich V, Okcuoglu A, Tarcon Y, Arcasoy A, Cin S, Yorukoglu O, Renda F, Demirag B: Pica in Turkey: II. Effect of clay upon iron absorption. Am J Clin Nutr 21:78, 1968

Mitelman F, Strombeck B, Ursing B: No cytogenetic effect of metronidazole. Lancet 1:1249, 1980

Monheit AG: Maternal and fetal cardiovascular effects of nicotine infusion in pregnant sheep. Am J Obstet Gynecol 145:290, 1983

Murphy JF, Dauncey M: Employment in pregnancy. Lancet 1:1163, 1984

Naeye R: Weight gain and the outcome of pregnancy. Am J Obstet Gynecol 135:3, 1979

Naeye RL, Peters EC: Working during pregnancy: Effects on the fetus. Pediatrics 69:724, 1982

Nakano R: Post-term pregnancy. Acta Obstet Gynecol Scand 51:217, 1972

Paintin DB, Thomson AM, Hytten FE: Iron and the haemoglobin level in pregnancy. J Obstet Gynaecol Br Commonw 73:181, 1966

Perkins RP: Failure of pyridoxine to improve glucose tolerance in gestational diabetes mellitus. Obstet Gynecol 50:370, 1977

Pharoah POD, Buttfield IH, Hetzel BS: Neurological damage to the fetus resulting from severe iodine deficiency during pregnancy. Lancet 1:308, 1971

Pirani BBK, MacGillivray I: Smoking during pregnancy: Its effects on maternal metabolism and fetoplacental function. Br J Obstet Gynaecol 52:257, 1978

Pitkin RM: Calcium metabolism in pregnancy: A review. Am J Obstet Gynecol 121:724, 1975

Poskitt EME, Hensey OJ, Smith CS: Dev Med Child Neurol 24:596, 1982

Prentice AM, Whitehead RG, Watkinson M, Lamb WH, Cole TJ: Prenatal dietary supplementation of African women and birth-weight. Lancet 1:489, 1983

Pritchard JA, Hunt CF: A comparison of the hematologic responses following the routine prenatal administration of intramuscular and oral iron. Surg Gynecol Obstet 106:516, 1958

Pritchard JA, Scott DE: Iron demands during pregnancy. In Hallberg L, Harwerth H-G, Vannotti A (eds): Iron Deficiency: Pathogenesis, Clinical Aspects, Therapy. New York, Academic, 1970

Pritchard JA, Whalley PJ: High risk pregnancy and reproductive outcome. In Gluck L (ed): Modern Perinatal Medicine. Chicago, Year Book, 1974

Pritchard JA, Scott DE, Whalley PJ: Folic acid requirements in pregnancy induced megaloblastic anemia. JAMA 208:1163, 1969

Pugh WE, Fernandez FL: Coitus late in pregnancy. Obstet Gynecol 2:636, 1953

Quaranta P, Currell R, Redman CWG, Robinson JS: Prediction of small-for-date infants by measurements of symphysial-fundal height. Br J Obstet Gynaecol 88:115, 1981

Recommended Dietary Allowances, 9th ed. Food and Nutrition Board, Washington, DC, National Research Council, National Academy of Sciences, 1979

Ribeiro MD, Stein Z, Susser M, Cohen P, Neugut R: Prenatal starvation and maternal blood pressure. Am J Clin Nutr 35:535, 1982

Robinson M: Salt in pregnancy. Lancet 1:178, 1958

Rosett HL, Weiner L, Lee A, Zuckerman B, Dowling E, Oppenheimer E: Patterns of alcohol consumption and fetal development. Obstet Gynecol 61:539, 1983

Rush D: Lower weight gain among smokers explains most of the effect of smoking on birthweight. Pediatr Res 8:450, 1974

Sauberlich HE: Vitamin indices. In Laboratory Indices of Nutritional Status in Pregnancy. Washington DC, National Research Council Committee on Nutrition of the Mother and Preschool Child, National Academy of Sciences, 1978, p 109

Saurel MJ, Kaminski M: Pregnant women at work. Lancet 1:475, 1983

Schaumburg H, Kaplan J, Windebank A, Vick N, Rasmus S, Pleasure D, Brown MJ: Sensory neuropathy from pyridoxine abuse. N Engl J Med 309:445, 1983

Seligman PA, Caskey JH, Frazier JL, Zucker RM, Podell ER, Allen RH: Measurements of iron absorption from prenatal multivitamin-mineral supplements. Obstet Gynecol 61:356, 1983

Scott DE, Pritchard JA, Saltin A-S, Humphreyes SM: Iron deficiency during pregnancy. In Hallberg L, Harwerth H-G, Vannotti A (eds): Iron Deficiency: Pathogenesis, Clinical Aspects, Therapy. New York, Academic, 1970

Shapiro S, Monson RR, Kaufman DW, Siskind V, Heinonen OP, Slone D: Perinatal mortality and birth-weight in relation to aspirin taken during pregnancy. Lancet 1:1375, 1976

Slone D, Heinonen OP, Kaufman DW, Siskind V, Monson RR, Shapiro S: Aspirin and congenital malformations. Lancet 1:1373, 1976

Smith CA: Effects of maternal undernutrition upon the newborn infant in Holland (1944–1945). Am J Obstet Gynecol 30:229, 1947

Smithells RW, Sheppard S, Schorah CJ, Seller MJ, Nevin NC, Harris R, Read AP: Possible prevention of neural-tube defects by periconceptual vitamin supplementation. Lancet 1:339, 1980

Smithells RW, Sellar MJ, Harris R, Fielding DW, Schorah CJ, Nevin NC, Sheppard S, Read AP, Walker S, Wild J: Further experience of vitamin supplementation for prevention of neural tube defect recurrences. Lancet 1:1027, 1983

Socol ML, Manning FA, Murata Y, Druzin ML: Maternal smoking causes fetal hypoxia: Experimental evidence. Am J Obstet Gynecol 142:214, 1982

Sokol RJ, Rosen MG, Stojkov J, Chik J: Clinical application of high-risk scoring on an obstetric service. Am J Obstet Gynecol 128:652, 1977

Soules MR, Hughes CL Jr, Garcia JA, Livengood CH, Prystowski MR, Alexander E III: Nausea and vomiting of pregnancy: Role of human chorionic gonadotropin and 17-hydroxyprogesterone. Obstet Gynecol 55:696, 1980

Stein Z, Susser M, Rush D: Prenatal nutrition and birth weight: Experiments and quasi-experiments in the past decade. J Reprod Med 21:287, 1978

Stein Z, Susser M, Saenger G, Marolla F: Nutrition and mental performance. Science 178:708, 1972

Stockman JA III: Infections and iron: Too much of a good thing? Am J Dis Child 135:18, 1981

Swanson CA, King JC: Gestational hypozincemia. Obstet Gynecol 1983, in press

Talkington KM, Gant NF, Scott DE, Pritchard JA: Effect of ingestion of starch and some clays on iron absorption. Am J Obstet Gynecol 108:262, 1970

Task Force Report. Am College Obstet Gynecol Assessment of Maternal Nutrition. Chicago, American College of Obstetricians and Gynecologists, 1978

Taylor DJ, Lind T: Haemotological changes during normal pregnancy: Iron induced macrocytosis. Br J Obstet Gynaecol 83:760, 1976

Taylor DJ, Mallen C, McDougall N, Lind T: Effect of iron supplementation on serum ferritin levels during and after pregnancy. Br J Obstet Gynaecol 89:1011, 1982

Turner G, Collins E: Fetal effects of regular salicylate ingestion in pregnancy. Lancet 2:338, 1974

Underwood PB, Hester LL, Lafitte T Jr, Gregg KV: The relationship of smoking empirically related to pregnancy outcome. Obstet Gynecol 29:1, 1967

Whalley PJ, Scott DE, Pritchard JA: Maternal folate deficiency and pregnancy wastage: I. Placental abruption. Am J Obstet Gynecol 105:670, 1969

White JA, Moffa AM: Periconceptional supplementation of folic acid and the incidence of open neural tube defects in golden hamster embryos. Presented before the Society for Gynecological Investigation, San Francisco, March 21–24, 1984

Whyte RK, Hussain Z, deSa D: Antenatal infections with *Candida* species. Arch Dis Child 57:528, 1982

Worthen N, Bustillo M: Effect of urinary bladder fullness on fundal height measurements. Am J Obstet Gynecol 138:759, 1980

Yerushalmy J: Infants with low birth weight born before their mothers started to smoke cigarettes. Am J Obstet Gynecol 112:277, 1972

Yerushalmy J, Milkovich L: Evaluation of the teratogenic effect of meclizine in man. Am J Obstet Gynecol 93:553, 1965

Yip R, Mohandas N, Clark MR, Jain S, Shohet SB, Dallman PR: Red cell membrane stiffness in iron deficiency. Blood 62:99, 1983

Zlatnik FJ, Burmeister LF: Dietary protein in pregnancy: Effect on anthropometric indices of the newborn. Am J Obstet Gynecol 146:199, 1983

14
Techniques to Evaluate Fetal Health

The Fetus as a Patient

Until relatively recently, the intrauterine sanctuary of the embryo and fetus was held to be inviolate. The mother was the patient to be cared for; the fetus was but another, albeit transient, maternal organ. The philosophy prevailed that "good maternal care" would automatically provide what was best for the products of conception. Ideally, labor would not occur until the fetus weighed more than 2500 g (once the widely accepted definition of fetal maturity), except in instances of gross developmental abnormality when, it was hoped, the embryo or nonviable fetus might be expelled spontaneously. If, however, spontaneous abortion did not ensue, society decreed the only alternative to be that the parents, or at times some governmental agency, must try to care for the subsequently liveborn but malformed offspring.

During the past two decades, remarkably intimate knowledge of the human fetus and his or her immediate environment has accumulated (see Chapter 8). As did maternal health earlier in this century, fetal health, or fetal medicine, has come to be appreciated not merely as an exciting arena for research but as a clinical discipline with great potential for favorably influencing the quality of human offspring. Indeed, the fetus is no longer dealt with as a maternal appendage ultimately to be shed at the whim of biologic forces beyond control. Instead, the fetus has achieved the status of the second patient, a patient who usually faces much greater risks of serious morbidity and mortality than does the mother.

It is now possible not only to identify but to quantify with some precision physical abnormalities and functional derangements that afflict the fetus. Moreover, in some instances treatment can be implemented—surgical as well as medical—while the fetus continues to mature in utero.

The many advances in diagnosis and treatment which now clearly establish the fetus as a patient have also contributed remarkably to legal considerations involving the fetus. Fetal legal rights are emerging; for example, in some courts, the fetus has been allowed to file suit. Moreover, law enforcement officials and the judiciary are now more inclined to think of the fetus as a person deserving protection against criminal acts performed against him. Interestingly, not too long ago in Dallas a fetus killed in a motor vehicle accident a few minutes before birth at term was not a victim of manslaughter in the eyes of the law enforcement officials; in fact, the fetus could not even qualify as a traffic fatality.

DIAGNOSTIC MODALITIES

A variety of techniques that may be of value for appraising the health of the embryo and fetus are considered, especially, but certainly not only, in this chapter: (1) amniocentesis, amnioscopy, and fetoscopy; (2) ultrasonography; (3) radiography, including amniography and fetography; (4) measurements of certain hormones and enzymes in maternal plasma, urine, or both; (5) antepartum surveillance of well-being using fetal heart "stress" and "nonstress" tests; and (6) intrapartum surveillance of fetal heart action, uterine contractions, and physicochemical properties of fetal blood.

The use of newer biochemical, biophysical, and electronic procedures should be regarded, *as their value is proved,* as worthy additions to existing clinical procedures already available to help identify the fetus at risk. It is emphasized at the outset that these procedures may impose some risk of morbidity and mortality to the fetus and the mother, or impose significant expense, or both. Therefore, their use should provide benefits that clearly outweigh both the potential risks and the costs. Certainly the physician who orders them must be prepared to acknowledge the results and to use them objectively.

There is no doubt that pregnancy outcomes have improved during the time that most, if not all, the techniques described in this chapter have been available to try to identify the presence or absence of fetal well-being. In 1969, for the first time, the perinatal death rate dropped below 30 per 1000. It has continued to fall and in 1980 was estimated to be 17.7 per 1000 births. Although tempting, it is inappropriate to ascribe the dramatic decrease solely to the availability of more techniques to evaluate fetal health. A multiplicity of important factors have undoubtedly contributed to this accomplishment:

1. Less unplanned and unwanted pregnancies as the consequence of federally funded family planning programs and the legalization of elective abortion.

2. Pregnant women taking greater advantage of antepartum care.

3. The prevention or selective abortion of some pregnancies in which the fetus or neonate would have been at increased risk of dying.

4. More liberal use of hospitalization in an attempt to prolong gestation safely.

5. Greater attention paid to the fetus, including the use of a variety of techniques to try to monitor fetal condition.

6. Increased use of cesarean delivery to try to minimize fetal trauma and asphyxia.

7. Availability of excellent neonatal care.

8. As was emphasized by Schifrin (1979), Factor X, or *tender loving care* for mother and fetus-neonate.

AMNIOCENTESIS

The ability to enter the amnionic sac without appreciable risk to the mother or fetus has influenced obstetric care remarkably. The aspiration of a sample of amnionic fluid provides for a variety of diagnostic tests that are indicative of fetal well-being or lack thereof. A very comprehensive listing of abnormalities of the fetus that are amenable to detection with the aid of appropriate analysis of amnionic fluid has been provided by Roberts and co-workers (1983) and is presented in modified form in Table 14-1.

Techniques

Beginning early in the second trimester, after the exocoelomic space between amnion and chorion has been obliterated, the chorion laeve has fused with the uterine decidua, and the uterus is enlarged sufficiently to be easily palpated above the symphysis, amnionic fluid may be aspirated transabdominally. After locally anesthetizing the abdominal wall, a 20- or 22-gauge needle 3 to 6 inches long, depending upon the thickness of the abdominal wall, the size of the uterus, and the site of puncture, is carefully inserted into the amnionic sac. When cells from amnionic fluid are desired for culture, up to 30 ml of amnionic fluid is withdrawn at 15 to 18 weeks gestation.

Risks. The three major risks from amniocentesis are readily deduced: (1) trauma to the fetus, to the placenta, or, less often, to the umbilical cord or to maternal structures; (2) infection; and (3) abortion or premature labor. Surgical asepsis is mandatory to avoid infection not only in the mother and fetus but also in the aspirated amnionic fluid, especially when it is to be used for cell culture or microbiologic studies.

As well as causing hemorrhage into the placenta and into the amnionic sac (Fig. 14-1), perforation of the placenta may lead to significant transfer of fetal blood to the mother, which may incite or enhance maternal

isoimmunization and, in turn, hemolytic disease in the fetus. Therefore, sonographic localization of the placenta before amniocentesis is recommended. Sonographic localization of the placenta before amniocentesis does reduce the likelihood of perforating the placenta during insertion of the needle, but, unfortunately, it does not always preclude fetal to maternal bleeding. Consequently, anti-Rho(D) globulin is commonly administered to nonsensitized Rh(D) negative women at the time of amniocentesis (see Chapter 38, p. 773).

Freda (1973) pointed out that late in pregnancy there is little risk of perforating the placenta if the transabdominal puncture is performed suprapubically, as shown in Figure 14-2. The experiences of Leach and co-workers (1978) further attest to the suprapubic site being the most favorable one for amniocentesis performed late in pregnancy. Whether such a low puncture site enhances the risk of a leak of amnionic fluid is not clear. It has been our experience that, if late in pregnancy the fetus can be easily palpated immediately beneath the proposed site of transabdominal puncture, the placenta is implanted elsewhere. If, however, fetal parts cannot be easily palpated immediately beneath the proposed site of puncture, sonographic localization of the placenta is indicated.

Trauma to the umbilical cord is more likely if the cord is around the neck of the fetus and entry into the amnionic space is attempted adjacent to the fetal head and shoulder. Injury to the fetus is more common when the volume of amnionic fluid is small compared to the size of the fetus, or when the amnionic fluid is thick and does not flow freely through the needle. These later conditions are more likely to be encountered late in pregnancy and especially in the postterm pregnancy. Whenever the possibility exists of placenta implanted beneath the proposed site of puncture, or when amnionic fluid volume appears to be restricted, amniocentesis should be performed with the aid of direct sonographic guidance. Repeated taps after failure to obtain amnionic fluid increase the risk of trauma to the fetus.

After amniocentesis, the fetus who is sufficiently mature to have reasonable potential for survival if delivered should be closely evaluated for evidence of deterioration by closely monitoring the fetal heart rate, especially if the tap was thought possibly to be traumatic. Immediately after delivery all infants should be carefully examined for any evidence of needle puncture. For example, death can be prevented from pneumothorax by detecting at birth a needle wound in the thorax and initiating appropriate treatment immediately.

Several attempts have been made to identify the overall risk of amniocentesis performed near midpregnancy for the purpose of detecting hereditary disease or congenital defects in the fetus. In one study (National Institute of Child Health and Human Development, 1976), no significant differences were found in fetal loss rate, birth weights, birth defects, neonatal complications, or growth and development at 1 year of age. The overall fetal loss was 3.5 percent for the amniocentesis group

TABLE 14-1. SOME DISORDERS DIAGNOSABLE BY AMNIONIC FLUID (AF) ANALYSIS

	Prenatal Diagnosis Possible by Amnionic Fluid Analysis
I. CHROMOSOMAL ANOMALIES*	
All chromosomal disorders	Karyotype of AF cells.
Trisomy 21 (Down syndrome)	Karyotype (AFP elevated).
Trisomy 13	Karyotype (AFP elevated).
Trisomy 18	Karyotype (AFP elevated).
Triploidy	Karyotype (AFP elevated).
II. SKELETAL DISORDERS	
Osteogenesis imperfecta (AR) or congenita (AD)	Increased pyrophosphate.†
Osteogenesis imperfecta tarda (AD)	Increased pyrophosphate.†
Robert syndrome (AR)	Chromosomes have poorly defined centromeres with G-banding and puffed-out centromeres with C-banding.†
III. FETAL INFECTIONS	
Cytomegalovirus	Recovery of cytomegalovirus from AF.
Herpes simplex (fetal liver necrosis)	Increased AFP in maternal serum.†
Rubella	Recovery of rubella virus.
IV. CENTRAL NERVOUS SYSTEM	
Anencephaly	See text.†
Meningocele	See text.†
X-linked aqueductal stenosis	Male karyotype.†
V. HEMATOLOGIC DISORDERS†	
Erythroblastosis fetalis	Increased bilirubin levels.†
Glucose phosphate isomerase deficiency (AD)	Reduced glucose phosphate isomerase activity in cultured AF cells.
Hemoglobin H disease and α-thalassemia	Molecular hybridization of DNA from cultured AF cells with α-globin with DNA to determine number of α-genes.
Sickle-cell anemia	DNA analysis in AF cells by restriction endonuclease digestion.
β-thalassemia	Linkage analysis of polymorphic restriction endonuclease sites and the β-thalassemia gene on amniocyte DNA.
VI. INBORN ERRORS OF METABOLISM	
A. *Amino acid metabolism and organic acid metabolism*	
Argininosuccinic aciduria (AR)	Elevated levels of ^{14}C argininosuccinic acid in cultured amnionic fluid cells or unlabeled argininosuccinic acid in amnionic fluid.
Argininosuccinate synthetase deficiency (citrullemia) (AR)	Elevated levels of citrulline in amnionic fluid fibroblasts.
Hyperargininemia (AR)	Deficient arginase in amnionic fluid.
Hyperornithinemia (gyrate atrophy of the choroid and retina) (AR)	Type I–deficient ornithine decarboxylase. Type III–deficient ornithine ketoacid transaminase.
Hyperlysinemia (AR)	Deficient lysine-ketoglutarate reductase in AF fibroblasts.
Cystinosis (AR)	Accumulation of ^{35}S-cystine in cultured AF cells.
Cystinuria (AR)	Elevated cystine in AF.
Glutaric acidemia (AR)	Glutaric acid in AF-deficient glutaryl-CoA dehydrogenase activity in cultured AF cells.
Homocystinuria (AR)	Increased methionine and homocystine or deficient cystathionine β-synthetase activity in AF cells.
Maple syrup urine disease (AR)	Deficient branched-chain ketoacid decarboxylase activity in cultured AF cells.
Hypervalinemia (AR)	Deficient valine transaminase.
Isovaleric acidemia (AR)	Increased isovaleric acid-deficient isovaleryl-CoA in cultivated AF cells.
β-methylcrotonic aciduria (AR)	Increased β-hydroxyisovaleric acid isovaleryl glycine and tiglic acid. Deficient β-methylcrotonyl-CoA carboxylase.
Methylmalonic aciduria (AR)	Deficient methylmalonyl CoA mutase activity in cultured and uncultured amnionic fluid cells.

(continued)

TABLE 14-1. *(continued)*

	Prenatal Diagnosis Possible by Amnionic Fluid Analysis
β-ketothiolase deficiency (AR)	Elevated levels of methylmalonate in amnionic fluid. Elevated levels of methylcitrate in amnionic fluid. Deficient enzyme.
Proprionyl CoA carboxylase deficiency (AR) (ketotic hyperglycemia)	Deficient proprionyl CoA carboxylase activity in AF cells and methylcitrate in AF.
Sulfite oxydase deficiency (AR)	Deficient sulfite oxidase. Accumulation of sulfite, thiosulfite and ^{35}S-sulfocysteine.
Histidinemia (AR)	Deficient histidase in cultivated AF fibroblasts.
Hyperphenylalaninemia, type V (AR) (PKU variant)	Deficient dihydropteridine reductase in cultivated AF cells. Increased phenylalanine in amnionic fluid.
Nonketotic hyperglycemia (AR)	Elevated glyceine/serine ratio in AF.

B. *Carboyhdrate metabolism*

Aspartylglucosaminuria (AR)	Deficient aspartylglycosylamine amniohydrolase in cultivated AF fibroblasts.
Fucosidosis (AR)	Deficient α-fucosidase in cultivated AF fibroblasts.
Galactosemia, classic form (AR)	Deficient galactose-1-phosphate uridyl transferase activity in cultured amnionic fluid cells.
Galactokinase deficiency (AR)	Deficient galactokinase in cultured amnionic fluid cells.
Gycogen storage disease, type II (AR) (Pompe disease)	Deficient α-1, 4-glucosidase activity in cultured AF cells.
Mannosidosis (AR)	Deficient α-mannosidase in amnionic fluid.
Pyruvate decarboxylase deficiency (AR)	Deficient pyruvate decarboxylase in cultured AF cells.
Pyruvate carboxylase deficiency (AR)	Deficient pyruvate carboxylase in cultured AF cells.

C. *Mucolipidoses*

Mucolipidoses, type II (AR) (I-cell disease)	Decreased activity of several lysosomal enzymes in cultured AF cells; increased lysosomal enzyme activity in AF. Cytoplasmic inclusions in electron micrograph of cultured AF cells.
Mucolipidoses, type III (AR) (pseudo-Hurler polydystrophy)	Multiple lysosomal enzyme deficiencies in cultured AF fibroblasts.
Mucolipodoses, type IV (AR)	^{35}S mucopolysaccharide incorporation in cultured AF cells and cytoplasmic inclusions of cultured AF cells on electron microscopy.

D. *Lipid metabolism*

Cholesteryl ester storage disease (AR)	Deficient acid cholesteryl ester hydrolase in cultured AF skin fibroblasts.
Fabry disease (XR) (diffuse angiokeratoma)	Deficient α-galactosidase activity in cultured and uncultured amnionic fluid cells and AF. Cytoplasmic lipid storage bodies on electron microscopy of cultured AF cells.
Familial hypercholesterolemia (homozygous form) (AD)	Absent or defective LDL cell surface receptors on cultured AF cells.
Farber disease (AR) (familial lipogranulomatosis)	Deficient acid ceramidase activity in cultured AF cells.
Gaucher disease, infant and adult type (AR)	Deficient glucocerebrosidase activity in cultured AF cells.
GM$_1$ gangliosidosis, type I (infantile) (AR)	Absent β-galactosidase activity in cultured AF cells and in AF.
GM$_1$ gangliosidosis, type II (juvenile) (AR)	No β-galactosidase activity in cultured AF cells.
GM$_2$ gangliosidosis, type I (AR) (Tay–Sachs disease)	Deficient β-N-acetyl-hexosaminidase A activity in cultured AF cells and AF.
GM$_2$ gangliosidosis, type II (AR) (Sandhoff disease)	Deficient β-N-acetyl-hexosaminidase A and B activity in cultured AF cells and AF.
GM$_2$ gangliosidosis, type III (juvenile Tay–Sachs disease) (AR)	Deficient hexosaminidase A in cultured AF cells.
GM$_3$ gangliosidosis (sphingolipodystrophy) (AR)	Deficient acetylgalactose acetylgalactos-aminyltransferase in cultured AF cells.
Krabbe disease (AR) (globoid cell leukodystrophy)	Deficient cerebroside β-galactosidase activity in cultured AF cells.
Metachromatic leukodystrophy (AR)	Deficient arylsulfatase A activity in cultured AF cells and AF. Cytoplasmic inclusions on electron microscopy of cultured AF cells.

(continued)

TABLE 14-1. (*continued*)

	Prenatal Diagnosis Possible by Amnionic Fluid Analysis
Multiple sulfatase deficiency (AR)	Deficient arylsulfatases A, B, and C and steroid sulfatases in cultured AF cells.
Niemann–Pick disease (AR)	Deficient sphingomyelin activity in cultured AF cells.
Refsum syndrome (AR)	Deficient phytanic acid α-hydroxylase in cultured AF cells.
Wolman disease (AR)	Deficient acid lipase (acid cholesteryl ester hydrolase) in cultured AF cells.
E. *Mucopolysaccharide (MPS) metabolism*	
MPSIH: Hurler syndrome (AR)	Decreased α-L-iduronidase activity in cultured AF cells.
MPSIS: Scheie syndrome (AR)	Decreased α-L-iduronate sulfatase activity in cultured AF cells.
MPS II: Hunter syndrome (XR)	Deficient iduronate sulfatase activity in cultured AF cells.
MPS III: Sanfilippo syndrome A(AR)	Deficient heparan N-sulfatase activity in cultured AF cells.
MPS III: Sanfilippo syndrome B(AR)	Deficient N-acetyl-α-glucosaminidase activity in cultured AF cells.
MPS IV: Maroteaux–Lamy syndrome (AR)	Deficient arylsulfatase B activity in cultured AF cells.
MPS VII: β-glucuronidase deficiency (AR)	Deficient β-glucuronidase activity in AF cells.
MPS VIII: glucosamine-6-sulfate (AR)	Deficient glucosamine-6-sulfate sulfatase activity in AF cells.
VII. MISCELLANEOUS METABOLIC DISORDERS	
Combined immunodeficiency disease (AR and XR)	Deficient adenosine deaminase activity in cultured AF cells.
Congenital adrenal hyperplasia (AR) (deficient 21-hydroxy-lase)	Elevated 17α-hydroxyprogesterone, Δ^4-androstenedione and pregnanetriol levels in AF.
Congenital sialidosis (mucolipidosis I) (AR)	Deficient neuraminidase activity, increased bound neuraminic acid and ultrastructural abnormalities in AF cells. Increased sialooligosaccharides in AF.
Glutathione synthase deficiency (AR)	Deficient glutathione synthase activity.
γ-Glutamylcysteine synthetase deficiency (AR)	Deficient γ-glutamylcysteine.
5-Oxoprolinuria (pyroglutamic aciduria) (AR)	Deficient glutathione.
Methylene tetrahydrofolate reductase deficiency (AR)	Deficient enzyme in AF cells.
Tetrahydrofolate methyltransferase deficiency (AR)	Deficiency enzyme in cultured AF cells.
Hypophosphatasia (AR)	Deficient bone/liver alkaline phosphatase isoenzyme activity in cultured AF cells and AF deficiency of total alkaline phosphatase activity in cultured AF cells.
Lesch-Nyhan syndrome (XR)	Deficient hypoxanthine-guanine phosphoribosyl transferase activity in cultured AF cells.
Lysosomal acid phosphatase deficiency (AR)	Deficient phosphatase in the lysosomes of cultured AF cells.
Orotic aciduria (AR)	Deficient orotate phosphoribosyltransferase and orotine-5-phosphate decarboxylase.
A. *Porphyrias*	
Congenital erythropoietic porphyria (AR)	Large amounts of uroporphyrin-1 and copro-porphyrin-1 in reddish-brown AF.
Hereditary coproporphyria (AD)	Deficient coproporphyrinogen oxidase activity.
Acute intermittent porphyria (AD)	Decreased activity of uroporphyrinogen-1-synthetase in cultured AF cells.
Protoporphyria (AD)	Deficient heme synthetase activity in AF.
Saccharopinuria (AR)	Decreased activity of aminoadipic semialdehyde-glutamate dehydrogenase.
Xeroderma pigmentosum (AR)	Absent DNA excision repair synthesis by autoradiography in cultured AF cells.
Placental steroid sulfatase deficiency (XR)	Increased dehydroepiandrosterone sulfate in AF.
Primary pituitary dysgenesis (AR)	Deficient prolactin in AF cells.
Fetal sex determination	Chromosomal analysis of AF cells.
Fragile-X syndrome (XR) (X-linked mental retardation)	Chromosomal analysis of cultured amnionic fluid cells.
Xeroderma pigmentosum (AR)	Defective ultraviolet-induced DNA repair in cultured AF cells.

* AF = amnionic fluid, AR = autosomal recessive, AD = autosomal dominant, XR = X-linked recessive.
† Tests suggestive but not confirmatory.
(*Adapted from Roberts and co-workers, 1983.*)

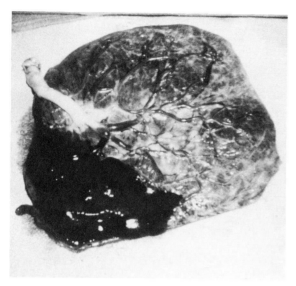

Figure 14-1. Hemorrhage from perforation of a fetal vessel in the placenta at the time of amniocentesis.

fetal loss rate—2.6 percent—was identified in the amniocentesis group, compared to an unusually low value of 1.1 percent in the control group. Of concern, there was an apparent increase in certain abnormalities in the newborn infants, especially respiratory problems at birth and orthopedic postural deformities. These abnormalities suggest that amniocentesis, at times, resulted in loss of amnionic fluid volume sufficient to restrict pulmonary excursion and to create abnormal fetal postures. In all studies, complications were greater when a large needle (18- gauge or larger) was used and when more than two taps were needed to obtain fluid.

Poreco and co-workers (1983), at a center in San Diego, analyzed the outcomes for more than 2300 pregnancies in which midtrimester amniocentesis was performed and estimated the procedure-related loss to have been 0.6 to 0.9 percent. Gillberg and associates (1982) evaluated 62 children at 5 to 7 years of age whose mothers had undergone amniocentesis at midpregnancy and for this small group identified no increase in neurodevelopmental disorders, orthopedic problems, or respiratory abnormalities.

and 3.2 percent for the control group. The overall accuracy of prenatal diagnosis was 99.4 percent. Similar results were obtained in a Canadian study (Simpson and colleagues, 1976). However, in a British study (Working Party on Amniocentesis, 1978), a significantly higher

Bloody Tap. Blood contaminating the amnionic fluid may complicate appreciably the techniques for study and the interpretation of the results. Erythrocytes may inhibit the replication in culture of fetal cells from amnionic fluid. Moreover, blood may change the apparent level of various constituents of amnionic fluid under

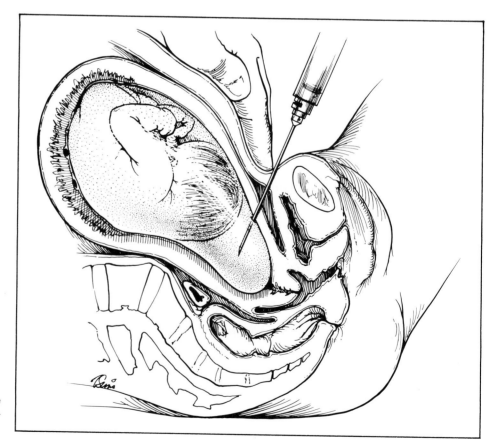

Figure 14-2. Amniocentesis late in pregnancy, performed suprapubically.

study, especially α-fetoprotein from fetal blood. Gibbons and co-workers (1974) have studied the effects of adding up to 4 percent maternal blood to fresh amnionic fluid which was then promptly centrifuged. The addition to amnionic fluid of blood concentrations of 1 percent or more produced a lowering of the lecithin-to-sphingomyeline (L/S) ratio, a direction of change that would lead to the prediction of a less mature fetus for reasons considered below. Buhi and Spellacy (1975) identified maternal serum to have a L/S ratio of 1:3 to 1:5, and they found that its addition to amnionic fluid influenced the ratio accordingly; meconium also lowered the L/S ratio somewhat. In general, if the "hematocrit" of the spun amnionic fluid exceeds 3 percent, the sample should be considered unsatisfactory for measurement of L/S ratio. *Minute amounts of fetal, but not maternal, blood can lead to falsely high levels of α-fetoprotein in amnionic fluid.* Therefore, if the amnionic fluid appears bloody, it should not be used for such analysis if the red cells are of fetal origin.

Amnionic Fluid Surfactant

Amniocentesis was initially employed primarily to estimate the concentration of bilirubin or bilirubin-like pigment in amnionic fluid and thereby to identify hemolytic disease in the fetus (see Chapter 38, p. 775). Currently, it is still probably used most often to determine the relative concentration of surfactant-active phospholipids to try to identify the fetus that is at risk of developing respiratory distress if delivered at that time.

So-called type II pneumonocytes of fetal lung alveoli produce surface-active phospholipids that are essential for the maintenance of effective respiration immediately after birth (see Chapter 8, p. 154). Without appropriate surfactant activity, the lung literally collapses with each expiration because of the high surface tension at air–fluid interfaces, and the syndrome of idiopathic respiratory distress develops (see Chapter 38, p. 769).

The specific lecithin dipalmitoyl phosphatidylcholine plus phosphatidylinositol and especially phosphatidylglycerol are critically important in the formation and stabilization of the surface-active layer that prevents alveolar collapse and the development of respiratory distress. These compounds are contained in lamellar bodies that are released from the type II cell into the alveolar space from which appreciable amounts are transported to the surrounding amnionic fluid. An important consequence of the containment of most of the surfactant in the lamellar bodies is that after too vigorous centrifugation the precipitate is likely to contain most of the lecithin, with most of the sphingomyelin remaining in the supernatant and thus giving a falsely low lecithin-to-sphingomyelin ratio.

Lecithin-to-Sphingomyelin (L/S) Ratio

Measurement of the L/S ratio demands a well-monitored laboratory, since slight variations in technique can appreciably affect the accuracy of the results.

Especially critical steps are centrifugation at appropriate speed, acetone precipitation, and densitometric measurement of the charred lecithin and sphingomyelin. If the analysis is not to be performed promptly, the specimen should be refrigerated.

Before 34 weeks gestation, lecithin and sphingomyelin are present in amnionic fluid in similar concentrations. At about 34 weeks, the concentration of lecithin relative to sphingomyelin begins to rise (Fig. 14-3).

It was shown by Gluck and co-workers (1971), and soon confirmed by others, that for pregnancies of unknown duration, but otherwise uncomplicated, the risk of respiratory distress in the newborn is very slight whenever the concentration of lecithin in amnionic fluid is at least twice that of sphingomyelin, whereas there is increased risk of respiratory distress when the L/S ratio is below 2. Harvey and colleagues (1975) combined the data from 25 reports in which L/S ratios were measured by similar techniques on amnionic fluid collected within 72 hours of delivery; their results are shown in Table 14-1. With an L/S ratio greater than 2.0, the risk of respiratory distress was found to be slight unless the mother had diabetes (see Chapter 28, p. 603). If the L/S ratio was 1.5 to 2.0, respiratory distress was identified in 40 percent, and if below 1.5, in 73 percent. Although 73 percent of infants developed respiratory distress when the L/S ratio was below 1.5, it proved fatal in but 14 percent (Table 14-1).

The experiences at Parkland Memorial Hospital have been that respiratory distress did not develop in some instances in which the L/S ratio was as low as 0.6. Moreover, infants for whom the L/S ratio in amnionic fluid was as low as 0.3 have survived after suffering respiratory distress (Herbert and colleagues, 1979). When the L/S ratio was greater than 0.5, deaths from respiratory distress were actually quite low. Obviously, there

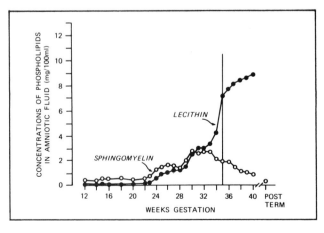

Figure 14-3. Changes in mean concentrations of lecithin and sphingomyelin in amnionic fluid during gestation in normal pregnancy. (*From Gluck and Kulovich: Am J Obstet Gynecol 115:541, 1973.*)

are times when the risk to the fetus from a hostile intra-uterine environment will be greater than the risk of death from respiratory distress even though the L/S ratio is less than 2.

Unfortunately, with some pregnancy complications, for example, class A and B maternal diabetes (Quirk and Bleasdale, 1984), or erythroblastosis fetalis, or most any event that causes the infant to be metabolically seriously compromised at birth, an L/S ratio of 2 does not necessarily preclude the development of respiratory distress.

Phosphatidylglycerol. Surfactant action insufficient to prevent respiratory distress, even though the L/S ratio is 2.0, is thought to be due in part to lack of phosphatidylglycerol and the enhancement of surface-active properties that phosphatidylglycerol provides. The identification of phosphatidylglycerol in amnionic fluid provides considerable assurance, but not necessarily an absolute guarantee, that respiratory distress will not develop (Whittle and co-workers, 1982).

Phosphatidylglycerol has not been detected in blood, meconium, or vaginal secretions; consequently, these contaminants do not confuse the interpretation. Importantly, the absence of phosphatidylglycerol is not necessarily a strong indicator that respiratory distress is likely to develop after delivery; its absence serves to indicate only that the infant *may* develop respiratory distress.

A rapid (15 minutes) immunologic agglutination test (Amniostat-FLM) to identify phosphatidylglycerol in amnionic fluid samples is available commercially. Its accuracy for identifying phosphatidylglycerol, and, in turn, the improbability of the neonate developing respiratory distress syndrome, has been found satisfactory by Garite and associates (1983) and by Halvorsen and Gross (1984).

Foam Stability (Shake) Test. To reduce the time and effort inherent in precise measurement of the L/S ratio, the foam stability test, or so-called shake test, was introduced by Clements and associates (1972). The test depends upon the ability of surfactant in amnionic fluid, when mixed appropriately with ethanol, to generate stable foam at the air–liquid interface. The technique takes no more than ½ hour to complete.

> Into one chemically clean 13″ × 100-mm glass tube with a Teflon-lined plastic screw cap are added 1.0 ml of recently collected amnionic fluid and 1 ml of 95 percent ethanol (prepared by diluting 19.0 parts absolute alcohol with 1 part of distilled water); 0.5 ml of amnionic fluid, 0.5 ml of 0.9 percent saline, and 1 ml of the 95 percent ethanol are added to another tube. Each tube is vigorously shaken for 15 seconds and placed upright in a rack for 15 minutes. The persistence of an intact ring of bubbles at the air-liquid interface after 15 minutes is considered a positive test.

If the ring of foam persists for 15 minutes, the risk of respiratory distress is very low. For example,

Schlueter and co-workers (1979) identified only 1 instance of respiratory distress developing out of 205 pregnancies in which the test was positive for amnionic fluid diluted with an equal volume of saline. There are, however, two problems with the test: (1) slight contamination of amnionic fluid, reagents, or glassware, or errors in measurement, may alter the test results markedly; and (2) a false negative test is rather common, that is, failure of the ring of foam to persist intact for 15 minutes in the tube containing diluted amnionic fluid is not necessarily predictive of respiratory distress. At least that is the experience at our institution.

Lumadex–FSI Test. This test represents a commercially available kit that utilizes the principle of foam stability to identify surfactant activity in amnionic fluid. It also has been found to be reliable (Sher and Stalland, 1983; Herbert and associates, 1984).

Fluorescent Polarization (Microviscometry). Another approach to the identification of surfactant activity in amnionic fluid has been evaluated by Blumenfeld and associates (1978), Elrad and colleagues (1978), and Golde and co-workers (1979). The microviscosity of lipid aggregates in the amnionic fluid may be assayed by mixing the fluid with a specific fluorescent dye that incorporates into the hydrocarbon region of the lipids in surfactant. The intensity of the fluorescence induced by polarized light is then measured. The technique is rapid and appears simple to perform but the instrument is expensive.

Amnionic Fluid Absorbence at 650 nm. The degree of absorbance of light of 650 nm wavelength has been reported to correlate well with the lecithin-to-sphingomyelin ratio in amnionic fluid (Sbarra and co-workers, 1977). Tsai and associates (1983) report the test to have been most informative at low absorbance and high absorbance; between these extremes, however, false positive and false negative values proved troublesome. Moreover, Khouzami and associates (1983) reported that differences in centrifugation altered appreciably light absorbance by the amnionic fluid.

Amnionic Fluid Bilirubin

Hemolysis yields bilirubin, most of which remains unconjugated by the fetus. How unconjugated bilirubin reaches the amnionic fluid from the fetus is uncertain, as there is essentially none in the fetal urine and the fetal skin appears to be impermeable to free bilirubin during the latter half of pregnancy. The respiratory tract and the amnion over the placenta and umbilical cord are possible but unproven pathways. The concentration of bilirubin in amnionic fluid normally falls progressively during the latter half of pregnancy, usually to become essentially zero as the fetus reaches maturity. Typically, the bilirubin levels and the rate of decrease during the last several weeks of pregnancy are so slight and problems inherent in analysis are sufficiently great to preclude its use as a sensitive test of fetal maturity. In case of fetal hemolytic disease, however, the concentration of bilirubin for any given fetal age usually reflects the intensity of the hemolysis (see Chapter 38, p. 775).

It is not always appreciated that bilirubin in the amnionic fluid need not be of fetal origin. An elevated maternal plasma concentration of free bilirubin, as, for example, with sickle cell anemia, is reflected in an elevation in the amnionic fluid.

Amnionic fluid supernatant is best analyzed for bilirubin using a continuous recording spectrophotometer. There is a characteristic absorption peak at 450 nm, the correct height of which, when measured as an increase in optical density above baseline, is proportional to the bilirubin concentration (Fig. 38-2, p. 775). In current symbolism, the value is usually expressed as Δ OD 450. Measurement of bilirubin by ordinary chemical methods is not satisfactory because of the low concentration in amnionic fluid.

Other Amnionic Fluid Indicators of Fetal Maturity

Evaluation of many other constituents or properties of amnionic fluid has been suggested to try to identify fetal maturity. Those that have been cited often are the concentration of creatinine, the osmolality, and the presence of appropriate amounts of cells that are lipid-stainable. Although these constituents or properties change as the fetus matures, the rate and the degree of change are often so slight or so variable that their measurements do not provide an acceptable level of precision for identification of fetal maturity. Moreover, results that imply functional maturity of one organ system should not be interpreted to imply functional maturity of another. For example, remarkable variation was demonstrated for quintuplets born at Parkland Memorial Hospital 222 days after the onset of the last menstrual period. Within the limits of measurement the creatinine concentration and the osmolality were identical in amnionic fluid from each sac, 2 mg/dl and 265 mOsm/L, respectively. These values implied fetal maturity as pointed out below. At the same time the L/S ratio in amnionic fluid from each sac ranged from less than 2 to greater than 5. Respiratory distress was associated with the low but not the high L/S ratios.

Amnionic Fluid Creatinine. During the latter half of pregnancy, the concentration of creatinine in amnionic fluid slowly rises until near term, when the increase is more rapid. The rise is the consequence of increased excretion of creatinine by the maturing fetal kidneys. A level of 2.0 mg/dl in amnionic fluid not treated to remove nonspecific chromogens most often indicates fetal maturity. There are two problems inherent in the test: (1) pulmonary function may prove to be mature even though the creatinine concentration is less than 2 mg/dl, (2) an increase in maternal plasma creatinine will cause an increase in the amnionic fluid creatinine although the fetus is not mature. If creatinine concentration is to be used, it is essential to ascertain that the mother's plasma creatinine level is not elevated. According to Teoh and co-workers (1973), measurement of uric acid offers no advantage over creatinine, while urea is even less reliable as an indicator of fetal maturity.

Amnionic Fluid Osmolality. Early in pregnancy, the osmolality of amnionic fluid and fetal serum are the same. From 20 weeks onward, however, the osmolality of amnionic fluid decreases at the rate of approximately 1 mOsm/L per week, presumably as the consequence of dilution by nonprotein nitrogen-rich, but hypotonic, fetal urine. The rate of decrease in osmolality, however, is too gradual and too variable to allow a precise prediction of fetal maturity.

Lipid-Staining of Cells in Amnionic Fluid. Staining of amnionic fluid aspirate with Nile blue sulfate discloses two categories of cells or cell particles. Blue-stained bodies represent shed fetal epithelial cells, while the orange-stained bodies originate from sebaceous glands. In the later stages of gestation, an increase in orange bodies appears to reflect maturity of the sebaceous glands. Two major problems arise from the use of the Nile blue sulfate technique to identify fetal maturity: (1) The orange-colored bodies tend to clump, which makes quantification difficult. (2) Lower percentages of orange-colored bodies do not necessarily indicate prematurity.

Amniocentesis to Identify Inherited Disorders

Amniocentesis allows retrieval of fetal somatic cells and fluid that can be used to identify the cytogenetic constitution of the fetus or to assess a variety of abnormal biochemical processes that are listed in Table 14-1.

To identify several genetic disorders in the fetus, chromosomal analysis can be employed. It is most often of value in the following circumstances:

1. Pregnancies in women 35 years of age or older.
2. A previous pregnancy that resulted in the birth of a chromosomally abnormal offspring.
3. Chromosomal abnormality in either parent, including
   a. balanced translocation carrier state
   b. aneuploidy
   c. mosaicism
4. Down syndrome or other chromosomal abnormality in a close family member.
5. Pregnancy after three or more spontaneous abortions.
6. A previous infant with multiple major malformations but no cytogenetic study was performed.
7. Fetal sex determination in pregnancies at risk of a serious X-linked hereditary disorder.
8. Biochemical studies in pregnancies at risk of a serious autosomal or X-linked recessive disorder.
9. A previous child or a parent with a neural tube defect or on routine screening maternal serum α-fetoprotein level is abnormally high.

The amnionic fluid is most often aspirated at 16 to 18 weeks of gestation when there are likely to be sufficient fetal cells present to allow successful cell culture. There is the possibility that the fluid collected at this time is urine from the maternal bladder rather than amnionic fluid. The two fluids can usually be quickly

TABLE 14-2. FREQUENCY OF SELECTED CHROMOSOME ABNORMALITIES IN THE NEWBORN

Trisomy 21	1 in 800–1000 births
Trisomy 18	1 in 8000 births
Trisomy 13	1 in 20,000 births
XXY	1 in 1000 male births
XYY	1 in 1000 male births
XXX	1 in 950 female births
XO	1 in 10,000 female biths

(*From Antenatal Diagnosis. NIH Publication Number 79–1973, April, 1979.*)

differentiated by the presence of crystallization when amnionic fluid is dried on a glass slide and examined microscopically under low power; moreover, amnionic fluid contains glucose and protein whereas urine usually does not.

The frequencies of the more common significant cytogenetic abnormalities in newborn infants in the United States are listed in Table 14-2. From these data, it is estimated that each year in the United States without cytogenetic studies at least 15,000 infants would be born with a chromosomal abnormality (Antenatal Diagnosis, 1979). Moreover, there are probably 175,000 spontaneous abortions of chromosomally abnormal fetuses annually.

The most common abnormality in the infant who is liveborn is trisomy 21, or Down syndrome (Table 14-2), even though it is estimated that two thirds of conceptuses with trisomy 21 do not survive the pregnancy. Whereas the risk of a liveborn offspring with Down syndrome is only 1 in 885 at maternal age 30, it increases to 1 in 365 at age 35, and to 1 in 109 at age 40, and 1 in 32 at age 45 (see Table 39-3, p. 801). The frequencies of most other trisomies and sex chromosome aneuploidies also increase with maternal age.

Cytogenetic studies are recommended for all women who are 35 or older, although any age limit is selected arbitrarily rather than being based on an immediate biologic difference that occurs once a woman has reached a certain age. The magnitude of the problem created by attempting to provide genetic counseling and cytogenetic screening of fetuses of all women who are 35 or older becomes readily apparent when it is appreciated that in one recent year there were 142,000 births by women 35 or older, compared to but 25,000 births by women who were 40 or older. Moreover, it has been predicted that soon the number of births by women 35 or older will exceed 200,000 annually.

When a parent is the carrier of a balanced chromosomal translocation, there is a 4 to 20 percent risk that the fetus will be abnormal (see Chapter 39, p. 801).

With X-linked recessive diseases for which no specific prenatal diagnostic test is readily available to differentiate affected from unaffected male fetuses, at least the sex of the fetus can be identified accurately, and when female and the father is not affected, the risk of an affected offspring is eliminated.

Fetal Sex

At 15 to 18 weeks of gestation, the sex of the fetus can be determined cytologically by demonstrating the nuclear sex chromatin mass (Barr body) and by Y chromosome staining of cells obtained from amnionic fluid, or more accurately by cell culture and karyotyping. With very careful studies to identify the presence or absence of nuclear sex chromatin in uncultivated, directly stained amnionic fluid cells, the overall accuracy is about 95 percent (Milunsky, 1973). Staining for the Y chromosome in uncultured cells from amnionic fluid, Valenti and co-workers (1972) reported an accuracy of about 97 percent. Thus, the test did not improve the accuracy significantly over the sex chromatin method, and when the prediction of sex is crucial, they recommend that confirmation be derived by karyotyping cultured amnionic fluid cells.

Identification of the sex of the fetus has been attempted by measuring testosterone and FSH in amnionic fluid. In one study, overlap of values for female and male fetuses was sufficient that in 7 percent neither determination was indicative of fetal sex (Belisle and colleagues, 1977).

High-resolution sonography, to be considered subsequently, can be applied to the identification of the sex of the fetus by visualizing the external genitalia, especially the penis (Fig. 14-4). Birnholz (1983) reported sonographic views were obtained sufficient to allow attempt at diagnosis in 69 percent of fetuses at 15 or more weeks of gestational age. For 590 fetuses sex was determined correctly 99 percent of the time. After 20 weeks of gestation, the genitalia were visualized in more than 90 percent of all fetuses examined.

Other Inheritable Disorders

A great variety of inheritable disorders of metabolic function have been detected by appropriate study of amnionic fluid contents. Listings of most such disorders are included in Table 14-1.

Approximately 75 recessively inherited X-sex chromosome-linked or autosomal metabolic disorders are now detectable in somatic cell systems and therefore are approachable in the fetus through amniocentesis. The risk of an autosomal recessive disorder in the fetus may have become apparent from either the previous birth of an affected infant or from screening of the parents for the carrier state. If both parents are carriers, the risk of the fetus being homozygous and therefore seriously affected is 25 percent, whereas for X-linked disease, if the mother is a carrier, the risk of male offspring being affected is 50 percent but for female offspring it is zero, unless the father is affected. Unfortunately, the carrier state for several recessive conditions cannot be detected except by birth of an affected infant. One that can be detected, however, is Tay–Sachs disease; screening programs have been established for Tay–Sachs disease, especially among Jewish couples, in whom it is 100 times more frequent. The affected fetus of heterozygous par-

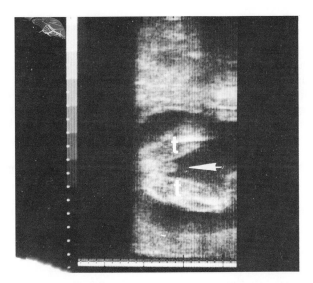

Figure 14-4. Sonographic caudal view of a male twin fetus at 24 weeks of gestation. The arrow points to the penis. t = thigh. (*Courtesy of Dr. R. Santos.*)

ents can be detected through biochemical studies on cells cultured from amnionic fluid.

Parents who are heterozygous for the gene for production of an abnormal hemoglobin or for β-thalassemia can be readily identified and the potential for an affected offspring thereby recognized. The fetus destined to develop a serious hemoglobinopathy or severe thalassemia can now be identified in utero through appropriate treatment of DNA in the cells in amnionic fluid (Table 14-1 and Chapter 28, p. 573).

Detection of Elevated α-Fetoprotein

The value of measurement of α-fetoprotein in amnionic fluid between 16 and 20 weeks of gestation to detect fetal abnormality, especially open neural tube defects, is now established.

The site of production of most, if not all, of the increased α-fetoprotein is the fetus. It is the major protein in serum of the embryo and early fetus. Initially, it is produced in the yolk sac but by the end of the first trimester it is nearly all of hepatic origin. In both fetal serum and amnionic fluid the concentration of α-fetoprotein is highest around the 13th week of gestation (Fig. 14-5). The concentration in fetal serum is about 150 times that in amnionic fluid. The normal source of the protein in amnionic fluid is fetal urine. Some of that protein, in turn, crosses the fetal membranes to enter the maternal circulation. The concentration of α-fetoprotein levels in maternal serum are only one hundredth to one thousandth those of fetal serum. The low maternal levels normally continue to rise slowly until late in pregnancy. *After 13 weeks the levels in both fetal serum and amnionic fluid normally decrease rapidly in essentially parallel fashion.* Because the levels decrease sharply,

correct interpretation of its concentration requires precise knowledge of gestational age.

The level of α-fetoprotein in amnionic fluid, maternal serum, or both, may be elevated in a great variety of circumstances. Several disorders are listed below:

1. Open neural tube defects (anencephaly, open spina bifida)
2. Congenital nephrosis
3. Bladder neck obstruction
4. Esophageal and duodenal atresia
5. Exomphalos
6. Sacrococcygeal teratoma
7. Pilonidal sinus
8. Turner syndrome (45, XO)
9. Potter syndrome (renal agenesis)
10. Fetal death
11. Fetal blood in amnionic fluid
12. Fetomaternal hemorrhage
13. Some low-birth-weight fetuses
14. Abdominal pregnancy

This list is by no means complete (Roberts and co-workers, 1983).

Open Neural Tube Defects. Experiences with screening for open neural tube defects are now considerable, especially in Great Britain, where neural tube defects are much more common. As one consequence, considerable enthusiasm has been generated for measuring near midpregnancy the level of α-fetoprotein in the serum of most

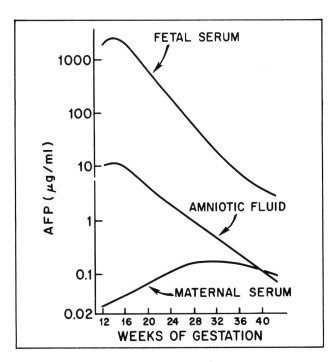

Figure 14-5. α-Fetoprotein (AFP) concentrations in fetal serum, amnionic fluid, and maternal serum throughout gestation. (*From Seppälä (ed): Amniotic Fluid, 2nd ed. New York, Excerpta Medica, 1978.*)

all women. When levels are sufficiently elevated to suspect the possibility of a neural tube defect, then amniocentesis is performed to look for distinctly elevated levels in amniotic fluid. Moreover, the fetus is usually carefully scanned sonographically for evidence of abnormality, especially anencephaly and spina bifida.

The appropriateness of routine screening of maternal serum for elevated levels of α-fetoprotein is still debated in the United States. For the pregnant woman with a family history of neural tube defects, as well as the woman in whom a previous pregnancy was similarly complicated, screening is certainly appropriate. Most laboratories do routinely test for elevated α-fetoprotein levels in all midtrimester amnionic fluid samples.

Congenital Nephrosis. Children with congenital nephrosis, although severely handicapped, may live for as long as 2 or 3 years. The abnormality is inherited as an autosomally recessive trait. In case of a previous infant born with congenital nephrosis, or a strong family history, an affected fetus may be identified through measurements of α-fetoprotein in maternal serum and especially in amnionic fluid (Aula and colleagues, 1978).

Amnionic Fluid Acetylcholinesterase Activity

Raised levels of acetylcholinesterase in amnionic fluid accompany most open neural tube defects. Moreover, by demonstrating the absence of an acetylcholinesterase band in amnionic fluid using a technique of slab gel electrophoresis, Milunsky and Sapirstein (1982) were able to reclassify correctly 89 percent of the normal pregnancies in which they had found spuriously high α-fetoprotein levels in the amnionic fluid. Acetylcholinesterase in amnionic fluid most likely comes from fetal neural tissue, that is, an open neural tube lesion; however, it has been found to be elevated at times in the absence of a neural tube defect.

BIOPSY OF CHORION

Recently there has been considerable enthusiasm displayed for biopsying the chorion very early in pregnancy to obtain fetal cells for genetic diagnosis. Fetal cells so obtained can be used in the same ways as cells obtained in amnionic fluid near midpregnancy are now used. By obtaining cells earlier, diagnosis can be made sooner; if pregnancy termination is to be performed, it can therefore be performed much more easily and with greater safety.

A variety of techniques have been applied to try to collect a small amount of villous material. Obtaining the tissue with a high degree of safety and free of contamination with maternal tissue are problems to be overcome (Liu and co-workers, 1983; Rodeck and associates, 1983; Elias and co-workers, 1984).

SONOGRAPHY

The impact of the use of ultrasonography on the practice of obstetrics has been profound! Given but one choice from the many biochemical and biophysical techniques that have been developed in more recent years to try to improve pregnancy outcome, sonography would seem the best. Methods for evaluating the health of the fetus that apply pulse–echo ultrasound are now widely employed for the very good reasons summarized below and illustrated frequently throughout this text. Sonographic techniques that are now available, when carefully performed and accurately interpreted, can supply vital information about the status of the fetus, with no known risks from ultrasound.

Intermittent high-frequency sound waves are generated by applying an alternating current to a transducer made of a piezoelectric material. The transducer is "connected" to the abdominal wall by placing a coupling agent—usually mineral oil—on the skin to diminish the loss of ultrasound waves at the interface between the transducer and the skin. In static systems the transducer so applied emits a pulse of sound waves that passes through soft tissue until an interface between the structures of different tissue densities is reached. When this occurs, some of the energy, proportional to the difference in densities at the interface, is reflected, or echoed, back to the transducer. This, in turn, stimulates the transducer while in the listening state to generate a small electrical voltage that is then amplified and displayed on a screen.

With *real-time* ultrasonography, the transducers employed generate multiple pulse–echo systems that are activated in sequence and thereby detect movement, including breathing, cardiac actions, and vessel pulsations.

Clinical Application

Sonography has proved valuable for monitoring the products of conception in a variety of ways that include the following:

1. Very early identification of intrauterine pregnancy.
2. Demonstration of the size and the rate of growth of the amnionic sac and the embryo, and, at times, resorption or expulsion of the embryo.
3. Identification of multiple fetuses, including conjoined twins.
4. Measurements of the fetal head, abdominal circumference, and femur, to help identify the duration of gestation for the normal fetus or, when measured sequentially, to help identify the growth-retarded fetus.
5. Comparison of fetal head and chest or abdominal circumference to identify hydrocephaly, microcephaly, or anencephaly.

6. Detection of fetal anomalies such as abnormal distention of the fetal bladder, ascites, polycystic kidneys, renal agenesis, ovarian cyst, intestinal obstruction, diphragmatic hernia, meningomyelocele, or limb defects.
7. Demonstration of hydramnios or oligohydramnios by comparing the size of the fetus to the amnionic space surrounding the fetus.
8. Identification of the location, size, and "maturity" of the placenta.
9. Demonstration of placental abnormalities such as hydatidiform mole, molar degeneration, and anomalies such as chorioangioma.
10. Identification of uterine tumors or anomalous development.
11. Detection of a foreign body such as an intrauterine device, blood clot, or retained placental fragment.

Fetal Motion

It is established unequivocally that the fetus breathes throughout most of pregnancy (see Chapter 8, p. 163). The movements can be witnessed with real-time sonography. Using real-time sonography fetal heart beat has been demonstrated as early as 7 weeks of gestation, trunk movement as early as 8 weeks, and limb movement as early as 9 weeks (Shawker and associates, 1980). Filling and intermittent emptying of the fetal urinary bladder are obvious with real-time sonography especially. Sonographic confirmation of fetal movement, fetal breathing, and the presence of normal amounts of amnionic fluid provides evidence that the fetus is behaving normally in utero. Echocardiography can be applied to the fetus and a variety of cardiac abnormalities thus detected. Real-time sonography especially has allowed surgical amelioration in utero of some defects identified sonographically, for example, hydrocephaly.

The already widespread use of sonography in obstetrics and its potential for identification of fetal abnormalities and for providing reassurance of fetal well-being have stimulated several questions that are difficult to answer at this time: Should sonography be used in all pregnancies and, if so, when should it be initiated, how often should it be repeated, and how vigorous an examination for possible fetal abnormalities should be carried out? Who should actually perform the examination? Who should directly supervise the examination? Who should interpret the results of the examination? What should be the responsibilities of the practicing obstetrician? In what circumstances should sonography be performed under the supervision of and interpreted by the certified obstetric specialist who is highly trained in sonography? When should these tasks be the responsibility of a radiologist who has been certified in sonography?

Person and Kullander (1983) have reported their extensive experiences with attempts at routine repetitive sonography in Malmö, Sweden, which included 43,000

routine examinations on 22,400 pregnancies. An examination was performed by a trained nurse during the 17th week and routinely repeated in the 33rd week. The first examination was directed at identifying the number of fetuses, fetal anatomy, cardiac activity, and placental site. The second examination emphasized detection of deviations in fetal growth and malformations. They attempted a cost–benefit analysis that suggested that large economic gains were realized by such screening. The costs of sonography seemed remarkably low when compared to the prices charged in the United States. Moreover, medicolegal expenses arising from misdiagnosis do not appear in their estimates.

RADIOGRAPHY, AMNIOGRAPHY, AND FETOGRAPHY

A variety of diagnostic radiologic techniques have been applied to try to evaluate the status of the fetus. It is of interest to note the reduction in the use of diagnostic x-ray that has taken place since the advent of sonography. Whitehouse and associates, for example, reported for their department in 1958 that more than half of the x-ray requests for obstetric conditions were for determination of fetal age or for placental localization. With the advent of sonography, both determinations are now performed sonographically with much greater precision and probably greater safety.

Simple Roentgenogram

A roentgenogram of the abdomen and pelvis after 16 weeks gestation will most often identify fetal skeletal parts. Usually during the latter half of pregnancy the presenting fetal part is easily identified, the number of fetuses can be quantified, and gross skeletal abnormalities such as anencephaly and marked hydrocephaly are obvious. During the second half of pregnancy characteristic x-ray changes in the fetus are usually evident some time after death (see Chapter 10, p. 219).

Neither the age nor the size of the fetus can be identified with precision by use of simple radiography. Studies that have shown the best correlation between fetal age and the time of appearance of *lower limb ossification centers* typically have evaluated the limb radiologically after birth. Identification of ossification centers radiologically while in utero is often difficult if not impossible.

Amniography

Radiopaque agents may be injected into the amnionic sac to identify certain characteristics of the amnionic fluid, fetus, and placenta. Amniography, using water-soluble, iodinated radiocontrast material such as Urografin or Hypaque to opacify the amnionic fluid, may be employed to demonstrate abnormal amounts of amnionic fluid, the abnormally located placenta, the soft-tissue silhouette of the fetus, and, after a few hours of swallowing, the fetal gastrointestinal tract.

Hydatidiform moles very often produce a diagnostic honeycombed x-ray pattern when water-soluble, iodinated contrast material is injected into the uterine cavity. However, sonography provides a simpler and usually more accurate technique for identification of a hydatidiform mole (Fig. 23-12, p. 451).

Fetography

Fetography involves the use of a heavily iodinated, lipid-soluble agent such as Ethiodol. When injected into the amnionic sac, the iodinated lipid adheres to the vernix on the skin of the almost-mature fetus and thereby may outline the fetus much more vividly than do water-soluble radiopaque agents.

Sonography carefully performed usually provides most of the information that may be afforded by amniography or fetography without using diagnostic x-rays, invading the amnionic sac, or injecting potentially harmful chemical agents.

AMNIOSCOPY

Saling (1973) has reported extensively on the visualization of amnionic fluid through the membranes when the cervix is sufficiently dilated. Amnioscopy to identify meconium staining of amnionic fluid may be of value in late pregnancy complicated by (1) maternal hypertension, (2) apparently prolonged pregnancy, (3) suspected fetal growth retardation, (4) previous unexplained stillbirth, and (5) lack of orderly cervical dilatation or descent of the presenting part during the first stage of labor. The following problems are associated with amnioscopy: (1) the cervix must be accessible for visualization, that is, neither too far posterior nor too far anterior; (2) the cervix must be dilated enough to visualize the membranes and the fluid behind them; (3) the membranes may be ruptured inadvertently during the examination; and (4) the intravaginal and intracervical manipulations may lead to infection of the products of conception and the upper genital tract. Amnioscopy to try to visualize amnionic fluid for meconium staining has not become very popular in the United States.

Use of an amnioscope to obtain fetal blood is described on page 288 and demonstrated in Figure 14-10.

FETOSCOPY

There is considerable interest in instrumentation that provides for direct visualization of the fetus and the placenta without the risk of disrupting the pregnancy. Hopefully, development of such a laparoamnioscope will allow more accurate detection of externally located fetal anomalies and will provide tissue from the fetus or fetal blood vessels in the placenta for identification of serious fetal disease without appreciable risk to the fetus or the mother. Fetoscopy must still be regarded as a research procedure because of the limitations of the fetoscope and the increased risks to the fetus and the mother compared to other methods of prenatal screening and diagnosis now available.

NUCLEAR MAGNETIC RESONANCE

Equipment essential for organ and body imaging using nuclear magnetic resonance is now available in several medical research centers. Once its safety during pregnancy has been established, major advancements that deal with both structure and function will be made rapidly! It is already being used to study abnormal states in the newborn infant. Nuclear magnetic resonance has provided intriguing observations made on the pregnancy products in utero (Smith and co-workers, 1983; Symonds and associates, 1984).

HORMONE AND ENZYME ASSAYS

Pregnancy-induced changes in a variety of hormones and enzymes have been extensively investigated with the hope of discovering practical tests to ascertain fetal age and fetal well-being.

Placental Lactogen and Estriol

Human placental lactogen (hPL) in maternal plasma and, especially, estriol in maternal plasma or urine have been claimed to provide important predictive information concerning fetal well-being or lack thereof. The use and abuse of measurements of these hormones are considered in Chapter 7 (pp. 122, 133), along with their production, distribution, metabolic functions, and clearance.

Chorionic Gonadotropin

This hormone, normally produced by trophoblast and of clinical value for identifying early pregnancy, is considered in Chapters 7 and 10, (pp. 120, 214, respectively). Its measurement to identify persistent trophoblastic neoplasia is discussed in Chapter 23 (p. 454).

Other Hormonal Tests

Raja and co-workers (1974) reported that estradiol-17β rose appreciably in peripheral plasma before the onset of premature labor, whereas progesterone levels showed no consistent trend. They suggested that the measurement of estradiol-17β might prove to be of value to identify pregnancies in which premature labor is likely to occur. Their observations await confirmation.

Measurements of *progesterone levels* in maternal plasma have uncovered no constant pattern of change in pregnancies complicated by hypertension, diabetes, Rh isoimmunization, fetal growth retardation, or impending fetal death.

Measurement of the increase in *urinary estriol* excretion following intravenous injection of dehydro-isoandrosterone has been evaluated as a test of placental function but has not been established to have clinical value.

The metabolic clearance rate of *dehydroisoandros-terone sulfate* for young women destined to develop pregnancy-induced hypertension is somewhat greater early in pregnancy and then significantly lower than in normal pregnant women (Gant and associates, 1971). Measurement of the metabolic clearance of dehydro-isoandrosterone sulfate has not been demonstrated to have practical clinical utility.

Enzymes in Maternal Serum

The activities of a number of enzymes change appreciably in maternal serum during pregnancy. Measurements of heat-stable and total alkaline phosphatase, oxytocinase, and diamine oxidase have been urged by some to monitor fetal well-being, or to identify fetal maturity, or to do both. Such measurements have, in general, provided little information of value clinically.

FETAL MOVEMENT AND WELL-BEING

Normally, throughout the second half of pregnancy expectant mothers are cognizant of frequent movement by the fetus. Ehrström (1979) identified fetal movements in normal pregnancies to increase from a median value of 86 per 12 hours in the 24th week to a maximum of 132 in the 32nd week. Activity then decreased to a median 12-hour value of 107 movements during the 40th week. It should be emphasized that there was considerable individual variation among the normal pregnancies that were studied.

Reduced Fetal Movements

The fetus who late in pregnancy is felt by the mother to move consistently is most often healthy. Conversely, a sudden decrease in fetal movements is an ominous sign of loss of fetal well-being. The absolute number of movements per day appears to be less important in prognosis than is the degree of change in the frequency of fetal movements. In the case of cessation of fetal movements, fetal heart sounds have been observed commonly to disappear within the next 24 hours. Sadovsky and Polishuk (1977) found loss of fetal movements to be more reliable than measurements of urinary estriol for predicting impending fetal death. Moreover, the test allows the

mother to participate actively in the monitoring of fetal well-being.

ELECTRONIC FETAL STRESS AND NONSTRESS TESTS

Two techniques have emerged in which subtle changes in the fetal heart rate are searched for to try to evaluate fetal well-being. One is commonly referred to as the contraction stress test and the other as the nonstress test, or fetal heart acceleration test.

Contraction Stress Test

Hammacher (1966) appears to be the first to suggest that the fetal heart rate response to uterine contractions be used antepartum as a test of fetal well-being. Subsequently, in this country, Ray and co-workers (1972), and many others since (see Huddleston and Freeman, 1977), have recommended the use of the contraction stress test, or oxytocin challenge test, for this purpose.

Technique. The contraction stress test usually takes 1 to 2 hours when performed as follows: With the mother lying on her back, but with her head and shoulders raised somewhat and turned toward her side, the fetal heart rate is recorded from an externally placed detector. Most often an ultrasound transducer (Fig. 14-6) is used because both phonocardiography and fetal electrocardiography when attempted through maternal tissue usually prove unsatisfactory (p. 285). Uterine activity is identified with an external tocographic transducer. As the uterus contracts and moves forward, a sensor pin attached to a strain gauge is pushed in by the change in shape of the abdominal wall. The change in electric current so generated is amplified and recorded. Although actual intrauterine pressure is not recorded, the onset, the time of maximum intensity, and the cessation of the contraction can be identified with reasonable precision. To try to detect any reduction in placental perfusion as the consequence of aortocaval compression by the pregnant uterus while the mother is recumbent and thereby avoid a false positive test, the maternal blood pressure is recorded initially and at least every 10 minutes thereafter during the procedure.

Baseline uterine activity and fetal heart rate are recorded for 15 to 30 minutes. If, by chance, spontaneous uterine contractions that last 40 to 60 seconds and recur approximately three times in 10 minutes are detected, the response of the fetal heart rate to the contractions is evaluated as described below. In the absence of demonstrable spontaneous uterine activity usually oxytoxin is administered intravenously. The initial rate of infusion of 0.5 mU per minute through a constant-speed infusion pump is doubled every 15 to 20 minutes until uterine contractions lasting 40 to 60 seconds with a frequency of three per 10 minutes are established.

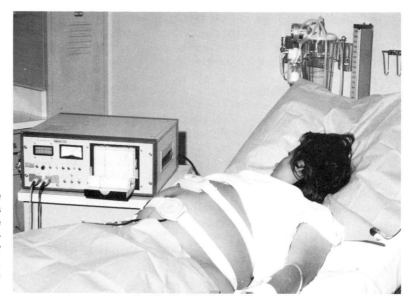

Figure 14-6. External tococardiography. The upper detector strapped to the abdomen senses uterine contractions from the change in the curvature of the abdomen. The lower one detects fetal heart rate action using the doppler principle and ultrasound. During the monitoring, the mother should not be restricted to the supine position.

Nipple Stimulation Test. To avoid the difficulties associated with the intravenous infusion of oxytocin, yet stimulate the uterus to contract somewhat, the breast stimulation, or more correctly, the *nipple stimulation test,* has been employed (Oki, 1983). The basis for the test presumably was that tactile stimulation of the nipple would stimulate the release of exogenous oxytocin from the neurohypophysis, although Ross and co-workers (1984) were unable to detect a surge of oxytocin into the plasma of women whose uterus contracted in association with nipple stimulation.

Indications and Contraindications

The following conditions may contraindicate the use of oxytocin—and perhaps nipple stimulation—to perform a contraction stress test: (1) threatened preterm labor, (2) placenta previa, (3) hydramnios, (4) multiple fetuses, (5) rupture of the membranes, (6) previous preterm labor, (7) and previous classical cesarean section. Otherwise, the proponents of the contraction stress test recommend that it be implemented during the third trimester whenever the fetus is suspected of being in jeopardy. If the test is negative, it has usually been repeated weekly thereafter as long as it remained negative.

Interpretation. Freeman (1975) has categorized the results of the contraction stress test as follows:

- *Positive:* There is consistent and persistent late deceleration of the fetal heart rate, that is, slowing of the heart rate develops sometime after the onset of the uterine contraction, the nadir for the heart rate is reached after the peak of uterine contraction, and recovery occurs after the contraction is completed (p. 287 and Fig. 14-7).

- *Negative:* At least three contractions in 10 minutes, each lasting at least 40 seconds, are identified without late deceleration of the fetal heart rate.
- *Suspicious:* There is inconstant late deceleration that does not persist with subsequent contractions.
- *Hyperstimulation:* If uterine contractions are more frequent than every 2 minutes, or last longer than 90 seconds, or persistent uterine hypertonus is suspected, late deceleration does not necessarily indicate uteroplacental disease.
- *Unsatisfactory:* The frequency of contractions is less than three per 10 minutes or the tracing is poor.

False Negative Tests. It is now apparent that a negative contraction stress test *usually, but not always,* is compatible with uteroplacental function sufficient to maintain the fetus alive in utero for at least another week. For example, in one study Evertson and associates (1978) identified the fetal death rate from all causes to be 7 out of 680, or 1 percent, within the next 7 days after a negative contraction stress test; in another study, Gal and co-workers (1979) reported 3 antepartum fetal deaths among 584 pregnancies within 1 week of a negative oxytocin challenge test. We have documented fetal death within 48 hours after the completion of the third 8-hour infusion of oxytocin administered to try to effect labor. The 24 hours of infusion were electronically monitored continuously. Careful review of all tracings failed to provide any evidence compatible with a positive test (Chapter 37, Figure 37-7).

False Positive Tests. The high false positive rate with the contraction stress test is troublesome. To avoid pre-

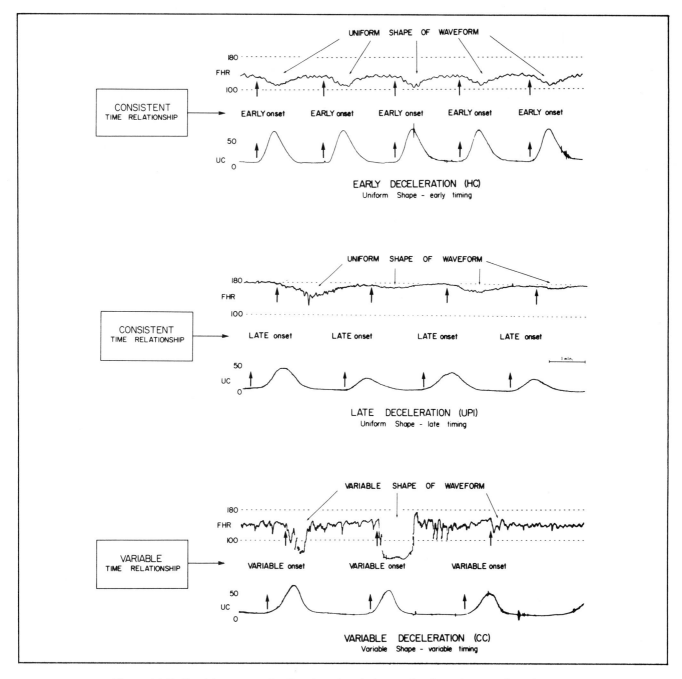

Figure 14-7. Fetal heart rate decelerations in relation to the time of onset of uterine contractions. (*From Hon: An Atlas of Fetal Heart Rate Patterns. New Haven, CT, Harty, 1968.*)

maturely interrupting pregnancy when the test is positive, most advocates of the test recommend the application of other tests, including measurements of amnionic fluid L/S ratio, urinary or plasma estriol, and, more recently, real-time sonographic evaluations of fetal breathing, fetal body movements, fetal tone, and amnionic fluid volume, to try to identify more precisely the status of the fetus.

Nonstress Test

Fetal movement typically is accomplished by transient acceleration of the fetal heart rate. This phenomenon, observed and reported by Hammacher and associates (1968), Kubli and co-workers (1969), and by many others, serves as the basis for the "nonstress test" or fetal heart acceleration test.

Technique. An ultrasonic transducer to detect the fetal heart beat is placed as described for the oxytocin test. Each time fetal movement is felt by the mother she presses a button to record the instant of movement on the same moving paper strip that the heart rate is recorded.

Interpretation. The test is generally considered normal when three or more fetal movements are accompanied by acceleration of the fetal heart rate of 15 beats per minute or more. Lack of acceleration with fetal movement is considered abnormal. No fetal movement is considered unsatisfactory for testing but, if lacking for a prolonged period, it is in itself ominous.

Several investigators have reported that acceleration of the fetal heart rate during and immediately after fetal movement is as good a prognosticator of fetal well-being as a negative contraction stress test but even more have not. Observations reported to date imply that acceleration of the fetal heart with fetal movement most often, *but certainly not always,* indicates that the fetus will survive in utero for at least one more week.

"Simplified" Antepartum Fetal Heart Assessment

Baskett and co-workers (1981) have listened to the fetal heart rate using a simple doppler device that translated each fetal heart beat into sound. In this fashion they detected 94 percent (82 out of 87) of reactive nonstress tests measured as described above. Moreover, in no case was a nonreactive stress test falsely called reactive by the listening observer.

Value of Antepartum Tests Concerned with Fetal Heart Rate

These tests are now widely applied at least in the United States. However, arguments persist as to the relative merits of the contraction stress test and the nonstress test to identify the fetus whose well-being might be deteriorating in utero. The nonstress test appears to be favored by many because it is easier to perform.

It is not always fully appreciated that considerable obstetric art in other forms has been applied by the proponents of either test to achieve the excellent fetal outcomes that they most often have reported to try to validate the importance of the test in pregnancy management. Therefore, it is not surprising that a few groups have reported that failure to use either test imposed no detectable penalty upon the fetus or neonate even though the pregnancy was high risk (Brown and co-workers, 1982; Lumley and associates, 1983). Interestingly, in one institution subsequent to a controlled study in which no benefits from antenatal fetal heart monitoring were identified, there was a 16-fold increase in antenatal monitoring (Lumley and associates, 1983). Importantly, earlier recommendations that included performance of fetal heart rate testing at weekly intervals in pregnancies considered to be high risk are no longer valid, especially in case of diabetes or retarded fetal growth, as emphasized by Barrett and associates (1981) and others.

In summary, the following statements seem appropriate: (1) A week can prove to be a dangerously long time in the life of a fetus! (2) Anything that focuses attention on the fetus is likely to improve care. (3) No test of fetal well-being, including cardiotocographic tests, provides complete reassurance.

Other Antepartum Fetal Heart Rate Tests

Read and Miller (1977) reported that sound of 105 to 120 decibels intensity delivered for 5 seconds through a microphone closely applied to the lower abdomen of the mother evoked acceleration of the fetal heart rate in instances where the oxytocin challenge test was negative. However, no response to the sound was frequently associated with a suspicious or positive oxytocin challenge test. Serafini and associates (1984) have reported similar results from acoustic stimulation studies. Harrigan and Marino (1978) have claimed that acceleration of the fetal heart rate in response to insertion of the needle during transabdominal amniocentesis is a favorable sign of fetal well-being, with the reverse usually being true for decelerations that accompany amniocentesis. More "fetal fright tests," using other stimuli noxious to the fetus, at least, are likely to be described.

INTRAPARTUM SURVEILLANCE OF THE FETUS

A goal to be constantly strived for during labor is the preservation of fetal well-being by early detection and relief of fetal distress. To monitor means simply to watch or check on a person or thing. In the minds of many people in obstetrics, however, the word "monitor" has come to mean specifically surveillance of the fetal heart and uterine activity by some sort of an electronic detecting and recording device. It is sometimes forgotten that clinical monitoring has produced meritorious results when conscientiously applied during labor and delivery by appropriately trained individuals (Haverkamp and colleagues, 1976, 1979).

Electronic Monitoring of Fetal Heart Rate and Uterine Contractions

With each uterine contraction, there is a temporary variable reduction in the flow of oxygenated maternal blood through the placental intracotyledonary spaces. Hon (1974) aptly pointed out that labor is a stress test for the fetus who may be handicapped by (1) intrinsic fetal disease, (2) placental disease, (3) cord compression, (4) maternal disease, (5) drugs administered for analgesia and anesthesia, or (6) maternal hypotension from the supine position, conduction anesthesia, or both. To detect fetal distress during labor, he and others urged that continuous beat-to-beat recording of the fetal heart rate

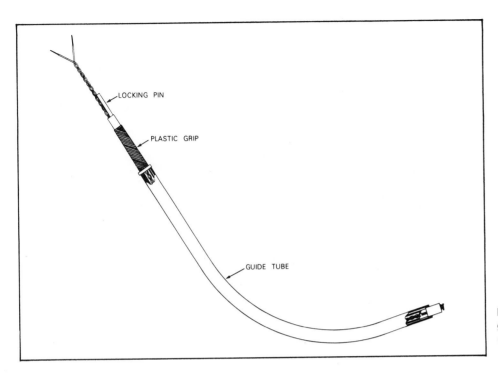

Figure 14-8. Spiral electrode with guide tube. (*From Hon co-workers: Obstet Gynecol 40:362, 1972.*)

be made concomitant with the pressure changes generated by the uterine contractions. To this end, Hon and others perfected sophisticated electronic detection and recording equipment that is widely used for monitoring the fetal heart and uterine contractions (Fig. 14-6).

Internal Monitoring of Fetal Heart

The fetal heart rate may be identified beat by beat by attaching a unipolar electrode directly to the fetus and another electrode to the mother and, after appropriate filtration and amplification, recording each contraction of the fetal heart on a time-calibrated moving-strip recorder.

The spiral electrode in common use, developed by Hon and associates (1972), is shown in Figure 14-8. Electrical contact with the fetus is established by twisting the driving tube, which propels the spiral electrode through the skin. To be able to attach the electrode to the fetus, the cervix must be dilated at least 1 cm, and, of course, the membranes above the cervix must be ruptured. It is important that the electrode be attached to the fetus at a relatively benign site, avoiding such critical areas as the fontanels and suture lines of the head, as well as the face and genitalia. Thus it is imperative that not only the presenting part be identified but that the site of attachment be precisely known.

The electrocardiographic signal picked up by the electrode inserted through the fetal skin is amplified sufficiently that typically the fetal R wave can be identified by a threshold detector that excludes all artifacts of lesser intensity. Good electrode placement that provides a high-amplitude fetal electrocardiographic signal yields the best "signal-to-noise" ratio. In practice, each detected R wave (and any electronic noise of equal intensity) is recorded on a calibrated moving paper strip.

Intrauterine Pressure Measurements

Measurements of intrauterine pressure, that is, the pressure of amnionic fluid, between and during contractions, are made by directly coupling the fluid to some sort of recording device. In clinical practice, a fluid-filled plastic catheter is positioned in utero so that the distal tip is located in amnionic fluid above the presenting fetal part (Fig. 14-9A, B). First, a plastic catheter guide that contains the distal portion of the catheter is inserted just through the cervical internal os; the fluid-filled catheter is then gently pushed beyond the guide into the uterine cavity. To minimize risk to the placenta from the catheter tip, Patel (1979) has recommended that when the site of placental implantation is known, the tip of the catheter inserter be positioned so that the catheter is likely to be inserted away from the placental site. The opposite end of the catheter, filled with saline, is connected to a strain-gauge pressure sensor adjusted to the same level as the catheter tip in the uterus. The amplified electrical signal produced in the strain-gauge by variations in pressure within the fluid system is recorded on a calibrated moving paper strip, usually simultaneously with the recording of the fetal heart rate. Free communication between amnionic fluid and fluid in the catheter is essential for meaningful pressure measurements. If the catheter tip becomes obstructed, it usually can be relieved by injecting a small volume of sterile saline from a syringe through the catheter. To avoid dam-

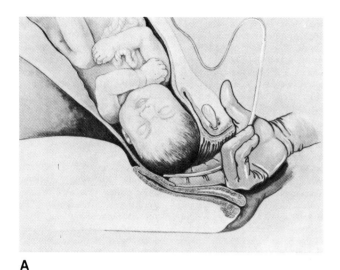

A

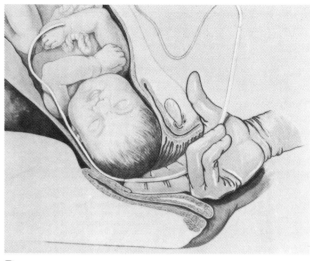

B

Figure 14-9. A. A sagittal view demonstrating placement of the catheter guide and catheter just within the cervix. **B.** A sagittal view showing the catheter inserted beyond the guide and within the amnionic sac. (*From Chan, Paul, Toews: Obstet Gynecol 41:7, 1973.*)

age to the transducer, it must be isolated from the system during this maneuver.

External (Indirect) Electronic Monitoring

The necessity for rupture of the membranes and invasion of the uterus may be avoided by use of external detectors to detect fetal heart action and to identify uterine activity (Fig. 14-6). External monitoring does not provide the precision of measurement of fetal heart rate afforded by internal monitoring or any quantification of uterine pressure.

The fetal heart rate may be detected in a number of ways through the maternal abdominal wall overlying the uterus. The easiest technique to use during the antepartum and early intrapartum periods employs the *ultrasound doppler principle.* Ultrasonic waves undergo a shift in frequency as they are reflected from moving fetal heart valves and from fetal blood cells ejected in pulsatile fashion by cardiac systole. The unit for detecting fetal heart action consists of a transducer that emits ultrasound, typically with a frequency of 2 megahertz, and a sensor to detect a shift in frequency of the reflected sound. The detector is placed on the abdomen at a site where fetal heart action is best detected. A coupling gel must be applied to the maternal skin, since air conducts ultrasound poorly. The device is held in position by an abdominal belt (Fig. 14-6).

Phonocardiography using a sensitive microphone may be tried to detect the sound generated by fetal heart action. Unfortunately, in clinical practice, extraneous sounds often create technical difficulties that limit the utility of this technique. The fetal *electrocardiogram* may, at times, be detected through electrodes attached to the maternal abdomen. The signal strength is typi-

cally quite weak and therefore is difficult to separate from extraneous electrical interference, including the maternal electrocardiogram.

Remote Display from Electronic Monitors. Observation of the fetal heart rate and uterine contraction patterns of laboring women by means of centrally located electronic display units is becoming popular. Although this enables one individual to observe these recorded functions at a distance from the laboring women, other aspects of intrapartum surveillance that are equally important may be neglected as a consequence.

Terminology To Describe Fetal Heart Rate

Since the fetal heart rate is rarely fixed, but, instead, shows frequent periodic variations, standardized terminology has been proposed to try to describe more precisely both baseline activity and periodic variations from the baseline (ACOG Technical Bulletin No. 32, 1975):

Baseline fetal heart rate refers to the modal rate that prevails apart from any periodic accelerations or decelerations associated with uterine contractions. A baseline rate between 120 and 160 beats per minute is considered *normal,* a rate of 100 to 120 *mild bradycardia,* and a rate of less than 100 *marked bradycardia.* Tachycardia is considered *mild* if the baseline rate is between 161 and 180 beats per minutes and *marked* if 180 or more.

Periodic fetal heart rate refers to deviations from baseline that are related to uterine contractions. *Acceleration* refers to an increase in fetal heart rate above baseline and *deceleration* to a decrease below the baseline rate. Three major patterns of deceleration are described: (1) *Uniform patterns of deceleration* reflect the shape of the simultaneously recorded uterine contractions. With the uniform pattern of *early deceleration,* the onset, nadir, and recovery of the fetal heart rate to baseline coincide with the onset, peak, and end of the uterine contraction. Early decelerations, sometimes referred to as Type I or early dips, are usually attributed to compression of the fetal head, although the stimulus to early deceleration may be more ominous. With the other uniform pattern, that of *late deceleration,* the onset of slowing occurs as the contraction intensity peaks, the nadir in heart rate is reached well after the peak, and recovery is not achieved until after the uterine contraction has terminated (Fig. 14-7). Late decelerations, also called Type II or late dips, are likely to be the consequence of uteroplacental insufficiency. (2) *Variable patterns of deceleration, or nonuniform decelerations,* are characterized by a decrease in heart rate beginning at no fixed time in relation to the uterine contractions and by wave forms that differ in shape from those of the uterine contractions and from each other, and may be nonrepetitive (Fig. 14-7). Variable decelerations may be the consequence of cord compression. (3) *Combined (mixed) patterns of deceleration,* as the term implies, exhibit the characteristics of both of the patterns described above.

The *pattern of early deceleration,* characterized by slowing of the heart rate at the onset of the contraction (Fig. 14-7), is likely to be the consequence of a transient increase in intracranial pressure from head compression, which stimulates the vagus nerve, thereby slowing the heart. Early decelerations may, however, have a more ominous origin. Mendez-Bauer and co-workers (1978), for example, have demonstrated early deceleration to be, at times, the consequence of compression of the umbilical cord. Prompt sterile vaginal examination to identify the status of the cervix and the presenting part, and to rule out prolapsed cord, is indicated. Treatment includes ascertaining that the mother is reclining comfortably on her side and checking the monitor, especially if external, to ensure that it is functioning properly. Early decelerations from head compression may be eliminated by the administration of atropine to the mother. Early decelerations that are severe and prolonged or persistent, and certainly if accompanied by gross meconium staining of the amnionic fluid, must not be ignored.

The *pattern of late deceleration* (Fig. 14-7) is likely to be the consequence of hypoxia and associated metabolic derangement from uteroplacental insufficiency. After termination of the uterine contractions, the heart rate may return to or rise transiently above normal baseline in the less severely affected fetus, or remain low in the severely affected fetus. The fetus stressed to an intermediate degree may demonstrate tachycardia between contractions. Delivery can be safely delayed only if the uteroplacental insufficiency is promptly corrected, as, for example, the relief of uterine overactivity by immediately stopping oxytocin stimulation or by correcting maternal hypotension and thereby improving uteroplacental perfusion. Otherwise, most often prompt delivery is indicated.

The *pattern of variable deceleration (nonuniform deceleration)* is likely to be the consequence of compression of the umbilical cord. Vaginal examination should be undertaken promptly to search for cord prolapse and determine the degree of cervical dilatation and the station and position of the presenting part. The position of the mother should then be changed so that she is laying on her side or turned to the opposite side. If decelerations persist, either immediate measurement of fetal scalp blood pH (p. 288) or prompt delivery is indicated.

It is becoming apparent that these various deceleration patterns just described do not always reflect the causes ascribed to them. Although the classification presented has served as a guide to the interpretation of various patterns of fetal heart response during labor, its rigid application, unfortunately, has led, at times, to erroneous diagnosis and treatment.

Beat-to-Beat Variation in Fetal Heart Rate. Later in pregnancy there is normally a beat-to-beat variation in the fetal heart rate, that is, the time interval between the same locus, for example, the R wave, in consecutive electrical systoles is not fixed. The variation was attributed by Hon (1974) to the continuous interaction of sympathetic and parasympathetic nerve action on the heart. However, Dalton and associates (1983) have demonstrated that in the sheep fetus, at least, sympathetic blockade has little effect on fetal heart rate variability and, although parasympathetic blockade reduces variability, it does not abolish it.

Absence of beat-to-beat variability in some circumstances late in pregnancy may be indicative of fetal compromise. In fact, Boehm (1977) maintained that fetal heart rate variability has become the most important aspect of the overall clinical evaluation of the fetus in utero. It should be emphasized, however, that an otherwise normal premature fetus or the fetus who is "asleep" may not demonstrate beat-to-beat variability. Moreover, medications in doses commonly used during labor and in preparation for delivery may ablate beat-to-beat variability. These include meperidine, morphine, alphaprodine, barbiturates, general and conduction anesthesia, diazepam, phenothiazines, atropine, scopolamine, and perhaps magnesium sulfate in large doses (Babaknia and Niebyl, 1978; Boehm, 1977; Cohen and Schifrin, 1977). Unfortunately, recordings made with externally applied detecting devices are unreliable for identifying the presence or absence of beat-to-beat variation.

Sinusoidal Fetal Heart Rate Pattern. A sinusoidal fetal heart rate pattern, especially when marked, can prove to be an ominous sign of fetal deterioration. For example, Katz and co-workers (1983) observed that with sinusoidal oscillations of more than 25 beats per minute, death of the fetus or newborn infant was very common (six out of nine died), but when the sinusoidal oscillations were less than 25 per minute, the outcome was very much better (82 out of 83 survived). A marked sinusoidal pattern of fetal heart rate has been identified frequently in fetuses who were severely anemic. Gray and associates (1978) observed the development of a sinusoidal fetal heart rate pattern in nearly one half of pregnancies in which the mothers received alphoprodine (Nisentil) for relief of labor discomfort. In this particular circumstance fetal outcome, in their experience, did not appear to be adversely affected by the presence of a sinusoidal heart rate pattern. Epstein and associates (1982) described a sinusoidal fetal heart rate pattern following maternal administration of meperidine, with reversal of the pattern when naloxone was administered.

Persistent Fetal Tachycardia or Bradycardia. Tachycardia without deceleration may be the consequence of febrile illness, a response to hypoxia, or rarely to fetal thyrotoxicosis.

Mild bradycardia without deceleration or acceleration is not necessarily caused by fetal distress. Young and associates (1979) found no evidence of acidosis during labor and delivery in several fetuses who demonstrated persistent bradycardia in the range of 100 to 120 beats per minute, and the neonatal outcomes were good. Interestingly, an occiput posterior or transverse position was identified in each instance. They ascribed the moderate bradycardia to a vagal response induced by persistent head compression in the occiput posterior position.

More severe bradycardia may be the consequence of congenital heart lesions or severe hypoxia. An association has recently been identified between heart block in the fetus and newborn infant and maternal collagen vascular diseases, especially lupus erythematosus (Chapter 28, p. 619). Viral infections of the fetus may also cause congenital heart block (Lewis and co-workers, 1980). We have also observed that fetal bradycardia accompanies marked maternal hypothermia; the heart rate rose from 90 to 136 when the mother became euthermic. Fetal bradycardia has also been associated with sudden lowering of the blood pressure from excessive administration of antihypertensive drugs to severely hypertensive women.

An important cause of presumed fetal bradycardia is fetal death, with the *maternal* heart rate being recorded by the monitor but erroneously considered to be the fetal heart rate (Odendaal, 1976). An illustration of this phenomenon is seen in Figure 21-9 (p. 403). Maternal tachycardia, as occurs with sepsis or with concealed hemorrhage from abruptio placentae, may, at times, spuriously provide a recording of what appears to be a normal fetal heart rate even though the fetus is dead. *Especially before performing any heroic treatment on the basis of electronic monitoring data, it is always wise to listen carefully to the fetal heart with an appropriate stethoscope while simultaneously checking the maternal pulse rate.*

Fetal Cardiac Arrhythmias. Intermittently recurring cardiac arrhythmias of ectopic origin may cause concern. The experience of Sugarman and associates (1978), as

well as the earlier reports of others, however, indicate that the arrhythmias are likely to be innocuous and that the generally favorable neonatal outcome is not improved by pregnancy intervention or attempts at pharmacologic treatment in utero.

Normal Fetal Heart Rate Pattern. The absence of an ominous fetal heart rate pattern is generally, but not absolutely, predictive of a good fetal outcome. Hayashi and Fox (1975) and others more recently have documented cardiac arrest and death of the fetus without detecting a preceding ominous fetal heart rate pattern.

Fetal Blood Sampling

Measurements of the pH of appropriately collected capillary blood may help to identify the fetus in serious distress. A suitably illuminated endoscope is inserted through the sufficiently dilated cervix and ruptured membranes so as to press firmly against fetal skin, usually the scalp (Fig. 14-10). The skin is wiped clean with a cotton swab; it may be sprayed with ethyl chloride to induce hyperemia, and coated with a silicone gel to cause the blood to accumulate as discrete globules. An incision is made through the skin to a calibrated depth with a special blade on an appropriately long handle. As a drop of blood forms on the surface, it is immediately collected into a heparinized glass capillary tube and the pH of the blood is promptly measured. The pH of fetal capillary blood usually is lower than arterial blood and approaches that of venous blood.

Saling (1964) initially proposed a pH of 7.20 as the critical value for identification of serious fetal distress, while Mann (1978) and some others recommended immediate delivery whenever scalp blood pH was 7.25 or less. Zalar and Quilligan (1979) have recommended the following protocol to try to confirm fetal distress through use of fetal scalp sampling: If the pH is greater than 7.25, labor is observed. If the pH is between 7.20 and 7.25, the pH measurement is repeated within 30 minutes. If the pH is less than 7.20, another scalp blood sample is immediately collected and the mother is taken to an operating room and prepared for surgery. Cesarean section is promptly performed if the low pH is confirmed. Otherwise, labor is allowed to continue and scalp blood samples are repeated periodically. The obstetrician must be careful not to allow time for repetition of laboratory tests to lead to dangerous clinical procrastination.

Adhering too closely to a critical pH value may in actual practice prove disadvantageous, since it will tend to allay suspicion of early hypoxic acidosis. A fall in pH is a relatively late effect of hypoxia and, when samples of fetal blood are obtained intermittently, detection of hypoxia of rapid onset may be unduly delayed. It must also be kept in mind that the pH of fetal capillary blood need not accurately reflect the degree of hypoxia in the fetus, since the pH will be influenced appreciably by that of the mother. The severely hypoxic fetus becomes overtly acidotic, which is reflected by a low blood pH except

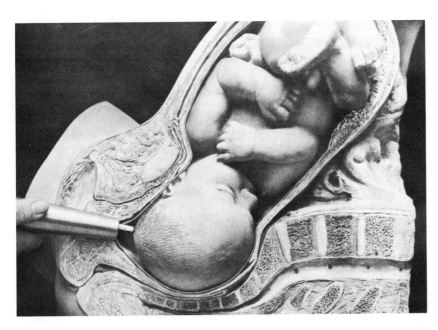

Figure 14-10. The technique of fetal scalp sampling utilizing an amnioscope. Note end of endoscope displaced from fetal vertex approximately 2 cm to show disposable blade against the fetal scalp before incision. (*From Hamilton and McKeown. In Wynn RM (ed): Obstetrics and Gynecology Annual: 1973. New York, Appleton, 1974.*)

when the mother is alkalotic, for example, from hyperventilation. Conversely, the fetus may have a low blood pH without being remarkably hypoxic if the mother is acidotic. Rooth and associates (1973) emphasized the impact of maternal pH on fetal scalp blood pH. They suggested that clinically important fetal acidosis be identified by demonstrating the value for the fetus to be at least 0.20 pH units less than that of the mother.

Measurements of blood Po_2 and Pco_2 require more blood but probably do not provide enough additional information to justify their determination. In fact, hypoxic danger to the fetus is better assessed by pH determinations, which reflect metabolic reactions to hypoxia, than by isolated measurements of blood gases, which may vary rapidly and remarkably with transient circulatory changes.

Continuous transcutaneous monitoring of fetal oxygen has been described and continues to be evaluated. Through a cervix dilated at least 3 cm, an electrode about 2 cm in diameter was attached by a tissue glue to a shaved region of the fetal scalp. The electrode was integrally heated to 44°C to effect vasodilatation. Among early studies using this technique, Huch and co-workers (1978) reported a number of observations of clinical interest: Fetal transcutaneous Po_2 rose when the mother was given oxygen. It fell, however, during maternal hypoventilation subsequent to hyperventilation, and it fell during uterine contractions when the mother was kept supine. Moreover, they reported that the Po_2 so measured was low when severe decelerations of the fetal heart rate were evident and low when the basal fetal heart rate was less than 100 or greater than 180 beats per minute. Unexpectedly, loss of baseline variability of fetal heart rate was not always accompanied by a low transcutaneous Po_2. Disturbingly, Willcourt and co-workers (1981) observed that transcutaneous Po_2 values varied remarkably during late decelerations of the fetal heart, which they interpreted to be suggestive of different mechanisms involved in their production.

Complications from Internal Electronic and Physicochemical Monitoring

There are potential dangers inherent in monitoring the fetal heart rate by direct application of an electrode to the fetus, measuring uterine pressure by inserting an indwelling catheter into the uterine cavity, or incising the fetal scalp to measure blood pH. A strong orientation toward universal use of internal monitoring techniques is likely to predispose to *early amniotomy* and its potential dangers, including cord prolapse, infection, and possibly more stress to the fetus when not cushioned by amnionic fluid during labor. In this regard the studies performed on late pregnant monkeys by Gabbe and associates (1976) and similar studies in sheep serve to reemphasize the protective cushion against cord compression provided by amnionic fluid. Acute reduction in amnionic fluid volume was accompanied by periodic fetal heart rate decelerations variable in pattern. Restoration of the amnionic fluid volume eliminated the abnormal pattern.

Another potential morbidity is *trauma*. Injury to the fetal scalp induced by the electrode is rarely a major problem, although application at some other site, for example, the eye in case of a face presentation, can prove serious. A fetal vessel in the placenta may be ruptured inadvertently by the placement of the catheter. Trudinger and Pryse-Davies (1978) observed four such accidents, two of which led to death of the fetus or newborn infant from exsanguination. Moreover, they identified one instance of severe cord compression from entanglement with the intrauterine catheter. Others have had similar experiences. Penetration of the placenta causing hemorrhage and perforations of the uterus during insertion of the catheter for pressure recording do occur and have led to serious morbidity, as well as spurious recordings that resulted in inappropriate management of labor and delivery.

Both the fetus and the mother may be at increased risk of *infection* as the consequence of internal electronic monitoring. Scalp wounds from the electrode may become infected by organisms of the vaginal flora (Okada and associates, 1977). Infection of the newborn infant with *Herpes hominis* type 2 virus has been identified following the use of scalp electrodes; systemic viral disease, as well as chronic scalp infection, resulted. Infants born after internal electronic monitoring appear more likely to have been colonized by maternal group B streptococcus.

An increase in maternal infections following the use of internal electronic monitoring has not been a common finding. Perhaps a decrease in the frequency and therefore the number of vaginal examinations for the woman who is being so monitored offsets the risk imposed by rupture of the membranes and the placement and persistence of the catheter and wires in utero.

Although external monitoring techniques obviate the necessity of ruptured membranes and invasion of the uterus, as well as direct trauma to the fetus, their use, unless meticulously guarded against, commonly results in the mother lying in the supine position most of the time so as to protect the placement of the external detectors. The supine position, by causing aortocaval compression, is likely to be deleterious to the fetus if the fetus is already in jeopardy for other reasons, fetal or maternal.

Three troublesome complications resulting from fetal scalp blood sampling are infection, blade breakage, and bleeding. If vaginal bleeding is encountered at any time following scalp blood sampling, fetal bleeding must be ruled out. Marked deficiencies of vitamin K–dependent coagulation factors have been implicated in the genesis of such hemorrhage in some infants (Hull, 1972), and hemophilia has been subsequently diagnosed in a few others. The negative pressure from use of a vacuum extractor to effect delivery after scalp blood sampling may incite troublesome hemorrhage.

ASSESSMENT OF RESULTS FROM ELECTRONIC MONITORING

In the United States, Hon, Quilligan, Paul, and Freeman are prominent among the names of obstetricians who have long championed continuous electronic recording of the fetal heart during labor. They observed somewhat lower perinatal mortality rates at Los Angeles County Hospital for labors in which the fetal heart rate was continuously recorded, despite the fact that the group so monitored was selected because of pregnancy complications recognized to predispose to a poorer outcome for the fetus (Paul and colleagues, 1977). Beard (1974) of Great Britain considered electronic monitoring limited only to so-called high-risk pregnancies to be unsound, and urged that electronic monitoring be used for all

labors. In his experience, in terms of the number of fetuses who became acidotic during labor, there was little difference between the identified high-risk pregnancies and those considered normal. He emphasized that only by so monitoring all labors will intrapartum asphyxial damage be eliminated.

Although many groups have stated, or at least implied, that fetal mortality rates were reduced significantly as the consequence of continuous electronic monitoring, some studies have demonstrated similarly good outcomes for pregnancies using systematic clinical monitoring. For example, in one series of studies in Denver, trained nursing personnel clinically monitored the mother and fetus in a standardized fashion throughout labor until the actual delivery of the infant (Haverkamp and co-workers, 1976, 1979). The fetal heart was routinely checked every 15 minutes during the first stage, every 5 minutes during the second stage, and more often if an abnormality was suspected. Uterine contractions were frequently evaluated by palpation and the mother was observed continuously. In the group so monitored clinically, the Apgar scores were as high as in the group routinely subjected to continuous electronic monitoring, while the cesarean section group was appreciably lower.

In Oxford, England, the results of two systems of obstetric care for apparently low-risk pregnancies* have been compared and the conclusion drawn that care of one mother by one midwife during labor and delivery without electronic fetal monitoring produced results as good or better than were achieved with electronic monitoring and a consultant team of obstetricians directly responsible for intrapartum management (Klein and co-workers, 1983). They were favorably impressed by the simplicity, yet safety, of delivery of low-risk parturients that could be achieved in labor management. (Those of us who were born before the era of electronic monitoring, or even the Apgar score, need not necessarily feel cheated!)

It cannot be overemphasized that the techniques for continuous recording of fetal heart rates and uterine pressures do not by themselves provide continuous surveillance of the fetus. Appropriately trained personnel must be immediately available to activate the electronic techniques, to inspect and analyze almost continuously the data that are being recorded, and to act sufficiently promptly on the findings.

For many, but not all, obstetric services the increasing use of electronic fetal monitoring has been accompanied by an appreciable increase in cesarean section rate (Antenatal Diagnosis, 1979). Whether the two phenomena are directly related is not clear in many instances. However, in the case of the two studies by Haverkamp

---

* *The following abnormalities were not identified before labor: Past history—previous cesarean delivery, perinatal death, or low-birth-weight infant. Current status—significant medical history, hemoglobin below 10 g/dl, abnormal antibodies, breech presentation, multiple fetuses, fetal weight less than 2500 g, blood pressure above 140/85 mm Hg.*

and co-workers cited above, cesarean section with electronic monitoring of labor, when compared to clinical monitoring carried out as described, was either two times or three times as high, depending upon whether or not scalp sampling to measure fetal blood pH was performed in conjunction with electronic monitoring.

CLINICAL MONITORING

The status of the fetus can often be satisfactorily monitored clinically by appropriately trained individuals who closely adhere to the guidelines that follow and are reemphasized in Chapter 17 (p. 335). In summary, the fetal heart rate is carefully determined at close intervals during and immediately after a uterine contraction until the infant is actually delivered; the frequency and intensity of uterine contractions are carefully estimated; and the rates of cervical dilatation and descent of the presenting part are determined periodically.

Normally, the fetal heart rate between contractions will average about 140 and will range from no less than 120 to no more than 160 beats per minute. Typically, the fetal heart rate drops somewhat with the onset of a uterine contraction but recovers promptly as the contraction ends. The fetal heart rate may be determined using a specialized stethoscope or an instrument that utilizes the doppler principle with ultrasound to detect fetal heart action.

INTRAPARTUM SURVEILLANCE OF THE FETUS AT PARKLAND MEMORIAL HOSPITAL

In two thirds of labors, the fetus is monitored clinically as described above and in Chapter 17. Continuous electronic monitoring currently is reserved for the following circumstances:

1. Variations in the fetal heart rate detected by auscultation *and for which immediate delivery is not considered necessary.*
2. Meconium in amnionic fluid.
3. Induction or augmentation of labor with oxytocin.
4. Previous cesarean delivery.
5. Increased likelihood of uteroplacental insufficiency or compromised fetus:
   a. Hypertension.
   b. Bleeding.
   c. Preterm and postterm pregnancies.
   d. Small fetus, probably growth-retarded.
   e. Abnormal presentations.
   f. Previous unexplained stillbirth.
   g. Sickle cell hemoglobinopathies.
   h. Hemolytic disease of the fetus.
   i. Diabetes.

Although the application of continuous electronic monitoring cannot by itself be credited for any remark-

able reduction in intrapartum or neonatal mortality at Parkland Memorial Hospital, it has provided an elegant means of demonstrating to physicians in training, medical students, nurses, physician's assistants, and others the normal and abnormal forces of labor and the cardiac responses of the fetus during this important event.

REFERENCES

ACOG Technical Bulletin No. 32. Fetal heart Rate Monitoring. Guidelines for Monitoring, Terminology and Instrumentation. Chicago, American College of Obstetricians and Gynecologists, 1975

Antenatal Diagnosis. Report of a Consensus Development Conference Sponsored by the National Institute of Child Health and Human Development, NIH Publication Number 79—1973. Washington, D.C., U.S., Gov Print Off, 1979

Aula P, Rapola J, Karjalainen O, Lindgren J, Hartikainen AL, Seppälä M: Prenatal diagnosis of congenital nephrosis in 23 high-risk families. Am J Dis Child 132:984, 1978

Babaknia A, Niebyl JR: The effect of magnesium sulfate on fetal heart rate baseline variability. Obstet Gynecol 51 (Suppl):2, 1978

Barrett JM, Salver SL, Boehm FH: The nonstress test: An evaluation of 1,000 patients. Am J Obstet Gynecol 141:153, 1981

Baskett TF, Boyce CD, Lohre MA, Manning FA: Simplified antepartum fetal heart assessment. Br J Obstet Gynaecol 88:395, 1981

Beard RW: The detection of fetal asphyxia in labor. Pediatrics 53:157, 1974

Belisle S, Fencl MD, Tulchinsky D: Amniotic fluid testosterone and follicle-stimulating hormone in the determination of fetal sex. Am J Obstet Gynecol 128:514, 1977

Birnholz JC: Determination of fetal sex. N Engl J Med 309:942, 1983

Blumenfeld TA, Stark RI, James LS, George JD, Dyrenfurth I, Freda VJ, Shinitzsky M: Determination of fetal lung maturity by fluorescence polarization of the amniotic fluid. Am J Obstet Gynecol 102:782, 1978

Boehm FH: FHR variability: Key to fetal well-being. Contemp Ob/Gyn 9:57, 1977

Brown VA, Sawers RS, Parsons RJ, Duncan SLB, Cooke ID: The value of antenatal cardiotocography in the management of high-risk pregnancy: A randomized controlled trial. Br J Obstet Gynaecol 89:716, 1982

Buhi WC, Spellacy WN: Effect of blood or meconium on the determination of the amniotic fluid lecithin/sphingomyelin ratio. Am J Obstet Gynecol 121:321, 1975

Clements JA, Platzker ACG, Tierney DF, Hobel CL, Creasy RK, Margolis AJ, Thibeault DW, Tooley WH, Oh W: Assessment of the risk of respiratory distress syndrome by a rapid test for surfactant in amniotic fluid. N Engl J Med 286:1077, 1972

Cohen WR, Schifrin BS: Diagnosis and treatment of fetal distress. In Bolognese RJ, Schwarz RH (eds): Perinatal Medicine. Baltimore, Williams & Wilkins, 1977, p. 131

Dalton KJ, Dawes GS, Patrick JE: The autonomic nervous system and fetal heart rate variability. Am J Obstet Gynecol 146:456, 1983

Ehrström C: Fetal movement monitoring in normal and high-risk pregnancy. Acta Obstet Gynecol 80 (Suppl), 1979

Elias S, Martin AO, Simpson JL: Chorionic villus biopsies: Techniques and cytogenetic analysis. Presented before the Society for Gynecological Investigation, San Francisco, March 21–24, 1984

Elrad H, Beydoun SN, Gagen JH, Cabalum MT, Aubry RH, Smith C: Fetal pulmonary maturity as determined by fluorescent polarization of amniotic fluid. Am J Obstet Gynecol 132:681, 1978

Epstein H, Waxman A, Gleicher N, Lauersen NH: Meperdine-induced sinusoidal fetal heart rate pattern and its reversal with naloxone. Obstet Gynecol 59 (Suppl):22, 1982

Evertson LR, Gauthier RJ, Collea JV: Fetal demise following negative contraction stress tests. Obstet Gynecol 51:671, 1978

Freda V: Hemolytic disease. Clin Obstet Gynecol 16:72, 1973

Freeman RK: The use of the oxytocin challenge test for antepartum clinical evaluation of utero-placental respiratory function. Am J Obstet Gynecol 121:481, 1975

Gabbe SG, Ettinger BB, Freeman RK, Martin CB: Umbilical cord compression associated with amniotomy: Laboratory observations. Am J Obstet Gynecol 126:353, 1976

Gal D, Neuhoff S, Lilling MI, Tancer ML: False negative oxytocin challenge test: Report of three cases. Am J Obstet Gynecol 133:111, 1979

Gant NF, Hutchinson HT, Siiteri PK, MacDonald PC: Study of the metabolic clearance rate of dehydroisoandrosterone sulfate in pregnancy. Am J Obstet Gynecol 111:555, 1971

Garite TJ, Yabusaki KK, Moberg LJ, Symons JL, White T, Itano M, Freeman RK: A new rapid slide agglutination test for amniotic fluid phosphatidylglycerol. Am J Obstet Gynecol 147:681, 1983

Gibbons JM Jr, Huntley TE, Corral AG: Effect of maternal blood contamination on amniotic fluid analysis. Obstet Gynecol 44:657, 1974

Gillberg C, Rasmussen P, Wahlström J: Long-term follow-up of children born after amniocentesis. Clin Genetics 21:69, 1982

Gluck L, Kulovich MV, Borer RC Jr, Brenner PH, Anderson GG, Spellacy WN: Diagnosis of the respiratory distress syndrome by amniocentesis. Am J Obstet Gynecol 109:440, 1971

Golde SH, Vogt JF, Gabbe SG, Cabal LA: Evaluation of the FELMSA microviscometer in predicting fetal lung maturity. Obstet Gynecol 54:639, 1979

Gray JH, Cudmore DW, Luther ER, Martin TR, Gardner AJ: Sinusoidal fetal heart rate pattern associated with alphaprodine administration. Obstet Gynecol 52:678, 1978

Halvorsen P, Gross TL: Clinical evaluation of a rapid slide agglutination test for amniotic fluid phosphatidylglycerol. Presented at the annual meeting of the Society for Perinatal Obstetricians, San Antonio, TX, February 2–4, 1984

Hammacher K: Früherkennung intrauteriner gefahrenzustände durch electrophonokardiographie und fokographie. In Elert R, Hüter KA (eds): Prophylaxe Frühkindlicher Hirnshäden. Stuttgart, Georg Thieme, 1966, p 120

Hammacher K. Hüter KA, Bokelmann J, Werners PH: Foetal heart frequency and perinatal condition of the foetus and newborn. Gynaecologia 166:349, 1968

Harrigan JT, Marino JF: Fetal heart rate reaction to amniocentesis as an indicator of fetal well-being. Am J Obstet Gynecol 132:49, 1978

Harvey D, Parkinson CE, Campbell S: Risk of respiratory-distress syndrome. Lancet 1:42, 1975

Haverkamp AD, Thompson HE, McFee JG, Cetrulo C: The evaluation of continuous fetal heart rate monitoring in high-risk pregnancy. Am J Obstet Gynecol 125:310, 1976

Haverkamp AD, Orleans M, Langendoerfer S, McFee JG, Murphy J, Thompson HE: A controlled trial of the differen-

tial effects of intrapartum fetal monitoring. Am J Obstet Gynecol 143:399, 1979

Hayashi RH, Fox ME: Unforeseen sudden intrapartum fetal death in a monitored labor. Am J Obstet Gynecol 122:786, 1975

Herbert WNP, Tyson JE, Jimenez JM: Absence of hyaline membrane disease at low lecithin to sphingomyelin ratios. Pediatr Res 13:497, 1979

Herbert WNP, Chapman JE, Cefalo RC: Reliability of the foam stability index test in assessing fetal lung maturation. Presented at the annual meeting of the Society for Perinatal Obstetricians, San Antonio, TX, February 2–4, 1984

Hon EH: Fetal heart rate monitoring. In Gluck L (ed): Modern Perinatal Medicine. Chicago, Year Book, 1974

Hon EH, Paul RH, Hon RW: Electronic evaluation of fetal heart rate. XI. Description of spiral electrode. Obstet Gynecol 40:362, 1972

Huch A, Huch R, Schneider H, Lucey JF: Monitoring fetal arterial oxygen continuously during labor. Contemp Ob/Gyn 12:73, 1978

Huddleston JF, Freeman RK: The use of the oxytocin challenge test for the management of pregnancies at risk for uteroplacental insufficiency. In Bolognese RJ, Schwarz RH (eds): Perinatal Medicine. Baltimore, Williams & Wilkins, 1977, p. 68

Hull MGR: Perinatal coagulopathies complicating fetal blood sampling. Br Med J 3:319, 1972

Katz M, Meizner I, Shani N, Insler V: Clinical significance of sinusoidal fetal heart rate pattern. Br J Obstet Gynaecol 90:832, 1983

Khouzami VA, Beck JC, Sullivant H, Johnson JWC: Amniotic fluid absorbance at 650 nm: Its relationship to lecithin/sphingomyelin ratio and neonatal pulmonary sufficiency. Am J Obstet Gynecol 147:552, 1983

Klein M, Lloyd I, Redman C, Bull M, Turnbull AC: A comparison of low-risk pregnant women booked for delivery in two systems of care: Shared-care (consultant) and integrated general practice unit: II. Labour and delivery management and neonatal outcome. Br J Obstet Gynaecol 90:123, 1983

Kubli FW, Kaeser O, Hinselmann M: Diagnostic management of chronic placental insufficiency. In Pecile A, Finzi C (eds): The Foeto-Placental Unit. Amsterdam, Excerpta Medica, 1969, p 323

Leach G, Chang A, Morrison J: A controlled trial of puncture sites for amniocentesis. Br J Obstet Gynaecol 85:328, 1978

Lewis PE, Cefalo RC, Zaritsky AL: Fetal heart block due to cytomegalo-virus. Am J Obstet Gynecol 136:967, 1980

Liu DTY, Mitchell J, Johnson J, Wass DM: Trophoblast sampling by blind transcervical aspiration. Br J Obstet Gynaecol 90:1119, 1983

Lumley J, Lester A, Anderson I, Renou P, Wood C: A randomized trial of weekly cardiotocography in high-risk obstetric patients. Br J Obstet Gynaecol 90:1018, 1983

Mann L: Intrapartum fetal monitoring: Scalp blood pH is a useful tool. Contemp Ob/Gyn 11:25, 1978

Mendez-Bauer C, Ruiz Canesco A, Andujar Ruiz M, Menendez A, Arroya J, Gardi RD, Sastry V, Zamarriego Crespo J: Early decelerations of the fetal heart rate from occlusion of the umbilical cord. J Perinat Med 6:69, 1978

Milunsky A: The Prenatal Diagnosis of Hereditary Disorders. Springfield, IL, Thomas, 1973

Milunsky A, Sapirstein VS: Prenatal diagnosis of open neural tube defects using the amniotic fluid acethycholinesterase assay. Obstet Gynecol 59:1, 1982

National Institute of Child Health and Human Development,

National Registry for Amniocentesis Study Group: Midtrimester amniocentesis for prenatal diagnosis: Safety and accuracy. JAMA 236:1471, 1976

Odendaal HJ: False interpretation of fetal heart rate monitoring in cases of intra-uterine death. S Afr Med J 50:1963, 1976

Okada DM, Chow AW, Bruce VT: Neonatal scalp abscess and fetal monitoring: Factors associated with infection. Am J Obstet Gynecol 129:185, 1977

Oki EY: A protocol for the nipple-stimulation CST. Contemp Ob/Gyn Oct 157, 1983

Patel N: Personal communication, 1979

Paul RH, Huey JE Jr, Yaeger CF: Clinical fetal monitoring. Postgrad Med 61:160, 1977

Person P-H, Kullander S: Long-term experience of general ultrasound screening in pregnancy. Am J Obstet Gynecol 146:942, 1983

Poreco R, Young PE, Resnik R, Cousins L, Jones OW, Richards T, Kernahan C, Matson M: Reproductive outcome following amniocentesis for genetic indications. Am J Obstet Gynecol 143:653, 1983

Quirk JG, Bleasdale JE: Fetal lung maturation in the pregnancy complicated by diabetes mellitus. In DiRenzo GC, Hawkins PR (eds): Perinatal Medicine: Updates and Controversies. (in press)

Raja RLT, Anderson AMB, Turnbull AC: Endocrine changes in premature labor. Br Med J 4:67, 1974

Ray M, Freeman R, Pine S, Hesselgesser R: Clinical experience with the oxytocin challenge test. Am J Obstet Gynecol 114:1, 1972

Read JA, Miller FC: Fetal heart rate acceleration in response to acoustic stimulation as a measure of fetal well-being. Am J Obstet Gynecol 129:512, 1977

Roberts NS, Dunn LK, Weiner S, Godmilow L, Miller R: Midtrimester amniocentesis: Indications, techniques, risks and potential for prenatal diagnosis. J Reprod Med 28:167, 1983

Rodeck CH, Gosden CM, Gosden JR: Development of an improved technique for first-trimester microsampling of chorion. Br J Obstet Gynaecol 90:1113, 1983

Rooth G, McBride R, Ivy BJ: Fetal and maternal pH measurements. Acta Obstet Gynecol Scand 52:47, 1973

Ross MG, Leake RD, Ervin G, Sicon J, Fisher DA: Breast stimulation contraction test. Presented at the annual meeting of the Society of Perinatal Obstetricians, San Antonio, Texas, February 2–4, 1984

Sadovsky E, Polishuk WZ: Fetal movements in utero: Nature, assessment, prognostic value, timing of delivery. Obstet Gynecol 50:49, 1977

Saling EZ: Die Blutgasverhaltnisse und der saure Basen-Haushalt der Feten bei ungerstörtem geburtsablauf. Z Geburtsh Gynaekol 161:262, 1964

Saling EZ, Dudenhausen JW: The present situation of clinical monitoring of the fetus during labor. J Perinat Med 1:75, 1973

Sbarra AJ, Michlewitz H, Selvaraj RJ, Mitchell GW, Cetrulo CL, Kelley EC, Kennedy JL, Herschell MJ, Paul BB, Louis F: Relation between optical density at 650 nm and L/S ratio. Obstet Gynecol 50:723, 1977

Schifrin BS: The non-stress test. Presented at the Seventy-eighth Ross Conference on Pediatric Research (Obstetrical Decisions and Neonatal Outcome), San Diego, CA, May 30, 1979

Schlueter MA, Phibbs RH, Creasy RK, Clements JA, Tooley WH: Antenatal prediction of graduated risk of hyaline membrane disease by amniotic fluid foam test for surfactant. Am J Obstet Gynecol 134:761, 1979

Serafini P, Lindsay MBJ, Nagey DA, Pupkin MJ, Tseng P, Crenshaw C Jr: Antepartum fetal heart rate response to sound stimulation: The acoustic stimulation test. Am J Obstet Gynecol 148:41, 1984

Shawker TH, Schuette WH, Whitehouse W, Rifka SM: Early fetal movement: A real-time ultrasound study. Obstet Gynecol 55:194, 1980

Sher G, Statland BE: Assessment of fetal pulmonary maturity by the Lumadex foam stability index test. Obstet Gynecol 61:444, 1983

Simpson H, Dallaire L, Miller J, Simonovitch L, Hamerton J: Prenatal diagnosis of genetic disease in Canada: Report of a collaborative study. Can Med Assoc J 115:739, 1976

Smith FW, Adam AH, Phillips WDP: NMR imaging in pregnancy. Lancet 1:61, 1983

Sugarman RG, Rawlinson KF, Schifrin BS: Fetal arrhythmias. Obstet Gynecol 52:301, 1978

Symonds EM, Johnson IR, Kean DM, Worthington BS, Pipkin FB, Hawkes RC, Gyngell M: Imaging the pregnant human uterus with nuclear magnetic resonance. Am J Obstet Gynecol 148:1136, 1984

Teoh ES, Lau YK, Ambrose A, Ratnam SS: Amniotic fluid creatinine, uric acid and urea as indices of gestational age. Acta Obstet Gynecol Scand 52:323, 1973

Trudinger BJ, Pryse-Davies J: Fetal hazards of the intrauterine pressure catheter: Five case reports. Br J Obstet Gynaecol 85:567, 1978

Tsai MY, Josephson MW, Knox GE: Absorbance of amniotic fluid at 650 nm as a fetal lung maturity test: A comparison with the lecithin/sphingomyelin ratio and tests for disaturated phosphatidylcholine and phosphatidylglycerol. Am J Obstet Gynecol 146:963, 1983

Turner RJ, Read JA: Practical use and efficiency of amniotic fluid OD 650 as a predictor of fetal pulmonary maturity. Obstet Gynecol 61:551, 1983

Valenti C, Lin CC, Baum A, Masobrio M: Prenatal sex determination. Am J Obstet Gynecol 112:890, 1972

Whitehouse WM, Simmons CS, Evans TN: Reduction of radiation hazard in obstetric roentgenography. Am J Roentgenol 80:690, 1958

Whittle MJ, Wilson AI, Whitfield CR, Paton RD, Logan RW: Amniotic fluid phosphatidylglycerol and the lecithin/sphingomyelin ratio in the assessment of fetal lung maturity. Br J Obstet Gynaecol 89:727, 1982

Willcourt RJ, King JC, Indyk L, Queenan JT: The relationship of fetal heart rate patterns to the fetal transcutaneous P_{O_2}. Am J Obstet Gynecol 140:760, 1981

Working Party on Amniocentesis: An assessment of the hazards of amniocentesis: Report to the M.R.C. Br J Obstet Gynaecol 85 (Suppl):2, 1978

Young BK, Katz M, Klein SA, Silverman F: Fetal blood and tissue pH with moderate bradycardia. Am J Obstet Gynecol 135:45, 1979

Zalar RW, Quillivan EJ: The influence of scalp sampling on the cesarean section rate for fetal distress. Am J Obstet Gynecol 135:239, 1979

15
Physiology of Labor

CAUSE OF LABOR

It is believed that the majority of our permanently institutionalized persons are those who are mentally or physically disabled as the consequence of an untimely birth. To suffer the agony of lifelong mental and physical impairment is surely the greatest tragedy that can beset a person, his or her family, society, and even the economies of the world. There can be no graver or more profound insult to the quality of life. Indeed, we suggest that the disabilities that attend and are the sequelae of an untimely birth constitute the major health problem of the world today—aside from those which will accompany unbridled population growth. Surely, it follows that the problems of heart disease, cancer, and stroke of the aged pale in comparison with those that are the consequence of birth-related disorders when considering factors that affect the quality of life.

An untimely birth may portend grave and horrendous impositions on the most innocent and vulnerable of our society, the newborn, and the sequelae of the complications of an untimely birth may produce lifelong disabilities. Guarantee of quality of life in newborns, who should expect to enjoy 70 to 80 years of good health, must be a major goal of scientists, physicians, and economists who are concerned with the health care needs of all persons.

The factor or factors that lead to the onset of labor in women are not defined, however. At present, our understanding of the biomolecular events involved in the initiation of parturition in the human is incomplete; nevertheless, several hypotheses can be formulated to explain the nature of the underlying events that lead to the onset of labor. Indeed, there are elements of plausibility in each hypothesis; yet, each also seems to be deficient to some extent. Our inability to identify conclusively the more relevant or true set of events that culminate in parturition only emphasizes the need for further indepth and critical investigative endeavors. Nonetheless, several attractive theories concerned with the mechanisms involved in the onset of parturition in the human are, to varying degrees, still viable.

OXYTOCIN THEORY

The long-established use of oxytocin to induce labor in women at or near term has led to the general suspicion, if not belief, that there is a physiologic role for oxytocin in the initiation of parturition and that oxytocin is released by the neurohypophysis of pregnant women during labor. From the findings of a carefully conducted study of the oxytocin levels in maternal, fetal, and newborn plasma, however, Chard (1973) concluded that the physiologic significance of oxytocin release during labor is poorly defined. He argued that the pattern of release of oxytocin from the pituitary of pregnant women during labor and delivery suggests that the only role for this compound, if any, in the initiation of spontaneous labor, is permissive. In fact, the most specific role for oxytocin may be exerted during the expulsive phase of labor and thence postpartum to ensure contraction and full retraction of the uterus and, thereby, reduced blood loss once the fetus and placenta are delivered (and therein loss of capacity for prostaglandin formation, that is, in the fetal membranes).

There are several lines of evidence that mitigate against the likelihood of an active or essential role for oxytocin of maternal or fetal origin in the spontaneous onset of labor. These can be summarized as follows:

1. The occurrence of pregnancy in women with diabetes insipidus has been reported on many occasions; the consensus view is that diabetes insipidus in women is not associated with prolonged gestation.
2. Hypophysectomy of a variety of pregnant animals does not interfere with the spontaneous onset of labor at term on time.
3. Leake (1983) and Chard (1983), by use of highly specific antibodies against oxytocin, could find no increase in oxytocin levels in blood of pregnant women before or during labor until the second stage, namely, the expulsive phase. This also is true of all animal species studied to date.
4. The levels of oxytocin in urine of women in labor

are not increased even though it is known that when oxytocin is infused intravenously at rates as low as 1 mU per minute, an increase in urinary oxytocin levels is found.

5. High levels of oxytocin are found in the umbilical cord blood of newborns, but there is no evidence that the levels rise before the onset of labor.
6. Oxytocin does not cross the placenta.
7. Oxytocin levels remain elevated in blood of neonates for several days; thus, the stimulus for increased fetal secretion of oxytocin may be independent of its intrauterine environment.
8. Oxytocin treatment does not cause the development of gap junctions between myometrial cells (p. 305).

For a review of the role(s) of oxytocin in parturition, see Chard (1983) and Leake (1983).

The only evidence in support of a physiologic role of oxytocin in the spontaneous onset of labor is circumstantial and subject to a variety of alternate interpretations. The oxytocic properties of oxytocin as a pharmacologic agent in late pregnancy are well known. Oxytocin receptor concentrations in myometrial tissue of some animal species are increased near term and during labor, and oxytocin levels in amnionic fluid are increased during labor (for review, see Soloff, 1983).

All of these responses, however, may point to the importance of oxytocin in the final stages of labor (including expulsion of the placenta), in the maintenance of uterine contraction after delivery (to reduce blood loss), and the hypersecretion of oxytocin during infant suckling of the maternal breast may act to effect milk letdown in lactating women. Thus, we do not dismiss the importance of oxytocin in reproductive processes; rather, we suggest that the physiologic role for oxytocin is related to processes independent of the initiation of labor.

PROGESTERONE WITHDRAWAL THEORY

For many years, theories have been proposed that involve progesterone withdrawal as an important endocrine event in the initiation of the biomolecular processes of human labor. This theory evolved initially from observations made years ago on pregnant rabbits. In rabbits, withdrawal of progesterone is, indeed, followed promptly by evacuation of the contents of the pregnant uteri. Conversely, the administration of progesterone to pregnant rabbits will inhibit uterine evacuation long beyond the normal time for delivery. Moreover, in the animal species in which the molecular events of parturition are most clearly elucidated, viz., the sheep, the initiation of progesterone withdrawal is clearly an important event that heralds the spontaneous onset of labor in this species. From the results of most studies on women, however, considerable evidence has been pro-

vided that progesterone levels, at least in maternal blood, do not decrease before labor commences. *Nonetheless, in all likelihood, for reasons to be presented, progesterone does serve an important role, albeit indirect, in the control of the length of gestation, and, in turn, the timely onset of labor.*

ORGAN COMMUNICATION SYSTEM HYPOTHESIS

Teleologically, it is satisfying, even fascinating and tantalizing, to believe that the fetus provides a signal to his or her mother to commence labor after key maturational events in vital fetal tissues and organs are initiated or completed. If this were true, it follows that these maturational events might culminate in the biogenesis of a fetal signal that is communicated from the fetus to its mother by way of an Organ Communication System. If this were the case, it is important to define the components of such an Organ Communication System and the mechanism(s) whereby a fetal signal may arise, may be transmitted to, and thence received by mother, as well as to define the components of the response(s) to such a putative signal.

Within the context of an Organ Communication System for the transmittal of biochemical signals to initiate labor, it is important to consider the following:

Considerable evidence has been presented in favor of the proposition, which now is generally accepted, that prostaglandins serve a key role in the initiation of partu-

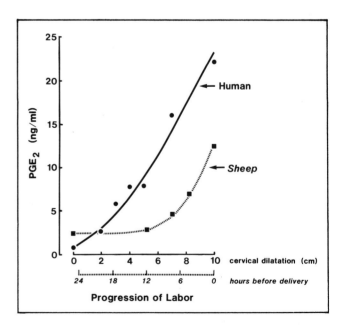

Figure 15-1. Concentration of PGE$_2$ in amnionic fluid of the human and sheep during labor, as a function of centimeters cervical dilatation or hours before delivery in women and sheep, respectively. (*Data from Mitchell, 1976. Illustration courtesy of Dr. L. Casey.*)

rition in mammalian species and similar processes are found even in other species. It has been demonstrated that prostaglandins (PGE_2 and $PGF_{2\alpha}$) will evoke myometrial contractions in women at any stage of gestation whether these substances are administered by instillation into the amnionic fluid, by intravenous infusion, or by extraovular injection (Karim, 1972). Moreover, Mitchell (1976) demonstrated that the levels of PGE_2 in amnionic fluid of the sheep and the human increase in a similar manner during labor (Fig. 15-1). In fact, Hertelendy has demonstrated that prostaglandins are physiologically important in oviposition, that is, laying of hard-shelled eggs by birds (for review, see Hertelendy, 1983).

The mechanism(s) by which the rate of formation of prostaglandins is regulated prior to the initiation of myometrial contractions is not understood. It is believed, however, that the enzymes that are important in the biosynthesis of, as well as the degradation of, prostaglandins are influenced by the steroid hormone milieu. Thus, we must consider the role of the fetus as a participant in the development of the hormonal milieu of pregnancy (Chapter 7) and in an Organ Communication System that could lead to increased prostanoid formation and thence the initiation and maintenance of labor.

ROLE OF THE FETUS IN INITIATION OF PARTURITION

Speigelberg, in 1882 (cited by Thorburn, 1983), put forward the proposition that the origin of the signal for the initiation of parturition in the human was the fetus. Indeed, the bovine fetus, the ovine fetus, and the human fetus each appear to participate in the timely onset of labor (for review, see Casey and co-workers, 1983; and Thorburn, 1983). Anomalies of the brain of the fetal calf, fetal lamb, and human fetus interfere with the timing of the onset of labor. When there is congenital absence of the pituitary in the bovine fetus, the gestation period is prolonged by several weeks. Adrenal hypoplasia in the bovine fetus also causes prolonged gestation. If, early in pregnancy, the ewe eats the foliage of a plant, *Veratrum californicum,* which grows wild in the northwestern United States, the fetal sheep develops a characteristic cyclopean deformity that is associated with abnormal vascularization of the pituitary from the hypothalamus. In a ewe with such a fetus, there is fetal adrenal hypoplasia and there is prolonged gestation. Indeed, the pregnancy goes far beyond term, and the sheep fetus continues to persist and ultimately dies in utero (for review, see Thorburn, 1983).

Fetal Cortisol and the Initiation of Labor. Among nonhuman species, the sheep is the experimental animal in which the biomolecular events of parturition have been elucidated most thoroughly. Even though the exact sequence of events and the nature of the signal(s) that leads to the onset of parturition in the ewe appear to dif-

fer from those in women, many of the fundamental biochemical events appear to be similar in most, if not all, species. In sheep, the origin of the signal for the initiation of parturition clearly seems to emanate from the fetus; in fact, for the timely, normal onset of labor, a functional fetal hypothalamus, pituitary gland, and adrenal gland, as well as a functional placenta, are required (Liggins and co-workers, 1973 and Liggins, 1973). The earliest well-defined event that may be regarded as a trigger for parturition in the sheep is a sharp increase in the rate of production of cortisol by the fetal adrenal. Fetal cortisol acts on the placenta in a manner that leads to reduced progesterone formation and possibly augmented estrogen secretion (Fig. 15-2), thereafter, and perhaps thereby, leading to increased production of prostaglandins (for review, see Flint, 1983). Moreover, there is much evidence in favor of the proposition that the accelerated production of prostaglandins, in the fetal membranes or uterine decidua vera, or both, is of signal importance in the initiation and maintenance of labor. We shall return to this issue.

The necessity of the functional integrity of fetal brain, pituitary, and adrenal in the timely onset of labor is demonstrated by several observations as follows: Hypophysectomy, transection of the pituitary stalk, or adrenalectomy in the fetal sheep leads to prolongation of pregnancy. Conversely, infusion of ACTH or a glucocorticosteroid into the sheep fetus causes premature parturition. From an evaluation of plasma ACTH and cortisol levels in the fetal sheep, it can be concluded that the rate of secretion of these hormones increases prior to the onset of parturition (Liggins and associates, 1973).

As stated, the increased secretion of cortisol in the sheep fetus is associated with an alteration in biosynthetic processes in the placenta; ultimately, these lead to an increased rate of placental estrogen production. It has been proposed that cortisol acts on the placenta to increase the activities of steroid 17α-hydroxylase and steroid 17,20-lyase (Fig. 15-3). Increased activities of these enzymes can lead to increased conversion of progesterone to 17α-hydroxyprogesterone and thence to androstenedione, a C_{19}-steroid that can serve as substrate for estrogen biosynthesis in placenta. In addition, it has been demonstrated that cortisol, in sheep placenta, acts to increase aromatization (estrogen formation) as well. Thus, the coordinated actions of cortisol in sheep placenta cause a precipitous decrease in progesterone secretion and thence a sharp rise in estrogen secretion (Figs. 15-2, 15-3) (for review, see Flint, 1983).

In 1898, Rea observed an association between anencephaly in the human fetus and prolonged gestation. In 1933, Malpas extended these observations on an association between anencephaly in the human fetus and prolonged gestation and concluded that this seemed to be attributable to anomalous brain–pituitary–adrenal function. These findings are suggestive that in the human, as in sheep, the fetal adrenal may serve an important role in the timely onset of labor. The adrenal glands of the anencephalic fetus are very small compared with those

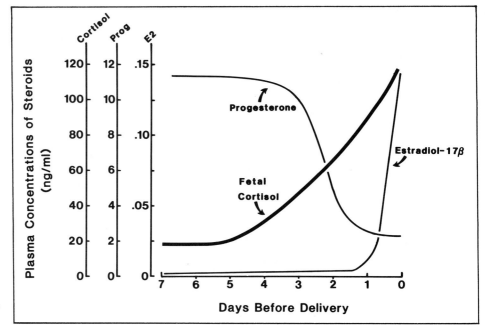

Figure 15-2. Endocrine events in the sheep that herald the onset of parturition. As the levels of fetal plasma cortisol rise, the levels of maternal plasma progesterone decline. Thereafter, there is an increase in estrogen production by the placenta. (*Illustration courtesy of Dr. L. Casey.*)

of normal fetuses (Chapter 7). Indeed, the adrenals of the anencephalic fetus at term may weigh only 5 to 10 percent of those of a normal fetus. The smallness of the gland is due largely to failure of development of the fetal zone—the structure that accounts for most of the mass of the human fetal adrenal (Chapter 7).

There is another corollary between the biomolecular events of parturition in the human and those in the sheep model. In the human pregnancy, in which there is a fetus with adrenal hypoplasia, there also may be prolonged gestation (for review, see Anderson and Turnbull, 1973). This condition is reminiscent of that in sheep in which the fetal adrenal has been rendered inactive either by hypophysectomy or adrenalectomy and in which there also is prolonged gestation.

On the other hand, at this point in the development

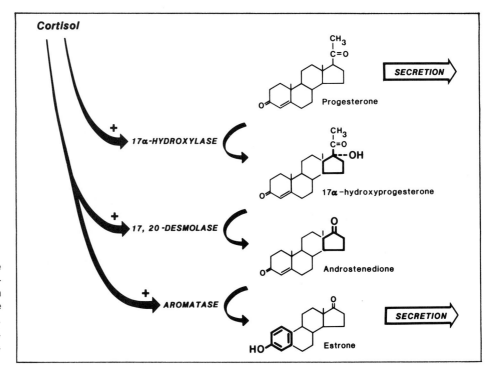

Figure 15-3. Regulation, by the action of fetal cortisol, of placental progesterone and estrogen biosynthesis just prior to the onset of parturition in the sheep. (*Data summarized by Flint, 1983. Illustration courtesy of Dr. L. Casey.*)

of analogies between the sheep and human models of parturition initiation, there is a divergence of considerable importance.

There is no clear-cut increase in cortisol concentration in fetal blood before the onset of parturition in the human—and no evidence of a decline in the concentration of progesterone, at least in maternal plasma, before or during labor.

Thus, the "cortisol hypothesis" with respect to the initiation of labor in the human does not appear to be as cogent as it is in the sheep model. In support of this interpretation, it is known that infusion of glucocorticosteroids or ACTH into the human fetus or amnionic fluid does not evoke premature parturition, as it does in the sheep (Katz and associates, 1978). Mati and colleagues (1973), however, reported the induction of labor in women beyond term after the intraamnionic injection of a large dose of betamethasone. On the other hand, in instances in which augmented fetal cortisol production is precluded, for example, in various forms of congenital adrenal hyperplasia, labor commences at term on time. Therefore, the hypothesis that fetal cortisol is important in the initiation of parturition does not appear to be verified in the human, as it is in the sheep. Nonetheless, considering the more common occurrence of prolonged gestation in women pregnant with an anencephalic fetus or with a fetus with adrenal hypoplasia than in women pregnant with a normal fetus, we suggest that a role for the fetal adrenal in the timely onset of parturition in women seems likely. If this is true, it would seem to follow that there must be a fundamental role for estrogen, derived from fetal adrenal precursors (Chapter 7), in the timely onset of labor in the human.

The mechanism(s) that is regulatory in the rate of formation and inactivation of prostaglandins, or related compounds, before parturition is not fully understood; yet, it would appear that major endocrine changes, such as increased cortisol secretion by the adrenals of the lamb fetus, lead to decreased placental secretion of progesterone and increased production of estrogen and, in turn, to an increase in prostaglandin levels in intrauterine tissues and uterine venous blood. Of these hormones, estrogen appears to be most closely related to the increased synthesis and release of prostaglandins within the uterus. Twenty-four hours after estrogen (stilbestrol, 20 mg in oil) is administered to the pregnant ewe, there is a marked increase in the concentration of prostaglandins in uterine venous blood (Liggins and colleagues, 1973). In women, estradiol-17β treatment also appears to facilitate cervical softening and effacement and, thereby, responsiveness to oxytocin (Pinto and co-workers, 1967).

Although progesterone withdrawal prior to the onset of labor is not observed in the monkey or in women, it still is possible that some form of progesterone deprivation is important in the initiation of labor in these two species. In the case of women, there may be an alternate means for progesterone deprivation. For example, Tul-

chinsky and Giannopoulos (1983) found lower levels of progesterone receptors in myometrium of pregnant women at term than in myometrium of nonpregnant women.

Nonetheless, there is a considerable body of evidence in support of the proposition that prostanoids serve a critical role during human pregnancy and in the final events that lead to the initiation of parturition. We emphasize again that PGE_2 and $PGF_{2\alpha}$ cause uterine contractions at any stage of pregnancy and also effect cervical softening and effacement (p. 306). In these respects, PGE_2 is five to ten times more potent than $PGF_{2\alpha}$. Ingestion of inhibitors of prostaglandin synthase activity by pregnant women leads to prolongation of gestation and lengthens the time interval between induction and abortion in pregnancies that are terminated by instillation of hypertonic saline. Inhibitors of prostaglandin synthase (specifically, inhibition of arachidonic acid cyclooxygenase activity) also are effective in suppressing preterm labor. There are striking increases in prostaglandin levels in amnionic fluid (Fig. 15-1) and maternal plasma during labor. These events are reminiscent of those that occur at the end of the ovulatory cycle in women when progesterone levels are falling. For all of these reasons, prostaglandins are considered to be important agents in the initiation of spontaneous labor and delivery in women.

A role for lipids in the initiation of parturition was suggested by the findings of Luukkainen and Csapo (1963), who demonstrated that the intravenous infusion of a lipid emulsion into pregnant rabbits caused an increase in the responsiveness of the myometrium to oxytocin. The active component of these emulsions was shown to be phosphatidylcholine that was enriched with linoleic acid, a precursor of arachidonic acid—the obligate precursor of PGE_2 and $PGF_{2\alpha}$. Nathanielsz and associates (1973) found that the intraaortic infusion of arachidonic acid into pregnant rabbits will induce labor, and Hertelendy (1972) found that the intrauterine injection of arachidonic acid will induce premature oviposition in quail.

In 1964, van Dorp and colleagues and Bergstrom and co-workers (1974) demonstrated that arachidonic acid is the obligate precursor for the biosynthesis of prostaglandins of the 2-series. Furthermore, Lands and Samuelsson (1968) and Vonkeman and van Dorp (1968) demonstrated that it is free arachidonic acid that is utilized for prostaglandin formation. Therefore, several pertinent questions can be asked.

By what mechanisms are arachidonic acid release and prostaglandin formation regulated during parturition? What is the tissue site of origin of the prostaglandins found in amnionic fluid? What is the tissue site of origin of prostaglandins that induce uterine contractions? It is evident that knowledge of the mechanism(s) that serves to regulate the rate of synthesis of prostaglandins is important for an understanding of the nature of the signal that initiates labor. For these reasons, detailed studies of the control of prostaglandin synthesis during labor have been conducted by a number of investigators around the world.

It seems reasonable to assume that in some way the fetus signals its mother by way of an Organ Communication System in a manner that will promote, ultimately, accelerated formation of prostaglandins. In consideration of the components of such a putative Organ Communication System, recall that there are a number of unique anatomical features of human pregnancy. During all of pregnancy, the human fetus exists in the aqueous environment of the amnionic fluid that is contained within the fetal membranes, i.e., the avascular amnion and the avascular chorion laeve.

Anatomically, the amnion is poised ideally to receive a fetal signal and to transmit a response to such a signal. This innermost, avascular fetal membrane is bathed by the amnionic fluid on one side and on the other side is contiguous with the chorion laeve, also a very thin membrane of fetal origin, which, in turn, is contiguous with the maternal decidua vera (parietalis). Direct communication between the fetus and avascular amnion is established by way of the amnionic fluid, which is comprised principally of fetal excretions or secretions from kidney (fetal urine), lung, and skin. At term, the fetal membranes occupy a large (~ 0.6 m^2) surface area in the uterine cavity. Thus, the fetus is in communication with its mother by way of the large surface area that is provided by the fetal membranes and thence maternal decidua, possibly by way of chorion laeve. Moreover, it would seem to be advantageous, teleologically, for prostaglandin formation to be initiated at a site removed from the placental implantation site because PGE$_2$ and PGF$_{2\alpha}$ are potent vasoconstrictive agents and thereby could lead to abruption of the placenta.

It has been known for many years that rupture, stripping, or infection of the fetal membranes, as well as instillation into the amnionic fluid of hypertonic solutions of NaCl, glucose, or urea, leads to the premature onset of labor. These observations, and others, have led some investigators to a consideration of the biochemical events in fetal membranes that may mediate the action of a signal that is transmitted from a mature fetus to mother and one that leads to increased prostaglandin synthesis and, thence, to the uterine contractions that are characteristic of labor.

As it is believed that the fetal membranes are of signal importance in the Organ Communication System that exists between the fetus and mother, it is imperative to evaluate the possible role of these tissues in the biochemical events that lead to prostaglandin formation.

These considerations led to an evaluation of the fetus–amnionic fluid–fetal membranes–decidua complex as a metabolically active unit that may, in fact, transmit and respond to signals that lead to the onset of labor in normal human pregnancy.

Prostaglandin biosynthesis in amnion, chorion laeve, and uterine decidua vera has been demonstrated by a number of techniques. (The general model of a glycero-

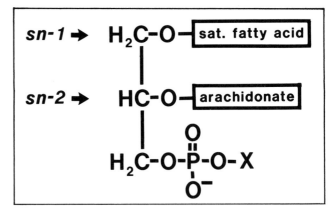

Figure 15-4. Schematic model (general) for a glycerophospholipid. The X is indicative of a specific substitution (e.g., choline, phosphatidylcholine; inositol, phosphatidylinositol; and, ethanolamine, phosphatidylethanolamine). Generally, there is a saturated fatty acid in the *sn*-1 position, for example, palmitate, and an unsaturated fatty acid in the *sn*-2 position. Almost always, the polyunsaturated, essential fatty acid, arachidonic acid, is esterified in the *sn*-2 position of glycerolipids. (*Illustration courtesy of Dr. L. Casey.*)

phospholipid, in which most tissue arachidonate is esterified, is presented in Figure 15-4 and the biosynthetic pathway of prostaglandin formation is given in Figure 15-5.) The biosynthesis and metabolism of prostaglandins in these tissues, however, are unique. By far, the major prostaglandin that is produced in amnion is PGE$_2$. Moreover, there is little or no 15-hydroxyprostaglandin dehydrogenase (PGDH) activity in amnion tissue; this is the enzyme that catalyzes the first and rate-limiting step in prostaglandin inactivation. Thus, PGE$_2$ can be formed in amnion in large quantities, but PGE$_2$ is not metabolized further in that tissue. In chorion, PGE$_2$ is also the major prostaglandin produced; but, in this tissue, PGDH activity is present. On the other hand, both PGE$_2$ and PGF$_{2\alpha}$ are biosynthesized, in large quantities, in uterine decidua vera tissue and PGDH activity is present in cytosolic fractions prepared from homogenates of this tissue. Again, all of these findings are suggestive of a unique role of the fetal membranes in the provision of arachidonic acid and in prostaglandin biosynthesis during labor (Fig. 15-6) (for review, see Casey and associates, 1983).

In addition, there are a number of lines of evidence to support the proposition that metabolic events that take place in amnion and chorion laeve are unique in the generation of prostaglandins; indeed, several considerations seem to be pertinent to the crucial role of the fetal membranes in human parturition: (i) the specific activity of prostaglandin synthase in amnion is greater than that in chorion laeve, decidua vera, myometrium, or placenta; (ii) the glycerophospholipids of amnion and chorion laeve are enriched with arachidonic acid, the obligate precursor of prostaglandins of the 2-series; (iii) the levels of free arachidonic acid, as well as those of PGE$_2$ and

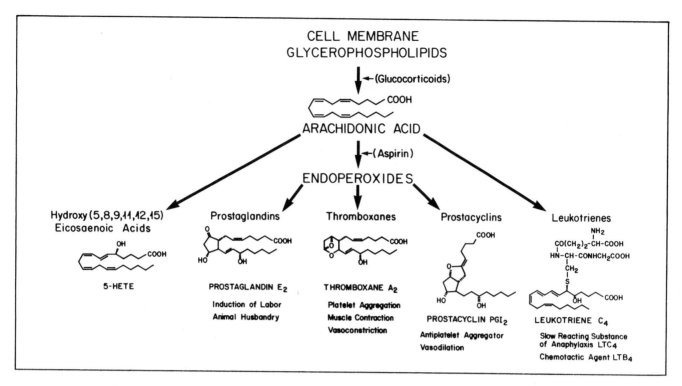

Figure 15-5. Pathways to prostanoid biosynthesis from the obligate precursor, arachidonic acid. A variety of actions ascribed to the various prostanoids are given. Glucocorticosteroids are believed to inhibit prostanoid formation by inhibiting the release of arachidonic acid from esterified stores; other agents, such as aspirin and indomethacin, act to inhibit arachidonate cyclooxygenase. (*Courtesy of Dr. J. Bleasdale.*)

$PGF_{2\alpha}$, in amnionic fluid increase strikingly during labor and as labor progresses; (iv) during early labor, there is a specific decrease in the arachidonic acid content of diacyl phosphatidylethanolamine and phosphatidylinositol of amnion and chorion laeve; (v) phospholipase A_2, with substrate specificity for phosphatidylethanolamines with arachidonic acid in the *sn*-2 position (Fig. 15-4) is present in fetal membranes (this enzyme catalyzes the release of arachidonic acid from phosphatidylethanolamine); (vi) phosphatidylinositol-specific phospholipase C activity is present in human amnion and chorion laeve (this enzyme catalyzes the hydrolysis of phosphatidylinositol to diacylglycerols); (vii) in turn, there is a diacylglycerol lipase in amnion and chorion laeve that catalyzes the release of the fatty acid from the *sn*-1 position of diacylglycerols, and this enzyme may be relatively specific for diacylglycerols with arachidonic acid in the *sn*-2 position; (viii) in turn, there also is a monoacylglycerol lipase in amnion and chorion laeve that catalyzes the release of the fatty acid in the *sn*-2 position of monoacylglycerols (there may be relative substrate specificity of this enzyme in fetal membranes for *sn*-2 arachidonoyl monoacylglycerols)—thus, in this coordinated manner, by three enzymatic reactions, arachidonic acid is released from phosphatidylinositol in the fetal membranes; (ix) the specific activities of phospholipases A_2 and C in human amnion increase strikingly late in gestation; (x)

diacylglycerols, the products of the reaction catalyzed by phosphatidylinositol-specific phospholipase C, accumulate in amnion during early labor; and, (xi) the activity of NAD^+-dependent 15-hydroxyprostaglandin dehydrogenase, the enzyme that catalyzes the first reaction in the inactivation of prostaglandins, is not detectable in human amnion tissue. (These studies were conducted in the laboratories of Dr. John M. Johnston; for reviews of the regulation of prostaglandin synthesis and metabolism in fetal membranes, see MacDonald and associates, 1978; Casey and co-workers, 1983; Bleasdale and colleagues, 1983; and Casey and MacDonald, 1984.)

It is believed, therefore, that by way of an Organ Communication System, the activities of these enzymes in amnion may be regulated in a manner such that the putative signal that emanates from the fetus acts to accelerate the rate of arachidonic acid release and thence to increase prostaglandin biosynthesis in the fetal membranes. The mechanisms of regulation of phospholipase A_2, phosphatidylinositol-specific phospholipase C, diacylglycerol lipase, and monoacylglycerol lipase activities in amnion and chorion have been studied in detail (Fig. 15-7). In addition to the substrate specificity of phospholipase A_2 of amnion for phosphatidylethanolamine that contains arachidonic acid in the *sn*-2 position, the activity of this enzyme in vitro is highly dependent on the concentration of Ca^{2+} (Fig. 15-7, reaction 1). The activity

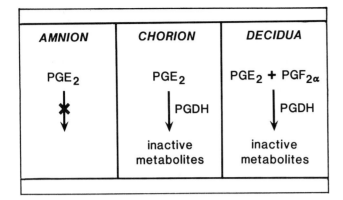

AMNION	CHORION	DECIDUA
PGE_2	PGE_2	$PGE_2 + PGF_{2\alpha}$
✗	↓ PGDH	↓ PGDH
	inactive metabolites	inactive metabolites

Figure 15-6. Comparison of prostaglandin biosynthesis and metabolism in amnion, chorion laeve, and decidua. The greatest prostaglandin synthase activity is in amnion in which only PGE_2 is formed; and, in amnion, PGE_2 is not metabolized. In chorion laeve, PGE_2 is the principal prostanoid produced; yet, in chorion laeve, there is considerable NAD^+-dependent 15-hydroxyprostaglandin dehydrogenase (PGDH) activity. In decidua, PGE_2 and $PGF_{2\alpha}$ are formed; and, PGDH is active in decidua. (*Illustration courtesy of Dr. L. Casey.*)

of phosphatidylinositol-specific phospholipase C is also Ca^{2+} dependent (Fig. 15-7, reaction 2). Diacylglycerol lipase catalyzes the relase of the *sn* −1 fatty acid of diacylglycerols. In this latter sequence of reactions, arachidonic acid is released, ultimately, from *sn*-2 arachidonoylglycerol in a reaction catalyzed by monoacylglycerol lipase (Fig. 15-7, reaction 4). On the other hand, the activity of diacylglycerol kinase, an enzyme that catalyzes the conversion of diacylglycerol to the glycerophospholipid precursor, phosphatidic acid, and an enzyme that is present in amnion, chorion, and decidua

vera tissue, is inhibited by Ca^{2+} (Fig. 15-7, reaction 5). The action of this enzyme serves to inhibit the release of arachidonic acid from diacylglycerols by recycling the diacylglycerols back to phospholipids (Fig. 15-7, reaction 5). Thus, Ca^{2+} may serve a role of signal importance in the regulation of arachidonic acid release and thence prostaglandin production in amnion and possibly chorion laeve and decidua vera. It is envisioned that an increase in the intracellular concentration of Ca^{2+} could lead to an increase in the rate of release of arachidonic acid from phosphatidylethanolamine by way of the reaction catalyzed by phospholipase A_2 as well as from phosphatidylinositol in a series of reactions that are catalyzed by phosphatidylinositol-specific phospholipase C, diacylglycerol lipase, and monoacylglycerol lipase. In addition, an increase in the intracellular concentration of Ca^{2+} could act to inhibit the utilization of diacylglycerol for glycerophospholipid biosynthesis by way of inhibition of the activity of diacylglycerol kinase, and, thereby, the release of arachidonic acid would be favored. Additional evidence has been obtained that is supportive of a role for Ca^{2+} in the regulation of PGE_2 synthesis in amnion. In enzymatically dispersed human amnion cells, prostaglandin production was decreased in the absence of calcium or in the presence of calcium channel blockers (Olson and co-workers, 1983), but prostaglandin production was increased in the presence of calcium or a calcium ionophore (for a review of the role of Ca^{2+} in the regulation of arachidonic acid metabolism in membranes and decidua, see Bleasdale and associates, 1983).

For the in vitro study of the regulation of PGE_2 synthesis by amnion, another model system that consists of human amnion cells maintained in primary monolayer culture has been employed (Okita and co-workers, 1983). In these cells in culture, the morphologic and biochemi-

Figure 15-7. Metabolism and enzymatic release of arachidonic acid in human amnion. A Ca^{2+} cycle is proposed, according to Dr. J.M. Johnston, whereby Ca_2^+, in increased concentrations, favors the release of arachidonate and prevents the recycling of arachidonate back into glycerophospholipids. (*For review, see Bleasdale and associates, 1983.*) (*Illustration courtesy Dr. L. Casey.*)

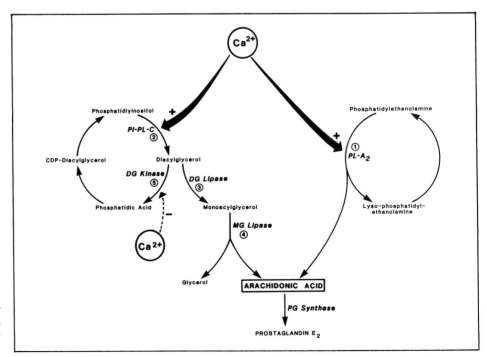

cal characteristics of amnion tissue are maintained. Specifically, PGE_2 is almost the exclusive prostanoid produced by these cells; PGE_2 is not metabolized by these cells; and phospholipase A_2, phosphatidylinositol-specific phospholipase C, diacylglycerol lipase, and monoacylglycerol lipase activities are present in these cells and the characteristics of these enzymes in these cells are similar to those of the same activities in amnion tissue. The efficacy of a host of compounds, which are known to be present in amniotic fluid or else are known to cause prostaglandin production in other tissues, on PGE_2 production by these human amnion cells in culture has been evaluated; none of the agents tested were effective in stimulating PGE_2 production. Thus, the original proposition was readdressed, viz., that an Organ Communication System is operative in the transmission of a signal from fetus to mother. With this in mind, the effect of human fetal urine, which was collected within 5 minutes of birth, on PGE_2 synthesis by amnion cells was evaluated (Casey and associates, 1983). Fetal urine stimulates PGE_2 production by amnion cells in a tissue-specific, concentration- and time-dependent manner. The PGE_2-synthesis stimulatory substance in fetal urine is proteinaceous, or else is closely associated with a protein, and is heat-stable. Evidence has also been obtained that the PGE_2-synthesis stimulatory substance is synthesized in fetal kidney and is not simply excreted by that organ (Casey and associates, 1983). Thus, fetal kidney and fetal urine appear to be important components in the Organ Communication System that is operative in the initiation and maintenance of labor in women.

With respect to the nature of the PGE_2-synthesis stimulatory substance in fetal urine, there are several observations that seemingly are important in defining the nature of the putative fetal signal in the initiation of human labor. First, there is no clear-cut, dramatic increase in the level of PGE_2-synthesis stimulatory activity in fetal urine or amnionic fluid as term is approached. Equally important, the PGE_2-synthesis stimulatory substance acts in a manner that is independent of the flux of extracellular Ca^{2+}; yet, the activity of PGE_2-synthesis stimulatory substance is facilitated if Ca^{2+} flux is effected by another agent, for example, a calcium ionophore. Therefore, during most of pregnancy, the fetal–renal PGE_2-synthesis stimulatory substance may act on amnion to effect PGE_2 synthesis in a manner that is principally involved in solute and H_2O transport from amnionic fluid and thus in the maintenance of amnionic fluid volume homeostasis. At term, however, the coordinated action of the PGE_2-synthesis stimulatory substance together with a calcium ionophore-like agent of fetal origin would lead to the striking increase in prostaglandin formation that is characteristic of labor.

Thus, it can be envisioned that increased synthesis of PGE_2 in amnion is the key event in the onset of labor. It can also be envisioned that the increase in prostaglandin synthesis in amnion occurs in response to a signal(s) that emanates from the fetus (by way of fetal urine and thence amnionic fluid). This fetal signal may act in amnion to cause an increase in the rate of release of arachi-

donic acid from glycerophospholipids or else to cause an increase in the activity of prostaglandin synthase (Strickland and co-workers, 1982) or both. In this manner, the human fetus may, indeed, be in control of its own destiny with respect to a timely birth.

Nonetheless, despite the data available, there are still many important gaps in our understanding of the involvement of prostaglandins in human parturition. In particular, the factors that regulate prostaglandin biosynthesis and release are not understood completely, and the mode of action of prostaglandins is not well defined.

It is anticipated, however, that in the near future rapid progress will be made in an elucidation of the molecular events that regulate parturition. Novy (1983) has made considerable progress in defining the sequence of events that are involved in the initiation of parturition in the rhesus monkey. Seron-Ferre and Jaffe (1981) have conducted elegant and detailed studies to define the regulation of fetal adrenal function in the rhesus.

In addition, exciting studies are being conducted to define the molecular events that are involved in myometrial contractions. Garfield (1983) is investigating, in detail, the regulation of development of gap junctions in myometrium of pregnant women. Krall and Korenman (1977) are conducting in-depth studies to define the regulation of adenylate cyclase activity and cyclic AMP levels in myometrial tissue. Indeed, progress is being made even in the prevention of preterm labor; Creasy (1980) has developed a scheme for the evaluation of factors likely to lead to preterm labor in women and has developed a very successful method for management of women at high risk for preterm labor (Creasy, 1983).

PHYSIOLOGY OF UTERINE CONTRACTIONS

Convincing evidence, which we now consider, has accrued that is indicative that the final event in initiating a myometrial contraction is the release of calcium from its repository form in the sarcoplasmic reticulum. The consequence of this event is to elevate the concentration of intracellular free calcium, which is believed to be of signal importance in the biomolecular events that give rise to uterine contractions; on the other hand, the ATP–energy-dependent translocation of calcium to a stored form in the sarcoplasmic reticulum is associated with uterine relaxation.

THE UTERINE ELEMENTS

The body of the uterus and the cervix, although parts of the same organ, are required to respond to the signal(s) that initiates parturition in quite different ways. During implantation of the blastocyst and most of pregnancy, it is essential that the myometrium be dilatable and remain quiescent. On the other hand, the cervix must remain rigid and unyielding. Coincident with the events that are involved in the initiation of parturition, on the other hand, the cervix must soften, yield, and dilate. The

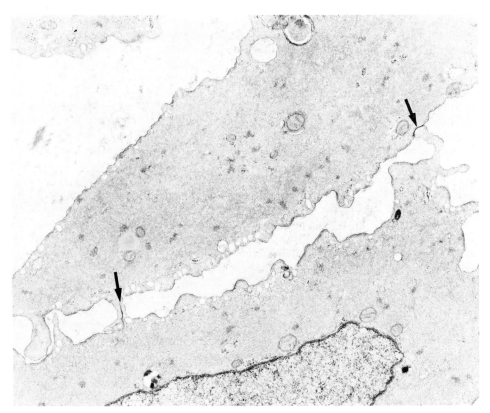

Figure 15-8. Electron photomicrograph of gap junctions in human myometrial cells. Tissue obtained after labor commenced. (*Courtesy of Dr. R. Garfield.*)

fundus must be transformed from the relaxed, quiescent organ characteristic of most of pregnancy to one of thunderous contractions of sufficient force and efficiency to drive the fetus through the yielding cervix and on through the birth canal. Failure of a timely interaction between the functions of cervix and fundus portends an unfavorable pregnancy outcome. Nevertheless, despite the apparent reversal of roles between cervix and fundus from before to during labor, there is evidence that both processes are regulated by common agents.

Myometrium

In the fundus, the myometrial smooth muscle cells are embedded in an extracellular matrix that is comprised principally of collagen fibers. This matrix is believed to facilitate the transmission of forces generated by the contraction of myometrial cells and also may serve to integrate the contractile forces of these cells.

Gap Junctions of Myometrium. Gap junctions are cell-to-cell contacts that are believed to be composed of symmetric portions of the plasma membranes of two apposing cells (Fig. 15-8). It is believed that communication between cells may be accomplished by way of gap junctions. The proteins within the membranes of the cells in apposition are aligned and, thereby, are believed to create pores between the cytoplasms of the two cells (cf. Garfield, 1983). Thus, a means can be established whereby a pathway is formed between coupled cells to facilitate the passage of current (electrical or ionic coupling) or metabolites (metabolite coupling) between cells. Only recently, however, has it been possible to demonstrate gap junctions in myometrial tissue (cf. Garfield, 1983). From the elegant studies of Garfield and associates, we now know that gap junctions between myometrial cells do develop during labor. In the study of a number of species, including the human, it was found that gap junctions are absent (or very nearly so) throughout pregnancy until term. At term, the frequency of gap junctions increases and these continue to increase in number and size during labor. The gap junctions begin to disappear within 24 hours of delivery. Gap junctions are present in premature labor, whether the onset of labor is spontaneous or induced.

The factor(s) that prevents the appearance of gap junctions between myometrial cells (e.g., prostacyclin) may be important in the maintenance of uterine quiescence. On the other hand, the rapid appearance of gap junctions at term may facilitate the coordinated contractions of the uterus that are characteristic of labor.

Therefore, the regulation of gap junction formation is a subject of considerable importance. Evidence has been obtained, by in vitro and in vivo studies of experimental animals, that progesterone prevents and estrogen promotes the formation of gap junctions. It is known that protein synthesis is required for the formation of gap junctions. Prostaglandins also are believed to be important in gap junction formation. Inhibition of prostaglandin synthesis inhibits gap junction formation in vitro. Some prostanoids, for example PGE_2, $PGF_{2\alpha}$, and thromboxanes and possibly endoperoxides, stimulate gap junction formation, whereas others, for example, prostacyclin, may inhibit gap junction formation. Interestingly (see p. 296), oxytocin does not act to increase gap junction formation (Garfield, 1983).

Cellular Organization of Myometrium. There are unique anatomic features of myometrial smooth muscle (and other smooth muscle) compared with skeletal muscle. Huszar (1983) and Huszar and Roberts (1982) point out that these differences come to create a peculiar advantage with respect to myometrial contractions and the successful delivery of the fetus. First, the degree of shortening in smooth muscle cells may be one order of

magnitude greater in smooth than in striated muscle cells with contraction. Second, in smooth muscle cells forces can be exerted in any direction, whereas the contraction force generated by skeletal muscle is such as to always be aligned with the axis of the muscle fibers; moreover, smooth muscle is not organized in the same manner as skeletal muscle. In myometrium, the thick and thin bundles of filaments are found in long, random bundles throughout the cells. This arrangement is such as to permit the greater shortening and force generating capacity of smooth muscle (Huszar, 1983). Other advantages include the fact that multidirectional force generation in smooth muscle permits versatility in expulsive force directionality that can come to bear irrespective of the lie or presentation of the fetus.

Molecular Regulation of Smooth Muscle Contractions. The protein of primary importance in muscle contraction is myosin (~500,000 daltons); the myosin molecule is about 1600 Å in length and is laid down in thick monofilaments (cf. Huszar, 1983).

Functionally, there is a "head" and a "tail" part of myosin. The globular-shaped head portion is (i) the site of the actin-combining site, where the interaction of myosin and actin occurs, and, thereby, force is generated, (ii) the site of ATPase—where ATP is hydrolyzed and chemical energy is converted to physical force, and (iii) the site of the low-molecular-weight (20,000) myosin light chains, the phosphorylation of which is the key reaction in contractile regulation, namely, the actin–myosin interaction in smooth muscle.

In this context, it is important to remember that calcium ion (Ca^{2+}) flux is essential to the generation of muscular contraction. Ca^{2+} is sequestered in intracellular vesicles of the sacroplasmic reticulum. In smooth muscle, the interaction of myosin and actin is regulated by enzymatic phosphorylation (or dephosphorylation) of the myosin (20,000 daltons) light chains (Stull and colleagues, 1980). Specifically, the actin–myosin interaction in myometrial cells can take place only after phosphorylation of the myosin light-chain. The phosphorylation of myosin light-chain is catalyzed by the enzyme myosin light-chain kinase—importantly, this enzyme is activated by Ca^{2+} (Fig. 15-9A). By contrast, dephosphorylation of the myosin light-chain by the action of myosin light-

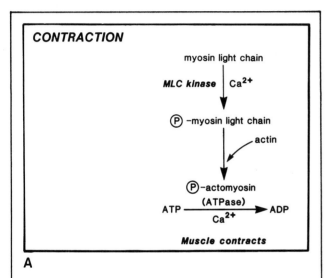

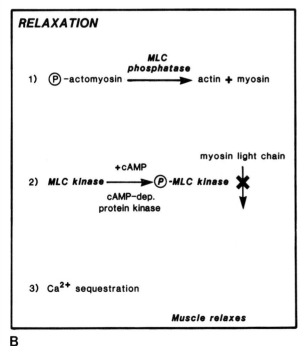

Figure 15-9. Metabolic regulation of smooth muscle contraction **A.** and relaxation **B.** Phosphorylation of myosin light chains by way of myosin light chain kinase (a reaction activated by Ca^{2+}) is essential for the association of myosin and actin to give rise to phosphorylated actomyosin, which is an enzyme that catalyzes the conversion of ATP to ADP, a reaction that gives rise to energy that can be converted to force in uterine contractions.

Relaxation is promoted if (a) phosphorylated actomyosin is dephosphorylated by the action of myosin light-chain phosphatase, (b) the action of enzyme myosin light-chain kinase is inhibited by phosphorylation of the enzyme in a reaction catalyzed by a cAMP-dependent protein kinase, and (c) by ATP-dependent sequestration of calcium in the sarcoplasmic reticulum. (*Illustration courtesy of Dr. L. Casey.*)

chain phosphatase gives rise to muscle relaxation (Fig. 15-9B). Actin and dephosphorylated myosin do not interact. In this context, another phosphorylation mechanism becomes important; namely, phosphorylation of the enzyme myosin light-chain kinase causes inactivation of this enzyme and thereby the phosphorylation of myosin light-chains is inhibited (Fig. 15-9B). Importantly, the phosphorylation of myosin light-chain kinase (the enzyme) is mediated by way of a cyclic AMP (cAMP)–dependent protein kinase. The decrease in activity, upon phosphorylation of the enzyme, is attributable to a decrease in the affinity of the phosphorylated enzyme for calmodulin, a calcium-dependent regulatory protein, by way of which the action of calcium commonly is modulated. The association of calmodulin with myosin light-chain kinase is mandatory for the expression of the activity of this enzyme.

Therefore, it can be envisioned that the regulation of myometrial contractions at the cellular level is attributable to the action of myosin light-chain kinase activity, which is modulated in large measure by calcium, the affinity of the calcium–calmodulin complex for the enzyme, and cAMP-dependent phosphorylation of the enzyme by a protein kinase. On balance, the dephosphorylation of myosin light-chain kinase by way of myosin light-chain kinase phosphatase also must be taken into consideration (Fig. 15-9B). The relationships between these processes are illustrated in Figures 15-9A,B. Thus, activation of contraction is accomplished by way of the interaction of phosphorylated myosin and actin to give phosphorylated actomyosin.

Cervix

In the cervix, there are three principal structural components—smooth muscle, collagen, and connective tissue, namely, the ground substance. In the ground substance, important constituents of cervix, the glycosaminoglycans, that is, dermatan sulfate and hyaluronic acid, are formed. The smooth muscle content of cervix varies upward–downward from 25 percent to only 6 percent. There is, however, in the human, no apparent role for smooth muscle in the cervical "ripening" process; rather, this process appears to involve changes that occur in collagen and connective tissue; thus, with "ripening," cervical flexibility increases as collagen and protein concentrations decrease. It is clear that the loss of collagen is accounted for by proteolytic digestion by the action of collagenase and thence elimination of the soluble products of collagen breakdown.

The glycosaminoglycans are also believed to be important in the processes leading to cervical ripening. Thus, cervical ripening is believed to be associated with two principal events—(1) collagen breakdown, and (2) an alteration in the relative amounts of the various glycosaminoglycans. Hyaluronic acid is a substance that is associated with the capacity of a tissue to retain water. Near term, there is a striking increase in the relative amount of

hyaluronic acid in cervix, together with a decrease in cervical dermatan sulfate.

Regulatory Factors in Myometrial Contractions and Cervical Ripening

The role of hormones and other factors in the appearance of gap junctions between myometrial cells is discussed on p. 305. There appears to be a unique response system whereby gap junctions in myometrial cells, activation of contractions, and cervical ripening can occur in a coordinated manner. Ultimately, it seems that prostaglandins occupy a crucial role in these processes. Consider the following: prostaglandins (E_2 and $F_{2\alpha}$) inhibit the ATP-dependent sequestration of calcium in sarcoplasmic reticulum, and thereby act to increase the concentration of cytosolic Ca^{2+}, a process that leads to activation of myosin light-chain kinase, phosphorylation of myosin, and, thereby, the interaction of phosphorylated myosin and actin (Carsten and Miller, 1983). At the same time, PGE_2 and $PGF_{2\alpha}$ act to cause the rapid appearance of myometrial gap junctions whereas prostacyclin inhibits gap junction formation. PGE_2 and $PGF_{2\alpha}$ act to induce the maturational changes of cervical ripening, that is, activation of collagenase(s) and an alteration in the relative concentration of the glycosaminoglycans. In some species, these same events can be recapitulated in response to an alteration in the effective endogenous estrogen-to-progesterone ratio by manipulations that favor estrogen (cf. Huszar, 1983). Thus, as stated earlier, (p. 299) estrogen appears to be most closely related, hormonally, to accelerated prostaglandin synthesis. Nevertheless, other compounds may serve as active participants in the activation or orchestration of these coordinated events. For example, relaxin acts to facilitate cervical ripening while maintaining the uterus in a quiescent state, possibly by accelerating prostacyclin formation in myometrium (Casey and associates, personal communication). Much remains to be learned with respect to the biomolecular events of parturition, but much insight into the very fundamental biochemical aspects of these processes has been acquired in the past 20 years.

THREE STAGES OF LABOR

Customarily, labor is, and for good clinical reasons, divided into three distinct stages.

The first stage of labor commences when uterine contractions (myometrial forces) of sufficient *frequency, intensity,* and *duration* to bring about readily demonstrable effacement and dilatation of the cervix are attained. The first stage of labor ends when the cervix is fully dilated, that is, when the cervix is sufficiently dilated to allow passage of the fetal head. The first stage of labor, therefore, is related primarily to the stage in which *cervical effacement* and *dilatation* occurs.

The *second stage of labor* begins when dilatation of

the cervix is complete and ends with delivery of the infant. The second stage of labor is the stage of *expulsion of the fetus.*

The third stage of labor begins with delivery of the infant and ends with the delivery of the placenta and fetal membranes. The third stage of labor is the stage of *separation and expulsion of the placenta.*

In addition to these classic three stages of labor, some obstetricians categorize a period of *prelabor* and a *latent phase of labor* that precede the first stage, and a *fourth stage of labor* that follows delivery of the placenta. Hendricks (1970), for example, identified *prelabor* as the period of increased uterine activity that occurs for a few weeks before active labor. During this time, the increased uterine activity is believed to facilitate softening of the cervix, some cervical effacement, slight-to-modest cervical dilatation, and expansion of the lower uterine segment. Friedman (1955) described a *latent phase of labor* that preceded active labor by several hours (see Chapter 29, p. 642). During the latent phase, uterine contractions typically are infrequent, produce some discomfort, and may be irregular; nonetheless, these contractions apparently can generate sufficient force to facilitate slow effacement and dilatation if there have occurred biochemical changes that lead to ripening and softening of the cervix.

A fourth stage of labor has been identified by some obstetricians as that period of an hour or so after delivery of the placenta during which time myometrial contractions and retraction, along with vessel thrombosis, act effectively to control bleeding from the placental implantation site. Prelabor, that is, the latent phase of labor, and the fourth stage of labor lack the precision of definition and ease of identification that are characteristic of the three classic stages of labor, but are of undoubted importance in successful parturition in women.

CLINICAL COURSE OF LABOR

"Lightening"

A few weeks before the onset of labor, the abdomen of the pregnant woman commonly undergoes a change in shape. The fundal height decreases somewhat, and this event at times is described by the mother as follows: "the baby dropped." This phenomenon is the consequence of the development of a well-formed lower uterine segment, the descent of the fetal head to or even through the pelvic inlet, and to some degree to a reduction in the volume of amnionic fluid.

False Labor

For a variable time before the establishment of true or effective labor, women may experience so-called false labor. The uterine contractions of false labor are characterized by irregularity in occurrence and by brevity of duration, and most often the discomfort produced is confined to the lower abdomen and groin. In contrast, the discomfort produced by the uterine contractions that are characteristic of true labor begins first in the fundal region and then radiates over the uterus and through to the lower back.

Uterine irritability that causes discomfort but that does not represent true labor (in that cervical dilatation does not occur) may develop at any time during pregnancy. False labor is observed most commonly late in pregnancy and in parous women. It often stops spontaneously but may proceed rapidly to the effective contractions of true labor. Therefore, the report of relatively infrequent and short-lived, but uncomfortable, uterine contractions cannot be dismissed summarily. All too frequently when this is done, delivery takes place without benefit of the assistance of professional personnel or facilities essential for optimal care of the mother and fetus–infant.

"Show"

A rather dependable sign of the impending onset of labor (provided no rectal or vaginal examination has been performed in the preceding 48 hours) is "show," or "bloody show," which consists of the discharge from the vagina of a small amount of blood-tinged mucus, representing the extrusion of the plug of mucus that was filling the cervical canal during pregnancy. "Show" is a late sign, for labor usually ensues during the next several hours to a few days. Normally, only a few drops of blood escape with the mucus plug; more substantial bleeding is suggestive of an abnormal condition.

CHARACTERISTICS OF UTERINE CONTRACTIONS IN LABOR

Unique among physiologic muscular contractions, those of labor are painful. Therefore, the common designation in many languages for such a contraction is "pain." The cause of the pain is not known definitely, but several hypotheses have been suggested: (1) hypoxia of the contracted myometrium (as in angina pectoris); (2) compression of nerve ganglia in the cervix and lower uterus by the tightly interlocking muscle bundles; (3) stretching of the cervix during dilatation; and (4) stretching of the overlying peritoneum. Compression of nerve ganglia in the cervix and lower uterine segment by the contracting myometrium is an especially attractive hypothesis since paracervical infiltration with a local anesthetic typically produces appreciable relief of pain during subsequent uterine contractions (see Chapter 18, p. 360).

Uterine contractions are involuntary and, for the most part, independent of extrauterine control. Neural blockage from caudal or epidural anesthesia, if initiated quite early in labor, is sometimes associated with a reduction in the frequency and intensity of uterine contractions, but not after labor is well established.

Moreover, in paraplegic women, there are normal, though painless, contractions as in women after bilateral lumbar sympathectomy. Thus far, attempts to initiate labor in women by electrical stimulation have been only partially successful (Theobald, 1968).

Ivy and co-workers (1931) believed that there are pacemakers in the uterus that act to initiate uterine contractions and thereby control the rhythmicity of uterine contractions. As pointed out by Carsten (1968), however, in a comprehensive review of myometrial composition, growth, and activity, the cells that participate in the pacemaker activities, unlike those of the heart, do not differ anatomically from the surrounding myocytes. Pacemaker activity is not confined to a specific site (Wolfs and van Leeuwen, 1979); only a group of highly excitable myometrial cells are required and uterine activity may commence in a variety of sites. The contractile rhythm of one pacemaker may be such as to reinforce or even to block that of another. Since electric current does not flow easily from one myometrial cell to another, activation of individual myometrial cell membranes almost certainly serves to propagate the impulse throughout the myometrium, probably by way of myometrial cell gap junctions. In women, the pacemaker sites in the uterus most often appear to be near the uterotubal junctions.

Mechanical stretching of the cervix enhances uterine activity in several species, including the human. This phenomenon has been referred to as the *Ferguson reflex*. The exact mechanism by which mechanical dilatation of the cervix causes increased myometrial contractility is not clear. Release of oxytocin was suggested as the cause by Ferguson (1941), but this has not been proved. More recently, it was shown, in studies of sheep and women, that manipulation of the cervix caused a rapid and striking increase in prostaglandin $F_{2\alpha}$ metabolites in blood (Mitchell, 1976).

The interval between contractions diminishes gradually, from about 10 minutes at the onset of the first stage of labor to as little as 1 minute or less in the second stage. Periods of relaxation between contractions, however, are essential to the welfare of the fetus, since unremitting contraction of the uterus may interfere with uteroplacental blood flow of sufficient magnitude as to produce fetal hypoxia. In the active phase of labor, the duration of each contraction ranges from 30 to 90 seconds, averaging about 1 minute. There is appreciable variability in the intensity of uterine contractions during apparently normal labor, as emphasized by Schulman and Romney (1970). They recorded the amnionic fluid pressures generated by uterine contractions in women during spontaneous labor; the pressures averaged about 40 mm Hg but varied from 20 to 60 mm Hg.

Differentiation of Uterine Activity

With labor, the uterus differentiates into two distinct parts. On the one hand, the actively contracting upper segment becomes thicker as labor advances; on the other hand, the lower portion, comprising the lower segment of the uterus and the cervix, is relatively passive compared with the upper segment, and it develops into a much thinner-walled passage for the fetus. The lower uterine segment is analogous to a greatly expanded and thinned-out isthmus of the uterus of nonpregnant women, the formation of which is not solely a phenomenon of labor. The lower segment develops gradually as pregnancy progresses and then thins remarkably during labor (Figs. 15-10, 15-11). By abdominal palpation, even before rupture of the membranes, the two segments can be dif-

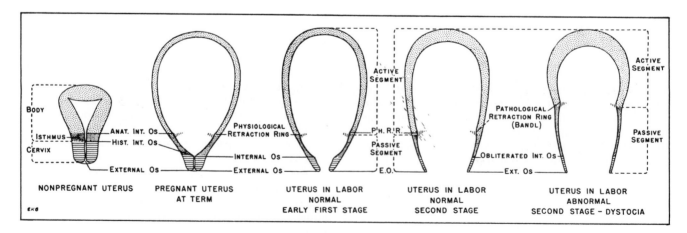

Figure 15-10. Sequence of development of the segments and rings in the uterus in pregnant women at term and in labor. Note comparison between the uterus of a nonpregnant woman, the uterus at term, and the uterus during labor. The passive lower segment of the uterine body is derived the isthmus; the physiologic retraction ring develops at the junction of the upper and lower uterine segments. The pathologic retraction ring develops from the physiologic ring. Anat. Int. Os = anatomic internal os; Hist. Int. Os = histologic internal os; Ph. R. R. = physiologic retraction ring; E.O. = external os.

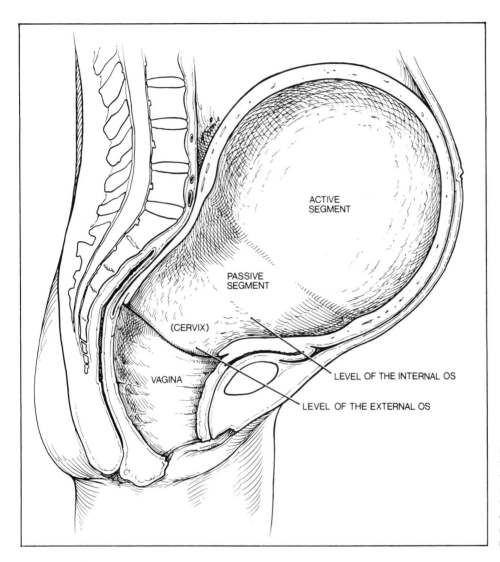

ACTIVE
SEGMENT

PASSIVE
SEGMENT

(CERVIX)

VAGINA

LEVEL OF THE INTERNAL OS

LEVEL OF THE EXTERNAL OS

Figure 15-11. The uterus at the time of vaginal delivery. The active upper segment of the uterus retracts about the fetus as the fetus descends through the birth canal. In the passive lower segment, there is considerably less myometrial tone.

ferentiated during a contraction. The upper uterine segment is quite firm or hard, whereas the consistency of the lower uterine segment is much less firm. The former represents the actively contracting part of the uterus; the latter is the distended, normally much more passive, portion.

If the entire sac of uterine musculature, including the lower uterine segment and cervix, were to contract simultaneously and with equal intensity, the net expulsive force would be decreased markedly. Therein lies the importance of the division of the uterus into an actively contracting upper segment and a more passive lower segment, which differ not only anatomically but also physiologically. The upper segment contracts, retracts, and expels the fetus; and, in response to the force of the contractions of the upper segment, the ripened lower uterine segment and cervix dilate and thereby form a greatly expanded, thinned-out muscular and fibromuscular tube through which the fetus can pass.

The myometrium of the upper uterine segment does not relax to its original length after contractions. Rather,

it becomes relatively fixed at a shorter length, with the tension, however, remaining the same as before the contraction. The purpose of the ability of the upper portion of the uterus, or active segment, to contract down on its diminishing contents with myometrial tension remaining constant is to take up slack, that is, to maintain the advantage gained with respect to expulsion of the fetus, and to maintain the uterine musculature in firm contact with the intrauterine contents. As the consequence of retraction, each successive contraction commences where its predecessor left off, so that the upper part of the uterine cavity becomes slightly smaller with each successive contraction. Because of the successive shortening of its muscular fibers with each contraction, the upper uterine segment (Fig. 15-10, Active Segment) becomes progressively thickened throughout the first and second stages of labor and tremendously thickened immediately after the birth of the baby. The phenomenon of retraction of the upper uterine segment is contingent upon a decrease in the volume of its contents. For its contents to be diminished, particularly early in labor when the entire uterus is virtually a closed sac with only a minute opening at the cervix, there is a requirement that the musculature of the lower segment stretch, permitting increasingly more of the intrauterine contents to occupy the lower segment. Indeed, the upper segment retracts only to the extent that the lower segment distends and the cervix dilates.

The relaxation of the lower uterine segment is by no means complete relaxation, but rather the opposite of retraction. The fibers of the lower segment become stretched with each contraction of the upper segment, after which these are not returned to the previous length but rather remain relatively fixed at the longer length; the tension, however, remains essentially the same as before. The musculature still manifests tone, still resists stretch, and still contracts somewhat on stimulation.

The successive lengthening of the muscular fibers in the lower uterine segment, as labor progresses, is accompanied by thinning, normally to as little as only a few millimeters in its thinnest part. As a result of the thinning of the lower uterine segment and the concomitant thickening of the upper, the boundary between the two is marked by a ridge on the inner uterine surface, the *physiologic retraction ring*. When the thinning of the lower uterine segment is extreme, as in obstructed labor, the ring is very prominent, forming, in extreme cases, a *pathologic retraction ring* (the ring of Bandl), an abnormal condition, the nature of which is illustrated in Figure 15-10 and one that is discussed further in Chapter 29 (p. 648).

From quantitative measurements of the difference in behavior of the upper and lower parts of the uterus during normal labor it was found that there is normally a gradient of diminishing physiologic activity from the fundus to the cervix. Several ingenious devices have been used to evaluate uterine forces, including the tokodynamometer, intrauterine receptors, and intramyometrial catheters.

In the tokodynamometer, three strain gauges set in heavy brass ring mountings are employed; the three gauges may be placed anywhere on the abdomen. When the uterus contracts, the increased convexity of the local arc of the uterus underlying the ring pushes upward on the gauge and applies a strain to its elements proportional to the local force of the uterine contraction. A record is obtained electrometrically, an example of which is shown in Figure 15-12. It is evident from these tracings that the intensity of each contraction is greater in the fundal zone than in the midzone, and greater in the midzone than lower down. Equally noteworthy is the differential in the duration of the contractions; those in the midzone are much briefer than those above, whereas the contractions in the lower zone are extremely brief and sometimes absent. This subsidence of contractions in the midzone at a time when the upper zone is still contracting indicates that the upper part of the corpus, throughout a substantial portion of each contraction, comes to exert pressure caudally on the more relaxed parts of the uterus. Occasionally, when labor is not progressing, this gradient is absent, and both the intensity and the duration of the contractions may be the same in all three zones.

These findings of Reynolds (1949) were confirmed by Karlson (1949) through the use of an entirely different apparatus. By his technique, the internal pressure in the uterus at any point was measured by means of so-called receptors (metal capsules about 12 mm long with a diameter of 4.5 mm), in the middle of which is a small aperture. On the inner side of this aperture, there is a membrane that is sensitive to pressure. Pressure exerted against the window is carried and registered electrometrically; an example of one of Karlson's tracings is shown in Figure 15-13. Here again there is a gradient of diminishing activity from the fundus to the lower uterine segment. Karlson's other tracings, like those of Reynolds, are indicative that in the absence of this gradient, that is, when the intensity of contraction of the lower segment equals or exceeds that of the fundus, cervical dilatation may cease. Similar results were obtained by Caldeyro-Barcia, Alvarez, and Reynolds (1950), who inserted either small intramyometrial balloons or open-ended catheters at various levels and recorded the pressures during contractions.

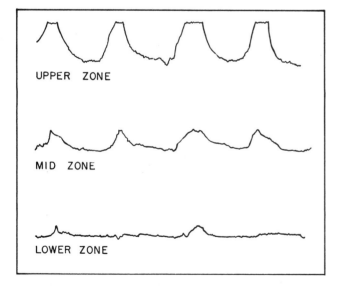

Figure 15-12. Uterine contractions in various parts of the uterus recorded by Reynolds tokodynamometer. The lower zone probably corresponds to the lower uterine segment. The woman studied was a primigravida in active labor, the cervix was 5 cm dilated, and contractions were occurring at about 3 minute intervals. The original tracings have been inked over for clearer reproduction. (*From Reynolds, Hellman, and Burns: Obstet Gynecol Surv 3:629, 1948.*)

Change in Uterine Shape

Each contraction produces an elongation of the uterine ovoid, with a concomitant decrease in horizontal diameters. By virtue of this change in shape, there are important effects on the process of labor:

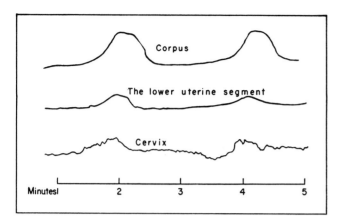

Figure 15-13. Uterine contractions in various parts of the uterus recorded by Karlson by means of intrauterine receptors. The woman studied was in early labor, but from the time this tracing was made, progress of labor was rapid. To permit clearer reproduction, the background of the original record has been eliminated and the tracings inked over. (*Modified from Karlson: Acta Obstet Gynecol Scand 28:209, 1949.*)

1. The decrease in horizontal diameter produces a straightening of the fetal vertebral column, pressing its upper pole firmly against the fundus of the uterus, whereas the lower pole is thrust farther downward and into the pelvis. The lengthening of the fetal ovoid thus produced has been estimated as between 5 and 10 cm. The pressure so exerted is known as fetal axis pressure.
2. With lengthening of the uterus, the longitudinal fibers are drawn taut; since the lower segment and cervix are the only parts of the uterus that are flexible, these are pulled upward over the lower pole of the fetus. This effect on the musculature of the lower segment and on the cervix is an important factor in cervical dilatation. The round ligaments also contain smooth muscle, which can contract and pull the uterus forward. These actions, however, are not essential for successful labor and delivery.

OTHER FORCES CONCERNED IN LABOR

Intraabdominal Pressure

After the cervix is dilated fully, the force that is principally important in the expulsion of the fetus is that produced by increased intraabdominal pressure created by contraction of the abdominal muscles simultaneously with forced respiratory efforts with the glottis closed. This is usually referred to as "pushing." The nature of the force produced is similar to that involved in defecation, but usually the intensity is much greater. The important role that is served by intraabdominal pressure in fetal expulsion is most clearly attested to by the labors of women who are paraplegic. Such women suffer no pain, although the uterus may contract vigorously. Cervical dilatation, in large measure the result of uterine contractions acting on a ripened cervix, proceeds normally, but expulsion of the infant is rarely possible except when the woman is instructed to bear down and can do so at the time that the obstetrician identifies uterine contractions. Although increased intraabdominal pressure is required for the spontaneous completion of labor, it is futile until the cervix is fully dilated. In other words, it is a necessary auxiliary to uterine contractions in the second stage of labor, but "pushing" accomplishes little in the first stage, other than fatiguing the mother.

Intraabdominal pressure may also be important in the third stage of labor, especially if the parturient is unattended. After the placenta has separated, its spontaneous expulsion is aided by the mother's bearing down, that is, by an increase in intraabdominal pressure.

Resistance

Labor is work; mechanically, work is the generation of motion against resistance. The forces involved in labor are those of the uterus and the abdomen that act to expel the fetus and those that must overcome the resistance offered by the cervix to dilatation and the friction created by the birth canal during passage of the presenting part. In addition, forces of resistance may be exerted by the muscles of the pelvic floor. The work involved in labor, according to Gemzell and colleagues (1957), is only a fraction of the maximal functional capacity of the normal woman.

Changes Induced in the Cervix

The effective force of the first stage of labor is the uterine contraction, which, in turn, exerts hydrostatic pressure through the membranes against the cervix and lower uterine segment. In the absence of intact membranes, the presenting part is forced directly against the cervix and lower uterine segment. As a result of the action of these forces, two fundamental changes, namely, effacement and dilatation, take place in the previously ripened cervix.

The Mechanism of Cervical Effacement

Effacement of the cervix ("obliteration" or "taking up") is the shortening of the cervical canal from a structure approximately 2 cm in length to one in which the canal is replaced by a mere circular orifice with almost paper-thin edges. This process takes place from above downward; it occurs as the muscular fibers in the vicinity of the internal os are pulled upward, or "taken up," into the lower segment, while the condition of the external os remains temporarily unchanged. As illustrated in Figures 15-14–15-17, the edges of the internal os are drawn upward several centimeters to become, functionally, part of the lower uterine segment. Effacement may be compared with a funneling process in which the whole length of a

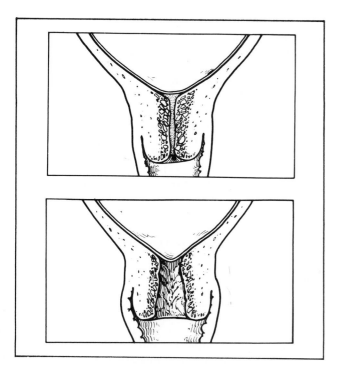

Figure 15-14. Cervix near the end of pregnancy but before labor. *Top,* primigravida; *bottom,* multipara.

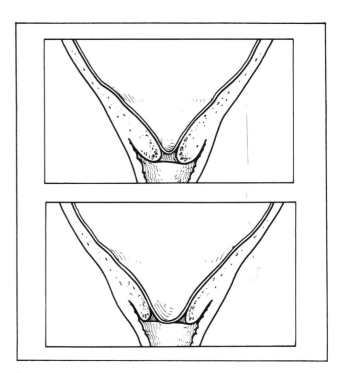

Figure 15-16. Further effacement of cervix. *Top,* primigravida; *bottom,* multipara.

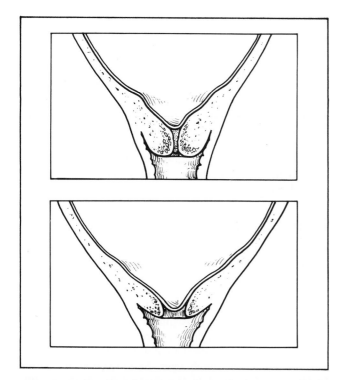

Figure 15-15. Beginning effacement of cervix. Note dilatation of internal os and funnel-shaped cervical canal. *Top,* primigravida; *bottom,* multipara.

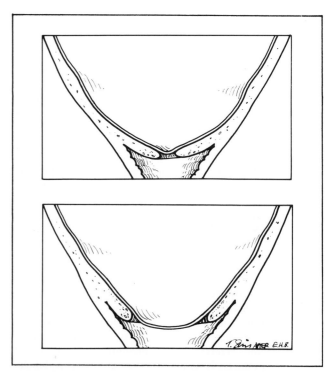

Figure 15-17. Cervical canal obliterated, i.e., the cervix is completely effaced. *Top,* primigravida; *bottom,* multipara.

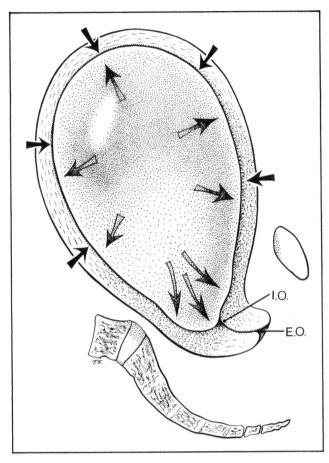

Figure 15-18. Hydrostatic action of membranes in effecting cervical effacement and dilatation. In the absence of intact membranes, the presenting part, applied to the cervix and forming the lower uterine segment, acts similarly. In this and the next two illustrations, note changing relations of the external os (E.O.), internal os (I.O.).

narrow cylinder is converted into a very obtuse, flaring funnel with only a small circular orifice for an outlet. As the result of increased myometrial activity during "pre-labor" or the "latent phase of labor," appreciable effacement of the ripened cervix is sometimes attained before true labor begins. Such effacement usually facilitates expulsion of the mucus plug from the cervical canal as the canal shortens.

The Mechanism of Cervical Dilatation

In order for the head of the average fetus at term to pass through the cervix, the canal must dilate to a diameter of about 10 centimeters. When sufficient dilatation is attained for the fetal head to pass through, the cervix is said to be "completely dilated" or "fully dilated."

Compared with the body of the uterus, the lower uterine segment and cervix are regions of lesser resistance. Therefore, during a contraction, these structures are subjected to distension, in the course of which a cen-

trifugal pull is exerted on the cervix (Figs. 15-18–15-20). As the uterine contractions act to cause pressure on the membranes, the hydrostatic action of the amnionic sac, in turn, dilates the cervical canal in the manner of a wedge. In the absence of intact membranes, the pressure of the presenting part against the cervix and lower uterine segment is similarly effective. Early rupture of the membranes ("dry birth") does not retard cervical dilatation so long as the presenting part of the fetus is positioned such as to exert pressure against the cervix and lower uterine segment.

The decidua of the lower uterine segment is thin and poorly developed. The slightest movement of the underlying muscle, therefore, might allow the fetal membranes to slip back and forth over the decidua. This loosening of the membranes in the lower segment is a normal feature of early labor and a prerequisite to successful cervical dilatation. Membranes that slide readily over the lower segment and partly through the cervix are much more efficacious dilators than are those that are more firmly attached. The physicochemical changes that accompany cervical dilatation are considered on page 306 and in Chapter 9.

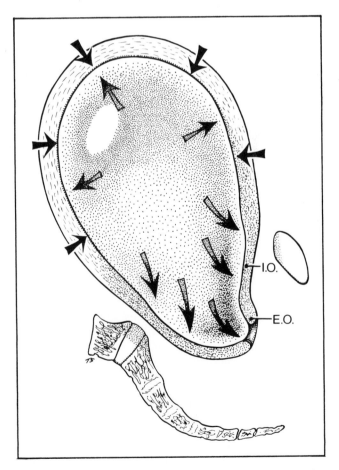

Figure 15-19. Hydrostatic action of membranes at completion of effacement.

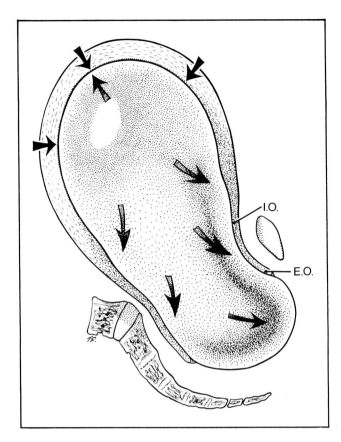

Figure 15-20. Hydrostatic action of membranes at full cervical dilatation.

There may be no fetal descent during cervical effacement, but, as a rule, the station of the presenting part descends somewhat as the cervix dilates. During the second stage, descent of the fetal presenting part typically occurs rather slowly but steadily in nulliparas. In multiparas, however, particularly those of high parity, descent may be very rapid.

Pattern of Cervical Dilatation

Friedman (1978), in his elegant treatise on labor, stated correctly that, "The clinical features of uterine contractions—namely, frequency, intensity, and duration—cannot be relied upon as measures of progression in labor nor as indices of normality.... Except for cervical dilatation and fetal descent, none of the clinical features of the parturient patient (woman) appears to be useful in assessing labor progression." The pattern of cervical dilatation that takes place during the course of normal labor takes on the shape of a sigmoid curve (Fig. 15-21). As depicted in Figure 15-21, two phases of cervical dilatation can be defined: the latent phase and the active phase. The active phase has been subdivided further into an acceleration phase, phase of maximum slope, and deceleration phase (Friedman, 1978). The duration of the

latent phase is more variable and subject to sensitive changes by extraneous factors and by sedation (prolongation of latent phase) and myometrial stimulation (shortening of latent phase). The duration of the latent phase has little bearing on the subsequent course of labor, whereas the characteristics of the acccelerated phase usually are predictive of the outcome of a particular labor. Friedman (1978) considers the maximum slope as a "good measure of the overall efficiency of the machine," whereas the nature of the deceleration phase is more reflective of fetopelvic relationships. The completion of cervical dilatation during the active phase of labor is accomplished by cervical retraction about the presenting part of the fetus. After complete cervical dilatation, the second stage of labor commences; thereafter, only progressive descent of the presenting fetal part is available to assess the progress of labor.

Patterns of Descent

In many nulliparas, engagement of the fetal head is accomplished prior to the onset of labor and further descent does not occur until late in labor. In others in whom engagement of the fetal head initially is not so extensive, further descent occurs during the first stage of labor. In the descent pattern of normal labor, a typical hyperbolic curve is formed when the station of the fetal head is plotted as a function of the duration of labor. Active descent usually takes place after cervical dilatation has progressed for some time. In nulliparas, increased rates of descent are ordinarily observed during the phase of maximum slope of cervical dilatation. At this time, the speed of descent increases to a maximum (Friedman, 1978), and this maximal rate of descent is maintained until the presenting fetal part reaches the perineal floor.

FIRST AND SECOND STAGES OF LABOR

Based upon the findings of a scholarly analysis of the labor patterns of a large number of women, Friedman (1978) also sought to select criteria that would delimit normal labor and thus enable us to identify significant abnormalities of labor. The limits, admittedly arbitrary, appear to be logical and clinically useful.

The group of women studied were nulliparas and multiparas, with no fetopelvic disproportion, no fetal malposition or malpresentation, no multiple pregnancy, and not treated with heavy sedation or conduction anesthesia, oxytocin, or operative intervention; all had normal pelves and were at term with vertex presentations and delivered average-size infants. From these studies, Friedman developed the concept of three functional divisions of labor—preparatory, dilatational, and pelvic—to describe the physiologic objectives of each phase (Fig. 15-22). He found that the preparatory division of labor may be sensitive to sedation and anesthesia. Although little cervical dilatation occurs during this phase, consid-

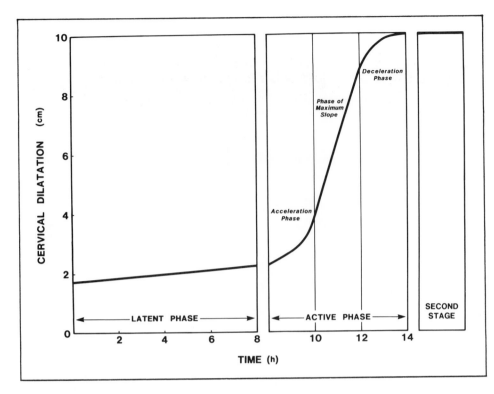

Figure 15-21. Composite of the average dilatation curve for nulliparous labor based on analysis of the data derived from the patterns traced by a large, nearly consecutive, series of gravidas. The first stage is divided into a relatively flat latent phase and a rapidly progressive active phase. In the active phase, there are three identifiable component parts—an acceleration phase, a linear phase of maximum slope, and a deceleration phase. (*Illustration courtesy of Dr. L. Casey, redrawn from Friedman, 1978.*)

erable changes take place in the ground substance, that is, collagen and other connective tissue components, of the cervix (Danforth et al., 1960). The dilatational division of labor, during which time dilatation is occurring at its most rapid rate, is principally unaffected by sedation or anesthesia that may be employed for analgesia. The pelvic division of labor commences with the deceleration phase of cervical dilatation. The classic mechanisms of

labor that involve the cardinal movements of the fetus take place principally during the pelvic division of labor. In actual practice, however, the time of onset of the pelvic division of labor is seldom clearly identifiable apart from the dilatational division of labor. Moreover, the rate of cervical dilatation does not always decelerate as full dilatation is approached; in fact, it may accelerate.

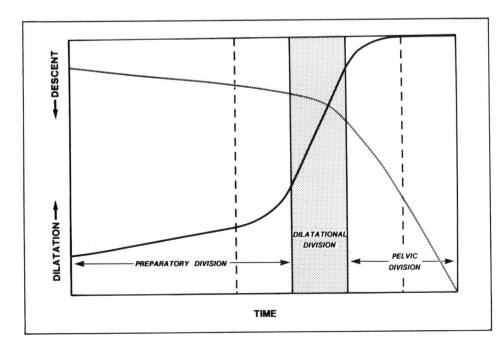

Figure 15-22. Labor course divided functionally on the basis of expected evolution of the dilatation and descent curves into (1) a preparatory division, including latent and acceleration phases, (2) a dilatational division, occupying the phase of maximum slope of dilatation, and (3) a pelvic division, encompassing both deceleration phase and second stage while concurrent with the phase of maximum slope of descent. Recognizing these distinctive functional divisions proves useful in clinical practice. (*Illustration courtesy Dr. L. Casey; redrawn from Friedman, 1978.*)

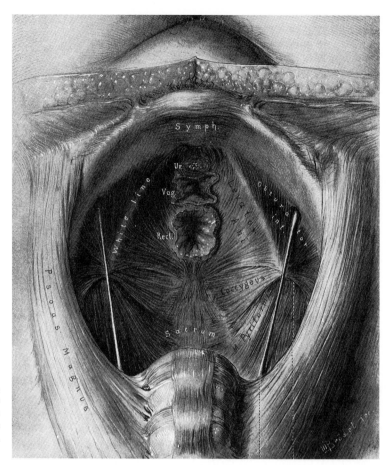

Figure 15-23. The pelvic floor seen from above. Uterus, tubes, ovaries, peritoneum, supporting ligaments, and internal fascial coverings have been removed. Symph = symphysis; Ur = urethra; Vag = vagina; Rect = rectum. (*From Kelly: Operative Gynecology. New York, Appleton, 1906.*)

Rupture of Membranes

Spontaneous rupture of the membranes most often occurs sometime during the course of active labor. Typically, rupture of the membranes is evident by a sudden gush of a variable quantity of normally clear or slightly turbid, nearly colorless fluid. Less frequently, the membranes remain intact until the time of delivery of the infant. If by chance the membranes remain intact until completion of delivery, the fetus is born surrounded by them, and the portion covering the head of the newborn infant is sometimes referred to as the *caul.*

Changes in the Vagina and Pelvic Floor

The birth canal is supported and is closed functionally by a number of layers of tissues that together form the pelvic floor. From within outward, these tissues are (1) peritoneum, (2) subperitoneal connective tissue, (3) internal pelvic fascia, (4) levator ani and coccygeus muscles, (5) external pelvic fascia, (6) superficial muscles and fascia, (7) subcutaneous tissue, and (8) skin.

Anatomy of the Pelvic Floor

Of these structures, the most impotant are the levator ani and the fascia covering its upper and lower surfaces, which for practical purposes may be considered as the pelvic floor (Fig. 2-6, p. 14). This muscle (or group of muscles) closes the lower end of the pelvic cavity as a diaphragm and thereby a concave upper and a convex lower surface are presented, as illustrated in Figures 15-23 and 15-24. On either side, the levator ani consists of a pubic and iliac portion. The former is a band 2 to 2.5 cm in width arising from the horizontal ramus of the pubis 3 to 4 cm below its upper margin and 1 to 1.5 cm from the symphysis pubis. Its fibers pass backward to encircle the rectum and possibly give off a few fibers that pass behind the vagina. The greater, or iliac, portion of the muscle arises on either side of the pelvis from the white line (the tendinous arch of the pelvic fascia) and from the ischial spine at a distance of about 5 cm below the margin of the pelvic inlet. The greater part of the muscle passes backward and unites with that from the other side of the rectum; the posterior portions meet in the tendinous raphe in front of the coccyx, with the most posterior fibers attached to the bone itself. The posterior and lateral portions of the pelvic floor, which are not filled out by the levator ani, are occupied by the piriformis and coccygeus muscles on either side (Fig. 2-6, p. 14).

The levator ani varies from 3 to 5 mm in thickness, though its margins encircling the rectum and vagina are somewhat thicker. During pregnancy, the levator ani usually undergoes hypertrophy. By vaginal examination,

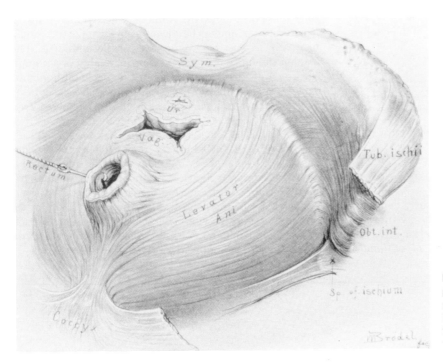

Figure 15-24. The deep muscles of the pelvic floor seen from below. Sym = symphysis; Ur = urethra; Vag = vagina; Sp. of Ishium = ischial spine; Obt. int. = obturator internus muscle; Tub. ischii = ischial tuberosity.

the internal margin of the muscle can be felt as a thick band that extends backward from the pubis and encircles the vagina about 2 cm above the hymen. On contraction, the levator ani draws both the rectum and vagina forward and upward in the direction of the symphysis pubis and thereby acts to close the vagina, for the more superficial muscles of the perineum are too delicate to serve more than an accessory function.

The internal pelvic fascia, which forms the upper covering of the levator ani, is attached to the margin of the pelvic inlet, where it is joined by the fascia of the iliac fossa, and the transverse fascia of the obturator internus and is attached firmly to the periosteum covering the lateral wall of the pelvis. The white line is indicative of its point of deflection from the periosteum. From there, the internal pelvic fascia spreads out over the upper surface of the levator ani and coccygeus muscles.

The inferior fascial covering of the pelvic diaphragm is divided into two parts by a line drawn between the ischial tuberosities. The posterior portion consists of a single layer, which, taking its origin from the sacrosciatic ligament and the ischial tuberosity, passes up over the inner surface of the ischial bones and the obturator internus to the white line, in the formation of which it takes part. From this tendinous structure, it is reflected at an acute angle over the inferior surface of the levator ani; the space included between the latter and the lateral pelvic wall forms the *ischiorectal fossa.* The structure filling out the triangular space between the pubic arch and a line joining the ischial tuberosities is known as the *urogenital diaphragm,* which, exclusive of skin and subcutaneous fat, consists principally of three layers of fascia: (1) the deep perineal fascia, which covers the anterior portion of the inferior surface of the levator ani muscle and is continuous with the fascia just described; (2) the middle perineal fascia, which is separated from the former by a narrow space in which are situated the pubic vessels and nerves; and, (3) the superficial perineal fascia, which, together with the layer just described, forms a compartment in which the superficial perineal muscles lie, with the exception of the sphincter ani, the rami of the clitoris, the vestibular bulbs, and the vulvovaginal glands (see Fig. 2-6, p. 14).

The superficial perineal muscles are comprised of the bulbocavernosus, the ischiocavernosus, and the superficial transverse perineal muscles. These muscles are delicately formed and are of no major obstetric importance except that the superficial transverse perineal muscles are always torn in the case of perineal lacerations.

In the first stage of labor, the membranes and presenting part of the fetus serve a role in dilating the upper portion of the vagina. After the membranes have ruptured, however, the changes in the pelvic floor are caused entirely by pressure that is exerted by the presenting part of the fetus. The most marked change consists of the stretching of the fibers of the levator ani muscles and the thinning of the central portion of the perineum, which becomes transformed from a wedge-shaped mass of tissue 5 cm in thickness to, in the absence of an episiotomy, a thin, almost transparent membranous structure that is less than 1 cm in thickness. When the perineum is distended maximally, the anus becomes dilated markedly and presents an opening, which varies from 2 to 3 cm in diameter, and through which the anterior wall of the rectum bulges.

The extraordinary number and size of the blood

vessels that supply the vagina and pelvic floor is such as to cause a great increase in the amount of blood loss when the tissues are torn.

THIRD STAGE OF LABOR

The third stage of labor, which begins immediately after delivery of the fetus, involves the separation and expulsion of the placenta.

The Phase of Placental Separation

As the baby is born, the uterus spontaneously contracts down on its diminishing contents. Normally, by the time the infant is completely delivered, the uterine cavity is nearly obliterated and the organ consists of an almost solid mass of muscle, the walls of which are several centimeters thick above the lower segment, and the fundus of which lies just below the level of the umbilicus. This sudden diminution in uterine size inevitably is accompanied by a decrease in the area of the placental implantation site (Fig. 15-25). In order for the placenta to accommodate itself to this reduced area, it increases in thickness, but because of limited placental elasticity, it is forced to buckle. The resulting tension causes the weakest layer of the decidua, the spongy layer or decidua spongiosa, to give way, and cleavage takes place at that site. Therefore, separation of the placenta results primarily from a disproportion created between the unchanged size of the placenta and the reduced size of the underlying implantation site. During cesarean section, this phenomenon may be observed directly when the placenta is implanted posteriorly.

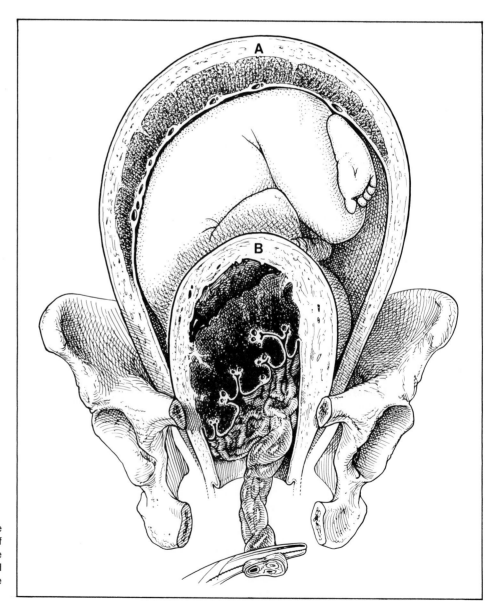

Figure 15-25. Diminution in size of placental site after birth of baby. **A.** Spatial relations before birth of the infant. **B.** Placental spatial relations after birth of the infant.

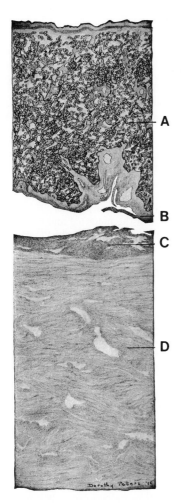

Figure 15-26. Separation of placenta with cleavage of the decidua. **A.** Placenta. **B.** Decidua cast off with placenta. **C.** Decidua retained in utero. **D.** Myometrium.

Cleavage of the placenta is greatly facilitated by the nature of the loose structure of the spongy decidua, which may be likened to the row of perforations between postage stamps. As separation proceeds, a hematoma forms between the separating placenta and the remaining decidua. Formation of the hematoma is usually the result, rather than the cause, of the separation, since in some cases bleeding is negligible. The hematoma may, however, accelerate the process of cleavage. Because the separation of the placenta is through the spongy layer of the decidua (see Chapter 6, p. 102), part of the decidua is cast off with the placenta, with the rest remaining attached to the myometrium (Fig. 15-26). The amount of decidual tissue retained at the placental site varies.

Most investigators have found that placental separation occurs within a very few minutes after delivery. Brandt (1933) and others, based on results obtained in combined clinical and roentgenographic studies, supported the idea that since the periphery of the placenta is probably the most adherent portion, separation

usually begins elsewhere. Occasionally, some degree of separation begins even before the third stage of labor commences, probably accounting for certain cases of fetal distress that occur just before expulsion of the infant.

Separation of Amnio-Chorion

The great decrease in the surface area of the cavity of the uterus simultaneously causes the fetal membranes (amnio-chorion) and the parietal decidua to be thrown into innumerable folds that increase the thickness of the layer from less than 1 to 3 to 4 mm. The lining of the uterus, as illustrated in Figure 15-27, early in the third stage, is indicative of the fact that much of the parietal layer of decidua vera is included between the folds of the festooned amnio-chorion laeve.

The membranes usually remain in situ until the separation of the placenta is nearly completed. These are then peeled off the uterine wall, partly by the further contraction of the myometrium and partly by traction exerted by the separated placenta, which lies in the flabby lower uterine segment or in the upper portion of the vagina. The body of the uterus at that time normally forms an almost solid mass of muscle, the anterior and posterior walls of which, each measuring 4 to 5 cm in thickness, lie in close apposition such that the uterine cavity is almost obliterated.

The Phase of Placental Extrusion

After the placenta has separated from its implantation site, the pressure exerted upon it by the uterine walls causes it to slide downward into the flaccid lower uterine segment or the upper part of the vagina. In some cases,

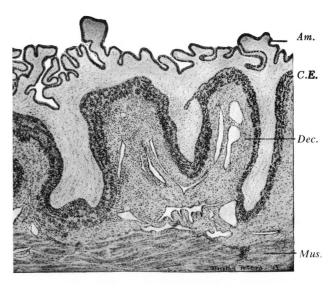

Figure 15-27. Folding of membranes as uterine cavity decreases in size. Am. = amnion; C.E. = epithelium of chorion laeve; Mus. = myometrium; Dec. = decidua vera.

the placenta may be expelled from those locations by an increase in abdominal pressure, but women in the recumbent position frequently cannot expel the placenta spontaneously. Therefore, an artificial means of completing the third stage generally is required. The usual method employed is alternate compression and elevation of the fundus, while minimal traction is exerted on the umbilical cord (see Chapter 17, p. 342).

Mechanisms of Placental Extrusion

When the central, or usual, type of placental separation occurs, the retroplacental hematoma is believed to push the placenta toward the uterine cavity, first the central portion and then the rest. The placenta, thus inverted and weighted with the hematoma, then descends. Since the surrounding membranes are still attached to the decidua, the placenta can descend only by dragging after it the membranes, which peel off its periphery. Consequently, the sac formed by the membranes is inverted, with the glistening fetal surface of the placenta presenting at the vulva. The retroplacental hematoma either follows the placenta or is found within the inverted sac. In this process, known as the *mechanism of Schultze* of placental expulsion, blood from the placental site pours into the inverted sac, not escaping externally until after extrusion of the placenta.

The other method of placental extrusion is known as the *Duncan mechanism,* in which separation of the placenta occurs first at the periphery, with the result that blood collects between the membranes and the uterine wall and escapes from the vagina. In this circumstance, the placenta descends to the vagina sideways, and the maternal surface appears first at the vulva.

REFERENCES

Anderson ABM, Turnbull AC: Comparative aspects of factors involved in the onset of labor in ovine and human pregnancy. In Klopper A, Gardner J (eds): Endocrine Factors in Labour. London, Cambridge University Press, 1973, p 141

Bergstrom S, Danielson H, Samuelsson B: The enzymatic formation of prostaglandin E_2 from arachidonic acid: Prostaglandins and related factors. Biochim Biophys Acta 90:207, 1964

Bleasdale JE, Okazaki T, Sagawa N, DiRenzo GC, Okita JR, MacDonald PC, Johnston JM: The mobilization of arachidonic acid for prostaglandin production during parturition. In MacDonald PC, Porter JC (eds): Initiation of Parturition: Prevention of Prematurity. Fourth Ross Conference on Obstetric Research. Columbus, OH, Ross Laboratories, 1983, p 129

Brandt ML: Mechanism and management of the third stage of labor. Am J Obstet Gynecol 25:662, 1933

Caldeyro-Barcia R, Alvarez H, Reynolds SRM: A better understanding of uterine contractility through simultaneous recording with an internal and a seven channel external method. Surg Gynecol Obstet 91:641, 1950

Carsten ME: Regulation of myometrial composition, growth, and activity. In Assali NS (ed): Biology of Gestation, Vol I, The Maternal Organism. New York, Academic, 1968

Carsten ME, Miller JD: Regulation of myometrial contractions. In MacDonald PC, Porter JC (eds): Initiation of Parturition: Prevention of Prematurity, Fourth Ross Conference on Ob-

stetric Research. Columbus, OH, Ross Laboratories, 1983, p 166

Casey ML, MacDonald PC, Mitchell MD: Stimulation of prostaglandin E_2 production in amnion cells in culture by a substance(s) in human fetal urine. Biochem Biophys Res Comm 114:1056, 1983

Casey ML, Winkel CA, Porter JC, MacDonald PC: Endocrine regulation of parturition. Clin Perinatol 10:709, 1983

Casey ML, MacDonald PC: Initiation of labor in women. In Huszar G (ed): The Biochemistry and Physiology of the Uterus and Labor. Cleveland, CRC Press, 1984, in press

Chard T: The role of the posterior pituitaries of mother and foetus in spontaneous parturition. In Comline KS, Cross KW, Dawes GS (eds): Foetal and Neonatal Physiology. Cambridge, Cambridge University Press, 1973, p 579

Chard T: The role of the maternal and fetal posterior pituitary gland in parturition. In MacDonald PC, Porter JC (eds): Initiation of Parturition: Prevention of Prematurity, Fourth Ross Conference on Obstetric Research. Columbus, OH, Ross Laboratories, 1983, p 121

Creasy RK: Premature Labor. Mead Johnston Symposium on Perinatal and Developmental Medicine, No. 15. Evansville, IN, Mead Johnson and Company, 1980, p 37

Creasy RK: Implications of treatment of preterm labor. In MacDonald PC, Porter JC (eds): Initiation of Parturition: Prevention of Prematurity, Fourth Ross Conference on Obstetric Research. Columbus, OH, Ross Laboratories, 1983, p 173

Danforth DN, Buckingham JC, Roddick JW: Connective tissue changes incident to cervical effacement. Am J Obstet Gynecol 80:939, 1960

Ferguson JKW: A study of the motility of the intact uterus at term. Surg Gynecol Obstet 73:359, 1941

Flint APF: Regulation of placental enzymes. In MacDonald PC, Porter JC (eds): Initiation of Parturition: Prevention of Prematurity, Fourth Ross Conference on Obstetric Research. Columbus, OH, Ross Laboratories, 1983, p 27

Friedman EA: Graphic appraisal of labor: A study of 500 primigravidas. Bull Sloan Hosp Women 1:42, 1955

Friedman EA: Labor: Clinical Evaluation and Management, 2nd ed. New York, Appleton, 1978

Gemzell CA, Robbe H, Stern B, Strom G: Observation on circulatory changes and muscular work in normal labor. Acta Obstet Gynecol Scand 36:75, 1957

Hertelendy F: Prostaglandin-induced premature oviposition in the coturnix quail. Prostaglandins 2:269, 1972

Hertelendy F: Regulation of oviposition. In MacDonald PC, Porter JC (eds): Initiation of Parturition: Prevention of Prematurity, Fourth Ross Conference on Obstetric Research. Columbus, OH, Ross Laboratories, 1983, p 79

Huszar G, Roberts JB: Biochemistry and pharmacology of the myometrium and labor: Regulation at the cellular and molecular levels. Am J Obstet Gynecol 142:225, 1982

Huszar G: Biology of the myometrium and cervix. In Washaw JB (ed): The Biological Basis of Reproductive and Developmental Medicine. New York, Elsevier, 1983, p 85

Ivy AC, Hartman, CG, Koff A: The contractions of the monkey uterus at term. Am J Obstet Gynecol 22:388, 1931

Karim SMM: The Prostaglandins. New York, Wiley, 1972

Karlson S: On the motility of the uterus during labour and the influence of the motility pattern on the duration of the labour. Acta Obstet Gynecol Scand 28:209, 1949

Katz Z, Lancet M, Levani E: The efficacy of intra-amniotic steroids for induction of labor. Obstet Gynecol 54:31, 1979

Krall JF, Korenman SG: Prevention of preterm labor. In

Knight J, O'Connor M (eds): The Fetus and Birth. Amsterdam, Elsevier, 1977, p 319

Lands WEM, Samuelsson B: Phospholipid precursors of prostaglandins. Biochim Biophys Acta 164:426, 1968

Leake RD: Oxytocin. In MacDonald PC, Porter JC (eds): Initiation of Parturition: Prevention of Prematurity, Fourth Ross Conference on Obstetric Research. Columbus, OH, Ross Laboratories, 1983, p 43

Liggins GC, Fairclough RJ, Grieves SA, Kendall JZ, Knox BS: The mechanism of initiation of parturition in the ewe. Rec Prog Horm Res 29:111, 1973

Liggins GC: Fetal influences on myometrial contractility. Clin Obstet Gynecol 16:148, 1973

Luukkainen TU, Csapo AI: Induction of premature labor in the rabbit after pretreatment with phospholipids. Fertil Steril 14:65, 1963

MacDonald PC, Porter JC, Schwarz BE, Johnston JM: Initiation of parturition in the human female. Semin Perinatol 2:273, 1978

Malpas P: Postmaturity and malformation of the fetus. J Obstet Gynaecol Br Emp 40:1046, 1933

Mati JKG, Horrobin DF, Bramley PS: Induction of labour in sheep and in human by single doses of corticosteroids. Br Med J 2:149, 1973

Mitchell MD: Studies on prostaglandins in relation to parturition in the sheep. D. Phil. thesis, Oxford University, 1976

Nathanielsz PW, Abel M, Smith GW: Hormonal factors in parturition in the rabbit. Foetal and Neonatal Physiology. Proceedings of the Sir J Bancroft Centenary Symposium. London, Cambridge University Press, 1973, p 594

Novy MJ: Endocrine control of parturition in rhesus monkeys. In MacDonald PC, Porter JC (eds): Initiation of Parturition: Prevention of Prematurity, Fourth Ross Conference on Obstetric Research. Columbus, OH, Ross Laboratories, 1983, p 62

Okita JR, Sagawa N, Casey ML, Snyder JM: A comparison of amnion cells in monolayer culture and amnion tissue. In Vitro 19:117, 1983

Olson DM, Opavsky MA, Challis JR: Prostaglandin synthesis by human amnion is dependent upon extracellular calcium. Can J Physiol Pharmacol 61:1089, 1983

Pinto RM, Leon C, Mazzocco N, Scasserra V: Action of estradiol-17β at term and at onset of labor. Am J Obstet Gynecol 98:540, 1967

Rea C: Prolonged gestation, acrania, monstrosity and apparent placenta praevia in one obstetrical case. J Am Med Assoc 30:1166, 1898

Reynolds SRM: Physiology of the Uterus with Clinical Correlations, 2d ed. New York, Hoeber, 1949

Sala NL, Schwarcz RL, Althabe O, Fisch L, Fuente O: Effect of epidural anesthesia upon uterine contractility induced by artificial cervical dilatation in human pregnancy. Am J Obstet Gynecol 106:26, 1970

Schulman H, Romney SL: Variability of uterine contractions in normal human parturition. Obstet Gynecol 36:215, 1970

Seron-Ferre M, Jaffe RB: The fetal adrenal gland. Ann Rev Physiol 43:141, 1981

Soloff MS: The role of oxytocin receptors in parturition. In MacDonald PC, Porter JC (eds): Initiation of Parturition: Prevention of Prematurity, Fourth Ross Conference on Obstetric Research. Columbus, OH, Ross Laboratories, 1983, p 160

Strickland DM, Saeed SA, Casey ML, Mitchell MD: Stimulation of prostaglandin biosynthesis by urine of the human fetus may serve as a trigger for parturition. Science 220:521, 1983

Stull JT, Blumenthal DK, Cooke R: Regulation of contraction by myosin phosphorylation. A comparison between smooth and skeletal muscles. Biochem Pharmacol 29:2537, 1980

Theobald GW: Nervous control of uterine activity. Clin Obstet Gynecol 11:15, 1968

Thorburn GD: Past and present concepts on the initiation of parturition. In MacDonald PC, Porter JC (eds): Initiation of Parturition: Prevention of Prematurity, Fourth Ross Conference on Obstetric Research. Columbus, OH, Ross Laboratories, 1983, p 2

Tulchinsky D, Giannopoulus G: Estrogen/progesterone receptors and parturition. In MacDonald PC, Porter JC (eds): Initiation of Parturition: Prevention of Prematurity, Fourth Ross Conference on Obstetric Research. Columbus, OH, Ross Laboratories, 1983, p 153

Van Dorp DA, Beerthuis RK, Nguteren DH, Vonkeman H: The biosynthesis of prostaglandins. Biochim Biophys Acta 90:204, 1964

Vonkeman H, van Dorp DA: The action of prostaglandin synthetase on 2-arachidonoyl-lecithin. Biochim Biophys Acta 164:430, 1968

Wolfs GMJA, van Leeuwen M: Electromyographic observations on the human uterus during labour. Acta Obstet Gynecol Scand Suppl 90, 1979

16
Mechanism of Normal Labor in Occiput Presentation

Occiput (vertex) presentations occur in about 95 percent of all labors.

DIAGNOSIS OF OCCIPUT PRESENTATION

The presentation of the fetus is most commonly ascertained during pregnancy by abdominal palpation and confirmed sometime before or at the onset of labor by vaginal examination. In the majority of cases, the vertex enters the pelvis with the sagittal suture in the transverse pelvic diameter.

Occiput Transverse Positions

For diagnosis by abdominal examination, the four maneuvers of Leopold are employed (see Fig. 12-10). With the fetus in the left occiput transverse position (LOT), the following findings are obtained by abdominal examination:

- *First maneuver:* Fundus occupied by the breech.
- *Second maneuver:* Resistant plane of the back felt directly to the examiner's right, readily palpated through the mother's left flank (see Fig. 12-10).
- *Third maneuver:* Negative if the head is engaged (biparietal diameter through the pelvic inlet); otherwise, the movable head is detected at or above the pelvic inlet.
- *Fourth maneuver:* Negative if head is engaged; otherwise cephalic prominence on the right.

In the right occiput transverse position (ROT) palpation yields similar information, except that the fetal back is in the mother's right flank and the small parts and cephalic prominence are on the left.

On vaginal examination, the sagittal suture occupies the transverse diameter of the pelvis more or less midway between the sacrum and the symphysis. In left occiput transverse positions (LOT), the smaller posterior fontanel is to the left in the maternal pelvis and the larger anterior fontanel is directed to the opposite side. In right occiput transverse positions, the reverse holds true. The fetal heart in right and left positions is usually heard in the right and left flank, respectively, at or slightly below the level of the mother's umbilicus.

Occiput Anterior Positions

In occiput anterior positions (LOA or ROA), the head either enters the pelvis with the occiput rotated 45 degrees anteriorly from the transverse position or subsequently does so. *This degree of anterior rotation produces only slight differences on abdominal examination* (see Figs. 12-5, 12-6). The mechanism of labor is usually very similar to that in transverse positions of the occiput.

Occiput Posterior Positions

The incidence of occiput posterior positions is approximately 10 percent and the right occiput posterior position (ROP) is much more common than the left (LOP). It appears likely from evidence obtained from radiographic studies that posterior positions more often are associated with a narrow forepelvis.

On vaginal or rectal examination in the occiput right posterior position (ROP), the sagittal suture occupies the right oblique diameter; the small fontanel is felt opposite the right sacroiliac synchondrosis; and the large fontanel is directed toward the left iliopectineal eminence (see Fig. 12-6). In the left position, the reverse is true (see Fig. 12-5). In many cases, particularly in the early part of labor, because of imperfect flexion of the head, the large fontanel lies at a lower level than in anterior positions and is more readily felt.

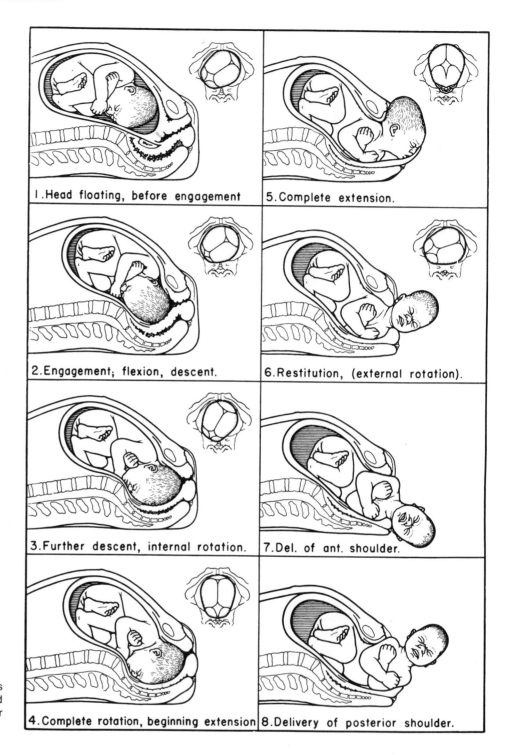

1. Head floating, before engagement

2. Engagement; flexion, descent.

3. Further descent, internal rotation.

4. Complete rotation, beginning extension

5. Complete extension.

6. Restitution, (external rotation).

7. Del. of ant. shoulder.

8. Delivery of posterior shoulder.

Figure 16-1. Principal movements in the mechanism of labor and delivery, left occiput anterior position.

CARDINAL MOVEMENTS OF A LABOR IN OCCIPUT PRESENTATION

Because of the irregular shape of the pelvic canal and the relatively large dimensions of the mature fetal head, it is evident that not all diameters of the head can necessarily pass through all diameters of the pelvis. It follows that a process of adaptation or accommodation of suit- able portions of the head to the various segments of the pelvis is required for completion of childbirth. These positional changes in the presenting part constitute the mechanism of labor. *The cardinal movements of labor are (1) engagement, (2) descent, (3) flexion, (4) internal rotation, (5) extension, (6) external rotation, and (7) expulsion.* These movements are illustrated in Figure 16-1.

For purposes of instruction, the various movements

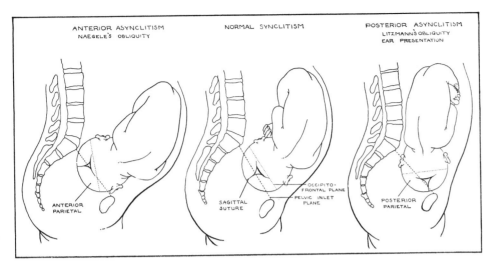

ANTERIOR ASYNCLITISM
NAEGELE'S OBLIQUITY

NORMAL SYNCLITISM

POSTERIOR ASYNCLITISM
LITZMANN'S OBLIQUITY
EAR PRESENTATION

ANTERIOR PARIETAL

SAGITTAL SUTURE

OCCIPITO-FRONTAL PLANE
PELVIC INLET PLANE

POSTERIOR PARIETAL

Figure 16-2. Synclitism and asynclitism.

are often described as though they occurred separately and independently. In reality, the mechanism of labor consists of a combination of movements that are going on at the same time. For example, as part of the process of engagement, there is both flexion and descent of the head. It is manifestly impossible for the movements to be completed unless the presenting part descends simultaneously. Concomitantly, the uterine contractions effect important modifications in the attitude, or habitus, of the fetus, especially after the head has descended into the pelvis. These changes consist principally of a straightening of the fetus, with loss of its dorsal convexity and closer application of the extremities and small parts to the body. As a result, the fetal ovoid is transformed into a cylinder with normally the smallest possible cross section passing through the birth canal.

promontory. The sagittal suture is frequently deflected either posteriorly toward the promontory or anteriorly toward the symphysis, as shown in Figure 16-2. Such lateral deflection of the head to a more anterior or posterior position in the pelvis is called *asynclitism*. If the sagittal suture approaches the sacral promontory, more of the anterior parietal bone presents itself to the examining fingers and the condition is called *anterior asynclitism*. If, however, the sagittal suture lies close to the symphysis, more of the posterior parietal bone will present and the condition is called *posterior asynclitism*. Moderate degrees of asynclitism are the rule in normal labor. Successive changes from posterior to anterior asynclitism facilitate descent by allowing the fetal head to take advantage of the roomiest areas of the pelvic cavity.

Engagement

As discussed in Chapter 11, the mechanism by which the biparietal diameter, the greatest transverse diameter of the fetal head in occiput presentations, passes through the pelvic inlet is designated *engagement*. This phenomenon may take place during the last few weeks of pregnancy or may not occur until after the commencement of labor. In many multiparous and some nulliparous women, at the onset of labor the fetal head is freely movable above the pelvic inlet into the iliac fossae. In this circumstance, the head is sometimes referred to as "floating." A normal-sized head usually does not engage with its sagittal suture directed anteroposteriorly. Instead, the fetal head usually enters the pelvic inlet either in the transverse diameter or in one of the oblique diameters.

Asynclitism. Although the fetal head tends to accommodate to the transverse axis of the pelvic inlet, the sagittal suture, while remaining parallel to that axis, may not lie exactly midway between the symphysis and sacral

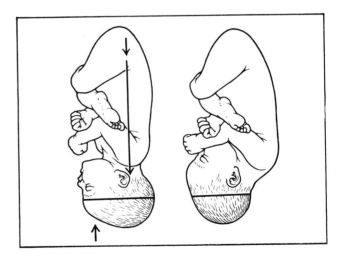

Figure 16-3. Lever action producing flexion of head; conversion from occipitofrontal to suboccipitobregmatic diameter typically reduces the anteroposterior diameter from nearly 12 cm to 9.5 cm.

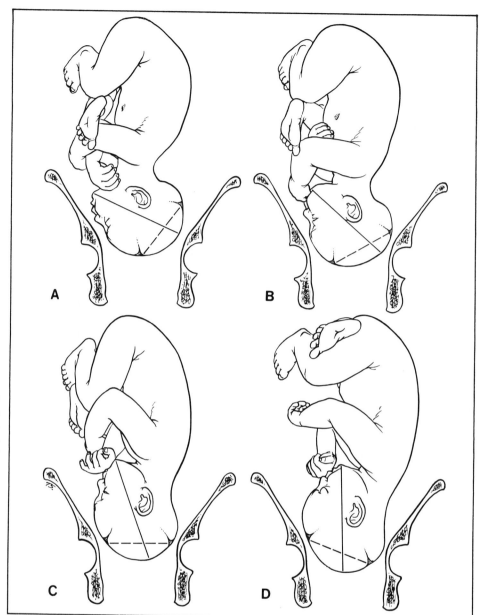

Figure 16-4. Four degrees of head flexion. Indicated by the solid line is the occipitomental diameter and the broken line connects the center of the anterior fontanel with the posterior fontanel: **A.** Flexion poor. **B.** Flexion moderate. **C.** Flexion advanced. **D.** Flexion complete. Note with flexion complete the chin is on the chest and the suboccipitobregmatic diameter, the shortest anteroposterior diameter of the fetal head, is passing through the pelvic inlet. (*Modified from Rydberg: The Mechanism of Labour. Springfield, IL., Thomas, 1954.*)

Descent

The first requisite for the birth of the infant is descent. With the nulliparous woman, engagement may occur before the onset of labor, and further descent may not necessarily follow until the onset of the second stage of labor. In multiparous women, descent usually begins with engagement. Descent is brought about by one or more of four forces: (1) pressure of the amnionic fluid; (2) direct pressure of the fundus upon the breech; (3) contraction of the abdominal muscles; and (4) extension and straightening of the fetal body.

Flexion

As soon as the descending head meets resistance, whether from cervix, the walls of the pelvis, or the pelvic floor, flexion of the head normally results. In this movement, the chin is brought into more intimate contact with the fetal thorax, and the appreciably shorter suboccipitobregmatic diameter is substituted for the longer occipitofrontal diameter (Figs. 16-3, 16-4).

Internal Rotation

This movement is a turning of the head in such a manner that the occiput gradually moves from its original position anteriorly toward the symphysis pubis or, less commonly, posteriorly toward the hollow of the sacrum (Figs. 16-5, 16-6). Internal rotation is essential for the completion of labor, except when the fetus is abnormally small. Internal rotation, which is always associated with descent of the presenting part, is usually not accom-

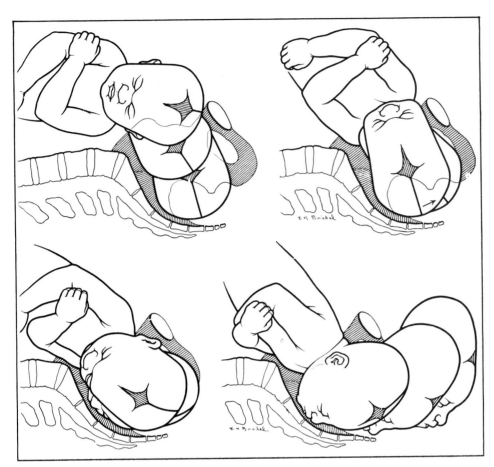

Figure 16-5. Mechanism of labor for left occiput transverse position, lateral view. Anterior asynclitism at the pelvic brim followed by lateral flexion, resulting in posterior asynclitism after engagement, further descent, rotation, and extension. (*From Steele and Javert: Surg Gynecol Obstet 75:477, 1942.*)

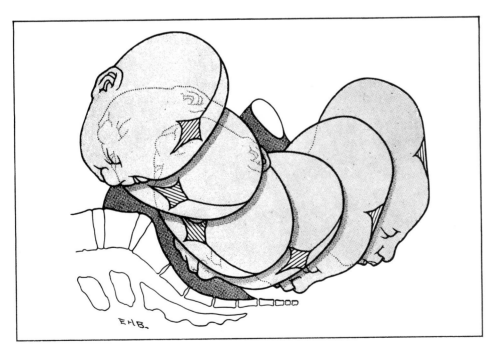

Figure 16-6. Mechanism of labor for left occiput anterior position.

plished until the head has reached the level of the spines and therefore is engaged.

> Calkins (1939) studied more than 5000 patients in labor to ascertain when internal rotation occurs. He concluded that in approximately two thirds of all women internal rotation is complete by the time the head reaches the pelvic floor; in about one fourth, internal rotation is completed very shortly after the head reaches the pelvic floor; and in about 5 percent, rotation to the anterior does not take place. When rotation fails to occur until the head reaches the pelvic floor, it takes place during the next one or two contractions in multiparas, and in nulliparas during the next three to five. Rotation before the head reaches the pelvic floor is definitely more frequent in multiparas than in nulliparas, according to Calkins.

Extension

When, after internal rotation, the sharply flexed head reaches the vulva, it undergoes another movement that is essential to its birth, namely, extension, which brings the base of the occiput into direct contact with the inferior margin of the symphysis pubis. Since the vulvar outlet is directed upward and forward, extension must occur before the head can pass through it. If the sharply flexed head, on reaching the pelvic floor, did not extend but was driven farther downward, it would impinge upon the posterior portion of the perineum and, if the force from behind were sufficiently strong, would eventually be forced through the tissues of the perineum. When the head presses upon the pelvic gutter, however, two forces come into play. The first, exerted by the uterus, acts more posteriorly, and the second, supplied by the resis-

tant pelvic floor and the symphysis, acts more anteriorly. The resultant force is in the direction of the vulvar opening, thereby causing extension.

With increasing distension of the perineum and vaginal opening, an increasingly large portion of the occiput gradually appears. The head is born by further extension as the occiput, bregma, forehead, nose, mouth, and finally the chin pass successively over the anterior margin of the perineum. Immediately after its birth, the head drops downward so that the chin lies over the maternal anal region.

External Rotation

The delivered head next undergoes restitution. If the occiput was originally directed toward the left, it rotates toward the left ischial tuberosity; if it was originally directed toward the right, the occiput rotates to the right. The return of the head to the oblique position (restitution) is followed by completion of external rotation to the transverse position, a movement that corresponds to rotation of the fetal body, serving to bring its bisacromial diameter into relation with the anteroposterior diameter of the pelvic outlet. Thus one shoulder is anterior behind the symphysis and the other is posterior. This movement is apparently brought about by the same pelvic factors that effect internal rotation of the head.

Expulsion

Almost immediately after external rotation, the anterior shoulder appears under the symphysis pubis, and the perineum soon becomes distended by the posterior

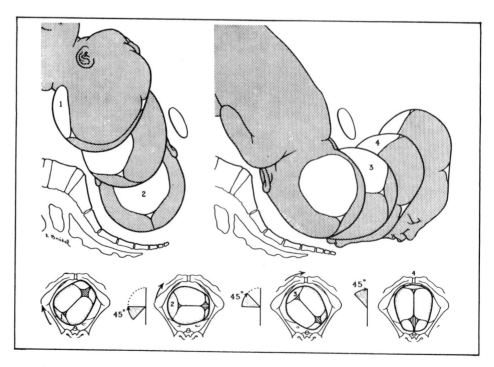

Figure 16-7. Mechanism of labor for right occiput posterior position, anterior rotation.

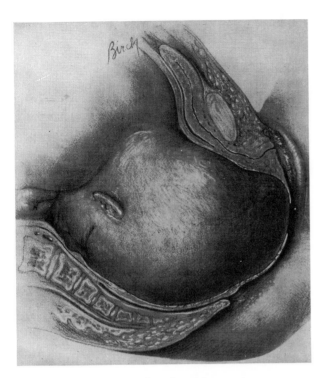

Figure 16-8. Formation of caput succedaneum.

shoulder. After delivery of the shoulders, the rest of the body of the child is quickly extruded.

Labor in Persistent Occiput Posterior Position

In the great majority of labors in the occiput posterior positions, the mechanism of labor is identical to that observed in the transverse and anterior varieties, except that the occiput has to rotate to the symphysis pubis through 135 degrees instead of 90 degrees and 45 degrees, respectively (Fig. 16-7).

With effective contractions, adequate flexion of the head, and a fetus of average size, the great majority of posteriorly positioned occiputs rotate promptly as soon as they reach the pelvic floor and labor is not appreciably lengthened. In perhaps 5 to 10 pecent of cases, however, these favorable circumstances do not occur. For example, with poor contractions or faulty flexion of the

head or both, rotation may be incomplete or may not take place at all, especially if the fetus is large. If rotation is incomplete, *transverse arrest* results. If rotation toward the symphysis does not take place, the occiput usually rotates to the direct occiput posterior position, a condition known as *persistent occiput posterior*. Both transverse arrest and persistent occiput posterior represent deviations from the normal mechanisms of labor and are considered further in Chapter 30.

CHANGES IN THE SHAPE OF THE FETAL HEAD

Caput Succedaneum

In vertex presentations, the fetal head undergoes important characteristic changes in shape as the result of the pressures to which it is subjected during labor. In prolonged labors before complete dilatation of the cervix, the portion of the fetal scalp immediately over the cervical os becomes edematous, forming a swelling known as the *caput succedaneum* (Fig. 16-8). It usually attains a thickness of only a few millimeters, but in prolonged labors it may be sufficiently extensive to prevent the differentiation of the various sutures and fontanels. More commonly, the caput is formed when the head is in the lower portion of the birth canal and frequently only after the resistance of a rigid vaginal outlet is encountered. Since it occurs over the most dependent portion of the head, in left occiput transverse position it is found over the upper and posterior extremity of the right parietal bone, and in right positions over the corresponding area of the left parietal bone. It follows that after labor the original position often may be ascertained by noting the location of the caput succedaneum.

Molding

Of considerable importance is the degree of molding that the head undergoes. Because the various bones of the skull are not firmly united, movement may occur at the sutures. Ordinarily the margins of the occipital bone, and more rarely those of the frontal bone, are pushed under those of the parietal bones. In many cases, one parietal

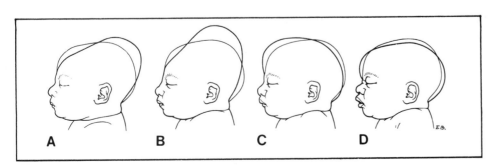

Figure 16-9. Molding of head in cephalic presentations. **A.** Occiput anterior. **B.** Occiput posterior. **C.** Brow. **D.** Face.

bone may overlap the other, the anterior parietal usually overlapping the posterior. These changes are of greatest importance in contracted pelves, when the degree to which the head is capable of molding may make the difference between successful vaginal delivery and a major obstetric operation (Fig. 16-9). Molding may account for a diminution in biparietal and suboccipitobregmatic diameters of 0.5 to 1.0 cm, or even more in prolonged labors.

REFERENCES

Calkins LA: The etiology of occiput presentations. Am J Obstet Gynecol 37:618, 1939

17
Conduct of Normal Labor and Delivery

PSYCHOLOGIC CONSIDERATIONS

The pregnant woman very often approaches labor with two major fears: "Will my baby be all right?" and "Will labor and delivery be very painful?" Her concerns should also be uppermost in the minds of everyone who participates in caring for the mother and her fetus. All things possible should be done to make the answer to the first question, "Yes" and to the second, "No."

Is labor easy because a woman is calm, or is she calm because her labor is easy? Is a woman pained and frightened because her labor is difficult, or is her labor difficult and painful because she is frightened? After scrutinizing many cases, the late British obstetrician Read concluded: "Fear is in some way the chief pain-producing agent in otherwise normal labor." Quite likely, fear may exert a deleterious effect on the quality of uterine contractions and on cervical dilatation.

It is not an easy task to dispel the age-old fear of pain during labor and delivery, but from the first prenatal visit a conscious effort should be made on the part of all persons involved in the care of the mother and her unborn child to make the point that labor and delivery are normal physiologic processes. Everyone who is involved in caring for the mother and her fetus must demonstrate professional competence but also instill the feeling that he or she is the mother's friend and friend of her unborn baby, sincerely desirous of sparing her all possible pain within the limit of safety for her and her child. Physicians, nurses, and students should note especially that the morale of a woman in labor may sometimes be destroyed by careless remarks or actions. Casual comments outside the labor room are often overheard by her and misinterpreted. Laughter is frequently interpreted as directed toward her.

Physiologic Childbirth

To eliminate the harmful influence of fear in labor, there has developed a school of thought that emphasizes the advantages of "natural childbirth" or "physiologic childbirth." Natural or physiologic childbirth entails antepartum education that emphasizes elimination of fear, exercises to promote relaxation, muscle control, and breathing, and adroit management throughout labor with a professional attendant skilled in reassurance of the mother constantly in attendance.

Most proponents of physiologic childbirth have never claimed that labor can be made devoid of pain or that delivery should be conducted without anesthetic aids. With natural childbirth, most women experience some pain, and analgesics and anesthetics are not withheld when they are indicated. Physiologic, or psychoprophylactic, childbirth is also considered in Chapter 18 (p. 364).

ADMITTANCE PROCEDURES

The woman should be urged to report early in labor rather than to procrastinate until delivery is imminent for fear that she might be experiencing false labor.

Identification of Labor

Although the differential diagnosis between false and true labor is difficult at times, it can usually be made on the basis of the following features:

Contractions of True Labor

- Occur at regular intervals
- Intervals gradually shorten
- Intensity gradually increases
- Discomfort in back and abdomen
- Cervix dilates
- Not stopped by sedation

Contractions of False Labor

- Occur at irregular intervals
- Intervals remain long
- Intensity remains same
- Discomfort chiefly in lower abdomen
- Cervix does not dilate
- Usually relieved by sedation

The general condition of the mother and her fetus must be quickly but accurately ascertained by means of history and physical examination. Inquiry is made as to the frequency and intensity of the uterine contractions and when they first became uncomfortable. The degree of discomfort that the mother displays is noted. The heart rate, presentation, and size of the fetus are evaluated abdominally. *The fetal heart rate should be checked especially at the end of a contraction and immediately thereafter to identify pathologic slowing of the fetal heart rate.* Inquiries, particularly about the status of the membranes, are made. The questions of whether fluid has leaked from the vagina, if so, how much, and when the leakage first commenced are also addressed.

Admittance Vaginal Examination

Most often, *unless there has been bleeding in excess of bloody show,* a vaginal examination under aseptic conditions is performed as described below. Careful attention to the following items is essential in order to obtain the greatest amount of information and to minimize bacterial contamination from multiple examinations:

1. *Amnionic fluid.* If there is question of rupture of the membranes, the vulva and vaginal introitus are cleansed, a sterile speculum is carefully inserted, and fluid is sought in the posterior vaginal fornix. Any fluid is observed for vernix or meconium and, if the source of the fluid remains in doubt, it is collected on a swab for further study as described below (p. 333).
2. *Cervix.* Softness, degree of effacement (length), extent of dilatation, and location of the cervix with respect to the presenting part and vagina are ascertained as described below. The presence of membranes with or without amnionic fluid below the presenting part often can be felt by careful palpation and the membranes visualized if they are intact and the cervix is dilated somewhat.
3. *Presenting part.* The nature of the presenting part should be positively determined and, ideally, its position as well, as described in Chapter 12 (p. 235).
4. *Station.* The degree of descent of the presenting part into the birth canal is identified as described below and, if the fetal head is high in the pelvis (above the level of the ischial spines), the effect of firm fundal pressure on descent of the fetal head is tested.
5. *Pelvic architecture.* The diagonal conjugate, ischial spines, pelvic sidewalls, and sacrum are re-evaluated for adequacy (see Chapter 11, p. 227).
6. *Vagina and perineum.* The distensibility of the vagina and the firmness of the perineum are assessed.

Cervical Effacement. The degree of effacement of the cervix is usually expressed in terms of the length of the cervical canal compared to that of an uneffaced cervix (see Chapter 15, p. 311). When the length of the cervix is reduced by one half, it is 50 percent effaced; when the

cervix becomes as thin as the adjacent lower uterine segment, it is completely, or 100 percent, effaced.

Cervical Dilatation. The amount of cervical dilatation is ascertained by estimating the average diameter of the cervical opening. The examining finger is swept from the margin of the cervix on one side to the opposite side, and the diameter traversed is expressed in centimeters. The cervix is said to be fully dilated when the diameter of the opening measures 10 cm, for the presenting part of a term-size infant usually can pass through a cervix so widely dilated (see Chapter 15, p. 311).

Position of Cervix. The relationship of the cervical os to the fetal head is categorized as posterior, midposition, or anterior. The posterior position is suggestive of premature labor.

Station. When conducting a vaginal examination, it is valuable to identify the level of the presenting fetal part in the birth canal. The ischial spines are about halfway between the pelvic inlet and the pelvic outlet. When the lowermost portion of the presenting fetal part is at the level of the ischial spines, it is designated as being at zero station. The long axis of the birth canal above the ischial spines is arbitrarily divided into thirds. If the presenting part is at the level of the pelvic inlet, it is at −3 station; if it has descended one third the distance from the pelvic inlet to the ischial spines, it is at −2 station; if it has reached a level two thirds the distance from the inlet to the spines, it is at −1 station. The long axis of the birth canal between the level of the ischial spines and the outlet of the pelvis is similarly divided into thirds. If the level of the presenting part in the birth canal is one third or two thirds of the distance between the ischial spines and the pelvic outlet, it is at +1 station or +2 station, respectively. When the presenting fetal part reaches the perineum, its station is +3. If the vertex is at 0 station or below, most often engagement of the head has occurred, that is, the biparietal plane of the head has passed through the pelvic inlet. *If the head is unusually molded, or if there is an extensive formation of caput, or both, engagement might not have taken place even though the vertex is at 0 station or even lower.* Progressive cervical dilatation with no change in the station of the presenting part implies fetopelvic disproportion.

An alternative method for designating the station of the fetal head has been used by some obstetricians (Friedman, 1978). Five levels, rather than three levels, are identified above and below the ischial spines. Each of the five levels differs from the adjacent level by approximately 1 cm. A change in station of 1 cm implies precision of mensuration that is not achievable in clinical practice. It is important that the two systems not be confused in the course of management of labor.

Detection of Ruptured Membranes. The pregnant woman should be well coached antepartum to observe for leakage of fluid from the vagina and to report such an occurrence promptly. Rupture of the membranes is significant for three reasons: First, if the presenting part is not fixed in the pelvis, the possibility of prolapse of the cord to cause cord compression is greatly increased. Second, labor is likely to occur soon if the pregnancy is at or near term. Third, if the fetus remains in utero upward of 24 hours or more after the rupture of the membranes, there is likelihood of serious intrauterine infection unless vigorous steps are taken to minimize invasion of the uterus by potentially pathogenic organisms.

A firm diagnosis of rupture of the membranes is not always easy to make unless amnionic fluid is seen or felt escaping from the cervical os by the examiner. Although several diagnostic tests for the detection of ruptured membranes have been recommended, none is completely reliable. Perhaps the most widely employed procedures involve testing the acidity or alkalinity of the vaginal fluid. The basis for these tests is the fact that normally the pH of the vaginal secretion ranges between 4.5 and 5.5, whereas that of the amnionic fluid is usually 7.0 to 7.5.

Nitrazine Test.

The use of the indicator nitrazine for the diagnosis of ruptured membranes was first suggested by Baptisi (1938) and is a simple and fairly reliable method. Test papers are impregnated with the dye, and the color of the reaction is interpreted by comparison with a standard color chart. The pH of the vaginal secretion is estimated by inserting a sterile cotton-tipped applicator deeply into the vagina and then touching it to a strip of the nitrazine paper and comparing the color of the paper with the chart. Color changes are interpreted as follows:

Probably Intact Membranes

- Yellow   pH 5.0
- Olive-yellow   pH 5.5
- Olive-green   pH 6.0

Ruptured Membranes

- Blue-green   pH 6.5
- Blue-gray   pH 7.0
- Deep blue   pH 7.5

Baptisi (1938) pointed out that a false reading is likely to be encountered in women with intact membranes who have an unusually large amount of bloody show, since blood, like amnionic fluid, is not acidic. A more extended study of the nitrazine test by a slightly different technique was made by Abe (1940), who found the nitrazine test to be correct in 98.9 percent of women with known rupture of membranes and in 96.2 percent of women with intact membranes. In clinical practice, however, these tests will not yield such accurate results because they are used in questionable cases in which the amount of fluid is small and therefore more susceptible to a change in pH by admixed blood and vaginal secretions.

Other Evaluations.

The maternal blood pressure, temperature, pulse, and respiratory rate are checked for any abnormality, and these are recorded. The Pregnancy Record is promptly reviewed to identify complications. Any problem identified previously during the antepartum period, as well as any that were anticipated, should be prominently displayed in the Pregnancy Record, along with the plan of management.

Preparation of Vulva and Perineum.

The woman is placed on a bedpan with her legs widely separated. While washing the region, the attendant holds a sponge to the woman's introitus to prevent wash water from running into the vagina. Scrubbing is directed from above downward and away from the introitus. Attention should be paid to careful cleansing of the vulvar folds during this procedure. As the scrub sponge passes over the anal region, it is discarded immediately. In many hospitals the hair on the lower half of the vulva and the perineum is removed either by shaving or by clipping.

Vaginal vs. Rectal Examinations.

Ideally, after the vulvar and perineal regions have been prepared properly, and the examiner has donned sterile gloves, the thumb and forefinger of one hand separate the labia widely to expose the vaginal opening and prevent the examining fingers from coming in contact with the inner surfaces of the labia. The index and second fingers of the other hand are then introduced into the vagina (Fig. 17-1A–C). During vaginal examination, a precise routine of evaluation as described in the section on Admittance Vaginal Examination should be followed. It is important not to withdraw the fingers from the vagina until the examination is entirely completed.

Rectal examinations were once considered to be much safer than vaginal because they were less likely to carry bacteria from the introitus into the cervix and then the uterus. A vaginal examination, *properly performed with appropriate preparation and care,* is probably not much more likely than a rectal examination to carry pathogenic bacteria through the dilating cervix into the uterus. In spite of past reports that vaginal examinations during labor do not contribute to morbidity, clinical experience in certain circumstances strongly suggests the opposite, especially in cases of early rupture of the membranes followed by repeated vaginal examinations casually performed by multiple examiners.

Enema.

Early in labor, a cleansing enema is generally given to minimize subsequent contamination by feces, which otherwise may be a problem, especially during delivery. A ready-to-use enema solution of sodium phosphates in a disposable container (Fleet enema) has proved satisfactory at Parkland Memorial Hospital. Enemas are not used to stimulate labor. The infamous "3H" enema ("High, Hot, and Hell of a Lot") has no place in obstetrics!

Laboratory.

When admitted in labor, most often the hematocrit, or hemoglobin concentration, should be re-

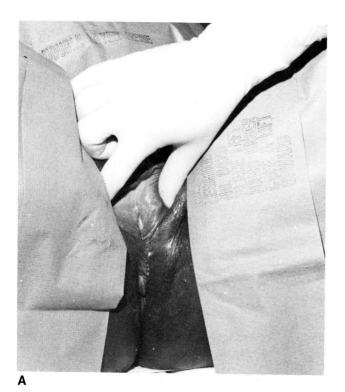

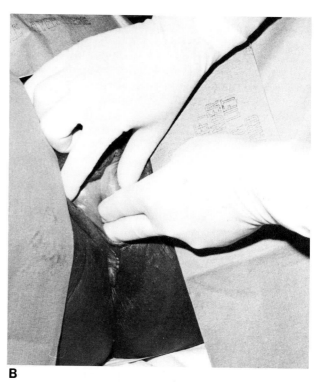

Figure 17-1. A. Vaginal examination. The labia are separated with a sterile gloved hand. **B.** Vaginal examination. The first and second fingers of the other sterile gloved hand are carefully inserted through the introitus.

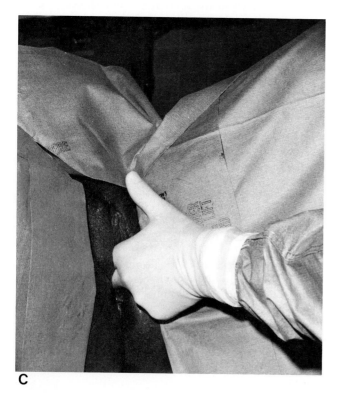

Figure 17-1. C. During vaginal examination, the fourth and fifth fingers should not contact the anus.

checked. The hematocrit can be measured easily and quickly. Blood may be collected in a plain tube from which a heparinized capillary tube is filled immediately. Employing a small microhematocrit centrifuge in the labor-delivery unit, the value can be obtained in 3 minutes. The labeled tube of blood is allowed to clot and is kept on hand for blood group and screen, if needed, or otherwise used for routine serology. A voided urine specimen, as free as possible of debris, is examined for protein and glucose.

SUBSEQUENT MANAGEMENT OF FIRST STAGE

As soon as possible after admittance, the remainder of the general physical examination is completed. The physician can reach a conclusion about the normalcy of the pregnancy only when all the examinations have been completed. The physician must then draw upon the information obtained from these results, as well as all information previously compiled during the antepartum period. A rational plan for monitoring labor can then be established based on the needs of the fetus and the mother. If no abnormality is identified or suspected, the mother should be assured that all is well. Although the average duration of the first stage of labor in nulliparous women is about 8 hours and in parous women about 5 hours, there is marked individual variation. Most often, therefore, any precise statement as to the duration of her labor is unwise. Obstetricians and others who venture to make precise statements will find that their predictions are likely to be faulty and the mother and family are made more anxious needlessly.

Monitoring Fetal Well-Being During Labor

The word *monitor* currently is equated in the minds of some only with continuous electronic recording of the fetal heart rate and intrauterine pressures. The desirability, let alone the necessity, of monitoring for *all* labors has certainly not been established, as pointed out elsewhere (see Chapter 14, p. 284).

It is mandatory, however, that for a good pregnancy outcome, a well-defined program be established that provides careful surveillance of the well-being of both the mother and the fetus. All observations must be appropriately recorded. The frequency, intensity, and duration of uterine contractions, and the response of the fetal heart rate to the contractions are of considerable concern. These features can be promptly evaluated in logical sequence.

Fetal Heart Rate. The heart rate of the fetus may be identified with a suitable stethoscope or any of a variety of doppler ultrasonic devices (Fig. 17-2A, B). Changes in the fetal heart rate that are most likely to be ominous almost always are detectable immediately after a uterine contraction. Therefore, it is imperative that the fetal heart be monitored by auscultation immediately after a contraction. To avoid confusing maternal and fetal heart actions, the maternal pulse should be counted as the fetal heart rate is counted. Otherwise, maternal tachycardia may be misinterpreted as a normal fetal heart rate.

Fetal distress, i.e., loss of fetal well-being, is suspected if the fetal heart rate immediately after a contraction is repeatedly below 120 per minute. Fetal distress very likely exists if the rate is heard to be less than 100 per minute, even though there is recovery to a rate in the 120 to 160 range before the next contraction. When decelerations of this magnitude are found after a contraction, the fetus may be in jeopardy and further labor, if allowed, is often best monitored electronically, as described in Chapter 14.

During the first stage of labor, in the absence of any abnormalities, the fetal heart is best checked immediately after a contraction at least every 15 minutes.

The findings of the study by Benson and associates (1968) have been quoted widely as evidence that auscultation of the fetal heart during labor is unreliable for detecting fetal distress save in an extreme degree. Their study by design ignored the determination of the fetal heart rate for at least the first 30 seconds after a contraction, a critical period for identifying ominous decelerations (see Chapter 14, p. 287). Moreover, the protocol for evaluating the fetal heart every 15 minutes during the first stage of labor and

every 5 minutes during the second stage frequently was not followed.

Uterine Contractions. The examiner with the palm of the hand lightly on the uterus determines the time of onset of the contraction. The intensity of the contraction is gauged from the degree of firmness the uterus achieves. At the acme of effective contractions, the finger or thumb cannot readily indent the uterus. Next, the time that the contraction disappears is noted. This sequence is repeated with the following contraction in order to evaluate the frequency, duration, and intensity of uterine contractions. It is inappropriate simply to describe ongoing uterine contractions, or labor, as "good." "Good" uterine contractions can be identified only retrospectively, that is, if the contractions produced orderly effacement and dilatation of the cervix with descent of the presenting part followed by uncomplicated delivery of an uncompromised infant. Then the contractions were good!

Attendance in Labor. Ideally, the person who performs these measurements is able to remain with the mother throughout labor to provide psychologic support as well as to discern promptly any fetal or maternal abnormalities. Haverkamp and co-workers (1976, 1979) have demonstrated that an equally satisfactory outcome for the fetus can be achieved without continuous electronic monitoring of the fetal heart rate, continuous intrauterine pressure recording, and fetal scalp blood pH measurement *if the mother and fetus are closely attended by appropriately trained labor room personnel.* Given a choice, many women would probably prefer the reassurance of the nearly continuous presence of the obstetrician or of a compassionate well-trained obstetric associate to that of a metal cabinet and its wires and tubes that invade her and her fetus.

Maternal Position During Labor. The normal mother and fetus need not be confined to bed early in labor prior to use of analgesia. A comfortable chair may be beneficial psychologically and perhaps physiologically. In bed, the mother should be allowed to assume the position she finds most comfortable, which will be lateral recumbent most of the time. She must not be restricted to lying supine.

Subsequent Vaginal Examinations. During the first stage of labor, the need for subsequent vaginal examinations to identify the status of the cervix and the station and position of the presenting part will vary considerably. When the membranes rupture, the examination should be repeated immediately if the fetal head was not definitely engaged at the previous vaginal examination. In any event, the fetal heart rate should be checked immediately and during the next uterine contraction to help detect cord compression.

Analgesia. Most often, analgesia is initiated on the basis of the woman's discomfort, a uterine contraction

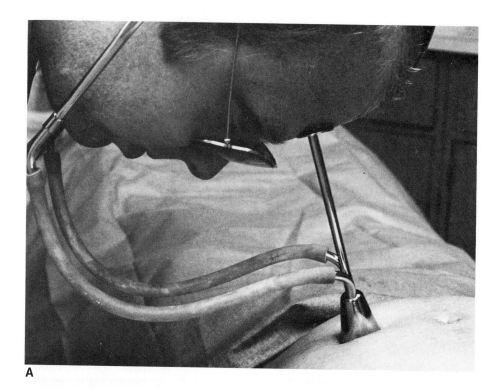

A

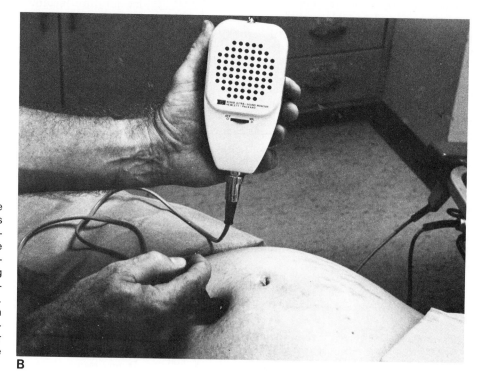

Figure 17-2. A. Monitoring the fetal heart rate with a DeLee-Hillis fetoscope. The bell of the stethoscope is firmly applied to the uterine wall to improve the transmission of sound. **B.** Monitoring the fetal heart rate by use of ultrasound and the doppler effect. The transducer may be held in an appropriate place on the abdomen by a comfortable rubber strap yet allow the mother to be free to move about.

B

pattern of established labor, and cervical dilatation of at least 2 cm. The kinds of analgesia, the amounts, and the frequency of administration should be based on the need to allay pain on the one hand and the likelihood of delivering a depressed infant on the other (see Chapter 18, p. 354).

The timing, the method of administration, and the size of initial and subsequent doses of systemically acting analgesic agents are based to a considerable degree on the anticipated interval of time until delivery. A repeat vaginal examination is often appropriate, therefore, before administering more analgesia. With the onset of symptoms characteristic of the second stage of labor, that is, an urge to bear down or "push," the status of the cervix and the presenting part should be reevaluated. A common tendency, especially at large, busy public institutions, has been too little "laying on of hands" to gauge the quality of labor and too much "putting in of hands" to identify cervical dilatation.

Maternal Vital Signs. The mother's temperature, blood pressure, and pulse are evaluated every 1 to 2 hours. The blood pressure is taken between contractions. The blood pressure normally rises during a contraction (Kjeldsen, 1979). If membranes have been ruptured for many hours before the onset of labor, or if there is a borderline elevation, the temperature should be checked hourly during labor. Moreover, with prolonged rupture of the membranes, the pregnancy should be considered high risk.

Amniotomy. If the membranes are thought to be intact, there is great temptation even during normal labor to perform amniotomy. The presumed benefits are more rapid labor, earlier detection of instances of meconium staining of amnionic fluid, and the opportunity to apply an electrode to the fetus and insert a pressure catheter into the uterine cavity. Amniotomy may shorten the length of labor slightly but there is no evidence that shorter labor is necessarily beneficial to the fetus or to the mother. Indeed, the reverse may be true (Caldeyro-Barcia and associates, 1974). If amniotomy is performed, aseptic technique should be attempted and the fetal head must not be dislodged from the pelvis to hasten the escape of amnionic fluid; to do so invites prolapse of the umbilical cord.

Oral Intake. In essentially all circumstances, food and oral fluids should be withheld during active labor and delivery. Gastric emptying time typically is remarkably prolonged once labor is established and analgesics are administered. As the consequence, ingested food and most medications remain in the stomach and are not absorbed. However, they can be vomited and aspirated!

Intravenous Fluids. Although it has become customary in many hospitals to establish an intravenous infusion system routinely early in labor, there is seldom any real need for such in the normally pregnant woman at least

until analgesia is administered. An intravenous infusion system is advantageous during the immediate puerperium in order to administer oxytocin prophylactically and at times therapeutically when uterine hypotonicity persists. Morever, with longer labors the administration of glucose, some salt, and water to the otherwise fasting woman at the rate of 60 to 120 ml per hour is efficacious to combat dehydration and acidosis.

Urinary Bladder Function. Bladder distension must be avoided, since it can lead both to obstructed labor and to subsequent bladder hypotonia and infection. In the course of each abdominal examination, the suprapubic region should be palpated in order to detect a filling bladder. If the bladder is readily palpated above the symphysis, the woman should be encouraged to void. At times she can ambulate with assistance to a toilet and successfully void, even though she could not void on a bedpan. If the bladder is distended and she cannot void, catheterization is indicated. It is likely, however, to be less traumatic to catheterize again during labor, if needed, than to leave an indwelling catheter in place.

MANAGEMENT OF SECOND STAGE

Identification

With full dilatation of the cervix, which signifies the onset of the second stage of labor, the woman typically begins to bear down and with descent of the presenting part she develops the urge to defecate. Uterine contractions and the accompanying expulsive forces may last 1½ minutes and recur at times after a myometrial resting phase of no more than a minute.

Duration

The median duration of the second stage (from complete dilatation of the cervix to delivery) is 50 minutes in nulliparas and 20 minutes in multiparas, but it can be highly variable. In a woman of higher parity with a stretched vagina and perineum, two or three expulsive efforts after the cervix is fully dilated may suffice to complete the delivery of the infant. Conversely, in a woman with a contracted pelvis or a large fetus, or with impaired expulsive efforts from conduction anesthesia or intense sedation, the second stage may become abnormally long.

Fetal Heart Rate. It is essential to good care that the status of the fetal heart rate be identified at 5-minute intervals during this critical period. Slowing of the fetal heart rate induced by compression of the fetal head is common during a contraction and the accompanying maternal expulsive efforts. If recovery of the fetal heart rate is prompt after the contraction and expulsive efforts cease, labor is allowed to continue. Not all instances of

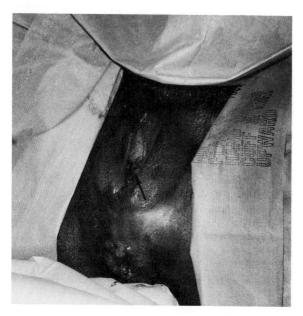

Figure 17-3. Scalp (arrow) appearing at vulva during a contraction.

slowing of the fetal heart during the second stage of labor are the consequence of head compression, however. The vigorous force generated within the uterus by its contraction and by the woman's expulsive efforts may reduce placental perfusion appreciably. Descent of the fetus through the birth canal towards the perineum and the consequent reduction in uterine volume may trigger some degree of premature separation of the placenta, with further compromise of fetal well-being. Descent of the fetus is even more likely to tighten a loop or loops of umbilical cord around the fetus, especially the neck, sufficiently to obstruct umbilical blood flow. Prolonged, uninterrupted expulsive efforts by the mother can be dangerous to the fetus especially in this circumstance. Maternal tachycardia, which is common during the second stage, must not be mistaken for a normal fetal heart rate.

Maternal Expulsive Efforts. In most cases, bearing-down is reflex and spontaneous in the second stage of labor, but occasionally the woman does not employ her expulsive forces to good advantage and coaching is desirable. Her legs should be half-flexed so that she can push with them against the mattress. Instructions should be to take a deep breath as soon as the next uterine contraction begins and, with her breath held, to exert downward pressure exactly as though she were straining at stool. She should not be encouraged to "push" beyond the time of completion of each uterine contraction. Instead, she and her fetus should be allowed to rest and recover from the combined effects of the uterine contraction, breath holding, and considerable physical effort.

Usually bearing-down efforts are rewarded by increasing bulging of the perineum, that is, by further de-

scent of the fetal head. The mother should be informed of such progress, for encouragement at this stage is very important. During this period of active bearing-down, the fetal heart rate auscultated immediately after the contraction is likely to be slow but should recover to normal range before the next expulsive effort.

As the head descends through the pelvis, small particles of feces are frequently expelled by the mother. As they appear at the anus, they should be sponged downward with large pledgets soaked in diluted soap solution. As the head descends still farther, the perineum begins to bulge and the overlying skin becomes tense and glistening. Now the scalp of the fetus may be visible through the slitlike vulvar opening (Fig. 17-3). At this time, or before in instances where little perineal resistance to expulsion is anticipated, the woman and her fetus are formally prepared for delivery.

Preparation for Delivery. Actual delivery of the fetus can be accomplished with the mother in a variety of positions. The most widely used and often the most satisfactory one is the dorsal lithotomy position on a delivery table with leg supports. In placing the legs in leg-holders, care should be taken not to separate the legs too widely or place one leg higher than the other. The popliteal region should rest comfortably in the proximal portion and the heel in the distal portion of the leg-holder. Too often the leg is forced to conform to the existing setting. Cramps in the leg may develop in the second stage of labor in part because of pressure by the fetal head on nerves in the pelvis. Such cramps may be relieved by changing the position of the leg or by brief massage, but leg cramps should never be ignored.

No one should be permitted in the delivery room without a scrub suit, a mask covering both nose and mouth, and a cap that completely covers the hair. Preparation for actual delivery entails thorough vulvar and perineal scrubbing and covering with sterile drapes in such a way that only the immediate area about the vulva is exposed (Fig. 17-4A, B).

Scrubbing and Gloving. Since sterile rubber gloves are punctured easily or tear occasionally, the necessity for meticulously cleaning the hands before putting on gloves is apparent. Even with these precautions, the possibility of disseminating bacteria within the genital tract is not eliminated entirely, since the organisms may be carried up from the vaginal outlet by the gloved finger.

SPONTANEOUS DELIVERY

Delivery of the Head

With each contraction, the perineum bulges increasingly and the vulvovaginal opening becomes more and more dilated by the fetal head (Fig. 17-5), gradually forming an ovoid and finally an almost circular opening. With the cessation of each contraction, the opening becomes

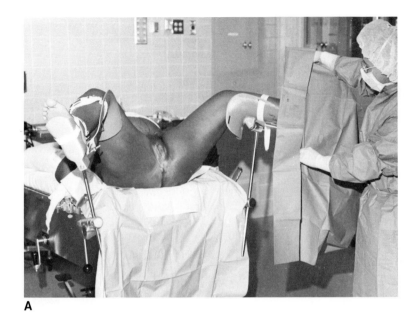

A

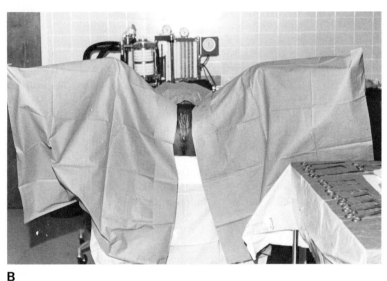

B

Figure 17-4. A. The vulva, perineum, and adjacent regions have been thoroughly scrubbed. Sterile disposable drapes are being applied. **B.** The field is sterile-draped in preparation for delivery.

smaller as the head recedes. As the head becomes increasingly visible, the vaginal outlet and vulva are stretched further until they ultimately encircle the largest diameter of the baby's head (Fig. 17-6). This encirclement of the largest diameter of the fetal head by the vulvar ring is known as *crowning*.

Unless an episiotomy has been made, as described on page 347, the perineum by now is extremely thin and, in the case of the nulliparous woman especially, is almost at the point of rupture with each contraction. At the same time the anus becomes greatly stretched and protuberant, and the anterior wall of the rectum may be easily seen through it. Failure to perform an episiotomy by this time invites perineal lacerations and some degree of permanent relaxation of the pelvic floor with its possible sequelae of cystocele, rectocele, and uterine prolapse.

Ritgen Maneuver. By the time the head distends the vulva and perineum during a contraction sufficiently to open the vaginal introitus to a diameter of 5 cm or so, it is desirable to drape a towel over one gloved hand to protect it from the anus and then exert forward pressure on the chin of the fetus through the perineum just in front of the coccyx, while the other hand exerts pressure superiorly against the occiput (Fig. 17-7). Although this maneuver is simpler than that originally described by Ritgen (1855), it is customarily designated the Ritgen maneuver, or the modified Ritgen maneuver. It allows the physician to control the delivery of the head. It also favors extension, so that the head is delivered with its smallest diameters passing through the introitus and over the perineum (Fig. 17-8). The head is delivered slowly with the base of the occiput rotating around the

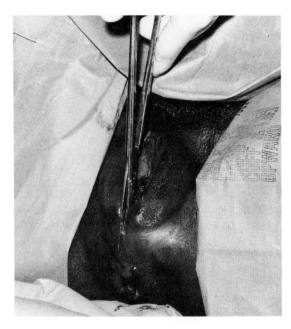

Figure 17-5. Vulva partially distended by fetal head. Midline episiotomy being made.

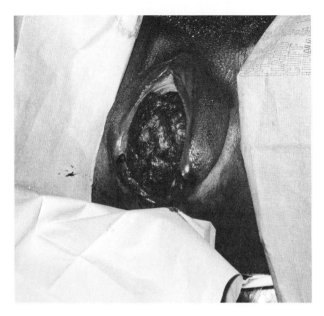

Figure 17-6. Birth of head. The occiput is being kept close to the symphysis by moderate pressure to the fetal chin at the tip of the maternal coccyx.

lower margin of the symphysis pubis as a fulcrum, while the bregma (anterior fontanel), brow, and face pass successively over the perineum (Fig. 17-9).

Clearing the Nasopharynx. To minimize the likelihood of aspiration of amnionic fluid debris and blood that might occur once the thorax is delivered and the infant can inspire, the face is quickly wiped and the nares and mouth are aspirated as demonstrated in Figure 20-1.

Nuchal Cord. Next the finger should be passed to the neck of the fetus to ascertain whether it is encircled by one or more coils of the umbilical cord (Fig. 17-10). Coils occur in about 25 percent of cases and ordinarily do no harm. If a coil is felt, it should be drawn down between the fingers and, if loose enough, slipped over the infant's head. If it is applied too tightly to the neck to be slipped over the head, it should be cut between two clamps and the infant delivered promptly.

Delivery of Shoulders

After its birth, the head falls posteriorly, bringing the face almost into contact with the anus. As described in Chapter 16, the occiput promptly turns toward one of the maternal thighs so that the head assumes a transverse position. The successive movements of restitution and external rotation indicate that the bisacromial diameter (transverse diameter of the thorax) has rotated into the anteroposterior diameter of the pelvis.

In most cases, the shoulders appear at the vulva just after external rotation and are born spontaneously. Oc-

casionally, a delay occurs and immediate extraction may appear advisable. In that event, the sides of the head are grasped with the two hands and *gentle* downward traction applied until the anterior shoulder appears under the pubic arch. Then, by an upward movement, the posterior shoulder is delivered and the anterior shoulder usually drops down from beneath the symphysis. An equally effective method entails completion of delivery of the anterior shoulder before that of the posterior (Fig. 17-11).

The rest of the body almost always follows the shoulders without difficulty, but in case of prolonged delay its birth may be hastened by *moderate* traction on the head and moderate pressure on the uterine fundus. Hooking the fingers in the axillae should be avoided, however, since it may injure the nerves of the upper extremity, producing a transient or possibly even a permanent paralysis. Traction, furthermore, should be exerted only in the direction of the long axis of the infant, for if applied obliquely it causes bending of the neck and excessive stretching of the brachial plexus.

Immediately after extrusion of the infant, there is usually a gush of amnionic fluid, often tinged with blood, but not grossly bloody.

Clamping the Cord

The umbilical cord is cut between two clamps such as pean clamps placed 4 or 5 cm from the abdomen, and, subsequently, about 2 or 3 cm from the abdomen, a formal cord clamp is applied. A plastic clamp that is safe, efficient, easy to sterilize, and fairly inexpensive is shown in Figure 17-12.

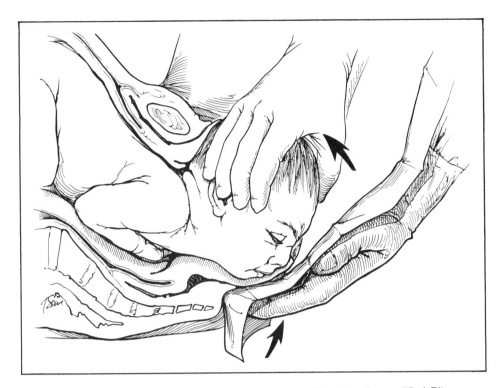

Figure 17-7. Near completion of the delivery of the fetal head by the modified Ritgen maneuver. Moderate upward pressure is applied to the fetal chin by the posterior hand covered with a sterile towel while the suboccipital region of the fetal head is held against the symphysis.

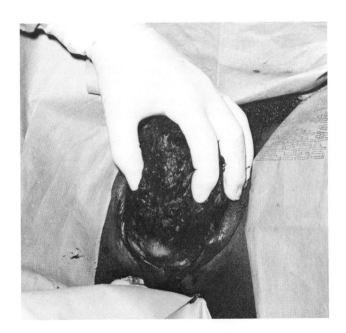

Figure 17-8. Pressure is applied through the towel covering the hand to the underside of the chin of the infant as soon as the occiput is beyond the symphysis. This extends the head. At the same time, the fingers of the other hand simultaneously elevate the scalp to help extend the head.

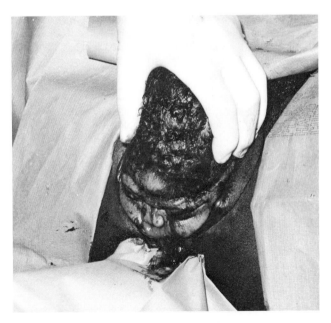

Figure 17-9. Birth of head; the mouth is appearing over perineum.

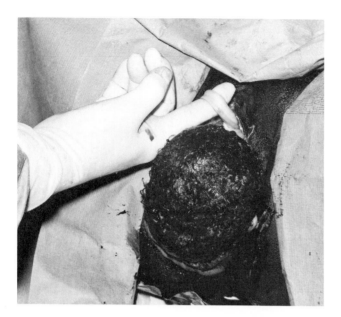

Figure 17-10. Cord identified around the neck. It readily slipped over the head.

Timing of Cord Clamping. If after delivery the infant is placed at the level of the vaginal introitus or below and the fetoplacental circulation is not immediately occluded by clamping the cord, as much as 100 ml of blood may be shifted from the placenta to the infant.

Yao and Lind (1969, 1974) measured the residual volume of placental blood in response to positioning the infant at precisely measured distances above or below the introitus for varying periods of time before clamping the cord. They observed that placing the infant within 10 cm above or below the introitus for 3 minutes before clamping the cord resulted in the shift of about 80 ml of blood from the placenta to the infant. Lowering to 40 cm below the introitus for only 30 seconds before clamping effected the same degree of transfer. If the infant was held at 50 or 60 cm above the introitus, however, transfer of blood to the infant was negligible even after 3 minutes.

One benefit to be derived from placental transfusion is the fact that the hemoglobin in 80 ml of placental blood that shifts to the fetus eventually provides about 50 mg of iron to the infant's stores and no doubt reduces the frequency of iron-deficiency anemia later in infancy. In the presence of accelerated destruction of erythrocytes, as occurs with maternal alloimmunization, the bilirubin formed from the added erythrocytes contributes further to the danger of hyperbilirubinemia (see Chapter 38, p. 776). Although theoretically the risk of circulatory overloading from gross hypervolemia is formidable, especially in premature infants, the addition of placental blood to the infant's circulation does not ordinarily cause difficulty.

Our policy is to clamp the cord after first thoroughly clearing the infant's airway, all of which usually takes upwards of 30 seconds. The infant is not elevated above the introitus at vaginal delivery nor above the maternal abdominal wall at cesarean section. The cord is then clamped.

MANAGEMENT OF THE THIRD STAGE

Immediately after delivery of the infant, the height of the uterine fundus and its consistency are determined. As long as the uterus remains firm and there is no unusual bleeding, watchful waiting until the placenta is separated is the usual practice. No massage is practiced; the hand is simply rested on the fundus frequently, to make certain that the organ does not become atonic and filled with blood behind a separated placenta.

Signs of Placental Separation

Since attempts to express the placenta prior to its separation are futile and possibly dangerous, it is most important that the following signs of placental separation be recognized:

1. The uterus becomes globular and, as a rule, firmer. This sign is the earliest to appear.
2. There is often a sudden gush of blood.
3. The uterus rises in the abdomen because the placenta, having separated, passes down into the lower uterine segment and vagina, where its bulk pushes the uterus upward.
4. The umbilical cord protrudes farther out of the vagina, indicating that the placenta has descended.

These signs sometimes appear within about a minute after delivery of the infant and usually within 5 minutes. When the placenta has separated, the physician first ascertains that the uterus is firmly contracted. The mother, if she is not anesthetized, may be asked to bear down, and the intraabdominal pressure so produced may be adequate to expel the placenta. If these efforts fail, or if spontaneous expulsion is not practicable because of anesthesia, the physician, again having made certain that the uterus is contracted firmly, exerts pressure with the hand on the fundus to propel the detached placenta into the vagina, as depicted and described in Figure 17-13.

Delivery of the Placenta

Placental expression should never be forced before placental separation lest the uterus be turned inside out. *Inversion of the uterus* is one of the grave accidents associated with delivery (see Chapter 34, p. 715). As pressure is applied to the body of the uterus (Fig. 17-13), the umbilical cord is kept slightly taut. The uterus is lifted cephalad with the abdominal hand. This maneuver is repeated until the placenta reaches the introitus.

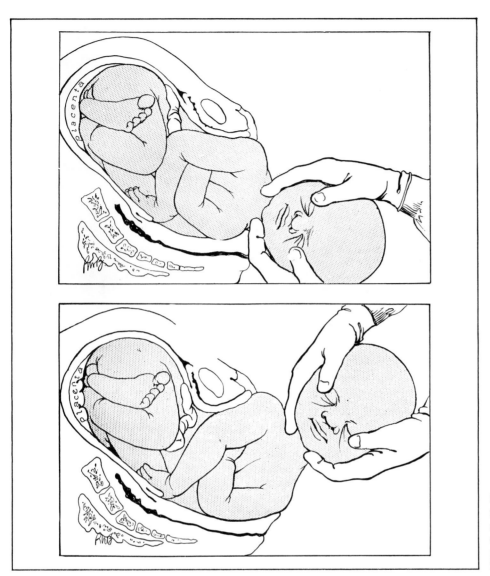

Figure 17-11. *Gentle* downward traction to bring about descent of anterior shoulder (top). Delivery of anterior shoulder completed; *gentle* upward traction to deliver the posterior shoulder (bottom).

Traction on the cord, however, must not be used to pull the placenta out of the uterus. As the placenta passes through the introitus, pressure on the uterus is stopped. The placenta is then gently lifted away from the introitus (Fig. 17-14). Care is taken to prevent the membranes from being torn off and left behind. If the membranes start to tear, they are grasped with a clamp and removed by gentle traction (Fig. 17-15). The placenta should be examined carefully to ascertain whether it has been delivered in its entirety from the uterine cavity.

Manual Removal of Placenta. If at any time there is brisk bleeding and the placenta cannot be delivered by these techniques, manual removal of the placenta is indicated, with all of the safeguards described in Chapter 34 (p. 709).

Occasionally, the placenta will not separate promptly. A question to which there is still no definite answer concerns the length of time that should elapse in the absence of bleeding before the placenta is manually removed. Manual removal of the placenta is rightfully practiced much sooner and more often than in the past. In fact, some obstetricians practice routine manual removal of any placenta that has not separated spontaneously by the time they have completed delivery of the infant and care of the cord. The majority, however, do not resort so promptly to manual removal of the placenta, although the procedure must be performed whenever bleeding is excessive.

Routine manual removal of the placenta has proved to be a safe procedure only in the following circumstances: (1) if few vaginal examinations were performed during labor and if they were accompanied by a minimum of bacterial contamination; (2) if the vulva, perineum, and adjacent regions were carefully prepared and draped prior to delivery; (3) if

344

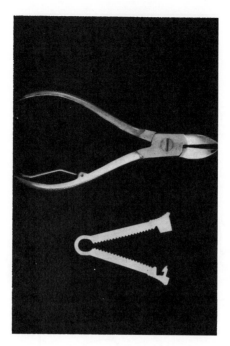

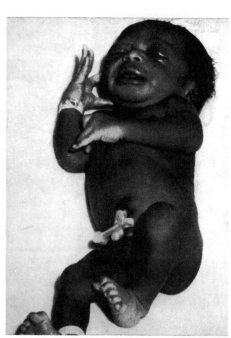

Figure 17-12. Plastic cord clamp. These clamps lock in place and cannot slip. They are removed on the second or third day simply by cutting the plastic at the loop, or they can be allowed to drop off with the cord.

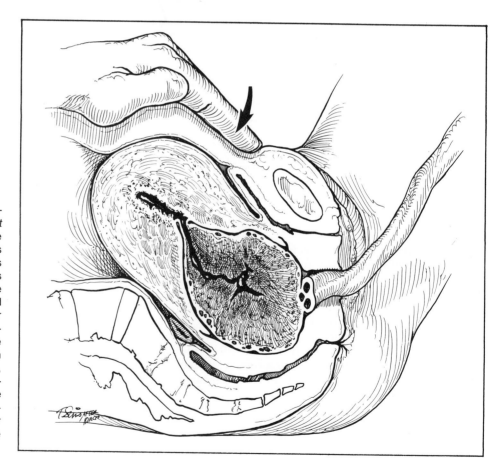

Figure 17-13. Expression of placenta. Note that the hand is *not* trying to push the fundus of the uterus through the birth canal! As the placenta leaves the uterus and enters the vagina, the uterus is elevated by the hand on the abdomen (arrow) while the cord is held in position. The mother can aid in the delivery of the placenta by bearing down. As the placenta reaches the perineum the cord is lifted, which, in turn, lifts the placenta out of the vagina. Adherent membranes are teased away from thin attachments so as to prevent their being torn off and retained in the birth canal.

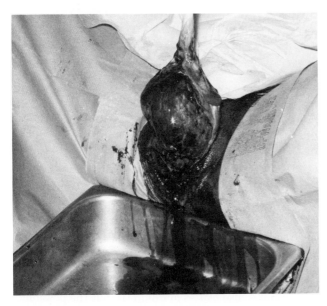

Figure 17-14. The placenta is removed from the vagina by lifting the cord.

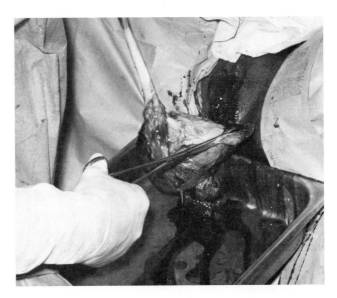

Figure 17-15. Membranes that were somewhat adherent to the uterine lining are separated by gentle traction with a ring forceps.

delivery was accomplished without contaminating the genital tract; and (4) if regional or general anesthesia is satisfactory. In other circumstances, since the risks of immediate manual removal of the placenta outweigh the advantages, the procedure should be restricted to instances in which hemorrhage threatens.

"Fourth Stage" of Labor

The placenta, membranes, and umbilical cord should be examined for completeness and for anomalies, as described in Chapter 23.

The hour immediately following delivery of the placenta is a critical period and has been designated by some obstetricians as the "fourth stage of labor." Even though oxytocics are administered, as described below, postpartum hemorrhage as the result of uterine relaxation is most likely to occur at this time. As emphasized in Chapter 19 (p. 374), it is mandatory that the uterus be evaluated very frequently throughout this period by a competent attendant, who places a hand frequently on the fundus and massages it at the slightest sign of relaxation. At the same time, the vaginal and perineal region is also inspected frequently to allow prompt identification of any excessive bleeding.

OXYTOCIC AGENTS

After the uterus has been emptied and the placenta has been delivered, the primary mechanism by which hemostasis is achieved at the placental site is vasoconstriction produced by a well-contracted myometrium (see Chapter 21, p. 391). Oxytocin (Pitocin, Syntocinon), ergonovine

maleate (Ergotrate), and methylergonovine maleate (Methergine) are employed in various ways in the conduct of the third stage of labor, principally to stimulate myometrial contractions and thereby reduce the blood loss.

Oxytocin

The synthetic form of the octapeptide oxytocin is commercially available in the United States as Syntocinon and Pitocin; 1 mg of oxytocin is equal to about 500 USP units. Each milliliter of injectable oxytocin contains 10 USP units of oxytocin, which is not effective by mouth. The half-life of intravenously infused oxytocin is very short, perhaps 3 minutes.

Before delivery, the spontaneously laboring uterus is very likely to be exquisitely sensitive to oxytocin. Even with an intravenous dose of a few milliunits per minute, the pregnant uterus may contract so violently as to kill the fetus, rupture itself, or both (see Chapter 29, p. 645). After delivery of the fetus, these dangers no longer exist. Nonetheless, at this time there are other potentially grave dangers from inappropriate use of oxytocin.

Cardiovascular Effects. Deleterious effects may on occasion follow the intravenous injection of a bolus of oxytocin. Hendricks and Brenner (1970), for example, demonstrated with the rapid intravenous injection of 5 units (0.5 ml) of oxytocin that the uterus contracted tetanically for several minutes but maternal blood pressure decreased simultaneously. In one dramatic instance of hypotension from uterine bleeding following delivery of twins, they noted that the injection of 5 units of oxytocin intravenously was followed promptly by a further de-

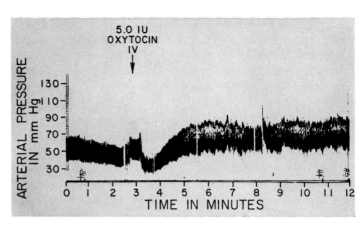

Figure 17-16. Adverse effect of the intravenous bolus of five units of oxytocin in a case of postpartum hemorrhage 18 minutes postdelivery. The hypotension worsened to a level of 44/26 mm Hg until saline was infused rapidly. (*From Hendricks and Brenner: Am J Obstet Gynecol 108:751, 1970.*)

crease in blood pressure from 70/42 to 44/26 mm Hg (Fig. 17-16). After rapid administration of 500 ml of saline, the blood pressure rose and the mother again became responsive.

Secher and co-workers (1978) consistently found in healthy women after an intravenous bolus of 10 units of oxytocin a transient but marked fall in arterial blood pressure that was followed rapidly by an abrupt increase in cardiac output. They too conclude that these hemodynamic changes could be dangerous to women whose circulation was already compromised by hypovolemia or who had cardiac disease that limits cardiac output or is complicated by right-to-left shunts. Oxytocin should not, therefore, be given intravenously as a large bolus, but rather as a much more dilute solution by continuous intravenous infusion as described on page 347, or be injected intramuscularly in a dose of 10 units.

Antidiuresis. Another important adverse effect of oxytocin is antidiuresis, caused primarily by reabsorption of free water. Abdul-Karim and Assali (1961) demonstrated clearly that in both pregnant and nonpregnant women oxytocin possesses antidiuretic activity. In women who are undergoing diuresis in response to the administration of water, the continuous intravenous infusion of 20 milliunits of oxytocin per minute usually produces a demonstrable decrease in urine flow. When the rate of infusion is raised to 40 milliunits per minute, urinary flow is strikingly reduced. With doses of this magnitude, it is possible to produce water intoxication if the oxytocin is administered in a large volume of electrolyte-free aqueous dextrose solution (Liggins, 1962; Whalley and Pritchard, 1963; Eggers and Fliegner, 1979).

The hyponatremic, hypoosmotic state is not limited to just the mother. Schwartz and Jones (1978), for example, described convulsions in both the mother and her newborn infant following the administration of 6.5 liters of 5 percent dextrose solution and 36 units of oxytocin predelivery. The concentration of sodium in cord plasma was 114 mEq/L.

In general, if oxytocin is to be administered at a relatively high rate of infusion for a considerable period of time, increasing the concentration of the hormone is preferable to increasing the rate of flow of the more di-

lute solution. The antidiuretic effect of intravenously administered oxytocin disappears within a few minutes after the infusion is stopped. Oxytocin injected intramuscularly in doses of 5 to 10 units (0.5 to 1 ml) every 15 to 30 minutes also causes antidiuresis, but the possibility of water intoxication is not nearly so great, since large volumes of electrolyte-free aqueous solution are not required as a vehicle (Whalley, Pritchard, 1963).

Ergonovine and Methylergonovine

Ergonovine is an alkaloid obtained either from ergot, a fungus that grows upon rye and some other grains, or synthesized in part from lysergic acid. Methylergonovine is a very similar alkaloid made from lysergic acid. The alkaloids are dispensed as the maleate (Ergotrate and Methergine, respectively) either in solution for parenteral use or in tablets for oral use.

Effects. There is no convincing evidence of any appreciable difference in the actions of ergonovine and methylergonovine; therefore, they will be considered together. Whether given intravenously, intramuscularly, or orally, ergonovine and methylergonovine are powerful stimulants of myometrial contraction, exerting an effect that may persist for hours. The sensitivity of the pregnant uterus to ergonovine and methylergonovine is very great. In pregnant women, an intravenous dose of as little as 0.1 mg, or an oral dose of only 0.25 mg, results in a tetanic contraction that occurs almost immediately after intravenous injection of the drug and within a few minutes after intramuscular or oral administration. Moreover, the response is sustained with little tendency toward relaxation. The tetanic effect of ergonovine and methylergonovine is effective for the prevention and control of postpartum hemorrhage but is very dangerous for the fetus and the mother prior to delivery.

The parenteral administration of these alkaloids, especially by the intravenous route, sometimes initiates transient but severe hypertension. Such a reaction is most likely to occur when conduction anesthesia is used for delivery and in women who are prone to develop hypertension. Browning (1974) has vividly described four instances of serious side effects postdelivery attributable to 0.5 mg of ergonovine administered intramuscularly. Two women promptly became severely hypertensive, the third became hypertensive and convulsed, and the fourth suffered a cardiac arrest. Because of the frequency of hypertension among our obstetric population, these alkaloids are not used routinely at Parkland Memorial Hospital.

Oxytocics During and After Delivery. Oxytocin, ergonovine, and methylergonovine are all employed widely in the conduct of the normal third stage of labor, but the timing of their administration differs in various institutions. Oxytocin and especially ergonovine given before delivery of the placenta will decrease blood loss somewhat. Of considerable concern, the use of oxytocin, and especially ergonovine or methylergonovine, before delivery of the placenta may entrap an undiagnosed and therefore undelivered second twin. This may prove injurious, if not fatal, to the entrapped fetus. In most cases following uncomplicated vaginal delivery, the third stage of labor can be conducted with reasonably small blood loss without using alkaloids of ergot.

If an intravenous infusion is in place, standard practice at Parkland Memorial Hospital has been to add 20 units (2 ml) of oxytocin per liter, which is administered after delivery of the placenta at a rate of 10 ml per minute for a few minutes until the uterus remains firmly contracted and the bleeding is controlled. Then the infusion rate is reduced to 1 to 2 ml per minute until the mother is ready for transfer from the recovery suite to the postpartum unit, when it is usually discontinued.

Lacerations of the Birth Canal

Lacerations of the vagina and perineum are classified as first, second, or third degree. Such lacerations most often are preventable with an appropriate episiotomy and avoidance of midforceps delivery.

First-degree lacerations involve the fourchet, the perineal skin, and vaginal mucous membrane but not the underlying fascia and muscle.

Second-degree lacerations (Fig. 17-17) involve, in addition to skin and mucous membrane, the fascia and muscles of the perineal body but not the rectal sphincter. These tears usually extend upward on one or both sides of the vagina, forming an irregular triangular injury.

Third-degree lacerations extend through the skin, mucous membrane, and perineal body, and involve the anal sphincter. Not infrequently, these third-degree lacerations may also extend a distance up the anterior wall of the rectum.

A so-called *fourth-degree laceration* is distinguished by some. This designation is applied to third-degree tears that extend through the rectal mucosa to expose the lumen of the rectum. The term fourth-degree laceration will not be used in the ensuing discussion. Instead, when third-degree lacerations with rectal wall extension are mentioned, they will be so designated. Tears in the region of the urethra are also likely to occur unless an

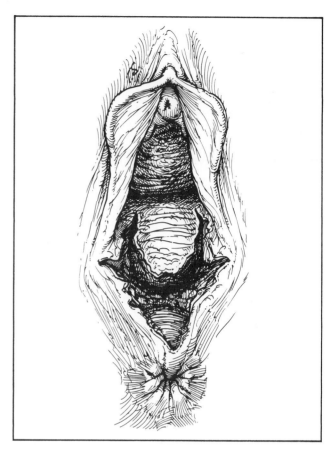

Figure 17-17. Deep second-degree laceration of perineum and vagina.

adequate episiotomy is performed, and they may bleed profusely.

Since the repair of perineal tears is virtually the same as that of episiotomy incisions, albeit often less satisfactory because of irregular lines of tissue cleavage, the technique of repairing lacerations is discussed in the following section.

EPISIOTOMY AND REPAIR

Episiotomy, in a strict sense, is incision of the pudenda. Perineotomy is incision of the perineum. In common parlance, however, episiotomy is often used synonymously with perineotomy, a practice that will be followed here. The incision may be made in the midline (median or midline episiotomy), or it may begin in the midline but be directed laterally and downward away from the rectum (mediolateral episiotomy).

Purposes of Episiotomy

Except for cutting the umbilical cord, episiotomy is the most common operation in obstetrics. The reasons for its popularity among obstetricians are clear. It substitutes a straight, neat surgical incision for the ragged laceration that otherwise frequently results. It is easier to repair and heals better than a tear. With mediolateral episiotomy, the likelihood of lacerations into the rectum is reduced.

More recently, the advantages provided by episiotomy have been questioned by some individuals (Thacker and Banta, 1983), as have most aspects of obstetric care. It can be said with certainty, however, that, since the era of in-hospital deliveries with episiotomy, there has been an appreciable decrease in the number of women subsequently hospitalized for treatment of symptomatic cystocele, rectocele, uterine prolapse, and stress incontinence!

The important questions for the obstetrician concerning episiotomy are:

1. How long before delivery should it be performed?
2. Should a median or mediolateral incision be made?
3. Should the incision be sutured before or after expulsion of the placenta?
4. What are the best suture materials and technique to employ?

Timing of Episiotomy. If episiotomy is performed unnecessarily early, bleeding from the gaping wound may be considerable during the interim between the incision and the birth of the baby. If episiotomy is performed too late, the muscles of the perineal floor already will have undergone excessive stretching, and one of the objectives of the operation is defeated. It is common practice to perform episiotomy when the head is visible during a contraction to a diameter of 3 to 4 cm (Fig. 17-5).

In this connection, the question arises whether episiotomy should be performed before or after the application of forceps. Application and articulation of forceps with widely separated shanks, as with Simpson forceps, may cause tearing of the introitus (see Chapter 41, pp. 838). The application of those with narrow overlapping shanks, such as Tucker McLane forceps, before episiotomy is not likely to be so traumatic. Although it is slightly more awkward to perform episiotomy with the forceps in place, blood loss from the episiotomy wound is somewhat less with this technique, since immediate traction on the forceps can be exerted, and the resultant tamponade of the perineal floor by the fetal head is effected earlier than could otherwise be achieved.

Median (Midline) vs. Mediolateral Episiotomy

The advantages and disadvantages of the two types of episiotomy may be enumerated as follows:

Median Episiotomy

1. Easy to repair
2. Faulty healing rare
3. Less painful in puerperium
4. Dyspareunia rarely follows
5. Anatomic end results almost always excellent

6. Blood loss smaller
7. Extension through the anal sphincter and into rectum is rather common

Mediolateral Episiotomy

1. More difficult to repair
2. Faulty healing more common
3. Pain in one third of cases for a few days
4. Dyspareunia occasionally follows
5. Anatomic end results more or less faulty in some 10 percent of cases (depending on operator)
6. Blood loss greater
7. Extension through sphincter is uncommon

With proper selection of cases, it is possible to secure the advantages of median episiotomy and at the same time reduce to a minimum its one disadvantage, the greater risk of third-degree extension. The size of the perineal body is related to the likelihood of third-degree laceration, since the accident is naturally more likely to occur if the perineal body is short. The possibility of extension of a median episiotomy into the rectal sphincter is also much greater when the fetus is large, when the occiput is posterior, in midforceps deliveries, and in breech deliveries. It is good practice, in general, to use mediolateral episiotomy in the circumstances mentioned but to employ the median incision otherwise. Even with this selection of cases, however, the total number of third-degree lacerations sustained with this policy is probably greater than with routine mediolateral episiotomy. In any case, sharply pointed scissors should not be used lest they inadvertently penetrate the rectum.

Benyon (1974) described her experiences with a policy of mandatory midline episiotomy. Of 1166 nulliparas who underwent a midline episiotomy, there was extension through the sphincter with involvement of *the rectum in 8.0 percent.* The technique of repair was similar to that described below. She emphasized that the episiotomies and repairs were performed primarily by house officers in training. Following repair, there was no special emphasis on bowel action. Suppositories, rectal tubes, and enemas were not allowed and rectal examinations were avoided. All were followed after primary repair and in only one woman was a rectovaginal fistula subsequently identified. Therefore, a third-degree laceration as the consequence of a median episiotomy need not be a major catastrophe. Despite its one drawback, the median episiotomy is a satisfactory procedure for most deliveries.

Timing of the Repair of Episiotomy. The most common practice is to defer repair of the episiotomy until after the placenta has been delivered. That policy permits the obstetrician to give undivided attention to the signs of placental separation and to deliver the organ just as soon as it has separated. Early delivery of the placenta is believed to decrease the loss of blood from the implantation site, since it prevents the development of exten-

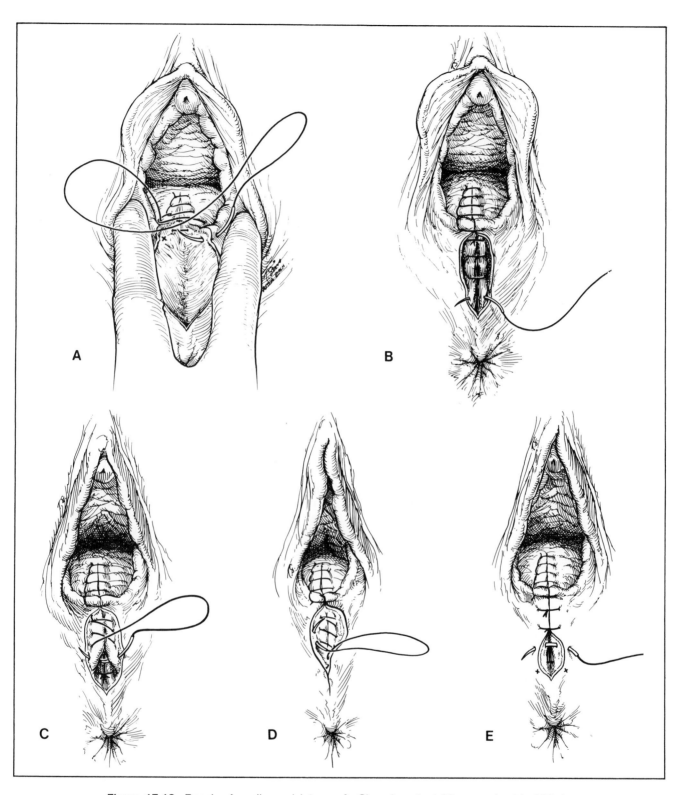

Figure 17-18. Repair of median episiotomy. **A.** Chromic catgut 00, or preferably 000, is used as a continuous suture to close the vaginal mucosa and submucosa. **B.** After closing the vaginal incision and reapproximating the cut margins of the hymenal ring, the suture is tied and cut. Next three or four interrupted sutures of 00 or 000 catgut are placed in the fascia and muscle of the incised perineum. **C.** A continuous suture is now carried downward to unite the superficial fascia. **D.** Completion of repair. The continuous suture is carried upward as a subcuticular stitch. An alternative method of closure of skin and subcutaneous fascia is illustrated in E. **E.** Completion of repair of median episiotomy. A few interrupted sutures of 000 chromic catgut are placed through the skin and subcutaneous fascia and loosely tied. This closure avoids burying two layers of catgut in the more superficial layers of the perineum.

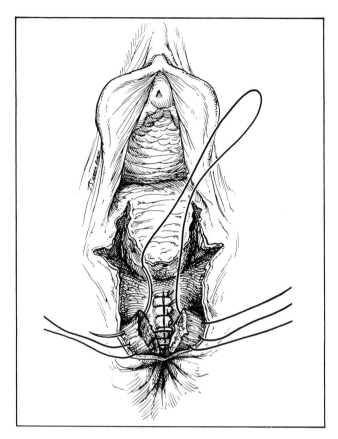

Figure 17-19. Repair of complete perineal tear. The rectal mucosa has been repaired with interrupted, fine chromic catgut sutures. The torn ends of the sphincter ani are next approximated with two or three interrupted chromic catgut sutures. The wound is then repaired, as in a second-degree laceration or an episiotomy.

sive retroplacental bleeding. A further advantage of this practice is that the episiotomy repair is not interrupted or disrupted by the obvious necessity of delivering the placenta, especially if manual removal must be performed.

Technique. There are many ways to close the episiotomy incision, but *hemostasis and anatomic restoration without excessive suturing are essential* for success with any method. A technique that is commonly employed in episiotomy repair is shown in Figure 17-18A–E. The suture material ordinarily used is 000 chromic catgut.

Third-Degree Laceration. The technique of repairing a third-degree laceration with extension into the wall of the rectum is shown in Figure 17-19. Here again various techniques have been recommended, but all emphasize careful approximation of the torn edges of the rectal wall with stitches about 0.5 cm apart, then covering this layer with a layer of fascia, and finally, careful isolation, approximation, and suture of the cut ends of the anal sphincter with two or three interrupted stitches. The re-

mainder of the repair is the same as for episiotomy. If the rectal mucosa was involved, stool softeners should be prescribed for a week. Enemas, of course, should be avoided. The value of prophylactic antibiotics has not been established.

Pain After Episiotomy. For the relief of episiotomy pain, a heat lamp has been a standard remedy, but during the summer months especially it may produce more discomfort than relief. An ice collar applied early tends to reduce swelling and allay discomfort. Aerosol sprays containing a local anesthetic are helpful at times. Analgesics such as codeine give considerable relief. *Since pain may be a signal of a large vulvar, paravaginal, or ischiorectal hematoma or abscess, it is essential to examine these sites carefully if pain is severe or persistent.* Management of these complications is discussed in Chapter 36.

REFERENCES

Abdul-Karim R, Assali NS: Renal function in human pregnancy: V. Effects of oxytocin on renal hemodynamics and water and electrolyte excretion. J Lab Clin Med 57:522, 1961

Abe T: The detection of the rupture of fetal membranes with the nitrazine indicator. Am J Obstet Gynecol 39:400, 1940

Baptisti A: Chemical test for the determination of ruptured membranes. Am J Obstet Gynecol 35:688, 1938

Benson RC, Shubeck F, Deutschberger J, Weiss W, Berendes H: Fetal heart rate as a predictor of fetal distress. A report from the Collaborative Project. Obstet Gynecol 32:259, 1968

Benyon CL: Midline episiotomy as a midline procedure. J Obstet Gynaecol Br Commonw 81:126, 1974

Browning DJ: Serious side effects of ergometrine and its use in routine obstetric practice. Med J Austral 1:957, 1974

Caldeyro-Barcía R, Schwarcz R, Belizán JM, Martell M, Nieto F, Sabatino H, Tenzer SM: Adverse perinatal effects of early amniotomy during labor. In Gluck L (ed): Modern Perinatal Medicine. Chicago, Year Book, 1974

Eggers TR, Fliegner JR: Water intoxication and syntocinon intoxication. Aust NZ J Obstet Gynaecol 19:59, 1979

Friedman EA: Labor, Clinical Evaluation and Management, 2nd ed. New York, Appleton, 1978

Haverkamp AD, Thompson HE, McFee JG, Cetrulo C: The evaluation of continuous fetal heart rate monitoring in high risk pregnancy. Am J Obstet Gynecol 125:310, 1976

Haverkamp AD, Orleans M, Langendoerfer S, McFee J, Murphy J, Thompson HE: A controlled trial of the differential effects of intrapartum fetal monitoring. Am J Obstet Gynecol 134:399, 1979

Hendricks CH, Brenner WE: Cardiovascular effects of oxytocic drugs used postpartum. Am J Obstet Gynecol 108:751, 1970

Kjeldsen J: Hemodynamic investigations during labour and delivery. Acta Obstet Gynecol Scand Suppl 89, 1979

Liggins GC: Treatment of missed abortion by high dosage syntocinon intravenous infusion. J Obstet Gynaecol Br Commonw 69:277, 1962

Ritgen G: (Concerning his method for protection of the perineum. Monatschrift für Geburtskunde 6:21, 1855.) See English translation, Wynn RM: Am J Obstet Gynecol 93:421, 1965

Schwartz RH, Jones RWA: Transplacental hyponatremia due to oxytocin. Br Med J 1:152, 1978

Secher NJ, Arnso P, Wallin L: Haemodynamic effects of oxytocin (Syntocinon) and methylergometrine (Methergin) on the systemic and pulmonary circulations of pregnant anaesthetized women. Acta Obstet Gynecol Scand 57:97, 1978

Thacker SB, Banta HD: Benefits and risks of episiotomy: An interpretive review of the English language literature, 1860–1980. Obstet Gynecol Survey 38:232, 1983

Whalley PJ, Pritchard JA: Oxytocin and water intoxication. JAMA 186:601, 1963

Yao AC, Lind J: Effect of gravity on placental transfusion. Lancet 2:505, 1969

Yao AC, Lind J: Placental transfusion. Am J Dis Child 127:128, 1974

18
Analgesia and Anesthesia

Labor may subject the nulliparous woman to the most pain that she has ever experienced. Fortunately, it often proves to be the most rewarding. The relief of pain in labor presents special problems, which may be best appreciated by reviewing the several important differences between obstetric and surgical anesthesia and analgesia:

1. In surgical procedures, there is but one patient to consider, whereas in parturition there are at least two, the mother and the fetus–infant. The respiratory center of the infant is highly vulnerable to sedative and anesthetic drugs and, since these agents, if given systemically, regularly traverse the placenta, they may jeopardize respiration after birth.
2. In major surgery, anesthesia is essential to the safe, satisfactory, and humane execution of the technical procedures. Whereas anesthesia is mandatory in many abnormal deliveries, it is not absolutely necessary in spontaneous vaginal delivery, because the baby can be born satisfactorily without any medication, although some mothers may suffer severe pain.
3. Surgical anesthesia is administered for the duration of the operation, which lasts in most cases for not more than an hour or two. Efficient pain relief in labor must cover not only the delivery ("obstetric anesthesia") but also a preceding period of from 1 to 12 hours or longer ("obstetric analgesia").
4. In both obstetric analgesia and anesthesia, it is important that the agents used exert little deleterious effect on uterine contractions and maternal voluntary expulsive efforts. If they do, the progress of labor may stop, or if uterine contractility is depressed immediately after delivery, postpartum hemorrhage is likely to occur.
5. In the majority of surgical operations, there is ample time to prepare the patient for anesthesia, especially by withholding food and fluids for 12 hours. Since most labors begin without warning, obstetric anesthesia is often administered within a few hours after a full meal. Moreover, gastric emptying is likely to be delayed appreciably during labor, especially after analgesics for pain re-

lief. Vomiting with aspiration of gastric contents is, hence, a frequent threat and a major cause of morbidity and mortality in obstetric anesthesia.

Because of these inherent difficulties, no completely safe and satisfactory method of pain relief in obstetrics has yet been developed. It is therefore sometimes falsely alleged that the hazards of pain relief in labor offset its advantages. On the contrary, vast experience has shown that obstetric analgesia and anesthesia, when judiciously employed by skilled personnel, are in general beneficial rather than detrimental to both baby and mother. Pain relief forestalls the importunities of the parturient and her family for premature operative interference. Formerly, premature and injudicious operative delivery so provoked constituted a common cause of trauma to both mother and infant. Such injuries were occasionally fatal to the mother and frequently so to the baby. The relief of pain itself, however, although desirable, does not justify the use of anesthetic procedures that are potentially lethal if administered by poorly trained individuals or with inadequate equipment.

Personnel and Facilities

The Joint Commission on Accreditation of Hospitals has urged that skilled personnel and appropriate equipment be immediately available to provide obstetric anesthesia: "Obstetric anesthesia must be considered as emergency anesthesia demanding a competence of personnel and equipment similar to or greater than that required for elective procedures." The societal benefits to be derived from modifying existing priorities for utilization of trained anesthesia personnel were stated succinctly by Jacoby (1974): "Young women with babies are far more important to society than old people with irreversible disease. If we cannot do justice to both, then we should concentrate on the obstetrical patients."

GENERAL PRINCIPLES

As stressed in another connection (see Chapter 17, p. 331), the proper psychologic management of the mother throughout the antepartum period and labor is a valuable basic tranquilizer. A woman who is free from fear and who has complete confidence in the obstetric staff that care for her usually enjoys a relatively comfortable first stage of labor and requires only a modest amount of analgesia.

Three essentials of obstetric pain relief are preservation of fetal homeostasis, simplicity, and safety. Fetal homeostasis must not be impaired by the analgesic or anesthetic method. Most important is the transfer of oxygen, which is dependent on the concentration of inhaled oxygen, transfer of oxygen across maternal alveoli, uterine blood flow, transfer of oxygen across the placenta, and umbilical blood flow. Impaired fetal oxygenation most often is the consequence of either compression of the umbilical cord or prolonged or repeated falls in placental perfusion. Prominent causes of reduced placental perfusion include hypertonic uterine contractions, severe pregnancy-induced hypertension, hemorrhage, premature separation of the placenta, and hypotension from spinal or epidural anesthesia.

The woman who receives any form of analgesia requires close supervision. If unattended and under heavy sedation, she may throw herself out of bed or against a wall, or she may vomit and aspirate the gastric contents. Numerous injuries and a few deaths as a result of such negligence are on record. Similarly, safe spinal and epidural anesthesia demands assiduous attention to the blood pressure and anesthetic levels.

It is practically impossible for an obstetrician to achieve expertise in the use of all the currently available techniques for obstetric analgesia and anesthesia. He should, however, master an effective method of systemic analgesia such as provided by meperidine (Demerol) plus promethazine (Phenergan), and become expert in local, pudendal, and low spinal ("saddle block") anesthesia. He should also have immediately available general anesthesia appropriate for laparotomy such as that produced by the combination of thiopental (Pentothal), nitrous oxide, and succinylcholine. Continuous lumbar or caudal epidural analgesia and anesthesia are niceties that, when skillfully administered in appropriately selected circumstances, provide elegant and safe relief from the discomfort of parturition. General anesthesia that will effectively and rapidly relax the uterus, such as provided by halothane (Fluothane), may be needed when intrauterine manipulation of the fetus is required to effect delivery or, even more rarely, when the acutely inverted uterus must be replaced.

ANALGESIA AND SEDATION DURING LABOR

Once labor is established, that is, once the cervix is dilating and the uterine contractions cause discomfort, medication for pain relief with a narcotic analgesic drug, such as meperidine, plus one of the tranquilizer drugs, such as promethazine, is usually indicated. With a successful program of analgesia and sedation, the mother should rest quietly between contractions, and although discomfort is felt at the acme of an effective uterine contraction, the pain is not unbearable. Finally, she does not recall labor as a horrifying experience. Appropriate drug selection and administration should accomplish these objectives for the great majority of women in labor without risk to them or their infants.

Meperidine and Promethazine

Meperidine, 50 to 100 mg, with promethazine, 25 mg, can be administered intramuscularly at intervals of 3 to 4 hours. In general, a small dose given more frequently is preferable to a larger one administered less often. Then, if delivery occurs during the next hour or so after injection, the infant is less likely to be depressed by the medication. The size of the mother must be taken into account in determining the size of the dose.

A more rapid but less prolonged effect is achieved by giving the agents as an intravenous bolus, but, in general, not more than 50 mg of meperidine or more than 25 mg of promethazine should be given at one time by this route. Whereas analgesia is maximal about 45 minutes after intramuscular administration, it develops much more rapidly, about 5 minutes, when given intravenously. The times for the depressant effect to develop in the fetus are not far behind. Some physicians advocate that the intravenous administration be made during the uterine contraction when, theoretically, blood flow to the uterus and, therefore, the amount of drug delivered to the placenta are reduced.

Effect of Meperidine on Labor. Fear has been expressed by some that administration of meperidine to provide obstetric analgesia might at times prolong or even arrest labor. Certainly, with the doses usually used for analgesia, there is no convincing evidence that this occurs. Riffel and co-workers (1973), for example, evaluated the effects of meperidine alone and meperidine plus promethazine on labor, and they observed not a decrease but a slight increase in uterine activity following their injection, confirming and extending the earlier observations by DeVoe and co-workers (1969).

Other Drugs for Relief of Labor Pain

Other narcotic analgesics, for example, alphaprodine (Nisentil), are used to provide pain relief during labor, but meperidine is most popular. A great variety of sedative and tranquilizer agents are administered with a narcotic analgesic or, at times, alone. It is important to recognize that all narcotics and tranquilizers cross the placenta to reach the fetus.

Morphine during labor has been nearly abandoned after a period of popularity in which it was used with scopolamine to produce so-called twilight sleep. The combination produced excellent analgesia and amnesia, but the mother sometimes became quite excited, delirious, and hallucinated. Moreover, at birth the infant was more likely to demonstrate apnea.

Narcotic Antagonists

The administration of meperidine or other narcotics to a woman in labor may impair respiratory function in the newborn infant. Naloxone hydrochloride (Narcan) is a narcotic antagonist capable of reversing respiratory depression induced by opioid narcotics by displacing the narcotic from specific receptors in the central nervous system. Unfortunately, it concomitantly inhibits the analgesia and the euphoria produced by the narcotic. In fact, withdrawal symptoms may be precipitated in recipients who are physically dependent on narcotics. The suggested dose for the newborn infant is 10 μg/kg injected into the umbilical vein. When so injected, naloxone usually acts within 2 minutes and its beneficial effects persist for at least 30 minutes. Since the depressant action of meperidine may persist beyond this time, the injection of naloxone may have to be repeated.

In the absence of narcotics, naloxone exhibits little, if any, adverse activity and thereby differs from levallorphan (Lorphan) and nalorphine (Nalline). The last two compounds may, in fact, enhance respiratory depression not caused by narcotic drugs. Therefore, naloxone is the drug of choice for treating narcotic depression in the newborn. Although narcotic antagonists may help relieve respiratory depression from opioid drugs in the newborn infant, it is best to avoid, as much as possible, the administration of narcotics to the mother in doses that cause serious respiratory depression in the newborn.

GENERAL ANESTHESIA

The placenta is not a barrier to general anesthetics. Without exception, all anesthetic agents that depress the central nervous system of the mother cross the placenta and depress the central nervous system of the fetus. Another constant hazard with any general anesthetic is aspiration of gastric contents. Particulate matter will, of course, obstruct airways. However, fasting before the time of anesthesia is not always an effective safeguard, since fasting gastric juice, even though free of particulate matter, is likely to be strongly acidic and thus can produce fatal aspiration pneumonitis. At the same time, endotracheal intubation is valuable to ensure a satisfactory airway and to minimize the risk of aspiration.

With inhalation anesthesia, the concentration of the anesthetic agent increases in the lungs of the pregnant woman somewhat more rapidly because the functional residual capacity and residual volume of the lungs are reduced (see Chapter 9, p. 196). For the same reason, the residual oxygen in the lung after expiration is appreciably less, a factor of importance when there is delay in intubation and oxygenation after injection of a muscle-paralyzing agent. Trained personnel and specialized equipment are mandatory for the safe use of general anesthesia. Airway obstruction and hypoxia must be avoided.

A unique use for acute obstruction of the airway of the laboring woman is cited by Vogel (1970) in his treatise

American Indian Medicine. Allegedly, the treatment of protracted labor in Indian women included binding a cloth tightly over the mouth and nose to bring on partial suffocation. From the struggles that ensued, "she was in a few seconds delivered." It is hoped that modern women and their infant are never so "aided," inadvertently or otherwise.

Gas Anesthetics

Only one anesthetic gas, nitrous oxide, is used currently in obstetrics.

Nitrous Oxide. Nitrous oxide is used to provide relief of pain during labor as well as at delivery. This agent produces analgesia and altered consciousness but by itself does not provide true anesthesia. Nitrous oxide does not prolong labor or interfere with uterine contractions. When appropriately administered, satisfactory analgesia is often obtained with a concentration of 50 percent nitrous oxide and 50 percent oxygen, but its satisfactory use requires that personnel be in close attendance. During the second stage of labor, when the woman indicates that a uterine contraction is beginning, a well-fitting mask is placed on her face and she is encouraged to take three deep breaths of the mixture and then to bear down. The concentration of nitrous oxide mixed with oxygen for analgesia should not exceed 70 percent, since concentrations higher than 70 percent may result in maternal as well as fetal hypoxia.

Cyclopropane

At one time cyclopropane was popular in obstetric practice. There are several disadvantages inherent in the use of cyclopropane for abdominal or vaginal delivery. *The gas is highly explosive and must always be given in a closed system.* It is not likely to relax the myometrium sufficiently to allow intrauterine manipulation of the fetus. Unless the time of anesthesia is kept very short, resuscitation of the infant is required.

Volatile Anesthetics

Of the volatile anesthetics, ether, halothane (Fluothane), methoxyflurane (Penthrane), and enflurane (Ethrane) merit consideration. These agents cross the placenta readily and are capable of producing narcosis in the fetus.

Ether. Since in the hands of inexperienced anesthetists the margin of safety was usually greater with diethyl ether than with any other general anesthetic, it enjoyed considerable popularity in former years but not now. Ether is unpleasant to the mother; it depresses the fetus-infant; it causes the uterus to relax, thereby enhancing hemorrhage immediately after delivery; and it is explosive. Therefore, it is little used.

Halothane. This potent, nonexplosive agent is of limited use for obstetric anesthesia. Halothane produces remarkable uterine relaxation and should be restricted to those very uncommon situations in which uterine relaxation is a requisite rather than a hazard. Therefore, it is the anesthetic agent of choice for the now very uncommon procedures of internal podalic version, for breech decomposition, and for replacement of the acutely inverted uterus. As soon as the maneuver has been completed, the administration of halothane should be stopped and immediate efforts made to promote myometrial contraction and retraction to minimize hemorrhage from the placental implantation site. Because of its cardiodepressant and hypotensive effects, halothane may intensify the adverse effects of maternal hypovolemia.

Methoxyflurane. This agent is pleasant to take and may be self-administered in low concentration to provide analgesia during the first and second stages of labor, and during delivery. Overdose may be a major complication when methoxyflurane is self-administered for analgesia. Unless the woman is kept under very close surveillance, she may, at times, cover the inhaler and her head with a pillow or sheet and thereby increase appreciably the concentration inhaled. Methoxyflurane, especially in higher concentrations, may depress myometrial contractility and thereby increase blood loss from the placental implantation site. There is also convincing evidence of dose-related methoxyflurane nephrotoxicity.

Enflurane. The dose of enflurane that provides analgesia is likely to cause unconsciousness. Also, like halothane, it may cause myometrial depression and increased hemorrhage. It should not be given to anyone suspected of impaired renal function.

Trichloroethylene

Although once quite popular, this compound is no longer available in this country. When a closed circuit system with soda lime was used to provide anesthesia, trichloroethylene formed toxic products. Moreover, deaths were recorded from trichloroethylene self-administered for analgesia during labor.

Intravenous Anesthesia

Thiopental (Pentothal) is widely used in conjunction with other agents for general anesthesia in obstetrics; ketamine is not.

Thiopental. Intravenous thiopental in obstetrics offers the advantages of ease and extreme rapidity of induction, ample oxygenation, ready controllability, minimal postpartum bleeding, and promptness of recovery without vomiting. The first and last of these advantages make it very popular with patients. Thiopental and similar compounds are poor analgesic agents, and the administration of enough of the drug alone to maintain anesthesia in the mother may cause appreciable depression of the newborn infant. Therefore, thiopental is not used as the sole anesthetic agent. Rather, it is ad-

ministered in a dose that induces sleep along with a muscle relaxant, usually succinylcholine, and nitrous oxide plus oxygen inhaled through an endotracheal tube. Some individuals are aware of the operation when these agents are used. Therefore, a low concentration of halothane (0.5 percent) may be administered before delivery to assure loss of consciousness. The concentration of halothane must be kept low to avoid myometrial depression and hemorrhage postpartum from the placental implantation site. As soon as the infant is delivered, halothane can be stopped and a narcotic—fentanyl, meperidine, or morphine—injected intravenously to prevent awareness of the procedure.

Induction of Anesthesia. General anesthesia should not be induced until all steps preparatory to actual delivery have been completed, so as to minimize transfer of the anesthetic agent to the fetus and, in turn, avoid respiratory depression in the newborn infant. General anesthesia need not cause appreciable depression of the newborn. For example, Zagorczyki and Brinkman (1982) have compared the status of infants immediately after cesarean delivery whose mothers received either epidural anesthesia or general anesthesia, the technique for which consisted of preoxygenation, thiopental (4 mg/kg), muscle relaxant, nitrous oxide (50 percent), and halothane (0.5 percent). No difference was found in Apgar scores at 1 and 5 minutes. No appreciable differences in mean scores or in the frequency of scores below 7 were evident.

When the time from induction of anesthesia to delivery is prolonged appreciably, there is increased possibility of the newborn infant being depressed. Often the delay is the consequence of obstetric difficulties that necessitate the manipulation of the uterus and the fetus, leading to fetal depression.

Ketamine. The intravenous injection of ketamine will produce appreciable anesthesia. It usually causes a rise in blood pressure, which is not desirable in the already hypertensive woman. Unpleasant delirium and hallucinations are commonly induced by this agent. Ketamine may cause respiratory depression in the newborn infant and hypertonus sufficient to impair efforts at ventilation.

ASPIRATION DURING GENERAL ANESTHESIA

Pneumonitis from inhalation of gastric contents has been the most common cause of anesthetic death in obstetrics. For example, a survey in Great Britain reported by Crawford (1972) identified inhalation of gastric contents to be associated with at least one half of all obstetric deaths. The aspirated material from the stomach may contain undigested food and thereby cause airway obstruction that, unless promptly relieved, may prove rapidly fatal. Fasting gastric juice is likely to be free of particulate matter but extremely acidic and thereby capable of inducing a lethal chemical pneumonitis. The aspiration of strongly acidic gastric juice is probably more common and perhaps more dangerous than is the aspiration of gastric contents that contain particulate matter but are buffered somewhat by the food.

Prophylaxis

Important to effective prophylaxis are (1) fasting for 12 hours before anesthesia, (2) use of agents to reduce gastric acidity during the induction and maintenance of general anesthesia, (3) skillful endotracheal intubation accompanied by pressure on the cricoid cartilage to occlude the esophagus, and (4) at completion of the operation, extubation with the mother awake and lying on her side with head lowered.

Fasting. Withholding food for 12 hours should rid the stomach of undigested food but not necessarily of acidic liquid. If general anesthesia is necessary soon after eating, the stomach contents may be emptied by provoking emesis. Many consider such prophylactic treatment to be cruel, yet it may protect the life of the mother and the fetus. Unfortunately, use of apomorphine as an emetic may cause respiratory depression and use of a nasogastric tube with suction to empty the stomach of particulate matter is unpleasant, time consuming, and not totally effective.

Antacids. Ingestion of antacids shortly before induction of anesthesia can appreciably reduce the acidity of the gastric juice. It is essential that the antacid disperse promptly throughout all of the gastric contents to neutralize the hydrogen ion effectively, but it is equally important that the antacid, if aspirated, not incite comparably serious pulmonary pathologic problems. A number of antacids are now being used. *Magnesium hydroxide suspension* (milk of magnesia) is an effective neutralizer (Wheatley and colleagues, 1979). Its laxative effect is usually not marked and therefore not a contraindication to its use. At Parkland Memorial Hospital, 30 ml of magnesium hydroxide suspension is given up to one-half hour before the anticipated time of induction of anesthesia. In theory, 1 ml of milk of magnesia will neutralize nearly 3 mEq of acid, or about 25 ml of gastric juice of pH 1. Its favorable effect persists long enough for cesarean section to be performed. We have observed no long-term adverse effects on the respiratory tract in those instances in which it was aspirated. The opaque white appearance of ingested milk of magnesia simplifies identification of gastric liquid in the pharynx and trachea.

A solution of 0.3 molar sodium citrate will usually mix rapidly with gastric juice and neutralize acid. If aspirated, it appears to be less irritating than colloidal antacid mixtures. A suitable dose is 30 ml, 10 to 45 minutes before surgery.

Cimetidine given sometime before general anesthesia for delivery has recently been recommended. Unfortunately, in emergency cases at least 60 minutes are required after parenteral administration to decrease gastric acidity to relatively safe levels if aspirated. Therefore, in an emergency situation either an antacid or antacid plus cimetidine has been recommended (Moir, 1983).

Intubation. Various positions have been tried to minimize aspiration before and during endotracheal intubation and inflation of the cuff, but the disadvantages from positions other than supine outweigh any advantages. Cricoid pressure from the time of induction of anesthesia until intubation is worthwhile but requires a trained associate. Intubation may be attempted with the mother awake, but to intubate without local anesthesia is barbaric; yet the use of local anesthesia may obtund the laryngeal reflex sufficiently to allow aspiration.

Extubation. At the completion of the procedure, the endotracheal tube may be safely removed only if the patient is conscious and has been placed in the lateral recumbent position with her head lowered.

Pathology

Aspiration pneumonia associated with obstetric anesthesia was clearly described by Mendelson in 1946. Teabeaut (1952) demonstrated experimentally that if the pH of aspirated fluid was below 2.5, severe chemical pneumonitis developed. It is of interest that in one study the pH of gastric juice of nearly one half of women tested intrapartum without treatment was below 2.5 (Taylor and Pryse-Davies, 1966).

The right main bronchus usually offers the simplest pathway for aspirated material to reach the lung parenchyma and therefore the right lower lobe is most often involved. In severe cases, there is bilateral widespread involvement.

Signs and Symptoms. The woman who aspirates may develop evidence of respiratory distress immediately or as long as several hours after aspiration, depending in part upon the material aspirated, the severity of the process, and the acuity of the attendants. Aspiration of a large amount of solid material causes obvious signs of airway obstruction. Smaller particles without acidic liquid may lead to patchy atelectasis and later to bronchopneumonia.

When highly acidic liquid is inspired, tachypnea, bronchospasm, rhonchi, rales, atelectasis, cyanosis, tachycardia, and hypotension are likely to develop. At the sites of injury, protein-rich fluid containing numerous erythrocytes exudes from capillaries into the lung interstitium and alveoli to cause decreased pulmonary compliance, shunting of blood and severe hypoxemia. Roentgenographic changes may appear relatively late and be quite variable. Therefore chest x-ray alone should not be used to exclude aspiration of a significant amount of strongly acidic gastric contents.

Treatment

In recent years, the methods recommended for treatment of aspiration have changed appreciably, indicating that previous therapy was not very successful. Suspicion of aspiration of gastric contents demands very close monitoring of the patient for evidence of any pulmonary damage.

Suction and Bronchoscopy. As much as possible of the inhaled fluid should be immediately wiped out of the mouth and removed from the pharynx and trachea by suction. Saline lavage, rather than being beneficial, probably further disseminates the acid throughout the lung. If large particulate matter is inspired, prompt bronchoscopy is indicated to relieve airway obstruction. Otherwise, bronchoscopy not only is unnecessary but may contribute to morbidity and mortality.

Corticosteroids. There has been considerable enthusiasm for administering corticosteroids in very lage pharmacologic doses in an attempt to maintain cell integrity in the presence of strong acid. There is no clinical evidence that such therapy is unequivocally beneficial (Bynum and Pierce, 1976), nor do experimental studies support the thesis that appreciable benefits accrue from the use of corticosteroids. Nonetheless, the clinical impression of some has been that the immediate intravenous administration of 500 mg of methylprednisolone sodium succinate (Solu-Medrol), with repeated doses of 250 mg every 8 hours for 24 hours, is beneficial.

Oxygen and Ventilation. Oxygen delivered through an endotracheal tube in increased concentration by intermittent positive pressure is often required to raise and maintain the arterial P_{O_2} at 60 mm Hg. Frequent suction is necessary to remove secretions including edema fluid. Mechanical ventilation that produces positive end-expiratory pressure may prove lifesaving by preventing on expiration the complete collapse of the now surfactant-poor lung and by retarding the outpouring of protein-rich fluid from pulmonary capillaries into the interstitium and alveoli.

Antibiotics. Although the likelihood of bacterial contamination and infection from aspiration is appreciable, the use of antibiotics prophylactically remains controversial (Bynum and Pierce, 1976). Bartlett and associates (1974) identified anaerobic bacteria in 50 of 54 cases of pneumonia that was caused by aspiration. They concluded that anaerobes play a key role in most cases of infection after aspiration and suggested the use of clin-

domycin or chloramphenicol for those anaerobes that are not sensitive to penicillin.

An extensive review of the aspiration syndrome has been provided by Cohen (1982).

Anesthetic Gas Exposure and Pregnancy Outcome

Sufficient data have accumulated to create concern over the welfare of the embryo and fetus of pregnant women who work in operating rooms where they are exposed chronically to anesthetic gases. In some reports, but not all, the abortion rate is about twice that for unexposed personnel and the malformation rate about less than one times greater (Knill-Jones and colleagues, 1975). In England and Wales, a comparison has been made between pregnancy outcomes of women doctors exposed to anesthetic gases during pregnancy and those working but not so exposed. Conception that occurred while the woman was actively engaged in anesthesiology resulted in possibly smaller babies (3347 vs. 3388 g), an increased frequency of cardiovascular malformation (1.4 vs. 0.4 percent), and of stillbirth (1.7 vs. 0.8 percent). Spontaneous abortions were the same (13.8 percent) in both groups (Pharoah and co-workers, 1977). Ericson and Källén (1979) found no differences in pregnancies of operating room workers in Sweden. Husum and co-workers (1938) in Denmark detected no indication of a mutagenic effect from long-term exposure to trace concentrations of waste anesthetic gases. Sister chromatid exchanges and structural chromosomal aberrations in lymphocytes were no more common in operating room personnel than in unexposed control subjects.

SENSORY INNERVATION OF GENITAL TRACT

Innervation of Uterus

Pain in the first stage of labor stems largely from the uterus. Visceral sensory fibers from the uterus, cervix, and upper vagina traverse from the uterus, travel through *Frankenhäuser's ganglion,* which lies just lateral and posterior to the cervix, into the pelvic plexus, and thence to the middle and superior hypogastric plexuses. From there, the fibers travel in the lumbar and lower thoracic sympathetic chains to enter the spinal cord through the white rami communicantes associated with the 10th, 11th, and 12th thoracic and 1st lumbar nerves. Early in the first stage of labor, the pain of uterine contractions is transmitted through predominantly the 11th and 12th thoracic nerves.

The motor pathways to the uterus leave the spinal cord at the level of the seventh and eighth thoracic vertebrae. Theoretically, any method of sensory block that does not also block the motor pathways to the uterus can be used for analgesia during labor.

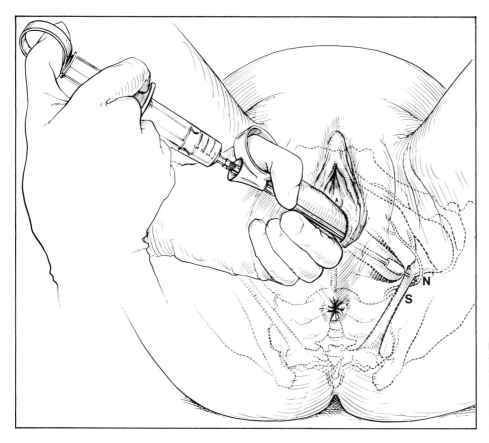

Figure 18-1. Local infiltration of the pudendal nerve. Transvaginal technique showing the needle extended beyond the needle guard and passing through the sacrospinous ligament (S) to reach the pudendal nerve (N).

Innervation of Lower Genital Tract

Although painful contractions of the uterus continue during the second stage of labor, much of the pain of vaginal delivery arises in the lower genital tract. Painful stimuli from the lower genital tract are transmitted in large part through the *pudendal nerve,* the peripheral branches of which provide sensory innervation to the perineum, anus, and the more medial and inferior parts of the vulva and clitoris. The pudendal nerve passes across the posterior surface of the sacrospinous ligament just as the ligament attaches to the ischial spine (Fig. 18-1). The sensory nerve fibers of the pudendal nerve are derived from the ventral branches of the second, third, and fourth sacral nerves.

REGIONAL ANALGESIA AND ANESTHESIA

Anesthetic Agents

A variety of compounds are currently used in obstetrics to produce local or regional analgesia and anesthesia. Although their appropriate use almost always proves to be safe for both the mother and the fetus-infant, the potential exists for toxic reactions that may prove life threatening. Perhaps the least common toxic reaction, but often terrifying, is the induction of convulsions from high circulating levels of the compound. Since convulsions may follow any route of administration, management of this complication is considered now.

Central Nervous System Toxicity. Symptoms include lightheadedness, dizziness, slurred speech, metallic taste, numbness of tongue and mouth, muscle fasciculation, loss of consciousness, and generalized convulsions. Quickly and simultaneously the convulsions should be controlled, an airway established, and oxygen delivered. Succinylcholine abolishes the peripheral manifestations of the convulsions and allows endotracheal intubation. Thiopental or diazepam acts centrally to inhibit convulsions. In those instances in which it has been tried at Parkland Memorial Hospital, magnesium sulfate administered according to our Eclampsia Regime (Chapter 27, p. 548) has also effectively controlled the convulsions. Maternal hypotension, if it develops, and impaired uteroplacental perfusion is combatted by turning the woman toward the left side to relieve aortocaval compression as well as the rapid intravenous administration of balanced salt solution and the intravenous administration of ephedrine. Fetal distress, manifested by either late decelerations of the heart rate or persistent bradycardia, may develop as the consequences of maternal hypoxia and lactic acidosis induced by the convulsions and of drug-induced impaired uteroplacental perfusion, fetal cardiac depression, and fetal hypotension. With arrest of the convulsions, the administration of oxygen and the application of the other supportive measures outlined above, the fetus is likely to recover more quickly in utero than if immediately delivered by cesarean section. Moreover, maternal well-being is usually better served by waiting until the intensity of the hypoxia and metabolic acidosis have diminished. Personnel and facilities for instituting cardiopulmonary resuscitation should be immediately available for both the mother and the infant.

Inadvertent intravenous injection of local anesthetic is likely to cause these adverse effects. Another mechanism is repeated injections of sizable doses of the drug at multiple sites, for example, epidural analgesia ineffective for vaginal delivery, followed by pudendal block, which was not satisfactory for repairing an episiotomy or lacerations, followed by local infiltration. The physician must be aware of the upper limit of safety for the local anesthetics he or she uses.

Local Infiltration

This technique is of negligible value for analgesia during labor but has been employed for delivery. Local infiltration is of especial value in the following circumstances: (1) before episiotomy and delivery, (2) after delivery into the site of lacerations to be repaired, and (3) around the episiotomy wound if adequate anesthesia from epidural or pudendal block is lacking. From the standpoint of safety, local infiltration anesthesia is preeminent. From the standpoint of effectiveness, too often the incision or repair is begun before the local anesthetic agent has had time to be effective!

Transvaginal Pudendal Block

Used to guide the needle into position over the pudendal nerve is a tubular director that allows 1.0 to 1.5 cm of a 15-cm-long, 22-gauge needle to protrude beyond its tip (Fig. 18-1). The end of the director is placed against the vaginal mucosa just beneath the tip of the ischial spine. The needle is pushed beyond the tip of the director into the mucosa and a mucosal wheal is made with 1 ml of 1 percent lidocaine solution or an equivalent dose of another local anesthetic with similar high tissue penetration and rapid action. Aspiration is attempted before this and all subsequent injections to guard against intravascular infusion. The needle is then advanced until it touches the sacrospinous ligament, which is infiltrated with 3 ml of the 1 percent lidocaine solution. The needle is advanced further through the ligament, and as it pierces the loose areolar tissue behind the ligament, the resistance of the plunger decreases (Fig. 18-1). Another 3 ml of the anesthetic solution is injected in the region. Next, the needle is withdrawn into the guide, the tip of the guide is moved to just above the ischial spine, and the needle is inserted through the mucosa. After again aspirating to avoid intravascular injection, the rest of the 10 ml of solution is deposited.

Within 3 to 4 minutes after injection, the successful pudendal block will allow pinching of the lower vagina and posterior vulva bilaterally without pain. It is often of benefit before pudendal block to infiltrate directly the fourchette, perineum, and adjacent vagina at the site where the episiotomy is to be made with 5 to 10 ml of 1 percent lidocaine solution. Then, if delivery occurs before pudendal block becomes effective, an episiotomy usually can be made without pain.

Pudendal block very often works well for spontaneous delivery but is not likely to provide adequate anesthesia for forceps delivery. Moreover, anesthesia limited to pudendal block is inadequate after delivery for complete visualization of the cervix and upper vagina or manual exploration of the uterine cavity. Under these circumstances, the addition of an intravenously administered narcotic analgesic, such as 50 mg of meperidine, may provide appreciable, although not total, relief from the pain of examination. *With such an approach, caution must be exercised not to give narcotics and sedatives in doses or combinations that might so obtund the woman that she would suffer airway obstruction or aspiration.*

Complications from Pudendal Block. The intravascular injection of the local anesthetic may cause serious systemic toxicity characterized by stimulation of the cerebral cortex, leading to convulsions as described above. A troublesome hematoma, the consequence of perforation of a blood vessel, is most likely to occur when there is defective coagulation such as that induced by heparin or by severe placental abruption. Rarely, a severe infection may originate at the injection site. The infection tends to spread to the region posterior to the hip joint, into the gluteal musculature, or into the retropsoal space (Svancarek and associates, 1977). Deaths and, in some survivors, severe permanent impairment have been recorded (Wenger and Gitchell, 1973).

Paracervical Block

This technique serves to relieve pain of uterine contractions, but inasmuch as the pudendal nerves are not blocked, additional anesthesia is required for delivery. Since the anesthetic is relatively short-acting, it may be necessary to repeat the paracervical block during labor.

Complications. While good to excellent pain relief is usually achieved from paracervical block during the first stage of labor, *fetal bradycardia* is a complication. Reports indicate a 10 to 70 percent incidence of this complication. Although several investigators stress that fetal bradycardia is not a sign of fetal asphyxia, since the bradycardia is usually transient and the newborns are in most instances vigorous at birth, there are reports in which fetal scalp blood pH and Apgar scores were found at times to be low, and a few fetuses have died. The effect on the fetus may be the consequence of transplacental transfer of the anesthetic agent or its metabolites and, in turn, a depressant effect on the heart. Greiss and co-workers (1976) and Fishburne and co-workers (1979), based on studies in pregnant ewes, believe that the fetal bradycardia results from the decreased placental perfusion as the consequence of drug-induced uterine vasoconstriction and myometrial hypertonus. Paracervical block should not be used in situations of potential fetal compromise.

Spinal Anesthesia

Introduction of a local anesthetic into the subarachnoid space to effect spinal anesthesia has long been used for uncomplicated cesarean section and for vaginal delivery of normal women of low parity. It must always be kept in mind that because of the smaller subarachnoid space during pregnancy, the same amount of anesthetic agent in the same volume of solution produces a much higher spinal blockade in the parturients than in nonpregnant women. The smaller subarachnoid space is most likely the consequence of engorgement of the internal vertebral venous plexus, which, in turn, is the consequence of compression by the uterus of the inferior vena cava and adjacent large veins.

Vaginal Delivery. A popular form of anesthesia for delivery is low spinal block with a level of anesthesia to the tenth thoracic dermatome (T10), which corresponds at the midline to about the level of the umbilicus. Blockade to T10 provides relief from the pain of uterine contractions. The term *saddle block* has been applied to this level of anesthesia, but incorrectly since the area of skin anesthetized is appreciably greater than that which would be in contact with a saddle.

Nearly all local anesthetic agents have been used for spinal anesthesia, but for many years one that has proved quite satisfactory for vaginal delivery is tetracaine (Pontocaine) in a dose of 4 mg already dissolved in 2 ml of 6 percent solution of dextrose in water. The anesthetic should not be administered for vaginal delivery until the cervix is fully dilated and all other criteria for safe forceps delivery have been fulfilled. Spinal anesthesia is not recommended before this time because of the frequency with which it disrupts orderly labor and, as the consequence, results in a complicated delivery that is traumatic to the infant and the mother. With 4 mg of tetracaine, satisfactory anesthetic in the lower vagina and the perineum persists for about 1 hour.

Cesarean Section. For cesarean section, a higher level of spinal sensory blockade is essential to at least the level of the eighth thoracic dermatome (T8), which is in the midline just below the xiphoid process of the sternum. Therefore, a somewhat larger dose of anesthetic agent *relative to that used for vaginal delivery* is necessary. This increases the frequency and the intensity of the complications just cited. Depending upon the mother's size, 8 to 10 mg of tetracaine is administered. Undue delay between intrathecal injection of anesthetic agent and delivery of the infant should be avoided if the dose of the anesthetic drug to be used is to be safe and yet have spinal anesthesia of sufficient intensity and duration to allow completion of abdominal delivery without serious discomfort. Therefore, catheterization of the bladder and the shaving of the operative field should be done before the anesthetic is administered.

Complications with Spinal Anesthesia

A number of complications may ensue.

Hypotension. Maternal hypotension may occur very soon after the injection of the anesthetic agent. The hypotension is the consequence of vasodilatation from sympathetic blockade compounded by obstructed venous return caused by compression by the uterus of the vena cava and adjacent large veins. Importantly, in the supine position, even in the absence of maternal hypotension as measured in the brachial artery, placental blood flow may be reduced significantly as the consequence of compression of the aorta. Important to prophylaxis and to treatment of spinal hypotension are (1) uterine elevation and displacement to the left of the abdomen, (2) acute hydration with a balanced salt solution, and (3) at the first sign of a decrease in blood pressure, the intravenous injection of 10 to 15 mg of ephedrine.

Total Spinal Blockade. Complete spinal blockade with respiratory paralysis may complicate spinal anesthesia. Most often total spinal blockade is the consequence of administration of a dose of anesthetic agent far in excess of that tolerated by pregnant women. Hypotension and apnea promptly develop and must be immediately treated to prevent cardiac arrest. The undelivered woman should be turned toward her left side. Effective ventilation is urged, through an endotracheal tube, when possible, to protect against aspiration. When the woman is hypotensive, ephedrine is urged. Elevation of the legs will increase venous return and help combat hypotension. Preparations should be made for cardiac resuscitation in the event of cardiac arrest.

Anxiety and Discomfort. It is imperative that everyone in the operating room remember at all times that the woman under regional anesthesia is awake. In every case, great care must be exercised over what is said and how the many activities associated with care of the mother and fetus are performed lest the mother interpret remarks or actions as an indication that she or her fetus is in jeopardy, or that there is inappropriate concern for her welfare. The woman is usually aware of the surgical manipulation, identifying each surgical maneuver as a feeling of pressure. She is painfully aware of any manipulation above the level of the spinal sensory blockade.

At times, the degree of pain relief from the spinal anesthetic is inadequate, making the operation a most unpleasant experience. In this circumstance, a significant measure of relief can be provided before delivery of the infant by administering 50 to 70 percent nitrous oxide with oxygen. Immediately after clamping the cord, a variety of techniques can be employed to provide effective analgesia. Morphine, meperidine, or fentanyl given intravenously at this time often provides excellent analgesia and euphoria as the operation is being completed.

Spinal (Postpuncture) Headaches. Leakage of cerebrospinal fluid from the site of puncture of the meninges is the major factor in the genesis of spinal headache. Presumably, when the woman sits or stands, the diminished volume of cerebrospinal fluid allows traction on pain-sensitive central nervous system structures. The likelihood of this unpleasant complication can be reduced by using a small-gauge spinal needle and avoiding multiple punctures of the meninges. Placing the woman absolutely flat on her back for many hours has been recommended to prevent postspinal headache, but there is no good evidence that this procedure is very effective. Hyperhydration has been claimed to be of value, without compelling evidence to support its use. Creation of a "blood patch" has been demonstrated to be efficacious; in this, a few milliliters of the woman's blood without anticoagulant is injected epidurally at the side of the spinal tap. Saline similarly injected in larger volumes has also been claimed to provide relief. Abdominal support with a girdle or abdominal binder does seem to afford relief and is worth trying. Typically, the headache is remarkably improved by the third day and absent by the fifth.

Bladder Dysfunction. With spinal anesthesia, bladder sensation is likely to be obtunded and bladder emptying impaired during the first few hours after delivery. As a consequence, bladder distension is a frequent complication of the puerperium, especially if appreciable volumes of intravenous fluid have been or are being administered. Combinations of (1) infusion of 1 liter or more of aqueous fluid, (2) neural blockade from epidural or spinal anesthesia (3) antidiuretic effect of oxytocin infused for a time after delivery and then stopped, (4) discomfort from a sizable episiotomy, (5) failure to observe the woman very closely for bladder distension, and (6) failure to relieve bladder distension promptly by catheterization are very likely to lead to quite troublesome bladder dysfunction and urinary tract infection.

Oxytocics and Hypertension. Paradoxically, hypertension from ergonovine (Ergotrate) or methylergonovine (Methergine) injected following delivery is most common in women who have received a spinal or epidural block.

Arachnoiditis and Meningitis. No longer are the ampules of local anesthetic stored in alcohol, formalin, or other highly toxic media. Needles and catheters are now rarely subjected to cleaning by chemical treatment so that they can be reused. Instead, one-time disposable equipment is used. These current practices, coupled with strict aseptic technique, have made meningitis and arachnoiditis rarities.

Continuous Spinal Anesthesia

Use of continuous spinal anesthesia, in which an indwelling catheter is inserted into the subarachnoid space, allows the anesthetic to be administered in fractional doses. This technique minimizes the likelihood of many of the serious adverse effects that may promptly follow a larger dose of anesthetic by single injection, especially total spinal block. Also, for longer procedures, the anesthetic drug can be replenished as needed. A hole through the meninges large enough initially for a needle containing the indwelling catheter and the perpetuation of the hole by the continued presence of the catheter are very likely to predispose to troublesome postspinal headache.

Contraindications to the Use of Spinal Anesthesia

The common serious complication from spinal anesthesia is hypotension. The supine position late in pregnancy commonly predisposes to a reduction in return of blood from veins below the level of the large pregnant uterus and, in turn, a reduction in cardiac output (see Chapter 9, p. 195). Moreover, sympathetic blockade from spinal anesthesia is usually extensive and leads to further pooling of blood in dilated blood vessels below the level of the blockade. Obstetric complications that in themselves predispose to maternal hypovolemia and hypotension are contraindications to the use of spinal anesthesia. *Severe falls in blood pressure can be predicted when spinal anesthesia is used in the presence of hemorrhage or of severe hypertension and associated hypovolemia induced or aggravated by pregnancy.*

The cardiovascular effects of spinal anesthesia in the presence of acute blood loss but in the absence of hemodynamic effects of pregnancy have been investigated by Kennedy and co-workers (1968). In 15 nonpregnant volunteers, spinal anesthesia to T5 sensory level was induced twice, the second time after a phlebotomy of 10 ml/kg. In the case of subarachnoid block without hemorrhage, the mean arterial blood pressure fell 10 percent, while cardiac output rose slightly. In the case of hemorrhage without subarachnoid block, the mean blood pressure fell to the same degree and again the cardiac output rose slightly. However, when there was subarachnoid block after the modest hemorrhage, the mean arterial pressure fell 29 percent and cardiac output fell 15 percent. Undoubtedly, the presence of a large pregnant uterus serves in the supine position to magnify appreciably these deleterious changes from spinal anesthesia after overt hemorrhage.

Disorders of coagulation and defective hemostasis preclude the use of spinal anesthesia. Spinal anesthesia is contraindicated when the skin or underlying tissues at the site of needle entry is infected, and neurologic disorders are usually considered to be a contraindication, if for no other reason than exacerbation of the neurologic disease might be attributed to the spinal anesthetic.

EPIDURAL (PERIDURAL) BLOCK

Relief from the pain of uterine contractions and delivery, vaginal or abdominal, can be accomplished by injecting a suitable local anesthetic agent into the epidural or peridural space. The epidural space, in effect, is a potential space that contains areolar tissue, fat, lymphatics, and the internal venous plexus, which becomes engorged during pregnancy so that it reduces appreciably the volume of the epidural space. It is limited peripherally by the ligamentum flavum and centrally by the dura mater, and it extends from the base of the skull to almost the end of the sacrum. The portal of entry into the epidural space for obstetric analgesia and anesthesia is through either a lumbar intervertebral space or through the sacral hiatus and sacral canal. The injection may be solitary or, much more often, repetitive through an indwelling plastic catheter.

Continuous Lumbar Epidural Block

Complete anesthesia for the pain of labor and vaginal delivery necessitates a block from T10 to S5. For abdominal delivery, a block is essential from at least T8 to S1. The spread of epidural anesthesia will depend upon the location of the catheter tip, the dose and volume of anesthetic agent used, and whether the woman is placed in the head-down, horizontal, or head-up position. It is important that the meninges not be perforated. Otherwise, the injected anesthetic enters the subarachnoid space, and in the dose used to achieve epidural anesthesia it will rapidly produce total spinal blockade.

Continuous Caudal Analgesia and Anesthesia

At the lower end of the sacrum, on its posterior surface, there is a foramen resulting from the nonclosure of the laminae of the last sacral vertebra. It is screened by a thin layer of fibrous tissue. This foramen, called the sacral hiatus, leads to the caudal canal or caudal space, which is actually the lowest extent of the epidural, or peridural, space. Through the caudal space, a rich network of sacral nerves passes downward after having emerged from the dural sac a few inches higher. The dural sac separates the caudal canal from the spinal cord and its surrounding fluid.

A suitable anesthetic solution that fills the caudal canal may abolish the sensation of pain carried via the sacral nerves and anesthetize the pelvis, producing anesthesia suitable for vaginal delivery. Higher levels with continuous caudal technique provide both analgesia in the first and second stages and anesthesia for delivery.

Complications. Both lumbar epidural and caudal epidural analgesia for labor and anesthesia for delivery may provide most pleasant relief from the pain of labor.

There are certain problems inherent in their use, however:

1. *Inadvertent Spinal Anesthesia.* Puncture of the dura along with inadvertent spinal anesthesia is always a potential complication, so personnel and facilities must be immediately available to manage the complications of high spinal anesthesia. Postspinal headache is a less serious but troublesome complication of inadvertent entry into the subarachnoid space.

2. *Ineffective Anesthesia.* The extent to which pain relief can be obtained with lumbar epidural analgesia varies. In the best of circumstances, according to Crawford (1979), about 85 percent of parturient women are free of pain, 12 percent experience partial relief, and 3 percent have no relief whatsoever. Nonetheless, establishment of effective pain relief with maximum safety takes time. Consequently, in case of rapid labor, the potential for pain relief during labor and for delivery is not realized. Therefore, epidural anesthesia for women of higher parity in active labor is likely to prove not worth the bother, risk, and expense.

   If the epidural anesthesia is allowed to dissipate before another injection of anesthetic drug, subsequent anesthesia may be delayed, incomplete, or both.

   At times, perineal anesthesia for delivery is difficult to obtain, especially with the lumbar epidural technique. When this condition is encountered, Akamatsu and Bonica (1974) recommend use of a second catheter to achieve low caudal block. Insertion of a second catheter, of course, increases many of the risks being described. For this problem, others have suggested addition of low spinal ("saddle block") anesthesia, pudendal block, or systemic analgesia or anesthesia.

3. *Hypotension.* Epidural anesthesia by blocking the sympathetic tracts may cause hypotension. In the nonhypertensive and normally hypervolemic pregnant women, hypotension induced by epidural anesthesia can usually be prevented by rapid infusion of balanced salt solution or treated successfully as described for spinal anesthesia. It is important that with each injection of anesthetic the blood pressure be followed closely for the next 20 minutes. Ueland and co-workers (1972) have confirmed by a number of physiologic measurements that hypotension with epidural anesthesia in *normal* pregnant women usually is modest and easily corrected.

4. *Central Nervous Stimulation.* Convulsions are an uncommon but serious complication, the immediate management of which has been described above. Tahir and co-workers (1975) have emphasized that late in pregnancy epidural veins are

thin walled and engorged, which predisposes to perforation by the catheter and intravenous injection of the anesthetic agent. Treatment is described above.

5. *Effect on Labor.* Epidural block induced prior to well-established labor may be followed by desultory labor. The precise role played by epidural anesthesia in this phenomenon is not clear, since this sequence of events is seen in the absence of epidural analgesia. Lowensohn and co-workers (1974) report significant depression of uterine activity for about 30 minutes following the epidural injection of lidocaine. Akamatsu and Bonica (1974) suggest that epinephrine injected with the anesthetic agent may impair labor. During the second stage of labor, epidural anesthesia that provides effective pain relief is likely to reduce appreciably maternal expulsive efforts. As a consequence, epidural anesthesia may lead to delay, or less frequently to failure, of the descent of the presenting part and spontaneous rotation to the most favorable position for delivery, that is, the occiput anterior position. Therefore, with epidural anesthesia there is likely to be an increased incidence of deliveries by use of midforceps, including forceps rotations.

Contraindications. As with spinal anesthesia, these include actual or anticipated serious *maternal hemorrhage, overt hypertension, infection* at or near the sites for puncture, and suspicion of *neurologic disease.*

Disagreements persist over the use of epidural anesthesia in the presence of *hypertension.* Some obstetric anesthesiologists urge regional analgesia and anesthesia for women with overt hypertension. Marx (1974), for example, has contended that, by use of regional anesthesia, maternal circulatory and cerebrospinal fluid pressure responses to painful uterine contractions are reduced and the hazard of hypertensive crisis is minimized. For slowly progressing labor, she recommends a double-catheter extradural block, but for labor with rapid progress, possibly a spinal block. The intrigue surrounding the use of regional anesthesia in hypertensive states complicating pregnancy undoubtedly stems from the fact that the mother is hypertensive and the blood pressure is very often lowered by the regional anesthetic. This attitude prevails even though the mechanism by which the blood pressure is lowered is probably no more physiologic than phlebotomy. Shnider and Levinson (1979) have emphasized "Sudden falls in blood pressure can rapidly produce fetal distress and demise as the uteroplacental circulation becomes further compromised." For these reasons, in over 250 consecutive cases of antepartum or intrapartum *eclampsia* at Parkland Memorial Hospital, regional anesthesia has been deliberately avoided. Instead, local or pudendal block plus nitrous oxide analgesia were used for easy vaginal deliveries and general anesthesia with thiopental, succinylcholine, and nitrous oxide was used for the occasional difficult vaginal deliv-

ery and for cesarean sections. Perinatal and maternal mortality rates have been very low in these pregnancies complicated by eclampsia (Pritchard and co-workers, 1984).

Psychoprophylaxis for Pain Relief

In 1944, Grantley Dick Read provided a text in which he emphasized that the intensity of pain with labor is related to a large degree to emotional tensions. He urged that women be well informed about the physiology of parturition and the various hospital procedures to which they would be subjected during labor and delivery. He also urged training in breathing and muscle relaxation be instituted well in advance of labor.

Subsequently, Lamaze (1970) described his psychoprophylactic method of childbirth, which emphasizes that childbirth is a natural physiologic process and that pain can be minimized by appropriate training in breathing and appropriate psychologic support.

Read and Lamaze, through their pioneer writings and the "satisfied customers" who have used their methods, have had considerable impact on the use of potent analgesic, sedative, and amnesic drugs during labor and general anesthesia for delivery. Undoubtedly, by minimizing fear, the discomfort from contractions is minimized. The presence of an involved, supportive father, of a conscientious labor attendant, and a considerate obstetrician who instills confidence contributes greatly to accomplishing this goal (see Chapter 17, p. 331).

Although psychoprophylaxis will not be completely successful in many women, it should be available for those who desire it and are willing to make the effort. At the same time, women who attempt psychoprophylaxis but find the discomforts of labor to be too great should not be denied relief provided by appropriate analgesics. It is not unusual for Lamaze-prepared women in the United States to receive some narcotic analgesia or even epidural anesthesia during labor. For delivery, local, pudendal, or epidural anesthesia has been employed commonly (Hughey and colleagues, 1978).

Abdominal Decompression

In 1959, Heynes introduced a large plastic shield that produced negative pressure when applied to the abdomen of the parturient. He claimed that the device reduced the pain and duration of labor and increased the oxygenation of the fetus, thus producing infants with high IQs. These claims have not been substantiated. Castellanos and colleagues (1968) were unable to show that the decompression apparatus relieved the pains of labor. Liddicoat (1968), in a controlled study, was unable to find a difference in IQs between children born to mothers who used the apparatus and those who did not.

Acupuncture

Although the contemporary American woman is likely to be subjected to a multitude of needle punctures during labor and delivery, there are few reports concerned with formal application of acupuncture. Bonica (1974) commented that in one small group of obstetric patients relief of pain was good in about one third, partial in a third, and poor in a third. Nineteen of the 21 laboring women studied by Wallis and co-workers (1974) regarded acupuncture as unsuccessful in providing analgesia for labor and delivery.

Conclusions

It is evident that no single method is entirely satisfactory for the alleviation of pain during labor and delivery. At the same time, demand by the laity persists for relief of suffering associated with childbirth. Such relief of pain is desirable, provided it carries no danger to mother or infant. Safety must remain the prime consideration!

REFERENCES

Akamatsu TJ, Bonica JJ: Spinal and extradural analgesia-anesthesia for parturition. Clin Obstet Gynecol 17:183, 1974

Bartlett JG, Gorbach SL, Finegold SM: The bacteriology of aspiration pneumonia. Am J Med 56:202, 1974

Bonica JJ: Acupuncture anesthesia in the People's Republic of China: Implications for American medicine. JAMA 229:1317, 1974

Bynum LJ, Pierce AK: Pulmonary aspiration of gastric contents. Am Rev Respir Dis 114:1129, 1976

Castellanos R, Aguero O, deSoto E: Abdominal decompression: A method of obstetric analgesia. Am J Obstet Gynecol 100:924, 1968

Cohen SE: The aspiration syndrome. Clin Obstet Gynecol 9:235, 1982

Crawford JS: Maternal mortality associated with anesthesia. Lancet 2:918, 1972

Crawford JS: Continuous lumbar epidural analgesia for labour and delivery. Br Med J 1:72, 1979

DeVoe SJ, DeVoe K Jr, Rigsby WC, McDaniels BA: Effects of meperidine on uterine contractility. Am J Obstet Gynecol 105:1004, 1969

Ericson A, Källén B: Survey of infants born in 1973 or 1975 to Swedish women working in operating rooms during their pregnancies. Anesth Analg 58:302, 1979

Fishburne JI Jr, Greiss FC Jr, Hopkinson R, Rhyne AL: Response of the gravid uterine vasculature to arterial levels of local anesthetic agents. Am J Obstet Gynecol 133:753, 1979

Greiss FC Jr, Still JG, Anderson SG: Effects of local anesthetic agents on the uterine vasculatures and myometrium. Am J Obstet Gynecol 124:889, 1976

Heyns OS: Abdominal decompression in the first stage of labor. Br J Obstet Gynaecol 66:220, 1959

Hughey MJ, McElin TW, Young T: Maternal and fetal outcome of Lamaze prepared patients. Obstet Gynecol 51:643, 1978

Husum B, Wulf HC, Norgaard I: Sister chromatid exchanges and structural chromosome aberrations in lymphocytes in operating room personnel. Acta Anaesthesiol Scand 27:262, 1983

Jacoby J: Anesthesia for normal vaginal delivery. Anesth Rev 1:11, 1974

Kennedy WF Jr, Bonica JJ, Akamatsu TJ, Ward RJ, Martin WE, Grinstein A: Cardiovascular and respiratory effects of subarachnoid block in the presence of acute blood loss. Anesthesiology 29:29, 1968

Knill-Jones RP, Newman BJ, Spence AA: Anaesthetic practice and pregnancy. Lancet 2:807, 1975

Lamaze F: Painless Childbirth: Psychoprophylactic Method. Chicago, Henry Regnery, 1970

Liddicoat R: The effects of maternal antenatal decompression treatment on infant mental development. S Afr Med J 42:203, 1968

Lowensohn RI, Paul RH, Fales S, Yet S-Y, Hon EH: Intrapartum epidural anesthesia: An evaluation of effects on uterine activity. Obstet Gynecol 44:388, 1974

Marx GF: Obstetric anesthesia in the presence of medical complications. Clin Obstet Gynecol 17:165, 1974

Mendelson CL: The aspiration of stomach contents into the lungs during obstetric anesthesia. Am J Obstet Gynecol 52:191, 1946

Moir DD: Ametidine, antacids, and pulmonary aspiration. J Anesthesiol 59:81, 1983

Pharoah POD, Alberman E, Doyle P: Outcome of pregnancy among women in anesthetic practice. Lancet 1:34, 1977

Pritchard JA, Cunningham FG, Pritchard SA: The Parkland Memorial Hospital protocol for treatment of eclampsia: Evaluation of 245 cases. Am J Obstet Gynecol, 148:951, 1984

Read GD: Childbirth Without Fear. New York, Harper, 1944, p 192

Riffel HD, Nochimson DJ, Paul RH, Hon EHG: Effects of meperidine and promethazine during labor. Obstet Gynecol 42:738, 1973

Schultz JH, Luthe W: Autogenic Training. New York, Grune & Stratton, 1959

Shnider SM, Levinson G: Anesthesia for Obstetrics. Baltimore, Williams and Wilkins, 1979

Svancarek W, Chirino O, Schaefer G Jr, Blythe JG: Retropsoas and subgluteal abscesses following paracervical and pudendal anesthesia. JAMA 237:892, 1977

Tahir AH, Adriani J, Naraghi M: Acute systemic toxicity from bupivicaine during epidural anesthesia in obstetric patients. South Med J 68:1377, 1975

Taylor G, Pryse-Davies J: The prophylactic use of antacids in the prevention of the acid pulmonary aspiration syndrome. Lancet 1:288, 1966

Teabeaut JR II: Aspiration of gastric contents: An experimental study. Am J Pathol 28:51, 1952

Ueland K, Akamatsu TJ, Eng M, Bonica JJ, Hansen JM: Maternal cardiovascular dynamics: I. Cesarean section under epidural anesthesia without epinephrine. Am J Obstet Gynecol 114:775, 1972

Vogel VJ: American Indian Medicine. Norman, OK, University of Oklahoma Press, 1970

Wallis L, Shnider SM, Palahniuk RJ, Spivey HT: An evaluation of acupuncture analgesia in obstetrics. Anesthesiology 41:596, 1974

Wenger DR, Gitchell RG: Severe infections following pudendal block anesthesia: Need for orthopaedic awareness. J Bone Joint Surg (Am) 55:202, 1973

Wheatley RG, Kallus FT, Reynolds RC, Giesecke AH: Milk of magnesia is an effective pre-induction antacid in obstetrical anesthesia. Anesthesiology 50:514, 1979

Zagorzycki MT, Brinkman CR III: The effect of general and epidural anesthesia upon neonatal Apgar scores in repeat cesarean section. Surg Gynecol Obstet 155:641, 1982

19

The Puerperium

Definition

Although the puerperium is defined literally as the period of confinement during and just after birth, it has come to include the subsequent weeks during which the reproductive tract returns to a normal nonpregnant state. The plan for follow-up care that has been generally practiced by most obstetricians, at least until recently, has resulted in the first 6 weeks commonly being considered the puerperium. During this time, the reproductive tract returns anatomically to a normal nonpregnant state, which includes those permanent structural changes in the cervix, vagina, and perineum that were acquired as the consequence of labor and delivery. Moreover, by 6 weeks after delivery, or not long thereafter, in most nonnursing mothers pituitary-ovarian synchrony will have been reestablished appropriate for ovulation.

INVOLUTION OF THE GENITAL AND URINARY TRACTS

Involution of the Body of the Uterus

Immediately after expulsion of the placenta, the fundus of the contracted body of the uterus is about midway between the umbilicus and symphysis, or slightly higher. The body of the uterus now consists of mostly myometrium covered by serosa and lined by basal decidua. The anterior and posterior walls, in close apposition, each measure 4 to 5 cm in thickness. Because its vessels are compressed by the contracted myometrium, the puerperal uterus on section appears ischmic when compared to the reddish purple hyperemic pregnant organ. During the next 2 days, the uterus remains approximately the same size and then shrinks, so that within 2 weeks it has descended into the cavity of the true pelvis and can no longer be felt above the symphysis. It normally regains its previous nonpregnant size within about 4 weeks. The rapidity of the process is remarkable. The freshly delivered uterus weighs approximately 1 kg. As the consequence of *involution* 1 week later it weighs about 500 g, decreasing at the end of the second week to about 300 g, and soon thereafter to 100 g or even less. The total number of muscle cells does not decrease appreciably; instead, the individual cells decrease markedly in size. The

mechanism by which the individual muscle cell divests itself of excess cytoplasm, including contractile protein, remains to be elucidated. The involution of the connective tissue framework occurs equally rapidly (Woessner, 1968).

Since the separation of the placenta and membranes involves primarily the spongy layer of the decidua, the basal portion of the decidua remains in the uterus. The decidua that remains presents striking variations in thickness, an irregular jagged appearance, and infiltration with blood, especially at the placental site.

Regeneration of Endometrium

Within 2 or 3 days after delivery, the decidua remaining in the uterus becomes differentiated into two layers. The superficial layer becomes necrotic, whereas the basal layer adjacent to the myometrium does not. The former is cast off in the lochia, and the latter, which contains the fundi of the endometrial glands, is the source of new endometrium. The endometrium arises from proliferation of the endometrial glandular remnants and the stroma of the interglandular connective tissue.

The process of endometrial regeneration is rapid, except at the placental site. Elsewhere, the free surface becomes covered by epithelium within a week or 10 days, and the entire endometrium is restored during the third week. Sharman (1953), in an extensive study of postpartum uteri, identified fully restored endometrium in all biopsy specimens obtained from the 16th day onward. The endometrium was normal except for occasional hyalinized decidual remnants and leukocytes. The so-called endometritis identified histologically in the reparative days of the puerperium is but part of the normal process of repair.

Involution of the Placental Site

According to Williams (1931), complete extrusion of the placental site takes up to 6 weeks. This process is of great clinical importance, for when it is defective, late puerperal hemorrhage may ensue. Immediately after delivery, the placental site is about the size of the palm of the hand, but it rapidly decreases in size. By the end of the second week, it is 3 to 4 cm in diameter. Very soon after termination of labor, the placental site normally consists

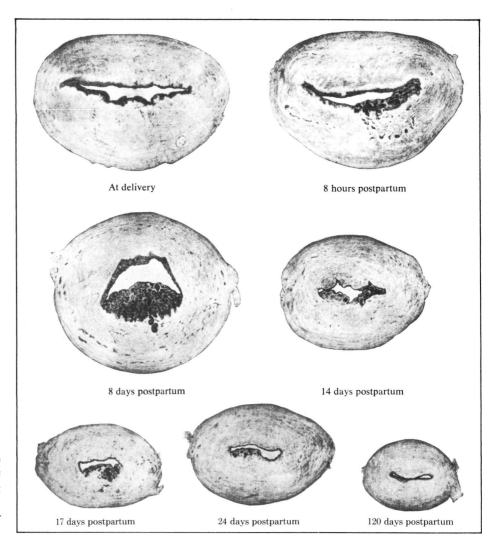

Figure 19-1. Cross sections of the uterus made at the level of the involuting placental site at varying times after delivery. (*From Williams: Am J Obstet Gynecol 22:664, 1931.*)

At delivery

8 hours postpartum

8 days postpartum

14 days postpartum

17 days postpartum

24 days postpartum

120 days postpartum

of many thrombosed vessels (Fig. 19-1) that next undergo typical organization of the thrombus.

If involution of the placental site comprised only these events, each pregnancy would leave a fibrous scar in the endometrium and subjacent myometrium, thus eventually limiting the number of future pregnancies. In his classic investigations, Williams (1931) explained involution of the placental site as follows:

> Involution is not effected by absorption in situ, but rather by a process of exfoliation which is in great part brought about by the undermining of the placental implantation site by the growth of endometrial tissue. This is affected partly by extension and down growth of endometrium from the margins of the placental site and partly by the development of endometrial tissue from the glands and stroma left in the depths of the decidua basalis after the separation of the placenta ... such a process of exfoliation should be regarded as very conservative, and as a wise provision on the part of nature; otherwise great difficulty might be experienced in getting rid of the obliterated arteries and organized thrombi which, if they remained in situ, would soon

convert a considerable part of the uterine mucosa and subadjacent myometrium into a mass of scar tissue with the result that after a few pregnancies it would unlikely be possible for it to go through its usual cycle of changes, and the reproductive career would come to an end.

Anderson and Davis (1968), on the basis of their studies of involution of the placental site, concluded that exfoliation of the placental site is brought about as the consequence of a necrotic slough of infarcted superficial tissues followed by a reparative process not unlike that which takes place on any denuded epithelium-covered structure.

Changes in the Uterine Vessels

A successful pregnancy requires a great increase in uterine blood flow. To provide for this, arteries and veins that transport blood to and from the uterus and those that convey blood within the uterus, especially to the placental site, enlarge remarkably, as do transport vessels to and from the uterus (Chapter 9, page 183). Within the uterus, growth of new vessels also provides for the marked increase in blood flow. After delivery the caliber of the extrauterine vessels decreases to equal, or at least closely approximate, that of the prepregnant state.

Within the puerperal uterus, for the most part, the blood vessels are obliterated by hyaline changes, and vessels that are smaller develop in their place. The resorption of the hyalinized residue is accomplished by processes similar to those observed in the ovaries subsequent to ovulation and corpus luteum formation. Minor vestiges, however, may persist for years, affording under the microscope a means of differentiating between the uteri of parous and nulliparous women.

Changes in the Cervix and Lower Uterine Segment

Immediately after the completion of the third stage of labor, the cervix and lower uterine segment are thin, collapsed, flabby structures. The outer margin of the cervix that corresponds to the external os usually is lacerated, especially laterally. The cervical opening contracts slowly. For a few days immediately after labor, it readily admits two fingers, but by the end of the first week, it has become so narrow as to render difficult the introduction of one finger. As the cervical opening narrows, the cervix thickens and a canal is reformed. At the completion of involution, however, the external os does not resume its pregravid appearance completely. It remains somewhat wider, and, typically, bilateral depressions at the site of lacerations remain as permanent changes that characterize the parous cervix (Fig. 2-11, page 17).

After delivery, the markedly thinned-out myometrium of the lower uterine segment contracts and retracts but not as forcefully as the body of the uterus. Over the course of a few weeks the lower segment is converted from a clearly evident structure large enough to contain most of the head of the term fetus to a barely discernible uterine isthmus located between the body of the uterus above and the internal os of the cervix below (Fig. 2-8, page 16).

Vagina and Vaginal Outlet

The vagina and vaginal outlet in the first part of the puerperium form a capacious, smooth-walled passage that gradually diminishes in size but rarely returns to the nulliparous dimensions. The rugae reappear by the third week. The hymen is represented by several small tags of tissue, which during cicatrization are converted into the myrtiform caruncles characteristic of parous women.

Changes in the Peritoneum and Abdominal Wall

As the myometrium contracts and retracts after delivery and for a few days thereafter, the peritoneum covering much of the uterus is thrown into folds and wrinkles.

The broad and round ligaments are much more lax than in the nonpregnant condition, and they require considerable time to recover from the stretching and loosening to which they have been subjected during pregnancy.

As a result of the rupture of the elastic fibers of the skin and the prolonged distention caused by the enlarged pregnant uterus, the abdominal walls remain soft and flabby for a while. The return to normal of these structures requires several weeks. Recovery is aided by exercise. Except for silvery striae, the abdominal wall usually resumes its prepregnancy appearance, but when the muscles are atonic, it may remain lax. There may be a marked separation, or diastasis, of the rectus muscles. In that condition, the abdominal wall in the vicinity of the midline is formed simply by peritoneum, attenuated fascia, subcutaneous fat, and skin.

Changes in the Urinary Tract

Cystoscopic examination soon after delivery shows not only edema and hyperemia of the bladder wall but, frequently, submucous extravasation of blood. In addition, the puerperal bladder has an increased capacity and a relative insensitivity to intravesical fluid pressure. Therefore, overdistention, incomplete emptying, and excessive residual urine must be watched for closely. The paralyzing effect of anesthesia, especially conduction anesthesia, and the temporarily disturbed neural function of the bladder are undoubtedly contributory factors. Residual urine and bacteriuria in a traumatized bladder, coupled with the dilated renal pelves and ureters, create optimal conditions for the development of urinary tract infection (Chapter 28, page 580). The dilated ureters and renal pelves return to the prepregnant state anywhere from 2 to 8 weeks after delivery (Chapter 9, page 198). The stretching and dilatation during pregnancy do not cause permanent changes in the renal pelves and ureters unless infection has supervened.

CHANGES IN MAMMARY GLANDS

Anatomy of the Breasts

The anlagen of the mammary glands are contained in the ectodermal ridges that form on the ventral surface of the embryo and extend from forelimb to hindlimb laterally. The multiple pairs of buds normally all disappear from the embryo except for one pair in the pectoral region that eventually develops into the two mammary glands (Fig. 19-2). At times, however, the buds elsewhere may not completely disappear but, instead, may participate to an amazing degree in the pattern of growth that characterizes the two normal mammary glands (Fig. 36-5).

At midpregnancy, each of the two mammary buds in the fetus destined to form the breasts begins to grow and divide, with the formation of 15 to 25 secondary buds that provide the basis for the duct system in the mature

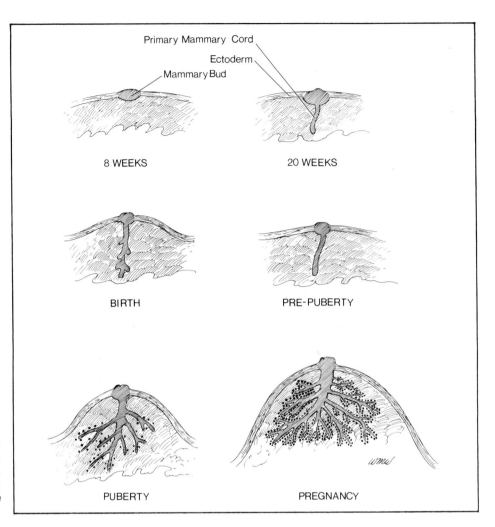

Primary Mammary Cord

Ectoderm

Mammary Bud

8 WEEKS

20 WEEKS

BIRTH

PRE-PUBERTY

PUBERTY

PREGNANCY

Figure 19-2. Sequential growth of the mammary gland is illustrated from 8 weeks embryonic age through puberty and during pregnancy. (*Courtesy of Dr. John C. Porter.*)

breast. Each secondary bud elongates into a cord, bifurcates, and differentiates into two concentric layers of cuboidal cells and a central lumen. The inner layer of cells eventually gives rise to the secretory epithelium which synthesizes the milk, while the outer layer becomes myoepithelium, which provides the mechanism for milk ejection (Fig. 19-3A, B).

Thelarche, the onset of rapid increase in breast size from estrogen stimulation, begins about the time of puberty when estrogen production rises. The previously infantile mammary glands respond to estrogen with growth and development of the mammary ducts and the deposition of fat. With the onset of ovulation, progesterone is produced, which stimulates development of the alveoli of the mammary glands and sets the stage for future lactation.

Anatomically, each mature mammary gland is made up of 15 to 25 lobes that arose from the secondary mammary buds described above. The lobes are arranged more or less radially and are separated from one another by a varying amount of fat. Each lobe consists of several lobules, which in turn are made up of large numbers of alveoli (Fig. 19-3A, B). Every alveolus is provided with a

small duct that joins others to form a single larger duct for each lobe (Fig. 19-3B). These lactiferous ducts make their way to the nipple and open separately upon its surface, where they may be distinguished as minute but distinct orifices. The alveolar secretory epithelium synthesizes the various constituents of the milk (Fig. 19-3C).

Lactation

By the second postpartum day, a modest amount of colostrum, the liquid secreted by the breasts for the first 5 days after birth of the infant, can be expressed from the nipples.

Colostrum. Compared with the mature milk that is ultimately secreted by the breasts, colostrum contains more protein, much of which is globulin, and more minerals but less sugar and fat. Colostrum, nevertheless, contains rather large fat globules in so-called colostrum corpuscles, which are thought by some to be epithelial cells that have undergone fatty degeneration and by others to be mononuclear phagocytes containing considerable fat. The secretion of colostrum persists for about 5 days, with gradual conversion to mature milk. Antibodies are

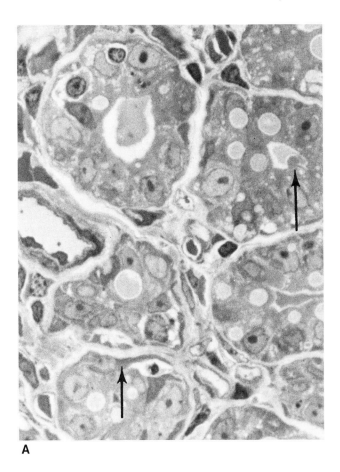

A

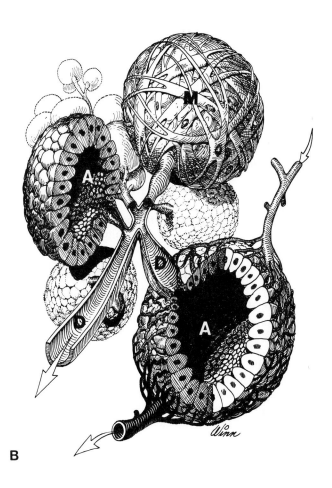

B

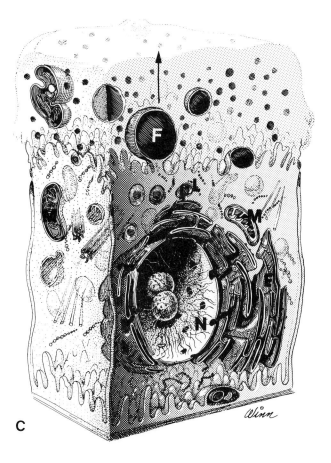

C

Figure 19-3. A. Histology of maternal breast at 32 weeks gestation in preparation for lactation. Secretions are evident in the lumen of each alveolus. Myoepithelial cells are evident around alveoli (*lower left arrow*). Secretions are being delivered by exocytosis into the lumen of one alveolus (*upper right arrow*). **B.** Graphic demonstration of alveolar and ductal system shown in **A.** Note the myoepithelial fibers (M) that surround the outside of the uppermost alveolus. The secretions from the glandular elements are extruded into the lumen of the alveoli (A) and ejected by the myoepithelial cells into the ductal system (D) which empties through the nipple. The arterial blood supply to the alveolus is identified by the upper right arrow and the venous drainage by the arrow beneath. **C.** Individual secretory cell. Two nucleoli are located within the nucleus (N). The endoplasmic reticulum (E) surrounds the nucleus. Mitochondria (M) are evident. Lactose granules (L) and fat droplets (F) migrate to the luminal margin of the cell and are there secreted by exocytosis into an alveolus (*arrow*). (*Courtesy of Dr. John C. Porter.*)

371

readily demonstrable in colostrum. Its content of immunoglobulin A may offer protection to the newborn infant against enteric infection, as described below. Other host resistance factors, as well as immunoglobulins, are present in human colostrum and milk. These include components of complement, macrophages, lymphocytes, lactoferrin, lactoperoxidase, and lysozyme.

Milk. The major components of milk are proteins, lactose, water, and fat. Milk is isotonic with plasma, with lactose accounting for half of the osmotic pressure. The major *proteins* in milk—α-lactalbumin, β-lactoglobulin, and casein—are synthesized in the rough endoplasmic reticulum of the alveolar secretory cell. The essential amino acids are derived from the blood, and nonessential amino acids are derived in part from the blood or synthesized in the mammary gland. Most of the proteins of milk are unique proteins not found elsewhere.

The synthesis of lactose from glucose in the alveolar secretory cells is catalyzed by lactose synthetase. Some lactose spills into the maternal circulation and may be excreted by the kidney and detected in the urine unless specific glucose oxidase is used in testing for glycosuria.

Fatty acids are synthesized in the alveoli from glucose. Fat droplets are secreted by an apocrine-like process (Fig. 19-3A).

All vitamins except vitamin K are present in human milk but in variable amounts (Committee on Nutrition, 1981). The levels of most vitamins in the milk are increased by maternal dietary supplementation. Since the mother does not provide for the vitamin K requirements of the breast-fed infant, vitamin K administration to the infant soon after delivery is beneficial to prevent hemorrhagic disease of the newborn (Chapter 38, page 783).

Human milk contains a low concentration of iron. However, iron in human milk is better absorbed than is iron in cow's milk. Maternal iron stores do not seem to influence the amount of iron in breast milk. The mammary gland, like the thyroid gland, concentrates iodine, which appears in the milk.

The approximate concentrations of the more important components of human colostrum, human mature milk, and cow's milk are presented in Table 19-1.

Endocrinology of Lactation

The precise humoral and neural mechanisms involved in lactation are obviously complex. Progesterone, estrogen, and placental lactogen, as well as prolactin, cortisol, and insulin, appear to act in concert to stimulate the growth and development of the milk-secreting apparatus of the mammary gland (Porter, 1974). With the delivery of the placenta, there is an abrupt and profound decrease in the levels of progesterone and estrogen, which somehow serves to initiate lactation. It is very likely that lactation is not initiated until the end of pregnancy because the high levels of estrogen and progesterone during pregnancy interfere with the lactogenic actions of prolactin and adrenal steroids.

TABLE 19-1. APPROXIMATE CONCENTRATIONS (PER DL) OF COMPONENTS OF HUMAN COLOSTRUM, HUMAN MATURE MILK, AND COW'S MILK

	Human Colostrum	Human Mature Milk	Cow's Milk
Water (g)	—	88	88
Lactose (g)	5.3	6.8	5.0
Protein (g)	2.7	1.2	3.3
Casein:lactalbumin ratio	—	1:2	3:1
Fat (g)	2.9	3.8	3.7
Linoleic acid	—	8.3% of fat	1.6% of fat
Potassium (mg)	55	55	58
Sodium (mg)	92	15	138
Chloride (mg)	117	43	103
Calcium (mg)	31	33	125
Magnesium (mg)	4	4	12
Phosphorus (mg)	14	15	100
Iron (mg)	0.09*	0.15*	0.10*
Vitamin A (μg)	89	53	34
Vitamin D (μg)	—	0.03*	0.06*
Thiamine (μg)	15	16	42
Riboflavin (μg)	30	43	157
Nicotinic acid (μg)	75	172	85
Ascorbic acid (μg)	4.4†	4.3†	1.6†

* Poor source.
† Just adequate.
(*From Edwards (ed): Res Reprod Vol 6, 1974.*)

In otherwise normal circumstances, the intensity and the duration of lactation are subsequently controlled in large part by the repetitive stimulus of nursing. Prolactin is essential for lactation; women with extensive pituitary necrosis, as in Sheehan's disease, do not lactate (Chapter 34, page 709). Although plasma prolactin falls after delivery to appreciably lower levels than during pregnancy, each act of suckling triggers a rise in prolactin levels (McNeilly and associates, 1983). Presumably a stimulus from the breast curtails the release of prolactin-inhibiting factor from the hypothalamus, which, in turn, induces transiently an increased secretion of prolactin by the pituitary.

The neurohypophysis in pulsatile fashion secretes oxytocin, which stimulates the expression of milk from a lactating breast by causing contraction of myoepithelial cells in the alveoli and small milk ducts. In fact, this mechanism has been utilized to assay oxytocin activity in biologic fluids. The ejection, or letting down, of milk is a reflex initiated especially by suckling, which stimulates the neurohypophysis to liberate oxytocin (McNeilly and associates, 1983). It may be provoked just by the cry of the infant or inhibited by fright or stress.

Immunologic Consequences of Breast-feeding

Antibodies are present in human colostrum and milk but are poorly absorbed, if at all, from the infant's gut. Indeed, no Rho (D) antibodies have been detected in the sera of infants fed milk containing a high titer of Rho antibodies. This circumstance, however, does not mitigate necessarily against the importance of at least some of the antibodies in breast milk. The predominant immunoglobulin in milk is secretory IgA, a macromolecule that is important in antimicrobial processes in the mucous membranes across which it is secreted. In this context, it is envisioned that secretory IgA contained in mother's milk may act locally within the infant's gastrointestinal tract. Human breast milk contains secretory IgA antibodies against *Escherichia coli,* and it is known that breast-fed babies are less prone to enteric infections than are bottle-fed babies. It has been suggested that IgA exerts its antimicrobial action by preventing attachment of bacteria to cells on mucosal surfaces, preventing their penetration into tissues.

In addition to the role of antibodies in human milk, much attention is being directed to an elucidation of the role of maternal lymphocytes in breast milk in fetal immunologic processes. It has been reported that human milk contains both T and B lymphocytes. Lymphocytes in colostrum undergo blastoid transformation in vitro following exposure to specific antigens. In studies of experimental animals, Beer and Billingham (1976) obtained evidence that there is transmission of viable lymphocytes from mother to infant through the breast milk.

The amounts of protective factors in human milk appear to vary appreciably, being much richer in the milk of young women compared to that of older women (Whitehead, 1983).

Nursing

An ideal food for the newborn child is the milk of the mother. Appropriately, the frequency of infant breast-feeding in recent years has increased considerably. In one recent survey in the United States carried out by a manufacturer of infant formula, nearly two thirds of women were breast-feeding their 1-week-old infants, compared to less than one third 25 years before.

In most instances, even though the supply of milk at first appears insufficient, it becomes adequate if suckling is continued. Nursing also accelerates involution of the uterus, since repeated stimulation of the nipples through release of oxytocin from the neurohypophysis leads to increased contractions of the myometrium.

Drugs Secreted in Milk. Most drugs given to the mother are secreted in the milk. Many factors influence their excretion, including the concentration of drugs in plasma, the degree of protein binding of the drug, plasma and milk pH, degree of ionization, lipid solubility, and molecular weight. Drugs are secreted in milk usually in concentrations no higher than in maternal plasma. Consequently, the amount of drug ingested by the infant typically is small. Platzker and co-workers (1980) have provided an extensive list of drugs and an appraisal of their compatibility with breast-feeding.

CLINICAL ASPECTS OF THE PUERPERIUM

Temperature

Breast engorgement, which is common on the third or fourth day of the puerperium, was once thought to cause a rise in temperature. This so-called milk fever was regarded as physiologic. Although no such entity is clearly recognized today, on occasion perhaps, extreme vascular and lymphatic engorgement may cause a sharp rise in fever, but it does not last more than 24 hours at the most. *Any rise of temperature in the puerperium implies an infection, most likely somewhere in the genitourinary tract.*

Afterpains

In primiparas, the puerperal uterus tends to remain tonically contracted unless blood clots, fragments of placenta, or other foreign bodies are retained in its cavity, causing hypertonic contractions in an effort to expel them. In multiparas especially, the uterus often contracts vigorously at intervals, the contractions giving rise to painful sensations that are known as "afterpains" and that occasionally are sufficiently severe to require an analgesic. In some mothers, they may last for days. Afterpains are particularly noticeable when the infant is put to the breast, presumably because of the release of oxytocin. Usually, they decrease in intensity and become quite mild by the third day after delivery.

Lochia

Early in the puerperium, there is a variable amount of uterine discharge, the lochia. Microscopically, the lochia consists of erythrocytes, shreds of decidua, epithelial cells, and bacteria. Microorganisms can always be demonstrated in lochia pooled in the vagina and are present in most cases even when the discharge has been obtained from the uterine cavity.

For the first few days after delivery, the content of blood in the lochia is sufficient to color it red, or *lochia rubra*. After 3 or 4 days, the lochia becomes progressively paler, or *lochia serosa*. After the 10th day, because of a marked admixture with leukocytes and a reduced fluid content, the lochia assumes a white or yellowish white color, or *lochia alba*. Foul-smelling lochia suggests, but does not prove, infection.

Adams and Flowers (1960) measured the lochia of 120 women during the first 5½ days after delivery. During this period, the lochial weight in nursing and nonnursing women averaged 251 and 277 g, respectively. Similar patients also received 0.2 mg of methylergonovine maleate (Methergine) orally every 4 hours for the first 3 days after delivery. There was no appreciable difference in the amount of lochia between the women who received methylergonovine maleate and those who did not. The morbidity rates during the puerperium were the same, and the height of the fundus was identical in both the treated and untreated groups. The only real observed difference related to the mother's discomfort. Those who received the drug suffered much more from uterine cramping. These investigators concluded that the routine use of such medication was unwarranted. Newton and Bradford (1961) similarly concluded that after the immediate period following delivery the routine administration of intramuscular oxytocin to normal women was of no value in decreasing blood loss or hastening involution of the uterus.

In many instances, a reddish color in the lochia is maintained for a longer period. When it persists for more than 2 weeks, however, it indicates either the retention of small portions of the placenta or imperfect involution of the placental site, or both.

Urine

Diuresis regularly occurs between the second and fifth days, even when intravenous fluids were not vigorously infused during labor and delivery. Normal pregnancy is associated with an appreciable increase in extracellular water. The puerperal diuresis represents a reversal of this process as the fluid-retaining stimuli of pregnancy-induced hyperestrogenism and elevated venous pressure in the lower half of the body are removed and as any residual hypervolemia is dissipated. In preeclampsia, both retention of fluid antepartum and diuresis postpartum may be greatly increased (Chapter 27, page 541).

Occasionally, substantial amounts of sugar may be found in the urine during the first weeks of the puerperium. The sugar most likely is lactose, which, fortunately, is nonreducing in test systems using glucose oxidase.

After a long labor, acetone may be identified in the urine as a consquence of starvation.

Blood

Rather marked leukocytosis occurs during and after labor, the leukocyte count sometimes reaching levels as high as 30,000 per μl (Chapter 9, page 193). The increase is made up predominantly of granulocytes. There is a relative lymphopenia and an absolute eosinopenia.

Normally, during the first few days after delivery, the hemoglobin, hematocrit, and erythrocyte count fluctuate moderately. In general, however, if they fall much below the level present just before or during early labor, the woman has lost a considerable amount of blood (Chapter 21, page 389). By 1 week after delivery, the blood volume has returned to near the usual nonpregnant level.

The pregnancy-induced changes in blood coagulation factors persist for variable periods of time after delivery. The elevation of plasma fibrinogen is maintained at least through the first week of the puerperium. As a consequence, the elevated sedimentation rate normally found during much of pregnancy normally remains high during the early puerperium.

Loss of Weight

In addition to the loss on the average of about 12 pounds as the consequence of evacuation of the contents of the uterus and normal blood loss, there is generally further loss of body weight during the puerperium of about 5 pounds. This weight loss is accounted for by fluid lost chiefly through urination, as described above. Chesley and co-workers (1959) demonstrated a decrease in the sodium space of about 2 liters, or nearly 5 pounds, during the first week after delivery.

CARE OF THE MOTHER DURING THE PUERPERIUM

Attention Immediately after Labor

After delivery of the placenta, the uterus should be firm, with its upper margin just below the umbilicus. As long as it remains in this condition, there is no danger of postpartum hemorrhage *from uterine atony.* To guard against such an occurrence, the uterus should be palpated through the abdominal wall at frequent intervals after the completion of the third stage of labor, that is, delivery of the placenta. If relaxation is detected, the uterus should be massaged through the abdominal walls until it remains contracted. Blood may accumulate within the uterus without external evidence of bleeding. This condition may be detected early by identifying uterine enlargement through frequent palpation of the fundus during the first few hours postpartum. *Even in normal cases, a trained attendant should remain with the mother for at least 1 hour after completion of the third stage of labor.*

Care of the Vulva

Shortly after completion of the third stage of labor and perineal repair, the draping and soiled linen beneath the mother are removed, provided there is no excessive bleeding or other reason to keep her in the lithotomy position on the delivery table. The external genitalia and buttocks are flushed with soap and water in such a way that all of the liquid drains from the vulva and perineum down over the anus, rather than in the reverse direction. A sterile vulvar pad is then applied over the genitalia and replaced by a clean pad as necessary. After each bowel movement and before any local treatment or examination, the external genitalia should be similarly cleansed.

Subsequent Discomfort

The discomfort from cesarean section, its causes, and its management are considered in Chapter 43 (page 867). During the first few days after vaginal delivery, the mother may be uncomfortable for a variety of reasons, including afterpains, episiotomy and lacerations, breast engorgement, and, at times, postspinal headache. It is prudent to provide codeine, 60 mg, or aspirin, 0.6 g, at intervals as frequent as every 3 hours during the first few days after delivery. Uterine contractions are commonly accentuated during nursing, giving rise at times to troublesome afterpains.

The repaired episiotomy or lacerations may be uncomfortable, as discussed in Chapter 17, page 350. Early application of an icebag to the perineum may minimize the swelling and discomfort. The majority of women also appear to obtain a measure of relief from the periodic application of a local anesthetic spray to the site of episiotomy or laceration. Severe discomfort may mean that a sizable hematoma has formed in the genital tract. Therefore, careful examination is warranted, especially whenever ordinary orally ingested analgesics do not provide appreciable relief. The episiotomy incision is normally firmly healed and nearly asymptomatic by the third week after delivery.

Depression

It is fairly common for a mother to exhibit some degree of depression a few days after delivery. The transient depression, or "postpartum blues," most likely is the consequence of a number of factors. Prominent in its genesis are (1) the emotional letdown that follows the excitement and fears that most women experience during pregnancy and delivery, (2) the discomforts of the early puerperium that have been described above, (3) fatigue from loss of sleep during labor and postpartum in most hospital settings, (4) anxiety over her capabilities for caring for her infant after leaving the hospital, and (5) fears that she has become less attractive to her husband. In the great majority of cases effective treatment need be nothing more than anticipation, recognition, and reassurance.

Early Ambulation

Immediately after World War II, important changes began to take place in the management of the puerperium in the direction of early ambulation. Women are now out of bed well within the first 24 hours after vaginal delivery. The many advantages of early ambulation are confirmed by numerous well-controlled studies. Women state that they feel better and stronger after early ambulation. Bladder complications and constipation are less frequent. Early ambulation has also reduced materially the frequency of thrombosis and pulmonary embolism during the puerperium. For the first ambulation, at least, an attendant should be present to help prevent injury if the woman were to become syncopal.

Abdominal Wall Relaxation

An abdominal binder is unnecessary, although it was formerly believed to aid involution and help restore the mother's figure. It is now the consensus that it has no effect on involution. If the abdomen is unusually flabby or pendulous, an ordinary girdle is often more satisfactory than an abdominal binder. Exercises to help restore tone to the abdominal wall may be started at any time after vaginal delivery and as soon as the abdominal soreness diminishes after cesarean section.

Diet

It was formerly customary to restrict the diet of the puerperal woman who has been delivered vaginally, but at present an attractive general diet is recommenced. If at the end of 2 hours after vaginal delivery there are no complications likely to necessitate an anesthetic, the patient should be given something to drink if she is thirsty and something to eat if she is hungry. The diet of the lactating mother, compared with that consumed during pregnancy, should be increased somewhat, especially in calories and protein, as recommended by the Food and Nutrition Board of the National Research Council (Table 13-1, page 251). If the mother does not breastfeed her infant, her dietary requirements are the same as for a normal nonpregnant woman. There is absolutely no rationale for restricting fluids for women who do not desire to nurse.

It is standard practice at Parkland Memorial Hospital to continue iron supplementation for 1 month after delivery. The hematocrit is also checked at the time of the postpartum check, which is performed routinely during the third week of the puerperium.

Bladder Function

The rate of accumulation of urine in the bladder after delivery may be quite variable. Currently, intravenous fluids are nearly always infused during labor and for an hour or so after delivery. Oxytoxin, in doses that are antidiuretic, is commonly infused in the intravenous fluid after the third stage of labor. As a consequence of the volume of fluid infused and the sudden withdrawal of the antidiuretic effect of oxytocin, rapid filling of the bladder is common. Moreover, both bladder sensation and the capability of the bladder to empty spontaneously may be appreciably diminished by anesthesia, especially conduction anesthesia, and by painful lesions in the genital tract, such as extensive episiotomy, lacerations, or hematomas. It is not surprising, therefore, that urinary retention with overdistention of the bladder is a nagging complication of the early puerperium. Once overdistention occurs, bladder function becomes further impaired, and ascending infection of the urinary tract is a likely consequence.

Prevention of overdistention demands close observation of the bladder after delivery to make sure that it does not overfill and that with each voiding it empties adequately. The bladder may be palpated as a cystic mass suprapubically, or the enlarged bladder may be evident abdominally only indirectly, the full bladder having elevated the uterine fundus to well above the umbilicus.

If the woman has not voided within 4 hours after delivery, it is likely that she cannot do so. Ambulation to a commode usually should be tried before resorting to catheterization. The woman who has trouble voiding initially is likely to have further trouble. At times, an indwelling catheter is necessary, as described in Chapter 36, page 739. The likelihood of hematomas of the genital tract must be kept in mind when the woman cannot void following delivery. Whenever the bladder has become overdistended, an indwelling catheter for a day, until the factors causing the retention have for the most part abated, is likely to be beneficial.

Bowels

At times, the lack of a bowel movement is no more than the expected consequence of an efficient cleansing enema administered a few hours before delivery and little food being eaten subsequently. With both early ambulation and early feeding of a general diet, constipation has become much less of a problem in the puerperium.

Care of the Breasts and Nipples

The nipples require little attention in the puerperium other than cleanliness and attention to fissures. Since dried milk is likely to accumulate and irritate the nipples, cleansing of the aerolae with water and mild soap is helpful before and after nursing. Occasionally, with irritated nipples, it is necessary to resort to a nipple shield for 24 hours or longer. A nursing brassiere that provides support without constriction is desirable. Suppression of lactation in the woman who does not nurse her infant is considered in Chapter 36, page 739.

Immunizations

The Rho negative woman who is not isoimmunized and whose baby is Rho(D) positive is given 300 μg of Rho-immune globulin shortly after delivery (Chapter 38, page 773). Women who are not already immune to rubella (Chapter 13, page 260) are excellent candidates for vaccination before discharge. At Parkland Memorial Hospital the mother also receives a tetanus toxoid booster injection at this time, unless it is contraindicated.

Time of Discharge

Puerperal women now are usually up and about shortly after the birth of their children and we certainly see no reason after vagnial delivery for hospitalization normally beyond 3 days. The price has become so great that women and their newborn infants frequently are sent home sooner.

Return of Menstruation and Ovulation

If the woman does not nurse her child, the menstrual flow will probably return within 6 to 8 weeks after labor. At times, however, it is difficult clinically to assign a specific date to the first menstrual period after delivery. A minority of women bleed small to moderate amounts in-

termittently, starting soon after delivery. Menses may not appear so long as the infant is nursed but great variations are observed, for in lactating women, the first period may occur as early as the second or as late as the 18th month after delivery.

Sharman (1966), by means of histologic dating of the endometrium, identified ovulation as early as 42 days after delivery, and Perez and associates (1972) did so as early as 36 days. Moreover, a corpus luteum has been observed 6 weeks after delivery at the time of sterilization (Chester, 1979). The necessity for avoiding delay in instituting contraceptive techniques by the sexually active woman is obvious.

It has long been appreciated that ovulation is much less frequent in women who nurse their infants compared to those who do not. Nonetheless, pregnancy can occur while lactating. Hefnawi and Badraoui (1977) have provided the following quantitative information for women who nurse: Of 340 lactating Egyptian women who used no contraception after delivery, one fourth had conceived again within the next 12 months. Of those who became pregnant, one fourth had never menstruated since delivery. Onset of menses increased from 8 percent the first month after delivery to 61 percent by 12 months. Among those who menstruated, ovulation, identified by examinations of cervical mucus and endometrial biopsies, rose from 3 percent at 1 month to 59 percent at 12 months.

It is generally thought that amenorrhea during the period of lactation is the consequence of lack of appropriate ovarian stimulation by pituitary gonadotropins. In keeping with this concept, as illustrated in Figure 19-4A and B, the levels of luteinizing hormone (LH) and follicle-stimulating hormone (FSH) in one carefully studied lactating woman were appreciably lower during the time of amenorrhea than they were after the resumption of menstruation (Madden and colleagues, 1978).

While Keettel and Bradbury (1961), in a much earlier study, noted very low pituitary gonadotropic activity, as anticipated, in the urine of some lactating women with amenorrhea, they also detected by bioassay normal or even elevated amounts of gonadotropins in the urine of others. They concluded that in the latter circumstance the absent or very limited estrogenic effect on the vaginal epithelium, as well as the amenorrhea and anovulation, resulted from the failure of the ovaries to respond to the gonadotropins. The studies of Bonnar and co-workers (1975) have provided an explanation for their observation. In some women in their study who were breast-feeding, plasma estrogens did not increase despite a rise in FSH. The lack of response was attributed to an inhibitory effect of the increased prolactin levels on follicular development.

Follow-up Care

By the time of discharge from the hospital after a vaginal delivery and a normal in-hospital puerperium, the mother can resume most activities, including bathing,

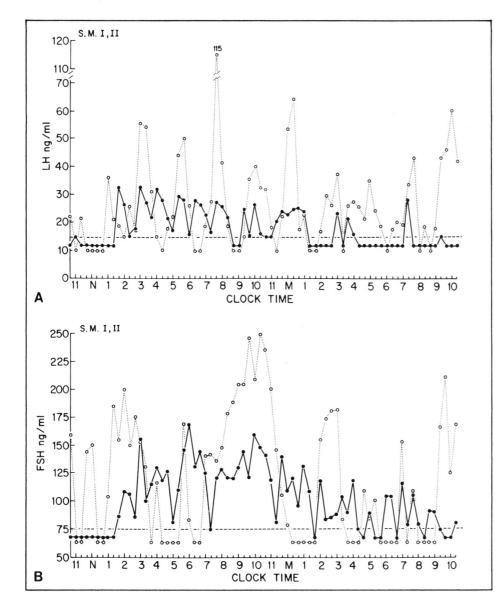

Figure 19-4. A. Comparison of the 24-hour secretory patterns of LH in the lactating woman. The closed circles denote plasma LH levels during the period of amenorrhea. The open circles correspond to the plasma LH concentrations after menses had resumed. **B.** Comparison of the 24-hour secretory patterns of FSH in the lactating woman. The closed circles denote plasma FSH levels during the period of amenorrhea. The open circles correspond to the plasma FSH concentrations after menses had resumed. (*From Madden and coworkers: Am J Obstet Gynecol 132:436, 1978.*)

driving, and household functions. Although it has been customary for some obstetricians to recommend that she not resume employment or return to school for several weeks, there is no evidence that to do so earlier causes any physical harm. Ideally, it would appear that much of the care and attention received by the very young infant should be provided by the mother, amply augmented by the father; for her to do so precludes early return by the mother to full-time work or school.

Recommendations as to the time of resumption of sexual intercourse have varied considerably. It is most unlikely that there are increased risks from intercourse as early as 2 weeks after delivery except perhaps for dyspareunia, which can be minimized by careful repair of the episiotomy (Richardson and associates, 1976). Delay of examination of the mother until 6 weeks postpartum became routine practice in obstetrics, but from

the standpoint of optimal clinical care, the reasons for selecting that time are not altogether clear. Since 1969, at Parkland Memorial Hospital, puerperal women typically have been given appointments for follow-up examination during the third week following delivery. The third week has proven quite satisfactory both to identify any abnormalities of the later puerperium and to initiate contraceptive practices. Estrogen plus progestin oral contraceptives started at this time have proved effective without increased morbidity. Moreover, the frequencies of uterine perforation, expulsions, and pregnancies when intrauterine devices were inserted during the third week postpartum were no greater than when the devices were inserted 3 months or more postpartum. Family planning technique and follow-up care are discussed further in Chapter 40, page 811.

REFERENCES

Adams H, Flowers CE: Oral oxytocic drugs in the puerperium. Obstet Gynecol 15:280, 1960

Anderson WR, Davis J: Placental site involution. Am J Obstet Gynecol 102:23, 1968

Beer AE, Billingham RE: The Immunobiology of Mammalian Reproduction. Englewood Cliffs, NJ, Prentice-Hall, 1976, p 198

Bonnar J, Franklin M, Nott PN, McNeilly AS: Effect of breast-feeding on pituitary-ovarian function after childbirth. Br Med J 4:82, 1975

Chesley LC, Valenti C, Uichano L: Alterations in body fluid compartments and exchangeable sodium in early puerperium. Am J Obstet Gynecol 77:1054, 1959

Chester D: Personal communication, 1979

Committee on Nutrition: Nutrition and lactation. Pediatrics 68:435, 1981

Hefnawi F, Badraoui MHH: The benefits of lactation amenorrhea as a contraceptive. Fertil Steril 28:320, 1977

Keettel WC, Bradbury JT: Endocrine studies of lactation amenorrhea. Am J Obstet Gynecol 82:995, 1961

Madden JD, Boyar R, MacDonald PC, Porter JC: Analysis of secretory patterns of prolactin and gonadotropins during twenty-four hours in a lactating woman before and after resumption of menses. Am J Obstet Gynecol 132:436, 1978

McNeilly AS, Robinson ICA, Houston MJ, Howie PW: Release of oxytocin and prolactin in response to suckling. Br Med J 286:257, 1983

Newton M, Bradford WM: Postpartal blood loss. Obstet Gynecol 17:229, 1961

Perez A, Vela P, Masnic GS, Potter RG: First ovulation after childbirth: The effect of breastfeeding. Am J Obstet Gynecol 114:1041, 1972

Platzker ACD, Lew CD, Stewart D: Drug "administration" via breast milk. Hosp Pract, Sept 1980, p 111

Porter JC: Hormonal regulation of breast development and activity. J Invest Dermatol 63:85, 1974

Richardson AC, Lyon JB, Graham EE, Williams NL: Decreasing postpartum sexual abstinence time. Am J Obstet Gynecol 126:416, 1976

Sharman A: Postpartum regeneration of the human endometrium. J Anat 87:1, 1953

Sharman A: Ovulation in the post-partum period. Excerpta Medica International Congress Series, No 133, 1966, p 158

Whitehead RG: Nutritional aspects of human lactation. Lancet 1:167, 1983

Williams JW: Regeneration of the uterine mucosa after delivery with especial reference to the placental site. Am J Obstet Gynecol 22:664, 1931

Woessner JF: Postpartum involution of the uterus connective tissue framework. Ob/Gyn Digest, July 1968, p 14

20

The Newborn Infant

The First Breath of Air

As the infant is born and the fetoplacental circulation ceases to function, the infant is subjected to rapid and profound physiologic changes (Chapter 8, p. 147). The baby's survival demands a prompt and orderly interchange of oxygen and carbon dioxide between his or her new environment and the pulmonary circulation. For efficient interchange, the fluid-filled alveoli of the lungs must fill with air, the air must be exchanged by appropriate respiratory motion, and a vigorous microcirculation must be established in close proximity to the alveoli.

Intrauterine Respiration. Until recently, it was widely taught that only at times of hypoxic stress did the fetus breathe in utero. This view was so strongly championed by some eminent fetal physiologists that observations to the contrary most often were promptly rejected as being the consequence of abnormal stimulation, most likely hypoxia, during the course of the experiment. In recent years, however, conclusive evidence of episodic respiratory movements in utero has been obtained during normal human pregnancy. Pressure changes during inspiration recorded in monkey fetuses by Martin and co-workers (1974) appear sufficiently intense to induce movement of amnionic fluid into and out of the fetal lungs, as demonstrated in both monkey and human fetuses by Duenhoelter and Pritchard (1976).

Initiation of Air Breathing

Very soon after birth, the breathing pattern shifts from one of shallow episodic inspirations that characterize fetal breathing to that of regular deeper inhalations. It is now apparent that aeration of the newborn lung is not the inflation of a collapsed structure but, instead, the rapid replacement of bronchial and alveolar fluid by air.

In the lamb, and presumably in the human infant, residual alveolar fluid after delivery is cleared through the pulmonary circulation and, to a lesser degree, through pulmonary lymphatics (Chernick, 1978). Delay in the removal of fluid from the alveoli probably contributes to the syndrome of *transient tachypnea of the newborn.*

As the fluid is replaced by air, there is considerable reduction in pulmonary vascular compression and, in turn, lowered resistance to blood flow. With the fall in pulmonary arterial blood pressure, the ductus arteriosus normally closes. Closure of the foramen ovale is more variable.

High negative intrathoracic pressures are required to bring about the initial entry of air into fluid-filled alveoli. Normally, from the first breath after birth, progressively more residual air accumulates in the lung, and with each successive breath, lower pulmonary opening pressure is required. In the mature normal infant, by about the fifth breath of air, the pressure-volume changes achieved with each respiration are very similar to those of the normal adult.

Alveolar Surface Tension and Lung Surfactant. The successful filling of the lungs with air and the rapid establishment of a physiologic pattern of pressure-volume changes on inspiration and expiration require the presence of surface-active material that will lower surface tension in the alveoli and thereby prevent the collapse of the lung with each expiration (Chapter 8, page 154). Lack of sufficient surfactant leads to the prompt development of the respiratory distress syndrome (Chapter 38, page 769).

The Stimuli to Breathe Air. Normally, the newborn infant begins to breathe and cry almost immediately after birth, indicating the establishment of active respiration. All the factors involved in the first breath of air have been difficult to elucidate, undoubtedly because many individually subtle stimuli contribute simultaneously. Some noteworthy explanations follow.

Physical Stimulation. The handling of the infant during delivery and contact with various relatively rough surfaces are believed to provoke respiration through stimuli reaching the respiratory center reflexly from the skin.

Compression of Fetal Thorax Incident to Delivery. The compression of the thorax during the second stage of labor forces some fluid from the respiratory tract. For example, Saunders (1978) found that considerable pressure is often produced by compression of the chest during vaginal delivery and estimated that lung

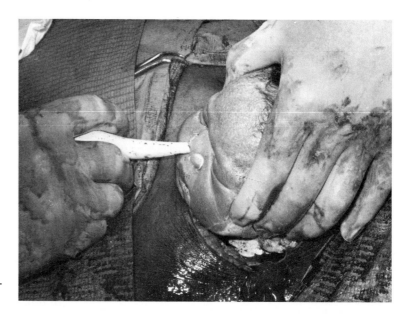

Figure 20-1. Aspirating the nose and mouth immediately after delivery of the head.

fluid is expelled equivalent to one fourth to one third of ultimate functional residual capacity. While babies born by cesarean section usually cry satisfactorily and sometimes just as quickly as babies born vaginally, they are likely to have more fluid and less gas in their lungs throughout the first 6 hours after birth (Milner and colleagues, 1978). The compression of the thorax incident to vaginal delivery and the expansion that follows delivery may, nevertheless, be an auxiliary factor in the initiation of respiration.

Deprivation of Oxygen and Accumulation of Carbon Dioxide. It was the opinion of Barcroft and associates (1939), based on animal experimentation, that lack of oxygen caused respiration after birth. Observations on both animals and human beings, however, have shown that profound lack of oxygen produces apnea. If minor degrees of hypoxia produce the first respiration after birth, certain observations become difficult to explain. For example, there is no relation between the concentration of oxygen in the blood at birth and the onset of respiration except possibly that infants with normal levels of oxygen breathe more readily than those with extremely low levels who are often apneic. Blood samples obtained from catheters implanted into fetal vessels of experimental animals for prolonged periods of time without interruption of the pregnancy have revealed that Po_2 is low by adult standards. A further decrease in Po_2 diminishes or abolishes fetal respiratory motion, whereas elevation of Pco_2 increases the frequency and magnitude of fetal breathing movements (Dawes, 1974). The fetus-infant most likely responds to hypoxia and to hypercapnea the same way in utero and after birth.

Immediate Care. As the head of the infant is delivered, either vaginally or by cesarean section, the face is immediately wiped and the mouth and nares suctioned (Fig.

20-1). A soft rubber ear syringe or its equivalent inserted with care is quite suitable for the purpose. Before clamping and severing the cord, while the infant is still being held head down, it may be beneficial to aspirate the mouth and pharynx again. Once the cord has been divided, as described in Chapter 17 (page 342), the infant is immediately placed supine with the head lowered and turned to the side in a heated unit with appropriate thermal regulation and equipped for immediate intensive care (Fig. 20-2). To minimize heat loss, the baby is wiped dry.

Evaluation of the Infant. Before and during delivery, careful consideration must be given to the following determinants of well-being for the infant: (1) health status of the mother, (2) fetal (gestational) age, (3) duration of labor, (4) duration of rupture of the membranes, (5) kinds, amounts, times, and routes of administration of analgesics, (6) kind and duration of anesthesia, and (7) degree of difficulty encountered in effecting delivery. The obstetrician is responsible for having this information available and effectively disseminating it. The obstetrician inspects the infant for any visible abnormalities during delivery and until the cord is severed, and the infant is handed over to a trained associate for further care.

The person immediately in charge of caring for the infant should observe respirations closely and identify the heart rate. The heart rate can be determined by auscultation over the chest or by palpating the base of the umbilical cord. A readily discernible heart beat of 100 or more is acceptable. Persistent bradycardia requires prompt resuscitation. The mouth, nares, and pharynx are carefully suctioned.

Most normal infants take a breath within a few seconds of birth and cry within half a minute. If respirations are infrequent, suction of the mouth and pharynx,

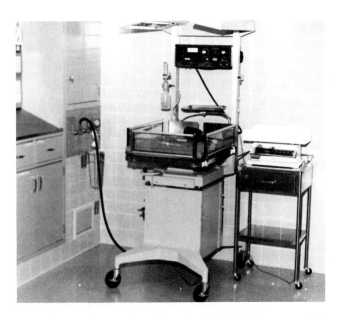

Figure 20-2. Thermostatically controlled infant care unit in delivery room.

score, up to a maximum of 10, the better is the condition of the infant. The 1-minute Apgar score determines the need for immediate resuscitation. Most infants at birth are in excellent condition, as indicated by Apgar scores of 7 to 10, and require no aid other than perhaps simple nasopharyngeal suction. *Mildly to moderately depressed infants* score 4 to 7 at 1 minute, demonstrating depressed respirations, flaccidity, and pale to blue color. Heart rate and reflex irritability, however, are good. *Severely depressed infants* score 0 to 4, with heart rate slow to inaudible and reflex response depressed to absent. Resuscitation, including artificial ventilation, should be started immediately. Often, babies who need immediate active intervention are obvious. They are flaccid, apneic, often covered with meconium, and the heart rate is below 100. There is no need for considering further the 1-minute Apgar score. Pharyngeal suction, endotracheal intubation, endotracheal suction, and positive pressure oxygenation should be instituted as soon as possible.

A low Apgar score at 5 minutes after birth is indicative of increased risk of infant mortality and morbidity.

followed by light slapping of the soles of the feet and rubbing of the back, usually together serve to stimulate breathing. Prolongation of these intervals beyond 1 and 2 minutes, respectively, indicates an abnormality. Continued lack of breathing indicates either marked central depression or mechanical obstruction and demands active resuscitation. "Tubbing," "jackknifing," and dilatation of sphincters are condemned as wasteful of valuable time and may cause serious injury.

Lack of Effective Respirations. Important causes of failure to establish effective respirations include the following: (1) fetal hypoxemia from any cause, (2) drugs administered to the mother, (3) gross immaturity of the fetus, (4) upper airway obstruction, (5) pneumothorax, (6) other lung abnormalities, either intrinsic (e.g., hypoplasia) or extrinsic (e.g., diaphragmatic hernia), (7) aspiration of amnionic fluid grossly contaminated with meconium, and (8) central nervous system injury.

Apgar Score

A useful aid in the evaluation of the infant is the Apgar scoring system applied at 1 minute and again at 5 minutes after birth (Table 20-1). In general, the higher the

ACTIVE RESUSCITATION

Although resuscitative measures beyond the stimulation provided by suctioning the mouth and nares, patting the feet, and rubbing the back are needed by only a small percentage of infants, more active measures, skillfully performed, are lifesaving for that small group. Common errors in the resuscitation of the newborn are listed:

1. Failure to check resuscitation equipment beforehand
   a. Damaged resuscitation bag
   b. Laryngoscope with dull or flickering light
   c. Unsterile umbilical catheter
2. Use of a cold resuscitation table
3. Unsuccessful intubation
   a. Hyperextension of neck
   b. Inadequate suctioning
   c. Excessive force
4. Inadequate ventilation
   a. Improper head position
   b. Improper application of mask
   c. Placement of tube into esophagus or right mainstem bronchus
   d. Failure to secure tube

TABLE 20-1. APGAR SCORING SYSTEM

Sign	0	1	2
Heart rate	Absent	Slow (below 100)	Over 100
Respiratory effort	Absent	Slow, irregular	Good, crying
Muscle tone	Flaccid	Some flexion of extremities	Active motion
Reflex irritability	No response	Grimace	Vigorous cry
Color	Blue, pale	Body pink, extremities blue	Completely pink

5. Failure to detect and determine cause of poor chest movement or persistent bradycardia
6. Failure to detect and treat hypovolemia
7. Failure to perform cardiac massage

Successful active resuscitation requires (1) skilled personnel who are immediately available, (2) a suitably heated, well-lighted, appropriately large work area (Fig. 20-2), (3) equipment to deliver oxygen by intermittent positive pressure through a face mask and to carry out endotracheal intubation with endotracheal suction and positive-pressure oxygenation (Fig. 20-3), and (4) drugs, syringes, needles, and catheters for possible intravenous administration of naloxone (Narcan), sodium bicarbonate, and, rarely, intracardiac injection of epinephrine. The site of every delivery, vaginal or abdominal, must be so equipped for resuscitation, and the equipment should be thoroughly checked before each delivery.

Ventilation by Mask

Inadequate respirations that persist much beyond a minute lead to a falling heart rate and decreased muscle tone and call for a quick but careful physical examination, especially of the mouth, nose, pharynx, neck, and chest, and the administration of oxygen. If the mouth and pharynx are free of liquid and foreign material and no physical obstruction to breathing is identified, oxygen may be delivered through a well-fitting mask at a pressure of about 20 cm of water in 1- to 2-second bursts to deliver oxygen into the bronchi. If this maneuver does not *promptly* stimulate breathing and correct the evidence of hypoxia, endotracheal intubation is necessary under direct visualization with an appropriate laryngoscope.

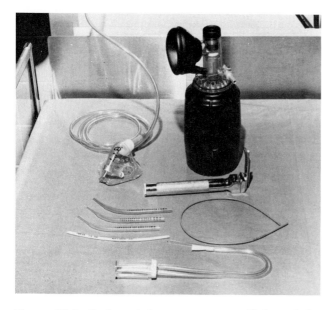

Figure 20-3. Equipment for emergency ventilation of the newborn infant.

Endotracheal Intubation

The head of the supine infant is kept level. The laryngoscope is introduced into the right side of the mouth and then directed posteriorly toward the oropharynx (Fig. 20-4). The laryngoscope is next gently moved into the space between the base of the tongue and the epiglottis. Gentle elevation of the tip of the laryngoscope will pick up the epiglottis and expose the glottis and the vocal cords. The endotracheal tube is entered through the right side of the mouth and is inserted through the vocal cords until the shoulder of the tube reaches the glottis. Care must be exercised to make sure that the tube is in the trachea and not in the esophagus. The laryngoscope is then removed. Any foreign material encountered is immediately removed by suction. Meconium, blood, mucus, and particulate debris in amnionic fluid or in the birth canal may have been inhaled in utero or in the vagina. The resuscitator fills his mouth from an oxygen line and repeatedly puffs oxygen-rich air into the endotracheal tube at 1- to 2-second intervals with force adequate to lift gently the infant's chest wall. Pressures of 25 to 35 cm of water are desired to expand the alveoli yet not cause pneumothorax or pneumomediastinum. Alternatively, intermittent positive-pressure ventilation with oxygen delivered from a bag connected to the endotracheal tube is used. If the stomach expands, the endotracheal tube is almost certainly in the esophagus rather than in the trachea. Once adequate spontaneous respirations have been established, the endotracheal tube can usually be removed safely.

Acidosis. Sodium bicarbonate, 1 mEq/kg, is injected through the umbilical vein of the severely depressed, hypoxic newborn infant who does not respond promptly to establishment of an airway and positive-pressure oxygen administration. This dose may be repeated if a favorable clinical response is not soon achieved. It is essential that the infant be ventilated effectively so that carbon dioxide from the bicarbonate can be dissipated. Otherwise, respiratory acidosis will develop, as well as a metabolic acidosis. Further administration of sodium bicarbonate is dependent upon results of measurements of blood gases and pH.

Depression from Opioid Drugs. Meperidine (Demerol) and similar drugs given to the mother an hour or less before delivery may cause respiratory depression in the newborn infant. If this appears to be the case, naloxone (Narcan) may be given in a dose of 10 µg/kg (Chapter 18, page 355).

Hypovolemia. Some severely depressed newborn infants are hypovolemic. Hypovolemia may occur without fetal hemorrhage having been detected, for example, with sepsis, fetal-to-maternal hemorrhage, trauma to the placenta, cord compression with obstruction of the umbilical vein and pooling of blood in the placenta, and twin-to-twin transfusion. At least partial restoration of

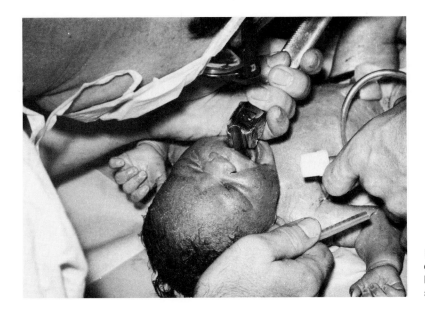

Figure 20-4. Use of laryngoscope to insert endotracheal tube under direct vision. Oxygen is being delivered from curved tube held by an assistant.

intravascular volume and correction of severe anemia are essential for improvement in the volume-depleted infant.

Cardiac Massage. If fetal heart action was present just before delivery but cannot be demonstrated after birth or if the heart stops after birth, external cardiac massage may be initiated. Immediately, the airway must be cleared, the trachea intubated, and adequate pulmonary ventilation established. External cardiac massage is effected with pressure from two fingers applied to the anterior chest wall in the lower midline at a rate of about 120 per minute. Four compressions of the chest are alternated with each inflation of the lung. A delay of several minutes in cardiac massage most likely will result in an unfortunate outcome, either death or permanent marked impairment of central nervous system function.

Epinephrine may be of value in resuscitating the arrested heart. Epinephrine, 0.1 ml/kg of a 1:10,000 dilution, is injected directly into the heart. A 22- or 24-gauge needle is inserted through the fourth intercostal space just to the left of the sternum, blood is aspirated to assure appropriate position of the needle tip, and the drug is injected as a bolus. Serious trauma from intracardiac injection is always a possibility, but an intravenous injection may never reach the heart.

Estimation of Fetal (Gestational) Age

A rapid yet rather precise estimate of gestational age of the newborn infant may be made very soon after delivery by examining (1) sole creases, (2) breast nodules, (3) scalp hair, (4) ear lobe, and (5) in the case of the male, testes and scrotum, as outlined in Table 20-2. A more definitive estimate can be made in a few days with the help of neurologic examination (Chapter 37, page 748).

Care of the Eyes

Because of the possibility of infection of the eyes of the newborn during passage through the vagina of a mother with gonorrhea, Credé, in 1884, introduced the practice of instilling into each eye immediately after birth one drop of a 1 percent solution of silver nitrate, which was later washed out with saline. This procedure led to a marked decrease in the frequency but not the elimination of *gonorrheal ophthalmia* and resulting blindness.

TABLE 20-2. RAPID ESTIMATION OF GESTATIONAL AGE OF THE NEWBORN

Sites	Gestational age		
	36 Weeks or Less	**37 to 38 Weeks**	**39 Weeks or More**
Sole creases	Anterior transverse crease only	Occasional creases anterior two thirds	Sole covered with creases
Breast nodule diameter	2 mm	4 mm	7 mm
Scalp hair	Fine and fuzzy	Fine and fuzzy	Coarse and silky
Ear lobe	Pliable, no cartilage	Some cartilage	Stiffened by thick cartilage
Testes and scrotum	Testes in lower canal, scrotum small, few rugae	Intermediate	Testes pendulous, scrotum full, extensive rugae

Technique for Using Silver Nitrate.

As a preliminary precaution, the region about each eye should be irrigated with sterile water applied to the nasal side of the eye and allowed to run off the opposite side. The lower lid should then be drawn down and the 1 percent silver nitrate solution dropped into the lower cul-de-sac. The silver nitrate produces a discernible chemical conjunctivitis in over half the cases, manifested by redness, edema, or discharge, which develops in 24 hours and lasts 2 to 3 days.

Antibiotic Prophylaxis. *Penicillin* serves as an alternate to silver nitrate in prophylaxis of gonococcal ophthalmia neonatorum. Penicillin ointment in the strength of 100,-000 units per g is placed in the eyes of the newborn baby, or penicillin is given parenterally. Some institutions, including ours, use a single dose of penicillin injected intramuscularly soon after delivery. Penicillin so administered to the neonate also reduces the frequency of sepsis from group B *Streptococcus*.

Tetracycline ointment containing the antibiotic in a concentration of 1 percent, liberally instilled into each eye with the lids held apart, affords effective prophylaxis. Tetracycline so administered in a single dose in our experience does not always prevent chlamydial conjunctivitis (Rettig and Patamasucon, 1981).

Permanent Infant Identification

Proper identification of each infant is of prime importance. A foolproof system must be operative at all hours. It should prevent separation of the infant from his or her mother until identification is complete, and it should provide a record easily recognized by the mother, such as an identification band or row of beads that spell the infant's name. It is crucial, furthermore, that a permanent record, such as footprints, be kept on file at the hospital (Fig. 20-5).

The definitive ridges on the palms, fingers, and feet of human beings begin to form several months before birth and remain throughout life. Most hospitals today use footprints rather than fingerprints or palmprints in identifying infants, because the ridges in the feet are more pronounced, and it is easier to obtain prints from them in newborn infants. For the footprint to be satisfactory, close attention must be paid to technique. Too often the ridges are not discrete and, therefore, the print is of no value (Clark and associates, 1981).

Temperature. The temperature of the infant drops rapidly immediately after birth. If the naked newborn is left exposed in the usual air-conditioned delivery room, chilling so produced incites shivering and increases oxygen requirements. Consequently, the infant must be cared for in a warm crib in which temperature control is regulated closely. During the first few days of life, the infant's temperature is unstable, responding to slight stimuli with considerable fluctuations above or below the normal level.

Vitamin K. Routine administration of vitamin K is urged, as described in Chapter 38 (page 783).

Umbilical Cord. Loss of water from Wharton's jelly leads to mummification of the cord shortly after birth. Within 24 hours, it loses its characteristic bluish white, moist appearance and soon becomes dry and black. Gradually the line of demarcation appears just beyond the skin of the abdomen, and in a few days the stump sloughs, leaving a small, granulating wound, which after healing forms the umbilicus. Separation usually takes place within the first 2 weeks after birth, most frequently around the 10th day but occasionally only after several weeks. The umbilical cord dries more quickly and sepa-

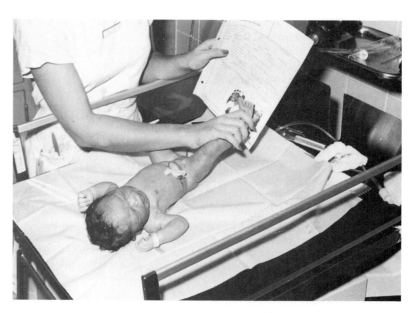

Figure 20-5. Making a permanent record of the newborn infant's footprints.

rates more readily when exposed to the air, and therefore a dressing is not recommended.

Formerly, disregard for asepsis in management of the cord frequently resulted in serious infection transmitted through the umbilical vessels. Even today serious umbilical infections are sometimes encountered, usually, but not always, indicating lack of care. The offending organisms often are *Staphylococcus aureus, Escherichia coli,* or group G *Streptococcus.* Since the umbilical stump in such cases may present no outward sign of infection, the diagnosis cannot be made with certainty except by autopsy. Strict aseptic precautions should, therefore, be observed in the immediate care of the cord.

Neonatal *tetanus* continues to kill infants in developing countries, as high as 145 per 1000 births in Haiti! Hygienic practices applied to the cutting and subsequent management of the umbilical cord serve to eliminate this serious complication. In addition, active immunization of the mother against tetanus with passage of antibody to the fetus can serve to reduce the risk to the infant appreciably (Editorial, 1983).

Care of the Skin. Infants should be promptly patted dry to minimize heat loss caused by evaporation. In most hospitals, not all the vernix caseosa is removed, but the excess, as well as blood and meconium, is gently wiped off. The vernix caseosa is readily absorbed by the baby's skin and disappears entirely within 24 hours. It is unwise to wash a newborn infant until his or her temperature has stabilized. Handling of the baby should be minimized.

Stools and Urine. For the first 2 or 3 days after birth, the contents of the colon are composed of soft, brownish green *meconium,* which is composed of desquamated epithelial cells from the intestinal tract, mucus, and epidermal cells and lanugo (fetal hair) that have been swallowed with the amnionic fluid. The characteristic color results from bile pigments. During intrauterine life and for a few hours after birth, the intestinal contents are sterile, but bacteria soon gain access. The passage of meconium and urine in the minutes immediately after birth or during the next few hours indicates patency of the gastrointestinal and urinary tracts. Of all newborn infants, 90 percent pass meconium within the first 24 hours; most of the rest do so within 36 hours. Voiding may not occur until the second day of life. Failure of the infant to eliminate meconium or urine after these times suggests a congenital defect, such as imperforate anus or a urethral valve.

After the third or fourth day, as the consequence of ingesting milk, the meconium disappears and is replaced by light yellow homogeneous feces with a characteristic odor. For the first few days, the stools are unformed, but soon thereafter they assume the cylindric shape.

Icterus Neonatorum. About one third of all babies, between the second and fifth day of life, develop so-called *physiologic jaundice of the newborn.* There is a hyper-

bilirubinemia at birth of 1.8 to 2.8 mg/dl of serum. It increases during the next few days but with wide individual variation. Between the third and fourth day, the bilirubin in mature infants commonly reaches somewhat more than 5 mg/dl of serum, the concentration at which jaundice usually becomes noticeable. Most of the bilirubin is free, or unconjugated. One cause, but not the sole cause, of the hyperbilirubinemia is immaturity of the hepatic cells, resulting in slight conjugation of bilirubin with glucuronic acid and reduced excretion of the conjugate in the bile (Chapter 38, page 776). Reabsorption of free bilirubin as the consequence of the enzymatic splitting of bilirubin glucuronide by intestinal conjugase activity in the newborn intestine also appears to contribute significantly to the transient hyperbilirubinemia. In premature infants, jaundice is more common and usually more severe and prolonged than in term infants because of greater hepatic enzymatic immaturity. Infants who are mature but small for gestational age, however, metabolize bilirubin in a manner similar to mature infants. Increased erythrocyte destruction from any cause contributes to hyperbilirubinemia.

Initial Loss of Weight. Because the infant may receive little nutriment for the first 3 or 4 days of life and at the same time produces a considerable amount of urine, feces, and sweat, he or she progressively loses weight until the flow of maternal milk or other feeding has been established. Premature infants lose relatively more weight and regain their birth weight more slowly than do term infants. Infants that are small for gestational age but otherwise healthy regain their initial weight more quickly when fed than do premature infants.

If the normal infant is nourished properly, the birth weight is usually regained by the end of the tenth day. Subsequently, the weight typically increases steadily at the rate of about 25 g a day for the first few months, to double the birth weight by the time the child is 5 months of age and to triple it by the end of the first year.

Feeding the Newborn. It is advisable, because of the stimulating effect of nursing on mother and baby, to commence regular nursing within the first 12 hours postpartum. Most mature infants thrive best when fed at intervals of about 4 hours. Premature or growth-retarded infants require feedings at shorter intervals. In most instances a 3-hour interval is satisfactory.

The proper length of each feeding depends on several factors, such as the quantity of breast milk, the readiness with which it can be obtained from the breast, and the avidity with which the infant nurses. It is generally advisable to allow the baby to remain at the breast for 10 minutes at first; 4 to 5 minutes are sufficient for some infants, however, and 15 to 20 minutes are required by others. It is satisfactory for the baby to nurse for 5 minutes at each breast for the first 4 days or until the mother has a supply of milk. After the fourth day, the baby nurses up to 10 minutes on each breast. A

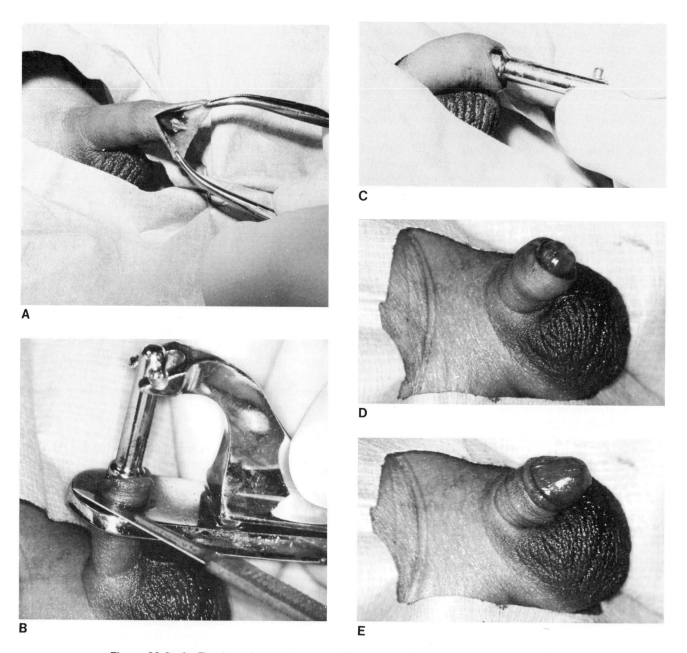

Figure 20-6. A. The foreskin has been carefully separated from the glans and incised superiorly. The length of the incision corresponds to the amount of foreskin to be removed. The cone of the Gomco clamp is now inserted (see **C**). **B.** The foreskin is excised immediately above the base of the Gomco clamp. Five minutes before excision, the cone of the clamp was placed between the foreskin and glans; the stem was then directed through the hole in the base; an appropriate amount of foreskin was carefully pulled over the cone through the hole in the base; the stem and fulcrum were engaged; and the nut on the opposite end of the clamp was firmly tightened. **C.** Approximately one half of the foreskin has just been excised and the clamp removed except for the cone still in position between the prepuce and glans. **D.** The cone has been removed. The foreskin that remains covers about one half of the glans. **E.** The foreskin is easily retracted to expose all of the glans.

baby receiving proper nourishment should increase steadily in weight.

Circumcision. There is no absolute medical indication for routine circumcision of the newborn, as emphasized in the report of the Ad Hoc Task Force on Circumcision to the American Academy of Pediatrics (1975). Nonetheless, this procedure has been very popular. For example, according to the Commission on Professional and Hospital activities, in 1974 the ratio of circumcisions of male infants (below 2 years of age) to the number of births of male infants was in excess of 0.8.

The following advantages are commonly claimed for circumcision of the newborn infant: (1) phimosis is prevented, (2) the incidence of balanitis is markedly reduced, (3) penile cancer is virtually eliminated, and (4) it has become traditional to circumcise male infants in the United States. None of these items justify routine circumcision. Lack of circumcision of the male sex partner does not appear to increase the risk of carcinoma of the cervix, as previously thought.

Circumcision, if it is to be done at all, should not be performed at delivery but rather a day or two later, after the infant has been demonstrated to be healthy. Prematurity, neonatal illness, most congenital anomalies of the penis, and coagulation defects are contraindications to circumcision.

Within the past few years, there has been a flurry of reports critical of routine circumcision. The adverse comments range from psychologic trauma to subsequent hypesthesia of the glans. The subjective nature of these allegations makes them difficult to prove. For example, Thompson (1983) cites at least 100 listings from the English-speaking literature referenced in *Index Medicus* from 1975 to 1983, 19 of which were in the journal *Pediatrics*. Perhaps 5 to 10 percent of males will be considered to need circumcision later in life when the cost, emotional trauma, and the risk from anesthesia will be greater. Routine circumcision of the male newborn is not performed at Parkland Memorial Hospital.

Objectively, operative complications can be minimized by attention to surgical technique. Proper use of the Gomco (Yellen) clamp (Fig. 20-6A–E) provides an additional safeguard against accidents.

Circumcision with Gomco Clamp

The healthy infant who has fasted for 4 hours is fastened supine to a clean, padded, rigid, x-shaped form of appropriate size using clean, soft fabric around the arms, legs, and abdomen. The genitalia and surrounding region are scrubbed and the operating field draped, usually using a small sterile towel with a central opening. The prepuce is very carefully separated from the glans penis. To do so, the margins of the opening of the prepuce are grasped bilaterally with two small hemostats, and a small curved hemostat is inserted between the inner surface of the foreskin and the glans, with particular care to avoid entering the urethral meatus. The jaws of the curved clamp are opened circumferentially. The prepuce, after being separated from the glans, is incised superiorly; the length of the incision

corresponds to the amount of foreskin to be removed (Fig. 20-6A). It is preferred by some to remove only one half to two thirds of the foreskin. The incised prepuce is next pushed back, and any adherence to the glans that might persist is relieved.

The cone of a Gomco clamp of appropriate size is inserted between the foreskin and glans, and the margins of the foreskin are drawn through the beveled hole in the platform of the clamp. *This maneuver is especially critical, since it is possible to pull skin that normally covers the shaft of the penis through the beveled hole and inadvertently denude much or all of the penis.* The opposite end of the cone and the elevator arm of the clamp are now engaged, and the nut is tightened firmly.

After 5 minutes to effect hemostasis, with the use of a scalpel the foreskin is excised immediately above the platform of the clamp (Fig. 20-6B). The clamp is disassembled, and the cone of the clamp is removed from over the glans (Fig. 20-6C). In the demonstration case provided in Figure 20-6, sufficient foreskin remains to cover part of the glans (Fig. 20-6D), yet can be easily pushed back to allow thorough cleansing (Fig. 20-6E). If there is no bleeding, and there should be none, the baby is returned to his crib with no dressing other than a diaper. Healing is normally prompt.

Anesthesia for Circumcision?

Kirya and Werthmann (1978) raised the question, "Why not anesthesia for neonatal circumcision?" and, in turn, described their experiences with regional nerve block from injected lidocaine. Perhaps a more pertinent question is, "Why routine neonatal circumcision in the first place?"

Rooming-in. Rooming-in involves keeping the infant in a crib at the mother's bedside rather than in the nursery, thus permitting the mother to take care of the baby. This practice stems in part from a trend to make all phases of childbearing as natural as possible and to foster proper mother–child relationships at an early date. By the end of 24 hours, the mother is generally fully ambulatory, and thereafter, with rooming-in, she can conduct for herself and for the infant practically all routine care. An advantage of this program is the mother's increased ability when she arrives home to assume full care of the baby.

Abnormalities of the Newborn Infant. These are considered throughout the text and especially in Chapters 37, 38, and 39.

REFERENCES

Barcroft J, Kramer K, Millikan GA: The oxygen in the carotid blood at birth. J Physiol 94:571, 1939

Chernick V: Fetal breathing movements and the onset of breathing at birth. Clin Perinatol 5:257, 1978

Clark DA, Thompson J, Cahill J, Salisbury B: Footprinting the newborn—cost effective? Pediatr Res 15:552, 1981

Credé CSF: Die Verhütung der Augenenzündung der Neugeborenen. Berlin, Hirschwald, 1884

388 WILLIAMS OBSTETRICS, 17TH EDITION

Dawes GS: Breathing before birth in animals or man. N Engl J Med 290:557, 1974

Duenhoelter JH, Pritchard JA: Fetal respiration: Quantitative measurements of amnionic fluid inspired near term by human and rhesus fetuses. Am J Obstet Gynecol 125:306, 1976

Editorial: Prevention of neonatal tetanus. Lancet 1:1253, 1983

Kirya C, Werthmann MW Jr: Neonatal circumcision and penile dorsal route nerve block—a painless procedure. J Pediatr 92:998, 1978

Martin CB Jr, Murata Y, Petrie RH, Parer JT: Respiratory movements in fetal rhesus monkeys. Am J Obstet Gynecol 119:939, 1974

Milner AD, Saunders RA, Hopkins IE: The effect of delivery by caesarean section on lung mechanics and lung volume in the human neonate. Arch Dis Child 53:545, 1978

Report of the Ad Hoc Task Force on Circumcision. Pediatrics 56:610, 1975

Rettig PJ, Patamasucon P: Postnatal prophylaxis of chlamydial conjunctivitis. JAMA 246:2321, 1981

Saunders RA: Pulmonary pressure/volume relationships during the last phase of delivery and the first postnatal breaths in human subjects. J Pediatr 93:667, 1978

Thompson HC: The value of neonatal circumcision. Am J Dis Child 137:939, 1983

21

Obstetric Hemorrhage

GENERAL CONSIDERATIONS

Mortality from Hemorrhage

Obstetrics is "bloody business." Even though the maternal mortality rate has been reduced dramatically by hospitalization for delivery and the availability of blood for transfusion, death from hemorrhage remains prominent in the majority of mortality reports. Obstetric hemorrhage is most likely to be fatal to the mother in circumstances in which whole blood or blood components are not immediately available. The establishment and maintenance of facilities that allow prompt administration of blood are absolute requirements for acceptable obstetric care. Bleeding from the maternal reproductive tract, including those cases in which the cause is unclear, is also dangerous to the fetus. For pregnancies complicated by bleeding during the second and third trimesters, the rate of premature delivery and perinatal mortality are at least quadrupled (Jouppilla, 1979).

Blood Loss at Parturition

Loss of 500 ml or more of blood after completion of the third stage of labor has persisted as the definition of postpartum hemorrhage (Hughes, 1972). Nonetheless, nearly one half of all women who are delivered vaginally and almost all who undergo cesarean delivery shed that amount of blood or more, when measured quantitatively, as emphasized by Newton (1966), by Pritchard and co-workers (1962) (Fig. 21-1A), and more recently by others.

The woman who develops a normal degree of pregnancy hypervolemia usually increases her blood volume by a factor of one third to two thirds, which for an individual of average size amounts to 1000 to as much as 2000 ml (Pritchard, 1965). Consequently, she will tolerate, without any remarkable decrease in hematocrit, blood loss at delivery that approaches the volume of blood she added during pregnancy (Fig. 21-1B). Data from a specific case that serve to dramatize the protective nature of pregnancy hypervolemia are presented in Table 21-1 and a brief case summary follows.

In spite of a blood loss of 2200 ml, incited by cesarean delivery plus radical hysterectomy and pelvic lymphadenec-

tomy performed on an otherwise normally pregnant woman, hypovolemia was effectively combatted with only 500 ml of blood augmented by sufficient lactated Ringer's solution to maintain urine output. Total blood loss was not much greater than the sum of the 500 ml of blood transfused plus the 1700 ml of blood she had added as pregnancy-induced hypovolemia. Instead of the hematocrit falling, the blood volume promptly did so to approximate closely her normal nonpregnant volume.

The tolerance to hemorrhage at parturition that is normally induced by pregnancy undoubtedly allowed the human race to survive before the era of hospitalization and blood banks. Nonetheless, deaths from hemorrhage were common because of the number of obstetric complications that predisposed to severe hemorrhage and, in turn, death in the absence of expert management, including appropriate blood replacement therapy.

Conditions That Predispose to Obstetric Hemorrhage

Listed below are the many clinical circumstances in which risk of obstetric hemorrhage is appreciably increased. It is apparent that serious obstetric hemorrhage may occur at any time throughout pregnancy and the puerperium. Moreover, more than one of the conditions listed may contribute either simultaneously or in sequence to the perpetuation of the hemorrhage.

A. Abnormal placental implantation or development
  1. Placenta previa
  2. Placental abruption
  3. Placenta accreta
  4. Ectopic pregnancy
  5. Midtrimester abortion
  6. Hydatidiform mole
B. Trauma during labor or delivery
  1. Vaginal delivery other than spontaneous or outlet forceps
  2. Cesarean section or cesarean hysterectomy
  3. Uterine rupture
    a. Previously scarred uterus
    b. High parity
    c. Hyperstimulation of myometrium
    d. Obstructed labor

389

e. Intrauterine manipulation to effect delivery (breech, version, destructive procedures on fetus)
C. Uterine atony
  1. Overdistended uterus
    a. Multiple fetuses
    b. Hydramnios
    c. Distended with blood (clots)
  2. Exhausted myometrium
    a. Vigorous (tumultuous) labor
    b. Prolonged labor
    c. Pharmacologically stimulated labor
  3. Anesthesia
    a. Ether and most halogenated agents
    b. Conduction anesthesia with hypotension
  4. Previous atony
D. Small maternal blood volume
  1. Small women
  2. Pregnancy hypervolemia not yet maximum
  3. Pregnancy hypervolemia obtunded
    a. Severe pregnancy-induced hypertension (especially eclampsia)
    b. Shrunken extracellular fluid volume (sodium restriction, diuretics, vomiting, diarrhea)
    c. Severe megaloblastic anemia

E. Coagulation defects
  1. Conditions predisposing to impaired coagulation
    a. Placental abruption
    b. Prolonged retention of dead fetus
    c. Amnionic fluid embolism
    d. Induced abortion
    e. Sepsis
    f. Gross intravascular hemolysis
    g. Massive hemorrhage treated with packed red cells plus electrolyte solution or old whole blood
    h. Eclampsia and severe preeclampsia
    i. Abnormalities of coagulation coincidental to pregnancy

The time of bleeding in pregnancy is widely used to classify obstetric hemorrhage, especially bleeding during the third trimester. The term *third trimester bleeding* serves only one useful purpose and that is to warn people *not* to proceed in routine fashion with pelvic examination on the bleeding woman, which would incite severe hemorrhage if there was a placenta previa. The term otherwise is so imprecise for describing gestational (fetal) age and, in turn, intelligent management of the pregnancy that it ought to be abandoned.

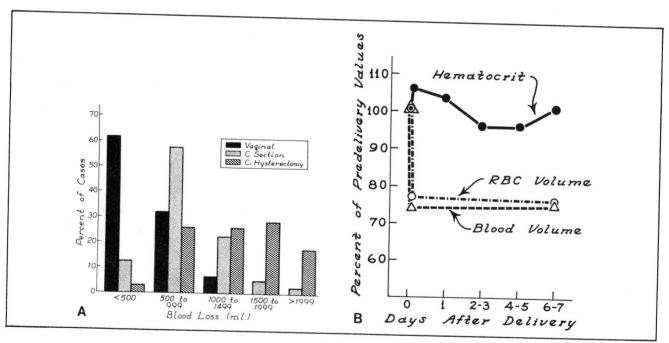

Figure 21-1. A. Blood loss associated with vaginal delivery, repeat cesarean section, and repeat cesarean section plus total hysterectomy. **B.** In a group of women undergoing cesarean section, the hematocrit postpartum changed insignificantly from the predelivery value in spite of an average blood loss of 1000 ml. At the same time, the blood volume and total erythrocyte volume dropped nearly 25 percent. (*From Pritchard and co-workers: Am J Obstet Gynecol 84:1271, 1962.*)

TABLE 21-1. PATIENT 37 WEEKS PREGNANT, CARCINOMA OF CERVIX, RADICAL HYSTERECTOMY AND PELVIC LYMPHADENECTOMY

Day	Hematocrit	Volume Blood	Volume RBC	Loss RBC	Loss Blood
−1	34.0	5444	1850		
Surgery		Transfused 500 ml blood			
+1	34.0	3835	1304	746*	2200
+2	30.5				
+4	30.5				
+6	29.0				
+8	31.0	4023	1247	813*	2400
+84	42.0	3755	1577		

* Includes 200 ml of transfused RBC.

Etiology of Obstetric Hemorrhage

Obstetric hemorrhage is the consequence of excessive bleeding from the placental implantation site or trauma to the genital tract and adjacent structures or both.

Bleeding from Placental Site. Near term, it is estimated that approximately 600 ml per minute of blood flows through the intervillous spaces that make up the maternal blood compartment of the placenta. With separation of the placenta, the many arteries and veins of the uterus that carry blood to and from the maternal compartment of the placenta are severed abruptly. Effective hemostasis demands that the patency of these vessels be quickly obliterated.

Elsewhere in the body hemostasis in the absence of surgical ligation depends upon intrinsic vasospasm and formation of blood clot locally. At the placental implantation site, most important for achieving hemostasis are contraction and retraction of the myometrium to compress the vessels and obliterate their lumens. Adherent pieces of placenta or large blood clots, and especially a hypotonic myometrium, will prevent effective contraction and retraction of the myometrium and thereby impair hemostasis at the implantation site. Fatal postpartum hemorrhage can occur from a hypotonic uterus while the maternal blood coagulation mechanism is quite normal. Conversely, if the myometrium at and adjacent to the denuded implantation site contracts and retracts vigorously, fatal hemorrhage *from the placental implantation site* is unlikely even though the blood coagulation mechanism may be severely impaired.

Bleeding from Sites of Trauma. Lacerated or incised blood vessels in the reproductive tract other than in the body of the uterus lack the unique mechanism for obliterating vessel patency that is provided by a vigorously contracting and retracting myometrium. Consequently, oxytocic drugs and uterine massage to stimulate vigorous myometrial contractility are ineffective in controlling hemorrhage if the hemorrhage is not of uterine origin. Therefore, following delivery of an intact placenta, hemorrhage from the genital tract that persists with the uterus firmly contracted and retracted is indicative almost certainly of bleeding from lacerations of the genital tract.

Management of Hemorrhage

Whenever there is any suggestion of excessive blood loss from the genital tract, irrespective of apparent cause, it is essential that steps be taken immediately to identify the presence of uterine atony, retained placental fragments, and trauma to the genital tract. It is imperative that at least one and, in the presence of frank hemorrhage, two intravenous infusion systems of large caliber be established immediately to allow rapid administration of aqueous electrolyte solutions and blood as one or both are needed. An operating room and surgical team, including an anesthesiologist, must be immediately available.

A number of techniques are employed to estimate the magnitude of the hemorrhage, most of which by themselves may yield grossly erroneous values, especially when hemorrhage is external but brisk or when hemorrhage is concealed, as with placental abruption or hemoperitoneum.

Visual Estimate. Visual inspection is resorted to most often but is notoriously inaccurate. In several reports the amount of blood estimated by inspection to have been lost was on average about one half the actual measured loss. The estimates may be greatly excessive but are more likely to be dangerously low. Furthermore, part or all of the hemorrhage may be concealed.

Blood Pressure and Pulse. Overt hypotension and tachycardia are, of course, signs of dangerous hypovolemia that cannot be ignored, but the converse is not necessarily true. These vital signs, if apparently normal, can be quite misleading. *A blood pressure reading in the normal range, or even hypertension, does not preclude imminently dangerous hypovolemia.* Hypertension, either pregnancy-induced or chronic, is not unusual in pregnant women, and therefore serious hemorrhage and the resultant hypovolemia may in this circumstance result in a fall in blood pressure only to normotensive levels. The normotensive reading may create a false sense of security, with delay in identification of compromised perfusion of vital organs.

The pulse rate may be equally misleading, since it may be elevated in circumstances in which the degree of hemorrhage is negligible, and normal, or even slow, in the presence of severe hypovolemia (Jansen, 1978).

"Tilt Test." The woman who has bled appreciably but whose blood pressure and pulse rate are normal when recumbent may, when placed in the sitting position, become hypotensive or develop tachycardia or both. This so-called "tilt test" should be applied and interpreted with caution for the following reasons: (1) For the woman who is already hypotensive when recumbent, the "tilt test" is needless and potentially dangerous. (2) The parturient who has not yet fully recovered from the sympathetic blockade of conduction anesthesia, especially spinal, may become hypotensive when placed in the sitting position without necessarily having suffered serious hemorrhage. (3) The normally hypervolemic pregnant woman may lose a large amount of blood before demonstrating orthostatic hypotension, as demonstrated in Figure 21-2.

The immediate effects from appreciable hemorrhage demonstrated in Figure 21-2 seem paradoxical. The woman with sickle cell–hemoglobin C disease near term underwent phlebotomy for exchange transfusion. Her measured blood volume was 6 liters and hematocrit 38. One liter of blood was removed over a period of 8 minutes while she was very carefully observed lying on her side. Her blood pressure and pulse, as well as the fetal heart rate, were monitored continuously. During the 20 minutes following hemorrhage, until infusion of packed erythrocytes was begun, she was observed first laterally recumbent, then supine, and finally sitting. Her blood pressure was unchanged until she sat up, when it rose moderately, as did the maternal and fetal heart rates. Thus the initial response to appreciable hemorrhage in the pregnant woman may be a rise in blood pressure similar to that observed at times in normal nonpregnant individuals.

Urine Flow. When carefully measured, the rate of urine formation *in the absence of potent diuretics or antidiuretics* reflects the adequacy of renal perfusion and, in turn, the perfusion of other vital organs, since renal blood flow is especially sensitive to changes in blood volume. With potentially serious hemorrhage, an indwelling catheter should be inserted promptly, first to empty the bladder completely and then to collect quantitatively all urine formed and thereby monitor its rate of formation. *Whenever urine flow through the catheter is very low to absent, the patency of the catheter must be investigated. Blood in the bladder may plug the catheter!*

Unfortunately, a potent diuretic, such as furosemide, is very likely to invalidate the relationship between urine

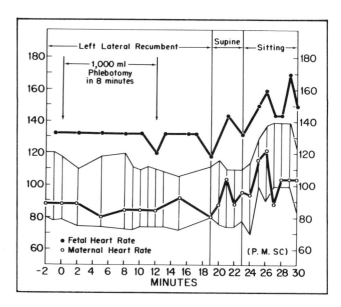

Figure 21-2. Responses late in pregnancy to phlebotomy and changes in posture following phlebotomy. Partial exchange transfusion was being carried out in a woman with sickle cell–hemoglobin C disease; her pregnancy-induced hypervolemia amounted to 1400 ml. Systolic and diastolic blood pressures are plotted as light lines and each reading is interconnected. The open circles connected by a heavy line demonstrate the maternal pulse rate, and the solid dots so connected are the fetal heart rates.

flow and renal perfusion. This need not be a problem in the management of the woman who is hemorrhaging, however, since there are no proven benefits to be derived from the use of furosemide in this setting. Actually, the reverse is true. There is potential for harm! An almost immediate effect of furosemide is venodilatation, which would further reduce venous return of blood to the heart and thereby further compromise cardiac output. The other dangerous effect is renal diarrhea, with loss of fluid and electrolyte from the already seriously depleted intravascular compartment.

The antidiuretic to which the hemorrhaging woman is likely to be exposed is oxytocin. However, with the infusion of isotonic electrolyte solution, such as lactated Ringer's solution, the amount of free water that is reabsorbed by the renal tubules is not greatly enhanced, and, therefore, *severe* oliguria does not develop as the consequence of oxytocin per se.

Measurements of Blood Volume. For identification of the magnitude of hemorrhage and the need for replacement therapy, measurements of blood volume have proven to be difficult to interpret for several reasons. For the individual woman, the ideal blood volume is not precisely known. This is especially true during the intrapartum or early postpartum period, since the size of the intravascular compartment normally undergoes remarkable change then as a consequence of delivery. Very important, in the presence of brisk hemorrhage, the blood volume changes so rapidly as to render any measurement invalid by the time it is completed.

Fluid Replacement for Hemorrhage

Treatment of serious hemorrhage demands prompt and adequate refilling of the intravascular compartment. Two general guidelines have proven to be most valuable for determining the amounts and kinds of fluids that are needed to combat hypovolemia from obstetric hemorrhage irrespective of cause: *Lactated Ringer's solution and whole blood are given in such amounts and in such proportions that (1) urine flow is at least 30 ml per hour and ideally approaches 60 ml per hour and (2) the hematocrit reading is maintained at 30 percent.*

Further support for the recommendation noted above that the hematocrit be raised to and kept at about 30 has been provided by Czer and Shoemaker (1978). In their series of 94 critically ill postoperative patients, mortality rates were lowest with hematocrit values maintained between 27 and 33.

Two precautions require emphasis: (1) Urine flow after administration of a potent diuretic does not necessarily bear any precise relationship to the level of renal perfusion. Therefore, if the rate of urine flow is to be used successfully to identify adequate perfusion of the kidney and, in turn, other vital organs, such diuretic agents as furosemide should not be given. (2) Insertion of catheters for monitoring central blood pressures may lead to troublesome bleeding at the site of venipuncture if significant coagulation defects exist. Hence, in circumstances where there may be coagulation defects, rather than insert a central venous pressure catheter into the subclavian vein, a vein in the antecubital fossa is preferable, since bleeding can be controlled by pressure and a dangerous hemorrhage avoided.

Whole Blood and Blood Fractions. Fresh compatible whole blood, rather than stored blood, would appear to be more nearly ideal for treatment of hypovolemia from serious acute hemorrhage, since stored blood soon suffers from loss of functional platelets especially. In spite of this disadvantage, the policy of the Obstetrics Service and the Blood Bank at Parkland Memorial Hospital, dictated by the practicalities of blood banking, is to treat hypovolemia from severe hemorrhage with any readily available whole blood that is compatible based on identification of the recipient's blood groups and the absence of abnormal red cell antibodies in the recipient's plasma. The panel of red cells used to identify abnormal antibodies has been enzyme-treated, and all incubations are performed at 37° C. Clinically significant antibodies have been detected only in 1 to 2 percent of cases. To date this so-called group and screen technique has been applied in nearly 80,000 cases without encountering dangerous incompatibility that was missed by group and screen but identified by subsequent crossmatch (E. Steene, personal communication).

If whole blood is lacking, packed red cells plus fresh frozen plasma, recently thawed, are administered. The so-called universal donor who has type O $Rh_o(D)$ negative erythrocytes plus low anti-A and anti-B serum titers is a rare individual, and therefore such blood is rarely available.

Blood Fractions. Fractionation of donor blood by blood banks to provide for component therapy is very common. One drawback to the use of blood component therapy in the treatment of severe obstetric hemorrhage is lack of prompt availability of reconstituted blood. Infusion of large volumes of packed red cells plus normal saline is not an appropriate substitute for the whole blood that is being rapidly shed in large quantity. The deleterious effects of saline infused in large volume on coagulation factors, plasma proteins, and, in turn, plasma oncotic pressure are shown in Table 21-2. In normally pregnant women the colloid oncotic pressure is already reduced, since the concentration of albumin in plasma is about 25 percent lower than when nonpregnant. Typically, with reconstituted blood the risk to the recipient of infection transmitted in the blood is increased, since the likelihood of the red cells and plasma coming from the same donor is extremely remote.

At times, after the infusion of many units of stored whole blood, generalized bleeding may develop as a consequence of intense thrombocytopenia or, less likely, from low levels of factors V and VIII. To treat hemorrhage believed to be the direct consequence of severe thrombocytopenia, platelets should be administered from 6 to 10 units of blood that has been obtained very recently from donors of the same blood type as the recipient. If the platelets from an Rh(D) positive donor are given to an $Rh_o(D)$ negative recipient who might conceive again, immune globulin containing $Rh_o(D)$ antibody should be administered promptly in amounts sufficient to provide circulating free antibody. Factor V

TABLE 21-2. RUPTURED UTERUS WITH MASSIVE HEMORRHAGE TREATED VIGOROUSLY WITH ELECTROLYTE SOLUTION CAUSING MARKED LOWERING OF COAGULATION FACTORS AND COLLOID ONCOTIC PRESSURE

	Plasma Proteins		Fibrinogen (mg/dl)	Platelets (μl)	Prothrombin (seconds)	Partial Thromboplastin (seconds)
	Total (g/dl)	Albumin (g/dl)				
Initial	6.4	3.4	324	187,000	11.3	28.3
Terminal	2.3	1.2	104	67,000	17.0	76.3

and VIII levels that are low after repeated transfusion with stored blood can be improved by administering fresh frozen plasma.

ACQUIRED COAGULATION DEFECTS

Gross derangement of the coagulation mechanism as the direct consequence of a variety of obstetric accidents, or less commonly as the result of a coincidental disease, may incite or enhance obstetric hemorrhage.

Pregnancy normally induces appreciable increases in the concentrations of coagulation factors I (fibrinogen), VII, VIII, IX, and X. Other plasma factors and platelets do not change so remarkably. Plasminogen levels are increased considerably, yet plasmin activity during the antepartum period is normally decreased compared to the nonpregnant state. Various stresses incite the conversion of plasminogen to plasmin, especially activation of the coagulation mechanism.

Investigations of a variety of accidents of pregnancy led many years ago to recognition of acquired intense intravascular coagulation, more recently referred to as "consumptive coagulopathy" or "disseminated intravascular coagulation" (DIC). During the 1950s, investigators in obstetric centers in Boston, San Francisco, Detroit, Cleveland, and Dallas provided many critical observations (Pritchard, 1973).

Pathologic Activation of Coagulation

The activation of the blood coagulation system has long been attributed primarily to activation of the extrinsic pathway by thromboplastin released at sites of tissue destruction and perhaps to the activation of the intrinsic pathway by collagen and other components of tissue to which plasma is exposed through loss of endothelial integrity. However, other mechanisms can be operational, including direct activation of factor X by an appropriate protease, as has been identified in some neoplasias, and by induction of procoagulant activity in lymphoid cells and leukocytes, as occurs with bacterial toxins.

Typically, coagulation incites the activation of plasminogen to plasmin, which can lyse fibrinogen, fibrin monomer, and fibrin polymer to form a series of fibrinogen–fibrin degradation products or split products. The degradation products, depending upon their size, may contribute to defective hemostasis by delaying fibrin polymerization (prolonged thrombin time) and by causing defective fibrin clot structure as a consequence of their incorporation into the fibrin polymer (impaired clot retraction and stability).

Significance of Consumptive Coagulopathy (DIC)

Observations of consumptive coagulopathy were initially confined almost totally to obstetric accidents but, more recently, have been made in most all branches of medicine. Management commonly recommended in obstetrics

and in other areas of medicine has unduly emphasized (1) heroic attempts to replace the deficient clotting factors, especially fibrinogen, (2) injection of heparin in the hope of blocking further intravascular coagulation, (3) administration of ε-aminocaproic acid to try to block fibrinolysis, or (4) some combination of these. Not infrequently, the precise nature of the underlying disease has not been considered thoroughly or has even been ignored. The use of heparin, for example, has been urged by some in circumstances in which the likelihood of benefit would appear to be slight but the risk of potentiating hemorrhage great. More specifically, a disease such as placental abruption, in which the process of intravascular coagulation ceases at delivery, if not before, rarely if ever justifies the use of heparin. It is perplexing that recommendations for treatment of obstetric hemorrhage with heparin have commonly been made in general medical textbooks and journals, as well as in those works concerned primarily with obstetrics, by authors who cite no significant data either personally accumulated or gleaned from the publications of others. This has been particularly true for placental abruption.

While the injection of coagulation factors, the blocking of fibrin formation with heparin, and the use of drugs to inhibit fibrinolytic activity have been unduly stressed, the value of vigorous restoration and maintenance of the circulation to combat intravascular coagulation has not received appropriate attention. With adequate perfusion of vital organs, activated coagulation factors and circulating fibrin and fibrin degradation products are much more promptly removed by the reticuloendothelial system. At the same time, synthesis of procoagulants is promoted, especially by the liver.

The likelihood of life-threatening hemorrhage in obstetric situations complicated by defective coagulation will depend not only on the extent of the coagulation defects but, of great importance, on whether or not the vasculature is intact or disrupted and, when it is disrupted, the magnitude of the disruption. With gross derangement of blood coagulation, there may be fatal hemorrhage when vascular integrity is disrupted, yet no hemorrhage as long as all blood vessels remain intact. Moreover, each category of disease must be considered separately, and for each case in any category the intensity of the intravascular coagulation and the dangers therefrom must be carefully measured before a decision is made to employ a therapy as potentially dangerous as heparin, fibrinogen, or ε-aminocaproic acid. It cannot be overemphasized that the laboratory identification of possible stigmas of intravascular coagulation, such as thrombocytopenia, fibrin degradation products in serum, or distorted erythrocytes in a blood smear suggesting microangiopathic hemolytic anemia, should *not* in themselves serve as indications for the prompt use of heparin, fibrinogen, or ε-aminocaproic acid. It also must be kept in mind that impaired synthesis or even dilution by vigorous treatment with electrolyte solutions, rather than abnormal consumption, may be the cause of pathologically low levels of some procoagulants.

Clinical Signs of Defective Hemostasis

Excessive bleeding at sites of modest trauma characterizes defective hemostasis. Persistent bleeding from venipuncture sites, nicks incurred from shaving the perineum or abdomen, trauma from insertion of a catheter, and spontaneous bleeding from the gums or nose serve to alert the physician to probable defects in the coagulation mechanism.

Hypofibrinogenemia. If serious *hypofibrinogenemia* is present, the clot formed from whole blood in a glass tube may be soft initially but not necessarily remarkably reduced in volume. Then, over the next one-half hour or so, it becomes quite small so that many of the erythrocytes are extruded and the volume of liquid clearly exceeds that of the clot. The addition of a drop of topical thrombin to hasten the conversion of circulating fibrinogen to fibrin has practical utility.

Thrombin Clot Test

One drop of fresh bovine thrombin, 5000 units/ml, is placed into each of a series of clean, small, plain glass tubes, which are then stoppered and promptly frozen. As needed, a frozen thrombin tube is obtained and about 2 ml of venous blood (a column about 1 inch high) is promptly ejected from a syringe into the tube without foam. The time is marked on the tube, which is then taped upright and inspected at intervals of 5 to 10 minutes over the next half hour or so. The important feature is the size of the clot that evolves and persists and not the rate with which the clot forms.

Thrombocytopenia. Serious thrombocytopenia is likely if petechiae are abundant or clotted blood fails to retract over a period of an hour or so, or if platelets are rare in a stained blood smear. Confirmation is provided by actual platelet count.

Prothrombin and Partial Thromboplastin Times. Prolonged partial thromboplastin time or prothrombin time may be the consequence, singly or in combination, of appreciable reductions in those coagulants essential for generating thrombin, of a fibrinogen concentration below a critical level of about 100 mg/dl, of appreciable amounts of circulating fibrinogen–fibrin degradation products, or of all three. Moreover, prolongation of the prothrombin time and partial thromboplastin time need not be the consequence of disseminated intravascular coagulation. For example, sepsis can derange vitamin K-metabolism sufficiently that vitamin K-dependent coagulation factors are reduced appreciably (Corrigan, 1984).

Thrombin Time. A long thrombin time may be the consequence of low fibrinogen, of appreciable amounts of fibrinogen–fibrin products, or of both. Moreover, in some cases of severe preeclampsia and especially eclampsia, the thrombin time may be prolonged for reasons not readily apparent (Pritchard and co-workers, 1976).

Uterine Bleeding Before Delivery

Slight bleeding through the vagina is common during active labor. This bleeding, or bloody show, is the consequence of effacement and dilatation of the cervix with tearing of small veins and, in turn, slight shedding of blood.

Uterine bleeding from a site above the cervix before delivery of the fetus is cause for concern! The bleeding may be the consequence of some separation of a placenta implanted in the immediate vicinity of the cervical canal, i.e., *placenta previa,* or from separation of a placenta located elsewhere in the uterine cavity, i.e., *abruptio placentae.* Rarely, the bleeding may be the consequence of velamentous insertion of the umbilical cord with rupture of a fetal blood vessel at the time of rupture of the membranes, i.e., *vasa previa,* with fetal hemorrhage (Chapter 23, Figure 23-18).

In actual practice, the source of uterine bleeding that originates above the level of the cervix is not always identified. In that circumstance, typically the bleeding occurs with little or no other symptomatology, then stops, and at delivery, days, weeks, or months later no anatomic cause is identified. Almost always the bleeding must have been the consequence of slight marginal separation of the placenta that did not expand. It is emphasized that the pregnancy in which such bleeding occurs remains at increased risk for a poor outcome even though the bleeding soon stops and placenta previa appears to have been excluded by sonography.

PLACENTAL ABRUPTION

Nomenclature

The separation of the placenta from its site of implantation in the uterus before the delivery of the fetus has been called variously placental abruption, abruptio placentae, ablatio placentae, and premature separation of the normally implanted placenta.

The term *premature separation of the normally implanted placenta* is most descriptive, since it differentiates the placenta that separates prematurely but is implanted some distance beyond the cervical internal os from one that is implanted over the cervical internal os, i.e., placenta previa. It is cumbersome, however, and hence the shorter term *abruptio placentae* or *placental abruption* has been employed. The Latin abruptio placentae, which means rending asunder of the placenta,

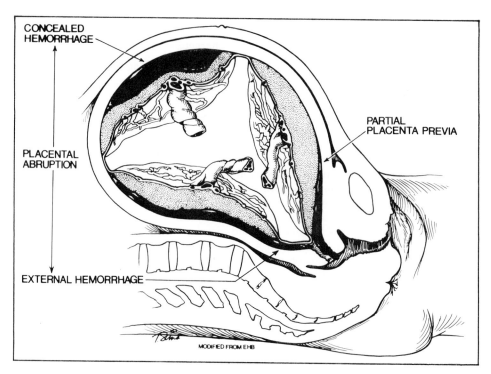

Figure 21-3. Hemorrhage from premature placental separation. (*Upper left*) Extensive placental abruption but with the periphery of the placenta and the membranes still adherent, resulting in completely concealed hemorrhage. (*Lower*) Placental abruption with the placenta detached peripherally and with the membranes between the placenta and cervical canal stripped from underlying decidua, allowing external hemorrhage. (*Right*) Partial placenta previa with placental separation and external hemorrhage.

denotes a sudden accident, a clinical characteristic of most cases of this complication. Ablatio placentae means a carrying away of the placenta, analogous to ablatio retinae; this term is not extensively used. The term frequently employed in Great Britain for this complication is *accidental hemorrhage*. The rationale for its use is that the condition is an accident in the sense of an event that takes place without expectation, in contrast to the unavoidable hemorrhage of placenta previa, in which bleeding is inevitable because of the anatomic relations between the placenta and dilating cervix. Since the term accidental hemorrhage may suggest an element of trauma, which is rarely a factor in these cases, it may be misleading and is seldom used in the United States.

Some of the bleeding of placental abruption usually insinuates itself between the membranes and uterus, then escapes through the cervix, and appears externally, causing an *external hemorrhage* (Fig. 21-3). Less often, the blood does not escape externally but is retained between the detached placenta and the uterus, leading to *concealed hemorrhage* (Figs. 21-3, 21-4). Placental abruption with concealed hemorrhage carries with it much greater maternal hazards not only because the likelihood of intense consumptive coagulopathy is increased but also because the extent of the hemorrhage is not appreciated. Consequently, with concealed hemorrhage blood replacement commonly has been too little and too late.

Frequency, Intensity, and Significance. The frequency with which abruptio placentae is diagnosed will vary since criteria employed for diagnosis differ. For example, especially during the second stage of labor as the fetus slowly is extruded from the uterus into the vagina, the placenta may separate partially and be diagnosed as placental abruption by some but not all obstetric units. This event alone will appreciably alter the recorded frequency. The intensity of the abruption often will vary depending on how fast the woman seeks and receives care following the onset of abdominal pain or vaginal bleeding or both. With delay, the likelihood of extensive separation causing death of the fetus is increased remarkably.

In recent years in the Dallas community, the frequency of diagnosis of placental abruption has been 1 in 86 deliveries. Applying the criterion of placental separation so extensive as to kill the fetus, the incidence at Parkland Memorial Hospital was 1 in 500 deliveries (Pritchard and Brekken, 1967). However, as the frequency of high parity in women cared for has decreased in more recent years and community-wide availability of emergency transportation has increased, the frequency of placental abruption fatal to the fetus has dropped to 1 in 750 deliveries.

Even so, as stillbirths from other causes have decreased appreciably, examples being maternal diabetes and maternal isoimmunization causing hydrops fetalis, stillbirth from abruptio placentae has become especially prominent. Of all third trimester stillbirths at Parkland Memorial Hospital during 1971 to 1980, 15 percent were the consequence of placental abruption, the same frequency as found by Hovatta and associates (1983).

At the perinatal center in Memphis, Tennessee, the frequency of placental abruption in recent years has been 1 in 89 deliveries (Abdella and associates, 1984). The perinatal mortality rate was 36.5 percent for all

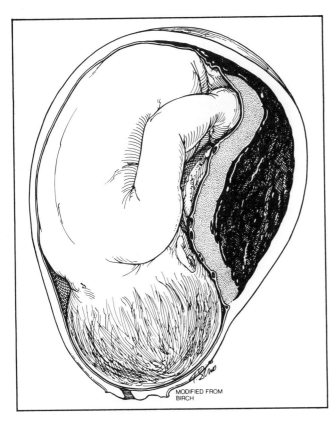

Figure 21-4. Total placental abruption with concealed hemorrhage. The fetus is now dead.

cases and 25.2 percent for infants who weighed 1000 g or more.

Hurd and co-workers (1983) in Cincinnati have observed a frequency for abruptio placentae of 1 case per 77 deliveries, with a perinatal mortality rate of 30.5 percent, about equally divided between stillbirths and neonatal deaths. Paterson (1979) in Birmingham, England, identified the perinatal mortality rate associated with placental abruption to be 35 percent.

It is quite obvious that placental abruption is a common obstetric problem that is especially dangerous to the fetus and newborn infant. Even though the fetus survives, the newborn infant may succumb. If the infant survives, he or she may be compromised. For example, of the 182 infants who survived placental abruption in the study by Abdella and associates (1984), 25 were identified to have significant neurologic deficits within the first year of life! While maternal mortality is now uncommon (none in the experiences cited above), morbidity is common and may be severe for reasons to be considered subsequently.

It is evident that placental abruption is a relatively common complication of pregnancy that certainly can jeopardize seriously the health of the mother and is likely to cause morbidity and even mortality in the fetus and newborn infant. For reasons not clear, in spite of

efforts by many organizations that are dedicated to research to try to minimize poor pregnancy outcomes, placental abruption has not received its deserved attention.

Etiology

The primary cause of placental abruption is unknown, but the following conditions have been suggested to be etiologic factors: trauma, shortness of the umbilical cord, sudden decompression of the uterus, uterine anomaly or tumor, pregnancy-induced or chronic hypertension, pressure by the enlarged uterus on the inferior vena cava, and dietary deficiency.

In the Parkland study of 201 cases of placental abruption so severe as to kill the fetus, maternal *hypertension* was apparent in nearly half of the cases once the depleted intravascular compartment was adequately refilled (Pritchard and co-workers, 1970). One half of the hypertensive women had chronic vascular disease; in the remainder, the hypertension appeared to be pregnancy-induced. So high a frequency of maternal hypertension in pregnancies complicated by placental abruption has been observed by some others (Abdella and co-workers, 1984) but not by all (Paterson, 1979). It appears that there is not an increased incidence of hypertension in pregnancies with lesser degrees of placental abruption, whereas severe placental abruption is much more likely to be associated with maternal hypertension.

External trauma, an unusually short cord, or a uterine anomaly or tumor could be implicated only rarely in cases of severe placental abruption cared for at Parkland Memorial Hospital. Hydramnios with sudden uterine decompression causing placental abruption was also uncommon (Pritchard and co-workers, 1970).

Lesser degrees of abruption may occur shortly before delivery of a singleton fetus when the amnionic fluid has drained from the uterus and the fetus has descended until the head is on the perineum. With twins, decompression following delivery of the first fetus may lead to premature separation of the placenta that endangers the second fetus (Chapter 26, p. 520).

Experimental obstruction of the inferior vena cava and ovarian veins was reported to produce placental abruption. There are, however, several recorded instances of ligation of ovarian veins and the inferior vena cava during the third trimester of pregnancy without subsequent placental abruption (Stone and colleagues, 1968).

Hibbard and Jeffcoate (1966) and some others contended that folic acid deficiency played an etiologic role in placental abruption (Chapter 13, p. 255). The hypothesis has been carefully examined by Whalley and associates (1969), Alperin and colleagues (1969), and others more recently. These investigators found no evidence to support such a relationship.

Marbury and colleagues (1983) suggest that maternal ethanol consumption (14 or more drinks per week), but not smoking, predisposes to placental abruption.

Recurrence

Of considerable importance to prognosis in women with a previous placental abruption, the risk of recurrence in a subsequent pregnancy is much higher than is the risk for the general population. Paterson (1979) noted a recurrence rate of 1 in 18 pregnancies, Pritchard and co-workers (1970) identified a recurrence rate of 1 in 10 pregnancies, and Hibbard and Jeffcoate (1966) observed the remarkably high rate of 1 in 6 pregnancies.

Indeed the likelihood of recurrence makes a subsequent pregnancy a high-risk pregnancy. Management of the subsequent pregnancy is made difficult by the fact that the placental separation may occur suddenly at any time, even remote from term. Beischer and associates (1970) found that normal levels of urinary estriol provided no assurance against imminent severe placental abruption. Moreover, Seski and Compton (1976) documented both normal acceleration of the fetal heart rate with fetal movement (normal nonstress test) and no abnormal deceleration of the fetal heart rate in response to uterine contractions (normal contraction stress test) when the tests were employed 4 hours before the onset of placental abruption so severe that it promptly killed the fetus.

Pathology

Placental abruption is initiated by hemorrhage into the decidua basalis. The decidua then splits, leaving a thin layer adherent to the myometrium. Consequently, the process in its earliest stages consists of the development of a decidual hematoma that leads to separation, compression, and ultimate destruction of function of placenta adjacent to it. In its early stage, there may be no clinical symptoms. The condition is discovered only upon examination of the freshly delivered organ, which will present on its maternal surface a circumscribed depression measuring a few centimeters in diameter covered by dark, clotted blood. Undoubtedly, it takes several minutes for these anatomic changes to materialize. Thus, a very recently abrupted placenta may appear no different than a normal placenta at delivery.

In some instances, a decidual spiral artery ruptures to cause a retroplacental hematoma, which, as it expands, disrupts more vessels to separate more placenta with more bleeding and, in turn, more separation. The area of separation rapidly becomes more extensive and reaches the margin of the placenta. Since the uterus is still distended by the products of conception, it is unable to contract sufficiently to compress the torn vessels that supply the placental site. The escaping blood may dissect the membranes from the uterine wall and eventually appear externally (Fig. 21-3) or may be completely retained within the uterus (Fig. 21-4).

Concealed Hemorrhage. Retained, or concealed, hemorrhage is likely to occur when (1) there is an effusion of blood behind the placenta but its margins still remain adherent, (2) the placenta is completely separated, yet the membranes retain their attachment to the uterine wall, (3) the blood gains access to the amnionic cavity after breaking through the membranes, and (4) the fetal head is so closely applied to the lower uterine segment that the blood cannot make its way past it. In the majority of such cases, however, the membranes are gradually dissected off the uterine wall, and blood sooner or later escapes from the cervix.

Chronic Placental Abruption. Most often, hemorrhage from the placental implantation site persists either until delivery, following which the blood vessels can be successfully constricted by the contracting and retracting myometrium, or until the woman dies. In a small minority of cases, however, hemorrhage with retroplacental hematoma formation is somehow completely arrested without delivery having taken place. We have been able to document this phenomenon by labeling maternal red cells with a chromium isotope. This technique served to demonstrate that red blood cells concealed as clot within the uterus at delivery some days later contained no chromium and therefore were shed long before, even though separation at the time of introduction of labeled red cells had been so massive as to kill the fetus (Cunningham, Pritchard, unpublished data).

Fetal-to-Maternal Hemorrhage. Severe fetal-to-maternal hemorrhage associated with placental abruption has been very uncommon in our experience but does occur. An example of massive bleeding from the fetus into the maternal circulation as the consequence of placental abruption is provided in Figures 21-5A and 21-5B.

At 33 weeks gestation, the mother was forcefully thrown against the steering wheel during an auto accident even though she was wearing an over-the-shoulder seat belt. The fetal heart was not heard when listened for 20 minutes later. Spontaneous labor developed 22 hours after the accident. At that time, the maternal blood contained at least 75 ml of fetal erythrocytes, or 115 ml of fetal blood, calculated from the percentage of red cells rich in fetal hemoglobin found in maternal blood (4.5 percent, as demonstrated in Fig. 21-5C), the maternal blood volume, and hematocrit. The macerated fetus weighed 2140 g. The placenta contained a long rent that extended to the chorionic plate. The clot adherent to the placenta at the site of partial placental abruption contained nearly all maternal red cells. Moreover, these red cells had been shed before the onset of labor, since they contained none of the labeled chromium used to measure the maternal blood volume at the onset of labor.

Clinical Diagnosis

It is emphasized that the signs and symptoms with abruptio placentae can vary considerably. For example, external bleeding can be profuse, yet placental separation not so extensive as to compromise the fetus directly, or there may be no external bleeding but the placenta is completely sheared off and the fetus dead as the direct consequence.

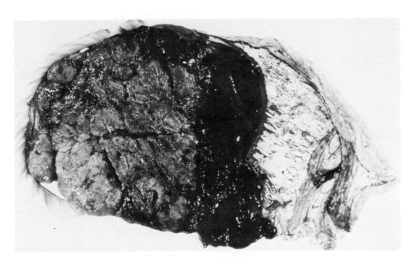

Figure 21-5. A. Partial placental abruption with adherent blood clot. The fetus died from massive hemorrhage chiefly into the maternal circulation.

Hurd and co-workers (1983), in a relatively small but impressive prospective study of abruptio placentae in which placenta previa was excluded by sonography, identified the frequency of a variety of pertinent signs and symptoms (Table 21-3). Note that in 15 percent of cases idiopathic premature labor was considered to be the diagnosis until subsequent fetal distress, including fetal death, serious bleeding, back pain, uterine tenderness, rapid uterine contractions, or persistent uterine hypertonus, were detected singly or more often in combination. They were able to recognize a retroplacental hematoma sonographically in only 1 of 59 cases. Negative sonography does not exclude life-threatening degrees of placental abruption!

Shock. It was long held that the shock sometimes seen in placental abruption was out of proportion to the amount of hemorrhage. An explanation proposed for this disparity was that thromboplastin from decidua and placenta entered the maternal circulation at the site of placental separation and incited intravascular coagulation

and, in turn, acute cor pulmonale. Admittedly, the sudden intravenous injection of large doses of thromboplastic material into experimental animals can cause profound shock, as shown by Schneider (1954), but, despite Schneider's observations, the weight of evidence is that the intensity of shock is seldom out of proportion to the maternal blood loss. Pritchard and Brekken (1967), for example, studied the blood loss in 141 gravidas with placental abruption so severe as to kill the fetus and found blood loss often to amount to one half of the pregnant blood volume (Fig. 21-6).

Neither hypotension nor anemia is obligatory in case of concealed hemorrhage even when the acute hemorrhage has achieved considerable magnitude. An example is cited:

P.P., 34 weeks pregnant, experienced continuous lower abdominal pain that became progressively more severe. When first seen 4 hours after the onset of the pain, fetal heart action was lacking, there was no external bleeding, her blood pressure was 150/100 mm Hg, and the hematocrit was 42, compared to 38 recorded 4 weeks before. She subsequently

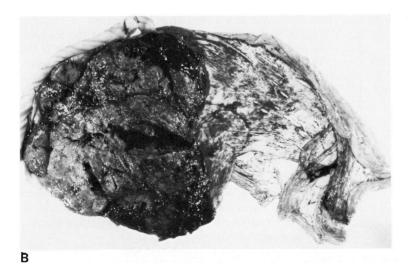

B

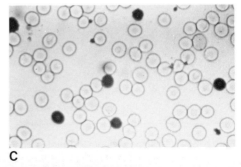

C

Figure 21-5. B. The adherent blood clot has been removed. Note the laceration of the placenta. **C.** Smear of maternal blood after fetal death. The dark cells are fetal red cells, whereas the empty cells are maternal in origin. Hemoglobin A has been eluted from the maternal cells by treatment with acid while hemoglobin F remains in the red cells of fetal origin.

TABLE 21-3. SIGNS AND SYMPTOMS WITH ABRUPTIO PLACENTAE (59 PROSPECTIVE CASES)

Sign or Symptom	Frequency
Vaginal bleeding	78%
Uterine tenderness or back pain	66%
Fetal distress	60%
High frequency contractions (17%)	
Hypertonus (17%)	34%
Idiopathic premature labor*	22%
Dead fetus	15%

* All treated with tocolytic agents.
(*From Hurd and associates: Obstet Gynecol 61:467, 1983.*)

expelled spontaneously a dead fetus, placenta, and blood clots plus liquid equivalent to 2 liters of blood! As well as total placental abruption, preeclampsia causing severe hypertension and hemoconcentration complicated the pregnancy and accounted for the hypertension and rise in hematocrit in spite of serious concealed hemorrhage. Prompt refilling of the intravascular compartment was accompanied by an appreciable rise in blood pressure, reestablishment of urine flow, and preservation of vital organ functions.

Oliguria caused by inadequate renal perfusion but responsive to vigorous treatment of hypovolemia is frequently observed in these circumstances. Fortunately, in this case the hypertension and high hematocrit initially were not misinterpreted as excluding serious concealed hemorrhage, and appropriate fluid replacement was initiated promptly.

Differential Diagnosis. The severe case of placental abruption is usually, but not always, marked by such classic signs and symptoms that the diagnosis is at once obvious, but the milder and more common forms are difficult to recognize with certainty, and the diagnosis is often made by exclusion. Therefore, with vaginal bleeding in the last trimester, it often becomes necessary to rule out placenta previa and other causes of bleeding by clinical inspection and sonographic study. It has long been taught, perhaps with some justification, that painful uterine bleeding means abruptio placentae, while painless uterine bleeding is indicative of placenta previa. Unfortunately, the differential diagnosis is not that simple. Labor accompanying placenta previa may cause pain suggestive of abruptio placentae. On the other hand, abruptio placentae may cause discomfort that mimics that of normal labor.

Unfortunately, there are neither laboratory tests nor diagnostic methods that will accurately detect lesser degrees of separation of the placenta. The cause of the vaginal bleeding at times remains obscure even after delivery.

Classic placental abruption with pain, shock, uterine rigidity, and absent fetal heart sounds may occur in the middle trimester of pregnancy. These cases present the same complications as do more advanced pregnancies and may cause the death of the woman unless she is appropriately treated.

Consumptive Coagulopathy with Placental Abruption. The most common cause of consumptive coagulopathy in pregnancy is placental abruption. Overt *hypofibrinogenemia* (less than 150 mg/dl of plasma), along with elevated levels of fibrinogen–fibrin degradation products and variable decreases in other coagulation factors, occurs in about 30 percent of cases with placental abruption severe enough to kill the fetus. Such coagulation defects may be found but are very uncommon in those cases in which the fetus survives. The experience at Parkland Memorial Hospital has been that serious coagulopathy, when it develops, often is evident by the time the symptomatic woman is hospitalized.

The major mechanism in the genesis of the coagulation defects of placental abruption almost certainly is the induction of coagulation intravascularly and, to a lesser degree, retroplacentally. Although an appreciable amount of fibrin is commonly deposited within the uterine cavity in cases of severe placental abruption and hypofibrinogenemia, the amounts are insufficient to account for all of the fibrinogen missing from the circulation (Pritchard and Brekken, 1967). Moreover, Bonnar and co-workers (1969) have observed, and we have confirmed, the levels of fibrin degradation products to be higher in serum from peripheral blood than in serum from blood contained in the uterine cavity. The reverse would be anticipated in the absence of significant intravascular coagulation.

An important consequence of intravascular coagulation is the activation of plasminogen to plasmin, which lyses microemboli of fibrin, thereby maintaining patency of the microcirculation. In every instance of placental abruption severe enough to kill the fetus, we have iden-

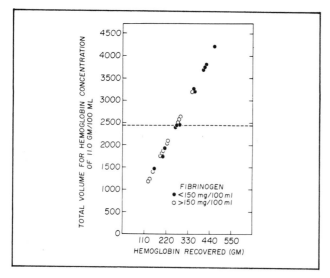

Figure 21-6. Volumes of hemorrhage concealed within the uterus until delivery in women with extensive placental abruption. The dotted line identifies the median value; the open circles represent cases with severe hypofibrinogenemia. (*From Pritchard and Brekken: Am J Obstet Gynecol 97:681, 1967.*)

tified clearly pathologic levels (> 100 μg/ml) of fibrinogen–fibrin degradation products in maternal serum. At the outset, severe hypofibrinogenemia may or may not be accompanied by overt thrombocytopenia. After repeated blood transfusions, however, thrombocytopenia is common.

Renal Failure. Acute renal failure that persists for any length of time is rare with lesser degrees of placental abruption but is seen in the severe forms when there is delayed or incomplete treatment of hypovolemia. Renal failure, usually renal cortical necrosis, was identified in 6 of 10 fatal cases of placental abruption reported by Krupp and associates (1970). However, the renal lesion more commonly encountered is that of acute tubular necrosis (Silke and associates, 1980). The precise cause of the renal damage that may be associated with placental abruption is not clear, but the major etiologic factors very likely are seriously impaired renal perfusion from both reduced cardiac output and intrarenal vasospasm as the consequence of massive hemorrhage and, at times, coexisting acute or chronic hypertensive disorders. Even when placental abruption is complicated by severe in-

travascular coagulation, prompt and vigorous treatment of hemorrhage with blood and electrolyte solution nearly always will prevent life-threatening renal dysfunction.

During nearly three decades at Parkland Memorial Hospital, more than 350 cases of placental abruption so severe as to kill the fetus have received fluid replacement therapy consisting of whole blood and lactated Ringer's solution, as discussed throughout this chapter. In no instance has dialysis for renal failure been necessary. Even among women who, unfortunately, suffered severe placental abruption and intense consumptive coagulopathy more than once, impaired renal function has not been a consequence.

Proteinuria is common, especially with more severe forms of placental abruption, but usually clears soon after delivery.

Uteroplacental Apoplexy (Couvelaire Uterus). In the more severe forms of placental abruption, widespread extravasations of blood often take place into the uterine musculature and beneath the uterine serosa (Figs. 21-7A and 21-7B). Such effusions of blood are also seen occa-

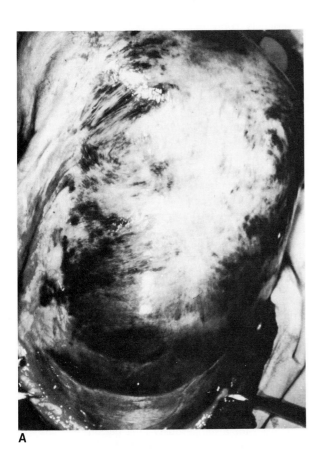
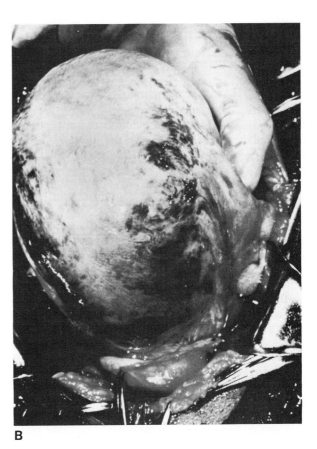

A   **B**

Figure 21-7. A. Couvelaire uterus; a uterus with total placental abruption before being emptied by cesarean section. Blood had markedly infiltrated much of the myometrium to reach the serosa. **B.** Same uterus as in Figure 21-7A after being emptied and closed. Note that it is well contracted even though there has been extensive hemorrhage into the myometrium.

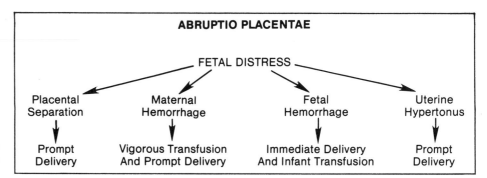

Figure 21-8. Various causes of fetal distress from placental abruption and their treatment.

sionally beneath the tubal serosa, in the connective tissue of the broad ligaments, and in the substance of the ovaries, as well as free in the peritoneal cavity, presumably from uterine bleeding through the oviducts.

The phenomenon *uteroplacental apoplexy,* first described by Couvelaire early in this century and now frequently called *Couvelaire uterus,* was thought at one time to impair uterine contractility after delivery, with severe postpartum uterine hemorrhage as the consequence. These myometrial hematomas seldom interfere with uterine contractions sufficiently to produce severe postpartum hemorrhage. Shown in Figure 21-7A is an example of Couvelaire uterus just before cesarean section early in the third trimester. In Figure 21-7B, the same uterus is seen well contracted after being emptied, appropriately sutured, and stimulated to contract with intravenous oxytocin. The infiltration of blood characteristic of Couvelaire uterus, therefore, is not an indication for hysterectomy. It is impossible to give a precise frequency of the incidence of Couvelaire uterus because the condition can only be demonstrated conclusively at laparotomy.

Management

Treatment will vary depending upon the status of the mother and of the fetus. With the development of massive external bleeding, intense therapy with whole blood plus electrolyte solution and prompt delivery to try to control the hemorrhage together are life-saving for the mother and, hopefully, for the fetus. In this circumstance the bleeding is more likely to be the consequence of placenta previa but may be from premature separation of a placenta that is located away from the cervical canal, i.e., abruptio placentae.

With blood loss occurring at a much slower rate, management will be influenced considerably by the status of the fetus. If the fetus is alive and there is no evidence of fetal distress, i.e., persistent bradycardia, ominous decelerations, or a sinusoidal heart rate pattern, and if maternal hemorrhage is not causing serious hypovolemia or anemia, procrastination with very close observation, coupled with facilities for immediate intervention, can be practiced. This is likely to prove most beneficial when the fetus is immature.

Sonography has served in some cases to identify a blood clot in the uterine cavity formed there as the consequence of placental abruption. *Failure to so identify such a clot does not exclude serious placental abruption.*

If the degree of separation is extensive, ominous decelerations in fetal heart rate are likely, especially when the myometrium contracts. Lack of ominous decelerations, however, does not guarantee the safety of the intrauterine environment for any period of time. The placenta may separate further at any instant and very soon seriously compromise the fetus and even kill the fetus unless delivery is performed immediately.

Some of the immediate causes of fetal distress from abruptio placentae are presented in Figure 21-8. It is very important for the welfare of the distressed fetus that steps be initiated immediately to correct maternal hypovolemia, anemia, and hypoxia so as to restore and maintain the function of any placenta that is still implanted and therefore capable of functioning. Little can be done to modify favorably the other causes that contribute to fetal distress except to remove the fetus promptly from the very unfavorable environment. For example, serious fetal hemorrhage, as demonstrated in Figure 21-5, cannot be treated effectively until the fetus is delivered. Moreover, we have not been able to decrease uterine hypertonicity significantly with parenterally administered magnesium sulfate (Hauth and Pritchard, unpublished). Ritodrine and other β-receptor agonists are not recommended, since they are likely to affect the maternal heart adversely and perhaps precipitate pulmonary edema in those circumstances in which serious hypovolemia is present or anticipated and vigorous fluid therapy will be required.

Åstedt (1982) has emphasized another potential risk from the use of β-receptor agonists to try to inhibit labor. In his experience the agonist can minimize the pain and uterine hypertonicity that typifies more extensive placental abruption, and the abruption may go unrecognized for a dangerously long period especially in the absence of external hemorrhage. Hurd and associates (1983) have encountered this same problem.

Cesarean Delivery. Rapid delivery of the fetus who is alive but in distress practically always means cesarean

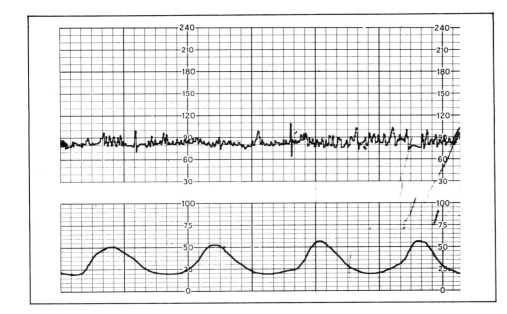

Figure 21-9. A recording of uterine pressures and presumed fetal heart rate in a case of placental abruption so severe as to have killed the fetus. The scalp electrode conducted the maternal EKG signal. Note the increased uterine basal tone. Commonly, in cases of severe placental abruption both the basal tone and the maximum uterine pressure are greater than illustrated here.

section. It is emphasized that an electrode applied directly to the fetus to record the fetal EKG may provide misleading information, as in the case of severe placental abruption illustrated in Figure 21-9. At first impression, at least, fetal bradycardia of 80 to 90 beats per minute with a degree of beat-to-beat variability seems evident. The fetus, however, was dead. There were no audible fetal heart sounds, and the maternal pulse rate was identical to that recorded through the fetal scalp electrode. Emergency cesarean section at this time might have proved especially dangerous to the mother, since she was profoundly hypovolemic in spite of no tachycardia, and she had developed severe hypofibrinogenemia. Moreover, because of a potentially dangerous antibody in her blood, compatible blood was not immediately available.

If the fetus is alive but cesarean delivery is not carried out promptly, the fetus must be monitored closely for evidence of distress and be delivered immediately whenever distress is detected. Therefore, appropriate facilities and staff for cesarean section must be continuously available whenever placental abruption is suspected.

Vaginal Delivery. If the separation is so severe that there is no evidence of fetal life, vaginal delivery is preferred unless hemorrhage is so brisk that it cannot be successfully managed even by vigorous blood replacement or there are other obstetric complications that prevent vaginal delivery.

Why vaginal delivery? The presence of serious coagulation defects is likely to prove especially troublesome when delivery is accomplished transabdominally, for reasons that do not apply to vaginal delivery. Vessels incised in the abdominal wall and the uterine incision are prone to bleed excessively when coagulation is seriously impaired. Avoidance of these incisions by vaginal deliv-

ery obviates this problem. Hemostasis at the placental implantation site depends primarily upon myometrial contraction and retraction to obstruct the many vessels that transport blood within the myometrium to and from the placental implantation site. Therefore, with vaginal delivery, stimulation of the myometrium pharmacologically and by uterine massage will cause these vessels to be constricted sufficiently that serious hemorrhage can be avoided even though defects in the coagulation mechanism persist. Moreover, bleeding that does occur is shed through the vagina, whereas with the incisions imposed by cesarean delivery, the blood is likely to accumulate as troublesome large hematomas.

Amniotomy. Rupture of the membranes as early as possible has long been championed in the management of placental abruption. The rationale for amniotomy is that the escape of amnionic fluid might both decrease bleeding from the implantation site and reduce the entry into the maternal circulation of thromboplastin and perhaps activated coagulation factors from the retroplacental clot. There is no evidence, however, that either is accomplished by amniotomy. If the fetus is reasonably mature, rupture of the membranes may hasten delivery. If the fetus is immature, the intact sac may be more efficient in promoting cervical dilatation than will a small fetal part poorly applied to the cervix.

Labor

With slight degrees of placental separation, uterine contractions usually are of normal frequency, duration, and intensity, and uterine tone between contractions is low. With extensive placental abruption, the uterus is likely to be persistently hypertonic. The baseline intra-amnionic pressure may be 25 to 50 mm Hg with rhythmic increases up to 75 to 100 mm Hg. Because of persistent hypertonus, it is difficult at times to determine by palpation if the uterus is contracting and relaxing to any degree, although periodic complaints by the woman of increased pain often signal cyclic increases in uterine activity.

Sher (1977, 1978) has emphasized that in his experience uterine inertia refractory to the usual therapy develops in about 1 of 5 cases of placental abruption complicated by severe consumptive coagulopathy. He claimed that in this circumstance the administration of Trasylol resulted in rapid recovery of uterine activity. Trasylol is an inhibitor of proteases, such as plasmin, and also possesses antithromboplastin and antikallikrein effects. In our extensive experiences with severe placental abruption, as well as those of many others, hypertonicity has characterized myometrial function in women with placental abruption complicated by gross disruption of the coagulation mechanism. Therefore, the need for Trasylol (which is not available for clinical use in the United States) is questioned. In fact, we and others have been looking for an agent that will safely decrease myometrial activity somewhat in these circumstances.

If severe placental abruption occurs before cervical effacement and dilatation, the subsequent pattern of change in the cervix typically is one of progressive effacement with little dilatation until effacement is complete. Dilatation is then usually rapid. Therefore, failure of the cervix to dilate while obviously effacing should not be considered as lack of progress.

Oxytocin. Uterine stimulation with oxytocin to effect vaginal delivery appears to provide benefits that override the risks. Care must be exercised not to provoke the uterus into self-destruction, especially in women of high parity or with fetopelvic disproportion. The use of oxytocin has been challenged on the basis that it might enhance the escape of thromboplastin into the maternal circulation and thereby initiate or enhance consumptive coagulopathy. There is no evidence to support this fear (Pritchard and Brekken, 1967).

Timing of Delivery After Severe Placental Abruption

In some of the earlier editions of this book, delivery within 6 hours was advocated. This recommendation arose from the general clinical impression that maternal morbidity and mortality were less when delivery was thus accomplished. Experiences at both the University of Virginia and Parkland Memorial Hospitals indicate that the outcome depends upon the diligence with which adequate fluid replacement therapy, especially blood, is pursued rather than the time to delivery (Brame and associates, 1968; Pritchard and Brekken, 1967). At the University of Virginia Hospital, women with severe placental abruption, who were transfused for 18 hours or more before delivery, experienced complications that were neither more numerous nor greater in severity than did the group in which delivery was accomplished

sooner. Serial observations at Parkland Memorial Hospital on one of the most severe cases in terms of the prolonged interval between the onset of symptoms and delivery and the necessity of transfusing a large volume of blood are summarized in Figure 21-10. She recovered rapidly after spontaneous delivery!

Hemorrhage and Hypovolemia

To combat hypovolemia successfully, blood must be available in large quantities, as demonstrated in Figure 21-10. More than 10 liters of blood were administered to a woman with severe placental abruption who recovered at Parkland Memorial Hospital.

The basic rule for treating obstetric hemorrhage is applied. Blood and balanced salt solution (lactated Ringer's solution) are infused in such proportions that the hematocrit is maintained at 30 percent or slightly higher and urine flow precisely measured is at least 30 ml per hour, and preferably 60 ml per hour, or 1 ml per minute. For the oliguric patient, the dangers from furosemide outweigh any advantages, actual or theoretical, that might accrue from its use. If *vigorous* fluid therapy does not relieve oliguria, the central venous pressure should be monitored as more fluids are administered. Since central venous pressure measurement might not detect early pulmonary congestion, the woman must simultaneously be observed for other signs, especially dyspnea, cough, and rales. If pulmonary congestion were to develop, furosemide would be beneficial!

Coagulation Defects

Much concern often has been expressed over the rate of development of coagulation defects, as well as their intensity. The extensive experiences at Parkland Memorial Hospital have been that coagulation defects most often occur within the first few hours after the onset of pain or bleeding and usually do not worsen subsequently, except for dilutional effects from vigorous transfusion with stored whole blood and lactated Ringer's solution. We have observed a fibrinogen level of only 40 mg/dl less than 3 hours after the onset of intermittent pain thought to be labor and less than 2 hours after the onset of constant pain. Moreover, sufficient placenta remained attached that the infant survived immediate delivery by cesarean section performed to try to save the distressed fetus (Table 21-4).

If the clot observation test yields a small or absent clot, the usual coagulation studies will be grossly abnormal and will provide very little immediately useful information, with the possible exception of a platelet count. Even though *platelet counts* have been recommended to identify disseminated intravascular coagulation, very low *fibrinogen* levels may develop with placental abruption, yet the platelet count simultaneously may be well above 100,000/mm^3, as was the case in Table 21-4. With extensive placental abruption, elevated levels of *fibrin degradation products* are so common as to be anticipated; therefore, their measurement provides

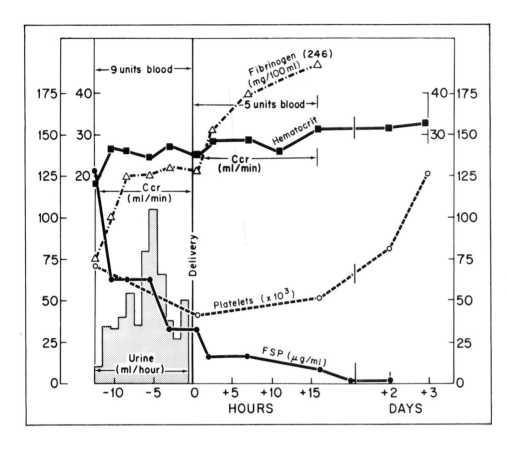

Figure 21-10. Serial data from a case of placental abruption so extensive as to kill the fetus and induce serious consumptive coagulopathy as well as severe anemia. Symptoms of abruption began 2 hours before hospitalization and 14 hours before delivery. Ccr = creatinine clearance; FSP = fibrin degradation products. Note the normal creatinine clearances. The patient left the hospital on the third postpartum day.

little immediate help in clinical management. Erythrocyte distortion or fragmentation characteristic of *fragmentation* or *microangiopathic hemolysis* is very uncommon unless renal failure supervenes.

Fibrinogen and Cryoprecipitate. Lyophilized fibrinogen had been used in cases of placental abruption with severe hypofibrinogenemia for years. Then, concern, mostly theoretic in origin, was expressed that the use of fibrinogen simply added fuel to the fire of disseminated intravascular coagulation, with the dire consequences of fibrin deposition and obstruction of the microcirculation in vital organs, especially the kidneys, adrenals, pituitary, and brain. There is no good evidence, however, that effective doses of 4 to 8 g of fibrinogen did so. For example, after 4 g of fibrinogen administered intravenously in less than 10 minutes to a woman with severe hypofibrinogenemia very soon before cesarean section, we observed no changes in central venous pressure, arterial blood pressure, pulse rate, or respiratory rate. Moreover, apprehension, a common occurrence with embolization to the lungs, did not develop. Typically, 4 g of fibrinogen proved to be an effective dose, raising the fibrinogen concentration in plasma by about 100 mg/dl.

The major problem from the use of lyophilized fibrinogen has been the likelihood of hepatitis, since each lot is prepared commercially from plasma from thousands of donors. For this reason especially, it is no longer available commercially.

Cryoprecipitate from several donors, rather than thousands, supplies fibrinogen with a very much lower risk of hepatitis. To supply 4 g of fibrinogen, 15 to 20 units of cryoprecipitate are required. Ness and Perkins (1979), for example, found an average fibrinogen content of 0.27 g of fibrinogen per unit of cryoprecipitate, but the content ranged from 0.06 to 0.42 g per bag.

For many years at Parkland Memorial Hospital, fibrinogen and cryoprecipitate have been used very infrequently. To avoid their use, trauma to the genital tract has been kept to a minimum through simple vaginal delivery, most often spontaneous. No episiotomy was made if the fetus was small or the perineum was relaxed; otherwise, a midline episiotomy was made and carefully repaired. The emptied and intact uterus was immediately stimulated with oxytocin, 100 to 200 milliunits per minute intravenously at the outset, and the uterine fundus was continuously monitored and massaged when not firmly contracted.

Uterine Massage

Effective uterine massage necessitates that the fundus of the uterus be clearly identified. If abnormally enlarged, the uterus is compressed to evacuate blood clots. Next a hand is placed over the anterior surface of the uterus with the fingers extending over the top of the fundus, and the uterus is now firmly rubbed to induce and maintain a contracted myometrium. An effective analgesic, such as meperidine, improves the mother's tolerance to this procedure.

TABLE 21-4. ABRUPTIO PLACENTAE WITH RAPID SEVERE DEFIBRINATION YET DELIVERY OF AN INFANT WHO SURVIVED

Time	Hematocrit	Fibrinogen (mg/dl)	Fibrin Split Products (µg/ml)	Platelets (µl)	Plasma Creatinine (mg/dl)
10/9					
0530		Onset of labor			
0630		Constant pain			
0805	34	43	1024	151,000	1.1
		Cesarean delivery at 0808			
0930	30	(Units 1 and 2 of whole blood started)			
1150	29	91	512		
		(Units 3 and 4 of whole blood infused)			
1425	32	166	128	87,000	1.6
1700	32	178	64	85,000	
10/10					
0500	26	263	8	95,000	2.2
10/11	25	—	—	124,000	2.1
10/12	24	—	—	198,000	1.8
10/16	24	—	—	638,000	1.1

Blood loss immediately postpartum may have been somewhat greater with this approach than if fibrinogen or cryoprecipitate had been given, but the overall risks and costs very likely were reduced.

With laparotomy for delivery, fibrinogen or cryoprecipitate has been given only if there was gross evidence of disruption of the coagulation mechanism, including uncontrolled bleeding from all sites of trauma. With lesser amounts of bleeding, ligation of all bleeding points with, at times, drainage of the abdominal incision subfascially with Penrose drains has proved statisfactory. Most often, however, delivery of the woman with severe placental abruption and a dead fetus has been accomplished vaginally.

Other Coagulation Factors. Factors V and VIII activities may be reduced and contribute to poor hemostasis. Also, their activities in stored whole blood decrease with time. Their activities can be maintained at a level sufficient for effective hemostasis by administering 1 unit of fresh frozen plasma with every 4 or 5 units of stored blood given.

Platelets may become sufficiently low (below 50,000/cu mm) as to contribute to defective hemostasis. Transfusion with 10 platelet packs that were appropriately collected and stored should provide adequate platelet function.

Following delivery, the coagulation defects repair spontaneously within 24 hours or so, except for platelets that, if very low, take 2 to 4 days to reach normal range (Fig. 21-10, Table 21-4).

Fibronectin

This opsonic protein normally present in plasma influences clearance of bloodborne particulate material that arises from intravascular coagulation. Fibronectin stimulates clearance of such debris from the blood by macrophages. Transfusion with blood should help replenish fibronectin, whose actions probably protect from ischemia vital organs of women suffering from intravascular coagulation. Cryoprecipitate is enriched with fibronectin.

Heparin. *The infusion of heparin to try to block disseminated intravascular coagulation associated with placental abruption is mentioned only to condemn its use.* Heparin should not be used for the following reasons: (1) No one has reported more than a few anecdotal experiences in which heparin did not appear to make hemorrhage worse. (2) The stimulus to active intravascular coagulation ceases after delivery. In fact, the intense phase of intravascular coagulation occurs most often during and very soon after the placental separation. (3) Heparin is a potent anticoagulant that can be predicted to aggravate hemorrhage when there has been gross disruption of the vasculature. (4) Excellent results have been achieved with the plan of management described above. For example, more than 350 cases so severe as to kill the fetus have been managed without renal impairment that necessitated dialysis.

Epsilon Aminocaproic Acid. This agent has been administered apparently to try to control fibrinolysis by inhibiting the conversion of plasminogen to plasmin and the proteolytic action of plasmin on fibrinogen, fibrin monomer, and fibrin polymer (clot). Failure to clear fibrin polymer from the microcirculation especially could result in organ ischemia and infarction, for example, renal cortical necrosis. Its use is *not* recommended.

Hysterectomy. In the presence of coagulation defects, the more extensive the surgery, the more likely the hemorrhage is to intensify. Therefore, hysterectomy to attempt prophylactically to minimize blood loss is unwise. At times, fortunately uncommon, the procedure must be performed because the uterus has been severely lacerated or simply will not contract to effect hemostasis at the implantation site. Supracervical hysterectomy, if the cervix is intact, will result in less blood loss than will total hysterectomy. For reasons already considered, the bruised Couvelaire uterus is of itself not an indication for hysterectomy.

Consumptive Coagulopathy in the Infant. Although we have never observed the phenomenon, changes in the coagulation mechanism of the newborn infant characteristic of those of intravascular coagulation have been described as accompanying placental abruption (Edson and colleagues, 1968; Nielsen, 1970). However, a variety of conditions predispose to the development of disseminated intravascular coagulation in the newborn in the absence of placental abruption. These include trauma, prematurity, hypoxia, and sepsis.

PLACENTA PREVIA

Definition

In placenta previa, the placenta, instead of being implanted in the body of the uterus well away from the cervical internal os, is located over or very near the internal os. Four degrees of the abnormality have been recognized:

1. Total placenta previa. The cervical internal os is covered completely by placenta (Fig. 21-11).
2. Partial placenta previa. The internal os is partially covered by placenta (Figs. 21-3 and 21-12).
3. Marginal placenta previa. The edge of the placenta is at the margin of the internal os.
4. Low-lying placenta. The placenta is implanted in the lower uterine segment such that the placental edge does not actually reach the internal os but is in close proximity to it.

The degree of placenta previa will depend in large measure on the cervical dilatation at the time of examination. For example, a low-lying placenta at 2 cm dilatation may become a partial placenta previa at 8 cm dilatation because the dilating cervix has uncovered placenta. Conversely, a placenta previa that appears to be total before cervical dilatation may become partial at 4 cm dilatation because the cervix dilates beyond the edge of the placenta (Figs. 21-12A and B). It is emphasized that digital palpation to try to ascertain these changing relations between the edge of the placenta and the internal os as the cervix dilates can incite severe hemorrhage!

In both the total and partial varieties, a certain degree of spontaneous separation of the placenta is an inevitable consequence of the formation of the lower uterine segment and the dilatation of the cervix. Such separation is associated with hemorrhage from blood vessels so disrupted.

Frequency. The zygote that implants very low in the uterine cavity is likely to form a placenta that at the outset lies in very close proximity to the internal os of the cervix. The placenta so located may then be aborted, or it may migrate toward the fundus, which it frequently

does, or it may remain in situ giving rise to placenta previa. Ultrasonic investigations of early pregnancies that subsequently aborted have disclosed an unexpectedly large number of low-lying embryos. Not all that do not abort eventuate in placenta previa, however. As the placenta and uterus both grow, the placenta is likely to

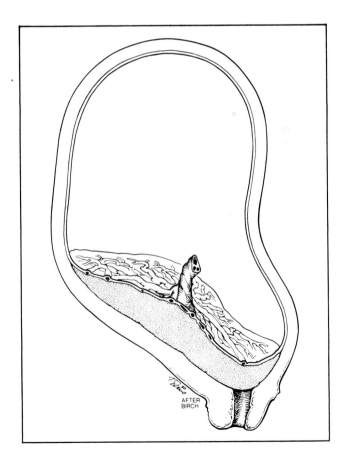

Figure 21-11. Total placenta previa. Even with the modest cervical dilatation illustrated, copious hemorrhage would be anticipated.

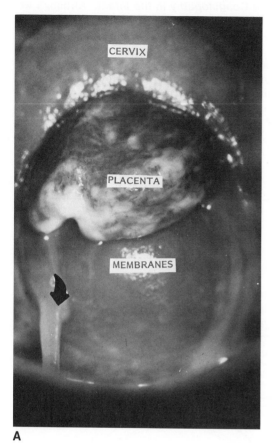

A

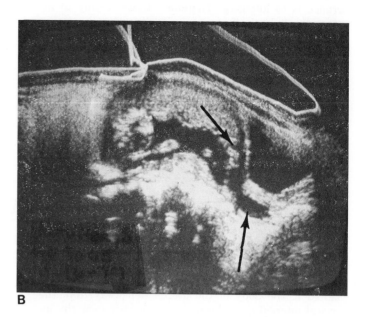

B

Figure 21-12. A. Partial placenta previa seen through a cervix 3 to 4 cm dilated at 22 weeks gestation. The arrow points to mucus dropping from the cervix. Uterine cramping was evident, but earlier intermittent bleeding had stopped 1 month before. The fetus weighed 410 g when delivered vaginally the next day. Blood loss was not massive. **B.** Gray scale longitudinal midline sonogram obtained the day after the photo in Figure 21-12 A. The upper arrow points to a partial placenta previa from an anteriorly implanted placenta. The lower arrow points to the amnionic sac bulging through the cervix. (*Courtesy of Dr. R. Santos.*)

migrate and eventually be located some distance from the cervix.

Placenta previa that becomes apparent clinically is a serious but uncommon complication. In the Dallas community, in recent years, placenta previa was diagnosed once in every 260 deliveries, or 0.4 percent. Brenner and co-workers (1978) identified during the latter half of pregnancy an incidence of placenta previa of 0.6 percent, or 1 per 167 pregnancies; 20 percent were of the complete, or total, variety. Contradictory statistics on the incidence of the various degrees of placenta previa reflect mostly the lack of precision in definition and identification for the reasons discussed above. A question difficult to answer is: "Should painless bleeding from focal separation of a placenta implanted in the lower uterine segment but away from a partially dilated cervical os be classified as placenta previa or placental abruption?"

Etiology

Multiparity, advancing age, and previous cesarean delivery increase the risk of placenta previa. Singh and associates (1981), for example, identified placenta previa in 3.9 percent of women who had undergone cesarean delivery compared to 1.9 percent for the whole obstetric population. One factor in the development of placenta previa is said to be defective vascularization of the decidua, the possible result of inflammatory or atrophic changes. Another is a large placenta, which spreads over a large area of the uterus, as seen with fetal erythroblastosis and with multiple fetuses. In such spreading, the lower portion of the placenta occasionally approaches the region of the internal os, completely or partially overlapping it.

Uncommonly, placenta previa is associated with *placenta accreta* or one of its more advanced forms, *placenta increta* or *percreta* (Chapter 34, p. 712). Such abnormally firm attachment of the placenta might be anticipated because of poorly developed decidua in the lower uterine segment.

Signs and Symptoms

The most characteristic event in placenta previa is painless hemorrhage, which usually does not appear until near the end of the second trimester or after. Many abortions, however, probably result from such an abnormal location of the developing placenta.

Character of the Hemorrhage. Frequently, the hemorrhage from placenta previa occurs without warning in a pregnant woman who appeared previously in perfect health. Occasionally, it makes its first appearance while she is asleep, and on awakening, she is surprised to find herself in a pool of blood. Fortunately, the initial bleeding is rarely so profuse as to prove fatal. It usually, but certainly not always, ceases spontaneously, only to recur when least expected. In some cases, particularly with placentas implanted near but not over the cervical os, bleeding does not appear until the onset of labor, when it may vary from slight to profuse hemorrhage.

The cause of the hemorrhage is reemphasized. When the placenta is located over the internal os, the formation of the lower uterine segment and the dilatation of the internal os result inevitably in tearing of placental attachments, followed by hemorrhage from the uterine vessels. The bleeding is augmented by the inability of the myometrial fibers of the lower uterine segment to contract and retract and thereby compress the torn vessels, as occurs normally when the placenta separates from the otherwise empty uterus during the third stage of labor.

As the result of abnormal adherence, i.e., placenta accreta, or an excessively large area of attachment, the process of placental separation is sometimes impeded, and then excessive hemorrhage is likely after the birth of the infant. Hemorrhage from the placental implantation site in the lower uterine segment may continue after delivery of the placenta, since the lower uterine segment is more prone to contract poorly than is the body of the uterus, and, as a consequence, there is less compression of the maternal vessels that traverse the lower segment. Bleeding may also result from lacerations in the friable cervix and lower uterine segment, especially with attempts at manual removal of a somewhat adherent placenta.

Coagulation Defects. Whereas coagulation defects characteristic of consumptive coagulopathy are rather common with placental abruption, they are rare with placenta previa even when extensive separation of the placenta from the implantation site has occurred. Presumably the incitors of intravascular coagulation that commonly characterize extensive abruptio placentae escape readily through the cervical canal rather than being forced into the maternal circulation. Of course, when very large volumes of stored donor blood have been transfused, thrombocytopenia and, less commonly, clinically significant deficiencies of factors V and VIII can be anticipated, since donor blood is variably deficient in these components.

Diagnosis

In women with uterine bleeding during the latter half of pregnancy, placenta previa or abruptio placentae should always be suspected. The possibility of placenta previa should not be dismissed until appropriate evaluation, in-

cluding sonography, has clearly proved its absence, in which case the diagnosis of placental abruption must be considered. The diagnosis of placenta previa seldom can be firmly established by clinical examination unless a finger is passed through the cervix and the placenta is palpated. **Such examination of the cervix is never permissible unless the woman is in an operating room with all the preparations for immediate cesarean section, since even the gentlest examination of this sort can cause torrential hemorrhage.** Furthermore, such an examination should not be made unless delivery is planned, for the trauma may cause bleeding of such a degree that immediate delivery becomes necessary even though the fetus is immature.

After the fetus has reached a gestational age of 37 weeks, the neonatal mortality rate is not greatly improved by further intrauterine development. In such cases, the cause of vaginal bleeding may be ascertained by pelvic examination but only under those conditions emphasized above. If placenta previa is identified, delivery should be accomplished forthwith.

Direct examination is withheld in women with premature fetuses for whom delay of delivery is advisable. In such instances, location of the placenta may be useful information, but it can be obtained by careful sonography. Moreover, it does not alter management remarkably, since those women who have bled must be carefully watched in any event. With proof that the placenta is normally located, the obstetrician may be more willing to discharge the mother from the hospital. However, whether at home or hospitalized, all women who have bled from the uterus are to be followed closely until delivery, as elaborated below.

Localization by Sonography. The simplest, most precise, and safest method of placental localization is provided by sonography, which can locate the placenta with considerable accuracy (Figs. 21-12B, 21-13, 21-14, and 21-15). Accuracies of as high as 98 percent have been obtained (Table 21-5). The false positive results very likely were contributed to by bladder distention. Therefore, the ultrasonic scans in apparently positive cases should be repeated after nearly emptying the bladder. An uncommon source of error has been identification of abundant placenta implanted in the uterine fundus but failure to appreciate that the placenta was large and extended downward all the way to the internal os of the cervix.

Placental Migration. Since the report of King (1973), the peripatetic nature of the placenta has come to be generally appreciated. Wexler and Gottesfeld (1977), for example, demonstrated sonographically that before the third trimester, up to one half of pregnancies were characterized by low-lying placenta. Young (1978) reached a similar conclusion upon localizing the placenta by means of arteriography. Therefore, placentas that lie close to the internal cervical os during the second trimester or even early in the third trimester are very likely to mi-

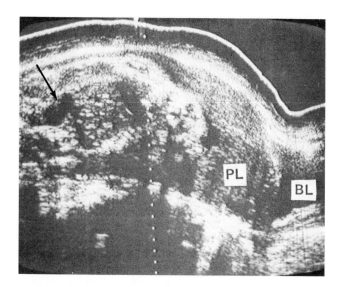

Figure 21-13. Gray scale sonogram of total placenta previa at 30 weeks gestation. (BL = partly filled maternal bladder; PL = total placenta previa; arrow on left points to full fetal bladder.) *(Courtesy of Dr. R. Santos.)*

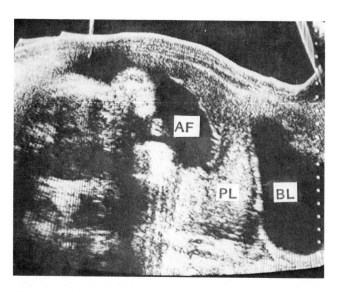

Figure 21-14. Gray scale sonogram of total placenta previa at 33 weeks gestation. (BL = maternal bladder; PL = total placenta previa; AF = somewhat excessive amnionic fluid.) *(Courtesy of Dr. R. Santos.)*

grate subsequently toward the fundus, with avoidance of the morbidity and mortality imposed by placenta previa. The low frequency with which placenta previa persists when it has been identified sonographically before the 30th week of gestation is shown in Table 21-6. It is apparent from these data, collected by Comeau and associates (1983), that in the absence of any other abnormality, sonography need not be repeated frequently simply to follow the migration of the placenta away from the cervix. Since the great majority of cases of asymptomatic placenta previa found early are cured by placental migration, restriction of activity need not be practiced unless the placenta previa persists beyond 30 weeks or becomes clinically apparent before that time.

Management

Women with placenta previa may be assigned to the following groups: (1) those in whom the fetus is premature but there is no pressing need for delivery, (2) those in whom the fetus is within 3 weeks of term, (3) those in whom labor is in progress, and (4) those in whom hemorrhage is so severe as to necessitate evacuation of the uterus despite the immaturity of the fetus.

Management of the pregnancy known to be complicated by placenta previa and a premature fetus, but no active bleeding, consists of procrastination in an environment that provides the greatest safety for both mother and fetus. Hospitalization, which provides close observation, a very sedentary lifestyle, avoidance of any intravaginal manipulation, and immediate availability of appropriate therapy, is ideal. Such therapy includes intravenous electrolyte solution, blood, cesarean delivery, and expert neonatal care from the time of delivery. How-

ever, in this practical world, compromises in care must be made at times and the mother and fetus not hospitalized. In this instance, the mother and her family must fully appreciate the problems of placenta previa and be prepared to transport her to the hospital immediately, where, in turn, her problem will be recognized immediately by hospital staff.

With delay of delivery, one of the benefits that may occur sometimes even relatively late in pregnancy is sufficient migration of the placenta away from the cervix so that placenta previa is no longer a major problem and vaginal delivery can be accomplished safely.

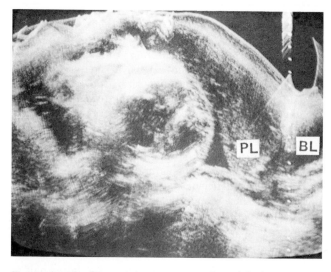

Figure 21-15. Gray scale sonogram of partial placenta previa at 37 weeks gestation. (BL = partly filled maternal bladder; PL = partial placenta previa.) *(Courtesy of Dr. R Santos.)*

TABLE 21-5. ACCURACY OF PLACENTAL LOCALIZATION BY ULTRASOUND

Authors	Year	Results
Gottesfeld et al. (Denver)	1966	112 cases: accuracy rate 97% 18 cesarean sections, 2 wrong predictions
Donald and Abdulla (Glasgow)	1968	613 cases: accuracy rate 94% 107 cesarean sections
Campbell and Kohorn (London)	1968	72 cases: accuracy rate 94% 9 cesarean sections 38 patients, no confirmation obtained 29 exploration of the uterus
Kobayashi et al. (Brooklyn)	1970	100 cases: accuracy rate 95% 92 cesarean sections, 4 errors 8 hysterotomies, 1 error
Sunden (Sweden)	1970	107 cases: accuracy rate 95.6% 45 cesarean sections, 2 wrong predictions
Santos et al. (Dallas)	1978	100 cases: accuracy rate 98% at cesarean section
Bowie et al. (Chicago)	1978	164 cases: accuracy rate 93% Missed 1 of 13 proven placenta previas

With placenta previa, the procedures available for delivery fall into two main categories: (1) cesarean delivery, the rationale for which is twofold: first, cesarean section, through immediate delivery of the fetus and placenta, allows the uterus to contract and to stop the bleeding, and second, cesarean delivery forestalls the possibility of cervical lacerations, a serious potential complication of vaginal delivery·in total and partial placenta previa; and (2) vaginal delivery, the rationale for which is, hopefully, to be able to press the detached placenta against the bleeding implantation site during labor and thereby tamponade the bleeding vessels sufficiently to prevent severe hemorrhage.

Cesarean Delivery. Cesarean section is the accepted method of delivery in practically all cases of placenta previa. In justifying cesarean section in the presence of a dead fetus, it is again necessary to understand that abdominal delivery is done for the welfare of the mother.

When the placenta lies far enough posteriorly that the lower uterine segment can be incised transversely without encountering placenta, and when the fetus is cephalic, the transverse incision is preferred. If, however, such an incision were to be made through the placenta, bleeding, both maternal and fetal, could be severe, and extension of the incision to involve one or both uterine arteries could occur with surprising ease. Therefore, with anterior placenta previa, a vertical uterine incision is often safer. When placenta previa is complicated by degrees of placenta accreta that render control of bleeding from the placental bed difficult by conservative means, total hysterectomy may be the procedure of necessity (Chapter 34, p. 715).

Vaginal Methods. There are four compression, or tamponade, methods for vaginal delivery, although only simple rupture of the membranes in case of partial or marginal placenta previa is now in general use. Willett forceps, insertion of a Voorhees bag, and Braxton Hicks version have all but disappeared from modern practice for a variety of good reasons that have been described in previous editions of this book.

Prognosis. A marked reduction in maternal mortality has been achieved, a trend that began in 1927 when Arthur Bill advocated adequate transfusion and cesarean section in the treatment of placenta previa. Since 1945, when Macafee and Johnson independently suggested expectant therapy for patients remote from term, a similar trend has been evident in perinatal loss. Half the patients are already near term when bleeding occurs, but prematurity still poses a formidable problem for the remainder, since not all women with placenta previa and a premature fetus can be treated expectantly. Delivery is forced by profuse hemorrhage in many instances and by labor in some.

Prematurity is a major cause of perinatal death even though expectant management of placenta previa is practiced. Moreover, for any fetal weight, perinatal mortality is likely to be somewhat greater with placenta previa than in the general population. Serious fetal malformations are also somewhat more common.

TABLE 21-6. SONOGRAPHIC IDENTIFICATION OF PLACENTA PREVIA AND SUBSEQUENT CLINICAL DISEASE

Gestational Age at Time of Sonography (Weeks)	Placenta Previa or Hemorrhage at Delivery (%)
< 20	2.3
20 to 25	3.2
25 to 30	5.2
30 to 35	23.9

(*Adapted from Comeau and associates: Obstet Gynecol 61:577, 1983.*)

FETAL DEATH AND DELAYED DELIVERY

In general, during the past two decades, the management for the woman whose fetus has died and who fails to go into labor spontaneously has changed from watchful waiting to more active intervention. Although most women will eventually go into labor spontaneously, the psychologic stress imposed upon the mother carrying a dead fetus, the dangers of blood coagulation defects that may develop, and the advent of more effective methods of induction of labor have increased the desirability of early delivery. Because the generally available methods for early diagnosis of fetal death still lack absolute certainty (Chapter 10, p. 219) and since the majority of women will deliver within 2 weeks (Goldstein and Reid, 1963; Tricomi and Kohl, 1957), it is recommended that, in the absence of other complications, attempts to evacuate the uterus may be delayed for that period of time but not much longer.

Coagulation Changes

Weiner and associates pointed out in 1950 that some isoimmunized Rh-negative women who carried a dead fetus developed coagulation defects. A prospective study indicated that gross disruption of the maternal coagulation mechanism rarely developed in less than 1 month after fetal death (Pritchard, 1959, 1973). If the fetus was retained for longer periods of time, however, about 25 percent of the cases demonstrated significant changes in the coagulation mechanism. Thus the old wives' tale that the dead baby would poison the mother, although scoffed at by physicians for a long time, proved to be true. Maternal isoimmunization with fetomaternal blood incompatibility is not essential to the development of the coagulation changes, as originally thought by Weiner and associates (1950). Extrauterine pregnancy with fetal death and delayed delivery may also be complicated by acquired hypofibrinogenemia (Dehner, 1972).

A few cases have been described with abrupt alterations in the plasma fibrinogen concentration, the values vacillating repeatedly between normal and very low over the course of a few days (Goldstein and Reid, 1963). Our experiences, however, have been that typically the fibrinogen concentration falls from levels that are normal for pregnancy to levels that are normal for the nonpregnant state, and in some cases the decrease continues to reach potentially dangerous concentrations of 100 mg/dl or less (Pritchard, 1973). The rate of decrease that was commonly found is demonstrated in Figure 21-16. Simultaneously, fibrin degradation products are elevated in serum. The platelet count tends to be reduced in these instances, but in our experience, severe thrombocytopenia does not necessarily develop, even though the fibrinogen level is quite low (Fig. 21-17A). Spontaneous correction of the coagulation defects can eventually occur before evacuation of the dead products of conception, but this happens quite slowly (Jennison and Walker, 1956; Pritchard, 1959). Apparently the access route for thromboplastin from the uterine contents through the vasculature of the implanation site bed is sealed eventually by fibrin deposited in the attached placenta (Figs. 21-17B and 21-19B).

Pathogenesis

A series of reports clearly establish that consumptive coagulopathy, presumably mediated by thromboplastin from the dead products of conception, is operational in these cases (Lerner and associates, 1967; Sherman and Middleton, 1958; Jimenez and Pritchard, 1968). As shown in Figure 21-18, heparin infused alone over a few days corrected the coagulation defects, but ϵ-aminocaproic acid did not. While these observations serve to establish the cause, they do not precisely identify the site where fibrinogen is converted to fibrin. The placenta from such a case commonly contains much insoluble protein (Fig. 21-17B) that can be made soluble by treatment with bovine fibrinolysin (Pritchard, 1973), but, most likely, considerably more fibrinogen has been converted to fibrin, presumably intravascularly, than can be recovered from the placenta.

Use of Heparin. Correction of coagulation defects has been accomplished using heparin under carefully con-

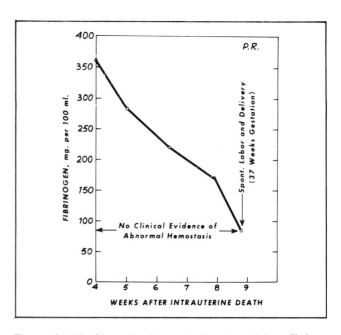

Figure 21-16. Slow development of maternal hypofibrinogenemia following fetal death and delayed delivery. (*From Pritchard: Obstet Gynecol 14:574, 1959.*)

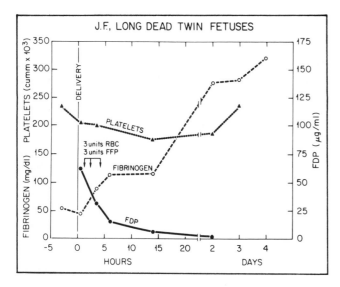

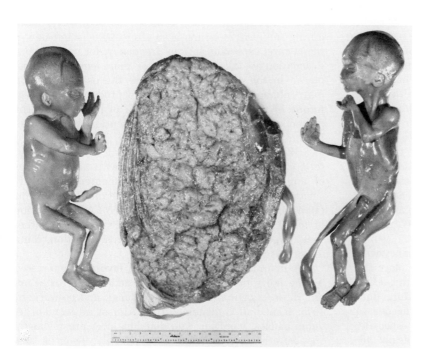

Figure 21-17. A. Data from a case of fetal death and delayed delivery treated on an emergency basis at Parkland Memorial Hospital. The twin fetuses had been dead for 8 weeks or more. Spontaneous delivery after spontaneous labor was followed by appreciable bleeding, which was treated with intravenous oxytocin, uterine massage, and blood transfusion. (Blood fractions were used because of nonavailability of type-specific blood.) Initially there was marked hypofibrinogenemia and elevation of fibrin degradation products without thrombocytopenia. Recovery was uneventful; the hematocrit at discharge was 29. In retrospect, hypofibrinogenemia was apparent from the very small clot in blood drawn for serology upon admittance to the hospital. (FDP = fibrin degradation products in maternal serum.)

trolled conditions *in women with an intact circulation.* Heparin appropriately administered can block further pathologic consumption of fibrinogen and other clotting factors and thereby allow the coagulation mechanism to repair spontaneously. Once correction has been accomplished and the heparin infusion is stopped, steps can be taken promptly to evacuate the dead products of conception (Jimenez and Pritchard, 1968). It is emphasized that for heparin to be used safely to block the consumptive coagulopathy, and thereby allow spontaneous repair of the coagulation mechanism, it is essential that the maternal circulatory system be intact. Otherwise, heparin most likely will incite or enhance hemorrhage. Im-

portantly, as soon as the dead products of conception have been evacuated, if not before, spontaneous repair will soon occur, so there is no good reason to give heparin at that time.

Fetal Death in Multifetal Pregnancy. As demonstrated in Figure 21-17, twin fetuses with death of both can cause severe hypofibrinogenemia. However, there is a paucity of reports in which an obvious derangement in coagulation has been detected in a mother pregnant with multiple fetuses, with some alive and some dead. Potentially dangerous coagulation defects have been described for one mother in the following circumstances: One of

Figure 21-17. B. Long-dead twin fetuses from case described in Figure 21-17A. The placenta contains much fibrin.

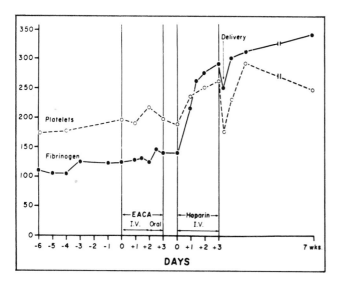

Figure 21-18. Coagulation defects with prolonged retention of a dead fetus. Fibrinogen concentration rose during intravenous infusion of heparin, 1500 units per hour, but not during administration of ε-aminocaproic acid (EACA). (*From Jimenez and Pritchard: Obstet Gynecol 32:449, 1968.*)

three fetuses died remote from term, and later a second fetus succumbed in utero, while a third fetus was born alive (Skelly and co-workers, 1982). In this case, following the first fetal death shortly after midpregnancy, consumptive coagulopathy was identified. Treatment with heparin intravenously reversed the hypofibrinogenemia. Even so, a second fetus died near 35 weeks of gestation. Cesarean section was performed very soon thereafter, and the third fetus survived.

We have observed, following death of one of twin fetuses and delayed delivery, a progressive but transient fall in maternal fibrinogen concentration and rise in fibrin split products. However, in the absence of therapy, these changes ceased spontaneously with normalization of the coagulation mechanism (Fig. 21-19A). The surviving fetus, when delivered near term, was healthy. The placenta of the long-dead fetus was filled with fibrin (Fig. 21-19B).

Even more dramatic was another instance of twin fetuses with one dead remote from term. The maternal fibrinogen level had dropped to less than 100 mg/dl when first measured, but as appropriate therapy was being debated, it rose spontaneously to normal levels, which persisted thereafter. The second fetus appeared healthy when delivered near term (Pritchard, unpublished).

Theoretically at least, in the case of pregnancy with two or more fetuses, death of one fetus might place the others in jeopardy of consumptive coagulopathy, especially when their circulations anastomose. More data carefully obtained in these circumstances are needed so as to be able to recommend optimal therapy, especially in regard to benefits versus risks from chronically ad-

ministered heparin, as well as the timing and route of delivery.

Treatment of Active Hemorrhage. If serious hemorrhage is encountered as the products of conception are being expelled or surgically removed and overt hypofibrinogenemia and associated coagulation defects are identified, treatment with heparin almost certainly will enhance the bleeding. In this circumstance, effective primary treatment is blood and lactated Ringer's solution, according to the guidelines for treatment of hemorrhage described under Fluid Replacement Therapy and as proved effective in the case demonstrated in Figure 21-17A. The consumptive coagulopathy stops once the products of conception are expelled, and repair soon takes place. If there is excessive bleeding from extensive trauma or surgery, cryoprecipitate, fresh frozen plasma, and platelet packs if thombocytopenia is a problem, coupled with ligation of all severed blood vessels, should prove effective. Although ε-aminocaproic acid has been recommended to block fibrinolysis (Pfeffer, 1966), its use seems irrational, potentially dangerous, and unsupported by sufficient clinical observations.

Pregnancy Termination with Dead Fetus

Near term, intravenously administered oxytocin usually is effective when given in a dose that stimulates uterine activity, although it may have to be repeated (Chapter 24, p. 482). Remote from term, however, it is less likely to prove effective unless given in high concentration and on more than one occasion. It is not unusual for the infused oxytocin to initiate some palpable contractions, which then abate even when the amount infused is increased. The oxytocin appears at times to influence the uterus to spontaneously contract subsequently, since during the next 24 hours or so after oxytocin infusion, it is not rare, especially late in pregnancy, for spontaneous evacuation to take place. One or more laminaria tents placed in the cervical canal before the use of oxytocin may enhance expulsion of the dead products. The magnitude of risk of infection from use of laminaria in the presence of dead products of conception has not yet been quantified.

Water intoxication as a consequence of the antidiuretic effect of oxytocin administered with large volumes of aqueous dextrose has been documented repeatedly since first described in these circumstances by Liggins (1962) and Whalley and Pritchard (1963). Administration of small volumes of lactated Ringer's solution, rather than large volumes of aqueous dextrose solution, minimizes this risk.

Numerous observers have been favorably impressed by the fairly prompt abortifacient action by prostaglandin E_2 as a vaginal suppository (Bailey and co-workers, 1975; Kent and Goldstein, 1976). Almost all women develop nausea, vomiting, and diarrhea after prostaglandin suppositories are inserted intravaginally; fever is also

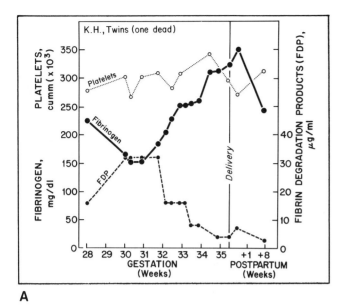

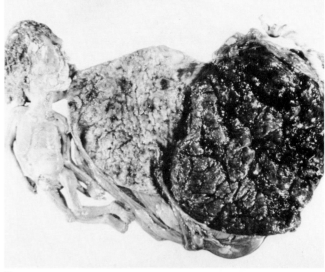

A   **B**

Figure 21-19. A. Death of one twin was confirmed sonographically at 28 weeks gestation. Coagulation studies initiated then demonstrated a somewhat low plasma fibrinogen concentration and distinctly abnormal amounts of fibrin degradation products (FDP) in maternal serum. The abnormalities in both became more intense 2 weeks later. Then, spontaneously, the fibrinogen concentration rose, and the fibrin degradation products fell in mirror fashion. The liveborn infant was healthy, and coagulation studies on cord plasma and serum were normal. **B.** The fibrin-filled placenta of the long-dead fetus is apparent. Presumably, the fibrin curtailed the escape of thromboplastin from the dead products into the maternal circulation.

common (Phelan and Cefalo, 1978). Apparently rare complications that have been reported include uterine rupture (Schulman and associates, 1979) and myocardial infarction (Patterson and colleagues, 1979).

Orr and co-workers (1979) have emphasized that failure of prostaglandin E₂ suppositories to expel the dead products of conception must raise the question of extrauterine fetal death and cite four such experiences. *Fetal death with delayed delivery should always pro-* *vide the stimulus for asking the question, "Is the pregnancy extrauterine?"*

The intrauterine injection of hypertonic saline is not recommended for evacuation of dead products of conception, since the volume of amnionic fluid is often reduced and the potentially highly toxic salt solution, therefore, is difficult to inject quantitatively into the sac. Coagulation defects may be induced or enhanced by intra-amnionic hypertonic saline.

AMNIONIC FLUID EMBOLISM

Pathogenesis

Entry of amnionic fluid into the maternal circulation in some circumstances may prove fatal. Essential to the development of amnionic fluid embolism are (1) a rent through the amnion and chorion, (2) opened uterine or endocervical veins, and (3) a pressure gradient sufficient to force the fluid into the venous circulation. Marginal separation of the placenta or laceration of the uterus or cervix serves to create an opening into the maternal circulation. Vigorous labor, including that induced with overdosage of oxytocin, is more likely to provide the

pressure. These events may also distress the fetus, leading to defecation of meconium in utero, thereby markedly potentiating the toxic nature of amnionic fluid if it should enter the maternal circulation.

In the typical case of amnionic fluid embolism, the woman is laboring vigorously, or has just done so, and is in the process of being delivered when she develops varying degrees of respiratory distress and circulatory collapse. If the woman does not die immediately, serious hemorrhage with severe coagulation defects is soon evident from the genital tract and all other sites of trauma.

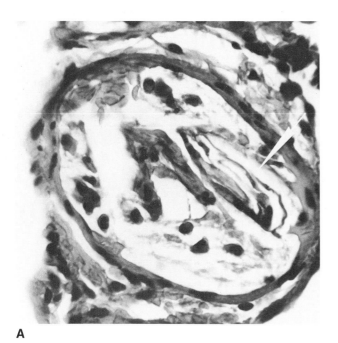

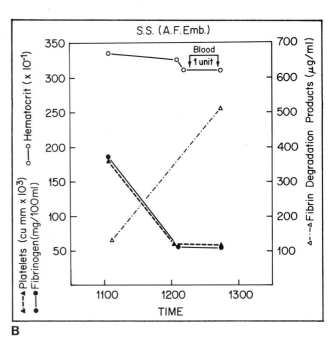

A   **B**

Figure 21-20. A. Fetal squames (arrow) packed into a small pulmonary artery from a fatal case of amnionic fluid embolism. Most of the empty spaces within the vessel were demonstrated by appropriate staining for lipid to have been filled with vernix caseosa. **B.** Levels of fibrinogen, fibrinogen–fibrin degradation products, and platelets during fatal amnionic fluid embolism.

Toxicity of Amnionic Fluid

The lethality of intravenously infused amnionic fluid appears to vary remarkably depending especially upon the particulate matter it contains. The suddenness and the intensity of cardiorespiratory problems that develop in many cases of amnionic fluid embolism and the histologic findings in the pulmonary vessels at autopsy strongly suggest, at least, that the likelihood of infused amnionic fluid proving lethal is greatest when it has been appreciably enriched with particulate debris. For example, severe amnionic fluid embolism seems to be more common in circumstances that lead to fetal distress with the escape of meconium from the fetal colon into the amnionic sac.

Schneider (1955) showed that the lethal nature of human amnionic fluid infused intravenously into dogs was enhanced very greatly by the addition of meconium. Under these circumstances, it is envisioned that the particulate matter shed previously into the amnionic fluid or contained in the meconium, including shed fetal squamous cells (squames) (Fig. 21-20A), fetal hairs (lanugo), vernix caseosa, and mucin, is pumped by a vigorous contraction from the disrupted amnionic sac into a maternal vein that drains the uterus. Severe pulmonary vascular obstruction from the particulate matter and possibly from fibrin formed intravascularly leads to *acute cor pulmonale* (Schneider and Henry, 1968). Abruptly, hypoxia and reduced cardiac output develop, and if they

are not immediately fatal, hemorrhage from coagulation defects is soon evident from disrupted blood vessels. Severe thrombocytopenia develops and the blood typically clots poorly when treated with thrombin, or, at most, there is formed a small, mushy clot that soon lyses completely. Plasma from such a patient, mixed with normal plasma and recalcified or with thrombin added to form a clot, has been observed by us to rapidly lyse, whereas the clotted normal plasma alone did not do so for days. Moreover, when fibrinogen was injected into the circulation, the thrombin–clottable protein promptly disappeared. These observations implicate intense fibrinolytic and even fibrinogenolytic activity, in some cases at least, as well as consumptive coagulopathy.

Coagulation Initiated by Amnionic Fluid. The clot-acccelerating activity of amnionic fluid is greater at term than early in the third trimester, an observation that led Hastwell (1974) to suggest its measurement as an index of fetal maturity. Even at term, however, the activity normally is not great. The clot accelerator principle appears to behave more like Russell's viper venom than tissue thromboplastin, in that factor VII is not essential for the clot-accelerating action of amnionic fluid (Courtney and Allington, 1972; Phillips and Davidson, 1972). Of significance, amnionic fluid at times contains appreciable amounts of mucus which, in case of amnionic fluid embolism, might incite or aggravate intravascular coagulation. Extracts of human mucus have been shown in vitro and in vivo to induce coagulation, apparently by activation of factor X (Pineo and co-workers, 1973).

Amnionic fluid contaminated with bacterial products, especially endotoxin, would almost certainly prove toxic if it were to enter the maternal circulation. The same is very likely to be true for amnionic fluid enriched with cytolytic products from a dead fetus.

Experimental Amnionic Fluid Embolism

Studies by Hanzlik and Karsner (1924) indicated that the intravenous injection of finely divided particulate matter, such as suspensions of charcoal particles or India ink, produced not only altered coagulability of the blood but also dramatic systemic phenomena, such as restlessness, tremors, marked dyspnea, convulsions, and often death. In the experiments of Halmagyi and co-workers (1962), after human amnionic fluid was injected into sheep, pulmonary hypertension, arterial hypoxia, and a marked fall in pulmonary compliance were noted. These changes, however, are similar to those found in pulmonary embolism of other cause, and, importantly, they failed to occur when the amnionic fluid was filtered. Moreover, they were not completely prevented by heparin. Adamson and associates (1971) and Stolte and co-workers (1967) could not produce the syndrome in monkeys, nor could Spence and Mason (1974) do so in rabbits. Attwood (1964) caused the death of only 5 of 15 dogs by the intravenous injection of 50 ml of amnionic fluid, and Pritchard and Capps (unpublished observations) noted an even lower mortality rate in dogs when sterile human amnionic fluid obtained at repeat cesarean section at or very near term was used. However, a suspension of human meconium injected into dogs has been shown to be highly lethal (Schneider, 1955).

Diagnosis. Fatal amnionic fluid embolism can be confirmed by the appearance of amnionic fluid debris, especially squames, vernix, mucin, and lanugo, widespread in small pulmonary blood vessels. Fatal amnionic fluid embolism has been encountered rarely at Parkland Memorial Hospital. A fairly typical case follows:

S.S., a young primigravida at term, felt no fetal movement for 12 hours before the onset of discomforts of labor. When first evaluated 2 hours later no fetal heart sounds were heard, but regular uterine contractions without uterine hypertonus or tenderness were identified clinically and electronically. The cervix was 2 cm dilated and 90 percent effaced. Neither amnionic fluid nor blood was visualized coming through the cervical canal until amniotomy when brown meconium-laden fluid escaped. She was moderately hypertensive and received magnesium sulfate prophylactically. The hematocrit was 34, and a blood clot of appreciable size formed in a thrombin tube. The platelet count, prothrombin time, and partial thromboplastin time were normal. Two hours after admittance her blood pressure began to fluctuate between 135/105 and 90/60 mm Hg. The hematocrit was now 29. She received 2 units of whole blood for presumed abruptio placentae, although uterine hypertonus and tenderness were lacking, there was no vaginal bleeding, and urine flow the previous hour was 60 ml per hour. She suddenly became very quiet and then unresponsive; her blood pressure was undetectable, and the apical pulse dropped to 60 and then to zero. Endotracheal intuba-

tion and cardiopulmonary resuscitation were initiated as a heavily meconium-stained, slightly macerated infant was delivered. The flattened placenta with the maternal surface covered with clot followed promptly.

The uterus contracted poorly and attempts at ventilation were thwarted by lack of pulmonary compliance. Cardiac function was maintained by closed chest compression, and hemorrhage from the flaccid uterus was combatted with blood transfusions. However, oxygenation was inadequate in spite of endotracheal intubation and mechanical ventilation. She was pronounced dead.

Histologically, small blood vessels in the lungs were plugged by debris, including squames, mucin, and vernix caseosa, which accounted for the inability to oxygenate the patient (Fig. 21-20A). Serial values for plasma fibrinogen, serum fibrinogen–fibrin degradation products, and platelets are presented in Figure 21-20B. Abnormalities suggestive of modest consumptive coagulopathy were present when she was hospitalized. These changes had become severe when she demonstrated loss of consciousness, hypotension, and bradycardia, and they persisted until death.

An unusual feature of this case is the presence of much meconium presumably from fetal distress associated with abruptio placentae. In our considerable experience, meconium is rarely found with extensive placental abruption even when severe enough to kill the fetus.

There almost certainly have been women who survived amnionic fluid embolism, although the diagnosis is always open to question without definite identification of obvious amnionic fluid debris within blood vessels in histologic sections of lung or at least in the buffy coat of blood from the right side of the heart.

Intriguing, but in some ways troublesome, observations have been reported in recent years in which the buffy coat of blood drawn from the right side of the maternal heart or pulmonary artery has been identified morphologically to contain amnionic fluid debris—typically squames or vernix caseosa—many hours to even days after suspected amnionic fluid embolism. Studies are needed to evaluate blood so collected and processed in the absence of suspicion of embolization. Tuck (1972) has described the identification of squames presumed to be from amnionic fluid in sputum stained with Nile blue sulfate. Confirmatory experiences with this technique are needed.

Treatment. Therapy for amnionic fluid embolism is notoriously unsuccessful. Moreover, when treatment is successful, the diagnosis may be challenged. Vigorous treatment of the hypoxia is mandatory and usually necessitates mechanical ventilation. Blood replacement therapy is equally essential (Resnik and co-workers, 1976), but the patient with cor pulmonale tolerates any deficit or excess in blood volume very poorly.

When amnionic fluid embolism is strongly suspected, use of a Swan-Ganz catheter, an intra-arterial line to facilitate the measurement of blood pressures and obtaining blood samples, and instrumentation to record systemic blood pressures, pulmonary artery and wedge pressures, cardiac output, and blood oxygenation are likely to prove beneficial, although invasion of large vessels in the presence of grossly defective hemostasis may in itself lead to dangerous hemorrhage. Use of fibrinogen and other blood component therapy, heparin, fibrinolytic agents, and antifibrinolytic agents has been described in various case reports, but it is very difficult to evaluate their efficacy (Chung and Merkatz, 1973; Gregory and Clayton, 1973; Kates and Schifrin, 1976; Pritchard and Dugan, 1956; Woodfield and colleagues, 1971).

HEMORRHAGE WITH ABORTION

Etiology of Hemorrhage

Remarkable blood loss, especially acute hemorrhage, but sometimes chronic, may occur as the consequence of abortion. Hemorrhage during the first trimester is less likely to be severe unless the abortion was induced and the procedure was traumatic. However, when the pregnancy is more advanced, the mechanisms responsible for the hemorrhage most often are the same as those described for placental abruption and placenta previa, i.e., the disruption of a large number of maternal blood vessels at the site of placental implantation without myometrial contraction and retraction appropriate for mechanical constriction of these vessels. At times, appreciable changes in the coagulation mechanism complicate abortion.

Coagulation Defects

Serious disruption of the coagulation mechanism as the consequence of abortion may develop in the following circumstances: (1) prolonged retention of a dead fetus, as described above, (2) sepsis, a notorious cause, (3) the intrauterine instillation of hypertonic saline or urea solutions, (4) medical induction with a prostaglandin, and (5) during instrumental termination of the pregnancy.

The kinds of changes in coagulation that have been identified with abortion induced with markedly *hypertonic solutions* imply, at least, that thromboplastin is released from placenta, fetus, decidua, or all three by the necrobiotic effect of the hypertonic solutions, which then initiates coagulation within the maternal circulation (Burkman and associates, 1977). Coagulation defects have been observed to develop rarely during induction of abortion with prostaglandin.

Gross disruption of the coagulation mechanism has been an uncommon but serious complication among women with *septic abortion* cared for at Parkland Memorial Hospital. The incidence of coagulation defects has been highest in those with *Clostridium perfringens* sepsis and intense intravascular hemolysis (Pritchard and Whalley, 1971). In the presence of gross intravascular hemolysis, plasma fibrinogen concentrations ranged from normal to low, as did the platelet counts, while fibrin degradation products in serum were variably elevated. It has long been recognized that intense intravascular hemolysis is capable of inciting disseminated intravascular coagulation, which, if the circulatory system is not intact, contributes significantly to serious hemorrhage.

Severe disruption of the coagulation mechanism, presumably by endotoxin, can develop with abortion complicated by gram-negative sepsis in the absence of intense intravascular hemolysis (Chapter 24, Table 24-2).

Prompt restoration and maintenance of the circulation and appropriate steps to control the infection, including evacuation of the infected products of conception, are most important for a successful outcome. There is no good evidence that routine hysterectomy, rather than prompt curettage to remove infected products of conception in an intact uterus, improves the outcome. Management is described further in Chapter 24, p. 484.

Midtrimester abortion induced by *dilatation and evacuation* has also served to induce severe consumptive coagulopathy. There has been an array of cases reported, especially in the last decade, in which midpregnancy abortions without prolonged fetal death have been complicated by severe consumptive coagulopathy (Guidotti and co-workers, 1981; White and colleagues, 1983). Usually the etiology has been ascribed to amnionic fluid embolism, although it has been our experience that amnionic fluid at or near midpregnancy contains very little particulate matter to obstruct the pulmonary microcirculation, and its capability for activating the coagulation mechanism is weak, at least in vitro.

We have observed four patients in whom dilatation of the cervix and mechanical evacuation of the pregnancy at 15 to 21 weeks gestation somehow induced severe comsumptive coagulopathy with fibrinogen levels that were low to undetectable and accompanied by high levels of fibrin degradation products. Three of the women were treated as described above for placental abruption and survived. One woman described below died:

> During attempts at dilatation and evacuation at an abortion clinic, she convulsed and suffered apparent cardiac arrest, which was treated immediately with closed chest cardiac compression plus artificial ventilation. Spontaneous cardiac activity was soon evident, and she regained consciousness once vigorous therapy with lactated Ringer's solution and whole blood was instituted and maintained.

Intense hypofibrinogenemia and markedly elevated levels of fibrinogen–fibrin degradation products were identified. However, pulmonary function was not impaired; arterial blood Po$_2$ was 151 mm Hg while receiving oxygen by mask. Severe hemorrhage from the superior portion of the liver and a torn hepatic vein, apparently traumatized during cardiopulmonary resuscitation, proved fatal. While this case has been ascribed to amnionic fluid embolism (Cates and associates, 1981), the results of histologic examinations of the lungs are equivocal (Pritchard, unpublished).

It seem plausible that in some of these cases, at least, rather than amnionic fluid debris being the culprit, mechanical separation of the placenta during the course of the abortion allowed thromboplastic materials from injured placenta and decidua to enter the maternal circulation at the implantation site, thereby triggering intense consumptive coagulopathy.

It seems unlikely that amnionic fluid per se is the major culprit, for reasons considered on page 416. In our experience, the coagulation defects are soon repaired and recovery is uneventful if perfusion of vital organs is maintained by appropriate refilling of the intravascular compartment, as described above for placental abruption, and the products of conception are removed from the uterine cavity.

COAGULATION DEFECTS POSSIBLY INDUCED BY HEMORRHAGE

Rarely, severe hemorrhage with overt disruption of the coagulation mechanism may develop in a woman without recognized evidence of any disease known to incite consumptive coagulopathy, as for example, an apparently uncomplicated repeated cesarean section. The experimental observations of Turpini and Stefanini (1959) support the thesis that severe hemorrhage of itself can induce consumptive coagulopathy. Animal studies by some other investigators, however, have not confirmed their observations (Herman and associates, 1972; Karayalcin and colleagues, 1973). In the case of massive fatal hemorrhage from rupture of the uterus considered in Table 21-2, the marked decrease in coagulation factors was primarily the consequence of hemodilution by electrolyte solution rather than intense intravascular coagulopathy. Prompt treatment with blood and lactated Ringer's solution and, at times, a concentrated source of fibrinogen (cryoprecipitate), fresh frozen plasma, and platelet packs, as described earlier in this chapter for placental abruption, has been effective in cases treated at Parkland Memorial Hospital.

OTHER COAGULATION DEFECTS

Coagulation defects caused by *eclampsia* or *severe preeclampsia* are discussed in Chapter 27. Rarely, a hemophilia-like state may be acquired during the postpartum period as a consequence of development of antibody to factor VIII. Treatment may require massive amounts of blood and cryoprecipitate. Attempts at immunosuppression with corticosteroids and plasmapheresis to try to remove antibody to factor VIII do not seem to have been of benefit.

Coagulation defects that coincide with pregnancy are considered in Chapter 28.

REFERENCES

Abdella TN, Sibai BM, Hays JM Jr, Anderson GD: Perinatal outcome in abruptio placentae. Obstet Gynecol, 63:365, 1984

Adamsons K, Mueller-Heubach E, Myers RE: The innocuousness of amniotic fluid infusion in the pregnant rhesus monkey. Am J Obstet Gynecol 109:988, 1971

Alperin JB, Haggard ME, McGanity WJ: Folic acid, pregnancy, and abruptio placentae. Am J Clin Nutr 22:1354, 1969

Åstedt B: Risk of β-receptor agonists delaying diagnosis of abruptio placentae. Acta Obstet Gynecol Scand [Suppl] 108:35, 1982

Attwood HD: A histological study of experimental amniotic-fluid and meconium embolism in dogs. J Pathol Bacteriol 88:285, 1964

Bailey CD, Newman C, Ellinas SP, Anderson GG: Use of prostaglandin E$_2$ vaginal suppositories in intrauterine fetal death and missed abortion. Obstet Gynecol 45:110, 1975

Beischer NA, Brown JB, Macafee J: Urinary estriol excretion before severe placental abruption. Obstet Gynecol 36:697, 1970

Bill AH: The treatment of placenta previa by prophylactic blood transfusion and cesarean section. Am J Obstet Gynecol 14:523, 1927

Bonnar J, McNicol GP, Douglas AS: The behavior of the coagulation and fibrinolytic mechanism in abruptio placentae. J Obstet Gynaecol Br Commonw 76:799, 1969

Bowie JD, Rochester D, Cadkin AV, Cooke WT, Kunzman A: Accuracy of placental localization by ultrasound. Radiology 128:177, 1978

Brame RG, Harbert GM Jr, McGaughey HS Jr, Thornton WN Jr: Maternal risk in abruption. Obstet Gynecol 31:224, 1968

Brenner WE, Edelman DA, Hendricks CH: Characteristics of patients with placenta previa and results of expectant management. Am J Obstet Gynecol 132:180, 1978

Burkman RT, Bell WR, Atienza MF, King TM: Coagulopathy with midtrimester induced abortion: Association with hyperosmolar urea administration. Am J Obstet Gynecol 127:533, 1977

Campbell S, Kohorn E: Placental localization by ultrasonic compound scanning. J Obstet Gynaecol Br Commonw 75:1007, 1968

Cates W Jr, Boyd C, Halvorson-Boyd G, Holck S, Gilchrest TF: Death from amniotic fluid embolism and disseminated intravascular coagulation after a curettage abortion. Am J Obstet Gynecol 141:346, 1981

Chung AF, Merkatz IR: Survival following amniotic fluid embolism with early heparinization. Obstet Gynecol 42:809, 1973

Comeau J, Shaw L, Marcell CC, Lavery JP: Early placenta previa and delivery outcome. Obstet Gynecol 61:577, 1983

Corrigan Jr JJ: Vitamin K-dependent coagulation factors in gram-negative septicermia. Am J Dis Child 138:240, 1984

Courtney LD, Allington M: Effect of amniotic fluid on blood coagulation. Br J Haematol 22:353, 1972

Czer LSC, Shoemaker WC: Optimal hematocrit value in critically ill postoperative patients. Surg Gynecol Obstet 147:363, 1978

Dehner LP: Advanced extrauterine pregnancy and the fetal death syndrome. Obstet Gynecol 40:525, 1972

Donald I, Abdulla U: Placentography by sonar. J Obstet Gynaecol Br Commonw 75:993, 1968

Edson JR, Blaese RM, White JG, Krivit W: Defibrination syndrome in an infant born after abruptio placentae. Pediatrics 72:342, 1968

Goldstein DP, Reid DE: Circulating fibrinolytic activity: A precursor of hypofibrinogenemia following fetal death in utero. Obstet Gynecol 22:174, 1963

Gottesfeld KR, Thompson HE, Holmes JH, Taylor ES: Ultrasound placentography: A new method for placental localization. Am J Obstet Gynecol 96:538, 1966

Gregory MG, Clayton EM Jr: Amniotic fluid embolism. Obstet Gynecol 42:236, 1973

Guidotti RJ, Grimes DA, Cates W Jr: Fatal amniotic fluid embolism during legally induced abortion, United States 1972 to 1978. Am J Obstet Gynecol 141:257, 1981

Halmagyi DR, Starzecki B, Shearman RP: Experimental amniotic fluid embolism: Mechanism and treatment. Am J Obstet Gynecol 84:251, 1962

Hanzlik PJ, Karsner HT: Anaphylactoid phenomena from the intravenous administration of various colloids, arsenicals and other agents. J Pharmacol Exp Ther 14:379, 1920; 23:173, 1924

Hastwell GB: Amniotic fluid thromboplastic activity as an index of fetal maturity: A preliminary report. Aust NZ J Obstet Gynaecol 14:196, 1974

Herman CM, Moquin RB, Horwitz DL: Coagulation changes of hemorrhagic shock in baboons. Ann Surg 175:197, 1972

Hibbard BM, Jeffcoate TNA: Abruptio placentae. Obstet Gynecol 27:155, 1966

Hovatta O, Lipasti A, Rapola J, Karjalainen O: Causes of stillbirth: A clinicopathological study of 243 patients. Acta Obstet Gynecol Scand 90:691, 1983

Hughes EC (ed): Obstetric-Gynecologic Terminology. Philadelphia, Davis, 1972, p 417

Hurd WW, Miodovnik M, Hertzberg V, Lavin JP: Selective management of abruptio placentae: A prospective study. Obstet Gynecol 61:467, 1983

Jansen RPS: Relative bradycardia: A sign of acute intraperitoneal bleeding. Aust AZ J Obstet Gynaecol 18:206, 1978

Jennison RF, Walker AC: Foetal death in utero with hypofibrinogenemia managed conservatively. Lancet 2:607, 1956

Jimenez JM, Pritchard JA: Pathogenesis and treatment of coagulation defects resulting from fetal death. Obstet Gynecol 32:449, 1968

Johnson HW: The conservative management of some varieties of placenta previa. Am J Obstet Gynecol 50:248, 1945

Jouppila P: Vaginal bleeding in the last two trimesters of pregnancy. A clinical and ultrasonic study. Acta Obstet Gynecol Scand 58:461, 1979

Karayalcin G, Kim KY, Aballi AJ: Coagulation changes after acute blood loss. Pediatr Res 7:357, 1973

Kates RJ, Schifrin BS: Self-limited acute defibrination in pregnancy: Case report. Am J Obstet Gynecol 124:432, 1976

Kent DR, Goldstein AI: Prostaglandin E₂ induction of labor for fetal demise. Obstet Gynecol 48:475, 1976

King DL: Placental migration demonstrated by ultrasonography. Radiology 109:163, 1973

Kobayashi M, Hellman L, Fillisti L: Placenta localization by ultrasound. Am J Obstet Gynecol 106:279, 1970

Krupp PJ Jr, Barclay DL, Roeling WM, Wegener G: Maternal mortality: A 20-year study of Tulane Department of Obstetrics and Gynecology at Charity Hospital. Obstet Gynecol 35:823, 1970

Lerner R, Margolin M, Slate WG: Heparin in the treatment of hypofibrinogenemia complicating fetal death in utero. Am J Obstet Gynecol 97:373, 1967

Liggins GC: Treatment of missed abortion by high dosage syntocinon intravenous infusion. J Obstet Gynaecol Br Commonw 69:277, 1962

Macafee CHG: Placenta previa: A study of 174 cases. J Obstet Gynaecol Br Emp 52:313, 1945

Marbury MC, Linn S, Monson R, Schoenbaum S, Stubblefield PG, Ryan KJ: The association of alcohol consumption with outcome of pregnancy. Am J Public Health 73:1165, 1983

Ness PM, Perkins HA: Cryoprecipitate as a reliable source of fibrinogen replacement. JAMA 241:1690, 1979

Newton M: Postpartum hemorrhage. Am J Obstet Gynecol 94:711, 1966

Nielsen NC: Coagulation and fibrinolysis in mothers and their newborn infants following premature separation of the placenta. Acta Obstet Gynecol Scand 49:77, 1970

Orr JW Jr, Huddleston JF, Goldenberg RL, Knox GE, Davis RO: Association of extrauterine fetal death with failure of prostaglandin E₂ suppositories. Obstet Gynecol [Suppl] 53:57, 1979

Paterson MEL: The aetiology and outcome of abruptio placentae. Acta Obstet Gynecol Scand 58:31, 1979

Patterson SP, White JH, Reaves EM: A maternal death associated with prostagladin E₂. Obstet Gynecol 54:123, 1979

Pfeffer RI: Hypofibrinogenemia in the dead fetus syndrome treated with aminocaproic acid. Am J Obstet Gynecol 95:1095, 1966

Phelan JP, Cefalo RC: A better approach to fetal demise—PGE₂ suppository. Contemp Ob/Gyn 11:93, 1978

Phillips LL, Davidson EC Jr: Procoagulant properties of amniotic fluid. Am J Obstet Gynecol 113:911, 1972

Pineo GF, Recoeczi E, Hatton MWC, Brain MC: The activation of coagulation by extracts of mucus: A possible pathway of intravascular coagulation accompanying adenocarcinomas. J Lab Clin Med 82:255, 1973

Pritchard JA: Fetal death in utero. Obstet Gynecol 14:573, 1959

Pritchard JA: Changes in the blood volume during pregnancy and delivery. Anesthesiology 26:393, 1965

Pritchard JA: Haematological problems associated with delivery, placental abruption, retained dead fetus, and amniotic fluid embolism. Clin Haematol 2:563, 1973

Pritchard JA, Brekken AL: Clinical and laboratory studies on severe abruptio placentae. Am J Obstet Gynecol 97:681, 1967

Pritchard JA, Dugan RJ: Presumed amniotic fluid embolism with recovery. Ohio State Med J 52:379, 1956

Pritchard JA, Ratnoff OD: Studies of fibrinogen and other hemostatic factors in women with intrauterine death and delayed delivery. Surg Gynecol Obstet 101:467, 1955

Pritchard JA, Whalley PJ: Abortion complicated by Clostridium perfringens infection. Am J Obstet Gynecol 11:484, 1971

Pritchard JA, Cunningham FG, Mason RA: Coagulation changes in eclampsia: Their frequency and pathogenesis. Am J Obstet Gynecol 124:855, 1976

Pritchard JA, Baldwin RM, Dickey JC, Wiggins KM: Blood volume changes in pregnancy and the puerperium. II. Red blood cell loss and changes in apparent blood volume during and following vaginal delivery, cesarean section, and cesarean section plus total hysterectomy. Am J Obstet Gynecol 84:1271, 1962

Pritchard JA, Mason R, Corley M, Pritchard S: Genesis of severe placental abruption. Am J Obstet Gynecol 108:22, 1970

Resnik R, Swartz WH, Plumer MH, Benirschke K, Stratthaus ME: Amniotic fluid embolism with survival. Obstet Gynecol 47:295, 1976

Santos R, Jimenez J, Duenhoelter J: Unpublished observations, 1978

Schneider CL: Obstetric shock: Some interdependent problems of coagulation. Obstet Gynecol 4:273, 1954

Schneider CL: Coagulation defects in obstetric shock: Meconium embolism and heparin; fibrin embolism and defibrination. Am J Obstet Gynecol 69:758, 1955

Schneider CL, Henry MM: Meconium embolism in vivo. Am J Obstet Gynecol 101:909, 1968

Schulman H, Saldana L, Lin C-C, Randolph G: Mechanism of failed labor after fetal death and its treatment with prostaglandin E$_2$. Am J Obstet Gynecol 133:742, 1979

Seski JC, Compton AA: Abruptio placentae following a negative oxytocin challenge test. Am J Obstet Gynecol 125:276, 1976

Sher G: Pathogenesis and management of uterine inertia complicating abruptio placentae with consumption coagulopathy. Am J Obstet Gynecol 129:164, 1977

Sher G: A rational basis for the management of abruptio placentae. J Reprod Med 21:123, 1978

Sherman E, Middleton EH: The management of missed abortion with hypofibrinogenemia. Maryland State Med J 7:300, 1958

Silke B, Carmody M, O'Dwyer WF: Acute renal failure in pregnancy. In Bonnar J, MacGillivray I, Symonds EM (eds): Pregnancy Hypertension. Baltimore, University Park Press, 1980

Singh PM, Rodrigues C, Gupta AN: Placenta previa and previous cesarean section. Acta Obstet Gynecol Scand 60:367, 1981

Skelly H, Marivate M, Norman R, Kenoyer G, Martin R: Consumptive coagulopathy following fetal death in a triplet pregnancy. Am J Obstet Gynecol 142:595, 1982

Spence MR, Mason KG: Experimental amniotic fluid embolism in rabbits. Am J Obstet Gynecol 119:1073, 1974

Stolte L, Seelen J, Eskes T, Wagatsuma T: Failure to produce the syndrome of amniotic fluid embolism by infusion of amniotic fluid and meconium into monkeys. Am J Obstet Gynecol 98:694, 1967

Stone SR, Whalley PJ, Pritchard JA: Inferior vena cava and ovarian vein ligation during late pregnancy. Obstet Gynecol 32:267, 1968

Sunden B: Placentography by ultrasound. Acta Obstet Gynecol Scand 49:179, 1970

Tricomi V, Kohl SG: Fetal death in utero. Am J Obstet Gynecol 74:1092, 1957

Tuck CS: Amniotic fluid embolism. Proc Royal Soc Med 65:2, 1972

Turpini R, Stefanini M: The nature and mechanism of the hemostatic breakdown in the course of experimental hemorrhagic shock. J Clin Invest 38:53, 1959

Weiner AE, Reid DE, Roby CC, Diamond LK: Coagulation defects with intrauterine death from Rh sensitization. Am J Obstet Gynecol 60:1015, 1950

Wexler P, Gottesfeld KR: Second trimester placenta previa: An apparently normal placentation. Obstet Gynecol 50:706, 1977

Whalley PJ, Pritchard JA: Oxytocin and water intoxication. JAMA 186:601, 1963

Whalley PJ, Scott DE, Pritchard JA: Maternal folate deficiency and pregnancy wastage: I. Placental abruption. Am J Obstet Gynecol 105:670, 1969

White PF, Coe V, Dworsky WA, Margolis A: Disseminated intravascular coagulation following midtrimester abortions. Anesthesiology 58:99, 1983

Woodfield DG, Galloway RK, Smart GE: Coagulation defect associated with presumed amniotic fluid embolism in the mid-trimester of pregnancy. J Obstet Gynaecol Br Commonw 78:423, 1971

Young GB: The peripatetic placenta. Radiology 128:183, 1978

22

Ectopic Pregnancy

GENERAL CONSIDERATIONS

Definition

In a normal intrauterine pregnancy, the blastocyst implants in the endometrium lining the uterine cavity. Implantation anywhere else is referred to as an ectopic pregnancy. Although more than 95 percent of ectopic pregnancies involve the oviduct, tubal pregnancy is not synonymous with, but rather a very common type of, ectopic gestation.

Etiology

The following have been implicated in the cause of ectopic pregnancy:

A. Conditions that prevent or retard the passage of the fertilized ovum into the uterine cavity
   1. *Salpingitis,* especially endosalpingitis, which causes agglutination of the arborescent folds of the tubal mucosa with narrowing of the lumen or formation of blind pockets. Reduced ciliation of the tubal mucosa as the consequence of infection may also contribute to tubal implantation of the zygote.
   2. *Peritubal adhesions* subsequent to postabortal or puerperal infection, appendicitis, or endometriosis, which cause kinking of the tube and narrowing of the lumen.
   3. *Developmental abnormalities of the tube,* especially diverticula, accessory ostia, and hypoplasia.
   4. *Previous operations on the tube,* either to restore patency or, occasionally, the failure of a deliberate attempt to disrupt tubal patency for sterilization (tubal constriction, partial resection, or fulgeration).
   5. *Tumors that distort the tube,* such as uterine myomas and adnexal masses.
   6. *External migration of the ovum* is probably not an important factor. There may be a slight increased risk of ectopic pregnancy for the woman with but one oviduct whenever she ovulates from the contralateral ovary. The delay in transport of the fertilized ovum

through the oviduct as the consequence of external migration increases invasive properties of the blastocyst while still within the oviduct. This is probably not an important factor in human ectopic gestation.
   7. *Menstrual reflux* has been suggested as a cause. Delayed fertilization of the ovum with menstrual bleeding at the usual time theoretically could either prevent the ovum from entering the uterus or flush it back into the tube. There is little supporting evidence for this phenomenon.

B. Increase in the receptivity of the tubal mucosa to the fertilized ovum
   1. *Ectopic endometrial elements* may enhance tubal implantation. Many observers have reported foci of endometriosis in fallopian tubes, but it is an uncommon finding.

Tubal pregnancy may rarely follow hysterectomy. Niebyl (1974) reviewed 21 such cases. In most instances, a very recently fertilized ovum was trapped in the oviduct at the time of hysterectomy, where it implanted and grew for a variable period. More rarely, an ovum was fertilized in the oviduct long after hysterectomy. In such cases, a fistula sufficient for passage of sperm had developed between the vagina and the severed end of the oviduct.

Incidence

A doubling of the number of ectopic pregnancies has occurred in more recent years. The number of ectopic pregnancies annually in the United States has been estimated at 40,000 for 1978 compared to less than 20,000 in 1970 (Rubin and associates, 1983). The causes of the increase are multiple and include the following: (1) increased prevalence of sexually transmitted tubal infection that damages tubal mucosa but not so severely as to cause complete occlusion, (2) popularity of contraception that prevents intrauterine but not extrauterine pregnancies, especially an intrauterine contraceptive device and possible low-dose progestational agents, (3) unsuccessful tubal sterilizations, especially laparoscopic coagulation procedures, (4) induced abortion followed by infection, (5) fertility induced by ovulatory agents, (6)

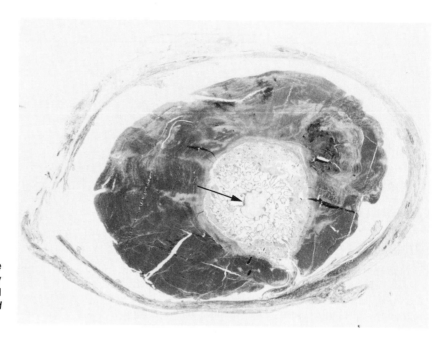

Figure 22-1. Early tubal pregnancy. The amnionic sac (*arrow*) is surrounded by chorionic villi, which, in turn, are encased in blood clot. (*Courtesy of Dr. Richard Voet.*)

previous pelvic surgery including salpingotomy for previous tubal pregnancy and tuboplasty, (7) exposure to stilbestrol in utero, and (8) better and earlier diagnostic techniques. It is estimated that, if left alone, from 10 to as many as 50 percent of ectopic pregnancies are either resorbed in situ or abort spontaneously.

Anatomic Considerations

The fertilized ovum may develop in any portion of the oviduct, giving rise to *ampullar, isthmic, and interstitial tubal pregnancies* (Fig. 2-17). In rare instances, the fertilized ovum may be implanted in the fimbriated extremity and occasionally even on the fimbria ovarica. The ampulla is the most frequent site of implantation and the isthmus the next most common. Interstitial pregnancy is very uncommon, occurring in only about 2.5 percent of all tubal gestations. From these primary types, certain secondary forms of tuboabdominal, tubo-ovarian, and broad ligament pregnancies occasionally develop.

Implantation of the Zygote. The fertilized ovum does not remain on the surface but promptly burrows through the epithelium. As the zygote penetrates the epithelium it comes to lie in the muscular wall, since the tube lacks a submucosa. At the periphery of the zygote is a capsule of rapidly proliferating trophoblast, which invades and erodes the subjacent muscularis of the tube. At the same time, maternal blood vessels are opened, and the blood pours out into the spaces of varying size, lying within the trophoblast or between it and the adjacent tissue, especially the covering tubal serosa.

The tube does not normally form an extensive decidua, although decidual cells can usually be recognized. The tubal wall in contact with the zygote offers but slight resistance to invasion by the trophoblast, which soon burrows through it, opening maternal vessels (Fig. 22-1).

The embryo or fetus in ectopic pregnancy is often absent or stunted.

Uterine Changes. In ectopic pregnancies, the uterus undergoes some of the changes associated with early normal intrauterine pregnancy, including softening of the cervix and isthmus and an increase in size. *These changes in the uterus do not, therefore, exclude an ectopic pregnancy.*

The degree to which the endometrium is converted to decidua is variable. The finding of uterine decidua without trophoblast certainly suggests ectopic pregnancy but is by no means an absolute indication. In 1954, Arias-Stella described, as had others before him, the following changes in the endometrium: The epithelial cells are enlarged and their nuclei are hypertrophic, hyperchromatic, lobular, and irregularly shaped. There is a loss of polarity, and the abnormal nuclei tend to occupy the luminal portion of the cells. The cytoplasm may be vacuolated and foamy, and occasional mitoses may be found. These endometrial changes have been collectively referred to as the *Arias-Stella reaction* (Fig. 22-2). The cellular changes in the Arias-Stella reaction are not specific for ectopic pregnancy but rather the blighting of the conceptus, either intrauterine or extrauterine.

The external bleeding seen commonly in cases of tubal pregnancy is uterine in origin and associated with degeneration and sloughing of the uterine decidua. Soon after the death of the fetus, the decidua degenerates and is usually shed in small pieces, but occasionally it is cast off intact, as a *decidual cast* of the uterine cavity. The absence of decidual tissue, however, does not exclude an ectopic pregnancy. Romney and co-workers (1950), for

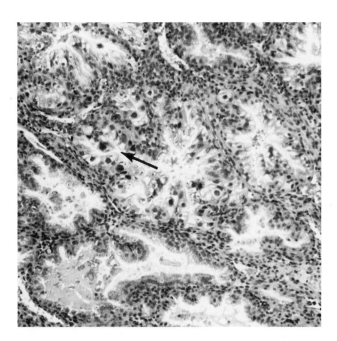

Figure 22-2. Arias-Stella reaction. Some of the nuclei are enlarged (*arrow*), hyperchromatic, and irregularly shaped. Some of the cytoplasm is vacuolated and foamy. (*Courtesy of Dr. Helen Graham.*)

example, identified secretory endometrium in 40 percent of cases of ectopic pregnancy, proliferative in 30 percent, and menstrual in 6 percent, while decidua was present in only 20 percent.

NATURAL HISTORY OF TUBAL PREGNANCY

Tubal Abortion

A common termination of tubal pregnancy is separation of the products of conception from the implantation site and extrusion of the abortus through the fimbriated end of the oviduct. The frequency of tubal abortion depends in great part upon the site of implantation of the zygote. In ampullary tubal pregnancy, it is common, whereas rupture of the tube is the usual outcome in isthmic pregnancy. The immediate consequence of the hemorrhage with tubal abortion is the further disruption of the connection between the placenta and membranes and the tubal wall, and if separation is complete, the entire products may be extruded through the fimbriated end into the peritoneal cavity. At that point, hemorrhage may cease and symptoms disappear.

In complete tubal abortion, when the zygote is retained within the oviduct and hemorrhage is moderate, the abortus may become infiltrated with blood and converted into a structure analogous to the blood mole observed in uterine abortion. Some bleeding usually persists as long as the products of conception remain in the oviduct, and the blood slowly trickles from the fimbriated end into the peritoneal cavity and typically pools

in the rectouterine cul-de-sac. If the fimbriated extremity is occluded, the fallopian tube may gradually become distended by blood, forming a *hematosalpinx*.

After incomplete tubal abortion, pieces of the placenta or membranes may remain attached to the tubal wall and, after becoming surrounded by fibrin, give rise to a *placental polyp*, as may occur in the uterus after an incomplete uterine abortion.

Tubal Rupture

The invading, expanding products of conception may rupture the oviduct at any of several sites. Many of the cases of tubal pregnancy end during the first trimester by intraperitoneal rupture. As a rule, whenever tubal rupture occurs in the first few weeks, the pregnancy is situated in the isthmic portion of the tube a short distance from the cornu of the uterus. When the fertilized ovum is implanted well within the interstitial portion of the tube, rupture usually does not occur until later.

The immediate cause of rupture may be trauma associated with coitus or a vigorous bimanual examination, although in the great majority of cases rupture occurs spontaneously. With intraperitoneal rupture, the entire products of conception may be extruded from the tube, or if the rent is small, profuse hemorrhage may occur without extrusion. In either event, commonly, the patient soon shows signs of collapse from hemorrhage and hypovolemia. If the woman is not operated upon and does not die from hemorrhage, the fate of the embryo or fetus will depend on the damage sustained by the products of conception and on the duration of the gestation. If an early conceptus is expelled essentially undamaged into the peritoneal cavity, it may reimplant almost anywhere, establish adequate circulation, and survive and grow, but this outcome is most unlikely because of damage during the transition. The products of conception, if small, may be resorbed or, if larger, may remain in the cul-de-sac for years as an encapsulated mass or even become calcified to form a *lithopedion*.

If only the fetus is extruded at the time of rupture, however, the effect upon the pregnancy will vary depending on the extent of injury sustained by the placenta. If the placenta is damaged appreciably, death of the fetus and termination of the pregnancy are inevitable, but if the greater portion of the placenta still retains its attachment to the tube, further development is possible. The fetus may then survive for some time, giving rise to an *abdominal pregnancy*. Typically, in such cases, a portion of the placenta remains attached to the tubal wall and the periphery grows beyond the tube and implants on surrounding structures.

Rupture into the Broad Ligament. When the original implantation of the zygote is toward the mesosalpinx, rupture may occur at the portion of the tube not immediately covered by peritoneum, and the contents of the gestational sac may be extruded into a space formed between the folds of the broad ligament. This condition is designated an intraligamentous or *broad ligament preg-*

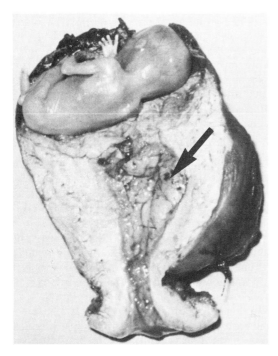

Figure 22-3. Right interstitial tubal pregnancy. The fetus weighed 55 g and measured 90 mm crown to rump (14 to 15 weeks gestational age). Note the abundant decidua (*arrow*) filling the uterine cavity. The patient sought medical help because of sudden severe abdominal pain with syncope following intercourse. Hysterectomy and blood tranfusion (2000 ml) were required.

nancy. It may terminate either in the death of the embryo or fetus and the formation of a *broad ligament hematoma* or in the further development of the pregnancy. Occasionally, the broad ligament sac ruptures at a later period, and the fetus is extruded into the peritoneal cavity while the placenta retains its position, forming an abdominal pregnancy.

Interstitial Pregnancy

When the fertilized ovum implants within the segment of the tube that penetrates the uterine wall, an especially grave form of tubal gestation, *interstitial pregnancy,* results (Fig. 22-3). Implantation at this site has also been referred to as a *cornual pregnancy.* Interstitial tubal pregnancy accounts for about 2.5 percent of all tubal gestations. Because of the site of implantation, no adnexal mass is palpable, but rather, there is variable asymmetry of the uterus that is often difficult to distinguish from an intrauterine pregnancy. Hence, the early diagnosis is even more frequently overlooked than in other types of tubal implantation. Because of the greater distensibility of the myometrium covering the interstitial portion compared to tubal wall not surrounded by myometrium, rupture of an interstitial pregnancy is likely to occur somewhat later, between the end of the second and the end of the fourth month. Because of the abundant blood supply from branches of both uterine and

ovarian arteries immediately adjacent to the implantation site, the hemorrhage that attends the rupture may be rapidly fatal. In fact, tubal pregnancies in which the woman dies before she can be brought to the hospital often fall into this group. Because of the large uterine defect, hysterectomy is commonly necessary. Very infrequently, an interstitial pregnancy may convert to a tubouterine pregnancy as described below.

Ectopic Multifetal Pregnancy

In rare instances, tubal pregnancy may be complicated by a coexisting intrauterine gestation, a condition designated as *combined pregnancy.* Combined pregnancy is quite difficult to diagnose clinically. Typically, laparotomy is performed because of a tubal pregnancy. At the same time, the uterus is congested, softened, and somewhat enlarged. Although these features are suggestive of intrauterine pregnancy, they are commonly induced by a tubal pregnancy alone. Gestational products should be demonstrable sonographically within the uterine cavity in practically all instances of combined pregnancy. Aspiration of the uterus for amnionic fluid has been recommended, but amnionic fluid may be difficult to obtain, especially if the chorion and amnion have not yet fused. Moreover, a blind aspiration to try to rule in or out with certainty the presence of amnionic fluid may be traumatic to the products of conception.

Combined pregnancy is rare. Five cases were observed relatively recently at one institution during which time 40,000 deliveries and 353 extrauterine gestations were cared for (Reece and associates, 1983). Simultaneous intrauterine and tubal pregnancy has followed induction of ovulation with either clomiphene therapy or menopausal gonadotropin.

The ultimate in combined pregnancies may have been reported by Funderburk (1974), who described a woman with a fetus in the right tube, a fetus in the left tube, and a fetus in the uterus. Since he preserved both oviducts, the potential for still another record persists.

Twin tubal pregnancy, at the same stage of development, has been reported with both embryos in the same tube, as well as with one in each tube. Arey (1923) considered the subject in detail and concluded that single-ovum twins form a far greater proportion of tubal than of uterine pregnancies. He postulated that difficulties in migration and implantation retard the growth of the zygote, which somehow stimulates to form two identical embryos. Simultaneous pregnancy in both fallopian tubes is the rarest form of double-ovum twinning.

Quadruplet tubal pregnancy in the same oviduct has been described by Fujii and associates (1981). The ruptured and hemorrhaging oviduct contained four amnionic sacs covered by a single chorion. Each of the sacs contained an embryo. There was appreciable difference in the size of the embryos, as is evident in Figures 22-4A and 4B, even though they arose almost certainly from a single fertilized ovum.

Tubal pregnancy with death of conceptus without

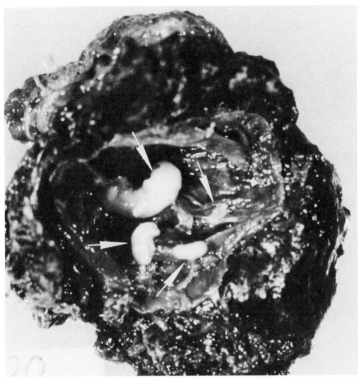

A

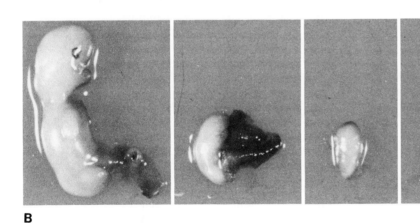

B

Figure 22-4. A. Ruptured, hemorrhaging oviduct containing four embryos (*arrows*), each in a separate amnionic sac, all enclosed by a single chorion. B. The four microscopically proven embryos arising from a single fertilized ovum differ markedly in size. (*From Fujii and associates: Am J Obstet Gynecol 141:840, 1981.*)

abortion or complete resorption may be followed by a tubal pregnancy in the opposite or the same oviduct or in the uterus.

Tubouterine, Tuboabdominal, and Tuboovarian Pregnancies

The so-called tubouterine pregnancy results from the gradual extension into the uterine cavity of products of conception that originally implanted in the interstitial portion of the tube. Tuboabdominal pregnancy is derived from a tubal pregnancy in which the zygote, originally implanted in the neighborhood of the fimbriated extremity, gradually extends into the peritoneal cavity. In such circumstances, the portion of the fetal sac projecting into the peritoneal cavity may form troublesome adhesions to the surrounding organs. As a result, removal of the sac is much more difficult. Both of these conditions are very uncommon.

The term tuboovarian pregnancy is employed when the fetal sac is adherent partly to tubal and partly to ovarian tissue. Such cases arise from the development of the zygote in a tuboovarian cyst or in a tube, the fimbriated extremity of which was adherent to the ovary at the time of fertilization or became so soon thereafter. Rarely, the fetus and placenta may achieve appreciable size before a catastrophe befalls the mother and fetus (Fig. 22-5).

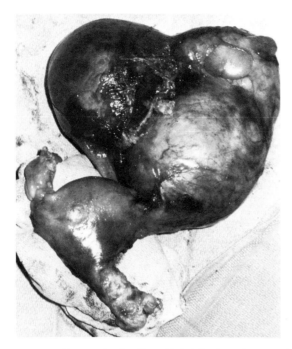

Figure 22-5. The markedly dilated left fallopian tube contains a recently dead fetus weighing 1850 g.

CLINICAL AND LABORATORY FEATURES OF TUBAL PREGNANCY

General Considerations

Before tubal rupture or abortion, the manifestations of a tubal pregnancy are diverse. Commonly, the woman believes she is normally pregnant or believes she is miscarrying an intrauterine pregnancy. Less often, she does not even suspect that she is pregnant. In the so-called textbook case of ruptured tubal pregnancy, normal menstruation is replaced by variably delayed slight vaginal bleeding, which is usually referred to as "spotting." Suddenly, the woman is stricken with severe lower abdominal pain, frequently described as sharp, stabbing, or tearing in character. Vasomotor disturbances develop, ranging from vertigo to syncope. Abdominal palpation discloses some tenderness, and vaginal examination, especially motion of the cervix, causes exquisite pain. The posterior fornix of the vagina may bulge because of blood in the cul-de-sac, or a tender, boggy mass may be felt to one side of the uterus. Symptoms of diaphragmatic irritation, characterized by pain in the neck or shoulder especially on inspiration, develop in perhaps 50 percent of patients in whom there is sizable intraperitoneal hemorrhage. This is caused by intraperitoneal blood reaching and irritating the cervical sensory nerves that supply the inferior surface of the diaphragm, especially on inspiration. The woman may or may not be hypotensive while lying supine. If she is not hypotensive when supine, she may become so when placed in a sitting position.

In cases of tubal pregnancy that present the afore-

mentioned clinical picture, there can be little question as to the diagnosis, but ideally the diagnosis should be made earlier. Even though the symptoms and signs of ectopic pregnancy often range from indefinite to bizarre before rupture or abortion, increasing numbers of women are seeking medical care before the classic clinical picture develops. *The physician must make every reasonable effort to diagnose the condition before catastrophic events occur, but the task may not be simple.* The following symptoms, signs, and laboratory studies must be carefully evaluated.

Pain. Pain may be unilateral or bilateral, in the lower abdomen or generalized, or just in the upper abdomen. In the presence of hemoperitoneum, pain from diaphragmatic irritation may be experienced. It has been generally assumed that the abdominal pain, often excruciating, associated with rupture of an ectopic pregnancy is caused by the escape of blood into the peritoneal cavity. Since there may be considerable pain in instances in which there is little hemorrhage and little pain with considerable hemorrhage, it is obvious that blood is not the sole cause of the pain. Nonetheless, appreciable blood in the peritoneal cavity may lead to a degree of peritoneal irritation and varying degrees of discomfort. Pritchard and Adams (1957) observed that 500 ml of blood in the peritoneal cavity more often than not caused abdominal tenderness, moderate intestinal distention, and especially pain in the top of the shoulder and the side of the neck from diaphragmatic irritation.

Amenorrhea. *The absence of a missed menstrual period by no means rules out tubal pregnancy.* A history of amenorrhea is not obtained in a quarter or more of cases. One reason is that the woman mistakes the uterine bleeding that frequently occurs with tubal pregnancy for a true menstrual period and so gives an erroneous date for the last menses. This important source of diagnostic error can be eliminated in many cases by a carefully obtained menstrual history. It is extremely important that the character of the last menstrual period be investigated in detail in respect to time of onset, duration, and amount of bleeding, and it is advisable to ask whether it impressed her as abnormal in any way.

Vaginal Spotting or Bleeding. As long as placental endocrine function persists, uterine bleeding is usually absent, but when endocrine support of the endometrium becomes inadequate, the uterine mucosa bleeds. The bleeding is usually scanty, dark brown, and may be intermittent or continuous. Although profuse vaginal bleeding is suggestive of an incomplete intrauterine abortion rather than an ectopic gestation, such bleeding can occur with tubal gestations.

Pregnancy Tests. The placenta, in cases of ectopic pregnancy, commonly secretes less chorionic gonatotropin than does the placenta of a normal intrauterine pregnancy of the same gestational age. Therefore, the generally used immunologic tests of limited sensitivity, as well as earlier biologic tests, have been reported as positive in as few as 50 percent of ectopic pregnancies (Hallatt, 1975). Radioimmunoassay for the β-subunit of chorionic gonadotropin is extremely sensitive, as well as specific, for the pregnancy hormone. Lack of availability of the assay and the time to carry out the procedure have deterred its use. In general, the more sensitive the test, the longer the test takes to be completed.

Because of the sensitivity of the assay for the β-subunit of chorionic gonadotropin, pregnancy may, at times, be confirmed so early that no macroscopic pathologic changes can be distinguished in the oviduct. Yaffe and associates (1979) described such a circumstance in which a tubal gestation was not identified at initial laparoscopy. The woman, 5 days overdue for a menstrual period, developed pelvic pain and chorionic gonadotropin was present in serum, but no lesion was seen at laparoscopy. When laparoscopy was repeated 7 days later because of persistent pain and vaginal bleeding, a mass was visible in the ampulla of the tube.

Blood Pressure and Pulse. The early response to moderate hemorrhage is no change in pulse and blood pressure or occasionally the same as that witnessed during the controlled phlebotomy of blood donation, namely, a slight rise in blood pressure (Fig. 21-1), or a vasovagal response with bradycardia and hypotension. In the otherwise healthy young woman with extrauterine pregnancy, only if bleeding continues and hypovolemia becomes intense can the blood pressure be counted upon to fall and the pulse rate to rise appreciably.

Hypovolemia. There are two simple means for detecting significant hypovolemia before development of hypovolemic shock. (1) The blood pressure and pulse rates of the patient in the sitting and the supine positions are compared. A distinct decrease in blood pressure and rise in pulse rate in the sitting position are indicative most often of a sizable decrease in circulatory volume. Unfortunately, such changes may not develop until there is serious hypovolemia. Thus, the test is informative only if the blood pressure falls or pulse rate rises when the patient is moved from the supine to the sitting position. (2) Urine flow is monitored carefully, since hypovolemia (in the absence of potent diuretic treatment) often causes oliguria before overt hypotension develops. The diagnosis and treatment of obstetric hemorrhage in general are considered in detail in Chapter 21, p. 389.

Anemia. After hemorrhage, the depleted blood volume is restored toward normal by hemodilution over the course of 1 or 2 days. Even after a substantial hemorrhage, therefore, the hemoglobin level or hematocrit reading may at first show only a slight reduction. For the first few hours after an acute hemorrhage, a decrease in the hemoglobin or hematocrit level while the patient is under observation is a more valuable index of blood loss than is the initial reading, unless the initial reading is low and the anemia is normocytic and, therefore, characteristic of recent blood loss. If the bleeding stops and the shed erythrocytes are free in the peritoneal cavity, their absorption may help repair the anemia over several days. Hyperbilirubinemia usually does not develop (Pritchard and Adams, 1957).

Pelvic Tenderness. Exquisite tenderness on vaginal examination, especially on *motion of the cervix,* is demonstrable in over three quarters of women with ruptured or rupturing tubal pregnancies but occasionally may be absent. Some degree of abdominal tenderness is present in about the same proportion of cases.

Pelvic Mass. A pelvic mass is palpable in about one half of the patients. The mass varies in size, consistency, and position, ranging as a rule between 5 and 15 cm in diameter, and is often soft and elastic. With extensive infiltration of the tubal wall with blood, however, it may be firm. It is almost always either posterior or lateral to the uterus. Pain and tenderness often preclude identification of the pregnant tube by palpation.

Uterine Changes. Because of the action of placental hormones, the uterus grows during the first 3 months of a tubal gestation to nearly the same size as it would in an intrauterine pregnancy. Its consistency, too, is similar as long as the fetus is alive. The uterus may be pushed to one side by the ectopic mass. In broad ligament pregnancies or when the broad ligament is filled with blood, the uterus may be greatly displaced. Uterine casts (decidual casts) are passed by a small minority of patients, possibly 5 or 10 percent. Their passage may be accompanied by cramps similar to those with spontaneous expulsion of an abortus from the uterine cavity.

Temperature. After acute hemorrhage, the temperature may be normal or even low. Temperatures up to 38°C, and perhaps related to hemoperitoneum, may develop, but higher temperatures are rare in the absence of infection. Fever is important, therefore, in distinguishing ruptured tubal pregnancy from acute salpingitis, in which the temperature is commonly above 38°C.

Leukocyte Count. The leukocyte count varies considerably in ruptured ectopic pregnancy. In about half the patients, it is normal, but in the remainder, varying degrees of leukocytosis up to 30,000 may be encountered.

Pelvic Hematocele. In many cases of ruptured tubal pregnancy, there is gradual disintegration of the tubal wall followed by a slow leakage of blood into the tubal lumen, the peritoneal cavity, or both. Signs of active hemorrhage are absent, and even the mild symptoms may subside, but gradually the trickling blood collects in the pelvis, more or less walled off by adhesions, and a pelvic hematocele results. In some cases, the hematocele is eventually absorbed, and the patient recovers without operation. In others, it may rupture into the peritoneal cavity, or it may become infected and form an abscess. Most commonly, however, the hematocele causes continued discomfort, and the physician is finally consulted weeks or even months after the original rupture. These cases present the most atypical manifestations.

Differential Diagnosis

Prompt diagnosis in ruptured tubal pregnancy is most important, yet there are few other disorders in the field of obstetrics and gynecology that present so many diagnostic pitfalls. The conditions most frequently confused with tubal pregnancy are (1) acute or chronic salpingitis, (2) threatened or incomplete abortion of an intrauterine pregnancy, (3) rupture of a corpus luteum or follicular cyst with intraperitoneal bleeding, (4) torsion of an ovarian cyst, (5) appendicitis, (6) gastroenteritis, and (7) discomfort from an intrauterine device.

Salpingitis. The disease most commonly mistaken for ruptured tubal pregnancy is salpingitis, in which there is often a history of similar attacks with usually no missed period. With salpingitis, abnormal bleeding is not nearly so common as the spotting characteristic of tubal gestation. Pain and tenderness are more likely to be bilateral in salpingitis. A pelvic mass in a tubal pregnancy, if palpable, is unilateral, whereas in salpingitis both fornices are likely to be equally resistant and tender. The temperature in acute salpingitis usually exceeds $38°$ C. In either condition, a negative hormonal test for pregnancy may be obtained with most rapid tests. Thus, a negative result will be of little diagnostic value.

Abortion of Intrauterine Pregnancy. In threatened or incomplete abortion of an intrauterine pregnancy, the uterine bleeding is usually more profuse, and shock from hypovolemia, when present, is usually in proportion to the extent of vaginal hemorrhage. In tubal pregnancy, however, hypovolemic shock is almost always far in excess of what might be expected from vaginal blood loss. The pain in uterine abortion is generally less severe, likely to be rhythmic, and located low in the midline of the abdomen, whereas in tubal pregnancy it is unilateral or generalized. If embryo or placenta is found in the vagina or at the external cervical os, the diagnosis of abortion of an intrauterine pregnancy is obvious. However, it should be remembered that shed decidua may be abundant with an ectopic pregnancy and might, unless carefully examined, be incorrectly considered products from an intrauterine pregnancy that is aborting. Moreover, combined extrauterine and intrauterine pregnancy may occur, albeit rarely. The marked histologic variations in the endometrium in cases of ectopic pregnancy are such that endometrial biopsy provides an often unreliable diagnostic criterion as well as the likelihood of being disruptive if the pregnancy was intrauterine.

Twisted Cyst or Appendicitis. In both torsion of an ovarian cyst and appendicitis, the signs and symptoms of pregnancy, including amenorrhea, are usually lacking and there is rarely a history of abnormal vaginal bleeding. The mass formed by a twisted ovarian cyst is more nearly discrete, whereas that of a tubal pregnancy is usually less well defined. With appendicitis, only rarely is there a mass found by vaginal examination, and pain on motion of the cervix is much less severe than in ruptured tubal pregnancy. The pain from appendicitis, furthermore, is often localized higher, over McBurney's point. If either appendicitis or a twisted ovarian cyst is mistaken for a tubal pregnancy, the error is not costly, since all three require prompt operation. Rupture of a follicular cyst or corpus luteum causing bleeding into the peritoneal cavity may be extremely difficult to distinguish from a ruptured tubal gestation. Identification of chorionic gonadotropin points to a tubal gestation.

Gastrointestinal Disturbance. In some women with a ruptured ectopic pregnancy, the prominent symptoms are diarrhea, nausea, and vomiting, along with abdominal pain. Inappropriate diagnosis and therapy have led to death.

Intrauterine Devices. Diagnosis of ectopic pregnancy is often more difficult in women who use an intrauterine device for contraception. The devices do not prevent ectopic pregnancies. Cramping pelvic pain and bleeding from the uterus, both common features of ectopic pregnancy, may be caused by an intrauterine device. Moreover, in some women the device predisposes to inflammation of the adnexa, which is typically unilateral.

Previous Tubal Sterilization. Such an operation does not absolutely preclude pregnancy. Failure of tubal sterilization results in tubal pregnancy nearly as often as intrauterine pregnancy.

Other Diagnostic Aids

Because of the difficulties in diagnosis of ruptured tubal pregnancy, a variety of diagnostic aids other than tests for chorionic gonadotropin have been utilized. These include culdocentesis, curettage, colpotomy (culdotomy), culdoscopy, laparoscopy, and sonography.

Sonography. In recent years, sonography has been applied to the diagnosis of tubal pregnancy. Identification of early products of conception in the fallopian tube by this means is difficult, but if a gestational sac is clearly identified within the cavity of the uterus, it is very unlikely that an ectopic pregnancy coexists. Moreover, the absence of any sonographic evidence of an intrauterine pregnancy but a positive pregnancy test and an abnormal pelvic mass nearly always is tantamount to ectopic pregnancy. Unfortunately, sonographic findings suggestive, at least, of early intrauterine pregnancy may be apparent in some cases of ectopic pregnancy. The sonographic appearance of a small sac (very early pregnancy) or a collapsed sac (dead products of conception) may actually be a blood clot or decidual cast. Conversely, demonstration of an adnexal or cul-de-sac mass by sonography is not necessarily helpful. Corpus luteum cysts and matted bowel can sometimes look like tubal pregnancies sonographically. However, the identification with real-time sonography of fetal heart action clearly outside the uterine cavity provides firm evidence of an ectopic pregnancy.

Culdocentesis. The simplest technique for identifying hemoperitoneum is culdocentesis, since it can be performed without hospitalization. As the cervix is pulled toward the symphysis with a tenaculum, a long 16- or 18-gauge needle is inserted through the posterior vaginal fornix into the cul-de-sac, whence fluid can be aspirated. Failure to aspirate any fluid can be interpreted only as unsatisfactory entry into the cul-de-sac. Fluid containing fragments of old clots or bloody fluid that does not subsequently clot is compatible with the diagnosis of hemoperitoneum resulting from an ectopic pregnancy. If the blood subsequently clots, it may have been obtained from an adjacent perforated blood vessel rather than from a bleeding ectopic pregnancy. The very important exception to this generalization is brisk bleeding from the site of rupture, in which case the blood may be aspirated from the cul-de-sac before it has had time to clot. With bleeding of such intensity, culdocentesis is rarely necessary to establish the diagnosis of an intra-abdominal catastrophe, one that demands immediate intravenous infusion of fluids, including whole blood, and prompt surgical intervention.

Culdocentesis may be unsatisfactory in women with previous salpingitis and pelvic peritonitis, since the cul-de-sac may have been obliterated.

Curettage. Differentiation between threatened or incomplete abortion of an intrauterine pregnancy and a tubal pregnancy may also be accomplished in many instances by curettage. If embryo, fetus, or placenta is identified, a simultaneous tubal pregnancy is very unlikely. When none of these structures is identified, tubal pregnancy is a probability. The identification of decidua alone in the uterine curettings strongly implies extrauterine pregnancy. Identification of secretory, proliferative, or menstrual-type endometrium, however, does not exclude ectopic gestation.

Colpotomy (Culdotomy). Direct visualization of the oviducts and ovaries can be accomplished by use of colpotomy unless pelvic inflammation, recent or remote, has obliterated the cul-de-sac or the tubes are adherent to the broad ligaments or uterus to a degree that they cannot be mobilized sufficiently to be drawn into the field of vision. The procedure requires an experienced operator, a scrubbed and gowned associate, an operating room, and surgical anesthesia. Salpingectomy may at times be successfully performed through the colpotomy opening. This approach to definitive therapy, while championed by a few, is not generally popular because of technical difficulties, especially if there are adhesions from chronic inflammation, and because of increased morbidity from infection.

Laparoscopy. This technique provides a means of diagnosing disease of the pelvic viscera, including ectopic pregnancy. Refined optic and electronic systems have overcome most of the objections that arose in the course of previous attempts to utilize transabdominal intraperitoneal lighted probes for visualization of organs. Nonetheless, successful and safe laparoscopy demands refined equipment, an experienced operator, an operating room, and, usually, surgical anesthesia. Complete visualization of the pelvis may be impossible in the presence of pelvic inflammation or recent or remote bleeding. At times, identification of an early unruptured tubal pregnancy may be difficult using the laparoscope, even though the tube is fully visualized. The tube may show little change in shape and minimal change in color if the pregnancy is early. Moreover, demonstration of tubal patency by the passage of dye through the tube does not exclude early tubal pregnancy (Yaffe and colleagues, 1976).

Culdoscopy. Visualization of pelvic organs through a culdoscope usually is more difficult than with a laparoscope. Culdoscopy, previously a popular procedure for visualizing the pelvic contents, requires entry through the cul-de-sac, with the patient in the knee-chest position.

Laparotomy. If any doubt remains, laparotomy should be performed, since an unnecessary operation is far less tragic than death contributed to by indecision or delay. There is remarkably little morbidity associated with surgery that is limited to a carefully made and repaired suprapubic incision. At the same time, diagnosis is often enhanced appreciably by the direct visualization and palpation of the pelvic organs that laparotomy allows. *It is imperative that laparotomy not be delayed while laparoscopy or colpotomy is performed on the woman with an obvious pelvic or abdominal catastrophe that requires immediate definitive treatment.*

Mortality

Between 1970 and 1978, the National Center for Health Statistics reported 437 deaths from ectopic pregnancy in the United States. It is somewhat gratifying that deaths per 1000 cases of ectopic pregnancy decreased from 3.5 in 1970 to 0.8 in 1979–1980 (Dorfman, 1983). Nonetheless, ectopic pregnancies still account for about 5 percent of deaths associated with reproduction (Rubin and associates, 1983). In one series of 300 plus cases, maternal mortality was nearly 1 percent (Helvacioglu and associates, 1979).

Treatment

Until recently, the treatment of tubal pregnancy most often has been salpingectomy to remove a shattered, bleeding oviduct with or without ipsilateral oophorectomy. Simultaneous blood transfusion is, of course, a necessity if either hypovolemia or severe anemia is present.

The response of most women to adequate blood replacement and hemostasis is dramatic.

Salpingectomy. In removing the oviduct, it is advisable to excise as a wedge certainly no more than the outer third of the interstitial portion of the tube (so-called cornual resection) in an effort to minimize the rare recurrence of pregnancy in the tubal stump but not weaken the myometrium at that site of excision. Resection so extensive as to reach the cavity of the uterus must be avoided, lest the defect created lead to uterine rupture in a subsequent intrauterine pregnancy.

Since the tubal lesions that predispose to ectopic pregnancy are commonly bilateral, a substantial number of women treated by salpingectomy are likely either to be sterile after one ectopic gestation or to develop another extrauterine pregnancy in the remaining tube. Probably one half or more of women who have had a tubal pregnancy fail to conceive again (Bronson, 1977; Kitchin and co-workers, 1979). When they do, there is a 10 to 15 percent risk of another ectopic pregnancy. Tragically, infertility subsequent to an ectopic pregnancy tends to be highest in nulliparous women.

Conservation of the Oviduct. Because of the strong likelihood of infertility following tubal pregnancy treated by salpingectomy, an alternative to removing the oviduct should be considered. The cumulative experiences in seven reports concerned with 352 women with ectopic pregnancies, on whom procedures to remove the pregnancy but preserve the tube had been performed, were that 119, or one third, subsequently became pregnant in utero. Twenty-one, or 15 percent of those who conceived again, had a repeat ectopic pregnancy (Hallatt, 1975).

One technique for conserving the oviduct involves incising the tube longitudinally over the implantation site, deftly shelling out the pregnancy products, procuring hemostasis at points of active bleeding, and approximating the cut edges with fine suture. With distal tubal implantations, simply squeezing the tube so as to abort the products through the ampulla may suffice. Alternatively, linear salpingostomy can be performed to remove the products of conception from the ampullary portion of the oviduct. Bleeding points are controlled, but the incision of about 2 cm is not closed. DeCherney and associates (1982) have observed successful pregnancies in 6 of 12 women so treated even though the opposite oviduct was missing. Two women had another tubal pregnancy.

Obviously, such procedures do not guarantee patency of the tube. Moreover, subsequent hemorrhage from the implantation site may necessitate reexploration and salpingectomy (Kelly and colleagues, 1979). Nonetheless, for the woman of very low or no parity especially, salpingotomy should be given strong consideration unless the oviduct is obviously destroyed.

Novy (1983) has provided descriptions and illustrations for performing salpingotomy and tuboplasty.

The intense desire of some women to procreate and the willingness of physicians to try to aid them in doing so is evident in a case reported by Kemmann and colleagues (1983). They outlined the obstetric history of one woman in whom the first pregnancy was tubal and was treated by laparotomy and right salpingectomy plus cornual resection. The second pregnancy was tubal and treated by laparotomy and milking the tube to abort the pregnancy from the isthmic-ampullary region. The third pregnancy was tubal and at laparotomy was removed through a linear salpingostomy. The fourth pregnancy was tubal and at laparotomy was removed by midsegment resection followed by tubal anastomosis. The fifth pregnancy terminated with a normal spontaneous delivery of a healthy baby!

Ipsilateral Oophorectomy. Removal of the adjacent ovary at the time of salpingectomy, as demonstrated in Figure 22-6, has been suggested as a possible means for both improving fertility and decreasing the likelihood of a subsequent ectopic pregnancy (Jeffcoate, 1967). Ovulation would thus always occur from the ovary immediately adjacent to the remaining oviduct. This should facilitate the pickup of the ovum by that tube and avoid the possibility of external migration of the ovum and the ectopic pregnancy that might result from such a peripatetic egg. The importance of this phenomenon in the genesis of ectopic pregnancy is not clear, although Hallatt (1975) identified the corpus luteum on the opposite ovary and, therefore, almost certainly, external migration of the ovum, in about 1 of every 5 tubal pregnancies. Even so, removal of an otherwise normal appearing ovary on these grounds seems hardly justifiable. Most gynecologists leave the ovary when possible and, to minimize ovarian dysfunction and cyst formation, preserve all the blood supply possible by clamping the vessels in the mesosalpinx as close to the oviduct as possible.

Sterilization. It is important that before surgical exploration for a suspected ectopic pregnancy the woman be asked about her wishes for future pregnancies. If the woman has a reasonable number of children and the ectopic pregnancy is the consequence of failed contraception, the decision usually is in favor of sterilization. If so, and her condition is good, hysterectomy may be considered. Otherwise, tubal sterilization usually can be performed very quickly without increased risk. Conversely, all organs possible should be conserved in the woman of low parity with a strong desire for future pregnancies in spite of the increased risk that she faces of a subsequent ectopic pregnancy.

Nonsurgical Management. Since some tubal pregnancies either abort or resorb without causing the woman serious debility, some authors have suggested, at least, that suspected early gestations may be simply watched closely to allow those that will terminate benignly to do so, especially those in whom the level of chorionic gonadotropin in urine or plasma appears not to be increasing (Mashiach and associates, 1982). Even methotrexate has been advocated to try to hasten resorption. There is little advantage to most women from such an approach, since methotrexate is extremely toxic, quantitative assays for chorionic gonadotropin are not always precise,

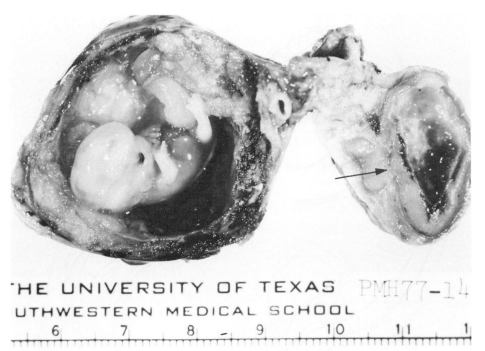

Figure 22-6. Right oviduct containing a fetus and placenta in the ampullary portion, and right ovary with corpus luteum of pregnancy (*arrow*). The woman had experienced vaginal spotting and intermittent dull pain for nearly a month. As she was refusing hospitalization the lower abdominal pain suddenly worsened and she became overtly hypotensive. At emergency laparotomy 1100 ml of free blood and clots were removed from the peritoneal cavity!

and the expanding tubal pregnancy may severely damage the tube so that it becomes unsuitable for successful salpingotomy.

Autotransfusion. In the face of serious blood loss, retransfusion of blood collected from the abdomen has, at times, been advocated. Although this procedure is effective in an emergency, we do not advise it as a routine because of the frequency of adverse reactions. Merrill and associates (1980), however, were enthusiastic in their recommendation of autotransfusion in this circumstance.

Some workers have recommended that free blood be left in the abdomen to benefit the patient. Pritchard and Adams (1957) demonstrated by means of suitably labeled erythrocytes that absorption of erythrocytes from the adult peritoneal cavity occurs over a period of days and is much too slow to be of significant help in combating either hypovolemia or severe anemia. Moreover, free blood in the peritoneal cavity at the completion of surgery makes it difficult to ascertain that hemostasis has been accomplished satisfactorily.

Rh negative Women. If the woman is Rh negative but not yet sensitized to Rh_o (D) antigen and the potential for reproduction persists, Rh_o immune globulin should be administered to protect against isoimmunization. Certainly, whenever Rh positive blood is administered inadvertently to the previously unsensitized Rh negative woman, sufficient immune globulin to protect her should be promptly administered. Moreover, if platelets were transfused, in all likelihood some contaminating Rh positive red cells were also included. Therefore, the Rh (D)

negative should also receive Rh_o (D) immune globulin soon after platelet transfusion.

ABDOMINAL PREGNANCY

Frequency

The incidence of abdominal pregnancy is influenced by the frequency of ectopic gestation in the population being cared for, by the availability of care early in pregnancy, and by the degree of suspicion of ectopic pregnancy exercised by those providing care. Almost all cases of abdominal pregnancy follow early rupture or abortion of a tubal pregnancy into the peritoneal cavity. An incidence for abdominal pregnancy of 1 in 3337 births at Charity Hospital in New Orleans was reported by Beacham and colleagues (1962), compared to 1 in 7931 births at Indiana University Hospital, noted by Strafford and Ragan (1977). At Parkland Memorial Hospital abdominal pregnancy has been an extreme rarity.

Etiology

Typically, the growing placenta, after penetrating the wall of the oviduct, maintains to a degree its tubal attachment but gradually encroaches upon and implants in the neighboring serosa. Meanwhile, the fetus, usually but not always surrounded by amnion, continues to grow within the peritoneal cavity. In such circumstances, the placenta is found in the general region of the oviduct, which eventually loses its identity as such, and over the

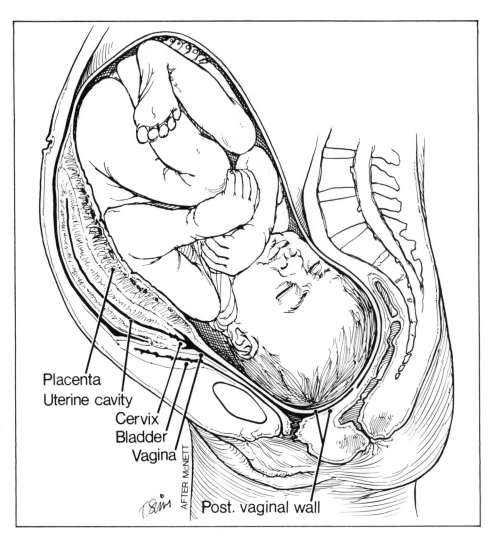

Figure 22-7. Abdominal pregnancy at term. The placenta is implanted on the posterior wall of the uterus and broad ligament. The enlarged, flattened uterus is located just beneath the anterior abdominal wall. The cervix and vagina are dislodged anteriorly and superiorly by the large fetal head in the cul-de-sac.

posterior aspect of the broad ligament and uterus (Fig. 22-7). In rarer instances, the conceptus appears to have escaped from the tube after rupture to reimplant elsewhere in the peritoneal cavity. Primary implantation of the fertilized ovum on the peritoneum is so rare that many authors have doubted its existence. Conclusive proof of a primary abdominal pregnancy, however, was provided by Studdiford's well-documented case (1942), which fulfills the following criteria upon which proof of such a pregnancy must rest: (1) normal tubes and ovaries with no evidence of recent or remote injury, (2) absence of any evidence of uteroplacental fistula, and (3) presence of a pregnancy related exclusively to the peritoneal surface and young enough to eliminate the possibility of secondary implantation following primary nidation in the tube.

King (1932) directed attention to a rare cause of abdominal pregnancy, namely, postoperative separation of the uterine wound of a previous cesarean section. In three of his four reported cases, the ovum had implanted upon omentum, over the uterine defect, whereas in the

fourth it had become attached to the abdominal wall. He believed that in each case the fertilized ovum escaped through the defect in the uterine wall and implanted as a primary abdominal pregnancy.

Status of Fetus

The condition of the fetus in abdominal pregnancy is exceedingly precarious, and consequently the great majority have succumbed. In a review of the world's literature, Ware (1948) cited a perinatal loss of 75.6 percent, but that figure may have been falsely low because of the tendency to report cases with happy results. Beacham and co-workers (1962) reported a perinatal loss in their own series of about 95 percent. Some authors, moreover, report an incidence of congenital malformation in the infants as high as 50 percent, though others disagree.

If the fetus dies after reaching a size too large to be resorbed, it may undergo suppuration, mummification, calcification, or formation of adipocere (see below). Bacteria may gain access to the gestational products, particularly when they are adherent to the intestines, with suppuration of the products. Eventually, the abscess ruptures at the point of least resistance, and if the patient does not soon die of septicemia, fetal parts may be extruded through the abdominal wall or more commonly into the intestines or bladder. Mummification and the formation of a lithopedion occasionally ensue, and the calcified products of conception may be carried for years without producing symptoms until they cause dystocia in a subsequent pregnancy or symptoms from pressure. There are instances in which a period of 20 to 30 years elapsed before removal of a lithopedion at operation or autopsy. Much more rarely, the fetus is converted into a yellowish, greasy mass to which the term *adipocere* is applied. The various bizarre terminations of abdominal pregnancy have been well discussed, with illustrative cases, by King (1954).

Diagnosis

Since early rupture or abortion of a tubal pregnancy is the usual antecedent of an abdominal pregnancy, in retrospect, a history suggestive of the accident can usually be obtained. The abnormalities likely to be recalled include spotting or irregular bleeding and abdominal pain, which usually was most prominent in one or both lower quadrants. Unexplained transient anemia early in pregnancy may accompany the rupture or abortion.

> In the one patient with a late abdominal pregnancy during the past 25 years cared for at Parkland Memorial Hospital throughout most of her pregnancy, anemia was identified when the woman was first evaluated near the end of the first trimester. The moderately severe normochromic, normocytic anemia was accompanied by reticulocytosis and hyperbilirubinemia, most of which was unconjugated. A careful evaluation uncovered no other abnormalities. Treatment of a presumed acquired hemolytic anemia with corticosteroids was followed by prompt correction that persisted after discontinuation of the steroids. She remained asymptomatic until she developed severe preeclampsia at term. A somewhat growth-retarded, recently dead fetus was delivered by laparotomy. The placenta implanted over the posterior surface of the uterus and right broad ligament was removed successfully. Recently, on the medical service in this hospital, similar hematologic changes were identified and attributed for a time to an acquired hemolytic anemia rather than to acute hemorrhage from an ectopic pregnancy, which resulted in hemoperitoneum, red cell destruction, and bone marrow hyperactivity to repair the anemia.

Symptomatology. Women with an abdominal pregnancy are likely to be uncomfortable but not sufficiently so to warrant thorough evaluation. Nausea, vomiting, flatulence, constipation, diarrhea, and abdominal pain may each be present in varying degrees. Multiparas may state that the pregnancy does not "feel right." Late in pregnancy, fetal movements may cause pain. Near term, the empty uterus has been alleged to go into spurious labor.

Physical Examination. By abdominal palpation, the abnormal position of the fetus, often a transverse or oblique lie, can frequently be confirmed. Ease of palpation of the fetal parts, however, is not a reliable sign, since they sometimes feel exceedingly close to the examining fingers in normal intrauterine pregnancies, especially in thin, multiparous women. *Massage of the abdomen over the pregnancy products does not stimulate the mass to become more firm, as it most always does with advanced intrauterine pregnancy.* The cervix is usually displaced (Fig. 22-7), depending in part on the position of the fetus, and it may dilate somewhat, but appreciable effacement is lacking. The uterus may be outlined over the lower part of the pregnancy mass. By palpation of the fornices, small parts or the fetal head clearly outside the uterus may be identified occasionally.

Oxytocin Stimulation. Cross and his collaborators (1951) emphasized that oxytocin could be a valuable aid in the diagnosis of abdominal pregnancy. If no evidence of uterine activity is detected using a sensitive strain gauge applied repeatedly to the maternal abdominal wall over the products of conception while oxytocin is infused intravenously in a sizable dose, the pregnancy almost certainly is extrauterine. Hertz and co-workers (1977) could detect no uterine activity while infusing oxytocin in excess of 50 milliunits per minute. In their case the empty uterus lay inferior and posterior to the fetus. If the uterus were anterior, as in Figure 22-7, it might contract in response to oxytocin and possibly lead to the false conclusion of intrauterine pregnancy.

In a case described by Orr and associates (1979), before the diagnosis of abdominal pregnancy was made, not only did the uterus presumably contract in response to oxytocin but also an oxytocin challenge test was interpreted as negative on two occasions. The growth-retarded fetus, who weighed 2000 g, expired undelivered 1 week later. The relationship between the abdominal wall, the uterus, and the extrauterine fetus was very similar to that depicted in Figure 22-7.

Radiographic Examination. A strong suspicion of abdominal pregnancy may be confirmed by x-ray examination with a probe or radiopaque material in the uterus. The fetus is then clearly shown to lie outside the uterine cavity. Unfortunately, such techniques are not safe diagnostic procedures if the fetus is intrauterine, especially if it is alive.

Isotope Localization. These techniques for localizing the placenta are likely to demonstrate only that the placenta is located in a region that is also appropriate for an intrauterine pregnancy. At times, gross discrepancy has been noted between the apparent location based on isotope studies and the actual implantation site. In one personal case described above, the placenta, on the basis of isotope studies, was reported to be implanted adjacent to the liver but was subsequently removed at laparotomy with difficulty from its implantation in the posterior cul-de-sac.

Sonography. In practice, sonographic findings with an abdominal pregnancy may not be so distinct as to allow an unequivocal diagnosis to be made. However, in some suspected cases, the sonographic findings may serve to identify the pregnancy as being extrauterine. For example, if the fetal head is seen to lie immediately adjacent to the distended maternal bladder with no interposed uterine tissue, a specific diagnosis of an abdominal pregnancy can be made, as in the case described by Kurtz and associates (1982).

Treatment

The operation for abdominal pregnancy may precipitate violent hemorrhage. Without massive blood transfusion, the outlook for many such patients is hopeless. Hence, it is mandatory that at least 2000 ml of compatible blood be on hand in the operating room, with more readily available in the blood bank. Preoperatively, two intravenous infusion systems, each capable of delivering large volumes of fluid at a rapid rate, should be functioning. At the same time, techniques for monitoring the adequacy of the circulation should be employed, as described in Chapter 21. Whenever time allows, the bowel should be prepared using both mechanical cleansing and antimicrobial agents, since the bowel is often intimately adherent to the placenta and membranes.

The massive hemorrhage that often occurs in the course of operations for abdominal pregnancy is related to the lack of constriction of hypertrophied opened blood vessels after placental separation. It has therefore been recommended that operation be deferred until the fetus is dead in anticipation of diminished vascularity to the placental site. However, procrastination may be dangerous and undesirable, since partial separation of the placenta with hemorrhage occasionally occurs spontaneously in the interval of waiting. Moreover, even though the fetus may have been dead several weeks, bleeding may still be torrential. For these reasons, operation is indicated as soon as the diagnosis has been established and the appropriate steps preparative for surgery have been completed.

Management of the Placenta. Since removal of the placenta in abdominal pregnancy always carries the risk of hemorrhage, one should be sure that the blood vessels supplying the placenta can be effectively ligated before attempting removal of the organ. Partial separation can develop spontaneously or, more likely, in the course of the operation from manipulation while attempting to locate the exact site of attachment of the placenta. Since massive hemorrhage can occur, it is, for the most part, best to avoid unnecessary exploration of the surrounding organs. In general, the infant should be delivered, the cord severed close to the placenta, and the abdomen closed.

Unfortunately, the placenta, if left in the abdominal cavity, commonly causes complications in the form of infection, abscesses, adhesions, intestinal obstruction, and wound dehiscence. In one case, evidence of consumptive coagulopathy, including overt hypofibrinogenemia, developed 2 months following laparotomy for delivery of the fetus but leaving the placenta. The coagulation defects cleared spontaneously before the placenta was delivered surgically 3 weeks later. Removal of the placenta in that case was prompted by right ureteral obstruction, which was relieved. *Although the complications of leaving the placenta are troublesome and usually lead to subsequent laparotomy, they may be less grave than the hemorrhage that sometimes results from placental removal during the initial surgery.*

Prognosis

Strafford and Ragan (1977) cite 6 percent maternal mortality and 91 percent perinatal mortality. Two of the 10 cases described more recently by Rahman and associates (1982) proved fatal.

Abdominal pregnancy is still one of the most formidable of obstetric complications. Detection and eradica-

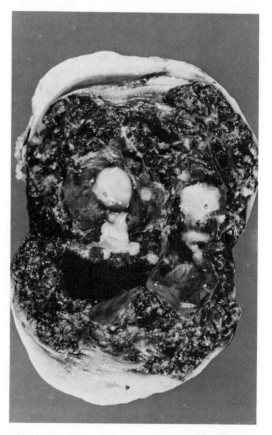

Figure 22-8. Ovarian pregnancy in a woman using an intrauterine device. There are twin embryos, each in a separate gestational sac. (*From Kalfayan and Gunderson: Obstet Gynecol 55:25 [Suppl.] 1980*).

tion of ectopic pregnancies during the first trimester continue to be the most effective means for avoiding these terrible risks!

OVARIAN PREGNANCY

In 1878, Spiegelberg formulated his criteria for diagnosis of ovarian pregnancy. He required that (1) the tube on the affected side be intact, (2) the fetal sac occupy the position of the ovary, (3) the ovary be connected to the uterus by the ovarian ligament, and (4) definite ovarian tissue be found in the sac wall.

Bobrow and Winkelstein (1956) were able to collect 154 cases from the literature and added 1 of their own that satisfied the criteria of Spiegelberg. Hallatt (1982) has described 25 cases of primary ovarian pregnancy, and Grimes and co-workers (1983) have described 24 more. It is not clear whether the use of an intrauterine contraceptive device predisposes to ovarian pregnancy, as in Figure 22-8. Gray and Ruffolo (1978), for example, have described 4 instances of ovarian pregnancy in which the woman conceived with a Cu-7 intrauterine device in situ.

Although the ovary can accommodate itself more readily than the tube to the expanding pregnancy, rupture at an early period is the usual termination. Nonetheless, there are recorded cases in which the ovarian pregnancy went to term, and a few produced infants that survived. For example, Williams and associates (1982), while attempting a cesarean delivery because of a transverse lie at 41 weeks gestation, were surprised to find an ovarian pregnancy. The infant, who weighed nearly 8 pounds, survived. The ovary, placenta, and membranes were resected, and the severed right ureter was reimplanted in the bladder.

The products of conception may degenerate early without rupture and give rise to a tumor of varying size, consisting of a capsule of ovarian tissue enclosing a mass of blood, placental tissue, and possibly membranes. The absence of a distinct decidua leads to direct invasion of the ovarian stroma by the trophoblast (Fig. 22-8).

Signs and Symptoms. The symptoms and physical findings are likely to mimic those of a tubal pregnancy or a bleeding corpus luteum. At the time of operation, early ovarian pregnancies are likely to be considered to be corpus luteum cysts or bleeding corpus luteum.

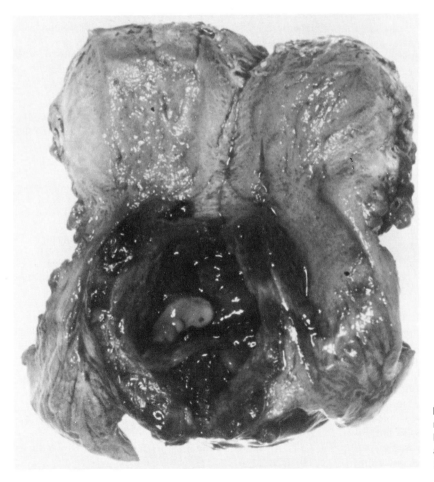

Figure 22-9. Cervical pregnancy in situ removed by hysterectomy nearly 3 months after last normal menstrual period and 1 month after onset of vaginal bleeding. (*Courtesy of Drs. D. Rubell and A. Brekken.*)

Management. Early ovarian pregnancies should be treated, when possible, by wedge resection or cystectomy; otherwise, oophorectomy is performed.

CERVICAL PREGNANCY

Cervical pregnancy is a rare form of ectopic gestation in which the ovum implants within the cervix below the internal os. Dees (1966) has estimated the incidence to be 1 in 18,000 pregnancies. The endocervix is eroded by the trophoblast, and pregnancy proceeds to develop in the fibrous cervical wall, as illustrated in Figure 22-9.

Signs and Symptoms

Usually, painless bleeding appearing shortly after nidation is the first sign. As pregnancy progresses, a distended thin-walled cervix with the external os partially dilated may be evident. Bleeding without pain is the common clinical characteristic. Above the cervical mass, a slightly enlarged uterine fundus may be palpated. Gabbe and co-workers (1975) reported 2 cases of cervical pregnancy with high fever that initially was erroneously attributed to septic intrauterine pregnancy.

Management

Cervical pregnancy rarely goes beyond the 20th week of gestation and is usually terminated surgically because of bleeding. Since attempts at removal of the placenta vaginally may result in profuse hemorrhage and even death of the patient, there should be little hesitation in performing hysterectomy to control the bleeding. Probably only in nulliparas very anxious to maintain fertility should conservative procedures be attempted. Bernstein and associates (1981) have successfully managed 2 cases of early pregnancy implanted in the cervical canal by placing a heavy silk ligature in and around the cervix above the implantation site similar to the McDonald cerclage technique (Chapter 24, p. 475) and then tying it quite snugly. The remaining products of pregnancy were then removed. Hemostasis was achieved, which persisted after removal of the ligature 8 and 10 days later.

OTHER SITES OF ECTOPIC PREGNANCY

A primary *splenic pregnancy* has been vividly described by Mankodi and associates (1977). The symptoms and signs that led to laparotomy included pain in the epigastrium and left shoulder, hypotension, tachycardia, syncope, and tenderness in the vaginal fornices. At laparotomy considerable hemoperitoneum but normal pelvic organs were found. A rent in the hilar surface of the spleen prompted splenectomy. Microscopically, chorionic villi were identified invading otherwise normal splenic tissue at the site of the rent. A few cases of primary hepatic pregnancy have been described, including

one with lithopedion formation (Luwuliza-Kirunda, 1978).

REFERENCES

Arey LB: The cause of tubal pregnancy and tubal twinning. Am J Obstet Gynecol 5:163, 1923

Arias-Stella J: Atypical endometrial changes associated with the presence of chorionic tissue. Arch Pathol 58:112, 1954

Beacham WD, Hernquist WC, Beacham DW, Webster HD: Abdominal pregnancy at Charity Hospital in New Orleans. Am J Obstet Gynecol 84:1257, 1962 (184 references cited)

Bernstein D, Holzinger M, Ovadia J, Frishman B: Conservative treatment of cervical pregnancy. Obstet Gynecol 58:741, 1981

Bobrow ML, Winkelstein LB: Intrafollicular ovarian pregnancy. Am J Surg 91:991, 1956

Bronson RA: Tubal pregnancy and infertility. Fertil Steril 28:221, 1977

Cross JB, Lester WM, McCain J: The diagnosis and management of abdominal pregnancy with a review of 19 cases. Am J Obstet Gynecol 62:303, 1951

DeCherney AH, Maheaux R, Naftolin F: Salpingostomy for ectopic pregnancy in the sole patent oviduct: Reproductive outcome. Fertil Steril 37:619, 1982

Dees HC: Cervical pregnancy associated with uterine leiomyomas. South Med J 59:900, 1966

Dorfman SF: Deaths from ectopic pregnancy, United States 1979 to 1980. Obstet Gynecol 62:344, 1983

Funderburk AG: Bilateral ectopic pregnancy with simultaneous intrauterine pregnancy. Am J Obstet Gynecol 119:274, 1974

Fujii S, Ban C, Okamura H, Nishimura T: Unilateral tubal quadruplet pregnancy. Am J Obstet Gynecol 141:840, 1981

Gabbe SG, Kitzmiller JL, Kosasa TS, Driscoll SG: Cervical pregnancy presenting as septic abortion. Am J Obstet Gynecol 123:212, 1975

Gray CL, Ruffolo EH: Ovarian pregnancy associated with intrauterine contraceptive devices. Am J Obstet Gynecol 132:134, 1978

Grimes HG, Nosal RA, Gallagher JC: Ovarian pregnancy: A series of 24 cases. Obstet Gynecol 61:174, 1983

Hallatt JG: Repeat ectopic pregnancy: A study of 123 consecutive cases. Am J Obstet Gynecol 122:520, 1975

Hallatt JG: Primary ovarian pregnancy: A report of twenty-five cases. Am J Obstet Gynecol 143:55, 1982

Helvacioglu A, Long EM Jr, Yang S-L: Ectopic pregnancy. An eight-year review. J Reprod Med 22:87, 1979

Hertz RH, Timor-Tritch I, Sokol RJ, Zador I: Diagnostic studies and fetal assessment in advanced extrauterine pregnancy. Obstet Gynecol 50:63 [Suppl], 1977

Jeffcoate TNA: Principles of Gynaecology, 3rd ed. New York, Appleton-Century-Crofts, 1967

Kelly RW, Martin SA, Strickler RC: Delayed hemorrhage in conservative surgery for ectopic pregnancy. Am J Obstet 133:225, 1979

Kemmann E, Grochmal SA, Harrigan JT: Term uterine pregnancy after four successive tubal pregnancies. JAMA 250:2673, 1983

King EL: Postoperative separation of the cesarean section wound, with subsequent abdominal pregnancy. Am J Obstet Gynecol 24:421, 1932

King G: Advanced extrauterine pregnancy. Am J Obstet Gynecol 67:712, 1954

Kitchin JD III, Wein RM, Nunley WC Jr, Thaigarajah S, Thornton WN Jr: Ectopic pregnancy: Current clinical trends. Am J Obstet Gynecol 134:870, 1979

Kurtz AB, Dubbins PA, Wapner RJ, Goldberg BB: Problem of abnormal fetal position. JAMA 247:3251, 1982

Luwuliza-Kirunda JMM: Primary hepatic pregnancy. Br J Obstet Gynaecol 85:311, 1978

Mankodi RC, Sankari K, Bhatt SM: Primary splenic pregnancy. Br J Obstet Gynaecol 84:634, 1977

Mashiach S, Carp JHA, Serr DM: Nonoperative management of ectopic pregnancy. A preliminary report. J Reprod Med 27:127, 1982

Merrill BS, Mitts DL, Rogers W, Weinberg PC: Autotransfusion. Intraoperative use in ruptured ectopic pregnancy. J Reprod Med 24:14, 1980

Niebyl JR: Pregnancy following total hysterectomy. Am J Obstet Gynecol 119:512, 1974

Novy MJ: Surgical alterations for ectopics: Is conservative treatment best? Contemp Ob/Gyn 21:91, 1983

Orr JW Jr, Huddleston JF, Knox GE, Goldenberg RL, Davis RO: False negative oxytocin challenge test associated with abdominal pregnancy. Am J Obstet Gynecol 133:108, 1979

Pritchard JA, Adams RH: The fate of blood in the peritoneal cavity. Surg Gynecol Obstet 105:621, 1957

Rahman MS, Al-Suleiman SA, Rahman J, Al-Sibai MH: Advanced abdominal pregnancy—observations in 10 cases. Obstet Gynecol 59:366, 1982

Reece EA, Petrie RH, Sirmans MF, Finster M, Todd WD: Combined intrauterine and extrauterine gestations: A review. Am J Obstet Gynecol 146:323, 1983

Romney SL, Hertig AT, Reid DE: The endometria associated with ectopic pregnancy. Surg Gynecol Obstet 91:605, 1950

Rubin GL, Peterson HB, Dorfman SF, Layde PM, Maze JM, Ory HW, Cates W Jr: Ectopic pregnancy in the United States: 1970 through 1978. JAMA 249:1725, 1983

Spiegelberg O: Casuistry in ovarian pregnancy. Arch Gynaekol 13:73, 1878

Strafford JC, Ragan WD: Abdominal pregnancy: Review of current management. Obstet Gynecol 50:548, 1977

Studdiford WD: Primary peritoneal pregnancy. Am J Obstet Gynecol 44:487, 1942

Ware HH: Observations on thirteen cases of late extrauterine pregnancy. Am J Obstet Gynecol 55:561, 1948

Williams PC, Malvar TC, Kraft JR: Term ovarian pregnancy with delivery of a live female infant. Am J Obstet Gynecol 142:589, 1982

Yaffe H, Navot D, Laufer N: Pitfalls in early detection of ectopic pregnancy. Lancet 1:277, 1979

Yaffe H, Sadovsky E, Beyth Y: Tubal pregnancy and tubal patency. Int J Gynaecol Obstet 14:265, 1976

23

Diseases and Abnormalities of the Placenta and Fetal Membranes

ABNORMALITIES OF PLACENTATION

Multiple Placentas with a Single Fetus

Occasionally, the placenta may be separated into lobes, most frequently two. When the division is incomplete and the vessels of fetal origin extend from one lobe to the other before uniting to form the umbilical cord, the condition is termed *placenta bipartita* or bilobed placenta (Figs. 23-1, Fig. 23-4C). The reported incidence of this placental anomaly varies widely, but in the experience of Fox (1978) it occurs in about 1 of 350 deliveries. If the two lobes are entirely separated and the vessels remain distinct, not uniting until just before entering the cord, the condition is designated *placenta duplex*. Sometimes both features are present. Occasionally, the organ may comprise three distinct lobes (*placenta triplex*). Rarely, more than three lobes are present.

Succenturiate Placenta

An important anomaly is the so-called *placenta succenturiata,* in which one or more small accessory lobes are developed in the membranes at a distance from the periphery of the main placenta, to which they ususally have vascular connection of fetal origin (Figs. 6-15, 6-16). Such an accessory lobe is of considerable clinical importance because it is sometimes retained in the uterus after expulsion of the main placenta and, when it separates subsequently, may give rise to serious maternal hemorrhage. If, on examination of the placenta, defects in the membranes are noted a short distance from the placental margin, retention of a succenturiate lobe should be suspected. The suspicion is confirmed if vessels extend from the placenta to the margins of the tear. In such cases, even if there is no hemorrhage at the moment, the retained lobe should be removed manually. The incidence of an accessory lobe is approximately 3 percent.

Ring-shaped Placenta

This is a very rare anomaly that occurs in less than 1 of 6000 deliveries. The placenta is annular in shape, and sometimes a complete ring of placental tissue is present,

but more commonly, because of atrophy of a portion of the tissue of the ring, a horseshoe shape is present. This placental abnormality appears to be associated with a greater likelihood of ante- and postpartum bleeding and fetal growth retardation. Fox (1978) considers this anomaly to be a variant of membranaceous placenta.

Membranaceous Placenta

In rare circumstances, all of the fetal membranes are covered by functioning villi, and the placenta develops as a thin membranous structure occupying the entire periphery of the chorion. This abnormality does not appear to interfere with nutrition of the fetus but occasionally gives rise to serious hemorrhage. Bleeding resembles that seen in central placenta previa, increasing in severity to necessitate interruption of the pregnancy by cesarean section, possibly followed by hysterectomy to control bleeding from the large area of implantation. During the third stage of labor, the placenta may not readily separate from its area of attachment. Manual removal is sometimes very difficult in such cases. Placenta membranacea is sometimes referred to as *placenta diffusa*. An interesting example has been described by Las Heras and associates (1982).

Fenestrated Placenta

This is a rare anomaly of the placenta in which the central portion of a discoidal placenta is missing. In some instances, there is an actual hole in the placenta, but more often the defect involves villous tissue only, the chorionic plate being present. The clinical significance of this anomaly is that the abnormality may be mistakenly considered to represent a missing portion that has been retained in the uterus.

Extrachorial Placenta

In these conditions, the chorionic plate, which is on the fetal side of the placenta, is smaller than the basal plate, which is located on the maternal side. If the fetal surface of such a placenta presents a central depression surrounded by a thickened, grayish white ring, which is sit-

441

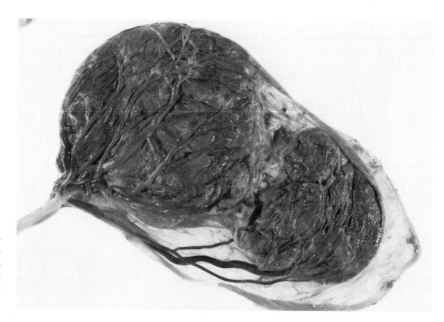

Figure 23-1. Placenta demonstrating bilobed structure, marginal insertion of umbilical cord, and partial velamentous insertion of cord (fetal vessels traversing membranes to reach smaller placental lobe on right).

uated at a varying distance from the margin of the organ, the placenta is classed as a *circumvallate placenta*. When the ring coincides with the placental margin, the condition is sometimes described as a *marginate* or *circummarginate placenta*. Within the ring, the fetal surface presents the usual appearance, gives attachment to the umbilical cord, and shows the usual large vessels, which instead of coursing over the entire fetal surface terminate abruptly at the margin of the ring. In a cir-

cumvallate placenta, the ring is composed of a double fold of amnion and chorion with degenerated decidua and fibrin in between. In a marginate placenta, the chorion and amnion are raised at the margin by interposed decidua and fibrin, without folding of the membranes. These relations are illustrated in Figure 23-2. The cause of circumvallate and circummarginate placentation is not understood. Antepartum hemorrhage, prematurity, perinatal deaths, and fetal malformations have

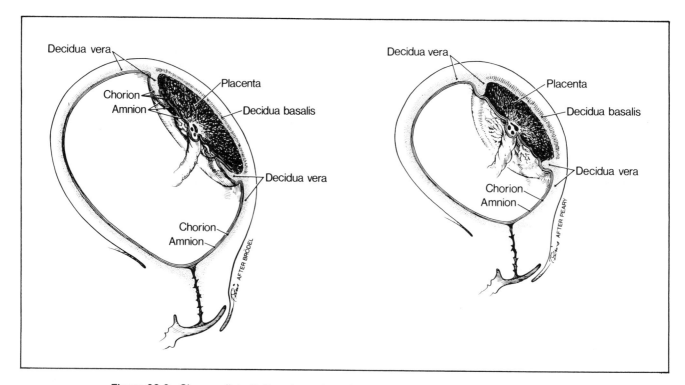

Figure 23-2. Circumvallate (*left*) and marginate (*right*) varieties of extrachorial placentas.

been reported to be increased for pregnancies with circumvallate placentas (Benirschke, 1974; Lademacher and co-workers, 1981).

Large Placentas

While the normal term placenta weighs on the average about 500 g, in certain diseases, such as syphilis, the placenta may weigh one fourth, one third, or even one half as much as the fetus. The largest placentas are usually encountered in cases of erythroblastosis fetalis, as demonstrated in Figure 38-5.

Placental Polyp

Occasionally, parts of a normal placenta or a succenturiate lobe may be retained after delivery. These may form polyps consisting of villi in varying stages of degeneration and covered by regenerated endometrium. The clinical sequelae are often subinvolution of the uterus and late postpartum hemorrhage (Chapter 36, p. 737).

CIRCULATORY DISTURBANCES

Infarcts

The most common lesions of the placenta, though of diverse origin, are referred to collectively as placental infarcts. The principal histopathologic features include fibrinoid degeneration of the trophoblast, calcification, and ischemic infarction from occlusion of spiral arteries.

Overclassification of placental infarcts has led to unnecessary confusion. Minute subchorionic and marginal foci of degeneration are present in every placenta. These lesions are of clinical significance only when they are abundant, in which case they may interfere with the function of a sufficiently large portion of the placenta to hamper seriously the nutrition of the fetus and on occasion cause fetal death. In simplest terms, degenerative lesions of the placenta have two etiologic factors in common: (1) changes associated with aging of the trophoblast and (2) impairment of the uteroplacental circulation causing infarction. Nutrition of the placental villi is derived more from the maternal than from the fetal circulation.

Although the placenta is by no means a dying organ at term (Chapter 6, p. 99), there are morphologic indications of aging. During the latter half of pregnancy, syncytial degeneration begins and syncytial knots are formed. At the same time, the villous stroma usually undergoes hyalinization. The syncytium may then break away and float off, exposing the connective tissue directly to maternal blood. As a result, clotting occurs, and propagation of the clot may result in the incorporation of other villi. Macroscopically, such a focus resembles closely an ordinary blood clot, but if it is not seen until it has become thoroughly organized, on section a firm, white island of tissue is revealed.

About the edge of nearly every term placenta there is a more or less dense, yellowish white, fibrous ring representing a zone of degeneration and necrosis, which is usually termed a *marginal infarct*. It may be quite superficial in places, but occasionally it extends 1 or 2 cm into the substance of the placenta. Underneath the chorionic plate, there are nearly always similar lesions, of more or less pyramidal shape, ranging from 0.2 cm to 2 or even 3 cm across the base, and extending downward with their apices in the intervillous space (subchorionic infarcts). Similar lesions are noted about the intercotyledonary septa, in which case the broadest portion rests upon the maternal surface and the apex points toward the chorionic plate. Occasionally, these lesions meet and form a column of cartilagelike material extending from the maternal surface to the fetal surface. Less frequently, round or oval islands of similar tissue occupy the central portions of the placenta (Fig. 23-3A, B).

The reported frequencies of placental infarction differ greatly for both normal and abnormal pregnancies. Fox (1978) has found that about one fourth of placentas from uncomplicated term pregnancies will demonstrate infarcts. In pregnancies complicated by hypertension, the frequency and size of infarcts are increased. In his experience, placentas in pregnancies complicated by severe hypertensive disease can be anticipated to be infarcted in about two thirds of cases.

Calcification of the Placenta. Small calcareous nodules or plaques are observed frequently upon the maternal surface of the placenta and are occasionally so abundant that the organ feels like coarse sandpaper. In view of the widespread degenerative changes in the term placenta, calcification is not surprising. In fact, the conditions for deposition of calcium in the aging placenta are almost ideal. Moderate degrees of calcification may be detected in at least half of all placentas examined roentgenographically. An extensive deposition of calcium is shown in Figure 23-4A, B, C. Tindall and Scott (1965), in a study of the placentas of 3025 pregnancies, concluded that calcification of the placenta is a normal process, with the amount of calcium deposited increasing in amount throughout the third trimester. Calcification of the placentas may be identified in vivo using sonography (Spirit and associates, 1982).

Clinical Significance of Degenerative Changes in the Placenta

In general, infarcts of the placenta, caused either by local deposition of fibrin or by the more acute process of intervillous thrombosis, have little clinical significance, probably because of a relatively large margin of safety for most placental functions. Nonetheless, in certain maternal diseases, notably severe hypertension, the reduction in functioning placenta through infarction, especially when coupled with reduced blood flow to the uterus, may be sufficient to cause fetal death.

Villous (fetal) vessels may show endarteritic thick-

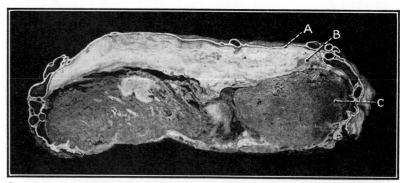

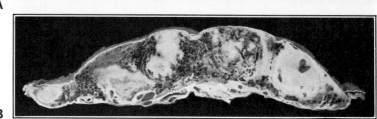

Figure 23-3. A. Placental infarcts. A, amnion and chorionic membrane. B, fibrin deposited locally beneath the chorion. C, unchanged placental tissue. (In this instance, the infarct was unusually extensive, most likely contributing to the death of the fetus.) B. Generalized fibrin deposition with little normal tissue remaining.

ening and obliteration in association with fetal death. When the placental villi are excluded from their supply of maternal blood by fibrin deposits, hematomas, or direct blockage of the decidual circulation, they necessarily become infarcted and die. Histologically, the compromised villi are characterized by fibrosis, obliteration of fetal vessels, and gradual disappearance of the syncytium.

Villous (Fetal) Arterial Thrombosis. Thrombosis of a fetal villous stem artery produces a sharply demarcated area of avascularity (Fig. 23-5). Fox (1978) found a single arterial thrombosis in 4.5 percent of placentas from normal pregnancies and in 10 percent of placentas of pregnancies involving diabetic women. He has estimated that thrombosis of a single fetal stem artery will deprive only 5 percent of the villi of their blood supply. However, he

also has observed a few placentas from fresh stillbirths in which 40 to 50 percent of the villi were deprived of their fetal blood supply.

Hypertrophic Lesions of the Chorionic Villi

Striking enlargement of the chorionic villi is seen commonly in association with erythroblastosis of the hydropic variety. It has also been described in diabetes and occasionally in severe fetal congestive heart failure.

Inflammation of the Placenta

Changes that are now recognized as various forms of degeneration and necrosis were formerly described under the term "placentitis." For example, small placental cysts with grumous contents were formerly thought to

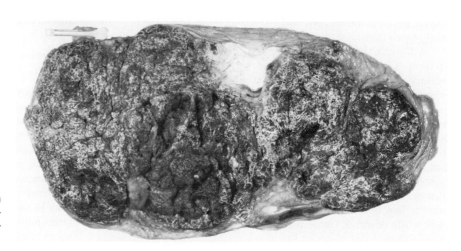

Figure 23-4. A. Placental calcification is evident as gray plaques on the maternal surface of the placenta, a common finding at term.

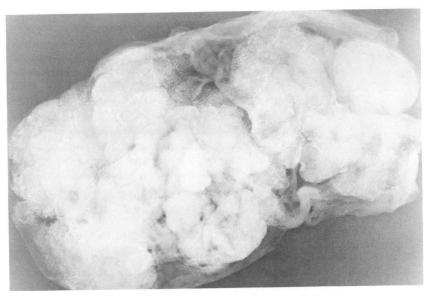

B

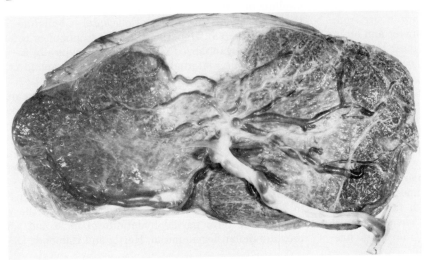

C

Figure 23-4. B. A roentgenogram of the same placenta emphasizing the extensive calcification. **C.** The fetal surface of this same calcified placenta demonstrates partial division and tendency toward the formation of two lobes, with some of the fetal vessels traversing the membranes. The placenta was firmly implanted on a considerably thinned-out preexisting vertical cesarean scar, which may account for the tendency toward a bilobed placenta. The newborn infant was healthy.

be abscesses. Nonetheless, especially in cases of prolonged rupture of the membranes, pyogenic bacteria do invade the fetal surface of the placenta and, after gaining access to the chorionic vessels, give rise to general infection of the fetus.

NEOPLASTIC TROPHOBLASTIC DISEASES

There are three general categories of neoplastic trophoblastic disease:

1. *Hydatidiform mole.* Hydatidiform moles are characterized by abnormalities of the chorionic villi consisting of varying degrees of proliferation of trophoblast and edema of the villous stroma.

Hydatidiform moles are subdivided into complete and incomplete, or partial, varieties.

2. *Invasive mole.* At times the villi, with their proliferating neoplastic covering, invade the uterus and adjacent structures or metastasize to distant organs or both. Invasion or metastasis by such villi characterizes an invasive mole. An invasive mole was formerly referred to as *chorioadenoma destruens.*

3. *Choriocarcinoma.* Neoplastic trophoblast without stroma may spread locally or disseminate far beyond the original site of zygote implantation and proliferate profusely to cause death from extensive organ destruction and hemorrhage. Such behavior by trophoblast is called choriocarcinoma. It was formerly called *chorionepithelioma.*

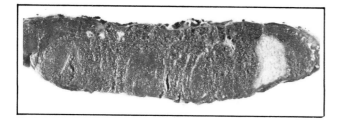

Figure 23-5. A localized area of pallor in a placenta that is due to fetal arterial thrombosis. (*From Fox: Pathology of the Placenta. Philadelphia, Saunders, 1978, Volume 7, page 131.*)

HYDATIDIFORM MOLES

Hydatidiform moles usually occupy the uterine cavity. However, they may rarely be located in the oviduct and even the ovary (Stanhope and associates, 1983).

Complete Hydatidiform Mole

The chorionic villi are converted into a mass of clear vesicles (Fig. 23-6, 23-12). The vesicles vary in size from barely visible to a few centimeters in diameter and often hang in clusters from thin pedicles. The mass may grow large enough to fill the uterus to the size occupied by an advanced normal pregnancy.

The histologic structure demonstrated in Figure 23-7 is characterized by (1) hydropic degeneration and swelling of the villous stroma, (2) absence of blood vessels in the swollen villi, (3) proliferation of the trophoblastic epithelium to a varying degree, and (4) absence of fetus and amnion.

Cytogenetic studies of complete molar pregnancies have identified the chromosomal composition most often, but not always, to be 46,XX with the chromosomes completely of paternal origin. This phenomenon is referred to as *androgenesis*. Typically, the ovum has

been fertilized by a haploid sperm, which then duplicates its own chromosomes after meiosis. The original chromosomes of the ovum are either absent or inactivated. However, not all complete hydatidiform moles are characterized by this chromosomal pattern. Infrequently, in a complete mole the chromosomal pattern may be 46,XY (Bagshawe and Lawler, 1982; Davis and associates, 1984). In this circumstance, two sperm have fertilized an ovum lacking chromosomes. Other variations have also been described, for example, 45,X. Thus, a morphologically complete hydatidiform mole can demonstrate a variety of chromosomal patterns. The trophoblast of a complete hydatidiform mole has a propensity to become malignant, i.e., to become a choriocarcinoma, as described subsequently.

Partial (Incomplete) Hydatidiform Mole

When the hydatidiform changes are focal and less advanced, and there is a fetus or at least an amnionic sac, the condition has been classified as a partial hydatidiform mole. There is slowly progressing hydatidiform swelling of some avascular villi, while other vascular villi that participate in the fetal-placental circulation are spared (Fig. 23-8). Hyperplasia of the trophoblast is focal rather than generalized. The karyotype typically is triploid, with one maternal but two paternal haploid complements (Jacobs and co-workers, 1982).

The risk of choriocarcinoma arising from a partial hydatidiform mole is slight. Szulman and co-workers (1981) reported a partial mole with demonstrated triploidy that was treated with chemotherapy because of persistence of chorionic gonadotropin after evacuating the partial mole, but such case reports have been rare.

Molar Degeneration. Difference of opinion remains as to when gross or histologic hydatid changes in the villi warrant the term partial hydatidiform mole and when they are molar degeneration. Hertig and Edmonds (1940)

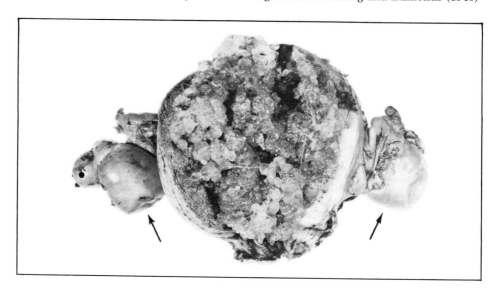

Figure 23-6. A complete hydatidiform mole characterized grossly by abundance of edematous enlarged chorionic villi but no fetus or fetal membranes. Note thecalutein cysts in each ovary (*arrows*).

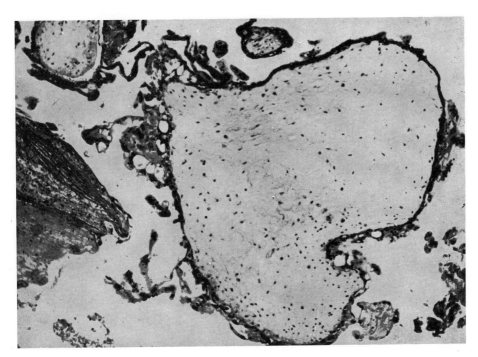

Figure 23-7. Example of hydatidiform mole with slight to moderate trophoblastic hyperplasia, confined to the syncytium and considered as probably benign. (*From Smalbraak: Trophoblastic Growths. Haarlem, Netherlands, Elsevier, 1957.*)

found that in two thirds of the aborted pathologic ova studied by them, there was early molar degeneration, i.e., moderate hydropic swelling of some villi without appreciable trophoblastic proliferation.

Histologic Diagnosis

Attempts to relate the histologic structure of individual hydatidiform moles that meet the criteria for complete moles to their subsequent malignant tendencies generally have been disappointing. Novak and Seah (1954), for example, were unable to establish precisely such a relation in 120 cases of hydatidiform mole or in the trophoblast-containing tissue submitted to them in 26 cases of choriocarcinoma following hydatidiform mole.

Ovarian Theca-Lutein Cysts

In many cases of hydatidiform mole, the ovaries contain multiple theca-lutein cysts (Fig. 23-6), which may vary from microscopic size to 10 cm and more in diameter. The surfaces of the cysts are smooth, often yellowish, and lined with lutein cells. The incidence of obvious cysts in association with a mole is reported to be from 25 percent to as high as 60 percent.

Lutein cysts of the ovaries are thought to result from overstimulation of lutein elements by large amounts of chorionic gonadotropin secreted by the proliferating trophoblasts. In general, extensive cystic change is usually associated with larger hydatidiform moles and a long period of stimulation. Lutein cysts are not limited to cases of hydatidiform mole. They may be associated with placental hypertrophy with fetal hydrops and with multifetal pregnancy.

Very large cysts especially may undergo torsion, infarction, and hemorrhage. However, oophorectomy should not be performed because of theca-lutein cysts alone. After delivery of the mole, the cysts eventually regress and disappear. At times, after evacuation of a mole, paradoxically, the cystic ovaries enlarge before they regress.

Incidence

Hydatidiform mole occurs approximately once in about 1500 to 2000 pregnancies in the United States and Europe but is much more frequent in some other parts of the world, especially in parts of Asia, where the frequency is at least 10 times that of the United States. A surprisingly high incidence has also been identified in Mexico and among native Alaskans.

Age. Age has an important bearing on the incidence of hydatidiform mole, as indicated by the relatively high frequency among pregnancies toward the end of the childbearing period. The most pronounced effect of age is seen in women older than 45, when the relative frequency of the lesion is more than 10 times greater than at ages 20 to 40. There are numerous authenticated cases of hydatidiform mole in women 50 years old and older, whereas normal pregnancy at such advanced ages is practically unknown (Jequier and Winterton, 1973).

Previous Mole. Recurrence of hydatidiform mole is uncommon but is seen in about 2 percent of cases. Wu (1973) described a case of nine consecutive molar pregnancies!

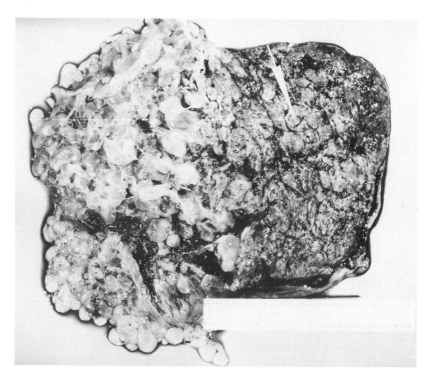

Figure 23-8. Molar placenta on the left and normal placenta (*white arrow*) on the right. The molar placenta was identified by sonography late in pregnancy when the mother developed preeclampsia. A healthy fetus was delivered near term by cesarean section. Most likely, this is a case of twins consisting of a placenta with a fetus from one ovum and a complete mole developing from the other ovum.

Clinical Course

In the very early stages of development of a mole, there are few characteristics to distinguish it from normal pregnancy, but later in the first trimester and during the second trimester the following noteworthy changes are often evident.

Bleeding. Uterine bleeding is the outstanding sign and may vary from spotting to profuse hemorrhage. It may occur just before abortion, or, more often, it occurs intermittently for weeks or even months. As the consequence of such bleeding, anemia is rather common. Moreover, a dilutional effect from appreciable hypervolemia has been demonstrated in some women with larger hydatidiform moles. At times, there may be considerable hemorrhage concealed within the uterus. Iron deficiency anemia is a common finding, and infrequently megaloblastic erythropoiesis is evident, presumably due to poor dietary intake as the consequence of nausea and vomiting, coupled with increased folate requirement imposed by rapidly proliferating trophoblast.

Uterine Size. The growing uterus often enlarges more rapidly than usual, the size clearly exceeding that expected from the duration of gestation in about one half of cases. Uterine size may be difficult to identify precisely by palpation in the nulliparous woman especially, because of the soft consistency of the uterus beneath a firm abdominal wall. At times, ovaries appreciably enlarged by multiple lutein cysts may be difficult to distinguish from the enlarged uterus. The ovaries are likely to be tender to palpation.

Fetal Activity. Even though the uterus is enlarged sufficiently to reach well above the symphysis, typically no fetal heart action can be detected even with sensitive instruments. Rarely, there may be twin placentas with a complete hydatidiform mole developing in one, while the other placenta and its fetus appear normal (Fig. 23-8). Very infrequently, there may be extensive but incomplete molar change in the placenta accompanied by a living fetus (Fig. 23-9). Six cases of a fetus with either an incomplete hydatidiform mole for a placenta or with a normal placenta plus a complete twin hydatidiform mole have been described by Block and Merrill (1982).

Pregnancy-induced Hypertension. Of special importance is the frequent association of pregnancy-induced hypertension with molar pregnancies that persist into the second trimester. Since the syndrome of pregnancy-induced hypertension is rarely seen before 24 weeks of gestation except in this circumstance, hypertension that develops before 24 weeks strongly suggests hydatidiform mole or extensive molar change.

Embolization. Variable amounts of trophoblast with or without villous stroma escape from the uterus in the venous outflow. Especially at the time of spontaneous expulsion or therapeutic evaluation of the large mole, the volume embolized may be sufficient to produce signs and symptoms of acute pulmonary embolism and even a fatal outcome (Fig. 23-10). Such fatalities are rare.

Much more often trophoblast with or without villous stroma will embolize to the lungs in volumes too small to produce overt blockade of the pulmonary vasculature, but subsequently they invade the pulmonary

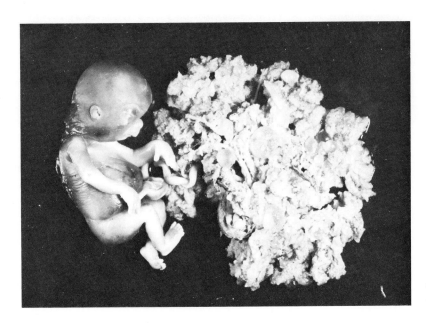

Figure 23-9. Extensive molar change and a fetus of 20 weeks gestation. The pregnancy was complicated further by eclampsia.

parenchyma to establish metastases that are evident roentgenographically. The lesions may consist of trophoblast alone (metastatic choriocarcinoma) or trophoblast with villous stroma (metastatic invasive mole). The subsequent course of such lesions is unpredictable. Some pulmonary lesions have been observed to disappear spontaneously either soon after evacuation of the uterus or even weeks to months later, while others proliferate and kill the woman unless she is effectively treated.

Disturbed Thyroid Function. Plasma thyroxine levels may be elevated appreciably, but clinically apparent hyperthyroidism is uncommon. Curry and associates (1975) identified hyperthyroidism in 2 percent of cases.

The elevation in plasma thyroxine concentration in cases of hydatidiform mole may be the effect primarily of estrogen, as in normal pregnancy, in which case free thyroxine levels are not elevated and the percentage of triiodothyronine bound by resin (T_3 uptake) is increased. Free thyroxine can become elevated as the consequence of the thyroid-stimulating effect of chorionic gonadotropin in high concentration and less likely from a thyroid-stimulating hormone produced by trophoblast.

Spontaneous Expulsion. Occasionally, hydatid vesicles, or grapes, are passed before the mole is aborted spontaneously or removed by operation. Spontaneous expulsion is most likely to occur around the fourth month and is rarely delayed beyond the seventh month.

Diagnostic Features

Persistent bleeding and a uterus larger than the expected size arouse suspicion of a mole (Fig. 23-11A, B). Consideration must be given to an error in menstrual data or a pregnant uterus enlarged by myomas, hydramnios, or multiple fetuses.

Sonography. The greatest diagnostic accuracy can be obtained from the characteristic ultrasonography of hydatidiform mole (Fig. 23-12A, B). The safety and precision of sonography make it the technique of choice. However, it must be kept in mind that some other structures may yield a sonogram similar to that of a hydatidiform mole, including a uterine myoma with early pregnancy and pregnancies with multiple fetuses. A careful review of the history, coupled with careful ultra-

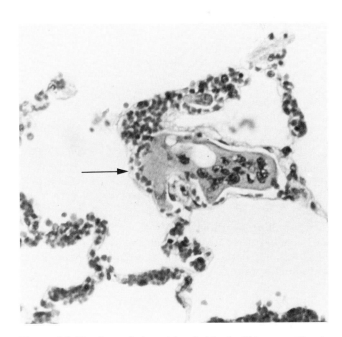

Figure 23-10. An embolus of trophoblast within a small pulmonary vein (*arrow*). The woman died from embolization of trophoblast and massive hemorrhage soon after abdominal hysterotomy was performed to evacuate a large hydatidiform mole.

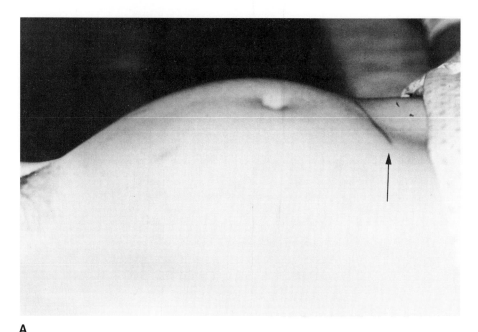

A

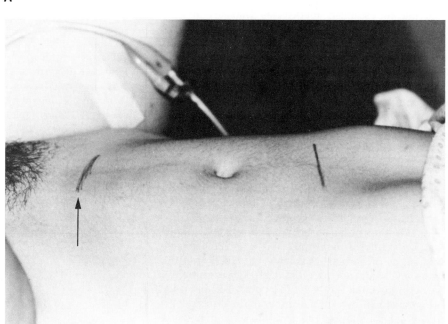

B

Figure 23-11. A. The uterine fundus (*arrow*) rises 27 cm above the symphysis in a woman with a complete hydatidiform mole 17 weeks after her last menstrual period. The hydatidiform mole causing the uterine enlargement is identified sonographically in Figures 23-12A and B. **B.** The uterine fundus (*arrow*) has decreased markedly immediately after evacuating the large hydatidiform mole by suction. Actual removal of the molar tissue is demonstrated in Figure 23-13A and B.

sonic scanning repeated in a week or two when necessary, should serve to avoid the incorrect sonographic diagnosis of hydatidiform mole when pregnancy products are actually normal.

Amniogram

Transabdominal intrauterine installation of a radiopaque substance, such as Hypaque, produces a characteristic roentgenogram in cases of hydatidiform mole. The woman is prepared and the uterine cavity is penetrated with the needle as for amniocentesis. Then 20 ml of Hypaque is in-

jected quickly, and 5 to 10 minutes later an anteroposterior roentgenogram is made of the lower abdomen and pelvis. A characteristic honeycombed x-ray pattern is produced by contrast material surrounding the chorionic vesicles. With a normal pregnancy, there is a slight risk of abortion from the intra-amnionic injection of hypertonic radiopaque contrast material. With the widespread availability of sonography this technique is seldom used.

Chorionic Gonadotropin Measurements. Tests for chorionic gonadotropin are useful if a reliable quantitative method of assay is used and the considerable variation

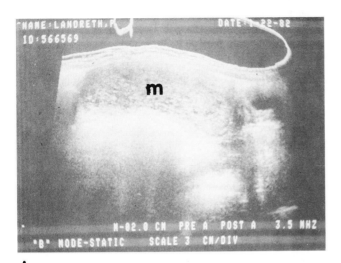

A

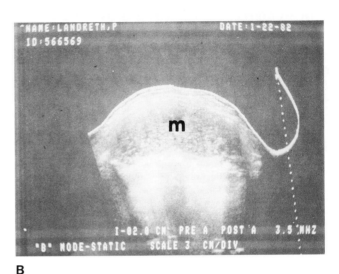

B

Figure 23-12. A. A longitudinal sonogram demonstrating a complete hydatidiform mole (m) that fills a uterus enlarged to well above the umbilicus. The woman had developed anemia, severe preeclampsia, and hyperthryroidism all induced by the hydatidiform mole. **B.** A transverse sonogram of the same hydatidiform mole (m). (*Courtesy of Dr. R. Santos.*)

in gonadotropin secretion in normal pregnancy is appreciated, especially the elevated levels that sometimes accompany pregnancy with multiple fetuses (Chapter 7, p. 122). Assays performed on serum are subject to fewer variables than are measurements of urinary chorionic gonadotropin. The results should be compared with the serum gonadotropin levels for normal pregnancy at the stage in question. If it is far above the normal range for that stage of pregnancy, a presumptive diagnosis of mole may be made. It is clear from the remarkably variable gonadotropin values for normal pregnancy that no *single value* can be established as the borderline between normal and abnormal pregnancy. High values in the first 2 or 3 months mean little, since they are encountered occasionally in normal pregnancy, especially with multiple fetuses. Beyond 100 days after the last menstrual period, however, there is in normal pregnancy a decline in chorionic gonadotropin, so that persistently high, and especially rising, levels after that time are strong evidence of abnormal growth of trophoblast. If the slightest doubt remains, one or more assays repeated at intervals of a week should be performed to observe the trend.

In summary, the diagnostic clinical features of a complete hydatidiform mole are:

1. Continuous or intermittent bloody discharge evident by about the 12th week of pregnancy, usually not profuse, and often more nearly brown rather than red.
2. Enlargement of the uterus out of proportion to the duration of pregnancy in about one half of the cases.
3. Absence of fetal parts on palpation and of fetal

heart sounds even though the uterus may be enlarged to the level of the umbilicus or higher.
4. Characteristic ultrasonographic pattern.
5. A very high chorionic gonadotropin level in the serum 100 days or more after the last menstrual period.
6. Preeclampsia-eclampsia developing before 24 weeks of gestation.

Prognosis

In a collective review of 576 cases, Mathieu in 1939 found an immediate mortality of 1.4 percent. Since then mortality has been reduced practically to zero by more prompt diagnosis and appropriate therapy.

About 10 to 20 percent of complete hydatidiform moles progress to invasive, potentially metastatic choriocarcinoma. Rarely, years may intervene between the occurrence of a hydatidiform mole and the development of choriocarcinoma. For example, Natsume and Takada (1961) reported a patient in whom choriocarcinoma developed 9 years after supravaginal hysterectomy for invasive mole (chorioadenoma destruens). From the subsequent course of 181 patients (Table 23-1) followed by Hertig and Mansell (1957) before the use of chemotherapy, it is evident that only a very small percentage of patients developed a lethal malignant tumor, although over a quarter did not initially have an entirely benign course. A sizable proportion regressed spontaneously or were cured by surgical procedures, including dilatation and curettage. It is precisely this spectrum of lesions, ranging from completely benign to highly malignant, with a rather unpredictable intermediate group, that has

TABLE 23.1 SUBSEQUENT COURSE OF 181 PATIENTS WITH HYDATIDIFORM MOLE AND NO CHEMOTHERAPY

Course	Percent
Initial spontaneous cure	73.5
Chorionephithelioma in situ*	3.5
Syncytial endometritis†	4.5
Chorioadenema destruens	16.0
Choriocarcinoma	2.5
Total	100.0

* Chorionepithelioma in situ: a term introduced by Hertig and Sheldon to describe a small, discrete mass of superficially invasive, apparently malignant trophoblast without villi found in uterine curettings in association with pregnancy, usually of molar type.
† Syncytial endometritis: a term that most pathologists agree refers to an accentuation of the morphologic features of the placental site. Endometrium and myometrium are infiltrated by trophoblastic cells with varying degees of inflammation, but the lesion is clinically benign (Hertig and Mansell, 1957).

produced dilemmas in diagnosis unmatched by any other tumor.

Treatment

The treatment for hydatidiform mole consists of two phases, the immediate evacuation of the mole and the later follow-up for detection of malignant change.

In the rare circumstance of twinning with a complete hydatidiform mole plus a fetus and placenta, the possibility of allowing the fetus to mature in utero must be considered. Neither the risks to the mother nor the likelihood of a healthy offspring have been established. Suzuki and associates (1980) reported a case in which the outcome was a healthy infant and healthy mother and cites several other previously reported instances. We have managed such pregnancies to favorable outcomes for both mother and fetus (Fig. 23-8).

Termination of Molar Pregnancy. Perhaps because of greater awareness, and certainly because of better techniques for diagnosis, especially sonography, moles now are terminated more often under controlled circumstances rather than the chaos commonly associated with their spontaneous abortion. Usually there is time for adequate evaluation of the woman with a mole, who may be anemic, hypertensive, fluid-depleted, or suffer from a combination of these abnormalities.

Prophylactic Chemotherapy. Prophylactic chemotherapy before evacuation is questioned because of the complications that are induced by or that accompany evacuation of a mole. These include hemorrhage, uterine perforation, and infection. At times, evacuation initiated vaginally eventuates in laparotomy. In these circumstances especially, the chemotherapeutic agents may contribute to morbidity and even mortality.

Goldstein (1974) and others have questioned the wisdom and necessity of administering toxic oncolytic agents to

women who, in the great majority of instances, will have a benign course subsequent to evacuation. The minority of women who will demonstrate persistent trophoblast may be treated chemotherapeutically quite successfully. Moreover, it is essential that women treated prophylactically be followed just as closely as if they had not been treated, since there is failure of prophylactic chemotherapy, albeit infrequently. Curry and associates (1975) concurred with Goldstein that the benefits from prophylactic chemotherapy so administered to women with hydatidiform moles do not justify the additional risks. They noted two deaths caused by toxicity from prophylactic chemotherapy.

Vacuum Aspiration. At least two, and preferably four, units of compatible whole blood are made ready and an intravenous infusion system is established suitable for rapid infusion of blood. Unless the cervix is long, very firm, and closed, which is very unlikely, dilatation can be safely accomplished under general anesthesia to a diameter sufficient to allow insertion of a plastic suction curet (Fig. 23-13A, B). Anesthetic agents that relax the uterus, such as halothane (Fluothane), should be avoided. Throughout the procedure, oxytocin is infused intravenously to contract the body of the uterus as its contents are being evacuated. This decreases bleeding from the implantation site and, as the myometrium retracts, thickens the uterine wall and thereby reduces the risk of perforating the uterus.

After the great bulk of the mole has been removed by aspiration and the myometrium has contracted and retracted, thorough *but gentle* curettage with a large sharp curet is usually performed. The tissue obtained by sharp curettage is so labeled and submitted separately for careful histologic examination. This specimen may possibly allow a better assessment of the malignant predisposition of the trophoblast and the subsequent biologic behavior of any tissue that persists in the uterus. Care must be taken neither to perforate the uterus nor to scrape so vigorously with the sharp curet as to invade deeply the myometrium and thereby weaken it. Facilities and personnel for immediate laparotomy are mandatory in case there is uncontrollable hemorrhage or serious trauma to the uterus.

Oxytocin, Prostaglandin, and Hypertonic Saline. Use of oxytocin without suction curettage to expel a large mole may prove unsatisfactory because either the uterus is not sufficiently stimulated to contract effectively or, more likely, during the time that the cervix is dilating and the mole is being extruded, hemorrhage becomes profuse. Prostaglandin E_2 has been used rather than oxytocin, but the same criticisms apply to both agents. Intrauterine instillation of hypertonic saline is mentioned only to condemn its use.

Hysterotomy. If for some reason not readily apparent suction curettage were not to be used to evacuate the large mole and the uterus is to be conserved, *hysterotomy* is the alternative. The incision should be large enough to evacuate the mole promptly but no larger.

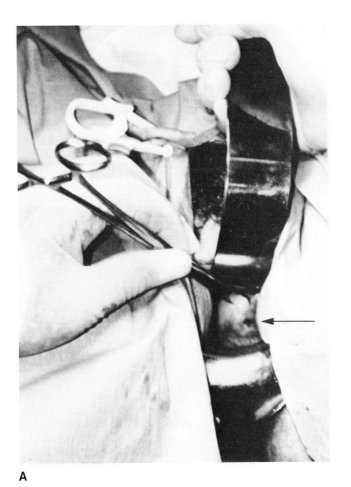

A

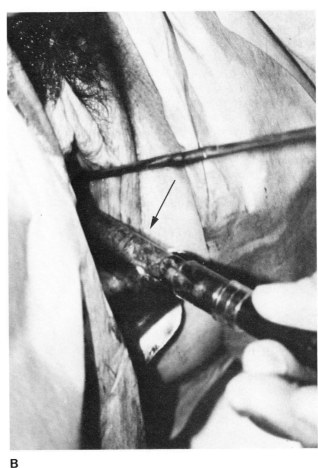

B

Figure 23-13. A. In the same case presented in Figures 23-11 and 23-12, the cervix (*arrow*) has been exposed and grasped with a tenaculum in preparation for dilatation and insertion of a suction curette. **B.** Molar tissue (*arrow*) is being rapidly removed from the uterine cavity by suction through the plastic curette.

Oxytocin is infused, and, after evacuation of the mole, sharp curettage is performed through the incision.

Hysterectomy. If the parity of the woman or her age is such that no further pregnancies are desired, *hysterectomy* may be preferred to suction curettage. Hysterectomy is a logical procedure in women of 40 or over, regardless of parity, and in women with three or more children, regardless of age, because of the frequency with which choriocarcinoma ensues in these age and parity groups. While hysterectomy does not eliminate trophoblastic disease, it does reduce appreciably the likelihood of such developing subsequently.

In 69 cases of hydatidiform mole, reported by Chun and associates (1964), in which initial hysterectomy was performed because of advanced age or parity, two women developed choriocarcinoma 2 to 3 years later, an incidence of 2.8 percent. In contrast, in 166 cases treated by evacuation of the molar tissue with conservation of the uterus, 14 women subsequently developed choriocarcinoma, a frequency of 8.4 percent. In any event, hysterectomy does not eliminate the necessity for careful follow-up. At laparotomy, it should be kept in mind that the ovaries often contain multiple theca-lutein cysts that need not be removed.

Follow-up Procedures

If the following extremely important procedures are not adhered to carefully, some women will die needlessly of choriocarcinoma. The prime objective of follow-up is prompt detection of any change suggestive of trophoblastic malignancy. To do so, it is necessary to rely on the chorionic gonadotropin values to detect persistent trophoblast. For this purpose, the test must be sufficiently sensitive and specific to detect very low levels of chorionic gonadotropin.

Chorionic gonadotropin levels should fall progressively to undetectable levels; otherwise viable trophoblast probably persists. An increase signifies proliferation of trophoblast that is most likely malignant unless the woman is again pregnant.

Estrogen–progestin contraceptives have been used commonly to prevent a subsequent pregnancy and to suppress pituitary luteinizing hormone that crossreacts with many tests for chorionic gonadotropin. Stone and co-workers (1976), however, reported the worrisome observation that the need for chemotherapy for trophoblastic tumor was increased significantly among women who took oral contraceptives starting shortly after evacuation of a hydatidiform mole. Moreover, oral contraceptives appeared to delay the fall in chorionic gonadotropin levels in women who did not require treatment with chemotherapy. More recently, Yuen and Burch (1983) have reported that neither the time that chorionic gonadotropin persisted after evacuating a mole nor the frequency of invasive complications was increased in women who used an oral contraceptive that contained 50 micrograms of estrogen or less per day.

A roentgenogram of the chest should be obtained during the first examination of the woman at least to serve as a baseline should future roentgenologic studies become necessary.

Although spontaneous disappearance of retained trophoblast is well known, the effectiveness of chemotherapeutic agents in the treatment of choriocarcinoma has led some to use these drugs in women with retained molar trophoblast to preclude the development of choriocarcinoma and to hasten the disappearance of the retained trophoblast. Since chemotherapeutic agents, such as methotrexate, are highly toxic and potentially lethal, the risk of chemotherapy must be weighed carefully against the chance of spontaneous regression.

Treatment of Persistent Trophoblast

In more recent times about 20 percent of women after evacuation of a hydatidiform mole have subsequently undergone further treatment for suspected persistent gestational trophoblastic disease (Lurain and co-workers, 1983). If the level of circulating chorionic gonadotropin has plateaued or is rising but there is no evidence of disease beyond the uterus, curettage, or hysterectomy if the uterus is not important for future reproduction, will effect a cure in some cases. Chorionic gonadotropin will disappear and the woman will remain well. If, however, the uterus is to be preserved or if there is roentgenographic evidence of lung lesions, chemotherapy is best started at this time with or without curettage. Therapy with methotrexate or actinomycin D, singly or in combination with other tumoricidal agents, most often has been successful in these circumstances.

Very small amounts of viable trophoblastic tumor can be detected by assaying for the β-subunit of chorionic gonadotropin. Once β-subunit activity has decreased to the limit of measurement, which is very low, therapy can be stopped safely without likelihood of recurrence. Treatment is best carried out in centers by highly interested and experienced individuals with all facilities for monitoring precisely chorionic gonadotropin levels as well as bone marrow, hepatic, and renal function.

A general method of follow-up is described:

1. Prevent pregnancy during the follow-up period.
2. Measure serum chorionic gonadotropin levels every 2 weeks using a specific radioimmunoassay. (Weekly assays have been recommended by some. However, no distinct benefit from so frequent assay has been demonstrated. Moreover, it has been difficult, at times, to obtain the results of the test within 1 week.)
3. Withhold therapy as long as the serum levels of chorionic gonadotropin continue to regress.
4. Once the level is normal, i.e., has reached the lower limit of measurement, test again 1 month later and then every 2 to 3 months for 1 year.
5. Follow-up may be discontinued and pregnancy allowed after 1 year.
6. A rise or persistent plateau in the serum level demands evaluation and usually treatment.

CHORIOCARCINOMA

Etiology

Except for rare cases arising in teratomas, choriocarcinoma in women develops during or, much more likely, after some form of pregnancy. Of 48 *fatal* cases of choriocarcinoma seen at the Brewer Trophoblastic Disease Center, 14 (29 percent) developed in association with a hydatidiform mole (Lurain and co-workers, 1982). The rest were associated with term or near term pregnancies, abortions, or ectopic pregnancies rather than hydatidiform moles.

Choriocarcinoma has been identified rarely in the placenta of a seemingly normal pregnancy. In a case described by Brewer and Majur (1981) widespread choriocarcinoma was evident at 18 weeks gestation. A primary choriocarcinoma of the placenta was detected! Choriocarcinoma in the mother that metastasized to the fetus has also been described (Kruseman and colleagues, 1977).

Pathology

This extremely malignant form of trophoblastic neoplasia may be considered a carcinoma of the chorionic epithelium, although in its growth and metastasis it often behaves like a sarcoma. The factors involved in malignant transformation of the trophoblast are unknown. In choriocarcinoma, the predisposition of normal trophoblast to invasive growth and erosion of blood vessels is greatly exaggerated. The characteristic gross picture is that of a rapidly growing mass invading both uterine muscle and blood vessels, causing hemorrhage and necrosis (Fig. 23-14A). The tumor is dark red or purple and ragged or friable. If it involves the endometrium, bleeding, sloughing, and infection of the surface usually occur

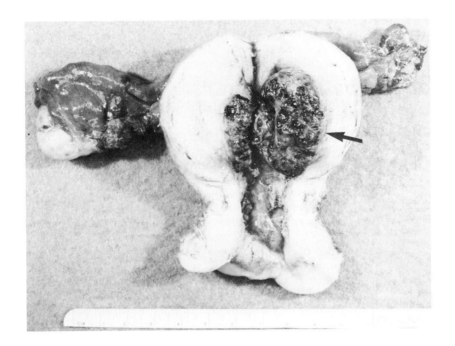

Figure 23-14. A. Choriocarcinoma (*arrow*) invading the uterus. Persistent trophoblastic disease was demonstrated by curettage subsequent to the expulsion of a hydatidiform mole. Chemotherapy was then instituted consisting of repeated courses of actinomycin D, then methotrexate, and finally triple therapy with actinomycin D, 5-fluorouracil, and cytoxan. When these failed to destroy the malignancy, hysterectomy and bilateral salpingo-oophorectomy were performed. The patient was known to be alive without detectable chorionic gonadotropin 10 years later.

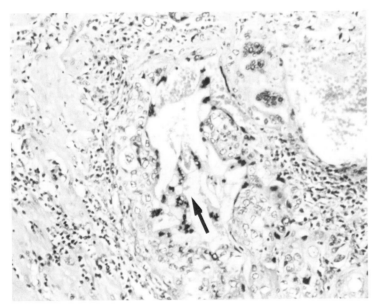

Figure 23-14. B. Histologic characteristics of the choriocarcinoma demonstrated in Figure 23-14A. Malignant syncytio- and cytotrophoblast without villous stroma invades the myometrium and vascular spaces, accompanied by necrosis and hemorrhage.

early. Masses of tissue buried in the myometrium may extend outward, appearing on the uterus as dark, irregular nodules that eventually penetrate the peritoneum.

Microscopically, columns and sheets of trophoblast penetrate the muscle and blood vessels, sometimes in plexiform arrangement and at other times in complete disorganization (Fig. 23-14B). An important diagnostic feature of choriocarcinoma, in contrast to hydatid mole or invasive mole, is absence of a villous pattern. Both cytotrophoblast and syncytial elements are involved, although one or the other may seem to predominate. Cel-

lular anaplasia exists, often in marked degrees, but is less valuable as a criterion of trophoblastic malignancy than in other tumors. The difficulty of cytologic evaluation is one of the factors leading to error in the diagnosis of choriocarcinoma from examination of uterine curettings. In fact, cells of normal trophoblast at the placental site have been diagnosed erroneously as choriocarcinoma.

Metastases often occur early and generally are blood-borne because of the affinity of trophoblast for blood vessels. The most common site of metastasis is the lungs (over 75 percent); the second most common is the vagina (about 50 percent). The vulva, kidneys, liver, ovaries, and brain also contain metastases in many cases. Lutein cysts of the ovary occur in over one third of the cases.

Clinical History

Choriocarcinoma may follow hydatid mole, abortion, ectopic pregnancy, or normal pregnancy. The most common, though not constant, sign is irregular bleeding after pregnancy termination in association with uterine subinvolution. The bleeding may be continuous or intermittent, with sudden and sometimes massive hemorrhages. Perforation of the uterus by the growth may cause intraperitoneal hemorrhage. Extension into the parametrium may cause pain and fixation that is suggestive of inflammatory disease.

In many cases, the first indication of the condition may be the metastatic lesions. Vaginal or vulvar tumors may be found. The woman may complain of cough and may produce bloody sputum arising from pulmonary metastases. In a few cases, it has been impossible to find choriocarcinoma in the uterus or pelvis, the original lesion having disappeared, leaving only distant metastases growing actively.

If unmodified by treatment, the course of choriocarcinoma is rapidly progressive, death occurring usually within a few months in the majority of cases. The most common cause of death is hemorrhage in various locations.

Diagnosis

Recognition of the possibility of the lesion is the most important factor in diagnosis. All cases of hydatidiform mole should be under suspicion and followed as described. Any case of unusual bleeding after term pregnancy or abortion should be investigated by curettage but especially by measurements of chorionic gonadotropin, since absolute reliance cannot be placed on the findings of examination of curettings. Malignant tissue may be buried within the myometrium, inaccessible to the curet, or hidden in a site of metastasis.

Solitary or multiple nodules present in a roentgenogram of the chest that cannot be otherwise explained are suggestive of the possibility of choriocarcinoma and warrant an assay for chorionic gonadotropin. It should be kept in mind, however, that some nontrophoblastic tumors secrete small amounts of chorionic gonadotropin (Shane and Naftolin, 1975).

Persistent or rising titers of gonadotropin in the absence of pregnancy are indicative of trophoblastic neoplasia. Of course, results of assays should be confirmed before resorting to medical or surgical therapy.

Treatment

Current treatment of choriocarcinoma is very much more successful than that of the past. Formerly, the only hope for cure was hysterectomy or, even more remote,

resection of a metastatic lesion. In 1956, Li and colleagues successfully treated a woman with a metastatic gestational trophoblastic neoplasm by using methotrexate. Since then, methotrexate and other agents effective against malignant tumors, especially actinomycin D, have been widely used with considerable success. The pharmacology and clinical use of methotrexate have been reviewed extensively by Jolivet and colleagues (1983).

The overall cure rate in recent years for persistent gestational trophoblastic neoplasia of all severities has been about 90 percent (Lewis, 1980). Patients in a low-risk category, therefore having a good prognosis, have been cured virtually 100 percent of the time. Low-risk category is identified as excreting in urine less than 100,000 IU of hCG per 24 hours, duration of the disease of less than 4 months, and no metastases to the brain or liver. Cure usually has been achieved for low-risk patients following treatment with a single chemotherapeutic agent. Treatment with a single agent reduces serious treatment toxicity. Fortunately, in those instances in which single agent therapy proved ineffective, prompt treatment with combination chemotherapy and, at times, irradiation therapy most often has provided a cure.

Patients who can be classified as high risk because of their poorer prognosis for cure have been identified. They excreted more than 100,000 IU of hCG per day, had their disease for more than 4 months, had previous chemotherapy, had metastases to the liver or brain, or had choriocarcinoma in association with a term pregnancy. In this group, combination chemotherapy, in spite of increased toxicity, has produced the highest cure rate.

In the past, cerebral metastases proved to be uniformly fatal. However, high-voltage irradiation, coupled with methotrexate and other chemotherapeutic agents, may eradicate such lesions on occasion. An extensive analysis of treatment failures in gestational trophoblastic disease has been provided by Lurain and co-workers (1982).

INVASIVE MOLE

Invasive mole (*chorioadenoma destruens*) occupies an intermediate position between benign hydatidiform mole and highly malignant choriocarcinoma. The incidence of the condition, like that of choriocarcinoma, is very low.

Diagnosis

The distinguishing features of invasive mole are excessive trophoblastic overgrowth and extensive penetration by the trophoblastic elements, including whole villi, into the depths of the myometrium, sometimes involving the peritoneum or the adjacent parametrium or vaginal vault (Fig. 23-15). Such moles are locally invasive but

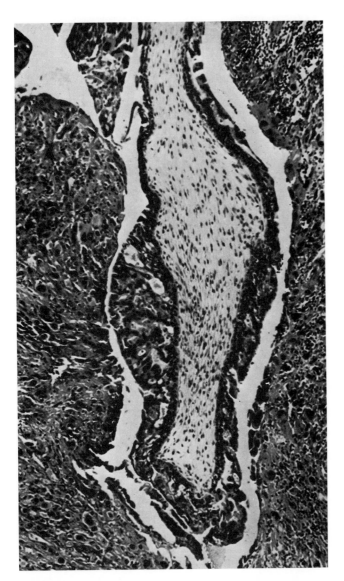

Figure 23-15. Invasive hydatidiform mole (chorioadenoma destruens), showing molar villus with hyperplastic trophoblast penetrating deeply into myometrium. (*Courtesy of Dr. Ralph M. Wynn.*)

generally lack the pronounced tendency to widespread metastasis that is characteristic of choriocarcinoma. As contrasted with the typically benign hydatidiform mole, with an invasive mole microscopically large fields of trophoblast are usually found, accompanied by some villous stroma.

Treatment

Chemotherapy with methotrexate without hysterectomy has brought about a complete remission in some cases. However, treatment may require hysterectomy because of uterine perforation by the tumor and massive intraabdominal hemorrhage.

Pregnancy After Trophoblastic Disease

Women who have suffered gestational trophoblastic disease and have been successfully treated with chemotherapy do not appear to be at increased risk of developing trophoblastic disease again with another pregnancy. Also, of considerable importance, they can anticipate a reproductive outcome with risks not much different from those for the general population (Berkowitz and colleagues, 1981; Rustin and associates, 1984).

OTHER TUMORS OF THE PLACENTA

Chorioangioma (Hemangioma) of Placenta

Various angiomatous tumors of the placenta ranging widely in size have been described. Because of the resemblance of their components to the blood vessels and stroma of the chorionic villus, the term *chorioangioma* or *chorangioma* has been considered the most appropriate designation. The tumors are most likely hamartomas of primitive chorionic mesenchyme. Their incidence has been reported to be about 1 percent. Larger chorioangiomas may be strongly suspected, at least, on the basis of sonographic changes within the placenta. A dramatic example is provided by the case cited in Figures 23-16A, B, C.

Small growths are essentially asymptomatic, but the large tumors may be associated with hydramnios or antepartum hemorrhage. Fetal death and malformations are uncommon complications, although there may be a positive correlation with low birth weight. Severe iron deficiency anemia has been identified in the neonate as the consequence of chronic fetal-to-maternal hemorrhage associated with multiple small chorioangiomas (Cunningham and Pritchard, unpublished). Large chorioangiomas provide an arteriovenous shunt in the fetal circulation that can lead to heart failure with all of its complications. With a large chorioangioma, consumptive coagulopathy and microangiopathic hemolytic anemia have also been observed in the fetus–infant. In Figures 23-16A, B, C are displayed a placenta and a very large, discrete chorioangioma, which led to heart failure, consumptive coagulopathy, and microangiopathic hemolysis in the fetus–infant.

Tumors Metastatic to the Placenta

Metastases of malignant tumors are rare (Freedman and MacMahon, 1960; Horner, 1960). Malignant melanoma apparently is the most common, making up nearly one third of the reported cases. However, any tumor with hematogenous spread is a potential source of placental metastases, as borne out by the case of Ewing sarcoma metastatic to the placenta reported by Greenberg and associates (1982); the mother succumbed from metastatic disease, but the child remained healthy at 12 years of age.

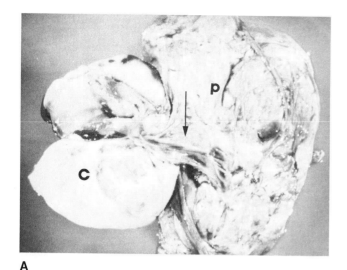

A

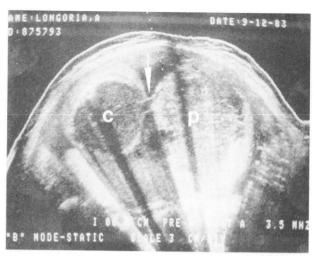

B

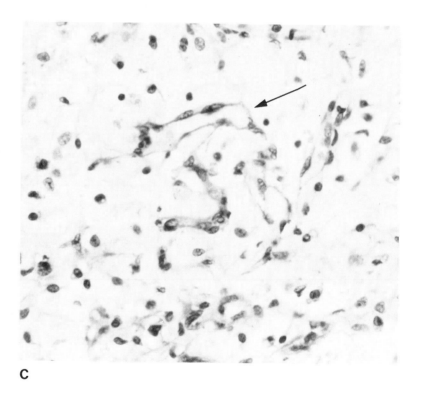

C

Figure 23-16. **A.** Placenta (p) and discrete very large (450 g) chorioangioma (c) connected to the placenta by a vascular stalk (*arrow*). The fetus of 34 weeks gestational age was identified by sonography to have marked hydrothorax. Demonstrated in cord blood were severe hypofibrinogenemia, thrombocytopenia, hypoprothrombinemia, and microangiopathic hemolysis. The infant suffered severe cardiomegaly, pleural effusion, and hepatomegaly. After several cardiac arrests the infant succumbed 3 days after birth. **B.** Sonogram of the same placenta (p) and chorioangioma (c) connected by a short pedicle (*arrow*). (*Courtesy of Dr. R. Santos.*) **C.** Microscopic section of the chorioangioma shown in Figures 23-16A, B. The tumor was quite vascular. The arrow points to one of the many vessels. (*Courtesy of Dr. Richard Voet.*)

ABNORMALITIES OF THE UMBILICAL CORD (FUNIS)

Abnormalities in Cord Length

Umbilical cord length varies appreciably, with the mean length being about 55 cm (Rayburn and associates, 1981). Extremes in cord length in abnormal instances range from apparently no cord (achordia) to lengths up to 300 cm. Vascular occlusion by thrombi and true knots are more common in excessively long umbilical cords, and such long cords are more likely to prolapse through the cervix. Rarely, excessively short umbilical cords may be instrumental in abruptio placenta and inversion of the uterus. They also may rupture with intrafunicular hemorrhage, which can cause fetal death.

An intriguing question is "What factors determine the length of the umbilical cord?" Studies performed on animals and experiments of nature in human pregnancy support the concept that the length of the cord is influenced positively by the volume of amnionic fluid present and by the mobility of the fetus. Miller and associates (1981) have identified the human umbilical cord to be appreciably shortened when there had been either chronic fetal constraint from oligohydramnios or decreased fetal movement because of limb dysfunction. Excessive cord length may be the consequence of nonlethal entanglement of cord and fetus and stretching of the cord during fetal movement.

Absence of One Umbilical Artery

Benirschke and Brown (1955) were principally responsible for drawing attention to the association between a single umbilical artery and its frequent association with fetal malformation. The absence of one umbilical artery, according to Benirschke and Dodds (1967), characterized 0.85 percent of all cords in singletons and 5 percent of the cords of at least one twin. A single umbilical artery was found in 2.5 percent of abortuses. About 30 percent of all infants with one umbilical artery missing had associated congenital anomalies.

Bryan and Kohler (1975) identified the umbilical cords of 143 infants, or 0.72 percent, to have a single artery out of nearly 20,000 examined. Among those 143 infants, the incidence of major malformations was 18 percent, retarded fetal growth 34 percent, and prematurity 17 percent. In the studies of Froehlich and Fujikura (1973) mortality was very high (14 percent) among infants with a single umbilical artery, but of those who survived infancy, serious anomalies were not much more common than in the control group. However, Bryan and Kohler (1975) followed beyond infancy 90 infants with a single umbilical artery and found previously unrecognized malformations in 10.

Peckham and Yerushalmy (1965) demonstrated that a single umbilical artery occurred twice as often in newborns of white women than in those of black women. The incidence is considerably increased in newborns of women with diabetes mellitus. Based on the finding of a high incidence of fetal malformations when a single umbilical artery exists, each umbilical cord should be examined carefully to ascertain the number of umbilical arteries present.

Abnormalities of Cord Insertion

The umbilical cord usually, but not always, is inserted at or near the center of the fetal surface of the placenta.

Marginal Insertion. Insertion of the cord at the margin of the placenta is sometimes referred to as a *battledore placenta*. Some have found that such insertion was more common in instances of premature labor but others have not (Robinson and co-workers, 1983).

Velamentous Insertion of Cord. The so-called velamentous insertion of the cord is of considerable practical importance (Figs. 23-17, 23-18). In this condition, the vessels of the cord separate in the membranes at a dis-

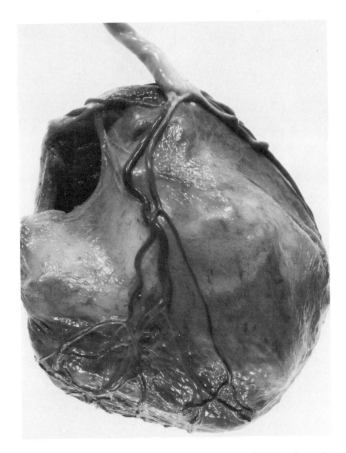

Figure 23-17. Velamentous insertion of cord. The placenta (*bottom*) and membranes have been inverted to expose the amnion. Note the large fetal vessels within membranes (*top*) and their proximity to the site of rupture of the membranes.

tance from the placental margin, which they reach surrounded only by a fold of amnion. This mode of insertion is noted in a little over 1 percent of singleton deliveries but much more frequently with twins, and it is almost the rule with triplets. With velamentous insertion of the cord, the likelihood of fetal deformity is increased (Robinson and co-workers, 1983).

Vasa Previa. Vasa previa results when with velamentous insertion some of the fetal vessels in the membranes cross the region of the internal os and present ahead of the presenting part of the fetus. At times, the careful examiner will be able to palpate a tubular fetal vessel in the membranes overlying the presenting part. Compression of the vessels between the examining finger and the presenting part is likely to induce changes in the fetal heart rate. At times, the vessels may be visualized directly by employing amnioscopy.

With vasa previa, there is considerable potential danger to the infant, for rupture of the membranes may be accompanied by rupture of a fetal vessel and lead to exsanguination of the infant (Fig. 23-18).

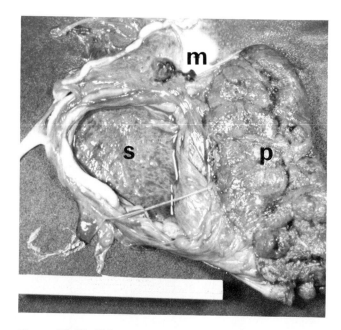

Figure 23-18. Velamentous insertion of the umbilical cord and ruptured vasa previa with rapidly fatal fetal hemorrhage. Milk injected through the umbilical vein of the cord escaped at the site of the rupture (m = milk; p = maternal surface of placenta; s = site of rupture of fetal membranes through which the fetus was delivered).

Whenever there is hemorrhage antepartum or intrapartum, the possibility of vasa previa and a ruptured fetal vessel exists. Unfortunately, the amount of fetal blood that can be shed without killing the fetus is relatively small compared to the volumes of blood that usually cause concern with antepartum or intrapartum hemorrhage of maternal origin. Blood can be ascertained to be of fetal origin by demonstrating resistance of hemoglobin to denaturation with alkali. A quick, readily available approach is to smear the blood on glass slides, stain the blood smears with Wright stain, and examine for nucleated red cells. Nucleated red cells are normally present in cord blood but are rarely so in maternal blood.

The pessimism expressed by Kouyoumdjian (1980) for improving fetal salvage with vasa previa once a vessel is ruptured is probably justified. The likelihood of a poor outcome for the fetus in spite of vigorous therapy is made evident by the following case of vasa previa and fetal hemorrhage with prompt intervention:

> Spontaneous premature rupture of the membranes at 36 weeks gestation was not promptly followed by spontaneous labor. In preparation for oxytocin stimulation of the myometrium, an electrode was applied to the fetal scalp through a cervix dilated 2 cm. This was followed immediately by bleeding through the cervix into the vagina. There had been no bleeding before this. The previously normal fetal heart rate soon dropped to 70 per minute and delivery of the fetus by cesarean section was performed less than 10 minutes after the application of the electrode. The infant

was treated intensively but unsuccessfully with cardiopulmonary resuscitation, saline, sodium bicarbonate, and O-negative blood. The large fetal vessel lacerated by the scalp electrode is evident in Figure 23-18.

Cord Abnormalities Capable of Impeding Blood Flow

Several mechanical and vascular abnormalities of the umbilical cord are capable of impairing fetal-placental blood flow.

Knots of the Cord. False knots, which result from kinking of the vessels to accommodate to the length of the cord, should be distinguished from true knots, which result from active movements of the fetus. In some 17,000 deliveries in the Collaborative Study on Cerebral Palsy, Spellacy and co-workers (1966) found an incidence of true knots of the umbilical cord of 1.1 percent, with a perinatal loss of 6.1 percent in the presence of true knots. The incidence of true knots in the cord is especially high in monoamnionic twins.

Loops of the Cord. The cord frequently becomes coiled around portions of the fetus, usually the neck. In 1000 consecutive deliveries studied by Kan and Eastman (1957), the incidence of coiling of the umbilical cord around the fetal neck ranged from one loop in 21 percent to three loops in 0.2 percent of deliveries. Coiling of the cord around the neck is an uncommon cause of fetal death. Typically, as labor progresses and the fetus descends in the birth canal, the cord tightens during a contraction to compress the cord and vasculature and, in turn, cause deceleration of the fetal heart rate, which persists until the contraction ceases. Recognition and prompt delivery will minimize the risk of fetal death or severe morbidity in the infant. In monoamnionic twinning, however, a significant fraction of the high perinatal mortality rate is attributed to entwining of the umbilical cords before labor (Fig. 26-12).

Torsion of the Cord. As a result of fetal movements, the cord normally becomes twisted. Occasionally, the torsion is so marked that the fetal circulation is compromised. Extreme degrees of torsion probably occur only after the death of the fetus by a mechanism that is not understood.

Stricture of the Cord. Most, but not all, infants with cord stricture are stillborns, and it seems that the stricture plays a role in producing fetal death (Fig. 23-19). Cord stricture, for unknown reasons, is associated with an extreme focal deficiency in Wharton's jelly. Stricture is commonly associated, causally, with torsion.

Hematoma of the Cord. Hematomas occasionally result from the rupture of the varix, usually of the umbilical vein, with effusion of blood into the cord (Fig. 23-20). Sonographic visualization of a large cord hematoma and

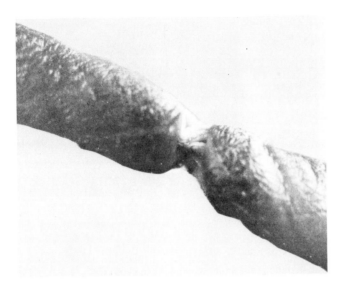

Figure 23-19. A sharply localized stricture in a cord from a stillborn infant. (*From Fox: Pathology of the Placenta. Philadelphia, Saunders, 1978, Volume 7, page 442.*)

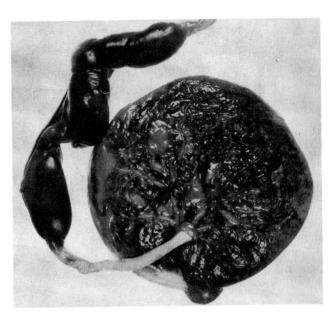

Figure 23-20. Hematoma of the umbilical cord.

a dead fetus has been described (Ruvinsky and associates, 1981). Fox (1978), who has reviewed the subject carefully, believes it unwise to attribute fetal death to a cord hematoma until other causes of death have been excluded.

Cysts of the Cord. Cysts occasionally occur along the course of the cord and are designated true and false, according to their origin. True cysts are quite small and may be derived from remnants of the umbilical vesicle or of the allantois. False cysts, which may attain considerable size, result from liquefaction of Wharton's jelly. Such cysts may be detected by sonography but may be difficult to identify precisely. For example, the cord cyst demonstrated in Figure 23-21A, B was thought possibly to be a meningocele when detected by sonography, since the cyst maintained a close and constant relationship over time with the lower spine of the fetus.

Edema of the Cord. This condition rarely occurs by itself but is frequently associated with edema of the fetus. It is very common with macerated fetuses.

DISEASES OF THE AMNION

Meconium Staining

The brownish green discoloration of the fetal membranes from meconium staining is characteristic. The amnion may be slippery from mucus discharged in the meconium. Meconium staining is relatively common; Benirschke (1974) identified it in 13 percent of 2000 con-

secutive placentas examined. He reported that in the majority of cases no other evidence of fetal distress was identified, and the subsequent course of the newborn infant was normal. Fujikura and Klionsky (1975) identified meconium staining of the membranes or fetus in 10.3 percent of 43,000 liveborn infants in the Collaborative Study of Cerebral Palsy and Other Disorders. The neonatal mortality rate was 3.3 percent in the stained group compared to 1.7 percent in the nonstained group.

Inflammation of the Amnion

Since amnionitis is a manifestation of an intrauterine infection, it is associated frequently with prolonged rupture of the membranes and long labors. When mononuclear and polymorphonuclear leukocytes infiltrate the chorion, the resulting lesion is properly designated *chorioamnionitis*. Organisms commonly found are those present in the vagina and in maternal feces.

Cysts of Amnion

Small cysts lined by typical amnionic epithelium are formed occasionally. The common variety results from fusion of amnionic folds, with subsequent retention of fluid.

Amnion Nodosum

These nodules in the amnion are sometimes called *squamous metaplasia* of the amnion or *amnionic caruncles.* They occur most commonly in the amnion in contact with the chorionic plate, but they may also be seen else-

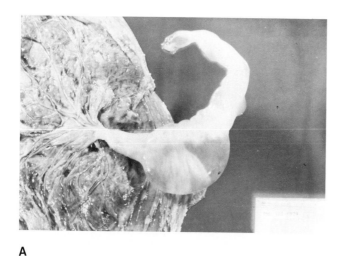

A

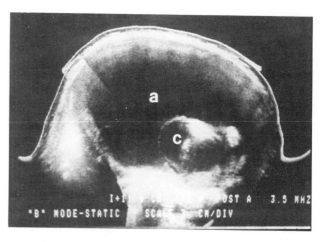

B

Figure 23-21. A. Cyst of umbilical cord at 27 weeks gestation in a monoamnionic twin pregnancy further complicated by symptomatic acute hydramnios and marked discordance in size of the fetuses. (*Courtesy of Dr. K. Leveno.*) **B.** Sonogram from the same case demonstrating the cyst of the cord (c) and marked hydramnios (a). The possibility that the cyst was a meningocele was considered originally. In spite of removal of fluid by amniocentesis and intravenous ritodrine, labor progressed. (*Courtesy of Dr. R. Santos.*)

where. They usually appear near the insertion of the cord as multiple, rounded or oval, shiny, grayish yellow, opaque elevations that vary from less than 1 mm up to 5 mm in diameter. Bartman and Driscoll (1968) reported an association between amnion nodosum and multiple congenital abnormalities, especially hypoplastic kidneys with oligohydramnios. The nodules most likely are made up of fetal ectodermal debris, including vernix caseosa.

Amnionic Bands

Disruption of the amnion may lead to formation of bands or strings of amnion that adhere to the fetus and impair growth and development of the involved structure. Some of the conditions that appear to be the consequence of this phenomenon, including intrauterine amputations, are considered in Chapter 39.

DISORDERS OF THE AMNIONIC FLUID

Hydramnios

Hydramnios, sometimes called *polyhydramnios,* is an excessive quantity of amnionic fluid. Normally, the volume of amnionic fluid increases to about 1 liter, or somewhat more, by 36 weeks but decreases thereafter. Postterm, there may be only a few hundred ml or even less. Somewhat arbitrarily, more than 2000 ml of amnionic fluid is considered excessive, or hydramnios. In rare instances, the uterus may contain an enormous quantity of fluid, with reports of as much as 15 liters on record. In most instances, the increase in amnionic fluid is gradual, or

chronic hydramnios. When the volume increases very suddenly, the uterus may become markedly distended within a few days, or *acute hydramnios.* The fluid in hydramnios is usually similar in appearance and composition to the amnionic fluid in normal conditions.

Incidence. Minor to moderate degrees of hydramnios, 2 to 3 liters, are rather common, but the more marked grades are not. Because of the difficulty of complete collection of the amnionic fluid, the diagnosis is usually based on clinical impression or sonographic estimation. Therefore, the frequency of the diagnosis varies appreciably with different observers. It is not surprising that the published data on the incidence have varied widely, ranging from 1 in 62 deliveries to 1 in 754. Hydramnios sufficient to cause clinical symptoms (generally in excess of 3000 ml of amnionic fluid) probably occurs about once in 1000 pregnancies, exclusive of twins. The incidence of hydramnios associated with fetal malformations, especially those of the central nervous system and gastrointestinal tract, is high. For example, hydramnios accompanies about half of cases of anencephalus and most all cases of atresia of the esophagus. The incidence of hydramnios is also markedly increased in pregnancies complicated by diabetes and in the hydropic variety of erythroblastosis. Excessive amnionic fluid in one of the amnionic sacs is common in twin pregnancies and is more frequent and usually more intense in monozygotic than in dizygotic twinning (Fig. 23-21B).

Etiology. The volume of amnionic fluid undoubtedly is controlled in a number of ways. Early in pregnancy, the amnionic cavity is filled with fluid very similar in composition to extracellular fluid. During the first half of pregnancy, transfer of water and other small molecules takes place not only across the amnion but through the fetal skin. Lind and Hytten (1970) considered amnionic fluid to be an extension of the fetal extracellular fluid space during the first half of pregnancy.

During the second trimester, the fetus begins to urinate, to swallow, and to inspire amnionic fluid (Abramovich and colleagues, 1979; Duenhoelter and Pritchard, 1976; Pritchard, 1966). These processes almost certainly have a significant modulating role in the control of amnionic fluid volume. Although the major source of amnionic fluid most often has been assumed to be the amnionic epithelium, no histologic changes in the amnion or chemical changes in the amnionic fluid in cases of hydramnios have been found.

Since the fetus normally swallows amnionic fluid, it has been assumed that this mechanism is one of the ways by which the volume of the fluid is controlled. The theory gains validity by the nearly constant presence of hydramnios when swallowing is inhibited as, for example, in cases of atresia of the esophagus. Fetal swallowing is by no means the only mechanism for preventing hydramnios, for both Pritchard (1966) and Abramovich (1970) have measured quantitatively amnionic fluid swallowing and found in some instances of gross hydramnios appreciable volumes of fluid being swallowed.

In cases of anencephalus and spina bifida, increased transudation of fluid from the exposed meninges into the amnionic cavity may be an etiologic factor. Another possible explanation of hydramnios in anencephalus when swallowing is not impaired is excessive urination brought about by either stimulation of cerebrospinal centers that have been deprived of their protective coverings or possibly the lack of antidiuretic hormone.

In hydramnios associated with monozygotic twin pregnancy, the hypothesis has been advanced that one fetus usurps the greater part of the circulation common to both twins and develops cardiac hypertrophy, which, in turn, results in increased urine. Naeye and Blanc (1972) have identified in this syndrome dilated renal tubules, enlarged bladder, and an increased urinary output in the early neonatal period, suggesting that increased fetal micturition is responsible for the hydramnios. Conversely, donor members of parabiotic transplacental transfusion pairs had contracted renal tubules with oligohydramnios.

The hydramnios that rather commonly develops with maternal diabetes during the third trimester remains unexplained. Wladimiroff and co-workers (1975) identified sonographically the rate of fetal urine formation in such a case to be in the normal range.

Naeye and Blanc (1972) have described hypoplastic lungs commonly in neonates with hydramnios and question their role in the genesis of the hydramnios. The observations of Duenhoelter and Pritchard (1976) on both monkey and human fetuses establish that normal fetal lungs have the potential, at least, for the exchange of relatively large volumes of fluid as the consequence of the inspiration of amnionic fluid. Hypoplastic lungs may compromise this pathway for removal of amnionic fluid.

The weight of the placenta tends to be high in some cases of hydramnios. The enlarged placenta may contribute to the increase in amnionic fluid. Prolactin has been suspected to have a role in the control of amnionic fluid volume. The concentration of prolactin in amnionic fluid is increased compared to that of maternal plasma. Prolactin receptors have been identified in amnion from pregnancies with a normal volume of amnionic fluid. However, in cases of idiopathic hydramnios, receptor binding was impaired compared to normal (Healy and co-workers, 1982).

Symptoms. The major symptoms accompanying hydramnios arise from purely mechanical causes and result chiefly from the pressure exerted within and around the overdistended uterus upon adjacent organs. The effects on maternal respiratory functions may be striking. When distention is excessive, the mother may suffer from severe dyspnea, and in extreme cases she may be able to breathe only in the upright position. Edema, the consequence of compression of major venous systems by the very large uterus, is common, especially of the lower extremities, the vulva, and the abdominal wall. Rarely, severe oliguria may result from obstruction of the urinary tract by the very large uterus. When the accumulation of fluid takes place gradually (*chronic hydramnios*) the patient may tolerate the excessive abdominal distention with relatively little discomfort. In *acute hydramnios*, however, the distention may lead to disturbances sufficiently serious to threaten the life of the mother. Acute hydramnios tends to occur earlier in pregnancy than does the chronic form, often as early as the fourth or fifth month, and it may rapidly expand the hypertonic uterus to enormous size. Without treatment, pain is likely to become intense and the dyspnea so severe that the woman is unable to lie flat. As a rule, acute hydramnios leads to labor before the 28th week, or the symptoms become so severe that intervention is mandatory. In the majority of cases of chronic hydramnios, and thus differing from acute hydramnios, the amnionic fluid pressure is not appreciably higher than in normal pregnancy.

Diagnosis of Hydramnios. Usually, uterine enlargement in association with difficulty in palpating fetal small parts and in hearing fetal heart tones is the main diagnostic sign of hydramnios. In severe cases, the uterine wall may be so tense that it is impossible to palpate any part of the fetus (Fig. 23-22). Such findings call for prompt sonographic examination of the abdomen to identify multiple fetuses or fetal abnormalities and to try to verify fetal age.

Sonography. The differentiation between hydramnios, ascites, and a large ovarian cyst can usually be made without difficulty with sonography. Large amounts of

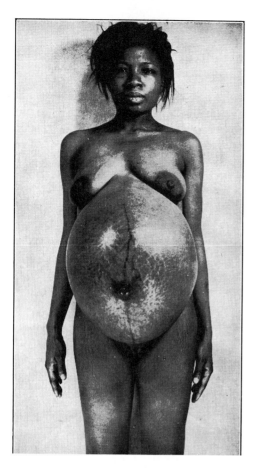

Figure 23-22. Advanced degree of hydramnios; 5500 ml of amnionic fluid was measured at delivery.

amnionic fluid can nearly always be readily demonstrated as an abnormally large echo-free space between the fetus and the uterine wall or placenta (Fig. 23-21B). At times, a fetal abnormality may also be demonstrated, such as anencephaly or other neural tube defects or an anomaly of the gastrointestinal tract.

Radiography. A large radiolucent area around the fetal skeleton suggests hydramnios, although a soft tissue mass, such as a sacrococcygeal tumor, may do the same. Most often, anencephaly and other gross skeletal defects are easily diagnosed. *Amniography,* using a contrast material such as Hypaque, may help identify excess amnionic fluid, soft tissue tumors projecting from the fetus, and the presence or absence of fetal swallowing.

Prognosis. In general, the more severe the hydramnios, the higher is the perinatal mortality rate, so that the outlook for the infant in pregnancies with major degrees of hydramnios is poor. Even though the sonogram and roentgenogram show an apparently normal fetus, the prognosis must be guarded. The incidence of fetal malformations is 20 percent (Queenan and Gadow, 1970). There is a further increase in perinatal mortality from

prematurity, since the frequency of premature births in association with hydramnios is more than twice the overall rate.

The hazards imposed by hydramnios on the mother are significant but can usually be combatted without serious threat to her life. The most frequent maternal complications are placental abruption, uterine dysfunction, and postpartum hemorrhage. Extensive premature separation of the placenta sometimes follows escape of massive quantities of amnionic fluid because of the decrease in the area beneath the placenta as the uterus empties. Uterine dysfunction and postpartum hemorrhage are the results of the uterine atony consequent upon overdistention. Abnormal presentations are more common, and operative interference is more frequently required.

Treatment of Hydramnios. Minor degrees of hydramnios rarely require treatment. Even moderate degrees of the complication, including cases in which there is some discomfort, can usually be managed without intervention until labor starts or until the membranes rupture spontaneously. If there is dyspnea or abdominal pain, or if ambulation is difficult, hospitalization becomes necessary. There is no satisfactory treatment for symptomatic hydramnios other than removal of some of the amnionic fluid. Bed rest with sedation may make the situation endurable, but it rarely has any effect on the accumulation of fluid. Diuretics and restriction of water and salt are likewise ineffective and potentially dangerous.

Amniocentesis. The chief purpose of amniocentesis is relief of the mother's distress, and to that end it is successful transiently. At times, amniocentesis appears to initiate labor even though only a part of the fluid is removed; hence, relief of the patient's distress may not enable her to continue with the pregnancy. The volume of fluid removed at one time appears to be critical. Queenan (1970) and Pitkin (1976) have described cases of recurrent severe hydramnios treated by amniocentesis. Whereas removal of a large volume of fluid at one time during the first pregnancy was soon followed by delivery of a very immature infant that succcumbed, repeated amniocenteses with the frequent removal of smaller volumes during the next pregnancy was not and, therefore, resulted in delivery of an infant sufficiently mature to survive.

The disadvantages inherent in rupture of the membranes through the cervix are the possibility of prolapse of the cord and especially of placental abruption. Very slow removal of the fluid helps to obviate these dangers but is very difficult to accomplish through the cervical canal, since even a small nick in the membranes is usually quickly converted into a large rent. The slight dangers of abdominal amniocentesis in the presence of hydramnios are puncture of a fetal vessel and bacterial infection. Sonography is useful not only to identify hydramnios and associated fetal anomalies but to locate the placenta and thereby perform amniocentesis so as to avoid puncturing the placenta. Careful aseptic technique should prevent infection.

Technique of Amniocentesis for Hydramnios. To remove amnionic fluid from women with hydramnios, a commercially available plaster catheter that tightly covers an 18-gauge needle (Angiocath) may be inserted through the locally anesthetized abdominal wall into the amnionic sac, the needle withdrawn, and an intravenous infusion set connected to the catheter hub. The opposite end of the tubing is dropped into a graduated cylinder placed at floor level, and the rate of flow of amnionic fluid is controlled with the screw clamp so that about 500 ml per hour is withdrawn. After about 1500 to 2000 ml of amnionic fluid has escaped, the uterus usually has decreased in size sufficiently that the plastic catheter has pulled out of the amnionic sac and the flow ceases. At the same time, maternal relief is dramatic, and the danger of placental separation from decompression is very slight. Using strict aseptic technique, this procedure can be repeated as necessary to make the woman comfortable.

Oligohydramnios

In some instances, the volume of amnionic fluid may fall far below the normal limits and occasionally be reduced to only a few ml of viscid fluid. The cause of this condition is not completely understood. Very small amounts of amnionic fluid may be found relatively often with pregnancies that have continued for weeks beyond term. The risk of cord compression and, in turn, fetal distress is increased as the consequence of the scant volume of fluid. Oligohydramnios is practically always evident when there is either obstruction of the fetal urinary tract or renal agenesis. Therefore, anuria almost certainly has an etiologic role in such cases of oligohydramnios. A chronic leak from a defect in the membranes may reduce the volume of amnionic fluid appreciably, but most often labor soon ensues.

When oligohydramnios occurs early in pregnancy, it is attended by serious consequences to the fetus, since adhesions between the amnion and parts of the fetus may cause serious deformities, including amputation. Moreover, subjected to pressure from all sides, the fetus assumes a peculiar appearance, and musculoskeletal deformities, such as clubfoot, are frequently observed. Typically, in cases of oligohydramnios, the skin of the fetus appears dry, leathery, and wrinkled.

When amnionic fluid is scant, *pulmonary hypoplasia* is very common. The possibilities to account for the hypoplasia are (1) compression of the thorax by the uterus in the absence of amnionic fluid, which prevents chest wall excursion and lung expansion, (2) lack of fluid to be inhaled into the terminal air sacs of the lung and, as a consequence, inhibition of lung growth, and (3) an intrinsic lung defect with failure of the lung to excrete fluid essential to maintenance of amnionic fluid volume. The appreciable volumes of amnionic fluid demonstrated by Duenhoelter and Pritchard (1976) to be inhaled by the fetus normally is suggestive of a role for the inspired fluid in expansion and, in turn, the growth and development of the lung.

REFERENCES

Abramovich DR: Fetal factors influencing the volume and composition of liquor amnii. J Obstet Gynaecol Br Commonw 77:865, 1970

Abramovich DR, Garden A, Jandial L, Page KR: Fetal swallowing and voiding in relation to hydramnios. Obstet Gynecol 54:15, 1979

Bagshawe KD, Lawler SD: Commentary: Unmasking moles. Br J Obstet Gynaecol 89:255, 1982

Bartman J, Driscoll SG: Amnion nodosum and hypoplastic cystic kidneys. Obstet Gynecol 32:700, 1968

Benirschke K, Brown WH: A vascular anomaly of the umbilical cord: The absence of one umbilical artery in the umbilical cords of normal and abnormal fetuses. Obstet Gynecol 6:399, 1955

Benirschke K, Dodds JP: Angiomyxoma of the umbilical cord with atrophy of an umbilical artery. Obstet Gynecol 30:99, 1967

Benirschke K, Driscoll SG (eds): The Pathology of the Human Placenta. New York, Springer-Verlag, 1974

Berkowitz RS, Goldstein DP, Bernstein MR: Management of nonmetastatic trophoblastic tumors. J Reprod Med 26:219, 1981

Block MF, Merrill JA: Hydatidiform mole with coexistent fetus. Obstet Gynecol 60:129, 1982

Brewer JI, Majur MT: Gestational choriocarcinoma: Its origin in the placenta during a seemingly normal pregnancy. Am J Surg Pathol 5:267, 1981

Bryan EM, Kohler HG: The missing umbilical artery. II. Paediatric follow-up. Arch Dis Child 50:714, 1975

Chun D, Braga C, Chow C, Lok L: Clinical observations on some aspects of hydatidiform moles. Br J Obstet Gynaecol 71:180, 1964

Curry SL, Hammond CB, Tyrey L, Creasman WT, Parker RT: Hydatidiform mole: Diagnosis, management, and long-time follow-up of 347 patients. Obstet Gynecol 45:1, 1975

Davis JR, Surwit EA, Garay JP, Fortier KJ: Sex assignment in gestational trophoblastic neoplasia. Am J Obstet Gynecol 148:722, 1984

Duenhoelter JH, Pritchard JA: Fetal respiration: Quantitative measurements of amnionic fluid inspired near term by human and rhesus fetuses. Am J Obstet Gynecol 125:306, 1976

Fox H: Pathology of the Placenta, Monograph. Philadelphia, Saunders, 1978, Vol 7

Freedman WL, MacMahon FJ: Placental metastasis: Review of the literature and report of a case of metastatic melanoma. Obstet Gynecol 16:550, 1960

Froehlich LA, Fujikura T: Follow-up infants with single umbilical artery. Pediatrics 52:22, 1973

Fijikura T, Klionsky B: The significance of meconium staining. Am J Obstet Gynecol 121:45, 1975

Goldstein DP: Prevention of gestational trophoblastic disease by use of antinomycin D in molar pregnancy. Obstet Gynecol 43:475, 1974

Greenberg P, Collins JD, Voet RL, Jariwala L: Ewing's sarcoma metastatic to the placenta. Placenta 3:191, 1982

Healey DL, Herington AC, O'Herlihy C: Chronic idiopathic polyhydramnios: Evidence for a defect in the chorion laeve receptor for lactogenic hormones. J Clin Endocrinal Metab 56:520, 1983

Hertig AT, Edmonds HW: Genesis of hydatidiform mole. Arch Pathol 30:260, 1940

Hertig AT, Mansell H: Tumors of the Female Sex Organs. I.

Hydatidiform Mole and Choriocarcinoma. Washington, D.C., Armed Forces Institute of Pathology, 1957

Hertig AT, Sheldon WH: Hydatidiform mole: A pathologico-clinical correlation of 200 cases. Am J Obstet Gynecol 53:1, 1947

Horner EN: Placental metastases. Case report: Maternal deaths from ovarian cancer. Obstet Gynecol 15:566, 1960

Jacobs PA, Szulman AE, Funkhowser J, Matsura JS, Wilson CC: Ann Hum Genet 46:223, 1982

Jequier AM, Winterton WR: Diagnostic problems of trophoblastic disease in women age 50 or more. Obstet Gynecol 42:378, 1975

Jolivet J, Cowan KH, Curt GA, Clendeninn NJ, Chabner BA: The pharmacology and clinical use of methotrexate. N Engl J Med 309:1094, 1983

Kan PS, Eastman NJ: Coiling of the umbilical cord around the foetal neck. Br J Obstet Gynaecol 64:227, 1957

Kouyoumdjian A: Velamentous insertion of the umbilical cord. Obstet Gynecol 56:737, 1980

Kruseman AC, Lent MV, Blom AH, Lauw GP: Choriocarcinoma in mother and child, identified by immunoenzyme histochemistry. Am J Clin Pathol 67:279, 1977

Lademacher DS, Vermeulen RCW, Harten JJVD, Arts NFT: Circumvallate placenta and congenital malformation. Lancet 1:732, 1981

Las Heras J, Harding PG, Haust MD: Recurrent bleeding associated with placenta membranacea partialis: Report of a case. Am J Obstet Gynecol 144:480, 1982

Lawler SD, Pickthall VJ, Fisher RA, Povey S, Evans MW, Szulman AE: Genetic studies of complete and partial hydatidiform moles. Lancet 2:580, 1979

Lewis JL Jr: Treatment of metastatic gestational trophoblastic neoplasms. Am J Obstet Gynecol 136:163, 1980

Li MC, Hertz R, Spencer DB: Effect of methotrexate therapy upon choriocarcinoma and chorioadenoma. Proc Soc Biol Med 93:361, 1956

Lind T, Hytten FE: Relation of amniotic fluid volume to fetal weight in the first half of pregnancy. Lancet 1:1147, 1970

Lurain JR, Brewer JI, Mazur MT, Torek EE: Fatal gestational trophoblastic disease: An analysis of treatment failures. Am J Obstet Gynecol 144:391, 1982

Lurain JR, Brewer JI, Torek EE, Halpern B: Natural history of hydatidiform mole after primary evacuation. Am J Obstet Gynecol 145:591, 1983

Mathieu A: Hydatidiform mole and chorio-epithelioma: Collective review of literature for years 1935, 1936, and 1937. Int Abstr Surg 68:52, 181, 1939

Miller ME, Higginbottom M, Smith DW: Short umbilical cord: Its origin and relevance. Pediatrics 67:618, 1981

Naeye RL, Blanc WA: Fetal renal structure and the genesis of amniotic fluid disorders. Am J Pathol 67:95, 1972

Natsume M, Takada J: Choriocarcinoma: An unusual case recurring nine years after subtotal hysterectomy and followed by spontaneous regression of pulmonary metastases. Am J Obstet Gynecol 82:654, 1961

Novak E, Seah CS: Choriocarcinoma of the uterus. Am J Obstet Gynecol 67:933, 1954

Peckham CH, Yerushalmy J: Aplasia of one umbilical artery: Incidence by race and certain obstetric factors. Obstet Gynecol 26:359, 1965

Pitkin RM: Acute polyhydramnios recurrent in successive pregnancies. Obstet Gynecol 48:425, 1976

Pritchard JA: Fetal swallowing and amniotic fluid volume. Obstet Gynecol 28:606, 1966

Queenan JT: Recurrent acute polyhydramnios. Am J Obstet Gynecol 106:625, 1970

Queenan JT, Gadow EC: Polyhydramnios: Chronic versus acute. Am J Obstet Gynecol 108:349, 1970

Rayburn WF, Beynen A, Brinkman DL: Umbilical cord length and intrapartum complications. Obstet Gynecol 57:450, 1981

Robinson LK, Jones KL, Benirschke K: The nature and structural defects associated with velamentous and marginal insertion of the umbilical cord. Am J Obstet Gynecol 146:191, 1983

Rustin GJS, Booth M, Dent J, Salt S, Rustin F, Bagshawe KD: Pregnancy after cytotoxic chemotheraphy for gestational trophoblastic tumours. Br Med J 288:103, 1984

Ruvinsky ED, Wiley TL, Morrison JC, Blake PG: In utero diagnosis of umbilical cord hematoma by ultrasonography. Am J Obstet Gynecol 140:833, 1981

Shane JM, Naftolin F: Abberant hormone activity by tumors of gynecologic importance. Am J Obstet Gynecol 121:133, 1975

Spellacy WN, Gravem H, Fisch RO: The umbilical cord complications of true knots, nuchal coils and cords around the body. Am J Obstet Gynecol 94:1136, 1966

Spirit BA, Cohen WN, Weinstein HM: The incidence of placental calcification in normal pregnancies. Radiology 142:707, 1982

Stanhope CR, Stuart GCE, Curtis KL: Primary ovarian hydatidiform mole: Review of the literature and report of a case. Am J Obstet Gynecol 145:886, 1983

Stone M, Dent J, Kardana A, Bagshawe KD: Relationship of oral contraception to development of trophoblastic tumor after evacuation of a hydatidiform mole. Br J Obstet Gynaecol 83:913, 1976

Suzuki M, Matsunobu A, Wakita K, Nishijima M, Osanai K: Hydatidiform mole with a surviving coexisting fetus. Obstet Gynecol 56:384, 1980

Szulman AE, Surti U, Berman M: Patient with partial mole requiring chemotherapy. Lancet 2:1099, 1978

Szulman AE, Wong LC, Hsu C: Residual trophoblastic disease in association with partial hydatidiform mole. Obstet Gynecol 57:392, 1981

Tindall R, Scott JS: Placenta calcification: A study of 3025 singleton and multiple pregnancies. Br J Obstet Gynaecol 72:356, 1965

Tow WSH: The classification of malignant growths of the chorion. Br J Obstet Gynaecol 73:1000, 1966

Wladimiroff JW, Barentsen R, Wallenburg HCS, Drogendijk AC: Fetal urine production in a case of diabetes associated with polyhydramnios. Obstet Gynecol 46:100, 1975

Wu FY: Recurrent hydatidiform mole: A case report of nine consecutive molar pregnancies. Obstet Gynecol 41:2000, 1973

Yuen BH, Burch P: Relationship of oral contraceptives and the intrauterine contraceptive devices to the regression of concentrations of the beta subunits of human chorionic gonadotropin and invasive complications after molar pregnancy. Am J Obstet Gynecol 145:214, 1983

24

Abortion

Abortion is the termination of pregnancy by any means before the fetus is sufficiently developed to survive. When abortion occurs spontaneously, the term *miscarriage* has been applied by laypersons.

U.S. Supreme Court Decision

Until the decision of the United States Supreme Court (Roe vs. Wade) in January, 1973, abortion in most states could be performed only to save the life of the mother and was referred to as *therapeutic abortion.* All non-therapeutic, induced abortions, therefore, were *criminal abortions.* Since the Supreme Court decision, *elective* or *voluntary abortion* performed at the request of the woman has emerged as the largest, by far, of the categories of abortion.

The Supreme Court decision voided the abortion statute of the State of Texas, but, as the consequence, nearly all state laws relative to abortion were affected. Moreover, the Court's decision went on explicitly to define the extent to which the States might regulate abortion:

> (a) For the stage prior to approximately the end of the first trimester, the abortion decision and its effectuation must be left to the medical judgment of the pregnant woman's attending physician.
>
> (b) For the stage subsequent to approximately the end of the first trimester, the State, in promoting its interest in the health of the mother, may, if it chooses, regulate the abortion procedures in ways that are reasonably related to maternal health.
>
> (c) For the stage subsequent to viability the State, in promoting its interest in the potential of human life, may, if it chooses, regulate, and even proscribe, abortion, except where necessary, in appropriate medical judgment, for the preservation of the life or health of the mother.

Viability

The term *viable* is widely used to identify a reasonable potential for subsequent survival if the fetus were to be removed from the uterus. Termination of pregnancy before 38 weeks gestation but after the fetus has achieved some potential for survival is referred to as preterm delivery of a premature infant. The gestational age at which the fetus upon delivery ceases to be an abortus and becomes an infant is most difficult to define. In many states, a birth certificate is prepared for any pregnancy at 20 weeks gestational age or more, or for any fetus that weighs 500 g or more.

The United States Supreme Court in its ruling on the legality of abortion used the term *viability* but did not define it. Moreover, the Court states,

> We need not resolve the difficult question of when life begins. When those trained in the respective disciplines of medicine, philosophy, and theology are unable to arrive at any consensus, the judiciary, at this point in the development of man's knowledge, is not in a position to speculate as to the answer.

The smallest surviving infant has been considered by some to be the one reported to Munro (1939). The infant was alleged to weigh about 400 g. The precision of measurement of the infant's weight on the village grocer's scales and the duration of gestation, which was said to be "2 months premature," are suspect. In very recent times infants have been reported, at least by newspapers and television, to have survived although their birth weight was somewhat less than 500 g (see Chapter 37, p. 749).

Infants that weigh 500 to 999 g are sometimes classified as *immature* rather than *premature,* although the degree of immaturity or prematurity should be based upon fetal age rather than weight. Although weight can be determined quite precisely, the duration of gestation at times cannot. Prematurity and fetal growth retardation are considered especially in Chapter 37.

SPONTANEOUS ABORTION

Incidence

The incidence of spontaneous abortion has commonly been quoted as 10 percent of all pregnancies (Tietze, 1953; United Nations, 1954). This figure has been derived from data that had at least two areas of instability, namely, failure to include early and therefore unrecognized abortions and the inclusion of illegally induced abortions that were claimed to be spontaneous.

The incidence of spontaneous abortion is difficult to determine precisely. First, agreement has to be reached as to when pregnancy actually begins. Does penetration of the ovum by a sperm constitute a pregnancy? Does cellular division of the fertilized ovum to form a blastocyst signal the onset of a pregnancy? Or does pregnancy begin with the invasion of the endometrium by the blastocyst? Second, the precision of the techniques that are used to identify a pregnancy are of obvious importance. With the use of a test that can detect minute amounts of human chorionic gonadotropin (hCG), the frequency of abortion will be higher than if the diagnosis is dependent upon histologic confirmation of shed trophoblast.

Most investigators have identified a substantial pregnancy loss very early in pregnancy. For example, Edmonds and associates (1982) identified small but significant amounts of hCG measured as beta subunit, in urine during 118 of 198 (60 percent) ovulatory cycles in healthy women who were attempting to conceive. However, 67 of the 118 early pregnancies, or nearly 60 percent, so identified failed before being recognized clinically. To the contrary, Whittaker and co-workers (1983), in an apparently similar study, reported only 8 percent of pregnancies identified by the presence of hCG were lost before the women were aware that conception has occurred.

Etiology

In the very early months of pregnancy, spontaneous expulsion of the ovum is nearly always preceded by death of the embryo or fetus. For this reason, etiologic considerations of early abortion involve ascertaining the cause of fetal death. In the subsequent months, on the contrary, the fetus frequently does not die in utero before expulsion and other explanations for its expulsion must be invoked. Fetal death may be caused by abnormalities in the ovum itself or in the generative tract, or by systemic disease of the mother, and, rarely perhaps, of the father.

Abnormal Development of Zygote

The most common morphologic finding in early spontaneous abortions is an abnormality of development of the embryo, the early fetus, or at times, the placenta. In an analysis of 1000 spontaneous abortions, Hertig and Sheldon (1943) observed pathologic ("blighted") ova in which the embryo was degenerated or absent in 49 percent (Fig. 24-1).

Poland and co-workers (1981) have morphologically identified disorganization of growth in 40 percent of abortuses (both embryos and fetuses) that were expelled spontaneously before 20 weeks of pregnancy. Among embryos (less than 30 mm crown–rump length), the frequency of abnormal morphologic development was 70 percent. Of the embryos on which tissue culture and chromosomal analyses were performed, 60 percent were demonstrated to have a chromosomal abnormality. For fetuses (30 to 180 mm crown–rump length) the frequency was 25 percent.

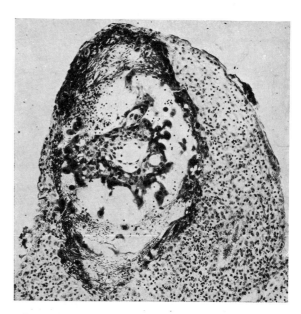

Figure 24-1. Abnormal ovum. A cross section of a defective ovum showing an empty chorionic sac embedded within a polypoid mass of endometrium. (*From Hertig and Rock: Am J Obstet Gynecol 47:149, 1944.*)

It is now appreciated that chromosomal abnormalities are common among embryos and early fetuses that are aborted spontaneously and account for much or most of early pregnancy wastage. From several studies it is apparent that 50 to 60 percent of early spontaneous abortions are associated with a chromosomal anomaly of the conceptus.

Abnormalities in the number of chromosomes are much more common than are structural abnormalities of chromosomes. Structural abnormalities can be transmitted by one of the parents who is a balanced chromosome carrier or the structural abnormality can arise de novo. The causes of the numeric errors include anomalous meiotic division of the gamete from either parent, dispermy at the time of fertilization, and abnormalities of early mitotic divisions.

With all of these numerical abnormalities of the chromosomes of the zygote, the parents most often have a normal chromosomal constitution. Monosomies, trisomies, and polypoidies are the most frequent abnormalities of number. Most monosomic zygotes are 45,X. The missing chromosome in monosomic zygotes is rarely an autosome, but the extra chromosome in trisomic zygotes is nearly always an autosome. It is apparent from the use of banding techniques that in early abortuses trisomies of all autosomes may be found, thus emphasizing the highly lethal nature of most autosomal trisomies.

Pregnancy destined to abort because of a chromosomally abnormal zygote may, on the one hand, go unrecognized because the products of conception are aborted with little or no delay in the onset of menstruation, or, on the other, may continue for some time after the embryo or early fetus has died. This latter phenomenon accounts for the markedly degenerated or absent embryo or early fetus commonly observed in the studies of Hertig and Sheldon referred to above.

The age of the gametes, sperm and egg may influence the spontaneous abortion rate. Guerrero and Rojas (1975) noted an increased incidence of abortion relative to successful pregnancies when insemination occurred 4 days before or 3 days after the time of shift in basal body temperature. They have concluded, therefore, that aging of the gametes within the female genital tract before fertilization increases the chance of abortion. Animal experiments have also shown that aging of spermatozoa and ova before fertilization is accompanied by an increased rate of abortion.

A suboptimal uterine environment, through its effects on implantation and early fetal nutrition, would be expected to lead to a defective conceptus. The appropriate hormonal control of tubal and uterine peristalsis, the multiple endocrine factors associated with appropriate maturation of the endometrium and formation of the decidua, the correct signal to and response of the blastocyst to implantation, and the cellular relation of trophoblast and endometrium must all be integrated to achieve nidation. It is remarkable that successful implantation occurs as often as it does. Immediately after implantation, furthermore, the trophoblast must obtain nutrition from the decidua and later tap maternal blood vessels, prior to the development of the villous circulation. If any of these mechanisms fail, survival of the ovum is jeopardized and abortion is likely to occcur.

Many factors may affect both the intrauterine environment and the embryo. Some are well recognized, such as radiation, viruses, and chemicals. Because they can also produce malformations, these factors are called *teratogens.*

Maternal Factors in Abortion

Structural chromosomal abnormalities in the mother and, in turn, the ovum, are considered subsequently. A variety of infectious diseases, chronic wasting diseases, endocrine abnormalities, nutritional deficiencies, alcohol and tobacco, deformity of the uterus or cervix, immunologic similarities and dissimilarities of the parents, and trauma—emotional as well as physical—have been implicated in abortion, although the evidence for such correlations has not always been convincing.

Infections. Some chronic infections have been either implicated or strongly suspected of causing abortion. In particular, *Brucella abortus,* well known as a cause of chronic abortion in cattle, has been implicated. Many investigators studied this organism and concluded that it has no significance in human abortion.

Listeria monocytogenes (Rappaport and colleagues, 1960) and *Toxoplasma* (Ruffolo and associates, 1962) can be etiologic agents in abortion, although they appear to be less important in this country than perhaps in other parts of the world. Presented in Figures 24-2A and 24-2B are sonograms that demonstrate a pregnancy lacking an embryo in a woman who had symptomatic *Listeriosis* proven by blood culture. She aborted spontaneously 5 days later.

The isolation of *Mycoplasma hominis* and *Ureaplasma urealyticum* (formerly called T mycoplasmas) from the genital tract of some women who have aborted

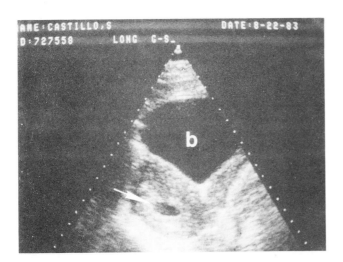

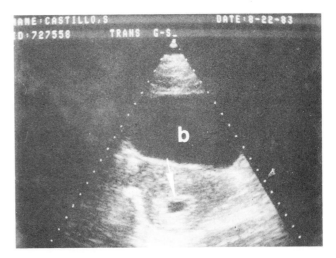

A   **B**

Figure 24-2. A. Longitudinal sector scan 7 weeks after the last menstrual period showing a gestational sac (*arrow*) devoid of any evidence of an embryo (b = bladder). *Listeria monocytogenes* was cultured from the blood of the febrile patient. **B.** Transverse sector scan demonstrating the same empty gestational sac (*arrow*) shown in A (b = bladder). She aborted spontaneously 5 days later. (*Courtesy of Dr. R. Santos.*)

has led to the hypothesis that mycoplasma infections involving the genital tract may be abortifacient. Serologic evidence supportive of a role for the organisms in the genesis of abortion has been provided by Quinn and co-workers (1983). They have also reported improvement in pregnancy outcome following treatment with erythromycin especially. Their success rate, however, of 83 to 85 percent is similar to what has been achieved repeatedly with widely varied treatment regimens.

Syphilis was formerly considered to be a common cause of abortion, but syphilis rarely, if ever, causes an abortion.

Chronic Debilitating Diseases.

In early pregnancy, chronic wasting diseases such as tuberculosis or carcinomatosis seldom have caused abortion; the patient often died undelivered. In later pregnancy, premature labor may be induced by severe systemic maternal illness. Hypertension is seldom associated with abortion before 20 weeks gestation, but rather may lead to fetal death and to premature delivery. Maternal diabetes has been found by some, but not others, to predispose to spontaneous abortion.

Endocrine Defects.

Abortion has often been attributed, perhaps without adequate reason, to deficient secretion of progesterone by first the corpus luteum and then the trophoblast. Since progesterone maintains the decidua, its relative deficiency would theoretically interfere with nutrition of the conceptus and thus contribute to its death.

It has been suggested that abnormal levels of one or more hormones might help to forecast abortion or even serve as therapeutic guides. Today, however, it is believed that, even though the values may be low or may fail to rise, the levels of chorionic gonadotropin (except perhaps very early), placental lactogen, progesterone, estrogens, and thyroid hormone are not of great clinical utility in predicting the outcome of a particular pregnancy or of any value in determining hormone replacement therapy. Reduced levels of these hormones usually are the consequence rather than the cause of irreversible damage to the fetoplacental unit (Salem and co-workers, 1984).

Nutrition.

At this time, it appears most likely that only very severe general malnutrition predisposes to increased likelihood of abortion. There is no conclusive evidence, however, that dietary deficiency of any one nutrient or moderate deficiency of all nutrients is an important cause of abortion. The nausea and vomiting that develop rather commonly during early pregnancy, and any inanition so induced, rarely are followed by spontaneous abortion. In fact, the reverse is more likely to be true (see Chapter 13, p. 261).

Most of micronutrients have been reported at one time or another to appear to have been of value in reducing the risk of spontaneous abortion. However, the evidence presented in support of such claims has been weak to nonexistent.

Alcohol and Tobacco.

Women who smoke have been identified to abort spontaneously more often than women who do not (Harlap and Shiono, 1980; Kline and associates, 1977).

Similarly, alcohol has been implicated in increasing the risk of spontaneous abortion even when consumed "in moderation" (Harlap and Shiono, 1980; Kline and co-workers, 1980). It may be that some of the risk of spontaneous abortion attributed to smoking was the consequence of alcohol also consumed during the pregnancy.

Immunologic Factors.

Both antigenic similarities and dissimilarities between sexual partners have been implicated by some as the genesis of spontaneous abortion. For example, women with antibodies against sperm have been reported not only to fail frequently to conceive, but also, when they do conceive, to abort much more often.

Although maternal isoimmunization and subsequent fetal–maternal Rh incompatibility may cause stillbirth from erythroblastosis, these events only occasionally lead to late abortion. An increase of questionable significance in the frequency of abortions among ABO-incompatible matings has been reported but not confirmed.

It has also been claimed that women who share an unusually large number of major antigens of the histocompatibility complex with their sex partners abort much more often (Beer and co-workers, 1981, 1984). The mechanism proposed is that blocking antibodies formed in response to paternal antigens are not synthesized by the mother sufficiently to protect the embryo and fetus against maternal lymphocytes. Beer and co-workers have been attempting immunization of such women using repeated injections of paternal lymphocytes intradermally. These attempts at therapy are experimental.

Laparotomy.

The trauma of laparotomy may occasionally provoke abortion. In general, the nearer the site of surgery is to the pelvic organs, the more likely is abortion to occur. Ovarian cysts and pedunculated myomas may, however, be removed during pregnancy most often without interfering with the gestation. Peritonitis increases the likelihood of abortion. The administration of progesterone or other progestational agents for the first week or 10 days after operation have been prescribed to diminish the probability of abortion, although the efficacy of these agents remains questionable.

Abnormalities of the Reproductive Organs.

Local abnormalities and disease of the generative tract are infrequent causes of abortion. Adnexal chronic inflammation and tumors of the uterus may result in sterility but rarely cause abortion.

Even large and multiple *myomas* of the uterus do not necessarily cause abortion. The location of the myoma in relation to the endometrium is more important in this regard than the size of the tumor. Submucous, but not intramural or subserous, myomas are likely to cause abortion. Uterine myomas can be regarded as the etiologic factor in abortion only if the remainder of the clinical investigation, including evaluation of the abortus, is negative and the hysterogram demonstrates a true deformity of the endometrial cavity. Myomectomy to remove an offending submucous myoma may weaken the uterus to the extent that rupture may ensue during a subsequent pregnancy, especially with labor. The only sure way to judge the behavior of a myoma in pregnancy is to allow a clinical test.

An important lesion of the generative tract in contributing to abortion is the *incompetent cervix,* discussed further on page 475.

Uncomplicated displacements of the uterus should not cause abortion. *Incarceration of the uterus* in the pelvis, however, may culminate in late abortion unless the uterus is freed from the pelvis (see Chapter 25, p. 499).

Faulty müllerian duct development, either idiopathic or from intrauterine exposure to stilbestrol, may result in increased frequency of abortion (see Chapter 25, p. 497).

Physical and Emotional Trauma. Both physicians and laymen are inclined to seek a simple explanation for commonplace medical phenomena. They may relate the abortion to a recent fall or blow or perhaps a fright. Multiple examples of trauma that failed to interrupt the pregnancy are forgotten. Only the particular event apparently related temporally to the abortion is remembered. Most spontaneous abortions, however, occur some time after death of the embryo or fetus. If abortion were caused typically by trauma, it would likely not be a very recent accident but an event that had occurred some weeks before the abortion, as a rule.

In a review of personality factors associated with habitual abortion, Tupper and Weil (1962) found that there were two types: the basically immature woman and the independent, frustrated woman. Results suggest that supportive therapy is as effective—or as ineffective—as anything else in preventing subsequent pregnancy loss.

Paternal Factors

Even less is known about the role of the paternal factors in the genesis of spontaneous abortion. Certainly, chromosome translocations in sperm can lead to a zygote with too little or too much chromosomal material, resulting in abortion.

Pathology

Hemorrhage into the decidua basalis and necrotic changes in the tissues adjacent to the bleeding usually accompany abortion. The ovum becomes detached in part or whole and, presumably acting as a foreign body in the uterus, stimulates uterine contractions that result in expulsion. When the sac is opened, fluid is commonly found surrounding a small macerated fetus, or, alternatively, there may be no visible fetus in the sac, the so-called *blighted ovum.* Visualized through the dissecting microscope, the placental villi often appear thick and

distended with fluid, the ends of the villous branches resembling little sausage-shaped sacs. Such fluid-filled villi are undergoing molar degeneration with the imbibition of tissue fluid (Chapter 23, p. 446).

Blood or carneous mole is an ovum that is surrounded by a capsule of clotted blood. The capsule is of varying thickness, with degenerated chorionic villi scattered through it. The small, fluid-containing cavity within appears compressed and distorted by the thick walls of old blood clot. This type of specimen is associated with an abortion that occurs rather slowly, so that blood is allowed to collect between the decidua and chorion and to coagulate and form layers.

Tuberous mole and *tuberous subchorial hematoma of the decidua* are names applied to the same lesion. The characteristic feature is a grossly nodular amnion resulting from its elevation by localized hematomas of varying size between the amnion and the chorionic membranes.

In abortions occurring after the fetus has attained considerable size, several outcomes are possible. The retained fetus may undergo *maceration.* In such circumstances, the bones of the skull collapse, the abdomen becomes distended with a bloodstained fluid, and the entire fetus takes on a dull reddish color. At the same time, the skin softens and peels off in utero or at the slightest touch, leaving behind the corium. The internal organs degenerate and necrose, becoming friable and losing their capacity for taking up the usual histologic stains. The amnionic fluid may be absorbed when the fetus becomes compressed upon itself and desiccated to form a *fetus compressus* (Fig. 24-3). Occasionally, the fetus eventually becomes so dry and compressed that it resembles parchment, the so-called *fetus papyraceus.* This

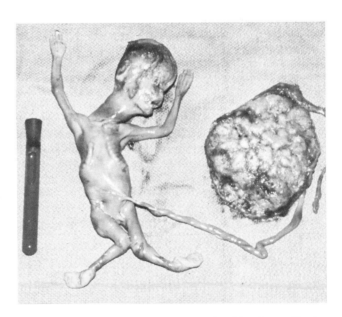

Figure 24-3. Immature fetus retained dead in utero with placenta for many weeks. Characteristic thick, opaque amnionic fluid is contained in the stoppered tube.

latter outcome is relatively frequent in twin pregnancy, if one fetus has died at an early period and the other has gone on to full development.

CATEGORIES OF SPONTANEOUS ABORTION

It is convenient to consider the clinical aspects of spontaneous abortion under five subgroups: threatened, inevitable, incomplete, missed, and habitual abortion.

Threatened Abortion

A threatened abortion is presumed when any bloody vaginal discharge or vaginal bleeding appears during the first half of pregnancy. A threatened abortion may or may not be accompanied by mild cramping pain resembling that of a menstrual period or by low backache. This definition of threatened abortion makes it an extremely commonplace occurrence, since one out of four or five pregnant women have vaginal spotting or heavier bleeding during the early months of gestation. Of those women who so bleed in early pregnancy, one half or even less actually abort. The bleeding of threatened abortion is frequently slight, but it may persist for days or weeks. Unfortunately, an increased risk of suboptimal pregnancy outcome in the form of prematurity, low birth weight, and perinatal death persists (Funderburk and colleagues, 1980; Batzofin and associates, 1984). However, the risk of birth of a malformed infant does not appear to be increased significantly.

Some bleeding about the time of expected menses may be physiologic, analogous to the *placental sign* described by Hartman (1929) in the rhesus monkey. In these animals, there is always at least microscopic bleeding. The blood apparently makes its way from ruptured blood vessels and eroded uterine epithelium into the uterine cavity. Bleeding begins most commonly 17 days after conception, or about 4½ weeks after the last menses. In many of Hartman's animals, this bleeding could be observed grossly for several days. In the woman, furthermore, lesions of the cervix are likely to bleed in early pregnancy, especially postcoitum. Polyps presenting at the external cervical os as well as decidual reaction in the cervix tend to bleed in early gestation. Lower abdominal pain and persistent low backache does not accompany bleeding from these causes.

Since most physicians consider any bleeding in early pregnancy to be indicative of threatened abortion, any treatment of so-called threatened abortion has considerable likelihood of apparent success. Most women who are in fact actually threatening to abort probably progress into the next stage of the process no matter what is done. If, however, the bleeding is attributable to one of the unrelated causes mentioned above, it is likely to disappear, regardless of treatment.

Inevitable Abortion

Inevitability of abortion is signaled by gross rupture of the membranes in the presence of cervical dilatation. Under these conditions, abortion is almost certain. Rarely, a gush of fluid from the uterus occurs during the first half of pregnancy without serious consequence. The fluid may have previously collected between the amnion and chorion to escape with rupture of the chorion while the initial defect in the amnion has completely healed. Most often, however, either uterine contractions begin promptly, resulting in expulsion of the products of conception, or infection develops.

Incomplete Abortion

The fetus and placenta are likely to be expelled together in abortions occurring before the tenth week, but separately thereafter. When the placenta, in whole or in part, is retained in the uterus, bleeding ensues sooner or later, to produce the main sign of incomplete abortion. With abortions of pregnancies that are more advanced, bleeding is often profuse and may occasionally be massive to the point of producing profound hypovolemia. If the placenta is partly attached and partly separated, the splint-like action of the attached portion of the placenta interferes with myometrial contraction in the immediate vicinity. The vessels in the denuded segment of the placental site, deprived of the constriction provided by the contraction and retraction of the myometrium, bleed profusely.

Missed Abortion

A missed abortion refers to the prolonged retention of a fetus who died during the first half of pregnancy. A missed abortion has been defined as the retention of dead products of conception in utero for 8 weeks or more. The rationale for a time period of 8 weeks as the sine qua non for the diagnosis of a missed abortion is not clear. It certainly serves no useful clinical purpose. In the typical instance, early pregnancy appears to be normal, with amenorrhea, nausea and vomiting, breast changes, and growth of the uterus. Upon death of the ovum there may or may not be vaginal bleeding or other symptoms denoting a threatened abortion. For a time, the uterus then seems to remain stationary in size but usually the mammary changes regress. The patient is likely to lose a few pounds in weight. Thereafter, from careful palpation and measurement of the uterus, it becomes apparent that it has not only ceased to enlarge but is becoming smaller, as result of absorption of amnionic fluid and maceration of the fetus. Many patients have no symptoms during the period except persistent amenorrhea. If the missed abortion terminates spontaneously, and most do, the process of expulsion is quite the same as in any ordinary abortion. The product, if retained several weeks after fetal death, is a shriveled sac containing a greatly macerated embryo (Fig. 24-2).

Occasionally, after prolonged retention of the dead products of conception, serious coagulation defects develop, especially when the gestation had reached the second trimester before the fetus died. The woman may note troublesome bleeding from the nose or gums and especially from sites of slight trauma. The pathogenesis and treatment of the coagulation defects and any attendant hemorrhage in instances of prolonged retention of a dead fetus are considered in Chapter 21 (p. 412).

The reason why some abortions do not terminate after death of the fetus, while others do, is not clear. The use of more potent progestational compounds to treat threatened abortion, however, may contribute to a missed abortion. For example, Piver and colleagues (1967) treated 57 women for threatened abortion with Depo-Provera (injectable medroxyprogesterone acetate), following which more than one third of the women retained a dead fetus for more than 8 weeks. Moreover, Smith and co-workers (1978) observed that 73 percent of women who were given hormonal support because they threatened to abort did abort, but on the average 20 days later, whereas 67 percent of those who received no hormonal support aborted on the average 5 days later. They concluded that the progestational agents did not improve the outcome in threatened abortion. Instead, the hormones only prolonged the problem by delaying the inevitable.

Habitual Abortion

Repeated spontaneous abortion, its diagnosis, and possible treatment, are considered below.

TREATMENTS

Threatened Abortion

The woman should be instructed to notify her physician immediately whenever vaginal bleeding occurs during pregnancy. If the bleeding is slight, and no cause is ascertained through careful inspection of the vagina and cervix, she should be so informed. If an intrauterine device is still present and the "string" is visible, the device should be removed for the reasons cited in Chapter 40 (p. 822).

Usually, but not always, bleeding begins first, and cramping abdominal pain follows a few hours to several days later. The pain of abortion may be anterior and clearly rhythmic, simulating mild labor; it may be a persistent low backache, associated with a feeling of pelvic pressure; or it may be a dull, midline, suprasymphyseal discomfort, accompanied by a tenderness over the uterus. Whichever form the pain takes, the prognosis for continuation of the pregnancy in the presence of bleeding and pain is poor. However, in some women with pain who threaten to abort, the bleed ceases, the pain resolves, and a normal pregnancy results. It may therefore be reasonable not to intervene to complete the abortion

if the woman desires to continue the pregnancy. Little immediate harm should occur, but it is important to remember that the higher perinatal mortality rates are observed in women whose pregnancies were complicated early by threatened abortion.

Each woman should be examined thoroughly, for there is always the possibility that the cervix is already dilated and that abortion is inevitable, or that there is a serious complication such as extrauterine pregnancy or torsion of an unsuspected ovarian cyst. The patient may be kept at home in bed with analgesia to help relieve the pain, but, in general, if the symptoms are more severe, she should be hospitalized. If the bleeding persists, she must be reexamined and the hemoglobin concentration or hematocrit should be rechecked. If blood loss is sufficient to cause anemia, evacuation of the products of conception is generally indicated. If bleeding is so great as to cause hypovolemia, termination of the pregnancy is mandatory.

Women threatened with abortion have been treated by some physicians with progesterone intramuscularly or with a wide variety of synthetic progestational agents orally or intramuscularly. Some of the progestins, particularly those structurally related to testosterone, may result in virilization of the female fetus. Of even greater importance is the lack of evidence of effectiveness of progestational agents in preventing most abortions. "Success" from their use often is no more than a missed abortion, as already described. Even in a group of habitual aborters who excreted low levels of pregnanediol, indicating impaired progesterone production, Goldzieher (1964), in a well-controlled study, could not demonstrate a beneficial effect of exogenous progestational agents.

Occasionally, in threatened abortion, slight hemorrhage may persist for weeks. It then becomes essential to decide whether there is any possibility of continuation of the pregnancy. If quantitative measurements of chorionic gonadotropin over several days do not demonstrate an increase in concentration, the outlook is *almost* hopeless. Importantly, the presence of chorionic gonadotropin in blood or urine does not indicate whether the fetus is alive or dead. If the uterus, when accurately measured over a period of time, does not increase in size, or becomes smaller, it is safe to conclude that the fetus is dead. An increase in uterine size indicates that the fetus is still alive or that a hydatidiform mole is present (see Chapter 23, p. 446).

The demonstration by sonography of a distinct, well-formed gestational ring with central echoes from the embryo implies that the products of conception are reasonably healthy. A gestational sac with no central echoes from an embryo or fetus implies, but does not prove, death of the conceptus (Fig. 24-2). When abortion is inevitable, the mean diameter of gestational sac is frequently smaller than appropriate for the gestational age. Moreover, at 9 to 10 weeks gestation and thereafter fetal heart action should be discernible using real-time ultrasound. Most often, a single examination is insufficient, however, to determine the likelihood of abortion. Serial sonographic observations to document lack of fetal growth are essential. After death of conceptus, the uterus should be emptied. Some women may elect abortion, which is their privilege according to the U.S. Supreme Court, before it is absolutely certain that the fetus is dead, rather than face further uncertainty and procrastination.

If bleeding and pain persist unabated for 6 hours, it is probably best to face the inevitability of abortion and either perform a dilation and curettage during the first 14 weeks of pregnancy, or, if much more advanced, encourage its completion by stimulating uterine contractions with oxytocin or a prostaglandin until the bulk of the products of conception are expelled. All tissue passed should be carefully studied to determine whether the abortion is complete as well as to try to ascertain whether the abortion is related to defective germ plasm or to some factor that has caused the uterus to empty itself of a normal ovum. Unless all of the fetus and placenta can be positively identified, curettage is most often indicated.

Inevitable Abortion

With obvious gross rupture of the membranes during the first half of pregnancy, the possibility of salvaging the pregnancy is very unlikely. If in early pregnancy the sudden discharge of fluid, suggesting rupture of the membranes, occurs before any pain or bleeding, the woman may be put to bed and observed for further leakage of fluid, bleeding, cramping, or fever. If after 48 hours there has been no further escape of amnionic fluid, no bleeding or pain, and no fever, she may get up and, except for any form of vaginal penetration, continue her usual activities. If, however, the gush of fluid is accompanied or followed by bleeding and pain, or if fever ensues, abortion should be considered inevitable and the uterus emptied.

Incomplete Abortion

In instances of incomplete abortion, it is often unnecessary to dilate the cervix before curettage. In many cases, the retained placental tissue simply lies loose in the cervical canal and can be lifted from an exposed external os with ovum or ring forceps. The suction curettage technique, as described subsequently, is effective for evacuating the uterus, especially if the procedure is to be performed with only local cervical anesthesia and moderate systemic analgesia such as meperidine. A woman with a more advanced pregnancy or who is actively bleeding should be hospitalized and the retained tissue removed without delay. Hemorrhage from incomplete abortion is occasionally severe but rarely fatal. Treatment of such hemorrhage is described in Chapter 21 (p. 391). Fever is not a contraindication to curettage once appropriate antibiotic treatment has been started (see Septic Abortion, p. 484).

Missed Abortion

Because of the risks involved in terminating by dilatation and curettage a missed abortion in which the fetus did not die until well after the first trimester, the treatment formerly was expectant. This method of management is emotionally trying for the woman and her relatives. Moreover, procrastination sometimes leads to coagulation defects (see Chapter 21, p. 412). Other techniques for evacuation the fetus and placenta well beyond the first trimester at the time of death are described in Chapter 21 (p. 414) and below.

Habitual Spontaneous Abortion

Habitual spontaneous abortion has been defined by various criteria of number and sequence, but probably the most generally accepted definition today refers to three or more consecutive spontaneous abortions.

Repeated spontaneous abortions are likely to be chance phenomena in the majority of cases. Support for this view is provided by the observation that in the past the employment of any of a great variety of unrelated but presumed therapeutic modalities were followed by a successful pregnancy outcome 70 to 90 percent of the time.

It is important to differentiate spontaneous abortions that result from problems within the zygote from those much less common abortions that are due to maternal factors. In early abortions there is likely to be a nonrecurring cytogenetic abnormality of the conceptus that is responsible for the abortion. In late abortions fetal development is more likely to have been normal with a maternal abnormality causing the abortion. Boué and Boué (1978) have described the mean incidence of spontaneous abortion for all known pregnancies to be 15 percent. According to their observation, when the first pregnancy is a spontaneous abortion, the likelihood of the next pregnancy culminating in a spontaneous abortion is 15 percent, irrespective of the karyotype of the first abortus.

Several investigators now recommend karyotyping the parents after they have experienced two or three spontaneous abortions. When karyotyping is performed, chromosomal banding techniques should be applied.

Most of the proposed (but not necessarily proven) causes of spontaneous habitual abortion are considered in the section Spontaneous Abortion, Etiology (p. 468).

Prognosis. With the exception of the incompetent cervix, the apparent cure rate after as many as three spontaneous abortions will range between 70 and 85 percent no matter what treatment is used, unless the treatment is abortifacient. In other words, the loss rate will be higher, but not a great deal higher, than that anticipated for pregnancies in general.

There is no evidence that the woman who has habitually aborted spontaneously is at greatly increased risk, when she finally carries her pregnancy to term, of having an abnormal child.

INCOMPETENT CERVIX

Definition

The term incompetent cervix is applied to a rather discrete obstetric entity. It is characterized by painless dilatation of the cervix in the second trimester or early in the third trimester of pregnancy, with prolapse of membranes through the cervix and ballooning of the membranes into the vagina, followed by rupture of the membranes and subsequent expulsion of a fetus that is so immature that it is likely to succumb. Unless effectively treated, this same sequence of events tends to repeat itself in each pregnancy. Thus the presumptive diagnosis can usually be made if a woman has experienced spontaneous rupture of membranes and appreciable cervical dilatation without the usual discomfort of labor.

Etiology

Although the cause of cervical incompetence is obscure, previous trauma to the cervix, especially in the course of dilatation and curettage, conization, cauterization, or amputation, appears to be a factor in many cases. In other instances, abnormal cervical development, including that following exposure to stilbestrol in utero (p. 471), plays a role.

The cervical dilatation characteristic of this condition seldom becomes prominent before the 16th week, since before that time the products of conception are not sufficiently large to efface and dilate the cervix except when there are painful uterine contractions. Abortion from incompetence of the cervix is an entirely different and distinct entity from spontaneous abortion in the first trimester, since it results from different factors, presents a different clinical picture, and requires different management. Whereas spontaneous abortion in the first trimester is an extremely common complication of pregnancy, incompetence of the cervix is relatively rare.

Treatment

The treatment of the apparently incompetent cervix is surgical. The surgical treatment consists of reinforcing the weak cervix by some kind of purse-string suture. It is best performed after the first trimester but before cervical dilatation of 4 cm is reached, if possible. Bleeding and uterine contractions are contraindications to surgery.

Cerclage Procedures. Two main types of operation are in current use during pregnancy. One is a very simple procedure as recommended by McDonald (1963) and illustrated in Figure 24-4. The other is the more complicated Shirodkar operation (1955). There is less trauma and blood loss with the McDonald procedure during placement of the suture than with the Shirodkar procedure.

Success rates approaching 85 to 90 percent are being achieved with both the McDonald and the Shirodkar techniques (Kuhn and Pepperell, 1977). The success rate has been higher when cervical dilatation was slight and prolapse of the membranes was minimal to absent. This is due, in part at least, to the fact that some cases so treated were not truly cases of cervical incompetence.

Charles and Edwards (1981) have identified complications, especially infection, to be much less frequent when cerclage was performed by 18 weeks gestation. When cerclage was done much after 20 weeks there was a high incidence of premature rupture of the membranes, chorioamnionitis, and intrauterine infection. No evidence has been presented that the use of antibiotics around the time of the procedure reduces the risk of infection. Any suggestion of infection (fever, uterine tenderness, fetal or maternal tachycardia) should be investigated. They recommend amniocentesis to substantiate a diagnosis of chorioamnionitis before antibiotic therapy. With clinical infection, the suture should be cut and the uterus emptied.

There is no good evidence that prophylactic antibiotics to try to prevent infection, or either progestational agents or beta mimetic drugs to try to prevent uterine contractions, are of any adjunctive value (Thomason and co-workers, 1982). In the event that the operation fails and signs of imminent abortion or delivery develop, it is urgent that the suture be released at once, since failure to do so promptly may result in grave sequelae. Rupture of the uterus or the cervix may be the consequence of vigorous uterine contractions with the ligature in place. If the membranes rupture in the absence of labor, the likelihood of serious infection in the fetus or the mother is increased appreciably if the suture is left in situ and delivery is delayed (Kuhn and Pepperell, 1977).

Following the Shirodkar operation the suture can be left in place if it remains covered by mucosa, and cesarean section can be performed near term (a plan designed to prevent the necessity of repeating the cerclage procedure in subsequent pregnancies). Otherwise, the Shirodkar suture is released and vaginal delivery is permitted.

Treatment of an incompetent cervix by transabdominal cerclage placed at the level of the uterine isthmus has been recommended in some instances (Olsen and Tobiassen, 1982). The procedure requires laparotomy for placement of the suture and another laparotomy for its removal or for delivery of the pregnancy products or both. We have had no personal experience with this operation. Obviously, the potential for trauma, initially and subsequently, is very much greater with this procedure than with the McDonald procedure.

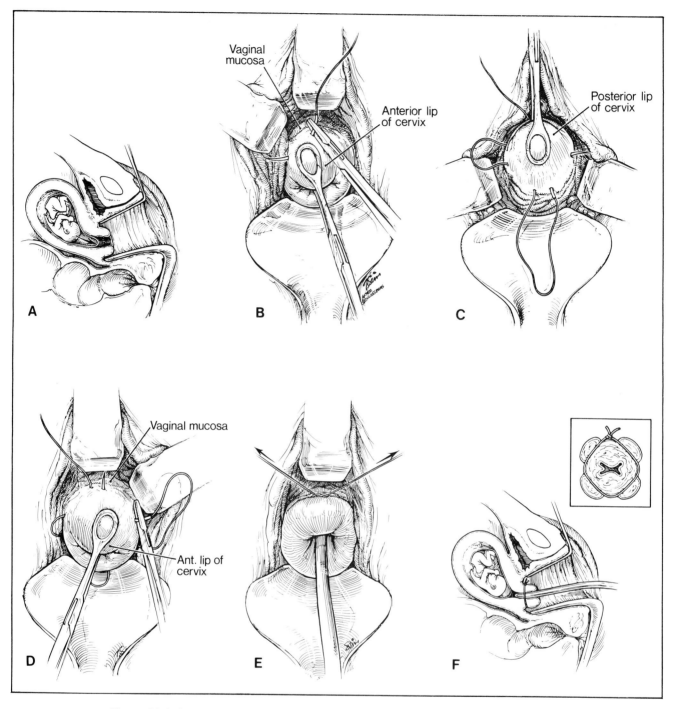

Figure 24-4. Incompetent cervix treated with McDonald cerclage procedure. **A.** Somewhat dilated cervical canal and beginning prolapse of membranes (*arrow*). **B.** Start of the cerclage procedure with a suture of number 2 monofilament proline being placed superiorly in the body of the cervix very near the level of the internal os. **C.** Continuation of the placement of the suture in the body of the cervix so as to encircle the os. **D.** Completion of encirclement. **E.** The suture is tightened around the cervical canal sufficiently to reduce the diameter of the canal to a few mm and is then securely tied. In the illustration the *small* dilator has been placed just through the level of ligation to maintain patency of the canal when the suture is tied. A second suture similarly placed but somewhat higher may be of value especially if the first is not in close proximity to the internal os. **F.** The effect of the suture placement on the cervical canal is apparent.

THERAPEUTIC ABORTION

Definition

The following definition of therapeutic abortion would appear to be acceptable to the majority of individuals, as well as being medically rational: Therapeutic abortion is *the termination of pregnancy before the time of fetal viability for the purpose of safeguarding the health of the mother.*

Legal Aspects

Until the United States Supreme Court decision of 1973 only therapeutic abortions could be legally performed in most states. The most common legal definition of therapeutic abortion until then was termination of pregnancy before the period of fetal viability for the purpose of saving the *life* of the mother. Not too long before the Supreme Court decision, a few states extended the law to read "to prevent serious or permanent bodily injury to the mother" or "to preserve the life or health of the woman." A very few states allowed abortion if the pregnancy otherwise was likely to result in the birth of an infant with grave malformation.

Contrary to popular belief, the stringent abortion laws that were in effect until 1973 were of fairly recent origin. Abortion before quickening (the term applied to the first definite perception of fetal movement, which most often occurs between 16 and 20 weeks of gestation), was either lawful or widely tolerated in both the United States and Great Britain until 1803. In that year, as part of a general restructuring of British criminal law, a basic criminal abortion statute was enacted that made abortion before quickening illegal. The Roman Catholic Church's traditional condemnation of abortion did not receive the ultimate sanction of universal law (excommunication) until 1869 (Pilpel and Norwich, 1969).

The British law of 1803 became the model for similar laws in the United States, but it was not until 1821 that Connecticut enacted the nation's first abortion law. Subsequently, throughout the nation abortion became illegal except to save the life of the mother. Since therapeutic abortion *to save the life of the woman* is rarely necessary or definable, it follows that the great majority of such operations previously performed in this country went beyond the letter of the law.

Indications

Some of the indications for therapeutic abortion are discussed with the diseases that commonly have led to the operation. A well-documented indication is persistent heart disease in the wake of previous cardiac decompensation. Another commonly accepted indication is advanced hypertensive vascular disease. Still another is invasive carcinoma of the cervix. Although it is impossible to predict what the future acceptable indications for therapeutic abortion will be, the therapeutic abortion policy formerly established by the American College of Obstetricians and Gynecologists seems most rational:

Therapeutic abortion may be performed for the following medical indications:

1. When continuation of the pregnancy may threaten the life of the woman or seriously impair her health. In determining whether or not there is such a risk to health, account may be taken of the woman's total environment, actual or reasonably foreseeable.
2. When pregnancy has resulted from rape or incest. In this case the same medical criteria should be employed in the evaluation of the patient.
3. When continuation of the pregnancy is likely to result in the birth of a child with severe physical deformities or mental retardation.

ELECTIVE (VOLUNTARY) ABORTION

Definition

Elective or voluntary abortion is the interruption of pregnancy before viability at the request of the women but not for reasons of impaired maternal health or fetal disease. The great majority of abortions now being done belong in this category. In 1983 nearly 1.3 million elective abortions were performed in the United States. That same year there were 3.6 million live births.

Legality

The legality of elective abortion was established by the United States Supreme Court in its decision in the case of Roe vs. Wade, discussed earlier on page 467. The pregnant woman, Ms. Roe, attempted to obtain an abortion in Texas in 1969, where the performance of any abortion was illegal by state law except when done to save the life of the mother. Ms. Roe's pregnancy was the consequence of a gang rape. In spite of millions of abortions that have been performed subsequently as the consequence of the Supreme Court ruling, Ms. Roe's pregnancy was not aborted. In fact, at the time of the Supreme Court decision the child was 4 years old.

The tenth anniversary of the Supreme Court decision of Roe vs. Wade served to emphasize the disagreement that persists in this country over abortion. On the tenth anniversary an estimated 26,000 people opposed to abortion marched past the White House in Washington, D.C. President Reagan was seen and heard widely through the news media to state that he considered the United States Supreme Court decision to be a tragedy and that he favored a constitutional amendment banning abortion. It can be assumed, at least, that the great majority of the millions of women who underwent elective abortion during that decade, as well as many others, have views quite contrary to those stated by the President. Ms. Roe a decade after the decision worked as a house painter in Dallas and Mr. Wade continued to be the Dallas District Attorney.

Attempts have been made by the passage of several local and state laws to obstruct the woman's constitutional right to reach and carry out decisions with her

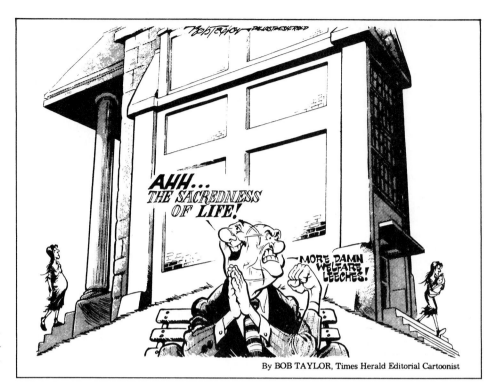

AHH...
THE SACREDNESS
OF LIFE!

MORE DAMN
WELFARE
LEECHES!

By BOB TAYLOR, Times Herald Editorial Cartoonist

Figure 24-5. A problem in desperate need of resolution. (*Courtesy of Bob Taylor and the* Dallas Times Herald.)

physician concerning abortion. However, the United States Supreme Court in 1983 reaffirmed the decision reached in Roe vs. Wade and declared most of such laws unconstitutional.

The opponents and proponents of elective abortion are influenced by a wide range of issues—ethical, moral, legal, and even the issue of national security. For example, Mumford (1982), after citing several internationally prominent political and military figures, concluded as follows: (1) world population growth is a threat to the security of all nations, (2) abortion is essential to effective control of population growth, (3) abortion is a national security issue, and (4) as availability of legal abortion in the United States grows, so does the availability of abortion in the developing world.

Whatever the feelings of the individual concerning abortion, the paradoxical, yet all too common, attitudes concerned with birth of another human being, and so clearly presented in Figure 24-5, must be resolved. If a child is to be born, means for providing appropriate care for that child *before and after* birth must be readily available. Fortunately, there are techniques for avoiding the birth of an unwanted child that are much more acceptable to most of us than is abortion. Hopefully, the opponents of abortion will support programs for providing effective contraception, and thereby avoid abortion, as discussed in Chapter 40. Unfortunately, strong opponents of abortion, all too frequently, have also opposed the dissemination and application of effective contraceptive techniques.

Counseling Before Elective Abortion

In some instances, the pregnant woman may well want to avoid abortion and allow the pregnancy to continue if social and economic problems can be resolved. Especially in these circumstances, knowledgeable, compassionate counselors are of great value.

TECHNIQUES FOR ABORTION

The various techniques for performing abortion currently in use are outlined and discussed below:

Techniques for Accomplishing Abortion

I. *Surgical*
    A. Cervical dilatation and evacuation of uterine contents
        1. Curettage
        2. Vacuum aspiration (suction curettage)
    B. Laparotomy
        1. Hysterotomy
        2. Hysterectomy
II. *Medical*
    A. Oxytocin intravenously
    B. Intra-amnionic hyperosmotic fluids
        1. 20 percent saline
        2. 30 percent urea
    C. Prostaglandins E_2, $F_{2\alpha}$, and prostaglandin analogues

1. Intra-amnionic injection
2. Extraovular injection
3. Vaginal insertions
4. Parenteral injection
5. Oral ingestion
D. Various combinations of the above

SURGICAL

The products of conception may be removed surgically through an appropriately dilated cervix or transabdominally by either hysterotomy or hysterectomy.

Transvaginal Evacuation

Surgical abortion through the vagina is performed by first dilating the cervix and then evacuating the products of conception by mechanically scraping out the contents (curettage) or by the technique of vacuum aspiration (suction curettage), or both. The likelihood of complications, including uterine perforation, cervical laceration, hemorrhage, incomplete removal of the fetus and placenta, and infection increases after the first trimester, and especially after about 16 weeks. For this reason, dilatation and curettage or vacuum aspiration is best performed before the duration of pregnancy has exceeded that limit.

In the absence of maternal systemic disease, the pregnancies are commonly terminated by dilatation and evacuation without hospitalization. When an abortion is not performed in a hospital setting, it is imperative that the capabilities for effective cardiopulmonary resuscitation be immediately available and that hospitalization can be promptly facilitated whenever needed.

Laminaria Tents. Mechanical dilatation of the "unripe," that is, firm and difficult to dilate, cervix at the time of abortion is a potentially traumatic procedure. The risk of trauma can be minimized by inserting into the cervical canal an agent that will slowly swell and thus slowly dilate the cervix. Laminaria tents, illustrated in Figure 24-6 are used commonly to help dilate the cervix for abortion. They are made from the stems of *Laminaria digitata* or *Laminaria japonica,* a brown seaweed obtained from northern ocean waters. The stems are cut, peeled, shaped, dried, sterilized, and packaged according to size (small, 3 to 5 mm in diameter; medium, 6 to 8 mm; and large, 8 to 10 mm). The strongly hygroscopic laminaria are thought to act by drawing water from proteoglycan complexes, causing them to dissociate and thereby allow the cervix to soften and dilate.

More recently, a synthetic hygroscopic dilator made of hydrogel polymer has become available. It is claimed to dilate the cervix more rapidly than those made of traditional seaweed (Chvapil and co-workers, 1982). Also, Lamicel, a polyvinyl alcohol polymer sponge impregnated with anhydrous magnesium sulfate ($MgSO_4$) has been used

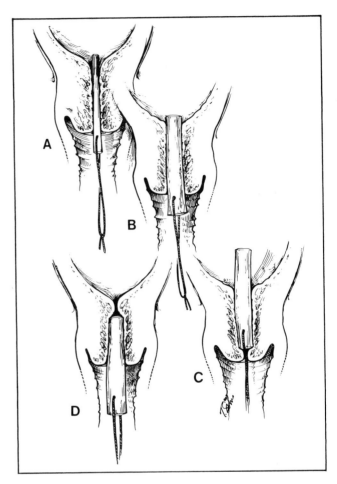

Figure 24-6. Insertion of laminaria prior to dilatation and curettage. **A.** Laminaria immediately after being appropriately placed with its upper end just through the internal os. **B.** The swollen laminaria and dilated, softened cervix about 18 hours later. **C.** Laminaria inserted too far through the internal os; the laminaria may rupture the membranes. **D.** Laminaria not inserted far enough to dilate the internal os.

recently as a synthetic laminaria tent and reported to be efficacious by Nicolaides and co-workers (1983). The magnesium levels in plasma described by them before and during its use are probably too low to be compatible with life, but presumably they are in error since no complications were noted in the subjects.

The cleansed cervix is grasped anteriorly with a tenaculum. The cervical canal is carefully sounded, without rupturing the membranes, to identify the length of the canal so as to gain some impression of its diameter and the resistance of the internal os. A laminaria of appropriate size is then inserted so that the tip passes just beyond the internal os using a uterine packing forceps or a radium capsule forceps (Fig. 24-6). Later, usually after 8 to 24 hours, the laminaria will have swollen and thereby dilated the cervix sufficiently to allow easier mechanical dilatation and curettage. The laminaria may cause cramping, which usually can be ame-

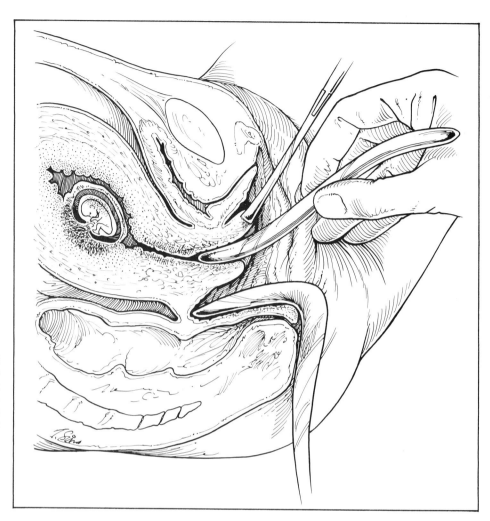

Figure 24-7. Dilatation of cervix with Hegar dilator. Note that the fourth and fifth fingers rest against the perineum and buttocks, lateral to the vagina. This maneuver is a most important safety measure because if the cervix relaxes abruptly, these fingers prevent a sudden and uncontrolled thrust of the dilator, a common cause of perforation of the uterus.

liorated with 0.6 g of aspirin or 60 mg of codeine orally every 3 to 4 hours.

Rather than using a laminaria to effect softening of the cervix and thereby minimize trauma to the cervix from mechanical dilatation, prostaglandin pessaries (suppositories) have been inserted into the vagina against the cervix 3 hours or so before attempting dilatation. Chen and associates (1983) have reported good results from so applying 1 mg of the prostin 16,16-dimethyl-trans-Δ_2 prostaglandin E_1 methyl ester.

Subsequent Dilatation and Evacuation. At the time of abortion the laminaria is removed by grasping the attached thread, and the vulva, vagina, and cervix are cleansed. The size and position of the uterus are carefully reevaluated through bimanual pelvic–abdominal examination. The anterior lip of the cervix is grasped with a multitoothed tenaculum and a local anesthetic is injected into the body of the cervix. Commonly, 5 ml of 1 or 2 percent solution of lidocaine is injected bilaterally. Alternatively, a paracervical block may be used (see Chapter 18, p. 360). The usual precautions for use of local anesthetics must be observed since

deaths have resulted from their use in abortion.

The uterus is *carefully* sounded to identify the status of the internal os, and to confirm the size of the uterus and the attitude of the fundus. The cervix is further dilated with Hegar or Pratt dilators until a vacuum aspirator suction curet of appropriate diameter can be inserted. As shown in Figure 24-7, the fourth and fifth fingers of the hand introducing the dilator should rest on the woman's perineum and buttocks as the dilator is pushed through the internal os. This provides a further safeguard against uterine perforation.

Suction curettage is then used to aspirate most, if not all, of the pregnancy products. The vacuum aspirator is moved over the surface systematically in order to cover eventually all the uterine cavity. Once this has been done and no more tissue is aspirated, the procedure is terminated. Gentle curettage with a sharp curet is then utilized if it is thought that any placenta or fetal fragments remain in the uterus. A sharp curet is more efficacious and its dangers need not be greater than those of the dull instrument. Perforations of the uterus rarely occur on the downstroke of the curet, but they may occur when any instrument is introduced into the

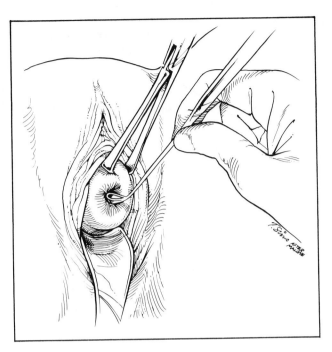

Figure 24-8. Introduction of the sharp curet. Note that the instrument is held merely with the thumb and forefinger; in the upward movement of the curet, only the strength of these two fingers should be used.

uterus. A curet, however, is a dangerous instrument if injudicious force is applied to it. As shown in Figure 24-8, the necessary manipulations should be carried out with the thumb and forefingers only.

It is reemphasized that morbidity, immediate and remote, will be kept to a minimum if (1) the cervix is adequately dilated (without trauma to the cervix) before attempting to remove the products of conception, (2) the removal of the products of conception is accomplished without perforating the uterus, and (3) all of the products of conception (but not the decidua basalis) are removed.

Perforation. Accidental perforation of the uterus may occur during sounding of the uterus, dilatation, or curettage. The reported incidence of uterine perforation associated with elective abortion varies. Two important determinants of this complication are the skill of the physician and the position of the uterus, with a much greater likelihood of perforation if the physician is inexperienced and the uterus is retroverted.

Generally, the accident of uterine perforation is easy to recognize, as the instrument passes without hindrance obviously further than it could have if uterine perforation had not occurred. Observation may be sufficient therapy if the rent in the uterus is small, as when produced by a uterine sound or narrow dilator. Such small defects often heal readily without complication.

Considerable damage intraabdominally can be caused by manipulation through a perforation of the uterus into the peritoneal cavity with a ring forceps,

sharp curet, or suction curet inserted unknowingly. In this circumstance, laparotomy to examine the abdominal contents, especially the bowel, is the safest course of action. We have recently cared for a woman transferred to us after much of her right ureter had been removed at the time of attempted abortion using suction curettage! Similar cases have been observed by others (Keegan and Forkowitz, 1982). Nonetheless, vacuum aspiration is generally preferable to mechanical curettage for abortion since it is quicker, has a lower perforation rate, induces somewhat less blood loss at operation, and there are fewer infections afterward. Especially in more advanced abortions, additional mechanical curettage as a second procedure may be necessary.

Some women may subsequently demonstrate cervical incompetence or uterine synechiae. The possibility of these complications should be explained to those contemplating abortion. In general, the risk of these complications is very slight, however. Very unfortunately, more advanced abortion performed by curettage may induce sudden, severe consumptive coagulopathy, which can prove fatal. This complication, with a demonstrative case, is considered further in Chapter 21 (p. 418).

Menstrual Aspiration. Aspiration of the endometrial cavity using a flexible 5- or 6-mm Karman cannula and syringe within 1 to 3 weeks after failure to menstruate has been variously referred to as menstrual extraction, menstrual induction, instant period, atraumatic abortion, and miniabortion. Problems include the woman not being pregnant, the implanted zygote being missed by the curet, the failure to recognize an ectopic pregnancy, and rarely, uterine perforation.

A positive pregnancy test will serve to eliminate a needless procedure on a nonpregnant woman whose period has been delayed for other reasons. Munsick (1982) recommends the following technique for identifying placenta in the aspirate: The syringe contents are placed in a clear plastic container and examined with back lighting. Tap water is added and the bloodstained liquid is decanted until tissue becomes visible. The tissue is then removed and immersed in clear water. Placenta is macroscopically, soft, fluffy, feathery, and villous. If there is doubt as to whether the tissue is placenta or decidua, microscopic examination of a small piece under a cover glass with high light contrast will allow differentiation. Placental villi are obvious.

Rh₀(D) Immunoglobulin. Treatment of Rh negative women after abortion with anti-Rh$_o$ (anti D) immunoglobulin is recommended, since about 5 percent of Rh negative women sustaining abortion otherwise become immunized.

Hysterotomy and Hysterectomy

In few circumstances, abdominal hysterotomy or hysterectomy for abortion is preferable to either dilatation and curettage or medical induction. If significant uterine disease is present, hysterectomy may provide ideal treatment. If sterilization is to be performed, either hysterotomy with interruption of tubal continuity or hysterectomy may on occasion be more advisable than curettage or medical induction followed by partial resection of the oviducts (see Chapter 40, p. 830). At times, hysterotomy or hysterectomy becomes necessary because of failure of medical induction during the second trimester.

The techniques employed for hysterotomy are similar to those for cesarean section (see Chapter 43, p. 879), except that the abdominal and uterine incisions are appreciably smaller. If further reproduction is anticipated, the smallest uterine incision that will allow removal of the fetus and placenta should be made away from the fundus, and the uterine wound carefully repaired.

Following abortion by abdominal hysterotomy, the potential for rupture during subsequent pregnancies is appreciable, especially during labor. Therefore, most obstetricians believe that in those women with previous hysterotomies, cesarean section is indicated for subsequent obstetric deliveries. After hysterotomy, Clow and Crompton (1973) identified 14 thin scars out of 31 evaluated in the subsequent pregnancy. Although Higginbottom (1973) believed that hysterotomy for abortion compared favorably with other methods of pregnancy termination, of the 242 cases reviewed by him, 12 required blood transfusion, 3 developed deep venous thrombosis, one had a pulmonary embolism, one had a repeat laparotomy for intestinal obstruction, and two subsequently required curettage for retained products of conception. Nottage and Liston (1975), based on a review of 700 hysterotomies, rightfully concluded that the operation is now outdated as a routine method for terminating pregnancy.

MEDICAL INDUCTION OF ABORTION

Very few effective, yet safe, abortifacient drugs have been discovered, although throughout history many naturally occurring substances have been tried by women desperate not to be pregnant. Serious systemic illness or even death, but not abortion, often was the result.

Oxytocin

Intravenously administered oxytocin during the second trimester is seldom effective in terminating the intact pregnancy of a healthy woman. In circumstances of severe maternal disease, however, especially vascular disease or diseases complicated by maternal hypoxia, intravenous oxytocin is much more likely to effect uterine contractions that will evacuate the uterus. For example, at Parkland Memorial Hospital, termination of pregnancy with intravenous oxytoxin was successful in five of eight eclamptic women pregnant with fetuses who weighed less than 1000 g (Pritchard and co-workers, 1984).

Once the cervix has undergone any degree of effacement and dilatation, either spontaneously or as the

consequence of some other agent such as a prostaglandin, intravenously administered oxytocin is much more likely to prove effective for evacuating the products of conception.

There are complications from the use of oxytocin. If appreciable volumes of electrolyte-free solution are administered along with oxytocin, water intoxication may develop (see Chapter 17, p. 346). Rupture of the uterus from oxytocin infused during the first half of pregnancy has been documented in women of high parity (Peyser and Toaff, 1972) but is very unlikely. Rupture of the cervix or isthmus is well documented in instances in which oxytocin was given after intra-amnionic prostaglandin $F_{2\alpha}$. A large bolus of oxytocin intravenously may produce troublesome hypotension (see Chapter 17, p. 346).

Prostaglandins

Because of the shortcomings of other medical methods of inducing abortion discussed below, prostaglandins are now widely used to terminate pregnancies, especially in the second trimester.

Mechanism of Action. Compounds commonly used are prostaglandins E_2, prostaglandin $F_{2\alpha}$, and certain analogues, especially 15-methyl-prostaglandin $F_{2\alpha}$ methyl ester. The probable mode of action of the prostaglandins on the uterus and cervix is considered in some detail in Chapter 15 (p. 306).

Technique. Prostaglandins can act effectively on the cervix and uterus when (1) placed in the vagina in the form of a suppository immediately adjacent to the cervix, (2) administered as a gel through a catheter into the cervical canal and lowermost uterus extraovularly, or (3) injected into the amnionic sac by amniocentesis (Embrey, 1981). These three approaches reduce appreciably, but do not eliminate, the unpleasant systemic effects, especially gastrointestinal, that accompany oral or parenteral administration of prostaglandins. At the same time these three routes of administration cause cervical softening, uterine contractions, cervical dilatation, and expulsion of the products of conception in the great majority of cases, although repeated doses of the prostaglandin may be required.

Prostaglandin vaginal suppositories applied to the cervix are also used by some in lower dose during the first and even early in the second trimesters to ripen, that is, soften and dilate somewhat, the cervix before terminating the pregnancy by curettage (MacKenzie and Fry, 1981; Niloff and Stubblefield, 1982). A troublesome feature with prostaglandin-induced abortions is the expulsion of a fetus with signs of life. The legal implications associated with expulsion of a living abortus may be profound. Although the purpose of abortion is to destroy the fetus before viability—a right of every pregnant woman, according to the United States Supreme Court—statutes continue to be enacted to protect the abortus. For example, one state law demands that an abortus with a heart beat or demonstrating any movement after expulsion from the mother be considered a living human child entitled to the same rights, powers, and privileges as a child born alive after the normal gestation period!

Consumptive coagulopathy and death have been reported rarely following use of prostaglandins to effect abortion (see Chapter 21, p. 418).

Intra-amnionic Hyperosmotic Solutions

In order to effect abortion during the second trimester, 20 to 25 percent saline, or 30 to 40 percent urea, has been injected into the amnionic sac to stimulate uterine contractions and cervical dilatation. Use of hypertonic dextrose has been abandoned because of its relative ineffectiveness as well as the occasional occurrence of serious infection, including *Clostridium perfringens* sepsis.

Mechanism of Action. The mechanism of action of the hyperosmotic agents when placed in the amnionic sac is not clear. Most often, but not always, the fetus is killed, but this does not explain their action nor does myometrial stretch from an increased intrauterine volume appear to be an important factor. Decidual damage induced by the hyperosmotic material probably incites the formation of prostaglandins which cause uterine contractions and cervical dilatation.

Hypertonic Saline. Intra-amnionically injected hypertonic saline was used as an abortifacient by the Japanese after World War II but later abandoned because of maternal morbidity and mortality. In spite of documented serious complications, hypertonic saline became popular in the United States for midtrimester abortion once the pregnancy has advanced beyond the 15th week and the amnionic sac could be entered by transabdominal amniocentesis. Serious complications, including death, have been documented. The specific complications are (1) hyperosmolar crisis following the entry of the hypertonic saline into the maternal circulation, (2) cardiac failure, (3) septic shock, (4) peritonitis, (5) hemorrhage, (6) disseminated intravascular coagulation, and (7) water intoxication. Moreover, myometrial necrosis has followed injection of hypertonic saline that apparently remained in contact with the myometrium; cervical and isthmic fistulas and lacerations have been described; and gross rupture of the body of the uterus has been described (Horwitz, 1974). Use of laminaria tents to prevent such cervical trauma has been recommended, but fistula formation has been documented following the use of such tents (Lischke and Gordon, 1974). Serious disruption of the coagulation mechanism characterized by the changes of disseminated intravascular coagulation have been reported repeatedly with use of hypertonic saline for abortion (see Chapter 21, p. 418).

Berger and colleagues (1975) have demonstrated that abortion occurs more promptly when oxytocin was administered intravenously within 8 hours after instillation of hypertonic saline, but the decrease in frequency of infection was accompanied by an increase in consumptive coagulopathy.

Hyperosmotic Urea. Urea, 30 to 40 percent, dissolved in 5 percent dextrose solution, has been injected into the amnionic sac, followed by intravenous oxytocin, about 400 milliunits per minute. Urea plus oxytocin is as efficacious an abortifacient as hypertonic saline, but less likely to be toxic. Urea plus prostaglandin $F_{2\alpha}$ injected into the amnionic sac is similarly effective.

Laminaria, Prostaglandin, Urea, and Oxytocin. Perhaps the ultimate in the use of multiple abortifacients was reported by Strauss and co-workers (1979), who first inserted a laminaria tent into the cervical canal, then 4 hours later injected intra-amnionically 20 mg of prostaglandin $F_{2\alpha}$ plus 80 g of urea, and followed this with oxytocin infused intravenously at the rate of 333 milliunits per minute. Complications were troublesome, but perhaps no more so than with medical inductions in general.

CONSEQUENCES OF ELECTIVE ABORTION

Maternal Mortality

It is apparent that serious morbidity and even mortality have followed some elective abortions. Nonetheless, legally induced abortion is a relatively safe surgical procedure, especially when performed during the first 2 months of pregnancy. The risk of death from abortion by dilatation and evacuation performed during the first 2 months is about 0.6 per 100,000 procedures. The relative risk of dying as the consequence of abortion is approximately doubled for each 2 weeks of delay after 8 weeks of gestation (MMWR, 1979). LeBolt and co-workers (1982) have estimated that during the 1970s, at least, the overall risk of death from legal abortion was no more than one seventh the risk from childbirth.

Impact on Future Pregnancies

The effects of elective abortion on subsequent pregnancies continues to be disputed. For example, a World Health Organization Task Force on Sequelae of Abortion (1979) reported a significantly higher risk of an adverse pregnancy outcome among women whose only previous pregnancy had been aborted than among women who were either primigravid or whose only previous pregnancy had ended in live birth. The adverse pregnancy outcomes took the form of midtrimester spontaneous abortions, preterm deliveries, and low-birth-weight infants. However, Cates (1979), who analyzed and tabulated 29 reports concerned with the apparent impact of previous abortions on subsequent pregnancies, concluded that the data did not support firm conclusions about induced abortion either causing or not causing any of a variety of the complications alleged to be more common in pregnancies subsequent to induced abortion. More recently Chung and co-workers (1982) and Linn and associates (1983) have reported that in their extensive studies previous induced abortion did not seem to increase the risk significantly of a subsequent adverse late pregnancy outcome.

Clinical experience in former years with the so-called incompetent cervix support the concept that this uncommon defect commonly followed induced abortion. Moreover, it seems likely that *forceful* dilatation of the cervix by surgical or medical techniques sufficient to allow evacuation or expulsion of more advanced products of conception will continue to predispose to cervical incompetency. Slater and associates (1981), who have provided supporting data, urge that women who undergo induced abortion should have it as early as possible to minimize cervical damage and its consequences.

Rupture of the uterus after hysterotomy, and less often after inadvertent uterine perforation at the time of abortion, may occur during a subsequent pregnancy, with a disastrous outcome for the fetus, the mother, or both.

Synechiae that compromise the uterine cavity as the consequence of abortion and vigorous curettage or infection have resulted in infertility. Treatment has been only partially successful for this phenomenon of posttraumatic intrauterine adhesions, sometimes referred to as *Asherman syndrome.* When infertility has been overcome, obstetric complications have been common. For example, in the experiences of Jewelewicz and associates (1976) only 18 of 36 women treated for Asherman syndrome subsequently conceived. Moreover, of those 18, only 10 were delivered of infants who survived. There were three instances of placenta accreta and one of cervical pregnancy.

RESUMPTION OF OVULATION

Ovulation may occur as early as 2 weeks after an abortion. Lähteenmäki and Luukkainen (1978) detected a surge of luteinizing hormone (LH) 16 to 22 days after abortion in 15 of 18 women studied. Moreover, the plasma progesterone level, which had plummeted after the abortion, increased soon after the LH surge. These hormonal events are in excellent temporal agreement with the histologic changes observed in endometrial biopsies and the rise in basal body temperature after abortion, as described previously by Boyd and Holmstrom (1972). Therefore, it is important that effective contraception be initiated soon after abortion. The use of various contraceptive techniques following abortion is discussed in Chapter 40.

SEPTIC ABORTION

Serious complications of abortion have been most often, but certainly not always, associated with criminal abortion. Severe hemorrhage, sepsis, bacterial shock, and acute renal failure have all developed in association with legal abortion but at a very much lower frequency.

Sepsis from abortion is most often caused by pathogenic organisms of the bowel and vaginal flora. Infection is most commonly confined to the uterus in the form of metritis, but parametritis, peritonitis (localized and general), and septicemia are by no means rare. Out of 300 cases of febrile abortions at Parkland Memorial Hospital shortly before the United States Supreme Court decision legalizing abortion, a positive blood culture was found in one fourth. The organisms that were identified are listed in Table 24-1.

Treatment of the infection included prompt evacuation of the products of conception. Although mild infections can be treated successfully with broad-spectrum antibiotics in the usual dosage, any serious infection should be attacked with great vigor from the very start.

For septic abortion complicated by persistent, apparently resistant infection, or with evidence of overwhelming sepsis, intravenous antibiotic therapy with penicillin, 20 million units per day, plus chloramphenicol, 3 to 4 g per day, has proved effective. Rather than chloramphenicol, clindamycin has been widely used in combination with gentamycin plus penicillin. Undoubtedly, newer antibiotics are also being used but extensive clinical experience in the treatment of septic abortion with these agents has not yet been achieved.

Septic Shock

Endotoxemia and exotoxemia are likely to cause severe and even fatal shock. Septic shock, which fortunately now is rare, was previously seen most often in women of reproductive age in connection with induced abortion, although it can occur as a result of infection in the genital or urinary tracts at any time during pregnancy or the puerperium.

Important pathophysiologic changes, especially to the cardiovascular system, induced by septic shock include widespread damage to vascular endothelium, in-

TABLE 24-1. BACTERIA PRESENT IN 76 CASES OF SEPTIC ABORTION WITH POSITIVE BLOOD CULTURES

Organisms Cultured	Frequency (%)
Anaerobic	63
Peptostreptococcus	
(anaerobic streptococcus)	41
Bacteroides	9
Both	9
Clostridium perfringens	4
Aerobic	37
Escherichia coli	14
Pseudomonas	9
β-hemoyltic streptococcus	4
Enterococcus	3
Combination	7

(From Smith, Southern, and Lehmann: Obstet Gynecol 35:704, 1970.)

appropriate vasomotor tone, and impaired myocardial function. These changes limit effective blood volume and cardiac output. As the consequence, septic shock is usually much more resistant to treatment than is hypovolemic shock from hemorrhage.

An outline of therapy that has proved successful in most cases in septic abortion at Parkland Memorial Hospital is presented.

Diagnosis and Treatment of Septic Shock

I. *Suspicion.* Whenever infection of the gravid uterus is suspected, blood pressure and urine flow should be closely monitored. Septic shock, as well as hypovolemic shock, should be considered whenever there is evidence of hypotension or oliguria.

II. *Recognition.* In the absence of other evidence of active hemorrhage, if hypotension and oliguria are not improved by the rapid administration of a liter or so of lactated Ringer's solution, it is likely that the shock is caused by infectious agents.

III. *Treatment.* Aggressive therapy is mandatory:
  A. Control of infection
    1. After obtaining anaerobic and aerobic cultures of blood and urine, as well as a smear for Gram stain from the cervix, or, better, the expelled products of conception, intensive broad-spectrum antibiotic therapy is begun as described above. The kinds of organisms commonly found in the blood are listed in Table 24-1. Cervical smears may be misleading except when there is an obvious abundance of pathogenic organisms, as for example, *Clostridium perfringens,* demonstrated in Figure 24-9.
    2. Once antibiotic therapy has been started and the condition of the woman suffering from septic abortion has been stabilized, the infected products of conception are promptly removed by curettage. Hysterectomy is seldom indicated unless the uterus has been lacerated or is obviously intensely infected (Figs. 24-10A, B). Evidence is lacking that hysterectomy in the absence of gross trauma to the uterus, including that induced by infection, improves the prognosis (Hawkins and colleagues, 1975; O'Neill and associates, 1972; Pritchard and Whalley, 1971; Smith and co-workers, 1978). Since bacterial shock can become clinically apparent after evacuation of the infected products from the uterus, careful monitoring, especially of blood pressure and urine flow, must be continued.
  B. Treatment of shock. The primary goal is to

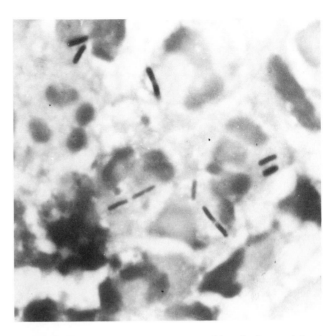

Figure 24-9. *Clostridium perfringens* evident in Gram stain of cervical smear.

reestablish effective perfusion of vital organs. The adequacy of the circulation may be ascertained by continuously monitoring urine flow.
    1. *Fluid therapy.* Red cells, or whole blood if there has been appreciable hemorrhage, are given in amounts that maintain the hematocrit at about 30. Electrolyte-containing fluids, such as lactated Ringer's solution, are given at a rate that maintains urinary flow at 30 ml per hour at least, and preferably about 60 ml per hour. Adequate filling of the intravascular compartment is desirable, but circulatory overload with pulmonary edema must be avoided. Pulmonary problems are much more likely to occur with vigorous fluid therapy given to treat septic shock than when administered to treat hypovolemic shock. Sepsis, as alluded to above, causes injury to the cardiovascular system, especially the microvasculature, which enhances the risk of serious fluid leakage into the lung and the development of not only pulmonary edema, but also so-called adult respiratory distress syndrome. At the same time, vigorous fluid therapy may be lifesaving. In these circumstances, frequent measurements of pulmonary artery wedge pressure, central venous pressure, cardiac output, and systemic blood pressure measured directly through an ar-

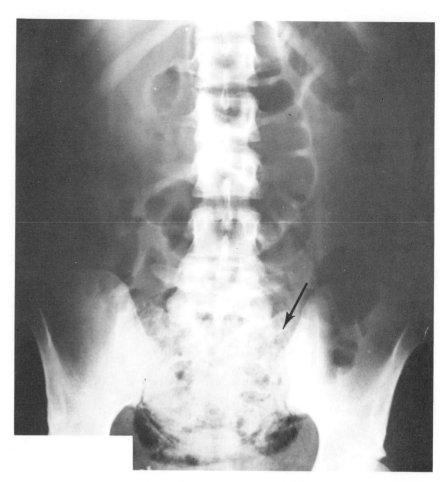

Figure 24-10. A. The honeycombed pattern of gas in the pelvis (*arrow*) was caused by gas in the myometrium of a fatal case of postabortal *Clostridium perfringens* sepsis.

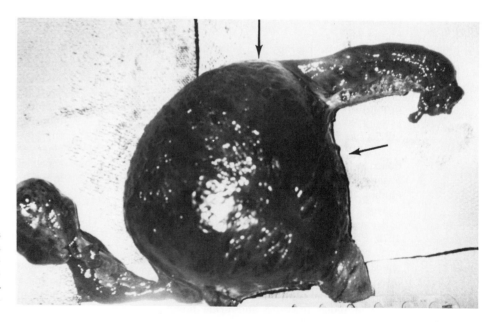

Figure 24-10. B. The numerous rents in the serosa of the uterus (*arrows*) were the consequence of gas formation plus intensive necrosis from *Clostridium perfringens*.

terial line can be of considerable help in directing further therapy.

2. *Adrenocortical steroids.* If control of the infection by antibiotics, and curettage, and the infusion of blood and aqueous fluids do not result in prompt improvement, large doses of corticosteroids are probably indicated. Lillehei and associates (1958) have recommended 10 g of hydrocortisone sodium succinate (Solu-Cortef) or its equivalent rapidly administered intravenously. We have used methylprednisolone sodium succinate (Solu-Medrol), 500 mg given as a bolus intravenously. Steroid therapy need not be continued beyond the acute phase, and most often can be stopped abruptly.

3. *Pressor agents.* These agents are not now used as widely as they were in the past, although selected ones, metaraminol and dopamine, may have value when used in conjunction with the treatment modalities outlined above, especially appropriate filling of the intravascular compartment. Both have a powerful inotropic effect on the heart and are much less likely to cause necrosis than is levarterenol bitartrate (Levophed). A rise in blood pressure is sought that reestablishes urine flow, which, in turn, indicates effective organ perfusion.

4. *Vasodilating agents.* Drugs such as isoproterenol were once recommended to relieve vasoconstriction. Their role in cases of septic abortion with endotoxic shock is questionable.

5. *Oxygenation.* Vigorous respiratory support may be required in the form of oxygen administration, effective pulmonary toilet, and even mechanical ventilation. Adult respiratory distress syndrome is a serious complication.

6. *Heparin.* Coagulation defects occur commonly in severe cases of septic shock. The genesis of these abnormalities is extremely complex and difficult to dissect in clinical studies. However, the concept that intravascular coagulation occludes the microcirculation in septic shock, as well as consumes coagulation factors and thereby causes hemorrhage, led to the recommendation by some that heparin be used in these circumstances. To date, no adequate clinical trial has been reported to show that the benefits from heparin outweigh the risks. Moreover, animal studies of gram-negative sepsis point out that inhibition of intravascular coagulation by heparin does not necessarily lower mortality (Corrigan and co-workers, 1974). Control of disseminated intravascular coagulation is dependent upon control of the inciting disease, in this circumstance sepsis!

Septic Abortion with Consumptive Coagulopathy. An illustrative case of septic abortion with intense but transient severe consumptive coagulopathy and not treated with heparin is summarized below and in Table 24-2.

TABLE 24.2 HEMATOLOGIC DATA AND RENAL FUNCTION IN A CASE OF SEPTIC ABORTION WITH INTENSIVE INTRAVASCULAR COAGULATION BUT NO GROSS HEMOLYSIS

Date and Time	Fibrinogen* (mg per dl)	Serum FDP† (µg per ml)	Thrombin Time‡	Platelets (mm³)	Hematocrit	Creatinine Clearance (ml per minute)	Comment
17 Jan							
1950	Large clot	8	—	—	35	—	
2300				Curettage			
18 Jan							
0600	No clot	—	—	—	31	—	Generalized bleeding
0700	20	1024	—	151,000	—	—	Hypotensive
1000	28	512	—	120,000	—	49	
1500	47	512	—	122,000	27	45	Afebrile
1930	67	512	—	158,000	—	36	Mild hypotension
19 Jan							
0900	172	128	18.7 (10.4)	118,000	27	14	
20 Jan	348	8	12.1 (10.2)	108,000	27	16	Normotensive
22 Jan	485	< 4	12.2 (10.1)	129,000	31	20	
24 Jan	432	< 4	13.0 (11.0)	172,000	27	35	
26 Jan	489	< 4	11.4 (10.3)	336,000	28	50	
20 Feb	288	< 4	12.0 (11.2)	—	37	119	

* Measured as thrombin clotable protein.
† Fibrin degradation products measured by tanned erythrocyte agglutination inhibition technique.
‡ Control value in brackets.

B.T., a 32-year-old multigravida, sought help because of loss of amnionic fluid, cramping, and vaginal bleeding following 3½ months of amenorrhea. She was febrile and the pregnant uterus palpable above the symphysis was tender. An intravenous infusion of oxytocin soon accomplished expulsion of the fetus and placenta.

Four hours later her temperature rose to 40.5° C. Seven hours after evacuation of the products of conception brisk bleeding from the vagina and obvious oozing from previous venipuncture sites were documented by a physician. The blood pressure was 90/50 mm Hg, pulse 120, urine output 20 ml for the previous hour, hematocrit 31 percent compared to 35 percent initially, and the leukocyte count had fallen from 13,000 to 7000 mm^3. Two milliters of her blood added to a tube that contained about 0.1 ml of thrombin yielded no visible clot.

Immediate treatment consisted of lactated Ringer's solution, 1 unit of whole blood and 2 units of thawed plasma, plus 2 units of packed erythrocytes. Urine flow was soon restored. Central venous pressure was monitored closely when the patient complained of a fullness in her chest and scattered rales were heard. Penicillin, kanamycin, and clindamycin were administered. During the next 12 hours the bleeding first decreased appreciably and then stopped. Her subsequent clinical course was benign except for a transient rise in plasma creatinine to 4.4 mg/dl. She was discharged 11 days after admittance.

A variety of interesting observations made on the coagulation mechanism and on renal function are summarized in Table 24-2: Platelets were abundant and a morphologic study of the erythrocytes yielded normal results in a blood smear made when she was first seen in the emergency suite. A large, stable clot was present in the tube of blood that had been routinely drawn before evacuation of the products of conception for blood typing. Serum removed later from that tube contained only 8 μg/ml of fibrin degradation products. Nine hours after admittance, she was bleeding excessively through the vagina and from sites of previous venipunctures. Severe hypofibrinogenemia was documented and the level of fibrin degradation products in serum had increased from 8 μg/ml or less to at least 1024 μg/ml, yet the platelet count was only slightly below normal.

The plasma fibrinogen concentration then rose and the serum fibrin degradation products fell. Erythrocyte deformity and some fragmentation of erythrocytes were observed to follow the consumptive coagulopathy.

Although severe oliguria did not persist after fluid therapy was started, the creatinine clearance fell to as low as 14 ml per minute 36 hours after the abortion had been completed. It then rose spontaneously to 50 ml per minute 1 week later and to 119 ml per minute when next checked 4 weeks after the abortion. Recovery of renal function occurred without the use of heparin even though the patient had chronic hypertension for which she had been subjected to thiazide therapy until the time of abortion and she was probably overtly hypotensive for several hours after the abortion before effective fluid therapy was instituted.

Acute Renal Failure

Persistent renal failure in abortion usually stems from multiple effects of infection and of hypovolemia. Less commonly, it has been induced by toxic compounds em-

ployed to produce abortion, such as soap, pHisoHex, or Lysol. Whereas very severe forms of bacterial shock are frequently associated with the intense renal damage, the milder forms rarely lead to overt renal failure. Early recognition of this very serious complication is most important. The word "serious" is used advisedly in connection with acute renal failure in abortion, for the maternal mortality before the extensive use of dialysis exceeded 75 percent (Knapp and Hellman, 1959).

Renal failure is likely to be most intense when the cause of the sepsis includes *Clostridium perfringens* with the production of a very potent hemolytic exotoxin. In our experience, whenever intense hemoglobinemia complicated clostridial infection, renal failure was the rule. At the outset, plans should be made to initiate effective dialysis early, before metabolic deterioration becomes severe.

REFERENCES

Andolesk L: The Ljubljana abortion study 1971–1973. Bethesda, MD, National Institutes of Health Center for Population Research, 1974

Batzofin JH, Fielding WL, Friedman EA: Effect of vaginal bleeding in early pregnancy on outcome. Obstet Gynecol 63:515, 1984

Beer AE, Quebbeman JF, Ayers JWT, Haines RF: Major histocompatibility complex antigens, maternal and paternal immune responses, and chronic habitual abortions in humans. Am J Obstet Gynecol 141:987, 1981

Beer AE, Quebbeman JF, Sempini AE, Smouse PE, Haines PF: Recurrent abortion: Analysis of the roles of parental sharing of histocompatibility antigens and maternal immunological responses to paternal antigens. Am J Obstet Gynecol, 1984, in press

Berger GS, Edelman DA, Kerenyi TD: Oxytocin administration, instillation to abortion time, and morbidity associated with saline instillation. Am J Obstet Gynecol 121:941, 1975

Boué A, Boué J: Chromosomal anomalies associated with fetal malformation. In Scrimgeour JB (ed): Towards the Prevention of Fetal Malformation. Edinburgh, University Press, 1978

Boyd EF Jr, Holmstrom EG: Ovulation following therapeutic abortion. Am J Obstet Gynecol 113:469, 1972

Cates W Jr: Late effects of induced abortion. Hypothesis or knowledge? J Reprod Med 22:207, 1979

Charles D, Edward WR: Infectious complications of cervical cerclage. Am J Obstet Gynecol 141:1065, 1981

Chen JK, Edler MG: Preoperative cervical dilatation by vaginal pessaries containing prostaglandin E$_1$ analogue. Obstet Gynecol 62:339, 1983

Chung CS, Smith RG, Steinhoff PG, Mi M-P: Induced abortion and spontaneous fetal loss in subsequent pregnancies. Am J Public Health 72:548, 1982

Chvapil M, Droegemueller W, Meyer T, Mascalka R, Stoy V, Suciu T: New synthetic laminaria. Obstet Gynecol 60:729, 1982

Clow WM, Crompton AC: The wounded uterus: Pregnancy after hysterotomy. Br Med J 1:321, 1973

Corrigan JJ, Kiornat JF, Pagel CJ: Experimental gram negative sepsis: Effect of heparin. Pediatr Res 8:399, 1974

Edmonds DK, Lindsay KS, Miller JF, Williamson E, Wood PJ: Early embryonic mortality in women. Fertil Steril 38:447, 1982

Embrey MP: Prostaglandins in human reproduction. Br Med J 283:1563, 1981

Funderburk SJ, Guthrie D, Meldrum D: Outcome of pregnancies complicated by early vaginal bleeding. Br J Obstet Gynaecol 87:100, 1980

Goldzieher JW: Double-blind trial of a progestin in habitual abortion. JAMA 188:651, 1964

Guerrero R, Rojas OI: Spontaneous abortion and aging of human ova and spermatozoa. N Engl J Med 293:573, 1975

Harlap S, Shiono PH: Alcohol, smoking, and incidence of spontaneous abortions in the first and second trimester. Lancet 2:173, 1980

Hartman CG: Uterine bleeding as an early sign of pregnancy in the monkey (Macaca rhesus), together with the observation on fertile period of menstrual cycle. Bull Hopkins Hosp 44:155, 1929

Hawkins DF, Sevitt LH, Fairbrother PF, Tothill AU: Conservative management of septic chemical abortion with renal failure. N Engl J Med 292:722, 1975

Hertig AT, Sheldon WH: Minimal criteria required to prove prima facie case of traumatic abortion or miscarriage: An analysis of 1,000 spontaneous abortions. Ann Surg 117:596, 1943

Higginbottom J: Termination of pregnancy by abdominal hysterotomy. Lancet 1:937, 1973

Horwitz DA: Uterine rupture following attempted saline abortion with oxytocin in a grand multiparous patient. Obstet Gynecol 43:921, 1974

Jewelewicz R, Khalaf S, Neuwirth RS, VandeWeile RL: Obstet complications after treatment of intrauterine synechiae (Asherman's syndrome). Obstet Gynecol 47:701, 1976

Keegan GT, Forkowitz MJ: A case report: Ureterouterine fistula as a complication of elective abortion. J Urology 128:137, 1982

Kline J, Stein ZA, Susser M, Warburton D: Smoking: A risk factor for spontaneous abortion. N Engl J Med 297:793, 1977

Kline J, Stein ZA, Shrout P, Susser M: Drinking during pregnancy and spontaneous abortion. Lancet 2:176, 1980

Knapp RC, Hellman LM: Acute renal failure in pregnancy. Am J Obstet Gynecol 78:570, 1959

Kuhn RPJ, Pepperell RJ: Cervical ligation: A review of 242 pregnancies. Aust NZ J Obstet Gynaecol 17:79, 1977

Lähteenmäki P, Luukkainen T: Return of ovarian function after abortion. Clin Endocr 8:123, 1978

LeBolt SA, Grimes DA, Cates W Jr: Mortality from abortion. Are the populations comparable? JAMA 248:188, 1982

Lillehei RC, MacLean LD: The intestinal factor in irreversible endotoxin shock. Ann Surg 148:513, 1958

Linn S, Schoenbaum SC, Monson RR, Rosner B, Stubblefield PG, Ryan KJ: The relationship between induced abortion and outcome of subsequent pregnancies. Am J Obstet Gynecol 146:136, 1983

Lischke JH, Gordon HR: Cervicovaginal fistula complicating induced midtrimester abortion despite laminaria tent insertion. Am J Obstet Gynecol 120:852, 1974

MacKenzie IZ, Fry A: Prostaglandin E$_2$ pessaries to facilitate first trimester aspiration termination. Br J Obstet Gynaecol 88:1033, 1981

McDonald IA: Incompetent cervix as a cause of recurrent abortion. J Obstet Gynaecol Br Commonw 70:105, 1963

MMWR: Abortion-related mortality—United States, 1977. Center for Disease Control Morbidity and Mortality Weekly Report 28:301, 1979

Mumford SD: Abortion: A national security issue. Am J Obstet Gynecol 142:951, 1982

Munro JS: Premature infant weighing less than one pound at birth who survived and developed normally. Can Med Assoc J 40:69, 1939

Munsick RA: Clinical test for placenta in 300 consecutive menstrual aspirations. Obstet Gynecol 60:738, 1982

Nicolaides KH, Welch CC, Koullapis EN, Filshie GM: Cervical dilatation by Lamicel—Studies on the mechanism of action. Br J Obstet Gynaecol 90:1060, 1983

Niloff JM, Stubblefield PG: Low-dose vaginal 15 methyl prostaglandin F$_{2\alpha}$ for cervical dilatation prior to vacuum curettage abortion. Am J Obstet Gynecol 142:596, 1982

Nottage BJ, Liston WA: A review of 700 hysterectomies. Br J Obstet Gynaecol 82:310, 1975

Olsen S, Tobiassen T: Transabdominal isthmic cerclage for the treatment of incompetent cervix. Acta Obstet Gynecol 61:473, 1982

O'Neill JP, Niall JF, O'Sullivan EF: Severe postabortal Clostridium welchii infections: Trends in management. Aust NZ J Obstet Gynecol 12:157, 1972

Peyser MR, Toaff R: Rupture of uterus in the first trimester caused by high-concentration oxytocin drip. Obstet Gynecol 40:371, 1972

Pilpel HF, Norwick KP: When should abortion be legal? New York, Public Affairs Committee Inc, No 429, 1969

Piver MS, Bolognese RJ, Feldman JD: Long-acting progesterone as a cause of missed abortion. Am J Obstet Gynecol 97:579, 1967

Poland BJ, Miller JR, Harris M, Livingston J: Spontaneous abortion. A study of 1961 women and their abortuses. Acta Obstet Gynecol Scand Suppl 102, 1981

Pritchard JA, Cunningham FG, Pritchard SA: The Parkland Memorial Hospital protocol for treatment of eclampsia: Evaluation of 245 cases. Am J Obstet Gynecol 148:951, 1984

Pritchard JA, Whalley PJ: Abortion complicated by Clostridium perfringens infection. Am J Obstet Gynecol 111:484, 1971

Quinn PA, Shewchuk AB, Shuber J, Lie KI, Ryan E, Chipman ML, Nocilla DM: Efficacy of antibiotic therapy in preventing spontaneous pregnancy loss among couples colonized with genital mycoplasmas. Am J Obstet Gynecol 145:239, 1983

Quinn PA, Shewchuck AB, Shuber J, Lie KI, Ryan E, Sheu M, Chipman ML: Serologic evidence of Ureaplasma urealyticum infection in women with spontaneous pregnancy loss. Am J Obstet Gynecol 145:245, 1983

Rappaport F, Rubinovitz M, Toaff R, Krocheck N: Genital listerosis as a cause of repeated abortion. Lancet 1:1273, 1960

Ruffolo EH, Wilson RB, Weed LA: Listeria monocytogenes as a cause of pregnancy wastage. Obstet Gynecol 19:533, 1962

Salem HT, Ghaneimah SA, Shaaban, Chard T: Prognostic value of biochemical tests in the assessment of fetal outcome in threatened abortion. Br J Obstet Gynaecol 91:382, 1984

Shirodkar VN: A new method of operative treatment for habitual abortions in the second trimester of pregnancy. Antiseptic 52:299, 1955

Slater PE, Davies AM, Harlap S: The effect of abortion method on the outcome of subsequent pregnancy. J Reprod Med 26:123, 1981

Smith C, Gregori CA, Breen JL: Ultrasonography in threatened abortion. Obstet Gynecol 51:173, 1978

Strauss JH, Wilson M, Caldwell D, Otterson W, Martin AO: Laminaria use in midtrimester abortions induced by intra-amniotic prostaglandin $F_{2\alpha}$ with urea and intravenous oxytocin. Am J Obstet Gynecol 134:260, 1979

Supreme Court of the United States Syllabus, *Roe et al. v. Wade,* District Attorney of Dallas County, Jan. 22, 1973

Thomason JL, Sampson MB, Beckman CR, Spellacy WN: The incompetent cervix. A 1982 update. J Reprod Med 27:187, 1982

Tietze C: Introduction to the statistics of abortion. In Engle ET (ed): Pregnancy Wastage. Springfield, IL, Thomas, 1953, p 135

Tupper C, Weil RJ: The problem of spontaneous abortion. Am J Obstet Gynecol 83:421, 1962

United Nations, Department of Social Affairs. Foetal, Infant, and Early Childhood Mortality: I. The Statistics. New York, United Nations, 1954

Whittaker PG, Taylor A, Lind T: Unsuspected pregnancy loss in healthy women. Lancet 1:1126, 1983

World Health Organization Task Force on Sequelae to Abortion: Gestation, birthweight, and spontaneous abortion in pregnancy after induced abortion. Lancet 1:142, 1979

25
Abnormalities of the Reproductive Tract

DISEASES OF THE VULVA AND VAGINA

Inflammation of Bartholin Glands

Gonococci or other pathogenic organisms may gain access to Bartholin glands and form abscesses. The labium majus on the side affected becomes swollen and painful, at and surrounding the collection of pus. Aside from causing pain and discomfort, such abscesses may be the starting point of a puerperal infection. For these reasons, drainage must be established whenever an abscess develops during pregnancy. After the contents have escaped, the cut edge of the abscess cavity, if actively bleeding, is sutured with fine chromic catgut. A gauze wick or Word catheter is inserted to keep the ostium open until granulation is complete. McCoy and Cunningham (1980) found in pus from Bartholin abscesses both aerobic and anaerobic bacteria in nearly 90 percent of cases. *Neisseria gonorrhoeae* was identified in only 4 of 353 cases. A broad-spectrum antibiotic to which *N. gonorrhoeae* is sensitive should be administered for 7 to 10 days.

The treatment of asymptomatic *Bartholin duct cysts,* which are frequently the sequelae of Bartholin gland abscesses, is best postponed until after delivery. Rarely is a labial cyst of sufficient size to cause difficulty at delivery. If this should occur, aspiration with a syringe and small needle will suffice as a temporary measure. Because of the hyperemia induced by pregnancy, excision should not be attempted. Definitive surgery, if necessary, should be postponed until later.

Urethral Diverticulae, Cysts, and Abscesses

Trauma to the urethra or infection of the periurethral glands may be followed by the formation of periurethral abscesses, cysts, and diverticulae. Abscesses usually resolve spontaneously, with, at times, cyst formation as a sequela. Most often, periurethral cysts are asymptomatic and are best not disturbed during pregnancy. A urethral diverticulum may fill with debris that empties intermittently through the urethra to give rise to proteinuria of obscure etiology until the diverticulum is recognized as the source. In general, an attempt at surgical excision should not be made during pregnancy.

Condylomas (Condylomata)

Condylomata acuminata, sometimes called *venereal warts,* are caused by a papilloma virus. Growth of the venereal warts is likely to be stimulated during pregnancy. Treatment during pregnancy is not very satisfactory. Local washing of the external genitalia, plus cleansing of the vagina by gentle douching (Chapter 13, p. 258), followed by thorough drying of the external genitalia, performed at least daily, may inhibit proliferation of the warts, as well as minimize discomfort.

A 20 percent solution of podophyllin in tincture of benzoin applied to the lesions has long been used to try to eradicate venereal warts. Its use during pregnancy is not likely to be highly effective, and considerable local discomfort may ensue! Rarely, topical application of podophyllin has proved to be extremely toxic. Slater and co-workers (1978) describe intense systemic toxicity with coma after its cutaneous application; it resolved after charcoal hemoperfusion. They also cited previously reported fatalities, including death of the fetus following topical application of podophyllin.

Infrequently, condylomata acuminata attain enormous size (Fig. 25-1) and may even necessitate cesarean section. If the woman is seen several weeks or more before the end of pregnancy, the large lesion sometimes can be removed by excision, fulguration, or both. Cryosurgery has not proven satisfactory in our experience. Considerable enthusiasm has been expressed for use of laser under anesthesia to remove large condylomata during pregnancy (Malfetano and co-workers, 1981). During and after the procedure the pain may be considerable.

Condylomata lata are small, flat excrescences that are highly infectious. *Treponema pallidum* is usually present on dark field examination. Treatment is described in Chapter 28, p. 623).

Vulvar Varices

Varicosities sometimes appear in the lower part of the vagina but are more common around the vulva. There they may attain considerable size and cause a sensation of weight and discomfort. Vulvar varices may rupture during labor or be torn or cut by lacerations or episiot-

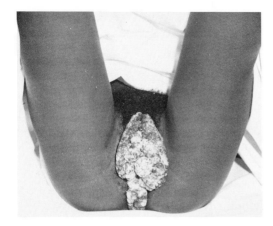

Figure 25-1. Enormous confluent condylomata acuminata complicating pregnancy. The lesion, attached to both labia majora by a relatively narrow base, was excised and the defect easily closed with chromic suture without excessive bleeding. Subsequent vaginal delivery was uneventful.

omy. Unless so traumatized, the varicosities in most instances become asymptomatic and decrease remarkably, or even disappear, after delivery. Vulvar varices are considered further in Chapter 13 (p. 261).

Cystocele and Rectocele

Attenuation of the fascial support that is normally interposed between the vagina and the bladder leads to prolapse into the vagina of the bladder, or cystocele. Attenuation between the vagina and the rectum results in a rectocele. In former years, vaginal delivery after a prolonged labor of a large infant without episiotomy, but with appreciable tearing of the lower genital tract, predisposed to the development of a cystocele and a rectocele. The more liberal use of cesarean section in cases of less than absolute cephalopelvic disproportion and of episiotomies for vaginal deliveries, especially when the fetus was large, coupled with generally lower parity, have made large symptomatic cystoceles and rectoceles very uncommon.

Urinary stasis associated with a large cystocele predisposes to urinary tract infection. A large rectocele may fill with feces, which, at times, can only be evacuated manually. Both lesions can block the normal descent of the fetus through the birth canal, unless they are emptied and pushed out of the way. Surgical repair of either should not be attempted during the antepartum or intrapartum periods. Rather, definitive repair, often with vaginal hysterectomy for associated uterine prolapse and sterilization, should be carried out after pregnancy-induced pelvic hyperemia has completely subsided.

Urinary Stress Incontinence

Infrequently, women may develop stress incontinence during pregnancy. Iosif and Ulmsten (1981), who studied

a group of such pregnant women, identified low urethral closing pressure that did not increase sufficiently to compensate for the progressive increase in bladder pressure induced by the enlarging uterus. Moreover, at the outset the urethra was shorter and did not increase in length during pregnancy in the group with stress incontinence, thereby differing from pregnant women who remained continent.

Vaginal Tumors. Vaginal cysts, the most frequent of benign vaginal tumors, may be discovered during pregnancy or sometimes not until the time of labor. Such cysts, usually embryologic rests (Gartner or müllerian duct), may be of sufficient size to cause serious dystocia. Treatment depends upon the size and location of the cyst, as well as the time at which it is first recognized. Rarely, drainage may be necessary to allow vaginal delivery to be completed. It is advisable to postpone surgical excision until after delivery and the puerperium when pelvic hyperemia has subsided.

CERVICAL NEOPLASIA

The effects of pregnancy and delivery on premalignant and malignant epithelial lesions of the cervix are not completely understood, and, therefore, disagreements persist in spite of the considerable interest displayed by numerous investigators for many years. In one study, at least, pregnancy did not seem to be a potent stimulus for progression of epithelial change from dysplasia to invasive neoplasia (Kiguchi and associates, 1981). The progression rate from dysplasia to invasive carcinoma (0.4 percent) after delivery was almost half that in the nonpregnant state (1 percent). Moreover, the regression rates of moderate and marked dysplasia within the 6-month period after delivery seemed much higher than those of dysplasia in the general population.

Screening for Cervical Cancer

As described in Chapter 13 (p. 347), all pregnant women should undergo examination that includes evaluation of the cervix cytologically as well as by visual inspection and palpation, except when there is active bleeding late in the second trimester or beyond and placenta previa is a possibility (Chapter 21, p. 408). Any visible fungating or ulcerating lesion should be evaluated by colposcopy or direct biopsy, since cytologic screening at times may fail to draw attention to a frankly invasive carcinoma.

Abnormal Cervical Cytology

If cytologic changes of mild dysplasia are identified and confirmed subsequently in another set of smears appropriately made from the cervix, further follow-up during pregnancy may consist of colposcopic evaluation. Simply repeating the cervical smears later in pregnancy to identify more serious cytologic changes, if any, should prove quite satisfactory. Cytologic changes in cervical smears compatible with severe dysplasia or neoplasia require confirmation and colposcopic evaluation to identify the responsible lesion. The cervix is examined and colposcopically directed biopsies made of any possibly malignant lesion. Colposcopy and directed focal biopsy during pregnancy has proved to be safe and reliable, thereby, in most cases, eliminating the need for conization (De Petrillo and associates, 1975; Kohan and co-workers, 1980).

If colposcopic examination is not available, multiple *punch biopsies* at the squamocolumnar junction should be obtained and evaluated histologically for carcinoma (Abitbol and colleagues, 1973; Selim and associates, 1973). Foci that do not stain with Lugol solution should be preferentially biopsied. The multiple biopsies need not all be made on one occasion. Instead, the squamocolumnar junction can be "mapped" and biopsies obtained systematically over a period of time without hospitalization. Bleeding from biopsy sites can usually be controlled by a vaginal pack well-applied to the cervix for a few hours. Occasionally, during pregnancy the cervix may bleed to the extent that a suture about the biopsy site must be used to effect hemostasis.

Conization of the cervix is less satisfactory during pregnancy than in its absence for three reasons: (1) The epithelium and underlying stroma within the cervical canal cannot be so extensively excised because of the risk to the fetal membranes adjacent to the internal os. (2) Blood loss from the cervix during and after conization is appreciable in pregnant women and at times may be severe. (3) There is some increased risk of abortion or premature delivery in the current pregnancy (Hannigan and associates, 1982), and probably subsequent ones as well (Larsson and co-workers, 1982). Fortunately, it has been the experience of most workers that colposcopic directed biopsies especially, or multiple punch biopsies of the squamocolumnar junction are an effective means of identifying invasive carcinoma, if present.

Because of the risks of hemorrhage and rupture of the membranes *endocervical curettage* should not be performed during pregnancy.

Dysplasia and Carcinoma in Situ

These epithelial lesions need no immediate treatment when detected during pregnancy. The pregnancy should be allowed to continue and delivery accomplished without regard to the presence of either lesion. In general, the cervix should be reevaluated for neoplastic disease after the puerperium. Appropriate therapy ranges from periodic reevaluation to hysterectomy, depending upon the lesion that persists and the parity. In general, cesarean hysterectomy to terminate the pregnancy and remove the affected cervix should be avoided unless there are other compelling indications for performing cesarean section. At times, it is difficult to be sure that all the cervix has been removed by cesarean hysterectomy.

For women who desire more children but have se-

vere dysplasia or carcinoma in situ that persists after the puerperium, conization that includes the removal of all of the squamocolumnar junction and the endocervical epithelium, including the immediately adjacent stroma, may be carried out and the specimen thoroughly studied histologically. Alternatively, the cervix may be carefully inspected with the colposcope and suspicious sites biopsied, followed by curettage of the endocervical canal. If only dysplasia or carcinoma in situ of the squamocolumnar junction and exocervix is identified, cryotherapy or laser therapy can be applied. If endocervical neoplasia is found, conization is performed and the excised tissue studied carefully. With no evidence of invasion the uterus can be conserved as long as carefully done cytologic evaluation is performed periodically and remains favorable. In the absence of stromal invasion, and with careful periodic follow-up, pregnancy can be encouraged.

Invasive Carcinoma

Pregnancy coexisting with invasive carcinoma of the cervix complicates both staging and treatment. Accurate identification of the extent of the cancer may be more difficult during pregnancy since induration of the base of the broad ligaments, which in nonpregnant women characterizes spread of tumor beyond the cervix, may be less prominent in the pregnant woman. Consequently, the extent of the tumor is more likely to be underestimated in the pregnant woman. Moreover, the decision between immediate interruption of the pregnancy and allowing the fetus to achieve several more weeks of maturity before interruption almost always is difficult.

Although few, if any, institutions have had great experience with the treatment of carcinoma of the cervix complicated by pregnancy, some generalizations can be made on the basis of some more recent reports, as well as the cumulative experiences at Parkland Memorial Hospital. Interestingly, the survival rate for invasive carcinoma of the cervix has not been profoundly different for pregnant and nonpregnant women within a given stage of disease. Moreover, the mode of delivery has not been shown to affect maternal survival significantly (Hacker and associates, 1982). Nonetheless, when frankly invasive carcinoma is known to exist, most clinicians favor hysterotomy or cesarean section for terminating pregnancy, rather than labor and vaginal delivery, if for no other reason than the cervix during labor might resist dilating and may lacerate severely.

Sufficient experience has accumulated to establish that for stage 1 invasive carcinoma complicated by pregnancy, extensive (radical) hysterectomy plus pelvic lymphadectomy is often the procedure of choice (Hacker and associates, 1982). Dissection is facilitated by the softening of uterine supportive structures induced by pregnancy, although blood loss is usually somewhat greater than in a nonpregnant woman, as is evident from Table 21-1.

For more extensive invasive cervical cancer, radiation therapy should be used. Early in pregnancy, external irradiation may be started. The pregnancy products usually will be expelled spontaneously or, if not, they can be removed by curettage. Sources of radiation are subsequently applied in standard fashion to the cervix and adjacent parts. If the uterus is enlarged sufficiently to be easily palpated above the symphysis (beyond the first trimester), hysterotomy with the uterine incision made remote from the cervix is performed to remove the pregnancy products. Care is taken to try to minimize adhesions, especially of the bowel. After a week or so, external irradiation is started, followed by intracavitary application of radiation sources.

There are no data with which to establish, with any degree of confidence, the risk to the mother from delay in treatment of frankly invasive carcinoma for many weeks while the fetus matures. In general, during the first half of pregnancy, at least, immediate treatment should be advised.

Other Tumors. *Adenocarcinoma of the endometrium* with an intrauterine pregnancy is rare. Sandstrom and associates (1978) have described a case and reviewed the few instances reported previously by others. The most common lesion was adenocanthoma.

Uterine myomas are relatively common and most often do not adversely affect the pregnancy. They are considered in detail in Chapter 32 (p. 689).

Carcinoma of the Oviduct. This malignancy has been rarely found complicating pregnancy. Schinfeld and Winston (1980) reported such a lesion encountered at the time of cesarean delivery for a breech presentation.

Ovarian Tumors. Such tumors, if large, may cause or contribute to dystocia and are considered in Chapter 32 (p. 690).

DEVELOPMENTAL ABNORMALITIES OF THE GENITAL TRACT

Although idiopathic developmental anomalies of the female genital tract are uncommon in obstetric practice, some do create serious fetal and maternal hazards.

Genesis

Because fusion of the two müllerian ducts to form a vagina, cervix, and uterine body in the human female takes place at three different levels at three different times, a variety of malformations can result. The three principal groups of deformities arising from three types of embryologic defects can be classified as follows:

1. The most common abnormality is the lack of or faulty midline fusion of the müllerian ducts. If there is complete lack of fusion, the result is the presence of two entirely separate uteri, cervices,

and vaginas. With incomplete fusion, the defect may arise at the level of vagina, cervix, or uterus or in combinations of any of these two levels (Fig. 25-2).
2. There may be unilateral maturation of the müllerian duct with incomplete or absent development of the duct on the opposite side. The resulting defects are often associated with abnormalities of the upper urinary tract.
3. There may be defective canalization of the vagina, resulting in a transverse vaginal septum or, in the most extreme form, absence of the vagina.

Various classifications of these anomalies have been proposed, but none is completely satisfactory. The terminology is often so complicated and replete with Latin words that the relative obstetric significance of the disorders is obscured. A simplified classification is outlined below in which five types of uteri are recognized:

1. *Single.* The normal symmetric uterus, resulting from normal fusion of the müllerian ducts.
2. *Septate.* Essentially normal uterus externally, with little or no external notching of the fundus. Internally, a septum of varying thickness extends part or all the way from fundus to cervix, dividing the uterine cavity into two more or less distinct compartments.
3. *Bicornuate.* The Y-shaped, forked uterus occurs in a wide range of varieties. Externally it may have only a shallow notch (arcuate uterus), or it may be cleaved so deeply as to be called a "double uterus." The internal septum may be partial, or it may extend down to the cervix, creating two separate cavities. The distinguishing characteristic of this uterus, regardless of the extent of fundal notching, is the cervix. The term "bicornuate" is limited to a forked uterus having a single cervix, rather than one having a double cervix.
4. *Double.* This designation is reserved for those instances of failure of midline fusion of the müllerian ducts, producing two hemiuteri, each having a distinct cervix. Complete reduplication of the uterus is also referred to as *uterus didelphys.* At times, development of one of the hemiuteri may be further distorted to yield a rudimentary structure lacking a cervix and, therefore, without vaginal communication or, less often, lacking even a uterine cavity.
5. *Single Hemiuterus.* There is maturation of but a single müllerian duct anlage, with complete failure of the other. The uterus is further characterized by having only one oviduct attached.

There are four types of cervices:

1. *Single.* The normal cervix.
2. *Septate.* A cervix consisting of a single muscular ring partitioned by a septum. The septum may be

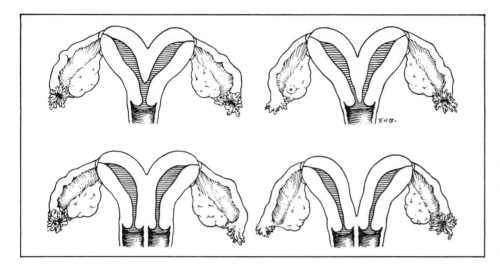

Figure 25-2. Varying degrees of faulty midline fusion of müllerian ducts. Upper uteri are bicornuate with partial septum on the left and complete septum on the right. Lower uteri are double with complete reduplication of cervices and uterine cavities.

confined to the cervix, or, more often, may be the downward continuation of a uterine septum or the upward extension of a vaginal septum.

3. *Double.* Two distinct cervices, each resulting from separate müllerian duct maturation. Both a septate and a true double cervix are frequently associated with a longitudinal vaginal septum, the result being that many septate cervices are erroneously classified as double. The diagnosis depends on careful visual and digital examination of the cervix and is of clinical importance.
4. *Single Hemicervix.* Arises from unilateral müllerian maturation.

The vagina may be classified as follows:

1. *Single.* The normal vagina.
2. *Longitudinally septate.* More or less complete longitudinal septum.
3. *Double.* It is often difficult to distinguish the double from the completely septate vagina. The true double vagina includes a double introitus and resembles a double-barreled shotgun, with each passage terminating in a distinct, separate cervix. At times with double vaginas, one may end blindly.
4. *Transversely septate.* Transverse vaginal septa are of different developmental origin, resulting from faulty canalization of the united müllerian anlage, rather than faulty longitudinal fusion.

Obstetric Significance

The significance of these defects can be anticipated. The various vaginal septa often are easily dilated, displaced, or surgically divided. The cervix, however, must undergo effacement and dilatation during labor. The septate cervix functions fairly well in these respects, but there is possible danger of rupture and consequent hemorrhage. The major obstetric difficulties arise from anomalies of the uterus. The uterus must dilate and hypertrophy suf-

ficiently to permit enlargement during pregnancy adequate to accommodate a term-sized fetus in a proper longitudinal lie and then, at the appropriate time, contract efficiently to expel the pregnancy products. The uterine defects resulting from maturation of only one müllerian duct or from complete lack of fusion often give rise to a hemiuterus that fails to dilate and hypertrophy appropriately, which, in turn, causes a host of possible difficulties, including abortion, prematurity, abnormal fetal presentation, uterine dysfunction, and even uterine rupture. Since lesser defects of fusion lead to proportionately less serious obstetric difficulties, women with the relatively more common minor abnormalities such as arcuate or partially septate uteri may be expected to have relatively normal deliveries.

Diagnosis

Some malformations are discovered by simple inspection, and others by bimanual examination. They are occasionally discovered first at cesarean section or during manual exploration of the uterine cavity after vaginal delivery. Fundal notching, palpated abdominally, is most often indicative of a malformed uterus. Without radiologic examination, high-resolution sonography, or direct visualization of the uterine cavity, it is difficult to distinguish the septate from the bicornuate uterus. *Hysterography* is of value to ascertain the configuration of the uterine cavity.

A high index of suspicion is important for a high rate of detection of uterine malformations. Green and Harris (1976) identified 80 uterine developmental anomalies during the course of 31,836 deliveries. They emphasized that detection was greatest during a period when one staff member was especially interested in the problem and espoused uterine exploration at delivery and, when an anomaly was suspected, suggested that hysterosalpingography be performed 6 to 8 weeks postpartum.

Sonography may be used to identify abnormal uterine development, although in some ways it lacks the pre-

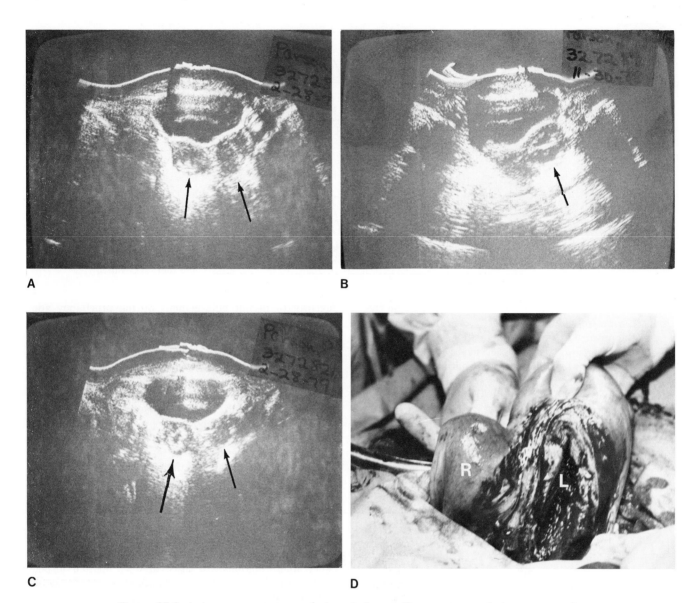

Figure 25-3. In transverse sonogram **A,** two uterine cavities are apparent above arrows. In sonogram **B,** a pregnancy ring, probably abnormal, is seen in the *left* uterine cavity above the arrow. In sonogram **C,** made 90 days later, a normal pregnancy ring is seen in the *right* uterine cavity above the larger arrow but not in the left uterine cavity above the smaller arrow. After seven abortions, a 2900-g healthy infant was delivered from the right uterus as a double footling breech by cesarean section at 38 weeks gestation. Necrotic placental villi from the missed abortion were expelled from the left uterus 2 days postpartum. **D.** Mother in Figure 25-3A–C conceived again 3 years later in the left uterus (L). A growth-retarded fetus who thrived after cesarean birth was delivered at 37 weeks through a vertical uterine incision. The small right uterus (R) is larger than when nonpregnant.

cision of diagnosis provided by hysterosalpingography. Especially during actual or suspected pregnancy, sonographic examination can be quite informative. In Figures 25-3A–C, for example, two separate uterine cavities are seen. A gestational ring, probably abnormal, was first identified in the left cavity. It subsequently degenerated but tissue was not expelled. Ninety days later, a pregnancy ring was identified in the right uterine cavity. The correct interpretation was a missed abortion in the left

hemiuterus and a normal appearing early pregnancy in the right hemiuterus. The latter conception produced a normal fetus who presented as a breech and was delivered at 38 weeks early in labor by cesarean section. The infant weighed 2900 g and thrived. At the time of surgery the left kidney was absent. She conceived again, this time in the left hemiuterus, and now has a second child. However, severe growth retardation was evident at birth. The infant weighed only 1690 g at 37 weeks gestation. The hemiuteri as they appeared immediately after cesarean delivery are presented in Figure 25-3D.

Urologic Evaluation

When asymmetric development of the reproductive tract is found, urologic evaluation is indicated because of the frequent association of anomalies of the urinary tract. Especially when there is uterine atresia on one side or one of double vaginas terminates blindly, an ipsilateral urologic anomaly is common (Toaff, 1974; Wiersma and associates, 1976; Woolf and Allen, 1953).

Prognosis

With minor uterine defects, the prognosis is excellent. Most published reports include only obvious major defects. In these situations also, except for uterine rupture, the prognosis for the mother is generally good. Cesarean section is, of course, required more frequently. With uterine anomalies, the occurrence of low-birth-weight infants is at least three times the normal rate, and, consequently, perinatal loss is increased. The abortion rate is also high. Among the 80 women with uterine developmental anomalies identified by Green and Harris (1976), overall fetal wastage was 55 percent.

Treatment

Abnormal fetal presentations, which are common in abnormal uteri, are generally treated in the same way as when they occur in normal uteri. Attempts at external podalic version are less likely to be successful and may prove dangerous. If uterine inertia occurs, it may be unwise to stimulate these defective uteri with oxytocin. Cesarean section is the safer treatment, but, unfortunately, the diagnosis is often unexpected.

Rarely, pregnancy occurs simultaneously in both hemiuteri (Fig. 25-4) or singly in a *rudimentary horn* (Fig. 25-5A and B). Rolen and colleagues (1966) reviewed the histories of 70 pregnancies in rudimentary uterine horns. Although few live births were reported, the duration of pregnancy before uterine rupture was usually 20 weeks or less. Intraperitoneal hemorrhage may be voluminous. Sometimes it is technically possible to remove the damaged rudimentary horn and preserve the larger horn.

Pregnancy in a rudimentary uterine horn 15 weeks after the last menstrual period is shown in Figure 25-5. There was no connection between the rudimentary horn and the opposite uterine horn or the vagina. The fertilizing sperm had to migrate out the oviduct attached to the patent uterine horn and cross transperitoneally to enter the oviduct attached to the rudimentary uterine horn. After she had missed three menstrual periods she was seen complaining of sudden, severe, cramping lower abdominal pain. A very tender mass was felt to the left of a somewhat enlarged uterus. Fetal heart action was identified in this mass with Doppler ultrasound. At laparotomy, about 200 ml of blood was free in the peritoneal cavity. A total hysterectomy and left salpingo-oophorectomy were performed. Her three pre-

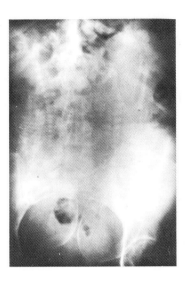

Figure 25-4. Roentgenogram in a case of a double uterus with a near-term fetus in each. Each was delivered by cesarean section. (*Courtesy of Dr. Jack Pearson.*)

vious pregnancies, all breech presentations, terminated with delivery of infants who weighed 750 g (expired), 1220 g (lived), and 2815 g (lived). The 2815-g infant was delivered by cesarean section. Although a rudimentary horn was identified at that time, tubal patency to that horn was not interrupted.

When a woman presents with a uterine anomaly and a poor obstetric history, for example, commonly repeated abortions not ascribable to some other cause, plastic repair of a septate or bicornuate uterus (*metroplasty*) may be justified. Musich and Behrman (1978) and Heinonen and associates (1982), on the basis of obstetric outcomes before and after metroplasty, concluded that women with septate or bicornuate anomalies and poor previous obstetric outcomes are very likely to have good outcomes after repair.

Cerclage has been attempted in some cases in which cervical incompetence has been suspected. If attempted, yet active labor supervenes, procrastination in severing the ligature must be avoided because of the increased risk of uterine rupture.

Progestational agents and β-mimetic drugs administered either acutely or chronically have been tried to prolong gestation. Their worth has not been established.

REPRODUCTIVE TRACT ANOMALIES FOLLOWING STILBESTROL EXPOSURE IN UTERO

For nearly a quarter of a century until the early 1970s stilbestrol (diethylstilbestrol), a synthetic, nonsteroidal estrogen, was prescribed for an estimated 3 million women in the United States. The enthusiastic endorsements provided in early uncontrolled reports from prestigous medical centers soon established it as the

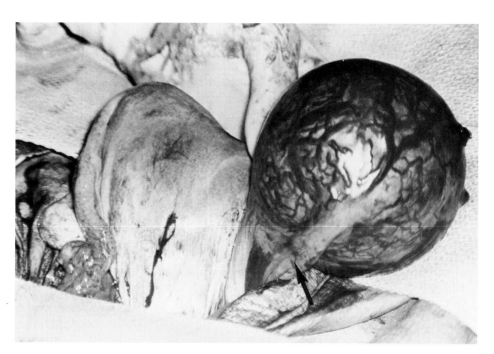

Figure 25-5. A. Pregnancy of 15 weeks gestational age in left rudimentary hemiuterus as seen at laparotomy. The tense, vascular rudimentary uterus was bleeding from veins over its extremely vascular surface. The attached oviduct (*arrow*) was patent and the adjacent left ovary contained the corpus luteum of pregnancy.

obstetrician's "magic bullet." It was claimed to be highly efficacious in the prevention of most forms of pregnancy wastage, including those resulting from abortion, preeclampsia and other hypertensive disorders, diabetes, and premature labor!

The first serious problem to be linked to the use of stilbestrol (other than it provided none of the miraculous powers attributed to it initially) was the identification of clear cell adenocarcinoma of the vagina in some daughters who were exposed in utero to stilbestrol (Herbst and co-workers, 1971). It has been established subsequently that the risk of malignancy is slight but real (from 0.14 to 1.4 per 1000 exposed daughters observed through the age of 24 years).

More recently, the reproductive performances of daughters exposed in utero to stilbestrol have been recognized to be impaired when compared to their unexposed sisters (Mangan and associates, 1982). Moreover, a variety of deformities of the reproductive tract of women exposed in utero have been identified.

Structural Abnormalities

One fourth to one half of women exposed in utero to stilbestrol demonstrate structural variations in the cervix and vagina, including transverse or circumferential ridges involving the vagina and cervix and the presence of hoods and collars over the cervix. The cervix may also be hypoplastic.

Anomalies of the uterine cavity are evident on hysterography in perhaps two thirds of exposed women (Kaufman and associates, 1980). Significantly smaller uterine cavities, shortened upper uterine segments, and T-shaped uterine cavities have been described (Fig. 25-6). About one half of those with uterine defects also have

cervical defects, especially a hypoplastic cervix. In at least one study, cervical intraepithelial neoplasia has been more common among women exposed to stilbestrol in utero (Fowler and associates, 1981). Finally, a variety of abnormalities of the oviduct have been described, including shortening, narrowing, and absence of fimbriae.

Reproductive Performance

Lower conception rates have been reported for women who were exposed to stilbestrol in utero. Of those who conceived, spontaneous abortions, ectopic pregnancies, and premature births were increased (Herbst and co-workers, 1981; Kaufman and associates, 1984). The risk seems greatest for those women with demonstrated structural abnormalities.

Treatment

The treatment of clear cell carcinoma of the vagina is gruesome, involving irradiation or radical extirpation. A case of clear cell carcinoma further complicated by pregnancy has been described. The mother was delivered by cesarean section followed immediately by radical hysterectomy, vaginectomy, and pelvic node dissection (Jones and co-workers, 1981).

Management of pregnancies in the presence of structural defects is empiric. The value of cervical cerclage for an incompetent cervix and of tocolytic therapy for premature labor are not known. Cerclage did not prove to be beneficial in the experiences of Kaufman and colleagues (1984). Therefore, they do not recommend routine cervical cerclage. Certainly, in this population especially, treatment first should do no harm!

Fortunately, these problems from in utero exposure

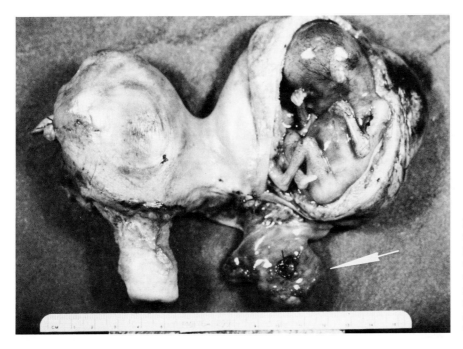

Figure 25-5. B. Hysterectomy specimen from Figure 25-5A, now with left hemiuterus opened to display the fetus and placenta. The inferior mass (*arrow*) consists of left tube and ovary. There is no cervix on the left and no communication with the right hemiuterus, which does have a cervix that communicated freely with the vagina.

to stilbestrol should eventually disappear since, hopefully, no one has been providing stilbestrol for pregnant women since the early 1970s at least.

UTERINE MALPOSITION

Anteflexion

Exaggerated degrees of anteflexion are frequently observed in the early months of pregnancy, but are without significance. In later months, particularly when the abdominal walls are very lax, the uterus may fall forward. The sagging occasionally is so exaggerated that the fundus lies considerably below the lower margin of the symphysis pubis. Even in less striking instances of so-called *pendulous abdomen,* the pregnant woman may complain of various annoying symptoms, especially dragging pains in the back and lower abdomen. Amelioration of symptoms is frequently effected by wearing a properly fitted abdominal support.

Retrodisplacement

Retroversion of the uterus is occasionally encountered during the first trimester, occurring in about 11 percent of women, according to Weekes and associates (1976). They noted not only a higher frequency of bleeding early in pregnancy in women with a retroverted uterus, but also an abortion rate of 16 percent, compared to 9 percent in women whose uterus was not retroverted. In their survey, perinatal mortality was slightly less, however, among women with a retroverted uterus. The biologic significance of these observations is not clear at this time. Most authorities no longer regard the retroverted

uterus per se to be a pathologic finding. Thus, it would need no treatment during pregnancy, except in the rare circumstance in which the growing retroverted uterus did not subsequently rise out of the pelvis by the end of the first trimester, but rather was incarcerated in the hollow of the sacrum, as shown in Figure 25-7. Women with a retroverted uterus should be evaluated frequently early in the second trimester, to make sure that the uterus is not incarcerated. If the uterus cannot be readily identified abdominally above the symphysis, pelvic examination is indicated.

The woman who becomes symptomatic with an incarcerated pregnant uterus is usually first seen complaining of abdominal discomfort and inability to void. As pressure from the full bladder increases, small amounts of urine are passed involuntarily, but the bladder never empties entirely (*paradoxical incontinence*). After the bladder has been emptied by catheterization, the uterus can usually be pushed out of the pelvis when the woman is placed in the knee–chest position; anesthesia is seldom necessary. A retention catheter should be left in place until bladder tone returns.

The urinary obstruction from an incarcerated gravid uterus can be so severe as to cause azotemia. With relief of the obstruction, there may be a marked diuresis with the loss of large amounts of sodium and potassium. Swartz and Komins (1977) have described such a case.

Sacculation of the Uterus

Continuation of pregnancy in the presence of a gravid uterus persistently entrapped in the pelvis involves sacculation, that is, extensive dilatation of the lower portion of the body of the uterus.

Rarely, the persistently entrapped retroverted

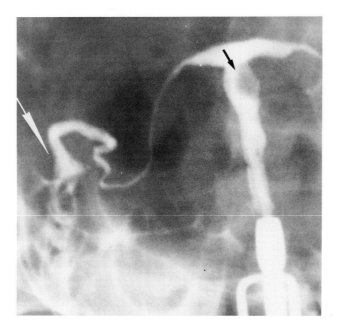

Figure 25-6. Hysterosalpingogram from a woman who was exposed in utero to stilbestrol. Note the T-shaped uterine cavity filled with contrast material which has also spilled from the end of the right oviduct (*white arrow*), demonstrating tubal patency. The filling defect within the uterine cavity (*black arrow*) probably is hyperplastic myometrium, the consequence of the stilbestrol exposure. She has since been pregnant successfully. (*Courtesy of Dr. Bruce R. Carr.*)

uterus produces few symptoms, and yet extensive dilatation of the lower portion of the body of the uterus, namely, the lower uterine segment, takes place to accommodate the fetus. In one case at Parkland Memorial Hospital, at the time of cesarean section, the Foley catheter bulb just above the urethra in the bladder lay at the level of the umbilicus. The cervix was at an equally high level. Most of the fetus (who was alive and weighed 2500 g), the amnionic fluid, and the fetal membranes were contained in a remarkably thin sacculation of the anterior wall of the lower segment. The fetal head was entrapped in the most superior part of the sacculation, along with three loops of cord, by a constricting ring of myometrium. The fundus of the uterus and the placenta were contained in the true pelvis beneath a sharp sacral promontory. After delivery, the uterus soon contracted and retracted to assume a more normal shape. Weissberg and Gall (1972) reviewed the relatively few published reports of sacculation of the pregnant uterus.

Prolapse of the Pregnant Uterus

Impregnation in a totally prolapsed uterus is very rare because of the difficulty of successful coitus, but impregnation when the uterus is only partially prolapsed is more common. In such cases, the cervix, and occasionally a portion of the body of the uterus, may protrude to a variable extent from the vulva during the early months of pregnancy. As pregnancy progresses, however, the body of the uterus usually rises gradually above the pelvis, and may draw the cervix up with it. If the uterus persists in its prolapsed position, symptoms of incarceration may appear during the third or fourth month of pregnancy.

For treatment of uterine prolapse during early pregnancy, the uterus should be replaced and held in position with a suitable pessary. If, however, the pelvic floor is too relaxed to permit retention of the pessary, the woman should be kept recumbent as long as possible until after the fourth month of pregnancy. When the cervix reaches or slightly protrudes from the vulva, scrupulous hygiene is mandatory. If much of the cervix persists outside the vulva and cannot be replaced, the pregnancy should be terminated.

When the vaginal outlet is markedly relaxed, the congested anterior or posterior vaginal walls may prolapse during pregnancy, usually along with bladder (cystocele) and rectum (rectocele), although the uterus may still remain in its normal position. This condition may give rise to considerable discomfort and interfere with locomotion, and it is not amenable to definitive treatment until after delivery. During labor, these structures may be forced down in front of the presenting part and interfere with its descent. In that event, they should be carefully cleansed and pushed back over the descending fetal presenting part.

MISCELLANEOUS CONDITIONS

Acute Edema of the Cervix

In rare instances, the cervix, particularly its anterior lip, may become so acutely edematous and enlarged during pregnancy that it protrudes from the vulva. This condition, if not associated with preexisting hypertrophy, may disappear with bed rest almost as suddenly as it developed.

Enterocele

In rare instances, an enterocele of considerable size filled with loops of intestine may complicate pregnancy. If this condition occurs during pregnancy, the protrusion should be replaced and the woman kept in the recumbent position. During labor, the mass may interfere with the advance of the fetal head. In such cases, it should be pushed up or held out of the way as well as possible, to allow delivery of the head past the mass.

Torsion of the Pregnant Uterus

Rotation of the pregnant uterus, most often to the right, is very common during pregnancy. However, torsion of the pregnant uterus of sufficient degree to arrest the uterine circulation and produce an acute abdominal catastrophe is a rare accident of human gestation. Laverson and co-workers (1984) have described a case at 20 weeks gestation and provided a review.

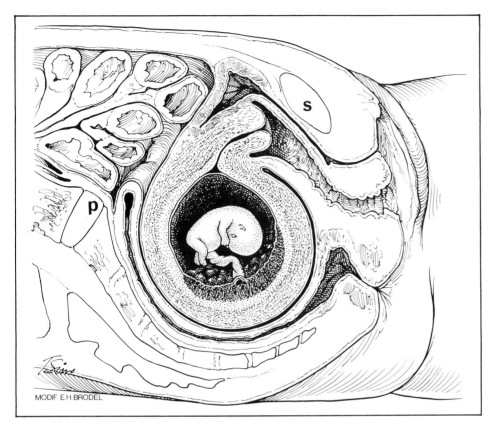

MODIF. E.H. BRODEL

Figure 25-7. Incarceration of retroflexed pregnant uterus.

Salpingitis and Tubo-Ovarian Abscess

Gonococcal salpingitis, salpingo-oophoritis, and pelvic peritonitis may develop during the first trimester of pregnancy by ascent of bacteria from the cervix to the endosalpinx. Once the chorion fuses with the decidua to obliterate completely the uterine cavity early in the second trimester, this pathway for ascending bacterial spread by way of the uterine mucosa is interrupted. Thereafter, primary acute inflammation of the tubes and ovaries is rarely, if ever, seen, although tubo-ovarian abscesses may form in previously damaged structures. Presumably, the organisms reach the previously damaged oviduct and ovary through lymphatics or the bloodstream. Jafari and associates (1977) described the successful outcome of a term pregnancy complicated by a tubo-ovarian abscess, as well as the few experiences of others that have been reported.

> In one of two instances of tubo-ovarian abscess complicating midpregnancy treated at Parkland Memorial Hospital during the past two decades, hysterectomy, as well as bilateral salpingo-oophorectomy, was carried out. The woman recovered after a very complicated postoperative course. In the other instance, the tubo-ovarian abscess was smaller and was mobilized intact. Therefore, only the affected tube and ovary were removed. The pregnancy subsequently proceeded normally, terminating in spontaneous vaginal delivery of a normal infant.

Even with extensive pelvic adhesions from previous pelvic infection, women usually suffer no adverse effects during pregnancy.

Hydrorrhea Gravidarum

Rarely, pregnant women may lose clear fluid from the uterus throughout much of pregnancy. The cause of this condition is not always obvious but may represent persistent *amniorrhea* following rupture of the membranes. Gregersen (1976) described a case with loss of fluid beginning about the tenth week of pregnancy and continuing until delivery at 31 weeks. Up to 200 ml of fluid per day was collected. The ruptured membranes may retract to such an extent as to create an *extramembranous* pregnancy with the fetus no longer contained within the amnionic sac. Extramembranous pregnancy involving a twin has also been described (Panayiotis, Grunstein, 1979). The membranes were diamnionic and dichorionic, with a single placenta in which there was appreciable circumvallate involvement on the side of the extramembranous fetus. That newborn quickly succumbed from anoxia. Pulmonary hypoplasia, presumably due to lack of amnionic fluid and the inability to inspire in utero, was evident at autopsy. In an era of frequent amniocentesis, this rare complication, fortunately, does not appear to have increased, although Vago and Chaukin (1980) described such a case.

Endometriosis

Since endometriosis is frequently associated with infertility, it is an uncommon complication of pregnancy. As emphasized in Scott's early report (1944), however, some women with endometriosis do become pregnant and, in the course of gestation, sometimes exhibit bizarre and vexing clinical symptoms.

A rare complication of ovarian endometriosis in pregnancy is rupture of an endometrial cyst, with clinical features that are suggestive of pyelonephritis, acute appendicitis, or tubal pregnancy (Rossman and associates, 1983). Another is an enlarging pelvic endometrioma that causes dystocia in labor. Many women with unrecognized endometriosis, however, doubtless do go through pregnancy and labor without complications.

Of the 12 cases of *adenomyosis* associated with pregnancy that Scott (1944) was able to collect from a review of the literature, 5 were complicated by uterine rupture, 3 by postpartum hemorrhage, and 2 by dystocia resulting from the adenomyoma.

REFERENCES

Abitbol MM, Benjamin F, Castillo N: Management of cervical smear and carcinoma in situ of the cervix during pregnancy. Am J Obstet Gynecol 117:904, 1973

DePetrillo AD, Townsend DE, Morrow CP, Lickrish GM, Di Saia PJ, Roy M: Colposcopic evaluation of the abnormal Papanicolau test in pregnancy. Am J Obstet Gynecol 121:441, 1975

Fowler WC Jr, Schmidt G, Edelman DA, Kaugman DG, Fenoglio CM: Risks of cervical intraepithelial neoplasia among DES exposed women. Obstet Gynecol 58:720, 1981

Green LK, Harris RE: Uterine anomalies: Frequency of diagnosis and associated obstetric complications. Obstet Gynecol 47:427, 1976

Gregersen E: Extramembranous pregnancy with amniorrhoea. Acta Obstet Gynecol Scand 55:69, 1976

Hacker NF, Berek JS, Lagasse LD, Charles EH, Moore JG: Carcinoma of the cervix associated with pregnancy. Obstet Gynecol 59:735, 1982

Hannigan EV, Whitehouse HH III, Atkinson WD, Becker SN: Cone biopsy during pregnancy. Obstet Gynecol 60:450, 1982

Heinonen PK, Saarikoski S, Pystynen P: Reproductive performance of women with uterine anomalies: An evaluation of 182 cases. Acta Obstet Gynecol Scand 61:157, 1982

Herbst AL, Ulfelder H, Poskanzer DC: Adenocarcinoma of the vagina. N Engl J Med 284:878, 1971

Herbst AL, Hubby MM, Azizi F, Makii MM: Reproductive and gynecologic surgical experiences in diethylstilbestrol-exposed daughters. Am J Obstet Gynecol 141:1019, 1981

Iosif S, Ulmsten U: Comparative urodynamic studies of continent and stress incontinent women in pregnancy and in the puerperium. Am J Obstet Gynecol 140:645, 1981

Jafari K, Vilovic-Kos J, Webster A, Steptoe R: Tubo-ovarian abscess in pregnancy. Acta Obstet Gynecol Scand 56:1, 1977

Jones WB, Woodruff JM, Erlandson RA, Lewis JL Jr: DES-related clear cell adenocarcinoma of the vagina in pregnancy. Obstet Gynecol 57:775, 1981

Kaufman RH, Adam E, Binder GL, Gerthoffer E: Upper genital tract changes and pregnancy outcome in offspring exposed in utero to diethylstilbestrol. Am J Obstet Gynecol 137:299, 1980

Kaufman RH, Noller K, Adam E, Irvine J, Gray M, Jeffries JJ, Hilton J: Upper genital tract abnormalities and pregnancy

outcome in DES-exposed progeny. Am J Obstet Gynecol 148:973, 1984

Kiguchi K, Bibbo M, Hasegawa T, Tsutsui F, Wied GL: Dysplasia during pregnancy. A cytologic follow-up study. J Reprod Med 26:66, 1981

Kohan S, Beckman EM, Bigelow B, Klein S, Douglas G: The role of colposcopy in the management of cervical intraepithelial neoplasia during pregnancy and postpartum. J Reprod Med 25:279, 1980

Larsson G, Grundsell H, Gullberg B, Svennerud S: Outcome of pregnancy after conization. Acta Obstet Gynecol Scand 61:461, 1982

Laverson PL, Hankins GDV, Leveno KJ: Torsion of the pregnancy uterus: Case report and literature review. Obstet Gynecol, in press, 1984

Malfetano JH, Marin AC, Malfetano JH Jr: Laser treatment of condylomata acuminata in pregnancy. Obstet Gynecol 26:574, 1981

Mangan CE, Borow L, Burtnett-Rubin MM, Egan V, Giuntoli RL, Mikuta JJ: Pregnancy outcome in 98 women exposed to diethylstilbestrol in utero, their mothers, and unexposed siblings. Obstet Gynecol 59:315, 1982

McCoy C, Cunningham FG: Unpublished observations

Musich J Jr, Behrman SJ: Obstetric outcomes before and after metroplasty in women with uterine anomalies. Obstet Gynecol 52:63, 1978

Panayiotis G, Grunstein S: Extramembranous pregnancy in twin gestation. Obstet Gynecol (Suppl) 53: 34S, 1979

Rolen AC, Choquette AJ, Semmens JP: Rudimentary uterine horn: Obstetric and gynecologic implications. Obstet Gynecol 27:806, 1966

Rossman F, D'Ablaing G III, Marrs RP: Pregnancy complicated by ruptured endometrioma. Obstet Gynecol 62:519, 1983

Sandstrom RE, Welch WR, Green TH: Adenocarcinoma of the endometrium in pregnancy. Obstet Gynecol (Suppl) 53:73S, 1979

Scott RB: Endometriosis and pregnancy. Am J Obstet Gynecol 47:608, 1944

Selim MA, So-Bosita JL, Blair OM, Little BA: Cervical biopsy versus conization. Obstet Gynecol 41:177, 1973

Schinfeld JS, Winston HG: Primary tubal carcinoma in pregnancy. Am J Obstet Gynecol 137:512, 1980

Slater GE, Rumack BH, Peterson RG: Podophyllin poisoning. Systemic toxicity following cutaneous application. Obstet Gynecol 52:94, 1978

Swartz EM, Komins JI: Postobstructive diuresis after reduction of an incarcerated gravid uterus. J Reprod Med 19:262, 1977

Toaff R: A major malformation—Communicating uteri. Obstet Gynecol 43:221, 1974

Vago T, Chavkin J: Extramembranous pregnancy: An unusual complication of amniocentesis. Am J Obstet Gynecol 137:511, 1980

Weekes ARL, Atlay RD, Brown VA, Jordan EC, Murray SM: The retroverted gravid uterus and its effect on the outcome of pregnancy. Br Med J 1:622, 1976

Weissberg SM, Gall SA: Sacculation of the pregnant uterus. Obstet Gynecol 39:691, 1972

Wiersma AF, Peterson LF, Justema EJ: Uterine anomalies associated with renal agenesis. Obstet Gynecol 47:654, 1976

Woolf RB, Allen WM: Concomitant malformations: Frequent simultaneous occurrence of congenital malformations of the reproductive and urinary tracts. Obstet Gynecol 2:236, 1953

26
Multifetal Pregnancy

Morbidity and mortality are increased appreciably in pregnancies with multiple fetuses. It is not an overstatement, therefore, to consider a pregnancy with multiple fetuses to be a complicated pregnancy. Many of the complications that occur more commonly with multiple fetuses and are of obvious clinical significance are listed below:

1. Abortion
2. Perinatal mortality
3. Low birth weight
   Prematurity
   Growth retardation
4. Malformations
5. Fetal–fetal hemorrhage
   Hypovolemia and anemia
   Hypervolemia and hyperviscosity
6. Pregnancy-induced or aggravated hypertension
7. Maternal anemia
   Acute blood loss
   Iron deficiency
   Folate deficiency
8. Placental accidents
   Placental abruption
   Placenta previa
9. Other maternal hemorrhage
   Uterine atony
10. Cord accidents
    Prolapse
    Entwinement
    Vasa previa
11. Hydramnios
12. Complicated labor
    Premature labor
    Ineffective labor
    Abnormal fetal presentation

ETIOLOGY OF MULTIPLE FETUSES

Twin fetuses more commonly result from fertilization of two separate ova (double-ovum, dizygotic, or "fraternal" twins). About one third as often, twins arise from a single fertilized ovum that subsequently divides into two similar structures, each with the potential for developing into a separate individual (single-ovum, monozygotic, or

"identical" twins). Either or both processes may be involved in the formation of higher numbers of fetuses. Quadruplets, for example, may arise from one, two, three, or four ova.

Fraternal vs. "Identical Twins"

Dizygotic twins are not in a strict sense true twins, since they result from the maturation and fertilization of two ova during a single ovulatory cycle. Newman (1923) wrote: "Strictly speaking, twainning is twinning or twoing—the division of an individual into two equivalent and more or less completely separate individuals." Also, monozygotic or identical twins are not always identical. As is pointed out below, the process of division of one fertilized zygote into two does not necessarily result in equal sharing of protoplasmic materials. In fact, dizygotic, or fraternal twins of the same sex, may *appear* more nearly identical at birth than do monozygotic twins; growth of monozygotic twin fetuses may be discordant and at times dramatically so.

Genesis of Monozygotic Twins

Valid hypotheses to explain single-ovum, or monozygotic twinning, are lacking. Monozygotic twins arise from division of the fertilized ovum at various early stages of development as follows:

1. If division occurs before the inner cell mass is formed and the outer layer of blastocyst is not yet committed to become chorion, that is, within the first 72 hours after fertilization, two embryos, two amnions, and two chorions will develop. There will evolve a *diamnionic, dichorionic,* monozygotic twin pregnancy. The frequency of two chorions with monozygotic twinning in various reports has ranged from 18 to 36 percent (MacGillivray, 1978). There may be two distinct placentas or a single fused placenta, as depicted in Figure 26-1A and 26-1B, respectively.
2. If division occurs between the fourth and eighth day, after the inner cell mass is formed and cells destined to become chorion have already differentiated but those of the amnion have not, two embryos will develop, each in separate amnionic

Figure 26-1. Placenta and membranes in twin pregnancies. **A.** Two placentas, two amnions, two chorions (from either dizygotic twins or monozygotic twins with cleavage of zygote during first 3 days after fertilization). **B.** Single placenta, two amnions, and two chorions (from either dizygotic twins or monozygotic twins with cleavage of zygote during first 3 days). **C.** One placenta, one chorion, two amnions (monozygotic twins with cleavage of zygote from the fourth to the eighth day after fertilization).

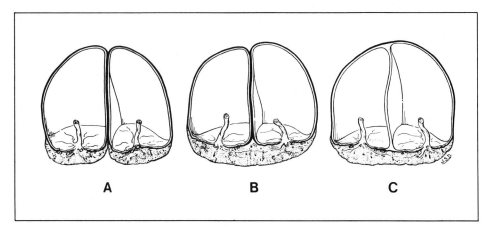

sacs. The two amnionic sacs will eventually be covered by a common chorion, thus giving rise to *diamnionic, monochorionic,* monozygotic twin pregnancy (Fig. 26-1C).

3. If, however, the amnion has already become established, which occurs about 8 days after fertilization, division will result in two embryos within a common amnionic sac, or a *monoamnionic, monochorionic,* monozygotic twin pregnancy.

4. If division is initiated even later, that is, after the embryonic disk is formed, cleavage is incomplete and conjoined twins are formed.

Frequency of Twins

The frequency of monozygotic twins appears to be relatively constant throughout the world at approximately one set of monozygotic twins per 250 births, and is largely independent of race, heredity, age, parity, and therapy for infertility. The incidence of delivery of dizygotic twins is influenced remarkably by race, heredity, maternal age, parity, and, especially, "fertility drugs."

It is now apparent through the use of sonography early in pregnancy that the incidence of twin conceptions is much higher than indicated by figures based on the delivery of two fetuses. Robinson and Caines (1977), for example, by means of sonography performed during the first trimester, identified twin conceptions in 30 women, only 14 of whom eventually gave birth to two infants. Eleven of the 16 women who did not do so were delivered of a single fetus and a blighted ovum. Four more were diagnosed as having twin blighted ova, and one a blighted ovum and a missed abortion. Varma (1979), and others more recently, have provided similar data. Undoubtedly, some "threatened" abortions have resulted in actual abortion of one embryo from an unrecognized twin gestation while the other embryo continued its growth and development.

Remarkably, fetal death occurring as late as the end of the first trimester can be followed by complete resorption of the fetus, leaving behind no gross evidence at delivery near term that twins ever existed. Sonographic demonstration of such a case is presented in Figures 26-2A–D.

Multiple embryos and fetuses may develop in varying degrees ectopically, that is, outside the uterus. Such multiple ectopic pregnancies, as well as *combined pregnancies* in which there are one or more embryos or fetuses extrauterine as well as one or more intrauterine, are considered in Chapter 22 (p. 426).

Race. The frequency of birth of multiple fetuses varies significantly among different races. For example, Myrianthopoulos (1970) identified in the Collaborative Cerebral Palsy Study the birth of twins in one out of every 100 pregnancies among white women, compared to one out of 79 pregnancies for black women. In some areas of Africa the frequency of twinning is very high. Knox and Morley (1960), in a survey of one rural community in Nigeria, found that twinning occurred once in every 19 births! Twinning among Orientals is less common. In Japan, for example, among more than 10 million pregnancies analyzed, twinning was identified only once in every 155 births. These marked racial differences are the consequence of variations in the frequency of dizygotic twinning.

Heredity. As a determinant of twinning, the genotype of the mother is much more important than that of the father. White and Wyshak (1964), in a study of 4000 records of the General Society of the Church of Jesus Christ of Latter-Day Saints, noted that women who themselves were a dizygotic twin gave birth to twins at the rate of one set per 58 births. However, women not a twin but whose husbands were a dizygotic twin, gave birth to twins at the rate of 1 set per 126 pregnancies. Moreover, in Bulmer's (1960) analysis of twins, 1 out of 25 (4 percent) of their mothers was also a twin but only 1 out of 60 (1.7 percent) of their fathers was a twin.

Maternal Age and Parity. The positive effects of increasing maternal age and parity on the incidence of twinning have been well demonstrated by Waterhouse

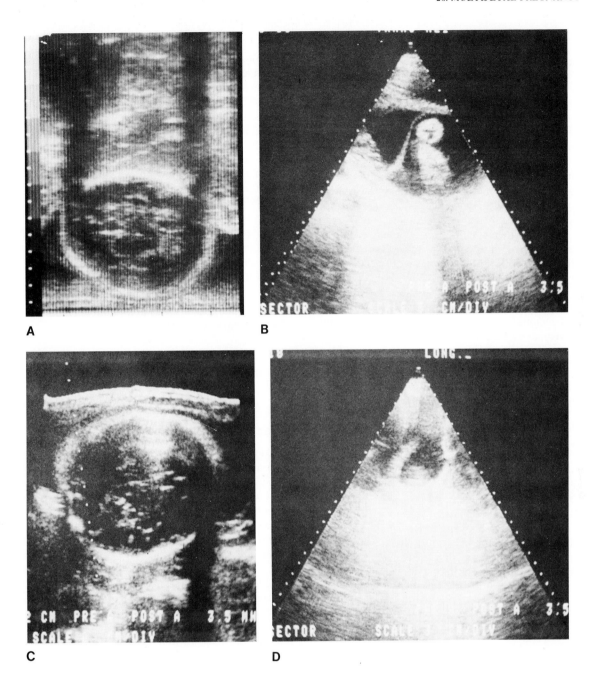

A

B

C

D

Figure 26-2. A. Sonography at 27 weeks gestation identified an appropriately grown fetus whose head is demonstrated in **A,** accompanied by **B.** a gestational sac containing a dead fetus of 12 weeks gestational age as estimated by crown–rump length. Four weeks later appropriate growth of one fetal head **C.** was ascertained and now resorption of the dead fetus **D.** had occurred leaving an empty gestational sac. Three weeks later that sac was no longer visible sonographically and at delivery by repeat cesarean section 1 week later no gross evidence of twins was found. (*Courtesy of Dr. R. Santos.*)

(1950). For any increase in age up to about 40, or parity up to 7, the frequency of twinning increased. Twin pregnancies were less than one third as common in women under 20 years of age with no previous children than in women 35 to 40 years of age with four or more previous children. In Sweden, Pettersson and associates (1976) confirmed the remarkable increase in multiple birth rate associated with increased parity. In first pregnancies, the frequency of multiple fetuses was 1.27 percent, compared to 2.67 percent in the fourth birth order.

In Nigeria, Azubuike (1982) identified the frequency of twinning to increase from 1 in 50 (2 percent) pregnancies among women pregnant for the first time to 1 in 15 (6.6 percent) for women pregnant six or more times!

Since the likelihood of twins increases with both parity and maternal age, it is not altogether surprising that a woman who at the age of 50 conceived for the ninth time had twins. The remarkable feature is that the pregnancy was completed successfully, with one infant weighing 8 pounds, 3 ounces at birth, and the other 7 pounds, 6 ounces (Dallas Times Herald, 1982).

Endogenous Gonadotropin. Benirschke and Kim (1973), in their excellent review, "Multiple Pregnancy," present intriguing reasons for implicating elevated levels of endogenous follicle-stimulating hormone in the genesis of spontaneous dizygous twinning. A higher rate of dizygous twinning has been described for women who conceived within 1 month after stopping use of oral contraceptives, but not during subsequent months (Rothman, 1977). One possibility to account for the apparent increase is release of pituitary gonadotropin in amounts greater than usual during the first spontaneous cycle after stopping contraception. Another is increased fecundity among very recent users of oral contraceptives.

Infertility Agents. The induction of ovulation by use of gonadotropins (follicle-stimulating hormone plus chorionic gonadotropin) or of clomiphene enhances remarkably the likelihood of ovulations of multiple ova. Multiple fetuses are common in pregnancies of women in whom ovulation was induced by injections of gonadotropins. The incidence of multiple fetuses following gonadotropin therapy is 20 to 40 percent, and in one instance as many as 11 fetuses were aborted (Jewelewicz, Vande Wiele, 1975). Nonuplet pregnancy with spontaneous labor 27 weeks after induction of ovulation with human pituitary gonadotropin has been described by Garrett and associates (1976). None of the nine infants survived. Two of octuplets survived in Italy. Sextuplets after gonadotropin therapy have survived in South Africa, as did five of the sextuplets born in Denver.

With clomiphene therapy, the likelihood of multiple fetuses is somewhat less than with human menopausal gonadotropin. Even so, among 2369 pregnancies following clomiphene, 165 (6.9 percent) were known to be twin, 11 (0.5 percent) triplet, 7 (0.3 percent) quadruplet, and 3 (0.13 percent) quintuplet (Merrell-National Laboratories Product Information Bulletin, 1972.) Harlap (1976) identified in smaller groups in Israel the frequency of multiple fetuses following clomiphene treatment to be 13 percent.

In Vitro Fertilization

Twinning is more common in pregnancies that result from in vitro fertilization, and several sets of triplets after in vitro fertilization have now been delivered. The practice of some groups of attempting fertilization of all the ova collected after inducing superovulation and then depositing in utero more than one blastocyst when available accounts, in part, at least, for the increased frequency of multifetal pregnancies. Liveborn quadruplets have been delivered in Australia and elsewhere following in vitro fertilization!

Sex Ratios with Multiple Fetuses

The percentage of male conceptuses in the human species decreases as the number of fetuses per pregnancy increases. Strandskov and co-workers (1946) found the sex ratio, or percentage of males, for 31 million singleton births in the United States to be 51.59 percent. For twins, it was 50.85 percent; for triplets, 49.54 percent; and for quadruplets, 46.48 percent. Two explanations have been offered: The differential fetal mortality between the sexes is well known, as it is for the newborn infant, child, and adult. Survival is always in favor of the female and against the male. The "population pressure" with multiple fetuses in utero may exaggerate the biologic tendency noted in singleton pregnancies. A second possible explanation is that the female-producing zygote has a greater tendency to divide into twins, triplets, and quadruplets.

DETERMINATION OF ZYGOSITY

With the advent of organ transplantation, the zygosity of multiple fetuses from a single pregnancy has assumed more than theoretical importance.

Examination of Placenta

A knowledgeably performed examination of the placenta and membranes serves to establish zygosity promptly in about two thirds of cases (Benirschke and Kim, 1973). Moreover, appropriate examination of the placenta and membranes often will serve to identify the zygosity of fetuses more firmly than will subsequent studies, which yield less precise information at considerable inconvenience and expense.

The following system for examination is recommended: As the first infant is delivered, one clamp is placed on the portion of the cord coming from the placenta. As the second infant is delivered two clamps are placed on the cord toward the placental side. Three clamps are used to mark the cord of a third infant, and so on as necessary. Until the delivery of the last fetus is completed, it is important that each segment of cord attached to the placenta remain clamped lest fetal hemorrhage occur through anastomosed fetal vessels in the placenta.

Delivery of the placenta should be accomplished with care to preserve the attachment of the amnion and chorion to the placenta since identification of the relationship of the membranes to each other is critical. With one common amnionic sac, which is a rare finding, or with juxtaposed amnions not separated by chorion arising between the fetuses, the infants are monozygotic. If adjacent amnions are separated by chorion, the fetuses may be monozygotic, but more often dizygotic (Figs. 26-1, 26-3, 26-4). If the infants are of the same sex, blood group studies to identify zygosity may be initiated at this time on samples of blood obtained from the umbilical

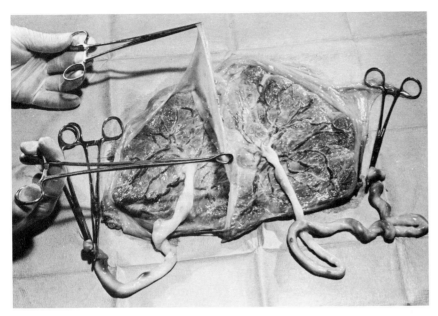

A

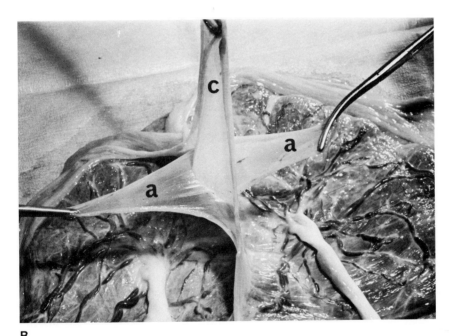

B

Figure 26-3. A. The membrane partition that separated twin fetuses is elevated. **B.** The membrane partition consists of chorion (c) between two amnions (a).

cords. A difference in major blood groups is indicative of dizygosity. If these simple procedures fail to identify zygosity, more complicated techniques, such as extensive blood and tissue antigen typing of the twins and their parents, may have to be used to look for differences.

Sex and Zygosity

Although twins of opposite sex are almost always dizygotic, monozygotic twins rarely may be discordant for phenotypic sex. Schmidt and co-workers (1974), for ex-

ample, described adolescent twins in whom concordance for 22 blood groups and other biochemical markers was demonstrated. The proband demonstrated classic features of Turner syndrome, including a single sex chromosome (karyotype 45, XO), in tissue cultures from streak gonads. The karyotype of the other twin, a normal-appearing male, was 46, XY. Pedersen and associates (1980) have summarized the salient features of 16 cases of monozygotic twins in whom one or both twins had gonadal dysgenesis and a 45, XO karyotype, at least in some cells.

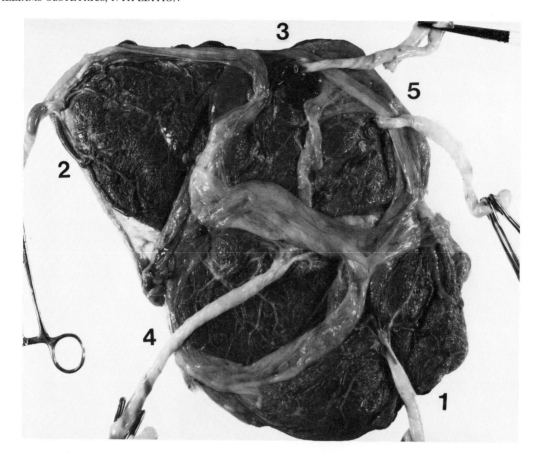

Figure 26-4. Quintuplet placenta with five separate amnionic sacs delivered at 32 weeks gestation. Amnionic sacs no. 3 and 5 were not separated by chorion and therefore those infants are identical. Infant birth weights ranged from a high of 1530 g (no. 1) to 860 g (no. 5). All of the infants survived.

CONJOINED TWINS

In the United States, united or conjoined twins are commonly referred to as Siamese twins, after Chang and Eng Bunker of Siam (Thailand), who were displayed worldwide by P.T. Barnum. If twinning is initiated after the embryonic disc and the rudimentary amnionic sac have been formed, and if division of the embryonic disc is incomplete, conjoined twins result. When each of the joined twins is nearly complete, the commonly shared body site may be (1) anterior (*thoracopagus*), (2) posterior (*pyopagus*), (3) cephalic (*craniopagus*), or (4) caudal (*ischiopagus*). The majority are of the thoracopagus variety (Figs. 26-5, 26-6).

When the bodies are only partly duplicated, the attachment is more often lateral. The incomplete division of the embryonic disc may begin at either or both poles and produce two heads; two, three, or four arms; two, three or four legs; or some combination thereof. The frequency of conjoined twins is not well established. At Kandang Kerbau Hospital in Singapore, Tan and co-workers (1971) identified seven cases of conjoined twins among somewhat more than 400,000 deliveries (1 in 60,000).

The diagnosis of conjoined twins at midpregnancy by sonography is demonstrated in Figure 26-6. The use of sonography to detect conjoined twins has been considered in some depth by Koontz and associates (1983).

Vaginal delivery of conjoined twins may occur, since the union most often is somewhat pliable, although dystocia is common. However, if mature, vaginal delivery may be traumatic. Surgical separation of conjoined twins may be successful when organs essential for life are not intimately shared.

HYDATIDIFORM MOLE

At times, twinning is expressed as a single fetus from one ovum plus a hydatidiform mole from another. (The development of a hydatidiform mole is described in Chapter 23.) Severe pregnancy-induced hypertension may develop at times before the 24th week, which is about as early as preeclampsia–eclampsia develops in the absence of a hydatidiform mole. The presence of a fetal heart and hypertension so early in pregnancy may cloud the etiology of the hypertension until the unsuspected mole is identified either by sonography or at delivery (see Chapter 27, p. 526).

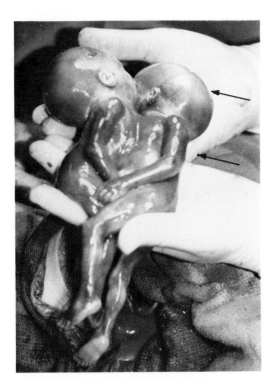

Figure 26-5. Conjoined twins at delivery by hysterotomy. The arrows indicate the approximate levels of the transverse sonograms depicted in Figure 26-6.

VASCULAR COMMUNICATIONS BETWEEN FETUSES

Frequently demonstrable in monochorionic placentas are vascular anastomoses, either artery to artery, artery to vein (arteries are recognized as crossing over veins), or vein to vein. The most troublesome interfetal vascular connection is artery to vein. Anastomoses are rarely demonstrable in dichorionic placentas (Robertson and Neer, 1983). Arteriovenous anastomoses may develop quite early in pregnancy and may vary appreciably in number and in size. As emphasized by Benirschke and Kim (1973), the arteriovenous communication often proceeds through the capillary bed of a placental cotyledon. As the consequence of such anastomoses blood is pumped from artery to vein, out of one fetus into the other.

Effects of Anastomotic Circulations

The effects from the arteriovenous anastomoses can be profound. One monozygous or "identical" twin may be very much smaller than the other as the consequence of chronic intrauterine malnutrition. The anatomic changes described by Naeye (1965), for example, in the underperfused twin resemble those found in growth-retarded singletons whose placentas were extensively infarcted. In monozygotic twins with anastomosed circulations, the

hemoglobin concentration may be 8 g/dl or less in the hypoperfused twin and as much as 27 g/dl in the other! Hypotension, microcardia, and generalized runting characterize the overtly affected hypovolemic "identical" donor twin, in contrast to hypertension and cardiac hypertrophy in the hypertransfused twin. Hydramnios, perhaps the consequence of increased renal perfusion and, in turn, increased urine formation, may accompany the hypervolemia and polycythemia in the typically larger recipient twin. At the same time, amnionic fluid

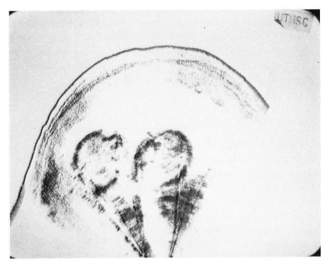

A

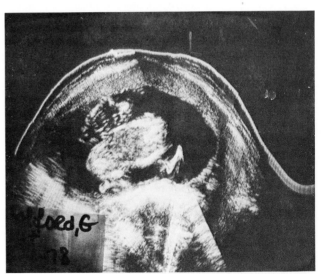

B

Figure 26-6. Transverse sonograms of the conjoined twins shown in Figure 26-5. Two fetal heads are seen in sonogram **A**. In sonogram **B**, made parallel to **A** but 5 cm below, the fused thoraces are evident. Below the thoraces are extremities and above are the umbilical cords. (*Courtesy of Dr. R. Santos.*)

may be scant to absent in the other sac, possibly as a result of marked oliguria in the underperfused donor twin. Death of one monozygotic fetus has been reported to precipitate serious consumptive coagulopathy in the other fetus (p. 513).

The neonatal period may be complicated by dangerous circulatory overload with heart failure if severe hypervolemia and blood hyperviscosity at birth are not promptly identified and treated by phlebotomy. Occlusive thrombosis is also much more likely to occur in this setting. Polycythemia may lead during the neonatal period to severe hyperbilirubinemia and, in turn, kernicterus (see Chapter 38, p. 781).

Viewed from the maternal side, one portion of the placenta often appears quite pale compared to the rest of the placenta when there is anemia in one twin and polycythemia in the other. The vascular anastomoses can usually be visualized directly after the overlying amnion is removed, especially after injecting milk into an umbilical artery.

Chimerism

A chimera is an individual with a mixture of genotypes from more than one ovum and sperm. Possible mechanisms include double fertilization of one ovum, and, in case of nonidentical fetuses, the transfer of genetic material from one across chorionic vascular anastomoses to the other. For example, the transfer of primitive blood cells from one dizygotic twin fetus through a vascular anastomosis to the other twin can lead to the production in the recipient of two populations of blood cells of quite dissimilar blood types, or *blood chimerism*. The "transfused" cells are not destroyed, since exposure of the recipient twin to the dissimilar antigens of the donor twin early in fetal development renders the recipient twin tolerant to the donor twin's tissues. Most commonly, blood chimerism has been discovered at the time of blood typing when discordant blood types are found (Benirschke, 1974).

Chimerism, in which cell lines are derived from different zygotes, is to be distinguished from *mosaicism*, in which two or more cell lines of different chromosomal composition arise from the same zygote as the consequence of nondisjunction during meiotic division.

DIAGNOSIS OF MULTIPLE FETUSES

It is unfortunate that the diagnosis of twins frequently has not been made until late in pregnancy, often as late as the time of parturition. Powers (1973), in his analysis of complications and treatment in twin pregnancy, ascertained from various reports that from 5 percent to more than 50 percent of the time twins were not diagnosed before labor. The identification of pregnancy complicated by multiple fetuses is missed not so much because it is unusually difficult but because the examiner fails to keep the possibility in mind.

History and Physical Examination

A familial history of twins by itself provides only a weak clue, but knowledge of recent administration of either clomiphene or pituitary gonadotropin provides a strong one.

Physical examination with accurate measurement of fundal height, as described in Chapter 13 (p. 249) is essential. *During the second trimester, a discrepancy develops between gestational age determined from menstrual data and that from uterine size. The uterus that contains two or more fetuses clearly becomes larger than with a single fetus!* In the case of the uterus that appears large for gestational age the obstetrician must carefully consider the following possibilities: (1) multiple fetuses, (2) the elevation of the uterus by a distended bladder, (3) inaccurate menstrual history, (4) hydramnios, (5) hydatidiform mole, (6) uterine myomas or adenomyosis, (7) a closely attached adnexal mass, and (8) fetal macrosomia late in pregnancy.

Diagnostic Aids

A variety of techniques are utilized to identify a multifetal pregnancy.

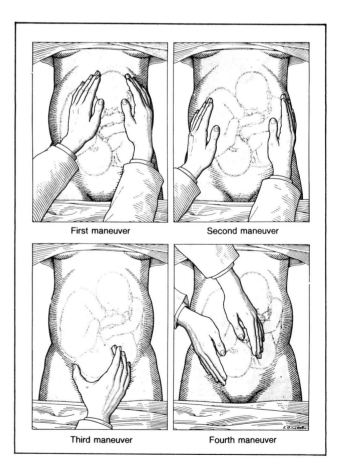

First maneuver

Second maneuver

Third maneuver

Fourth maneuver

Figure 26-7. Abdominal palpation in twin pregnancy. Cephalic presentation on the mother's right and frank breech on the left.

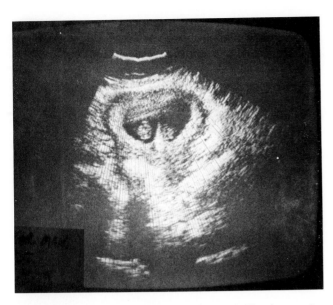

Figure 26-8. Transverse sonogram demonstrating two gestational sacs each containing a fetus of 10 weeks menstrual age. (*Courtesy of J. and J. Ackerman.*)

Fetal Parts. Before the third trimester, it is difficult to diagnose twins by palpation of fetal parts. It is apparent in Figure 26-7 that even late in pregnancy it may not always be possible to identify twins by transabdominal palpation, especially if the woman is obese or hydramnios is present.

Fetal Hearts. Late in the first trimester fetal heart action may be detected with generally available doppler ultrasonic equipment (see Chapter 10, p. 211). Sometime thereafter it becomes possible to identify the separate contractions of two fetal hearts if their rates are clearly distinct from each other as well as from that of the mother. It is possible by careful examination to identify fetal heart sounds with the usual aural fetal stethoscopes at 18 to 20 weeks gestation.

Sonography. By careful sonographic examination, separate gestational sacs can be identified very early in twin pregnancy (Fig. 26-8). Subsequently, the identification of each fetal head should be made in two perpendicular planes so as not to mistake a cross section of the fetal trunk for a second fetal head. A cross section of the fetal head remains nearly round in both planes, whereas the trunk does not. Carefully performed sonographic scanning should detect practically all sets of twins and even the presence of one amnionic sac or two (Fig. 26-9).

As the number of fetuses increases, the accuracy of diagnosis, both as to the number of fetuses and to the biparietal diameter of each head, decreases. In the case of quintuplets, demonstrated in the roentgenogram in Figure 26-10, only four fetuses were identified with certainty either by sonography or by roentgenography. It is not surprising that in the case of nonuplets studied by Kossoff and associates (1976), at 25 weeks gestational age only six of the nine fetuses were identified by sonography.

At times, sonographic examination will serve to identify conjoining of twins as demonstrated in Figures 26-6A, and 26-6B.

In multifetal pregnancies, there is a general slowing of the rate of fetal growth compared to singleton pregnancies. Moreover, individual growth in the same multifetal gestation may be discordant. Significant discordance can usually be detected by careful sonographic measurement of the abdominal circumference as well as the biparietal diameter. Measurements of the biparietal diameters solely may provide misleading information since dolichocephaly in one fetal head may suggest erroneously growth discordance.

Radiographic Examination. The indiscriminate use of x-ray should be avoided during pregnancy. Moreover, a roentgenogram of the maternal abdomen to try to demonstrate multiple fetuses in the following circumstances will provide no useful information and may be responsible for an incorrect diagnosis: (1) when taken during the first 18 weeks of pregnancy since the fetal skeletons are insufficiently radiopaque; (2) if the film is of poor quality from inappropriate exposure time or from malposition of the mother, so that her upper abdomen and the fetus beneath are excluded from the roentgenogram; (3) when the mother is obese; (4) when there is hydramnios; and (5) if one fetus moves during the exposure. There are times, however, when the importance of diagnosing the presence of multiple fetuses surely overrides the minimal risk associated with a carefully obtained and interpreted roentgenogram.

Biochemical Tests. The amounts of *chorionic gonadotropin* in plasma and in urine, on the average, are higher than those found with a singleton pregnancy but not so high as to allow a definite diagnosis (Thiery and coworkers, 1976). Neither are the amounts of chorionic go-

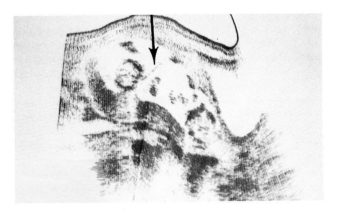

Figure 26-9. Longitudinal gray scale sonogram of twins at 15 weeks gestation. The arrow points to membranes that divide the two amnionic sacs. The fetal trunk and an extremity are seen in the upper sac. A fetal head and extremities are apparent in the lower. (*Courtesy Dr. R. Santos.*)

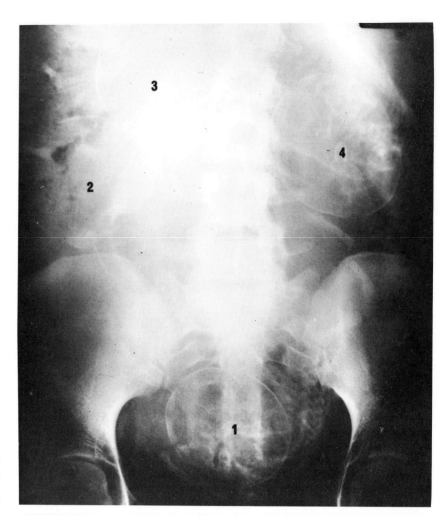

Figure 26-10. Roentgenogram at 27 weeks gestation that clearly demonstrates four fetal heads. A fifth fetus, not identifiable in this roentgenogram, weighed but 860 g when delivered 5 weeks later. (The placenta is demonstrated in Figure 26-4.)

nadotropin so low as to differentiate clearly between a twin pregnancy and a hydatidiform mole. *Placental lactogen* levels in maternal plasma average somewhat higher in a twin pregnancy than in a singleton pregnancy. Measurement of placental lactogen at 29 to 30 weeks gestation to screen for twins has been proposed (Magiste et al., 1976; Spellacy et al., 1978). Ideally, diagnosis of twins should be made somewhat before 29 to 30 weeks. Moreover, if the gestational age is known, clinical acumen alone should lead the obstetrician to suspect twins and to employ a technique for diagnosis that is far more precise than is the measurement of placental lactogen. The *α-fetoprotein level* in maternal plasma is commonly higher in pregnancies with twins than in those with a single fetus. Even though Keilani and co-workers (1978) found that in 40 percent of twin pregnancies the level was above the 95th percentile of the normal range for singleton gestations, the measurement provides little help in diagnosing twins over that provided by careful clinical evaluation. There are also somewhat higher maternal plasma levels on the average for *estrogens, alkaline phosphatase,* and *leucine aminopeptidase* ("oxytocinase"), and in urine for *estriol* and *pregnanediol.* So far, however, there is no biochemical test that in

any individual case will clearly differentiate between the presence of one and more than one fetus.

PREGNANCY OUTCOME

Abortion

Abortion is more likely to occur with multiple fetuses than with a single fetus. The demonstration sonographically of two gestational sacs with the subsequent disappearance of one or even both sacs is evidence that silent early abortion or resorption of one embryo is fairly common (p. 505). Both spontaneous abortion and surgically induced abortion have, on occasion, served to remove one embryo or fetus, with the pregnancy nevertheless continuing until the birth of another fetus who survived.

Death of One Fetus

On occasion, one fetus succumbs remote from term, but the pregnancy continues with one living fetus. At delivery, the dead fetus with placenta and membranes may be readily identified but may be appreciably compressed

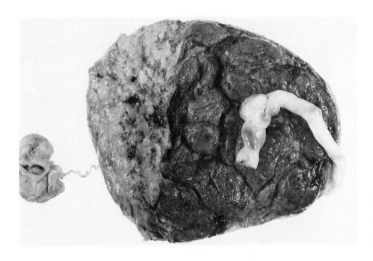

Figure 26-11. To the left are a papyraceous fetus that died at midpregnancy, its cord, and its pale placenta. To the right are the normal placenta and cord of the healthy, 3200 g, twin.

(*fetus compressus*) or may be remarkably flattened through loss of fluid and most of the soft tissue except skin (*fetus papyraceous*). A striking example is presented in Figure 26-11, in which the papyraceous fetus died at midpregnancy while the other fetus and placenta thrived. Sometimes the dead fetus will undergo complete resorption even though the conceptus had advanced well beyond the status of an embryo before succumbing, as demonstrated by serial sonography in Figures 26-2B and 26-2D).

Theoretically, at least, acquired coagulation defects (disseminated intravascular coagulation, consumptive coagulopathy) could be triggered in the mother by the death of one of multiple fetuses. However, we have documented dangerous maternal hypofibrinogenemia and troublesome hemorrhage at delivery only when both of twin fetuses were dead in utero for a prolonged period (Chapter 21, p. 413 and Figs. 21-17A and B). We have observed transient, spontaneously corrected consumptive coagulopathy when one fetus died and was retained in utero along with the other who was alive (see Chapter 21, p. 414). As concern mounted over the well-being of the mothers and their surviving fetuses, the fibrinogen concentration rose spontaneously and the level of serum fibrinogen–fibrin degradation products fell to normal. At delivery the portions of the placenta that supplied the living fetus appeared quite normal, whereas that which had once provided for the dead fetus was the site of massive deposition of fibrin. The fibrin deposition may have accounted directly for the fall in maternal fibrinogen and, in turn, an increase in fibrin degradation products, or it may have served to block the escape of thromboplastin from fetus and placenta into the maternal circulation and thereby prevented disseminated intravascular coagulation, or both mechanisms may have been operational until the extensive fibrosis had been achieved. The fetuses who were alive at the time of demise of the womb-mate continued to thrive in utero as they did after birth. At birth their plasma fibrinogen levels, serum fibrinogen–fibrin degradation products, and platelet counts were normal.

Romero and co-workers (1984) observed maternal hypofibrinogenemia to develop sometime after death of one of twin fetuses. The hypofibrinogenemia was soon corrected in the mother by heparin infusion. The first time heparin therapy was discontinued the hypofibrinogenemia recurred but the next time it was stopped it did not. Presumably, by the second time consumptive coagulopathy in the mother was arrested by the sealing off of the maternal vascular bed with fibrin. The liveborn infant appeared normal at 14 months of age.

The risk to a surviving fetus of development of serious consumptive coagulopathy may be enhanced if there are anastomoses between the fetal circulations, commonly found with monoamnionic twins, as emphasized by Benirschke and Kim (1973). So far, however, we have not identified consumptive coagulopathy in cord blood of the living monozygotic twin when the other had been long dead.

Perinatal Mortality

The perinatal mortality rate for pregnancies complicated by twin fetuses has been remarkably higher than for single fetuses. Perinatal loss with twins at many centers in the United States commonly has in the recent past ranged from 10 to 15 percent. For example, Kohl and Casey (1975) identified at several collaborative obstetric units in the United States a perinatal death rate of 10.9 percent (109 per 1000) for twins who weighed at least 500 g at birth. For twins who weighed 1000 g or more, the perinatal death rate was 6.2 percent, or three times that for singletons. Naeye and co-workers (1978), from data compiled through a prospective collaborative study in the United States, found that the perinatal death rate was 13.9 percent for twins compared to 3.3 percent for singletons.

The perinatal death rate for monozygotic twins was 2.5 times that for dizygotic twins. There is an extremely high fetal death rate with the relatively rare variety of monozygous twinning in which both fetuses occupy the same amnionic sac, that is, *monoamnionic twins*. A common cause of death is intertwining of their umbilical cords, which has been estimated to occur in 50 percent

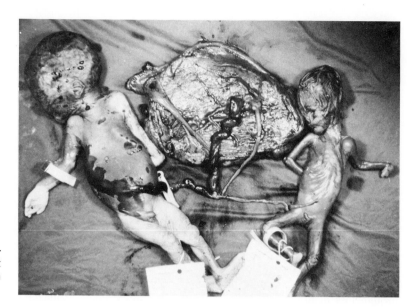

Figure 26-12. Monozygotic twins in a single amnionic sac; the smaller fetus apparently died first and the second subsequently succumbed when the umbilical cords entwined.

or more of cases (Benirschke, 1983). An example is provided in Fig. 26-12.

> When only one amnionic sac can be identified sonographically, because of the likelihood of death of one or both monoamnionic twins from cord entanglement, the destruction of one to try to protect the other has been considered by some. Following the death of the other twin, the possibility of an adverse effect on the "protected" twin, as a consequence of severe consumptive coagulopathy, has been raised (Benirschke, 1983).
>
> We have observed recently a case of monozygous, monoamnionic twins in which at 31 weeks gestation one twin was confirmed to be dead by real-time sonography while the other appeared to be thriving. Four weeks later, after a spontaneous labor, an apparently healthy infant was delivered whose Apgar score was 9 at 5 minutes. In cord blood the levels of fibrinogen, fibrin degradation products, and platelets were normal. The other fetus, badly decomposed and obviously dead in utero for more than 4 weeks, weighed 770 g. The two umbilical cords were in close proximity at their insertions into the single placenta. The cords were entwined for nine complete turns!
>
> In one recorded instance the cord of the twin who was delivered second was around the neck of the first-born. The cord was clamped and divided to facilitate vaginal delivery. Fortunately, the second twin whose cord had been severed was soon delivered and did survive (McLeod and McCoy, 1981).

Duration of Gestation

As the number of fetuses increases, the duration of gestation and birth weight decrease. McKeown and Record (1952) identified the mean duration of gestation for twins to be 260 days (37 weeks), and for triplets 247 days (35 weeks), compared to 281 days (40 weeks) for single fetuses. Caspi and associates (1976) ascertained precisely the time of ovulation for 111 pregnancies in women in

whom ovulation was induced with pituitary plus chorionic gonadotropins. As shown in Table 26-1, the average duration of gestation decreased dramatically as the number of fetuses increased.

Birth Weight

Powers (1973), in the several reports from the United States and Europe that he surveyed, noted the birth weight to be less than 2501 g in from 43 to 63 percent of twin infants. Retarded fetal growth, as well as premature delivery, is important in the genesis of low birth weight in multifetal gestations. After the second trimester, growth of the multiple fetuses, as determined either by sonographic measurements or by birth weight, is likely to be impaired somewhat compared to that of the singleton fetus. In general, the larger the number of fetuses, the greater the degree of growth retardation. Moreover, when two or more fetuses are derived from a single ovum, the degree of growth retardation is likely to be greater than when each fetus is derived from a different ovum. The differences in birth weight were dramatic in the Davis quintuplets presented in Figure 26-13A and

TABLE 26-1 AVERAGE LENGTH OF GESTATION FOR PREGNANCIES WITH KNOWN TIME OF OVULATION AND 20 OR MORE WEEKS GESTATION

No. of Fetuses	No. of Pregnancies	Weeks Completed*
Singleton	82	39
Twins	21	35
Triplets	5	33
Quadruplets	3	29

* Calculated from 2 weeks before ovulation.
(*From Caspi and co-workers: Br J Obstet Gynaecol 83:967, 1976.*)

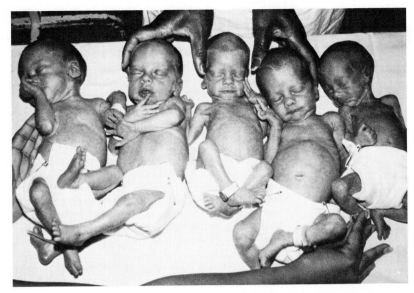

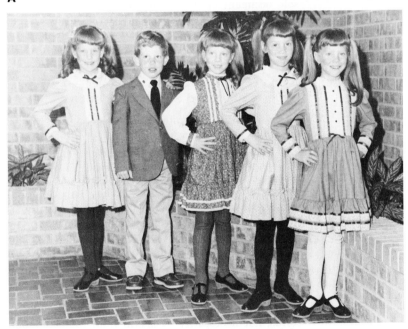

Figure 26-13. A. Davis quintuplets at 3 weeks of age. The first, second, and fourth infants from the left each arose from separate ova while the third and fifth infants are from the same ovum. **B.** Davis quintuplets at 8 years of age. (*Courtesy of Mr. Sidney Eads.*)

26-13B. When delivered at 31½ weeks gestation, the three infants from separate ova weighed 1420, 1530, and 1440 g, whereas the two derived from the same ovum weighed 990 and 860 g. Although the birth weights of these two monozygotic infants were nearly the same, remarkable differences have been observed. Marked discordance in size may also complicate pregnancies in which each fetus arose from a separate ovum. For example, dizygotic twins, one of whom weighed 2300 and the other 785 g, were delivered at Parkland Memorial Hospital (Fig. 26-14). Both survived but one remains appreciably smaller than the other.

Malformations

Kohl and Casey (1975) identified major malformations in 2.12 percent of twin infants, compared to 1.05 percent of singletons delivered during the same times and in the same institutions. The frequency of minor malformation was 4.13 percent in twins, compared to 2.45 percent in singletons. It appears, on the basis of the studies of Kohl and Casey, and others, that the frequency of malformations is nearly twice as great in twins as in singletons. Malformations are more common among monozygotic than dizygotic twins.

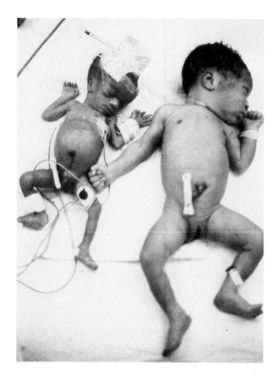

Figure 26-14. Marked discordance in dizygotic twins. The larger infant weighed 2300 g, appropriate for gestational age. The markedly growth-retarded smaller infant weighed only 785 g. Both thrived.

Genetic Amniocentesis. Several debilities are best detected by examination of amnionic fluid. Most often there are two amnionic sacs and ideally fluid should be obtained separately from each. The use of real-time sonography is recommended to identify a site for penetration into one amnionic sac adjacent to one fetus. After fluid is obtained a marker consisting of a few milliliters of dilute indigo carmine is injected. After a few minutes the second fetus is located sonographically and the procedure is repeated. The fluid, if from the second sac, is not discolored by indigo carmine. The complication rate in one series appeared to be minimal (Elias and co-workers, 1980).

Subsequent Development

Nilsen and associates (1984) in Norway evaluated the physical and intellectual development of male twins at 18 years of age. Compared to singletons, twice as many twins were found to be physically unfit for military service. They attributed this to preterm delivery rather than twinning per se. General intelligence did not appear to differ between twins and singletons.

The pattern of subsequent development of the growth-retarded infant from a multifetal pregnancy varies. Babson and Phillips (1973), for example, reported that in monozygotic twins whose birth weights differed on the average by 36 percent, the twin who was smaller

at birth remained so into adulthood. In their experience, height, weight, head circumference, and apparently intelligence often remained superior in the twin who weighed more at birth. Fujikura and Froelich (1974), however, failed to confirm a significant difference in mental and motor scores.

Baights and co-workers (1982) studied monozygotic twins who at age 17 had body frames that were quite similar but who were remarkably dissimilar in body weight, as they were at birth. The investigators documented hyperplasia of adipocytes in the heavier twin compared to her lighter sister. Their investigations excluded genetic differences (through identity of the HLA system and eight other genetic markers) and nutritional differences except for intra-uterine nutrition. They suggested that perhaps in human beings early (intrauterine) nutritional status helps to determine adipocyte numbers and the way the body evolves.

It seems reasonable to summarize that each fetus involved in a multifetal pregnancy is at some disadvantage from the outset compared to the fetus who is the sole occupant of the uterus. Those who do survive the newborn period may suffer some form of physical, intellectual, or psychologic handicap, with the smaller usually at greater risk. Fortunately, in most instances their handicap will be minimal.

Superfetation and Superfecundation

In superfetation, an interval as long or longer than an ovulatory cycle intervenes between fertilizations. Superfetation has not been unequivocally demonstrated in women, although it is theoretically possible until the uterine cavity is obliterated by the fusion of the decidua capsularis to the decidua vera. Thus, superfetation requires ovulation during the course of an established pregnancy, as yet unproven in humans, though known to occur in mares. Most authorities believe that the alleged cases of human superfetation result from marked inequality of growth and development of fetuses of the same gestational age, as described above.

Superfecundation refers to the fertilization of two ova within a short period of time, but not at the same coitus, nor necessarily by sperm from the same man. It may be that in many cases twin ova are not fertilized by sperm from the same ejaculate, but the fact can be demonstrated only in exceptional circumstances.

It is interesting that John Archer, the first physician to receive a medical degree in America, related in 1810 that a white woman after intercourse with both a white and a black man within a short period was delivered of twins, one of whom was white and the other mulatto. A similar instance of superfecundation, documented by Harris (1982), is demonstrated in Figure 26-15. The mother was raped on the tenth day of her menstrual cycle and had intercourse one week later with her husband. She went into labor very near term and was delivered vaginally of a mulatto infant whose blood type was A and a white infant whose blood type was O. The blood

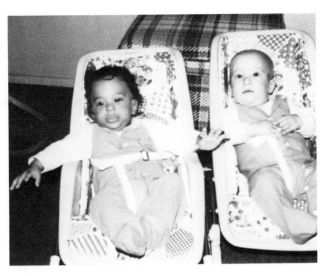

Figure 26-15. An example of dizygotic twin boys as the consequence of superfecundation. (*Courtesy of Dr. David Harris.*)

type of both the mother and her husband was O. HLA typing was not done. Terasaki and co-workers (1978) have described the use of HLA typing to establish that dizygotic twins were sired by different fathers.

Maternal Adaptation

In general, the degree of maternal physiologic change is greater with multiple fetuses than when there is a single fetus. For example, the average increase in maternal blood volume induced during pregnancy with twin fetuses is significantly larger (Pritchard, 1965; Rovinsky, Jaffin, 1966). Whereas the average increase in late pregnancy is about 40 to 50 percent with a single fetus, the mean increase amounts to about 50 to 60 percent with twins. Measurements in the same woman late in one pregnancy with a single fetus and at the same time in another pregnancy with twins are indicative that, typically, the maternal blood volume is about 500 ml greater with twins (Pritchard and Chase, unpublished). Interestingly, the average blood loss with vaginal delivery of 25 sets of twins averaged 935 ml, or nearly 500 ml more than with the delivery of a single fetus. Both the remarkable increase in maternal blood volume and the increased iron and folate requirements imposed by a second fetus predispose to a greater prevalence of maternal anemia.

The larger size of the uterus with multiple fetuses intensifies the variety of mechanical effects that occur during pregnancy. The uterus and its contents may achieve a volume of 10 liters or more and weigh in excess of 20 pounds! Especially with monozygotic twins, rapid accumulation of grossly excessive amounts of amnionic fluid, that is, *acute hydramnios,* may develop. In these circumstances, it is easy to envision appreciable compression and displacement of many of the abdominal viscera as well as the lungs by the elevated diaphragm.

The size and weight of the very large uterus may preclude more than a very sedentary existence for the woman pregnant with multiple fetuses.

At times, in pregnancies with multiple fetuses further complicated by hydramnios, maternal renal function may become seriously impaired, most likely as the consequence of obstructive uropathy. Quigley and Cruikshank (1977), for example, described two pregnancies with twin fetuses plus acute and severe hydramnios in which oliguria and azotemia developed. Maternal urine output and plasma creatinine levels promptly returned to normal after delivery. In case of gross hydramnios, transabdominal amniocentesis may be employed to provide relief for the mother and, hopefully, to allow the pregnancy to continue (see Chapter 23, p. 464). Unfortunately, the hydramnios is often characterized by acute onset remote from term and by rapid reaccumulation following amniocentesis.

The various stresses of pregnancy on the mother and the likelihood of serious maternal complications almost invariably will be greater with multiple fetuses than with a singleton. This should be taken into account, especially when counseling the woman whose health is compromised and who is recognized early in pregnancy to have multiple fetuses, or, for that matter, who is not pregnant but is considering treatment with agents used to induce ovulation.

MANAGEMENT OF PREGNANCIES WITH MULTIPLE FETUSES

To reduce perinatal mortality and morbidity significantly in pregnancies complicated by twins, it is imperative that (1) delivery of markedly premature infants be prevented, (2) failure of one or both fetuses to thrive be identified and fetuses so afflicted be delivered before they become moribund, (3) fetal trauma during labor and delivery be eliminated, and (4) expert neonatal care be provided continuously from the time of birth. The first major step in fulfilling these goals is to identify early the pregnancy complicated by multiple fetuses. As soon as multiple fetuses (or embryos) are identified, meaningful efforts should be directed toward providing the fetuses with the best intrauterine environment possible.

Diet

The requirements for calories, protein, minerals, vitamins, and essential fatty acids are further increased in women with multiple fetuses. The Recommended Dietary Allowances made by the Food and Nutrition Board of the National Research Council for uncomplicated pregnancy should not only be met but in most instances exceeded (see Chapter 13, p. 251). Therefore, consumption of energy sources should be increased by another 300 kcal per day. Failure of the mother to gain weight equal at least to the weight of the pregnancy products, both fetal and maternal, is clear proof that the diet being consumed is inadequate. Iron supplementation is essential; 60 to 100 mg per day is recommended. Folic acid, 1 mg per day, may prove beneficial, although a diet adequate in protein provided from a variety of sources should supply adequate amounts of folate. Rigid sodium restriction is not beneficial to the fetuses.

Maternal Hypertension

Pregnancy-induced and pregnancy-aggravated hypertension are much more likely to develop in pregnancies with multiple fetuses (see Chapter 27, p. 541). Hypertension not only occurs more often but tends to develop earlier and be more severe. In general, parous women never previously hypertensive are "immune" to the development of hypertension during a subsequent pregnancy. This does not hold true, however, for a subsequent pregnancy complicated by multiple fetuses. If women with twins are hospitalized far in advance of term, the onset of hypertension may be delayed and its severity reduced (Vedra, 1980).

Prevention of Prematurity

Several techniques have been applied to try to prolong gestation in multifetal pregnancy. These include considerable bed rest, especially through hospitalization, prophylactic administration of β-mimetic drugs, prophylactic cervical cerclage, and repeated injections of progestins.

Bed Rest. Several authors, but certainly not all, have claimed bed rest to be beneficial to twin fetuses, presumably by enhancing uterine perfusion and perhaps by reducing the physical forces that might act deleteriously on the cervix to hasten effacement and dilatation. Unfortunately, the benefits from bed rest are difficult to evaluate. Several of the experiences are summarized below:

> Laursen (1973) concluded from his study of 315 pregnancies with twins that rest in the hospital will prolong pregnancy, increase birth weights significantly, and reduce perinatal mortality. Komáromy and Lampé (1977), on the basis of a large study in Hungary, reached the same conclusions as Laursen. They identified the following differences between their hospitalized and nonhospitalized groups, respectively: mean gestational age at delivery 37.4 weeks compared to 35.0 weeks; mean birth weight 2581 g compared to 1972 g; and a frequency of weights below 2500 g of 43 percent compared to 77 percent. At any gestational age, the birth weights of twins whose mothers had been hospitalized averaged appreciably more than did the birth weights of those whose mothers were not hospitalized. Finally, perinatal mortality was 5.9 percent for twins in the hospitalized group compared to 21.7 percent in the nonhospitalized group.
>
> In Malmö, Sweden, during a 4-year period 88 percent of all twin pregnancies were identified by routinely scanning sonographically pregnant women during the second trimester. For those with twins, rest at home was prescribed until 28 weeks, at which time hospitalization was urged. The av-

erage hospital stay for the 86 women who participated was 55 days. If undelivered at 36 weeks, they were discharged from the hospital, provided that the course of pregnancy was completely normal. With few exceptions, the pregnancies were not allowed to go beyond 38 weeks gestation. The perinatal mortality rate was 0.6 percent, the same as for singleton pregnancies, whereas for twin gestations not so managed the perinatal mortality rate was 10.5 percent (Persson and colleagues, 1979). Similar decreases in perinatal mortality have been reported by Hartikainen-Sorri and co-workers (1983). They favor hospitalization by the 28th week at least and doubt if it is of much value begun after the 34th week.

The experiences of Jeffrey and co-workers (1974) in Denver were that bed rest promoted fetal growth but did not necessarily prolong gestation; however, twin fetuses of mothers at bed rest weighed somewhat more than did fetuses of comparable gestational age whose mothers remained ambulatory. Weekes and co-workers (1977), compared the outcomes of twin pregnancies treated by bed rest to those with no active treatment and found no remarkable differences in birth weights or gestational age at delivery. Perinatal mortality was 6.7 percent among those hospitalized and 5.6 percent for those not hospitalized.

O'Connor and co-workers (1981) have reported their experiences with twin pregnancies in which routine hospitalization during the last trimester was replaced by "intensive antenatal care" provided in a special clinic. The abolition of routine hospitalization was not followed by an increase in perinatal mortality, which was 4 percent, prematurity, or fetal growth retardation. Their program of intensive antenatal care did emphasize the importance of rest at home throughout pregnancy (at least 10 hours at night and 2 hours in the afternoon!). Moreover, "routine" hospitalization during the third trimester averaged only about 2 weeks per pregnancy, usually for pregnancy-induced or pregnancy-aggravated hypertension.

In recent years at Parkland Memorial Hospital, women with twins have been offered hospitalization on the High-Risk Pregnancy Unit hopefully as early as the onset of the third trimester. Although women so hospitalized lead a very sedentary life, they are not strictly confined to bed. In a preliminary audit 144 of 166 women so admitted stayed either until delivery or until they had completed 38 weeks gestation. The duration of stay was 2 weeks or more for 90 percent and 4 weeks or more for 68 percent. Perinatal mortality for the 288 fetuses was only 2.8 percent. Of the eight perinatal deaths, five were stillborn. Four of the five stillbirths were the consequence of fetal death at or very near 40 weeks gestation. The fifth dead fetus had expired remote from term before admittance to the hospital. Of the three neonatal deaths, only one was the consequence of prematurity. Another infant delivered at term died from a malformation incompatible with life (sirenomelia). The third infant born at 39 weeks died soon after birth with intracranial hemorrhage and renal cortical necrosis. The co-twin had died in utero some time before delivery, which may have triggered the apparent consumptive coagulopathy.

The fetal outcome was much poorer in the 22 instances in which the undelivered mothers soon left the High-Risk Pregnancy Unit. Seven of the 44 fetuses, or 15.9 percent, died!

It is our impression that especially for the typically socioeconomically deprived women cared for at Parkland Memorial Hospital the benefits to be derived from hospitalization during the third trimester of twin gestation include increased birth weight, decreased frequency of severe preeclampsia, and lowered perinatal mortality.

β-Mimetics. At least two double-blind trials of β-mimetics in twin pregnancies failed to demonstrate a significant reduction in the rates of premature birth (Marivate and associates, 1977, O'Connor and co-workers, 1979). However, Skjaerris and Åberg (1982) claimed a reduction in the frequency of threatened preterm labor among pregnant women with twins who were given oral terbutaline prophylactically. Six of 25 so treated were subsequently treated intravenously with terbutaline, compared to 15 of 25 who had not received any oral terbutaline.

Cerclage. No significant reduction in prematurity or perinatal deaths has been demonstrated from prophylactic cervical cerclage (Weekes, 1979; Dor and associates, 1982).

Progestin Administration. Serial injections of 17-hydroxyprogesterone caproate (Delalutin) to prevent premature delivery has been advocated by some. However, Hartikainen-Sorri and co-workers (1980) identified no benefits from its administration throughout the third trimester of pregnancy to women with twins. The length of gestation, birth weight, and neonatal outcomes were quite similar in the treated and the control groups.

Pulmonary Function. Although surfactant production, as reflected by the lecithin-sphingomyelin (L/S) ratio in amnionic fluid, and pulmonary function after birth usually are similar in twin gestation, they may differ markedly (Gluck, Kulovich, 1974). We have observed with quintuplets the L/S ratio in amnionic fluid to vary from less than 2 for the largest infant who weighed 1530 g at 32 weeks gestation and was of appropriate size for his gestational age, to greater than 5 for the severely growth-retarded smallest infant, who weighed 860 g. The largest infant developed appreciable respiratory distress, whereas the smallest infant did not.

Prolonged Gestation. Experiences at Malmö, Sweden, and at Parkland Memorial Hospital cited above under the section on Bed Rest suggest, at least, that twin fetuses may fail to thrive in utero when the pregnancy persists for 40 weeks or more. Unfortunately, there are not sufficient data to identify clearly the risks versus possible benefits from allowing a twin pregnancy to continue beyond 39 weeks.

DELIVERY OF MULTIPLE FETUSES

Labor

Many complications of labor and delivery, including premature labor, uterine dysfunction, abnormal presentations, prolapse of the umbilical cord, premature separation of the placenta, and immediate postpartum hemorrhage, occur much more often with multiple fetuses. Therefore, the conduct of labor and delivery with multiple fetuses is an excellent test of the skills of the obstetric team that provides care for the woman and her fetuses.

For women pregnant with multiple fetuses, to date the capability is limited for safely arresting premature labor once labor is established. Pulmonary edema associated with the use of β-mimetic agents, for example, has been observed much more frequently in twin gestations. Bed rest, if not already being used, should be instituted. The problems of premature labor and attempts to arrest it and of lack of fetal lung maturity and possible modification by corticosteroid therapy, are considered elsewhere (see Chapter 37, p. 751).

As soon as it is apparent that labor has been established, a number of steps are immediately taken to help assure a satisfactory outcome:

1. An appropriately trained obstetric attendant remains with the mother throughout labor. The fetal heart rates are monitored frequently, using any system of monitoring which, in that particular situation, will promptly identify significant changes in fetal heart rates. At times, continuous external electronic monitoring or, if the membranes are ruptured and the cervix dilated, evaluation of both fetuses by simultaneous internal and external electronic monitoring may prove quite satisfactory.
2. One liter of compatible whole blood or its equivalent in blood fractions is readily available.
3. A well-functioning intravenous infusion system capable of delivering fluid rapidly into the mother is established. (In the absence of hemorrhage or metabolic disturbance during labor, lactated Ringer solution alternated with aqueous dextrose solution is infused at a rate of 60 to 120 ml per hour.)
4. Two obstetricians are immediately available and both are scrubbed and gowned at delivery. At least one should be skilled in intrauterine identification of fetal parts and intrauterine manipulation of the fetus.
5. An experienced anesthesiologist is immediately available in the event that intrauterine manipulation or cesarean section is necessary.
6. For *each* fetus, two people, one of whom is skilled in resuscitation and care of newborn infants, are appropriately informed of the case and remain immediately available.
7. The delivery area is immediately operational and provides adequate space for all members of the team to work effectively. Moreover, the site is appropriately equipped to take care of all possible maternal problems plus resuscitation and maintenance of each infant.

Presentation and Position. With twins, all possible combinations of fetal positions occur. Either or both fetuses may present by the vertex, breech, or shoulder. Compound, face, brow, and footling breech presentation are relatively common, especially when the fetuses are quite small or there is excess amnionic fluid, or maternal parity is high. Prolapse of the cord is fairly common in these circumstances.

Often the presentation can be ascertained by real-time sonography. However, if any confusion about the relationship of the twins to each other or to the maternal pelvis persists, a single anteroposterior roentgenogram of the abdomen may be very helpful.

Induction or Stimulation of Labor. Even though labor, in general, is shorter with twins, both rupture of the membranes without effective labor and prolonged inefficient labor with or without previous rupture of the membranes do occur. These problems are often better handled by cesarean section unless there is little hope of salvaging the infants because of their gross immaturity. Occasionally, termination of pregnancy is desirable before the spontaneous onset of labor, as, for example, with severe pregnancy-induced hypertension. In these circumstances if the presenting part is well-fixed in the pelvis and the cervix dilated somewhat, amniotomy often will initiate labor and effect delivery. There is no reluctance by some obstetricians to give oxytocin by dilute intravenous infusion to initiate or to stimulate labor in pregnancies complicated by multiple fetuses. The risks compared to the benefits to mother and fetuses of oxytocin to initiate and maintain labor and delivery, compared with cesarean section, have not yet been adequately delineated in this circumstance.

Analgesia and Anesthesia. During labor and delivery of multiple fetuses, deciding what to use for analgesia and for anesthesia is unusually difficult because of the frequency of and, in turn, the problems imposed by (1) prematurity, (2) maternal hypertension, (3) desultory labor, (4) need for intrauterine manipulation, and (5) uterine atony and hemorrhage after delivery. There are undesirable effects from most forms of analgesia and anesthesia. Continuous epidural or caudal anesthesia in hypertensive women, or those who have hemorrhaged, may cause hypotension, with inadequate perfusion of vital organs, especially the placenta, which is dangerous to both the mother and her fetuses. The woman pregnant with multiple fetuses is even less tolerant of the supine position during labor and delivery. Moreover, conduction anesthesia may cause or further aggravate desultory or prolonged labor and will not provide adequate uterine relaxation for intrauterine manipulation when such is necessary. Use of narcotics, sedatives, and tranquilizers may lead to undue fetal depression if the fetuses are premature. Most forms of general anesthesia used for delivery will also depress the fetuses unless the anesthetic agents are carefully selected and skillfully administered, with little delay between induction of anesthesia and delivery. Paracervical block may cause transient fetal bradycardia.

The combination of thiopental, nitrous oxide plus oxygen, and succinylcholine, appropriately timed and in appropriate doses, has proved satisfactory at Parkland Hospital for cesarean section to deliver twins. For vaginal delivery, pudendal block skillfully administered along with nitrous oxide plus oxygen will provide appreciable relief of pain for spontaneous vaginal delivery. When intrauterine manipulation is necessary, as with internal podalic version, uterine relaxation is probably best accomplished with halothane. Although halothane provides effective relaxation for intrauterine manipulation, it also commonly leads to an increase in blood loss during the third stage of labor until the uterus regains its ability to contract (Chapter 18, p. 355).

Vaginal Delivery

More often, the presenting twin is the larger one. Typically, this twin bears the major brunt of dilating the cervix and the remaining soft tissues of the birth canal. Seldom with cephalic presentations are there unusual problems with delivery of the first infant. After appropriate episiotomy, spontaneous delivery, or delivery assisted by the use of outlet forceps, usually proves to be quite satisfactory.

When the first fetus presents as a breech, major problems are most likely to develop if (1) the fetus is unusually large and the aftercoming head taxes the capacity of the birth canal, (2) the fetus is quite small so that the extremities and trunk are delivered through a cervix inadequately effaced and dilated for the head to escape easily, or (3) the umbilical cord prolapses. When these problems are anticipated or identified, cesarean section would often be the better way to effect delivery, except in those instances in which the fetuses are so immature that they will not survive. Otherwise, breech delivery may be accomplished as described in Chapter 42 (p. 855).

The phenomenon of *locked twins* occurs rarely (once in 817 twin gestations, according to Cohen and coworkers, 1965). In order for locking to occur, the first fetus must present by the breech and the second by the vertex. With descent of the breech through the birth canal, the chin of the first fetus locks in the neck and chin of the second cephalic fetus. If unlocking cannot be effected, either cesarean section before the body is delivered or decapitation must be performed.

Delivery of Second Twin

This demands experience that includes for some cases intrauterine manual dexterity. As soon as the first twin has been delivered, the presenting part of the second twin, his size, and relationship to the birth canal are quickly determined by careful combined abdominal, vaginal, and, at times, intrauterine examination. If the vertex or the breech is fixed in the birth canal, moderate fundal pressure is applied and the membranes are ruptured. Immediately afterward, the examination is repeated to identify prolapse of the cord or other abnormality. Labor is allowed to resume while the fetal heart rate is monitored closely. With reestablishment of labor there is no need to hasten delivery, unless there is ominous deceleration of the fetal heart rate or persistent bradycardia, or bleeding from the uterus. Bleeding from the uterus indicates placental separation, which can be deleterious to both the fetus and the mother. If contractions do not resume within 10 minutes or so, dilute oxytocin may be used to stimulate appropriate myometrial activity, which will lead to spontaneous delivery or delivery assisted by outlet forceps.

If the occiput or the breech presents immediately over the pelvic inlet but is not fixed in the birth canal, the presenting part can often be guided into the pelvis with the vaginal hand while a hand on the uterine fundus exerts moderate pressure. Once the presenting part is fixed in the pelvic inlet, the membranes are ruptured and labor and delivery are conducted as described above.

If the occiput or the breech is not over the pelvic inlet and cannot be so positioned by gentle pressure on the presenting part, or if appreciable uterine bleeding develops, the problem of delivery of the second twin assumes serious dimensions. So as to take maximum advantage of the very recently dilated cervix before the uterus contracts and the cervix retracts, procrastination must be avoided. An obstetrician skilled in intrauterine manipulation of the fetus and an anesthesiologist skilled in providing anesthesia that will effectively relax the uterus are essential for vaginal delivery with a favorable outcome. Prompt delivery of the second fetus by cesarean section is the better choice if there is no one present who is skilled in the performance of internal podalic version (described below) or if anesthesia that will provide effective uterine relaxation is not immediately available.

Rarely, in the circumstances where one of the fetuses has been expelled quite prematurely and uterine activity then ceased, the pregnancy has been allowed to continue with delivery of another fetus days to even many weeks late. (A bizarre example is cited below.) Nonetheless, experiences would indicate that procrastination in the delivery of the second fetus has rarely proven advantageous to that fetus.

Maschiach and associates (1981) described a unique case of triplet pregnancy complicated further by uterus didelphys and previous cesarean delivery. Fetuses A and B were in the right uterine horn; fetus A was identified to be dead at 21 weeks gestation and at 27 weeks gestation was expelled. The descent of fetus B from the contracting right uterine horn through the birth canal was blocked mechanically by the head of fetus C, which was located in the left uterine horn. Fetus B, who weighed 1080 g at birth, was delivered from the right horn by cesarean section but succumbed 10 days later. The left horn was not contracting actively; ritodrine was administered intravenously.

At 37 weeks, or 72 days after delivery of fetuses A and B, a repeat cesarean section was performed and yielded a normal healthy girl who weighed 2490 g. Mother and daughter were discharged on the seventh postpartum day.

Internal Podalic Version

Through careful abdominal, vaginal, and intrauterine examinations, the various parts of the fetus are located. (Typically, if the buttocks and legs are toward the left side of the mother, or right side of the obstetrician, a sterile intrauterine examining glove that covers the gown to above the elbow is drawn over the right hand and arm.) The membranes are ruptured, both feet are accurately identified and grasped and only then are gently pulled toward the birth canal. With the other hand applied to the abdomen, the vertex is simultaneously gently elevated toward the mother's sternum. An episiotomy is made or extended whenever more room is needed for uterine and vaginal manipulation. The legs of the fetus are slowly drawn through the birth canal until the buttocks are visible anteriorly just beyond the maternal symphysis. A moist, warm towel is applied to the buttocks and gentle traction is continued until the lower thirds of both scapulas are visible. Next, the trunk is slowly rotated with gentle traction until the shoulder and arm on one side of the fetus are delivered. The rotation of the fetal trunk is now gently reversed to deliver the other arm and shoulder into the vagina. The aftercoming head may now be delivered either by simultaneous suprapubic external pressure to flex the head and gentle traction applied to the trunk, or by use of Piper forceps (see Chapter 42, p. 859).

The cord is clamped promptly with two clamps on the placental side to identify it as the cord of the second infant. The placenta or placentas are immediately delivered by manual removal, if necessary. The uterus is promptly explored for defects and for retained pregnancy products. As these steps are being carried out, the amount of uterine-relaxing anesthetic agent is rapidly decreased, and just as soon as uterine exploration has been completed, oxytocin is administered through the intravenous infusion system. Fundal massage, or, preferably, manual compression of the uterus with one hand in the vagina against the lower uterine segment and the other transabdominally over the uterine fundus, is applied to hasten and enhance myometrial contraction and retraction.

The cervix, vagina, periurethral region, vulva, and perineum are carefully inspected. Lacerations likely to bleed are repaired along with the episiotomy.

Cesarean Section

The recent trend in delivery of multiple fetuses at Parkland Memorial Hospital has been to use cesarean section much more often than in the past. For example, 44 percent of the twins cared for in the High-Risk Pregnancy Unit, as cited previously, were delivered by cesarean section. The most common indication was presentation other than cephalic by one or both fetuses. Other major indications were hypotonic uterine dysfunction, hypertension induced or aggravated by the pregnancy, fetal distress, gross discordance in the size of the fetuses, with the smaller fetus the first candidate for vaginal delivery, and prolapsed cord. Liberal use of cesarean section, when one or both twins present as a breech or are in a transverse lie, has been espoused by others (Cetrulo and associates, 1977; Taylor, 1976).

The use of cesarean delivery has been recommended by Barrett and associates (1982) for any twin expected to have a birth weight of less than 1500 g. However, not enough cesarean deliveries were performed among the pregnancy outcomes reviewed by them to verify unequivocally benefits from cesarean delivery. Welch and coworkers (1983) could demonstrate no improvement in neonatal outcome from cesarean section for delivery of infants who weighed less than 2000 g. Unfortunately, nearly one half of the cases were previously undiagnosed and overall twin mortality was 15.6 percent.

Twin fetuses create other unusual problems. The mother is likely to be even less tolerant of the supine position and therefore it is important to rotate her position so as to move the uterus and its contents to one side (see Chapter 18, p. 361). A vertical incision in the lower uterine segment may be advantageous. If a fetus lies transversely and the arms are inadvertently delivered first, it is much easier and safer to extend upward the vertical uterine incision than to extend a transverse incision.

It is important that the uterus be well contracted during completion of the cesarean section and thereafter. Remarkable blood loss from the uterus may be concealed within the uterus and vagina and beneath the operating drapes during the time taken to close the incisions.

At times, attempts to deliver the second twin vaginally, after vaginal delivery of first twin, may be not only unwise but even impossible, as, for instance, when the second fetus is much larger than the first and in the breech position or in a transverse lie; or, even more perplexing, when the cervix promptly contracts and thickens after delivery of the first infant and does not subsequently dilate. Prompt cesarean section may be performed in these circumstances and the infant saved. Undoubtedly, maternal and perinatal morbidity and mortality would be appreciably less if in these circumstances cesarean section had been used at the outset.

Three or More Fetuses

All of the problems of twin gestation are intensified remarkably by the presence of even more fetuses. With vaginal delivery the first infant is commonly born spontaneously or with little manipulation. However, subsequent infants are delivered according to the presenting part and may require complicated obstetric maneuvers, such as total breech extraction or internal podalic version, followed by breech extraction, or may necessitate the addition of cesarean delivery. Associated with malposition of the fetuses is an increased incidence of cord prolapse and fetal collision. Moreover, reduced placental perfusion and hemorrhage from separating placentas are

likely during the intrapartum period. Therefore, speed of delivery is very important.

Some of the kinds of complications that can arise from delivery of triplets are demonstrated by the following case:

Labor occurred spontaneously at 35 weeks gestation. (The obstetrician elected to attempt vaginal delivery on the basis primarily of previously observing the vaginal delivery of one set of triplets with a favorable outcome.) The first infant was delivered vaginally. The cervix rapidly contracted and thickened so a low transverse cesarean section was performed to deliver the second infant. The third fetus was then identified to be in a transverse lie and was delivered only after a vertical extension of the transverse incision was made to create a large inverted T-shaped defect in the uterus!

Itzkowicz (1979) has reviewed 59 triplet pregnancies born in four major obstetric hospitals. Most deliveries were accomplished vaginally. The perinatal mortality rate was 232 per 1000 (23.2 percent); 9 of the infants were stillborn and 32 who were born alive died during the neonatal period. Premature delivery and birth order were the most important identifiable factors in relation to neonatal death. Abnormal presentations frequently complicated the delivery of the second and especially the third fetus. The mortality rate for infants who were born last was double that for those who were born first and intermediate for those who were born second.

For all of the above reasons, we believe that delivery of pregnancies complicated by the presence of three or more fetuses is probably better accomplished by cesarean section, reserving vaginal delivery for those circumstances in which the fetuses are markedly immature or maternal complications make cesarean section hazardous to the mother.

Postpartum

The kinds of puerperal complications following the birth of multiple fetuses are not different from those after the birth of a single infant; their frequency and intensity, however, are often enhanced. The mother may be troubled by considerable physical fatigue and at times emotional depression from the increased physical work and other responsibilities associated with the care of two or more infants.

Troublesome uterine bleeding later in the puerperium seems to be increased. Perhaps this is the consequence of impairment of involution and of re-epithelialization of the larger placental implantation site. In general, supplemental iron should be continued for some weeks after delivery.

REFERENCES

Archer J: Observations showing that a white woman, by intercourse with a white man and a Negro man, may conceive twins, one of which shall be white and the other mulatto. Medical Repository, 3d Hexade 1:319, 1810

Azubuike JC: Multiple births in Igbo women. Br J Obstet Gynaecol 89:77, 1982

Babson SG, Phillips DS: Growth and development of twins dissimilar in size at birth. N Engl J Med 289:937, 1973

Baigts F, Dunica S, Fumeron F, Apfelbaum M: Birthweight difference in monozygous twins followed by differences in development of body weight. Lancet 2:274, 1982

Barrett JM, Staggs SM, Van Hooydonk JE, Growdon JH, Killam AP, Boehm FM: The effect of type of delivery upon neonatal outcome in premature twins. Am J Obstet Gynecol 143:360, 1982

Benirschke K: Personal communication, 1983

Benirschke K: Chimerism and mosaicism—Two different entities. In Wynn RM (ed): Obstetrics and Gynecology Annual. New York, Appleton, 1974, p 33

Benirschke K, Kim CK: Multiple pregnancy. N Engl J Med 288:1276, 1329, 1973

Bulmer MG: The familial incidence of twinning. Ann Hum Genet 24:1, 1960

Caspi E, Ronen J, Schreyer P, Goldberg MD: The outcome of pregnancy after gonadotropin therapy. Br J Obstet Gynaecol 83:967, 1976

Cetrulo CL, Freeman RK, Knuppel RA: Minimizing the risks of twin delivery. Contemp Ob/Gyn 9:47, 1977

Cohen M, Kohl SG, Rosenthal AH: Fetal interlocking complicating twin gestation. Am J Obstet Gynecol 91:407, 1965

Dallas Times Herald: 50-year-old Michigan woman thrilled by unexpected twins. Wednesday, Jan 6, 1982

Dor J, Shalev J, Masiach J, Blankstein J, Serr DM: Elective cervical suture of twin pregnancies diagnosed ultrasonically in the first trimester following induced ovulation. Gynecol Obstet Invest 13:55, 1982

Elias S, Gerbie AB, Simpson JL, Nadler HL, Sabagha RE, Shkolnik A: Genetic amniocentesis in twin gestations. Am J Obstet Gynecol 138:169, 1980

Fujikura T, Froelich LA: Mental and motor development in monozygotic co-twins with dissimilar birth weights. Pediatrics 53:884, 1974

Garrett WJ, Carey HM, Steven LM, Climie CR, Osborn RA: A case of nonuplet pregnancy. Aust N Z J Obstet Gynaecol 16:93, 1976

Gluck L, Kulovich MV: The evaluation of functional maturity in the human fetus. In Gluck L (ed): Modern Perinatal Medicine. Chicago, Year Book, 1974

Harlap S: Ovulation induction and congenital malformations. Lancet 2:961, 1976

Harris DW: Letter to the Editors. J Reprod Med 27:39, 1982

Hartikainen-Sorri AL, Kauppila A, Risto T: Inefficacy of 17α-hydroxyprogesterone caproate in the prevention of prematurity in twin pregnancy. Obstet Gynecol 56:692, 1980

Hartikainen-Sorri AL, Kauppila A, Tuimala R, Koivisto M: Factors related to improved outcomes for twins. Acta Obstet Gynecol Scand 62:23, 1983

Itzkowicz D: A survey of 59 triplet pregnancies. Br J Obstet Gynaecol 86:23, 1979

Jeffrey RL, Bowes WA Jr, Delaney JJ: Role of bed rest in twin gestation. Obstet Gynecol 43:822, 1974

Jewelewicz R, Vande Wiele RL: Management of multifetal gestation. Contemp Ob/Gyn 6:59, 1975

Keilani Z, Clarke PC, Kitau MJ: The significance of raised maternal plasma alpha-fetoprotein in twin pregnancy. Br J Obstet Gynaecol 85:510, 1978

Knox G, Morley D: Twinning in Yoruba women. J Obstet Gynaecol Br Emp 67:981, 1960

Kohl SG, Casey G: Twin gestation. Mt Sinai J Med 42:523, 1975

Komaromy B, Lampe L: The value of bed rest in twin pregnancies. Int J Gynaecol Obstet 15:262, 1977

Koontz WL, Herbert WNP, Seeds JW, Cefalo RC: Ultrasonography in the antepartum diagnosis of conjoined twins. J Reprod Med 28:627, 1983

Kossoff G, Garrett WJ, Radovanovich G: Ultrasonic examination of a nonuplet pregnancy. Aust N Z J Obstet Gynaecol 16:203, 1976

Laursen B: Twin pregnancy: The value of prophylactic rest in bed and the risk involved. Acta Obstet Gynecol Scand 52:367, 1973

MacGillivray I: Twin Pregnancies. In Wynn RM (ed): Obstetrics and Gynecology Annual. New York, Appleton, 1978, p 135

Marivate M, De Villiers KO, Fairbrother P: Effect of prophylactic outpatient administration of fenoterol on the time of onset of spontaneous labour and fetal growth rate in twin pregnancy. Am J Obstet Gynecol 128:707, 1977

McLeod FN, McCoy DR: Monoamniotic twins with an unusual cord complication. Br J Obstet Gynaecol 88:774, 1981

McKeown T, Record RG: Observations on foetal growth in multiple pregnancy in man. J Endocrinol 5:387, 1952

Mägiste M, Von Schenck H, Sjöberg NO, Thorell JI, Åberg A: Screening for detecting twins. Am J Obstet Gynecol 126:697, 1976

Mashiach S, Ben-Rafael Z, Dor J, Serr DM: Triplet pregnancy in uterus didelphys with delivery interval of 72 days. Obstet Gynecol 58:519, 1981

Myrianthopoulos NC: An epidemiologic survey of twins in a large prospectively studied population. Am J Hum Genet 22:611, 1970

Naeye RL: Organ abnormalities in a human parabiotic syndrome. Am J Pathol 46:829, 1965

Naeye RL, Tafari N, Judge D, Marboe CC: Twins: Causes of perinatal death in 12 United States cities and one African city. Am J Obstet Gynecol 31:267, 1978

Newman HH: The Physiology of Twinning. Chicago, Chicago University Press, 1923

Nilsen ST, Bergsjø P, Nome S: Male twins at birth and 18 years later. Br J Obstet Gynaecol 91:122, 1984

O'Connor MC, Arias E, Royston JP, Dalrymple IJ: The merits of special antenatal care for twin pregnancies. Br J Obstet Gynaecol 88:222, 1981

O'Connor MC, Murphy H, Dalrymple IJ: Double blind trial of ritodrine and placebo in twin pregnancy. Br J Obstet Gynaecol 86:706, 1979

Pedersen IK, Philips J, Sele V, Starup J: Monozygotic twins with dissimilar phenotypes and chromosome complements. Acta Obstet Gynecol Scand 59:459, 1980

Persson P-H, Grennert L, Gennser G, Kullander S: On improved outcome of twin pregnancies. Acta Obstet Gynecol Scand 58:3, 1979

Pettersson F, Smedby B, Lindmark G: Outcome of twin birth. Review of 1636 children born in twin birth. Acta Paediat Scand 64:473, 1976

Powers WF: Twin pregnancy: Complications and treatment. Obstet Gynecol 42:795, 1973

Pritchard JA: Changes in blood volume during pregnancy. Anesthesiology 26:393, 1965

Quigley MM, Cruikshank DP: Polyhydramnios and acute renal failure. J Reprod Med 19:92, 1977

Recommended Dietary Allowances, 9th rev ed. National Research Council, National Academy of Sciences, 1979

Robertson EG, Neer KJ: Placental injection studies in twin gestation. Am J Obstet Gynecol 147:170, 1983

Robinson HP, Caines JS: Sonor evidence of early pregnancy

failure in patients with twin conceptions. Br J Obstet Gynaecol 84:22, 1977

Romero R, Duffy TP, Berkowitz RL, Chang E, Hobbins JC: Prolongation of a preterm pregnancy complicated by death of a single twin in utero and disseminated intravascular coagulation. Effects of treatment with heparin. N Engl J Med 310:772, 1984

Rothman KJ: Fetal loss, twinning and birthweight after oral-contraceptive use. New Engl J Med 297:468, 1977

Rovinsky JJ, Jaffin H: Cardiovascular hemodynamics in pregnancy: III. Cardiac rate, stroke volume, total peripheral resistance, and central blood volume in multiple pregnancy. Synthesis of results. Am J Obstet Gynecol 95:787, 1966

Schmidt R, Nitowsky HM, Sobel EH: Monozygotic twins discordant for sex. Pediatr Research 8:395, 1974

Skjaerris J, Åberg A: Prevention of prematurity in twin pregnancy by orally administered terbutaline. Acta Obstet Gynecol Scand Suppl 108:39, 1982

Spellacy WN, Buhi WC, Birk SA: Human placental lactogen levels in multiple pregnancies. Obstet Gynecol 52:210, 1978

Strandskov HH, Edelen EW, Siemens GJ: Analysis of the sex ratios among single and plural births in the total "white" and "colored" U.S. populations. Am J Phys Anthrop 4:491, 1946

Tan KL, Goon SM, Salmon Y, Wee JH: Conjoined twins. Acta Obstet Gynecol Scand 50:373, 1971

Taylor ES: Editorial. Obstet Gynecol Surv 31:535, 1976

Terasaki PI, Gjertson D, Bernoco D, et al: Twins with two different fathers identified by HLA. N Engl J Med 299:590, 1978

Thiery M, Dhont M, Vandekerckhove D: Serum HCG and HPL in twin pregnancies. Acta Obstet Gynecol Scand 56:495, 1976

Varma TR: Ultrasound evidence of early pregnancy failure in patients with multiple conceptions. Br J Obstet Gynaecol 86:290, 1979

Vedra B: Pregnancy Hypertension. Baltimore, University Park Press, 1980

Waterhouse JAH: Twinning in twin pedigrees. Br J Soc Med 4:197, 1950

Weekes ARL, Menzies DN, DeBoer CH: The relative efficacy of bed rest, cervical suture, and no treatment in the management of twin pregnancy. Br J Obstet Gynaecol 84:161, 1977

Welch R, Mariona FC, Agronow SJ: Obstetrical outcome of very low and low birthweight twins. Proceedings of the Third Annual Scientific Meeting of the Society of Perinatal Obstetricians, San Antonio, TX, Jan 1983

White C, Wyshak G: Inheritance in human dizygotic twinning. N Engl J Med 271:1003, 1964

27

Hypertensive Disorders in Pregnancy

In some mysterious way the presence of chorionic villi in certain women incites vasospasm and hypertension. Moreover, to effect a cure the chorionic villi must be expelled or surgically removed. The vasospastic hypertensive state and related pathologic changes somehow induced by the presence of chorionic villi may not be so great that pregnancy need be terminated prematurely.

—Pritchard, 1978

SIGNIFICANCE

Pregnancy may induce hypertension in previously normotensive women or aggravate hypertension in women who are already hypertensive. Generalized edema, proteinuria, or both often accompany hypertension induced or aggravated by pregnancy. Convulsions may develop in association with the hypertensive state, especially in women whose hypertension is ignored.

The hypertensive disorders in pregnancy are common complications of gestation and form one of the great triad of complications that continue to be responsible for the majority of maternal deaths. Hypertensive disorders are an even more important cause of perinatal mortality and severe morbidity. How pregnancy per se incites or aggravates hypertensive vascular disease and associated complications remains unsolved despite decades of intensive research. These disorders remain among the most important unsolved problems in obstetrics.

The large toll of maternal and infant lives that may be taken by hypertension induced or aggravated by pregnancy is most often preventable. Good prenatal supervision followed by appropriate treatment will ameliorate many cases sufficiently that the outcome for baby and mother is satisfactory.

CLASSIFICATION AND DIFFERENTIAL DIAGNOSIS

Terminology

The unsatisfactory terms *toxemia of pregnancy* and *toxemias of pregnancy* have been applied variably to any or all disorders in which hypertension, proteinuria, or edema was present during pregnancy or the puerperium, and other disorders as well. The Committee on Terminology of the American College of Obstetricians and Gynecologists suggested, instead, the following defini-

tions and classification of hypertension that developed during pregnancy or the puerperium (Hughes, 1972). *Hypertension* is defined as a diastolic blood pressure of at least 90 mm Hg or systolic pressure of at least 140 mm Hg, or a rise in the former of at least 15 mm Hg or in the latter of 30 mm Hg. The blood pressures cited must be manifest on at least two occasions 6 hours or more apart. *Preeclampsia* is the development of hypertension with proteinuria, edema, or both, induced by pregnancy after the 20th week of gestation and sometimes earlier when there are extensive hydatidiform changes in the chorionic villi (Chapter 23, p. 448). *Eclampsia* is the occurrence of convulsions, not caused by any coincidental neurologic disease such as epilepsy, in a woman whose condition also fulfills the criteria for preeclampsia. *Superimposed preeclampsia or eclampsia* is defined as the development of preeclampsia or eclampsia in a woman with chronic hypertensive vascular or renal disease. *Chronic hypertensive disease* is defined as the presence of persistent hypertension, of whatever cause, before the 20th week of gestation in the absence of hydatidiform mole or extensive molar change, or persistent hypertension beyond 6 weeks postpartum.

Gestational hypertension is defined as hypertension that develops during the latter half of pregnancy or during the first 24 hours after delivery. It is not accompanied by other evidence of preeclampsia or hypertensive vascular disease, and it disappears within 10 days following parturition. *Gestational edema* is the generalized accumulation of fluid of greater than 1+ pitting edema after 12 hours bed rest or a weight gain of 5 pounds or more in a week. *Gestational proteinuria* is proteinuria during pregnancy in the absence of hypertension, edema, renal infection, or known renovascular disease; the existence of such an entity is questionable.

We have modified the classification of hypertension complicating pregnancy. The reason for this modification is to try to separate vasospasm and, in turn, hypertension generated by pregnancy from hypertension that merely coexists with pregnancy, yet emphasize that the presence of the latter enhances the frequency, and often the intensity, of the former.

  I. Hypertension induced by pregnancy (pregnancy-induced hypertension)
    A. Without proteinuria or generalized, gross edema
    B. With proteinuria or generalized edema (preeclampsia)
      1. Mild
      2. Severe
    C. Eclampsia
  II. Coincidental hypertension (chronic hypertension)
  III. Hypertension worsened by pregnancy (pregnancy-aggravated hypertension)
    A. Superimposed preeclampsia
    B. Superimposed eclampsia

PREGNANCY-INDUCED HYPERTENSION

Pregnancy-induced hypertension (PIH) is divided into three categories, (1) hypertension alone, (2) preeclampsia, and (3) eclampsia. The diagnosis of preeclampsia is based on the development of hypertension plus proteinuria, or edema that is generalized and overt. Eclampsia is characterized typically by the abnormalities just cited plus convulsions that are induced by the pregnancy-induced hypertension. Only rarely do these symptoms occur earlier than 20 weeks gestation, and then in cases of true hydatidiform mole or appreciable molar degeneration (Chapter 23, p. 448). Preeclampsia is almost exclusively a disease of the nulliparous woman. It more commonly affects the woman who is at the extremes of reproductive age, that is, a teenager or a woman more than 35 years of age. The disease is commonly seen, however, in the multipara with any of the following associated clinical conditions:

1. Multifetal pregnancy and fetal hydrops
2. Vascular diseases, including essential chronic hypertension and diabetes mellitus
3. Coexisting renal diseases

Diagnosis

The diagnosis of PIH is usually straightforward: The *blood pressure* is 140/90 or greater, or there has been an increase of 30 mm Hg systolic or 15 mm Hg diastolic over baseline values on at least two occasions 6 or more hours apart.

Although the diagnosis of preeclampsia has traditionally required the identification of PIH plus proteinuria *or* generalized edema, many authorities concur that edema, even of the hands and face, is such a common finding in pregnant women that its presence should not validate the existence of preeclampsia any more than its absence should deny the diagnosis. Indeed, although

Robertson (1971) found that one third of women developed generalized edema by the 38th week of pregnancy, he was unable to show a significant statistical correlation between edema and hypertension. In another study, Friedman and Neff (1976) identified perinatal mortality for women with edema alone to be one-third lower than for the general population. The edema of preeclampsia involves the face and hands and is present in the morning after arising. A useful indicator of nondependent edema is the woman's complaint that her rings have become "too tight."

Proteinuria is an important sign of preeclampsia. Proteinuria is defined as the presence of 300 mg or more of protein in a 24-hour urine collection or a protein concentration of 1 g/L or more in at least two random urine specimens collected 6 hours or more apart. It is important to note that the degree of proteinuria may fluctuate widely over any 24-hour period, even in severe cases. Therefore, a single random sample may fail to detect significant proteinuria.

The combination of proteinuria and hypertension during pregnancy markedly increases the risk of perinatal mortality. McCartney and co-workers (1971), in their extensive experience studying renal biopsy specimens of hypertensive pregnant women, invariably found that proteinuria was present when the glomerular lesion considered to be characteristic of preeclampsia was evident. It is important to recognize, however, that both proteinuria and alterations of glomerular histology develop late in the course of PIH. Evidence will be presented subsequently to show that preeclampsia becomes evident clinically only near the end of an often protracted, covert pathophysiologic process that may begin 3 to 4 months before hypertension appears. Therefore, even hypertension is a late manifestation in the pathophysiologic spectrum of preeclampsia—late enough, in fact, that once hypertension appears, the chance of perinatal survival is diminished.

The fact that *perinatal survival* is diminished by maternal hypertension is evident from an analysis of the large Collaborative Perinatal Project conducted by the Task Force on Toxemia of the National Institute of Neurologic and Communicative Disorders and Stroke (1976). From this 13-year prospective study of 58,806 obstetric patients, 38,636 cases were selected for analysis because they satisfied the following criteria: (1) antepartum care before the 28th week of pregnancy, (2) singleton fetus, (3) four or more antepartum visits before delivery, and (4) date of last mentrual period known.

In Table 27-1 the fetal death rate for these pregnancies is presented in relation to the presence or absence of hypertension, proteinuria, or both (Friedman and Neff, 1976). Note that hypertension alone, in the absence of proteinuria, was associated with a threefold rise in the fetal death rate (diastolic blood pressure greater than or equal to 95 mm Hg). Interestingly, proteinuria without associated hypertension had little overall influence on the frequency of fetal death. In an evaluation of the

TABLE 27-1. FETAL DEATH RATE PER 1000 BY DIASTOLIC PRESSURE AND PROTEINURIA COMBINATIONS

Diastolic Blood Pressure (mm Hg)	Proteinuria						
	None	*Trace*	*1+*	*2+*	*3+*	*4+*	*Total*
< 65	15.50*	13.64	6.20	—	—	—	13.60
65–74	9.30	8.06	5.58	32.86*	41.54	—	8.84
75–84	6.20	7.44	6.20	19.22*	—	—	6.80
85–94	8.68	9.30	23.56*	—	22.32	—	10.20
95–104	19.22*	17.36*	26.66*	55.80*	115.32*	143.22*	25.16
105 +	20.46*	27.90*	62.62*	68.82*	125.24*	110.98*	41.48*
TOTAL	8.60	9.46	12.94	23.22*	41.96*	56.76*	

* Statistically significant, $P < 0.01$.
(*From Freidman, Neff: In Lindheimer et al.* (eds): *Hypertension in Pregnancy. New York, Wiley, 1976.*)

causes of perinatal deaths in this study population, Naeye and Friedman (1979) concluded that 70 percent of the excess deaths were due to three disorders—large placental infarcts, markedly small placental size, and abruptio placentae. They further stated, "All three (disorders) display microscopic placental lesions (that) are the consequence of reduced uteroplacental perfusion...." Uteroplacental perfusion is considered at length later in this chapter.

When the blood pressure rises appreciably during the latter half of pregnancy it is perilous, to the fetus especially, not to take action simply because proteinuria has not yet developed. Many clinicians have witnessed the onset of *eclampsia* before the onset of overt proteinuria. Thus, from both pathophysiologic and epidemiologic perspectives, it is clear that hypertension is the sine qua non of preeclampsia and that from the moment blood pressure begins to rise, both the fetus and the mother are at increased risk. Once the blood pressure exceeds 140/90 mm Hg, the diagnosis of PIH should be made and the pregnancy managed accordingly. Proteinuria constitutes a sign of worsening hypertensive disease, and when the proteinuria is overt and persists, the risk to the fetus is increased even more.

SEVERITY OF PREGNANCY-INDUCED HYPERTENSION

Pregnancy-induced hypertension is classified as mild or severe according to the frequency and intensity of the abnormalities listed in Table 27-2. It is important to realize that an apparently mild case can rapidly become severe. Blood pressure alone is not always a dependable indication of severity, for an adolescent woman with a pressure of 145/85 mm Hg may develop convulsions, whereas some women with a blood pressure of 180/120 mm Hg do not. Fortunately, most women suffering from preeclampsia do not convulse. In some, the process is inherently mild and hence does not advance to the eclamptic stage. In others, suitable anticonvulsant treatment checks the process. In a third group, the termination of pregnancy either spontaneously or by in-

tervention, forestalls the development of convulsions, and the woman returns to normal after delivery.

Epigastric or right upper quadrant pain is presumed to be the result of hepatic edema and subcapsular hemorrhage, which stretches Glisson's capsule. Rarely, the pain presages rupture of the liver, a rare but catastrophic complication of PIH. Hence in this circumstance, prompt, definitive therapy is often indicated. Other signs of advanced PIH are overt *thrombocytopenia* and *hepatocellular dysfunction*, which are likely to coexist. The etiology of impaired liver function in severely preeclamptic patients is unclear. Pritchard and associates (1976) postulated that the thrombocytopenia results from platelet adherence to collagen exposed at sites of disrupted vascular endothelium. Brunner and Gavras (1975) demonstrated that induction of hypertension by angiotensin II infusion in experimental animals led to segmental constriction and dilatation of arterioles with disruption of the vascular endothelium, especially in the dilated segments. They also found platelet adherence

TABLE 27-2. INDICATORS OF SEVERITY OF PREGNANCY-INDUCED HYPERTENSION

Abnormality	Mild	Severe
Diastolic blood pressure	< 100 mm Hg	110 mm Hg or higher
Proteinuria	Trace to 1+	Persistent 2+ or more
Headache	Absent	Present
Visual disturbances	Absent	Present
Upper abdominal pain	Absent	Present
Oliguria	Absent	Present
Convulsions	Absent	Present
Serum creatinine	Normal	Elevated
Thrombocytopenia	Absent	Present
Hyperbilirubinemia	Absent	Present
SGOT elevation	Minimal	Marked
Fetal growth retardation	Absent	Obvious

and fibrin deposited at the sites of denuded subendothelium. Using the scanning electron microscope, Robertson and Khairallah (1972) clearly identified platelet aggregates and fibrin strands adherent to the exposed subendothelial layer in rabbits treated with angiotensin II. Fetal growth retardation is less common with pregnancy-induced hypertension than with pregnancy-aggravated hypertension, but when it is present, the physician should suspect that the disease process has been prolonged. The fetus in such a case can be in extreme jeopardy!

Eclampsia

In neglected or, less often, fulminant cases of pregnancy-induced hypertension, eclampsia may develop. The seizures are grand mal in character. Seizures of eclampsia may first appear before labor, during labor, or postpartum. Any seizure occurring more than 48 hours postpartum is more likely to be the consequence of some other lesion of the central nervous system.

COINCIDENTAL (CHRONIC) HYPERTENSION

All *chronic hypertensive disorders,* regardless of their cause, appear to predispose to the development of superimposed preeclampsia or eclampsia. These disorders can create a difficult problem of differential diagnosis and management in women who first present for obstetric care after the 20th week of gestation. The diagnosis of coincidental hypertension is supported by the following findings: (1) a history of hypertension (140/90 mm Hg or greater) antedating pregnancy or (2) discovery of hypertension (140/90 mm Hg or greater) before the 20th week of pregnancy (with the exception of molar pregnancy, noted above) or its persistence long after delivery. Additional historical factors that help support the diagnosis of coincidental hypertension are multiparity and the presence of hypertension in a previous pregnancy.

When the woman is not seen until the latter half of pregnancy, the diagnosis of chronic hypertension may be difficult to make because of the well-documented decrease in blood pressure that may occur during the second trimester and early in the third trimester of pregnancy in chronically hypertensive pregnant women. Thus, a patient with chronic vascular disease who is seen for the first time at the 20th week of pregnancy may have a blood pressure that is within the normal range. During the third trimester, however, her blood pressure usually increases to or toward its former hypertensive level, which presents a diagnostic problem: Is this chronic (coexistent) hypertensive disease, or is it pregnancy-induced hypertension? The physician is faced with a dilemma when a pregnant woman is not seen until the second half of pregnancy and at that time is normotensive but subsequently demonstrates hypertension during the third trimester.

There are many diseases and syndromes associated with hypertension that may be encountered in pregnant women. Sims (1970) proposed the following classification of hypertension, which is presented here with slight modifications.

I. Hypertensive disease
   A. Essential hypertension (hypertensive vascular disease)
      1. Mild
      2. Moderate
      3. Severe
      4. Accelerated (malignant)
   B. Renal vascular disease (renovascular hypertension)
   C. Coarctation of the aorta
   D. Primary aldosteronism
   E. Pheochromocytoma
II. Renal and urinary tract disease
   A. Glomerulonephritis
      1. Acute
      2. Chronic
      3. Nephrotic syndrome (may occur in several other diseases as well)
   B. Pyelonephritis
   C. Lupus erythematosus
   D. Scleroderma with renal involvement
   E. Periartitis nodosa with renal involvement
   F. Acute renal failure
      1. Acute renal insufficiency
      2. Cortical necrosis
   G. Polycystic disease
   H. Diabetic nephropathy

Essential hypertension is by far the most common of these diseases in pregnant women. McCartney (1964), in his study of renal biopsies from women with clinical preeclampsia, diagnosed chronic glomerulonephritis in 21 percent of the nulliparas and in 6.6 percent of the multiparas. Fisher and co-workers (1969), however, did not confirm a high prevalence of chronic glomerulonephritis in their own patients.

It must be remembered that chronic hypertension is a dangerous disease whether the patient is pregnant or not. Specifically, chronic hypertension may lead to cardiovascular deterioration, such as cardiac decompensation and cerebrovascular accidents. Finally, intrinsic renal damage may result from chronic hypertensive disease, or the hypertension itself may be the result of underlying chronic pyelonephritis or chronic glomerulonephritis. Additional dangers for chronically hypertensive pregnant women include worsening of the hypertensive disease processes (pregnancy aggravated hypertension or superimposed preeclampsia) and the risk of abruptio placentae. Placental abruption has been reported to occur in 5 to 10 perecent of all chronically hypertensive pregnant women.

The fetus of the woman with chronic hypertension is, of course, subjected to additional risks, including growth retardation and intrauterine death.

PREGNANCY-AGGRAVATED HYPERTENSION

Pregnancy-aggravated hypertension is the result of acute aggravation of the preexisting hypertension. With the development of proteinuria and often gross edema, a better term is superimposed preeclampsia. There may be a quick progression to eclampsia, which, unfortunately, may develop before the 30th week of gestation. Diagnostic criteria include the following:

1. Documentation that the woman has chronic hypertension
2. Evidence of a superimposed, acute process as demonstrated by elevation of systolic blood pressure at least 30 mm Hg or of diastolic blood pressure at least 15 mm Hg above baseline on two occasions at least 6 hours apart and development of proteinuria, gross edema, or both.

PATHOPHYSIOLOGY OF PREECLAMPSIA–ECLAMPSIA

Vasospasm

Vasospasm is basic to the disease process of preeclampsia–eclampsia. This concept, first advanced by Volhard (1918), is based upon direct observation of small blood vessels in the nail beds, ocular fundi, and bulbar conjunctivae, and it has been surmised from histologic changes that are seen in various affected organs. In preeclampsia, Hinselmann (1924) and later several others noted alterations in the size of the arterioles in the nail bed, with evidence of segmental spasm that produced alternate regions of contraction and dilatation. Even more striking changes have been identified in the bulbar conjunctivae; Landesman and co-workers (1954) described marked arteriolar constriction, even to the extent that capillary circulation was intermittently abolished. Further evidence that vascular changes play an important role in preeclampsia–eclampsia is afforded by the frequency with which spasm of the retinal arterioles, commonly segmental, is found in this disorder.

The vascular constriction imposes a resistance to blood flow and accounts for the development of arterial hypertension. Vasospasm most likely exerts a noxious effect on the blood vessels themselves as well as the organs they supply. Circulation in the vasa vasorum is impaired, leading to damage of the vascular walls. Alternating segmental dilatation that commonly accompanies the segmental arteriolar spasm probably contributes further to the development of vascular damage, since endothelial integrity may be compromised by stretch in the dilated segments. Moreover, angiotensin II appears to have a direct action on endothelial cells, causing them to contract. These events can create interendothelial leaks through which blood constituents, including platelets

and fibrinogen, can pass and be deposited subendothelially (Brunner and Gavras, 1975). The vascular changes, together with local hypoxia of the surrounding tissues, presumably lead to hemorrhage, necrosis, and other disturbances that have been observed at times with severe PIH. Deposition of fibrin is then likely to be prominent, as seen in fatal cases (McKay, 1965).

Increased Pressor Responses

Normally, pregnant women develop refractoriness to the pressor effects of angiotensin II (Abdul-Karim and Assali, 1961). Increased vascular reactivity to pressor hormones in women with early preeclampsia has been identified by Raab and co-workers (1956) and Talledo and colleagues (1968), using either angiotensin II or norepinephrine, and by Dieckmann and Michel (1937) and Browne (1946), using vasopressin. Subsequently, Gant and co-workers (1973) demonstrated that increased vascular sensitivity to angiotensin II clearly preceded the development of PIH. In the primigravid women studied by them, refractoriness to the pressor effect of infused angiotensin II characterized normal pregnancy (Fig. 27-1). However, those women destined to develop PIH subsequently demonstrated a loss of the normal pregnancy refractoriness to angiotensin II some time before the onset of hypertension. Of all the normotensive women studied who at 28 to 32 weeks gestation required more than 8 ng per kg per minute of angiotensin II to develop a standardized pressor response, 91 percent remained normotensive throughout the rest of the pregnancy. Conversely, among normotensive primigravid women who required for a pressor response less than 8 ng per kg per minute at 28 to 32 weeks, 90 percent subsequently be-

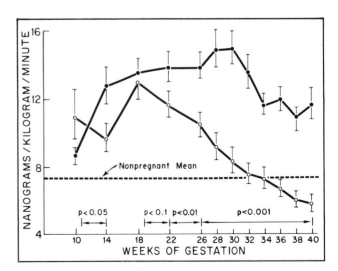

Figure 27-1. Comparison of the mean angiotensin II doses required to evoke a pressor response in 120 primigravidas who remained normotensive (*solid circles*) and 72 primigravidas who later developed pregnancy-induced hypertension (*open circles*). (*From Gant et al.: J Clin Invest 52:2682, 1973.*)

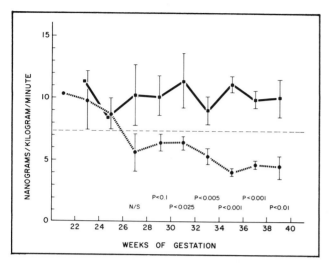

Figure 27-2. Comparison of angiotensin II responsiveness in 29 patients with uncomplicated essential hypertension and 34 patients with essential hypertension destined to develop superimposed preeclampsia. The dose of angiotensin II (ng/kg/minute) required to elevate resting diastolic blood pressure 20 mm Hg is shown on the vertical axis and is plotted as a function of weeks of gestation. The results obtained in gravidas with chronic hypertension alone are indicated by squares connected by a solid line. The results obtained in gravidas with chronic hypertension destined to develop superimposed preeclampsia are shown as dots connected by a broken line. The vertical bars represent the standard error of the mean. (*From Gant et al.: Am J Obstet Gynecol 127:369, 1977.*)

came overtly hypertensive. Similar results have been reported recently in 231 women studied by Öney and Kaulhausen in Germany (1982).

A similar prospective study of angiotensin II pressor responsiveness was also conducted in women whose pregnancies were complicated by coexistent (chronic) hypertension. In this study, 63 patients with chronic essential hypertension were studied throughout pregnancy. Two groups of patients were identified on the basis of clinical outcome and serial measurements of vascular reactivity to exogenously administered angiotensin II (Gant and associates, 1977). The first group consisted of 29 gravidas with chronic hypertension alone, and the second group was composed of 34 patients with chronic hypertension who were destined to develop pregnancy-aggravated hypertension. Both groups of hypertensive patients in this study were refractory to the pressor effects of infused angiotensin II between the 21st and 25th weeks of pregnancy, i.e., they required more than 7 ng per kg per minute to induce a 20 mm Hg increase in the baseline diastolic blood pressure. A clear separation between the two groups of women developed after the 27th week of gestation, and after the 30th week the difference between the means became significant (Fig. 27-2).

The pattern of angiotensin II responsiveness observed in these two groups of women with chronic hypertension is similar to that seen in the two groups of initially normotensive primigravid women whose results are illustrated in Figure 27-1. Indeed, from an inspection of the data ob-

tained between the 28th and 32nd weeks of pregnancy in the women with chronic hypertension, it is conceivable that pressor responsiveness to angiotensin II might be used as a screening technique to identify women with chronic hypertension who are destined to develop superimposed PIH, as is the case for normotensive primigravid patients destined to develop preeclampsia–eclampsia. However, caution must be exercised for several reasons before interpreting these data obtained in chronic hypertensive subjects in a manner analogous to that of the younger, normotensive primigravid women. First, both the number of patients and the number of infusions conducted in the study of chronically hypertensive gravidas are much smaller than reported in the earlier study of primigravid women. Second, in the chronically hypertensive woman the superimposition of a second vascular disease as the direct consequence of pregnancy is not always clearly evident except in retrospect.

Refractoriness to angiotensin II is not a generalized phenomenon, since aldosterone secretion is strikingly increased in pregnant women and increased aldosterone secretion is modulated by the action of angiotensin II on the cells of the zona glomerulosa of the adrenal cortex. Based on the findings of a number of studies, Gant and co-workers (1974a), Cunningham and associates (1975), and Everett and colleagues (1978a, 1978b) concluded that in pregnant women the blunted pressor response to angiotensin II was brought about by a specific decrease in responsiveness of the vasculature. Refractoriness to the pressor effects of angiotensin II begins early in pregnancy (Fig. 27-1), and in some women enormous amounts of angiotensin II are required to elicit a given pressor response. The refractoriness to angiotensin II appears to be mediated by the vascular tissue synthesis of a prostaglandin or prostaglandin-like substance, for example, prostacyclin or prostaglandin E_2. Indeed, the refractoriness to the pressor effect of angiotensin II in pregnant women can be abolished by the administration of the prostaglandin synthetase enzyme inhibitors, indomethacin and aspirin (Everett and colleagues, 1978a). In some tissues, angiotensin II action is mediated, at least in part, by promoting either the accelerated synthesis or the release of prostaglandins or by both mechanisms. It is interesting to speculate that pregnancy brings about an increased capacity for prostaglandin formation in vascular tissue, normally with relatively greater synthesis of prostaglandins that induce vasodilatation than of prostaglandins, e.g., prostaglandin $F_{2\alpha}$, that promote vasoconstriction.

A pressor response induced simply by the supine position, after lying in the lateral recumbent, has been demonstrated in some pregnant women by Gant and coworkers (1974b). They found that the majority of nulliparous pregnant women who demonstrated at 28 to 32 weeks an increase in diastolic blood pressure of at least 20 mm Hg when turned from side to back later became overtly hypertensive; conversely, most women who did not demonstrate such a rise did not become hypertensive. Those women who demonstrated a supine pressor

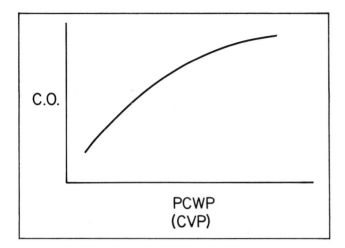

Figure 27-3. Ventricular function (Starling) curve for the normal heart. Pulmonary capillar wedge pressure (PCWP) or central venous pressure (CVP) represents fiber length, and cardiac output (CO) represents fiber shortening. (*Adapted from Hankins, et al.: Perinatol Neonatol 7:29, 1983.*)

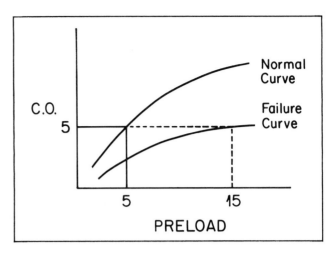

Figure 27-4. Ventricular function curve for heart failure. In order to maintain cardiac output (CO), the failing heart is required to function at higher preloads (PCWP or CVP). (*Adapted from Hankins et al.: Perinatol Neonatol 7:29, 1983.*)

response were also abnormally sensitive to angiotensin II, and vice versa. The mechanism by which the supine position may incite a rise in blood pressure is not clear, but it is another manifestation of intrinsic vascular hypersensitivity in women destined to develop PIH.

MATERNAL CONSEQUENCES OF PREGNANCY-INDUCED HYPERTENSION

Deterioration of function in a number of organs and systems, presumably in large part as the consequence of vasospasm, have been identified in severe preeclampsia and eclampsia. For descriptive reasons these effects will be separated into maternal and fetal consequences of PIH. However, it should be remembered that these alterations in maternal and fetal physiology are often occurring at the same time in both the maternal and fetal patient.

There are many possible maternal consequences of pregnancy-induced hypertension; however, for simplicity's sake, these maternal effects of hypertension can be considered through analysis of cardiovascular, hematologic, endocrine, fluid and electrolyte, renal, hepatic, and cerebral abnormalities.

CARDIOVASCULAR SYSTEM

Despite an increase in cardiac output in normal pregnant subjects, blood pressure does not increase but actually decreases as a consequence of decreased peripheral resistance (Chapter 9, p. 195). In the pregnant hypertensive patient, cardiac output does not usually decrease (Benedetti and associates, 1980; Phelan and Yurth, 1982; Hankins and co-workers, 1984), and because cardiac output does not decrease as arteriolar constriction and peripheral resistance increase, the blood pressure rises.

Clinical Assessment of Cardiac Function

In assessing cardiac function four areas must be addressed: (1) preload—end diastolic pressure and chamber volume, (2) afterload—intramyocardial systolic tension, i.e., resistance to ejection, (3) contractile or inotropic state of the myocardium, and (4) heart rate. An informative review of this subject was provided recently by Hankins and associates (1983).

Preload. Preload is determined by intraventricular pressure and volume, thus setting the initial myocardial muscle fiber length. Clinically, the right and left ventricular end diastolic filling pressures are assessed by central venous pressure (CVP) and pulmonary capillary wedge pressure (PCWP), respectively. By plotting cardiac output against CVP and PCWP, a cardiac function curve can be developed for the right and left heart chambers (Fig. 27-3). As illustrated in Figure 27-4, one can see that the failing heart requires a higher preload or filling pressure to achieve the same output. The preload can be increased by the administration of crystalloid, colloid, or blood and can be decreased by the use of diuretics, vasodilators (especially of the capacitance system), or phlebotomy, as might be indicated clinically.

Afterload. Afterload is defined as the ventricular wall tension during systole and is dependent on the end diastolic radius of the ventricle, the aortic diastolic pressure, and ventricular wall thickness. The extent to which the left intraventricular pressure will rise during systole depends primarily on the total systemic vascular resistance

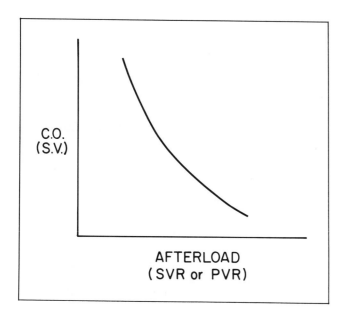

Figure 27-5. Relationship of afterload [systemic vascular resistance (SVR) or pulmonary vascular resistance (PVR)] to cardiac output (CO) or stroke volume (SV) at a constant preload. (*Adapted from Hankins et al.: Perinatol Neonatol 7:29, 1983.*)

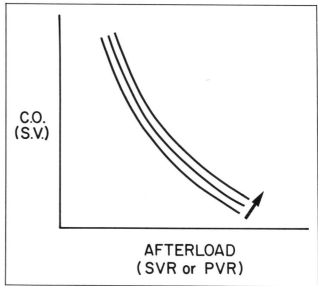

Figure 27-6. Relationship of afterload [systemic vascular resistance (SVR) or pulmonary vascular resistance (PVR)] to cardiac output (CO) or stroke volume (SV) at decreased, normal, and increased preloads as indicated by the arrow. (*Adapted from Hankins et al.: Perinatol Neonatol 7:29, 1983.*)

(Fig. 27-5). For practical purposes, the aortic or mean arterial pressure is a direct reflection of afterload. In the presence of heart failure, increases in afterload worsen the degree of failure by decreasing the stroke volume and, in turn, the cardiac output.

As with preload, afterload can be increased or decreased therapeutically as mandated by the clinical setting. Increases in afterload are mediated through modulation of the α-adrenergic system. Decreases in afterload, or systemic vascular resistance, can be achieved with a host of agents.

Intravenously administered hydralazine is the antihypertensive agent most commonly used in the treatment of severe preeclampsia and eclampsia. *The intermittent intravenous administration of small, incremental doses of hydralazine has been proven safe for both mother and fetus without the use of continuous arterial pressure monitoring.*

No evidence has been presented to support the hypothesis that volume expansion in the presence of increased afterload, as found in women with PIH, causes cardiac output or peripheral resistance to return to normal (Fig. 27-6). A transient fall in peripheral resistance and a slight increase in cardiac output has been observed by Groenendijk and co-workers (1984) after careful volume expansion. Importantly, they stress that women with PIH are unable to cope with a circulating volume necessary to maintain a cardiac output and a ventricular filling pressure considered to be normal for pregnancy. Volume expansion in patients with PIH may, in fact, cause a decrease in cardiac output and cardiac failure (Hankins and co-workers, 1984). Finally, vigorous

volume expansion as part of therapy contributed to the highest incidence of cerebrovascular accidents, pulmonary edema, and renal failure ever observed by López-Llera when his several treatment regimens were separated according to methods of treatment (Table 27-3).

Contractile State of the Heart. The third variable in the assessment of cardiac function is the contractile, or inotropic, state of the heart, defined as the force and velocity of ventricular contractions when preload and afterload are held constant. While cardiac output can be measured directly (Hankins and co-workers, 1983), the adequacy of the cardiac output may be assessed indirectly by acid-base status, arterial-venous oxygen differences, and urinary output. In cardiac failure with low output states, both preload and afterload should be optimized through previously mentioned therapeutic regimens. If these fail to restore the cardiac output to acceptable levels, attention should be directed to improving myocardial contractility. Beta-sympathomimetics, such as dopamine and isoproterenol, usually improve cardiac outputs acutely. Dependent on the cause of myocardial failure, either short-term or long-term therapy with digitalis alkaloids may be necessary.

Heart Rate. The final determinant of myocardial function is heart rate. Although heart block is rare in pregnant patients, cardiac output can be compromised by heart rates too slow to maintain adequate output. In this setting, treatment with either atropine or cardiac pacing

TABLE 27-3. RESULTS IN SOME PUBLISHED REPORTS OF MATERNAL MORTALITY FROM ECLAMPSIA

Authors	Treatment	Cases (No.)	Maternal Deaths (Percent)
Dewar and Morris (1947)	Tribromethanol	44	4.5
Browne (1950)	Thiopental	26	7.6
Shears (1957)	Lytic cocktail	124	8.8
Menon (1961)	Lytic cocktail*	402	2.2
Llewellyn-Jones (1961)	Lytic cocktail	150	6.6
Bryant and Fleming (1962)	Magnesium sulfate and veratrum alkaloids	253	1.6
Zuspan and Ward (1964)	Magnesium sulfate	59	3.4
López-Llera			
(1967) A	Lytic cocktail	108	10.2
(1970) B	Lytic cocktail	120	11.7
(1973) C	Diazepam + reserpine	137	17.5
(1976) D	Furosemide, reserpine + volume expansion (albumin) + antithrombotic	160	12.5
(1979) E	Barbiturates + magnesium sulfate + reserpine and/or isoxsuprine	179	16.2
		(704)	(13.9)
Lean and co-workers (1968)	Chlordiazepoxide	90†	3.3
	or diazepam	60‡	5.0
Kawathekar and associates (1973)	Diazepam	16	6.3
Mojadidi and Thompson (1973)	Morphine and magnesium sulfate	30	6.7
Sibai and associates (1981)	Magnesium sulfate + hydralazine	67	0
Pritchard and associates (1984)	Magnesium sulfate (hydralazine) and standardized treatment regimen	245	0.4

* Chlorpromazine, diethazine, and meperidine.
† Includes postpartum eclampsia (up to 14 days).
‡ Excludes eclampsia that developed postpartum.

is indicated. Alternatively, sustained tachycardia can lead to congestive heart failure due to shortened systolic ejection and diastolic filling times or myocardial ischemia. The cause of the tachycardia should be determined and corrected, i.e., fever, hypovolemia, pain, hyperthyroidism. Treatment with propranolol, digoxin, or calcium channel blockers, such as verapamil, is seldom required in the obstetric population.

HEMATOLOGIC CHANGES IN PREGNANCY-INDUCED HYPERTENSION

Important hematologic changes that have been identified at times in women with preeclampsia and eclampsia include (1) a decrease in, or actually an absence of, normal pregnancy hypervolemia (Chapter 9, p. 191), (2) alterations of the coagulation mechanism, and (3) evidence of increased erythrocyte destruction.

Blood Volume

Hemoconcentration in women with eclampsia was emphasized by Dieckmann (1952) in his lengthy monograph, *The Toxemias of Pregnancy*. More recently, Pritchard and co-workers (1984) reported measurements of the blood volume in women with eclampsia. Their findings are consistent with the view that in eclampsia, pregnancy hypervolemia most often is scant to absent (Table 27-4). The woman of average size can be expected to have a blood volume near 5000 ml during the last several weeks of a normal pregnancy compared to about 3500 ml in the nonpregnant state. With eclampsia, however, much or all of the added 1500 ml of blood normally present late in pregnancy can be anticipated to be missing.

The near absence of pregnancy-induced hypervolemia could be the consequence of generalized vasoconstriction, or it could result from increased vascular

TABLE 27-4. BLOOD VOLUMES IN FIVE WOMEN MEASURED (^{51}Cr) DURING ANTEPARTUM ECLAMPSIA, AGAIN WHEN NONPREGNANT, AND FINALLY AT A COMPARABLE TIME IN THEIR SECOND PREGNANCY UNCOMPLICATED BY HYPERTENSION

	Eclampsia	Nonpregnant	Normal Pregnant
Blood volume (ml)	3530	3035	4425
Change (%)	+ 16		+ 47
Hematocrit	40.5	38.2	34.7

(From Pritchard et al.: Am J Obstet Gynecol (in press), 1984.)

permeability, which would account for the classic features, when compared to normal pregnancy, of too little fluid intravascularly but a marked excess extravascularly. Both mechanisms could be involved.

It was taught by Dieckmann (1952), and more recently by others, that clinical improvement is characterized by hemodilution manifested by a fall in hematocrit. In our experience, however, a significant fall in hematocrit occurs most often only with delivery. Moreover, rather than directly reflecting clinical improvement, the fall may be the consequence of blood loss at delivery in the absence of the cushion of normal pregnancy hypervolemia or, much less commonly, may result from intense erythrocyte destruction, as described below, or both.

It is emphasized that in terms of capacity, the intravascular compartment in eclampsia in the absence of hemorrhage is usually not underfilled. Vasospasm has contracted the space to be filled, a reduction that persists until hours to a few days after delivery, when typically the vascular system dilates, the blood volume increases, and the hematocrit falls. The woman with eclampsia, therefore, is unduly sensitive to vigorous fluid therapy administered in an attempt to expand the contracted blood volume to normal pregnancy levels as well as to blood loss at delivery. Management of blood loss in these circumstances is considered in Chapter 21.

Coagulation

It has long been recognized that changes that might imply intravascular coagulation and, less often, pathologic erythrocyte destruction may further complicate cases of PIH, especially eclampsia (Pritchard and colleagues, 1954a, 1954b; Stahnke, 1922). In recent years, renewed interest in these changes has led to the concept by some investigators that not only is disseminated intravascular coagulation a characteristic feature of PIH but that it plays a dominant role in the pathogenesis of the syndrome. For example, Page (1972) theorized that many of the changes of preeclampsia were the consequence of fibrin deposited in vital organs as a product of slowly disseminated intravascular coagulation initiated by thromboplastin entering the maternal circulation from the placenta, while rapidly disseminated intravas-

scular coagulation and fibrin so formed caused cerebral vascular occlusion and the convulsions of eclampsia.

Since the early reports by Pritchard and co-workers (1954a, 1954b), we have continued to search for evidence of coagulopathy in eclamptic women. The results of these studies are presented in Table 27-5. Thrombocytopenia, infrequently severe, was the most frequent finding. The platelet count was below 150,000/mm^3 in 24 of 91 cases (26 percent) but below 100,000 in only 14 women (15 percent).

We have not identified overt thrombocytopenia in the cord blood from cases of severe preeclampsia–eclampsia (Pritchard and Cunningham, unpublished; Engle and Rosenfeld, 1984). It is difficult to reconcile these observations with those of Rote and associates (1984) who state that thrombocytopenia is often present in this disorder and suggest immunologic mechanisms are involved in the genesis of thrombocytopenia in mother and fetus.

Levels of fibrin degradation products in serum were clearly elevated very infrequently. Unless some degree of placental abruption had developed, fibrinogen in maternal plasma did not differ remarkably from levels found late in normal pregnancy. Interestingly, the thrombin time was somewhat prolonged in one third of the cases of eclampsia even when elevated levels of fibrin degradation products were not identified (Pritchard and colleagues, 1976). The reason for this elevation is not known. The various coagulation changes just described do occur in women with preeclampsia but are certainly no more common.

Our observations on eclampsia, as well as those reported by Kitzmiller and associates (1974) for pre-

TABLE 27-5. CHANGES IN COAGULATION FACTORS THAT IMPLY DISSEMINATED INTRAVASCULAR COAGULATION

	Intrapartum Primigravidas Normally Pregnant	Most Abnormal Value For Each Case of Eclampsia
Platelets*		
Mean (mm^3)	278,000	206,000
−2 standard deviations	150,000	—
<150,000	0/20	24/91
<100,000	0/20	14/91
< 50,000	0/20	3/91
Serum fibrin degradation products†		
8 µg per ml or less	17/20	51/59
16 µg per ml	3/20	6/59
>16 µg per ml	0/20	2/59
Plasma fibrinogen*		
mean, mg per dl	415	413
−2 standard deviations	285	—
<285 mg per dl	0/20	7/89
Fibrin monomer		
positive	1/20	1/14

* Lowest value identified for each case of eclampsia.
† Highest value identified for each case of eclampsia.

eclampsia, are most consistent with the concept that the coagulation changes are the sequelae of preeclampsia–eclampsia rather than the cause. Very likely, platelets aggregate and adhere to vessel walls whenever and wherever endothelial cells are discontinuous and variable amounts of fibrin are deposited there. For reasons presented subsequently, treatment with heparin is not inappropriate.

Erythrocyte Destruction

Evidence of increased erythrocyte destruction (microangiopathic hemolysis) in our studies has ranged from none to the very uncommon case of eclampsia with fulminant hemoglobinemia and hemoglobinuria accompanied by marked changes in erythrocyte morphology, including fragmented erythrocytes, basket cells, and, rarely, microspherocytes. Evidence of hemolysis, when present, most often clears soon after delivery.

ENDOCRINE AND METABOLIC CHANGES

Endocrine Changes

During normal pregnancy, plasma levels of renin, angiotensin II, and aldosterone are increased. Paradoxically, with pregnancy-induced hypertension, these substances commonly decrease toward the normal nonpregnant range (Weir and colleagues, 1973). With the development of sodium retention, hypertension, or both, the rate of renin release by the juxtaglomerular apparatus decreases. Since renin is the enzyme that catalyzes the conversion of angiotensinogen to angiotensin I (which is then transformed into angiotensin II by a converting enzyme), angiotensin II levels decline, and thence aldosterone secretion decreases. On the other hand, another potent mineralocorticoid, deoxycorticosterone (DOC), is strikingly increased in the plasma of women during the third trimester of pregnancy (Chapter 9, p. 204). Importantly, the increase in DOC concentration does not appear to rise as the consequence of increased secretion of DOC by the maternal adrenal glands. Treatment of pregnant women with the potent glucocorticosteroid, dexamethasone, to reduce ACTH secretion, does not bring about a reduction in plasma levels of DOC, and neither does ACTH treatment of near-term pregnant women cause an increase in plasma DOC levels. Since it has been shown that plasma progesterone is converted to DOC in nonadrenal tissues, it is reasonable to conclude that DOC formed in this manner is not subject to control by angiotensin II and thus the amount of DOC formed from plasma progesterone is not reduced by sodium retention or hypertension. Therefore, extra-adrenal DOC formation may play a crucial role in the pathogenesis or perpetuation of PIH.

Winkel and co-workers (1980) found that the fractional conversion of plasma progesterone to DOC varied widely among individuals (0.002 to 0.22). This finding is very intriguing, since, ordinarily, the fractional conversion of one steroid hormone to another is similar among normal persons. Thus, in near-term pregnant women producing 250 mg of progesterone per day, the amount of DOC produced from plasma progesterone could vary from 0.5 mg to 11 mg per 24 hours. Nonpregnant women produce, on average, 0.15 mg DOC per day. Given the progesterone produced in women with hyperplacentosis who are prone to develop preeclampsia, e.g., women with diabetes, multiple fetuses, fetal hydrops, and hydatidiform mole, the amount of DOC produced from plasma progesterone could be enormous.

The formation of DOC cannot be the only factor, however, in the development of PIH. DOC levels were measured throughout pregnancy by Parker and colleagues (1980). They found that the concentrations of DOC in the plasma of a group of primigravid women who ultimately developed preeclampsia were not greater than the concentrations of DOC in primigravid women who remained normotensive. Brown and co-workers (1972) had shown previously that the DOC levels in pregnant women who were already hypertensive were not greater than were those in normotensive gravidas. However, Winkel and co-workers (1983) reported that the conversion of progesterone into DOC was significantly increased in women who later developed PIH. It may be that the DOC produced has a local effect and is produced and metabolized within the kidney such that the plasma DOC concentration need not be different in hypertensive women. The possibility of a yet unidentified pressor hormone certainly persists.

Increased antidiuretic hormone activity to account for oliguria has been previously suggested but has not been established. In fact, low levels have been measured (Pritchard and Porter, unpublished). Chorionic gonadotropin levels in plasma have been found inconstantly to be elevated; conversely, placental lactogen has been found inconstantly to be reduced.

Necrosis of the adrenal and the pituitary has been identified in some fatal cases of eclampsia (McKay, 1965). In our experience, which is limited to nonfatal cases, compromised adrenal or pituitary function is rare.

Fluid and Electrolyte Changes

Commonly, the volume of extracellular fluid in women with severe preeclampsia–eclampsia has expanded appreciably beyond the increased volume that characterizes normal pregnancy. The mechanism responsible for the pathologic expansion is not clear. Edema is evident at a time when, paradoxically, aldosterone levels are reduced compared to the remarkably elevated levels of normal pregnancy. As noted above, however, DOC levels in plasma remain elevated but are not consistently greater than those in normotensive women. The electrolyte concentrations do not differ appreciably from those of normal pregnancy unless there has been vigorous diuretic therapy, dietary sodium restriction, or the administration of water with sufficient oxytocin to produce antidiuresis. Severe edema, by itself, is not indicative of a poor prognosis, nor does lack of appreciable edema

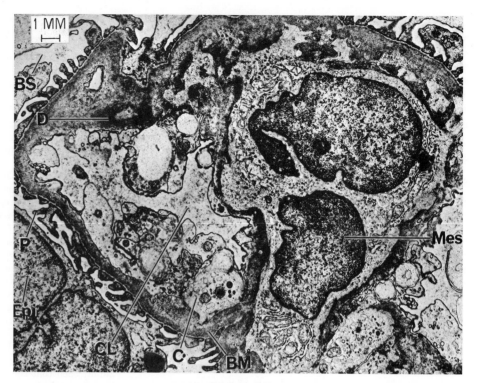

Figure 27-7. The glomerular capillary lesion of preeclampsia. BS = Bowman's space; D = electron-dense deposit, probably a derivative of fibrinogen; P = podocytes or foot processes of epithelial cell; Epi = nucleus of epithelial cell; CL = lumen of glomerular capillary; C = markedly swollen endothelial cytoplasm; BM = basement membrane (normal); MES = nucleus of mesothelial cell. (*From Chesley: Hypertensive Disorders of Pregnancy. New York, Appleton-Century-Crofts, 1978.*)

guarantee a favorable outcome for pregnancies complicated by preeclampsia–eclampsia.

Following a convulsion, the bicarbonate concentration is lowered as a consequence of the lactic acidosis and compensatory loss of carbon dioxide from plasma through the lungs. The intensity of the acidosis will relate to the amount of lactic acid produced and its rate of metabolism, as well as the rate at which carbon dioxide is exhaled.

ALTERATIONS IN ORGAN PERFUSION IN PREGNANCY-INDUCED HYPERTENSION

Renal Changes

During normal pregnancy, renal blood flow and the glomerular filtration rate are increased appreciably above nonpregnant levels (Chapter 9, p. 197), but with the development of pregnancy-induced hypertension, renal perfusion and glomerular filtration are variably reduced. Levels that are much below normal nonpregnant levels are the consequence of severe disease. Therefore, in milder cases the creatinine or urea concentration in plasma may not be appreciably elevated above normal nonpregnant values. The plasma uric acid concentration typically is elevated, especially in women with more severe disease. The elevation is a result primarily of decreased renal clearance of uric acid by the kidney, a decrease that exceeds the reduction in glomerular filtration rate and creatinine clearance (Chesley and Williams, 1945). Thiazide diuretics, if administered, contribute to

the increase in uric acid in plasma. In our experience, measurements of plasma uric acid levels are generally of little practical value for diagnosis or prognosis.

The experience at Parkland Memorial Hospital has been that after delivery, in the absence of underlying chronic vascular disease, complete recovery of renal function can be anticipated. This would not be the case, of course, if *renal cortical necrosis,* an irreversible but rare lesion, had developed.

Microscopic Changes. Changes identifiable by light and electron microscopy are usually found in the kidney. Sheehan (1950) observed that the glomeruli were enlarged by about 20 percent, often pouting into the neck of the tubule. The capillary loops are variably dilated and contracted. The endothelial cells are swollen, and deposited within and beneath them are fibrils that have been mistaken for thickening and reduplication of the basement membrane.

Sheehan's interpretations have been confirmed by electron microscopic studies of renal biopsies taken from women with preeclampsia. Most, but not all, of the electron microscopic studies are consistent with the view that the characteristic changes are glomerular capillary endothelial swelling, which Spargo and associates (1959) called "glomerular capillary endotheliosis," and subendothelial deposit of protein material. The endothelial cells are so swollen as to block partially, or even completely, the capillary lumens. Homogeneous deposits of an electron-dense substance are found between the basal lamina and the endothelial cell and within the cells themselves (Figs. 27-7, 27-8). Vassalli and co-workers

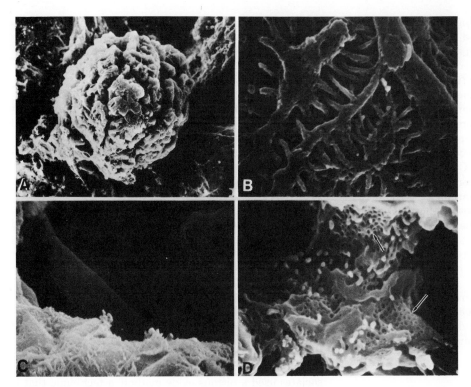

Figure 27-8. Scanning electron micrographs. **A.** Enlarged, swollen glomerulus × 500. **B.** Branching and interdigitation of terminal epithelial foot processes, usually normal in preeclampsia × 20,000. **C.** Interior of glomerular capillary. Endothelial fenestrae are not seen because of severe swelling of the cytoplasm × 5,000. **D.** Normal glomerulus for comparison; note polygonal endothelial fenestrae (*arrows*) × 5,000. (*Photographs by Ordóñoz: From Lindheimer and Katz: Renal Function and Disease in Pregnancy. Philadelphia, Lea & Febiger, 1977.*)

(1963), on the basis of immunofluorescent staining, considered the material to be a fibrinogen derivative and regarded its presence as characteristic of preeclampsia. This observation, in part, led to a theory that the renal lesions of PIH are the result of intravascular coagulation initiated by something, presumably thromboplastin, released from the placenta (Page, 1972). Lichtig and coworkers (1975), however, were able to identify fibrinogen or its derivatives so deposited in but 13 of 30 renal biopsy specimens from women considered, for good reasons, to have preeclampsia, and in only 2 of the 30 was the amount of fibrin graded as more than a trace. An alternative explanation for the renal lesion has been proposed by Petrucco and colleagues (1974), who detected IgM and IgG, and sometimes complement, in the glomeruli of women with preeclampsia in proportion to the severity of the disease. They suggested that an immunologic mechanism was active in the production of the glomerular lesion.

The renal changes identified by electron microscopy have been held out by some as being pathognomonic of preeclampsia, always present in that disease and specific for it. The uncertainties of clinical diagnosis are so great, however, as to preclude acceptance of such a one-to-one relation, except as an act of faith. The history of pathognomonic lesions in eclampsia engenders skepticism. One such pathognomonic lesion accepted in the past, but not now, was peripheral hemorrhagic necrosis of the hepatic lobules, as discussed below.

Tubular lesions are common in the kidneys of women with eclampsia, but what has been interpreted as degenerative changes may represent only an accumula-tion within the cells of protein reabsorbed from the glomerular filtrate. The collecting tubules may appear obstructed by casts from derivatives of protein, including, at times, hemoglobin.

Acute renal failure from *tubular necrosis* may develop, especially in neglected cases. Rarely, the major portion of the cortex of both kidneys undergoes necrosis. *Renal cortical necrosis* is characterized clinically by oliguria or anuria and rapidly developing azotemia. Although cortical necrosis of the kidney is known to have occurred in nonpregnant women and in men, in many institutions the lesion has been associated most often with pregnancy.

Hepatic Changes

With severe PIH there are, at times, alterations in tests of hepatic function, including delayed excretion of bromosulfonphthalein and elevation of serum glutamic oxaloacetic transaminase (SGOT, AST) levels (Combes and Adams, 1972). Severe hyperbilirubinemia is uncommon with PIH. In our experience with 134 women, including 45 with eclampsia, only 3 had a serum bilirubin greater than 1.2 mg/dl, with 2.3 mg/dl as the highest value. Much of the increase in serum alkaline phosphatase is usually in the form of heat-stable alkaline phosphatase, which most likely is of placental origin.

Hemorrhagic necrosis in the periphery of the liver lobule, identified commonly at autopsy, was long considered to be the characteristic lesion of eclampsia. However, the changes usually identified in fatal cases have seldom been demonstrated in liver biopsies of nonfatal cases (Combes and Adams, 1972; Ingerslev and Teilum, 1946). In our experience at Parkland Memorial Hospital, liver histology was normal in biopsies from 6 women with preeclampsia and 12 with otherwise uncomplicated eclampsia who were studied. Since the amount of tissue sampled by biopsy was small, some lesions may have been missed. Moreover, if the woman was thrombocytopenic, biopsy was avoided. This approach most likely excluded women with more marked hepatocellular damage, since a low platelet count is often accompanied by a high serum SGOT level (Pritchard and Cunningham, unpublished). Even so, the most characteristic feature of the hepatic lesion in eclampsia is its variability in both extent and severity. It is agreed by most authorities, therefore, that periportal necrosis can be the result but not the cause of eclampsia.

In rare instances, subcapsular hemorrhage in the liver may become so extensive as to cause rupture of the capsule, with massive hemorrhage into the peritoneal cavity. The mortality rate is high. Prompt surgical intervention with vigorous transfusion therapy can be lifesaving. One woman survived at Parkland Memorial Hospital after receiving blood and blood products from more than 200 donors!

Brain

McCall (1953) found that cerebral blood flow, oxygen consumption, and vascular resistance were not altered in women with preeclampsia, eclampsia, or essential hypertension; however, the possibility of focal hypoperfusion or hyperperfusion of the brain could not be excluded.

Nonspecific abnormalities in the electroencephalogram usually can be demonstrated for some time after eclamptic convulsions. An increased incidence of electroencephalographic abnormalities has been described for members of the families of women with eclampsia, a finding that is suggestive that some women who convulse as the consequence of PIH are by inheritance predisposed to do so (Rosenbaum and Maltby, 1943).

The main postmortem lesions that have been described in the brain of women who died with eclampsia are edema, hyperemia, focal anemia, thrombosis, and hemorrhage. Sheehan (1950) examined the brains of 48 eclamptic women very soon after their deaths. Hemorrhages, ranging from petechiae to gross bleeding, were found in 56 percent of the cases. According to Sheehan, if the brain is examined within an hour after death, most often it is as firm as normal and there is no obvious edema. Govan (1961) investigated the cause of death in 110 fatal cases of eclampsia and concluded that cerebral hemorrhage was responsible in 39. Forty-seven women died of cardiorespiratory failure; small hemorrhagic lesions were found in the brains of 85 percent of them. Govan described fibrinoid changes as a regular finding in the walls of the cerebral vessels. The lesions sometimes appear to have been present for some time, as judged from the surrounding leukocytic response and infiltration by pigmented macrophages, a finding that suggested that

the prodromal neurologic symptoms and the convulsions may be related to the lesions.

UTEROPLACENTAL PERFUSION

Compromised maternal placental perfusion is almost certainly a major culprit in the genesis of the increased perinatal morbidity and mortality associated with pregnancies complicated by pregnancy-induced or pregnancy-aggravated hypertension.

Measurements of Placental Perfusion

Attempts to measure human maternal placental blood flow have been hampered by several obstacles, including inaccessibility of the placenta, the complexity of its venous effluent, and the unsuitability of certain investigative techniques in humans.

Despite the formidable problems encountered in attempts to measure uterine blood flow, Assali and associates (1953), Browne and Veall (1953), and Metcalfe and co-workers (1955) attempted measurements of uterine blood flow in pregnant women and obtained reasonably consistent results. Both Assali and Metcalfe and their associates used a nitrous oxide method, a technique that is based on the Fick principle and required cannulation of a uterine vein. Total uterine perfusion is estimated rather than maternal placental blood flow. Browne and Veall estimated change in maternal placental flow through the use of a ^{24}Na clearance technique. This method required the insertion of a needle into the intervillous space. Both of these methods required technical proficiency, the use of invasive techniques in stressed subjects, and some risk to the mother and fetus. These investigators concluded from their studies that uterine blood flow in the normal, term pregnant woman is approximately 500 to 700 ml per minute.

Browne and Veall (1953) and, subsequently, Morris and colleagues (1956), Johnson and Clayton (1957), and Weis and associates (1958) observed that ^{24}Na, when injected into the intervillous space, was cleared two to three times more rapidly in normotensive pregnant women than in preeclamptic women, implying a two- to three-fold decrease in uteroplacental perfusion in the hypertensive subjects compared to normotensive gravidas.

Indirect Methods

The consistent results obtained in these early studies, as well as the conclusions these investigators drew from their data, continue to be supported by more recent studies using other methods of investigation. For instance, Brosens and associates (1972) reported that the mean diameter of myometrial spiral arterioles of 50 normal pregnant women was 500 μm. The same measurement in 36 women with preeclampsia was 200 μm.

Everett and colleagues (1980) have presented evidence that the rate of clearance of dehydroisoandrosterone sulfate and its conversion to estradiol-17β by the placenta is reflective of maternal placental perfusion. Normally, as pregnancy advanced, the placental clearance of maternal plasma dehydroisoandrosterone sulfate through the formation of estradiol-17β by the placenta increased greatly. Moreover, in women destined to develop PIH, the clearance rate of dehydroisoandrosterone sulfate was somewhat greater before the onset of hypertension than in control subjects, an intriguing observation in itself. The placental clearance rate then fell before the onset of overt hypertension (Worley and associates, 1975).

This placental clearance technique has been shown by Fritz and associates (1984) to parallel maternal placental perfusion in primates when the clearance technique was compared to direct measurements utilizing flow probe transducers.

Drugs and Placental Perfusion The placental clearance rate of dehydroisoandrosterone sulfate has been measured in a study of the effect of *thiazide diuretics* on placental function and perfusion (Shoemaker and co-workers, 1973). In this study, the placental clearance rate of dehydroisoandrosterone sulfate was computed for one woman with preeclampsia, another with chronic hypertension complicating pregnancy, and a third woman who had been hospitalized at 36 weeks gestation simply because of excessive weight gain. The placental clearance rate of dehydroisoandrosterone sulfate was markedly lowered during diuretic therapy in all three women, a result similar to that which had occurred in earlier studies in which the metabolic clearance rate of dehydroisoandrosterone sulfate was measured before and after thiazide diuretic therapy. A similar reduction in uteroplacental perfusion was noted following furosemide therapy (Gant and co-workers, 1976).

Gant and co-workers (1976) reported that the intravenous administration of hydralazine hydrochloride to eight chronically hypertensive women near term was followed by a decrease in the metabolic clearance rate of dehydroisoandrosterone sulfate by a mean of 23.5 percent, apparently as the result of the accompanying 37 percent decrease in diastolic blood pressure and, we presume, reduction in small vessel perfusion. Thus, even the intermittent administration of intravenous hydralazine with the goal of lowering diastolic blood pressure to no lower than 90 mm Hg can result in a decrease in uteroplacental perfusion. While the fetus in most normal pregnancies may tolerate an appreciable decrease in placental perfusion without suffering profoundly, the fetus in a pregnancy complicated by severe preeclampsia or eclampsia may not, since uteroplacental perfusion most likely is already compromised.

Histologic Changes in Placental Bed

Hertig in 1945 identified in preeclamptic pregnancies a lesion of the uteroplacental arteries characterized by prominent lipid-rich foam cells. Zeek and Assali in 1950 extended these observations and concluded that in pre-

eclampsia there is a pathognomonic lesion of the uteroplacental vessels, which they termed "acute atherosis." Most investigators are now in accord that a lesion occurs, but they do not necessarily agree on the precise nature of the lesion. On the basis of electron microscopic studies of uteroplacental arteries obtained by biopsy of the placental implantation site, DeWolf and co-workers (1975) reported as follows: Early preeclamptic changes include endothelial damage, insudation of plasma constituents into the vessel wall, proliferation of myointimal cells, and medial necrosis. Lipid accumulates first in the myointimal cells and then in macrophages.

INCIDENCE OF PREGNANCY-INDUCED HYPERTENSION

Pregnancy-induced hypertension most often affects nulliparas. Older nulliparas are at increased risk of having chronic hypertension, which predisposes to the superimposition of preeclampsia. Very young teenage primigravidas are also at appreciably greater risk (Duenhoelter and colleagues, 1975). Through ignorance and, at times, because of shame, an illegitimate pregnancy, they may not seek prenatal care until the disease is severe.

The incidence of preeclampsia is commonly stated to be about 5 percent, although remarkable variations are reported. At Parkland Memorial Hospital, for example, very close to 30 percent of the black nulliparous pregnant women cared for demonstrated during pregnancy or the early puerperium diastolic blood pressures of at least 90 mm Hg on two or more occasions 6 or more hours apart. Most of these nulliparous women had pregnancy-induced hypertension rather than coincidental chronic hypertension. Socioeconomically more affluent white women perhaps develop hypertension during pregnancy less often, but when it does develop it can be every bit as severe!

Eclampsia is usually preventable and, therefore, should become rare as more and more women receive appropriate prenatal care. The incidence nationwide is probably 1 in every 1000 to 1500 deliveries, but there are wide variations in different localities and countries. During the past 25 years and 170,000 deliveries, the incidence of eclampsia at Parkland Memorial Hospital has been close to 1 in 700; however, most of the emergency cases in Dallas and surrounding counties are brought to Parkland Memorial Hospital.

There is a familial tendency to pregnancy-induced hypertension. In a unique study of this question, Chesley and co-workers (1968) traced more than 96 percent of the grown daughters of women who had had eclampsia at the Margaret Hague Maternity Hospital. Among the 187 who carried pregnancies to viability, the incidence of preeclampsia in the first pregnancy was 26 percent. Moreover, 4 of the daughters, or 1 in 47, had eclampsia. A genetically determined predisposition has been implicated by Cooper and Liston (1979), as described below.

THEORIES OF CAUSE OF PREGNANCY-INDUCED HYPERTENSION

Any satisfactory theory must take into account that pregnancy-induced or aggravated hypertension is very much more likely to develop in the woman who (1) is exposed to chorionic villi for the first time, (2) is exposed to a superabundance of chorionic villi, as with twins or hydatidiform mole, (3) has preexisting vascular disease, or (4) is genetically predisposed to the development of hypertension during pregnancy. While chorionic villi are essential, they need not support a fetus nor need they be located within the uterus.

The possibility that immunologic as well as endocrine and genetic mechanisms are involved in the genesis of PIH is intriguing. The risk of PIH is enhanced appreciably in circumstances where formation of blocking antibodies to antigenic sites on the placenta *might* be impaired, such as during immunosuppressive therapy to protect a renal transplant during pregnancy (Chapter 28, p. 587) or effective immunization by a previous pregnancy is lacking, as in first pregnancies, or when the number of antigenic sites provided by the placenta is unusually great compared to the amount of antibody, as might be the case with multiple fetuses (Beer, 1978). Supporting this concept is the development of preeclampsia in multiparous patients who are impregnated by a new consort (Feeney and Scott, 1980). However, the concept of the "second husband" resulting in the development of preeclampsia has been challenged by Perkins and Mattox (1984). They presented evidence against this etiology based on the low incidence of hypertension observed to occur in pregnancies resulting from artificial insemination using semen from donors without repeated sexual acquaintanceships.

As pointed out by Chesley (1971), everyone from allergist to zoologist has proposed a theory and suggested "rational therapy" based upon his theory, including mastectomy, oophorectomy, renal decapsulation, trephination, alignment of the woman with the earth's magnetic field with her head pointing to the North Pole, and all sorts of medical regimens. Everything from watermelon season to infestation with a worm (*Hydatoxi lualba*) has been claimed to be of importance in the genesis of the disease. The interested reader is urged to examine the scholarly and entertaining review of various theories provided by Chesley in his elegant text, *Hypertensive Disorders in Pregnancy* (1978).

Cooper and Liston (1979) explored the possibility that susceptibility to PIH is dependent upon a single recessive gene. They calculated the frequencies to be expected in first pregnancies of daughters of women with eclampsia; daughters-in-law served as a control group. The frequencies calculated by them and those actually observed by Chesley and co-workers (1968) in daughters and daughters-in-law of women with eclampsia through his extensive long-term family studies are in remarkably close agreement.

Pregnancy-induced hypertension appears in some areas to have its highest incidence among indigent women, but, according to Chesley (1974), this has not always been the case. In the early years of the present century, eclampsia was believed to be most common in middle-class and upper-class women. Indeed, that observation led to the ready acceptance of the hypothesis that dietary restriction of protein (meat) accounted for the reduction in the incidence of eclampsia in Germany during World War I.

Although there are suggestions that dietary deficiencies might cause PIH, this hypothesis must be regarded as far from proven. Pregnancy-induced hypertension would be expected to be more common in multiparous women compared with nulliparous women if the hypothesis were correct. However, the opposite is true. Moreover, in a number of more recent studies in which dietary supplementation was provided, no reduction in the frequency of hypertension was demonstrated (Chapter 13, p. 255). Furthermore, Zlatnik and Burmeister (1983) have reported convincing evidence that in their patient population the incidence of preeclampsia is *not* directly related to the level of dietary protein.

Carefully controlled epidemiologic studies of pregnancy have been conducted in Aberdeen, Scotland, where for many years the relevant data have been available for nearly all deliveries. Baird (1969) found that the incidence of preeclampsia did not differ significantly among the five social classes, ranging from the professional and well-to-do (class I) through the unskilled laborers (class V), except for some slight increase in class III (skilled manual occupations).

CLINICAL ASPECTS OF PREECLAMPSIA

The two especially important signs of preeclampsia—hypertension and proteinuria—are abnormalities of which the pregnant woman is usually unaware. By the time she has developed symptoms, such as headache, visual disturbances, or epigastric pain, the disorder is almost always severe. Hence, the importance of prenatal care in the early detection and management of this complication becomes obvious.

Blood Pressure

The basic derangement in preeclampsia is vasospasm, especially of the arterioles. It is not surprising, therefore, that the most dependable warning sign of preeclampsia is a rise in blood pressure. The diastolic pressure is probably a more reliable prognostic sign than is the systolic, and any persisting diastolic pressure of 90 mm Hg or more is abnormal.

Weight Gain

Another sign of development of preeclampsia may be a sudden increase in weight. Indeed, excessive weight gain in some women is the first sign. Weight increase of about 1 pound per week is normal, but when weight gain exceeds much more than 2 pounds in any given week or 6 pounds in a month, incipient preeclampsia must be suspected. Characteristic of preeclampsia is the suddenness of the excessive weight gain rather than an increase distributed throughout gestation. Sudden and excessive weight gain in gestation is attributable almost entirely to abnormal retention of fluid and is demonstrable, as a rule, before visible signs of nondependent edema, for example, swollen eyelids and puffiness of the fingers. In cases of fulminating preeclampsia or eclampsia, waterlogging may be extreme, and in such women a weight gain of 10 pounds or more within a week is not unusual.

Proteinuria

Proteinuria varies greatly not only from case to case but also in the same woman from hour to hour. The variability points to a functional rather than an organic cause. In early preeclampsia, proteinuria may be minimal or entirely lacking. In the more severe forms, proteinuria is usually demonstrable and may be as much as 10 g/L. Proteinuria almost always develops later than the hypertension and usually later than excessive weight gain.

Headache

Headache is rare in milder cases but is increasingly frequent in the more severe grades. In women who develop eclampsia, severe headache is a frequent forerunner of the first convulsion. It is often frontal but may be occipital, and it is resistant to relief from ordinary analgesics.

Epigastric Pain

Epigastric or right upper quadrant pain often is a symptom of severe preeclampsia and is indicative of imminent convulsions. It may be the result of stretching of the hepatic capsule, possibly by edema and hemorrhage (p. 538).

Visual Disturbances

Visual disturbances ranging from a slight blurring of vision to blindness may accompany preeclampsia. Although such disturbances are thought by some to be of central origin, they are most likely attributable to retinal arteriolar spasm, ischemia, edema, and in rare cases actual retinal detachment. In general, the prognosis for such detachments is good, the retina reattaching, as a rule, within a few weeks after delivery. Hemorrhages and exudates are extremely rare in preeclampsia and when present are indicative most often of underlying chronic hypertensive vascular disease.

Immediate Prognosis

The prognosis for the mother and fetus is dependent to a considerable extent on the gestational age of the fetus, whether improvement follows hospitalization, when and how delivery is accomplished, and whether eclampsia supervenes.

The perinatal mortality rate is variably increased for pregnancies complicated by pregnancy-induced hypertension, as with the other hypertensive disorders. It is dependent primarily upon the time of onset and the severity of the disease. Much of the loss has been the consequence of prematurity, either from early spontaneous labor or because of therapeutic interruption necessitated by the development of severe preeclampsia.

PROPHYLAXIS AND EARLY TREATMENT

Early Detection

Because women seldom notice the signs of incipient preeclampsia, the early detection of the disease demands careful observation at appropriate intervals, especially in women known to be predisposed to preeclampsia. The major predisposing factors are (1) nulliparity, (2) a familial history of preeclampsia–eclampsia, (3) multiple fetuses, (4) diabetes, (5) chronic vascular or renal disease, (6) hydatidiform mole, and (7) fetal hydrops.

Rapid gain in weight any time during the latter half of pregnancy or an upward trend in the diastolic blood pressure while still in the normal range is ominous. Every woman should be examined at least weekly during the last month of pregnancy and every 2 weeks during the previous 2 months. At these visits, careful blood pressure measurements and weight checks of the woman are routine. Furthermore, all women should be advised verbally and, preferably, also by means of suitable printed instructions to report immediately any of the well-known symptoms or signs of preeclampsia, such as headache, visual disturbances, and puffiness of hands or face. The reporting of any such symptoms, of course, calls for an immediate examination to confirm or exclude preeclampsia.

Weight Gain. Obstetricians in the past often attempted to limit maternal weight gain to about 20 pounds, or even less, in the belief that preeclampsia can thereby be prevented. The total weight gained during pregnancy, however, probably has no relation to preeclampsia unless a large component of the gain is edema. Stringent restriction of weight gain is more likely to be detrimental rather than beneficial to both mother and fetus. The physician's scale, unfortunately, does not distinguish between the accumulation of edema fluid and the healthy deposition of fetal and maternal tissue.

Diuretics and Sodium Restriction. Natriuretic drugs, such as chlorothiazide and its congeners, have been severely overused. Although diuretics have been alleged to prevent the development of preeclampsia, the results of the studies of Kraus and co-workers (1966) and of others cast doubt on their real value. The women studied by Kraus and associates took either a placebo or 50 mg of hydrochlorothiazide daily during at least the last 16 weeks of gestation. The incidences of preeclampsia were identical (6.67 percent) in the primigravid subjects who received hydrochlorothiazide and those who took the placebo. Moreover, the frequency of development of hypertension was not altered in multiparous women. The failure of natriuretic drugs in the prevention of preeclampsia raises serious doubt about the efficacy of rigid dietary restriction of sodium.

Thiazide diuretics and similar compounds are not used in the treatment or prophylaxis of preeclampsia–eclampsia at Parkland Memorial Hospital. While there is no clear evidence that they are of any value, there is evidence that these agents can reduce renal perfusion as measured by creatinine clearance and, more important, reduce uteroplacental perfusion, as cited above (Gant and colleagues, 1975). The thiazide diuretics can induce serious depletion of both sodium and potassium. Minkowitz and associates (1964) and Menzies and Prystowsky (1967) reported the findings of depletion of electrolytes and hemorrhagic pancreatitis in women who died following treatment of preeclampsia with chlorothiazide. Rodriguez and associates (1964), moreover, found severe thrombocytopenia in some newborns whose mothers had received thiazide diuretics.

Objectives of Treatment

The basic objectives of management of any pregnancy complicated by PIH are (1) termination of the pregnancy with the least possible trauma to the mother and the fetus, (2) birth of an infant who subsequently thrives, and (3) complete restoration of the health of the mother.

In certain cases of preeclampsia, especially in women at or near term, all these objectives may be served equally well by one treatment, i.e., careful induction of labor and delivery. It cannot be emphasized too strongly, therefore, that the most important information that the obstetrician can possess for the successful management of pregnancy, and especially pregnancy that becomes complicated by hypertension, is precise knowledge of the age of the fetus (Chapter 13, p. 247).

Ambulatory Treatment

Ambulatory treatment has no place in the management of overt pregnancy-induced or pregnancy-aggravated hypertension. Excluding young nulliparas, some women whose systolic blood pressure does not exceed 135 mm Hg and whose diastolic pressure does not exceed 85 mm Hg and in whom proteinuria is absent may be managed tentatively at home as long as the disease does not become more severe and fetal growth retardation is not a problem. Bed rest throughout the greater part of the day is essential. Moreover, these women should be examined twice weekly rather than weekly and be instructed in detail about the reporting of symptoms. With minor elevations of blood pressure, the response to this regimen is often immediate, but the woman must be cooperative and the obstetrician wary.

Hospital Management

The indication for hospitalization of women with preeclampsia is a systolic blood pressure of 140 mm or above or a diastolic pressure of 90 mm or above. For an intelligent continuing appraisal of the severity of the disease, upon admittance to the hospital systematic study should be instituted that includes the following:

1. An appropriate history and general physical examination followed by daily search for the development of such signs and symptoms as headache, visual disturbances, epigastric pain, and rapid weight gain
2. Weight measured on admittance and every 2 days thereafter
3. Urine screened for protein on admittance and subsequently at least every 2 days
4. Blood pressure readings with an appropriate size cuff every 4 hours (except between midnight and morning, unless the midnight pressure has risen)
5. Measurements of plasma creatinine
6. Measurements of hematocrit, platelets, and serum SGOT
7. Frequent evaluation of fetal size by the same experienced examiner and by serial sonography if remote from term

Whenever observations so made serve to establish a diagnosis of severe preeclampsia (Table 27-2), further management is the same as described for eclampsia (p. 547).

Bed rest throughout much of the day is beneficial and ample, but not excessive, protein and calories should be included in the diet (Chapter 13, p. 252). Sodium and fluid intakes should be neither limited nor forced.

Phenobarbital administered in divided doses totaling 120 to 240 mg per day has been widely used for sedation. We do not do so. The possibility of adverse effects on the fetus from phenobarbital should be considered. The combination of phenobarbital and phenytoin given to the woman with epilepsy has been demonstrated to cause a reduction in vitamin K-dependent coagulation factors in some fetuses. Moreover, phenobarbital has been reported to delay lung maturation, at least in the rabbit fetus (Karotkin and colleagues, 1976).

The further management of a pregnancy complicated by preeclampsia will depend upon (1) its severity as gauged by the presence or absence of the conditions cited in Table 27-2, (2) the duration of gestation, and (3) the condition of the cervix. Fortunately, many cases prove to be sufficiently mild and near enough to term that they can be managed conservatively until labor commences spontaneously or until the cervix becomes favorable for induction of labor. Complete abatement of all signs and symptoms, however, is uncommon until after delivery. *Almost certainly, the underlying disease persists until after delivery!*

Occasionally, fulminant or neglected preeclampsia is

encountered, with blood pressure recordings in excess of 160/110 mm Hg, edema, and proteinuria. Headache, visual disturbances, or epigastric pain is indicative that convulsions are imminent; oliguria resulting from preeclampsia is another ominous sign. Severe preeclampsia demands anticonvulsant and usually antihypertensive therapy followed by delivery. Treatment is identical to that described subsequently for eclampsia (p. 547). The prime objectives are to forestall convulsions, to prevent intracranial hemorrhage or serious damage to other vital organs, and to deliver an infant who, hopefully, survives and subsequently thrives.

In a more severe case of preeclampsia, as well as eclampsia, magnesium sulfate administered parenterally is a most valuable anticonvulsant agent, as attested by the experience of many clinics over many years. Magnesium sulfate may be given intramuscularly by intermittent injection or intravenously by continuous infusion. At Parkland Memorial Hospital the dosage schedule for severe preeclampsia is the same as for eclampsia (p. 548). Since the period of labor and delivery is a more likely time for convulsions to develop, all women suspected to have PIH are treated at Parkland Memorial Hospital with intramuscular magnesium sulfate during labor and the early puerperium. Hydralazine (Apresoline), administered intravenously in appropriate doses intermittently, has proven to be an effective and safe antihypertensive agent; its use is discussed in more detail subsequently (p. 548).

To try to enhance fetal lung maturation, glucocorticoids have been administered by some to severely hypertensive pregnant women who need delivery and are thought to be remote from term. Several reports have appeared in which such treatment seemed not to worsen maternal hypertension, and a decrease in the incidence of respiratory distress and improved infant survival have been claimed. For example, Nochimson and Petrie (1979) administered β-methasone to 20 severely hypertensive women and observed no untoward effect. Perinatal survival was 85.7 percent. Similar results have been reported by Semchyshyn and associates (1983) and Ruvinsky and colleagues (1984).

We do not use corticosteroids in these circumstances for two reasons: (1) their administration poses potential risks to the mother and the fetus–infant, and (2) when the mother has severe pregnancy-induced hypertension requiring delivery, severe respiratory distress is uncommon in her neonate even remote from term.

Termination of Pregnancy

The cure for preeclampsia is the expulsion or removal of trophoblast, i.e., delivery. However, when the fetus is known or suspected to be premature, the tendency is widespread to temporize in the hope that a few more weeks in utero will reduce the risk to the infant of death or serious morbidity. Such a policy is justified in milder cases, but in severe preeclampsia, procrastination can prove to be ill-advised, since the preeclampsia itself may

kill the fetus. Even for the fetus remote from term, the probability of fetal survival may be greater in a well-operated neonatal intensive care unit than when the fetus is left in utero.

Assessments of fetal well-being and placental function have been attempted especially when there is hesitation to deliver the fetus because of prematurity. Serial measurements of plasma or urinary estriol or of placental lactogen or the oxytocin challenge (contraction) test or the fetal biophysical profile *may* produce abnormal results when the fetoplacental unit is compromised (Chapter 14). To date, these tests have not been clearly demonstrated to provide valuable information otherwise unavailable for intelligent management of the pregnancy complicated by preeclampsia.

Failure of the fetus to grow, as estimated clinically and by sonography, is an ominous sign of fetal jeopardy. Measurements of the L/S ratio in amnionic fluid may provide evidence of lung maturity, but it should be kept in mind during management of more severe cases that even when the L/S ratio is less than 2.0, respiratory distress may not develop and, when it does, most often it does not prove fatal (Chapter 14, p. 273; Chapter 38, p. 770).

With severe preeclampsia that does not improve after a few days of hospitalization as outlined above, termination of pregnancy is usually advisable for the welfare of both the mother and the fetus. Labor may be induced by administration of oxytocin. In severe cases, this procedure is often successful even when the cervix appears unfavorable for induction. Whenever it appears that induction of labor almost certainly will not succeed or attempts at induction of labor are not fruitful, cesarean delivery for the more severe cases is the procedure of choice. In cases of severe preeclampsia and eclampsia with subarachnoid or epidural block, hypotension detrimental to the fetus, as well as the mother, may occur (Chapter 18, p. 364)

For a woman near term, with a soft, partially effaced cervix, even milder degrees of preeclampsia probably carry more risk to the mother and her fetus–infant than does induction of labor by carefully monitored oxytocin stimulation. This is not likely to be the case, however, if the preeclampsia is mild but the cervix is firm and closed, indicating that abdominal delivery might be necessary if pregnancy is to be terminated. The hazard of cesarean delivery may be greater than that of allowing the pregnancy to continue *under close observation* in the hospital until the cervix is more suitable for induction.

High-Risk Pregnancy Unit

A high-risk pregnancy unit has been established at Parkland Memorial Hospital to provide care as just described. The results have been remarkable, as reported by Gilstrap and associates (1978). Of 576 nulliparous women, usually teenage and often black, admitted to the unit because of hypertension remote from term, 545 remained for care until the pregnancy was terminated; the perinatal mortality rate for this group was 0.9 percent. For the 31 who left the unit before delivery, although advised not to, the perinatal mortality was 13 percent! The mean birth weight of the infants whose mothers remained on the unit was 2974 g, with 83 percent weighing 2500 g or more. Through 1984 more than 2000 women with mild to moderate, early onset, pregnancy-induced hypertension have been so managed with equally good results! The cost of providing the relatively simple physical facility, modest nursing care, no drugs other than an iron supplement, and the very few laboratory tests that are essential is slight compared to the cost of neonatal intensive care. Moreover, the quality of the infant is very likely better.

Postpartum

After delivery there is usually rapid improvement, although, at times, the disease may worsen transiently. Eclampsia may develop any time during the first 24 hours after delivery. After 24 hours, eclampsia is rare in our now extensive experience. At Parkland Memorial Hospital magnesium sulfate therapy instituted before or during parturition is continued for 24 hours postpartum with parenterally administered hydralazine given intermittently, if needed, to lower a diastolic blood pressure of 110 mm Hg or higher.

The woman may be discharged, even though still hypertensive, if there is evidence that severe hypertension is abating and she is otherwise well. Unless the hypertension persists at high levels during the puerperium, antihypertensive agents are not prescribed; instead, the woman is reevaluated in 2 weeks. Typically, but not always, hypertension induced by pregnancy will have dissipated during this period. If so, the episode of PIH does not mitigate against the use of oral contraceptives (Chapter 40, p. 817).

CLINICAL ASPECTS OF ECLAMPSIA

Eclampsia is an acute disorder characterized by clonic and tonic convulsions that are caused in some way by hypertension induced or aggravated by pregnancy. It is better to limit the diagnosis of eclampsia to convulsive cases, regarding fatal nonconvulsive cases of pregnancy-induced or aggravated hypertension as exceedingly severe preeclampsia.

Clinical Course

Depending on whether the convulsion first appears before labor, during labor, or in the puerperium, eclampsia is designated as antepartum, intrapartum, or postpartum. Eclampsia occurs most often in the last third of pregnancy and becomes increasingly frequent as term approaches. Nearly all cases of postpartum eclampsia appear within 24 hours after delivery. In rare instances,

eclampsia is said to have begun as late as 1 week after delivery, but cases in which the first convulsion is observed more than 48 hours postpartum should be regarded with skepticism.

Almost without exception, preeclampsia precedes the onset of eclamptic convulsions. Isolated cases are occasionally cited in which an eclamptic convulsion is said to have occurred without warning in women who were apparently in good health. Usually such a woman had not been examined by her physician for some days or, more likely, weeks previously, and she had neglected to report symptoms of preeclampsia. Headache, visual disturbance, and epigastric or right upper quandrant pain are symptoms that should incite grave concern.

The convulsive movements usually begin about the mouth in the form of facial twitchings. After a few seconds, the entire body becomes rigid in a generalized muscular contraction. The face is distorted, the eyes protrude, the arms are flexed, the hands are clenched, and the legs are inverted. All the muscles of the body are now in a state of tonic contraction. This phase may persist for 15 to 20 seconds. Suddenly the jaws begin to open and close violently, and forthwith the eyelids also. The other facial muscles and then all the muscles of the body alternately contract and relax in rapid succession. So forceful are the muscular movements that the woman may throw herself out of her bed, and almost invariably, unless protected, the tongue is bitten by the violent action of the jaws (Fig. 27-9). Foam, often blood-tinged, exudes from the mouth. The face is congested, and the eyes are bloodshot. Few clinical pictures are so terrifying as this. This phase, in which the muscles alternately contract and relax, may last about a minute. Gradually, the muscular movements become smaller and less frequent, and finally the woman lies motionless. Throughout the seizure the diaphragm has been fixed, with respiration halted. For a few seconds the woman appears to be dying from respiratory arrest, but just when a fatal outcome seems almost inevitable, she takes a long, deep, stertorous inhalation, and breathing is resumed. Coma then ensues. She will remember nothing of the convulsion or, in all probability, of events immediately before and afterward.

Most often the first convulsion is the forerunner of other convulsions, which may vary in number from 1 or 2 in mild cases to 10 to 20, or even 100 or more, in untreated severe cases. In rare instances, they follow one another so rapidly that the woman appears to be in a prolonged, almost continuous convulsion.

The duration of coma after a convulsion is variable. When the convulsions are infrequent, the woman usually recovers some degree of consciousness after each attack. As the woman arouses, a semiconscious combative state may ensue. In very severe cases, the coma persists from one convulsion to another, and death may result before the patient awakens. In rare instances, a single convulsion may be followed by profound coma from which she never emerges, although, as a rule, death does not occur

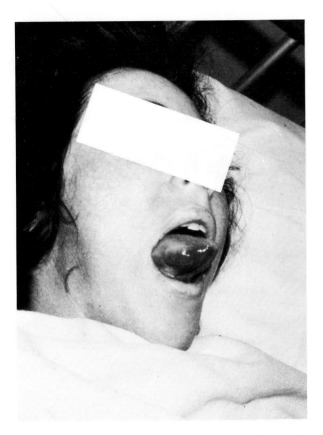

Figure 27-9. Hematoma of tongue from laceration during eclamptic convulsion. Thrombocytopenia may have contributed to the bleeding.

until after a frequent repetition of the convulsive attacks.

Respiration after an eclamptic convulsion is usually increased in rate and may be stertorous. The rate may reach 50 or more per minute in response presumably to hypercarbia from lactic acidemia, as well as varying intensities of hypoxia. Cyanosis may be observed in severe cases. Temperatures of 39.5° C or more are of very grave prognostic import. The cause of the fever is probably central.

Proteinuria is almost always present and frequently is pronounced. The output of urine is likely to be diminished appreciably and occasionally is entirely suppressed. Gross hemoglobinuria and hemoglobinemia may be observed rarely.

Some degree of edema is probably present in all women with eclampsia. Often, the edema is pronounced and, at times, massive, but it may be occult (Fig. 27-10A, B).

As with severe preeclampsia, after delivery, an increase in urinary output is usually an early sign of improvement. The proteinuria and edema ordinarily disappear within a week. In most cases, but certainly not all, the blood pressure returns to normal within 2 weeks after delivery. The longer the hypertension persists after delivery, the more likely the hypertension is the consequence of chronic vascular or renal disease.

In antepartum eclampsia, labor may begin spontaneously shortly thereafter and progress rapidly to completion, sometimes before the attendants are aware that the unconscious or stuporous woman is having effective uterine contractions. If the attack occurs during labor, the contractions may increase in frequency and intensity, and the duration of labor may be shortened.

Very uncommonly, convulsions cease, the coma disappears, labor does not commence, and the woman becomes completely oriented. This improved state may continue for several days or longer, a condition known as *intercurrent eclampsia*. It has been claimed that such pregnancies may often return entirely to normal with complete subsidence of the hypertension and proteinuria, but such an event appears to have been rare. Although convulsions and coma may subside entirely and the blood pressure and proteinuria may decrease somewhat, most women continue to show substantial evidence of disease and are likely to convulse again unless treated, including delivery. This second attack may be much more severe.

Pulmonary edema may develop in women with eclampsia, especially those treated vigorously with intravenous fluids, and is always a grave prognostic sign. Other signs of cardiac failure appear in the terminal stage of eclampsia, especially cyanosis, a rapid pulse rate, and a falling blood pressure.

In some women with eclampsia, death occurs suddenly, synchronously with or shortly after a convulsion, as the result of massive cerebral hemorrhage (Fig. 27-11); hemiplegia may result from a sublethal cerebral hemorrhage. Eclampsia is followed very infrequently by psychosis in which the mother may become violent. The psychosis ordinarily lasts for 1 or 2 weeks. Chlorpromazine in carefully titrated doses has proved effective in the few cases of posteclampsia psychosis seen at Parkland Memorial Hospital. The prognosis in general is good except when there is preexisting mental illness.

Very infrequently, the woman finds herself blind as she begins to arouse from her coma. The disturbed vision, sometimes preceding the attack, is caused mainly by retinal edema, which usually disappears spontaneously. The blindness is sometimes central in origin (Nishimura and Koller, 1982), possibly caused by intense vasospasm of the distal posterior cerebral arteries. Rarely, detachment of the retina is observed. Usually vision returns to normal within a week, and thus the prognosis for sight is good.

Differential Diagnosis

Generally, eclampsia is much more likely to be diagnosed too frequently rather than overlooked, because epilepsy, encephalitis, meningitis, cerebral tumor, acute porphyria, ruptured cerebral aneurysm, and even hysteria during late pregnancy and the puerperium may simulate it. Consequently, such conditions should be

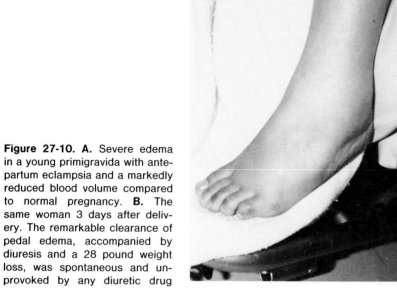
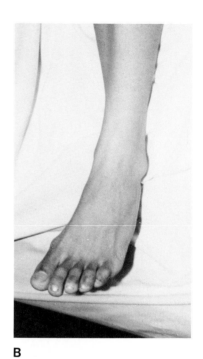

Figure 27-10. A. Severe edema in a young primigravida with antepartum eclampsia and a markedly reduced blood volume compared to normal pregnancy. **B.** The same woman 3 days after delivery. The remarkable clearance of pedal edema, accompanied by diuresis and a 28 pound weight loss, was spontaneous and unprovoked by any diuretic drug therapy.

A

B

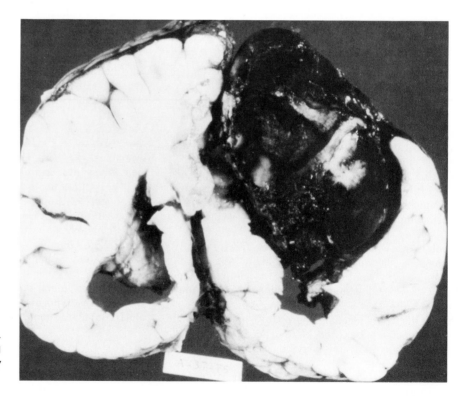

Figure 27-11. Massive fatal cerebral hemorrhage in a primigravid woman with eclampsia. (*Courtesy of Dr. K. Leveno.*)

borne in mind whenever convulsions or coma occur during pregnancy, labor, or the puerperium, and such conditions must be excluded before a positive diagnosis of eclampsia is made. Until eclampsia can be excluded, however, all pregnant women with convulsions should be considered to be eclamptic.

TREATMENT OF ECLAMPSIA

The basic treatment of eclampsia consists of (1) control of convulsions, (2) correction of hypoxia and acidosis, (3) lowering the blood pressure when markedly elevated, and (4) steps to effect delivery once the mother is free of convulsions and, hopefully, conscious. It is emphasized that once delivery is accomplished, the pathologic changes of eclampsia per se soon ameliorate and eventually are completely eradicated. This generalization holds true for the dysfunctions of the central nervous system, for the liver, for the kidneys, for hematologic abnormalities, including thrombocytopenia and intense hemolysis, and usually for subsequent pregnancies!

Prognosis

The prognosis is always serious, for eclampsia is one of the most dangerous conditions with which those caring for the pregnant woman and her fetus must deal, although the maternal mortality rate in eclampsia has fallen notably in the past three decades. The maternal mortality rate reported since World War II for various methods of treatment applied in several countries is summarized in Table 27-3. In these reports, the maternal mortality has ranged from zero to as much as 17.5 percent. At the same time, the perinatal mortality rate has ranged from 13 to 30 percent or more. Precise comparisons of perinatal mortality rates are difficult to make because of differences in the definition of stillbirth and neonatal deaths in different countries.

Historical Considerations

As a consequence of very poor outcomes from immediate delivery without medical stabilization, by the late 1920s the slogan became "Treat the eclampsia medically and ignore the pregnancy." Since then almost every drug suspected of having a sedative effect on the central nervous system, or a hypotensive effect, or a diuretic effect has been administered to the woman (and her fetus) with eclampsia. It became the custom to administer a large variety of drugs simultaneously. Often the convulsions were controlled, but the woman's coma persisted because of the medications rather than the disease. It was not unusual for the physician, and even the consultant, to have had little personal experience in managing such difficult cases. As a consequence, women with eclampsia have been, and in some circumstances still are, treated in a most variable way, especially in institutions where eclampsia is uncommon. Our extensive and well-controlled clinical experiences during the past 3 decades

have served as the basis for the report "How Should Hypertension During Pregnancy Be Managed: Experience at Parkland Memorial Hospital" (Cunningham and Pritchard, 1984) and are considered below. This report adjoins one, "How Should Hypertension During Pregnancy Be Managed: An Internist's Approach" (Ferris, 1984). The contrast between the regimes for management cited in the two reports is awesome!

PARKLAND MEMORIAL HOSPITAL ECLAMPSIA REGIMEN

Since 1955 a standardized treatment regimen has been used to manage women with eclampsia and their fetuses. The carefully analyzed results of treatment of 245 cases of eclampsia, typically the severest form of pregnancy-induced or aggravated hypertension, have been published recently (Pritchard and associates, 1984). The specific plan of management is summarized:

1. Control of convulsions with magnesium sulfate using an intravenously administered loading dose plus periodic intramuscular injections standardized as to the amount injected and the frequency of injections
2. Control of severe hypertension with intermittent intravenous injections of hydralazine to lower the blood pressure somewhat whenever the diastolic pressure is 110 mm Hg or higher
3. Avoidance of diuretics and hyperosmotic agents
4. Limitation of fluid intake unless fluid loss is excessive
5. Initiation of steps to effect delivery

Magnesium Sulfate to Control Convulsions

Magnesium sulfate is used to arrest and prevent the convulsions of eclampsia without producing generalized central nervous system depression in either the mother or the fetus–infant. (The drug is not given to treat hypertension!) Based on the studies of Borges and Gücer (1978) cited below, as well as extensive clinical observations, magnesium sulfate most likely exerts a rather specific anticonvulsant action on the cerebral cortex. Typically, the mother stops convulsing after the initial administration of magnesium sulfate, and within 1 or 2 hours regains consciousness sufficiently to be oriented as to place and time.

The magnesium sulfate dosage schedule is presented in Table 27-6, and the response in plasma magnesium levels is demonstrated in Figure 27-12A, B. Using this regimen, evidence of depression of the infants at birth from magnesium intoxication has been lacking.

In the unusual case in which magnesium sulfate in doses of 4 g intravenously plus 10 g intramuscularly has not arrested eclamptic convulsions, 2 g more, as a 20 percent solution, have been administered slowly intravenously, once if the woman was small, and twice, if needed, and the woman was larger. In only 5 of the 245

TABLE 27-6. MAGNESIUM SULFATE DOSAGE SCHEDULE FOR SEVERE PREECLAMPSIA AND ECLAMPSIA

1. Give 4 g of magnesium sulfate (MgSO$_4$•7H$_2$O USP) as a 20% solution intravenously at the rate of 1 g per minute.
2. Follow promptly with 10 g of 50% magnesium sulfate solution, one half (5 g) injected deeply in the upper outer quadrant of both buttocks through a 3-inch long, 20 gauge needle. (Addition of 1.0 ml of 2% lidocaine minimizes discomfort.)

   If convulsions persist after 15 minutes or so, give up to 2 g more intravenously as a 20% solution no faster than 1 g per minute; if the woman is large, up to 4 g may be given slowly.
3. Every 4 hours thereafter give 5 g of a 50% solution of magnesium sulfate injected deeply in the upper outer quadrant of alternate buttocks but only after ascertaining the following:
   a. The patellar reflex is present.
   b. Respirations are not depressed.
   c. Urine output the previous 4 hours was 100 ml or more.
4. Magnesium sulfate is discontinued 24 hours after delivery.

women with eclampsia was it necessary to use supplementary medication to control the convulsions. Then the slow intravenous administration of sodium amobarbital in doses up to 250 mg was effective. Maintenance magnesium sulfate therapy for eclampsia antepartum or intrapartum is continued intramuscularly every 4 hours for 24 hours after delivery. For eclampsia that develops postpartum, magnesium sulfate is administered for 24 hours after the onset of convulsions.

Parenterally administered magnesium is cleared almost totally by renal excretion, and magnesium intoxication is avoided by demonstrating before administering the next dose that (1) urine flow was at least 100 ml during the previous 4 hours, (2) the patellar reflex is

present, and (3) there is no respiratory depression. Eclamptic convulsions are almost always prevented by plasma magnesium levels maintained at 4 to 7 mEq/L. As discussed below, loss of patellar reflex occurs with plasma levels of 8 to 10 mEq/L and, importantly, severe respiratory depression and arrest at levels of 12 mEq/L or more. Calcium gluconate, 1 g intravenously, plus oxygen usually suffice for the treatment of respiratory depression. If respiratory arrest occurs, prompt endotracheal intubation and ventilation are lifesaving (McCubbin and associates, 1981).

Hydralazine to Control Severe Hypertension

At the time that this treatment regimen for eclampsia was formulated, it was appreciated that severe acute hypertension increased the maternal risk of intracranial hemorrhage (Fig. 27-11). Moreover, contrary to much of the teaching at that time, it was also apparent that severe hypertension frequently persisted or promptly recurred after parenteral administration of magnesium sulfate in doses that effectively arrested convulsions and prevented their recurrence. The likelihood that maternal hypertension helped maintain placental perfusion was also recognized. Thus there was concern, which since has proven to be appropriate, that aggressive treatment that promptly lowered the blood pressure to strictly normotensive levels might further compromise placental perfusion to the detriment of the fetus. From the outset, the regimen provided for intravenous injections of hydralazine whenever the diastolic blood pressure was 110 mm Hg or higher to be administered in 5 to 10 mg doses at 15 to 20 minute intervals until a satisfactory response was achieved. A satisfactory response antepartum or in-

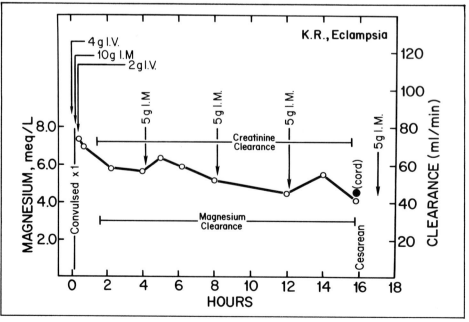

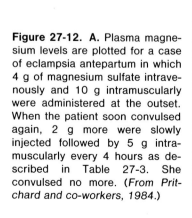

Figure 27-12. A. Plasma magnesium levels are plotted for a case of eclampsia antepartum in which 4 g of magnesium sulfate intravenously and 10 g intramuscularly were administered at the outset. When the patient soon convulsed again, 2 g more were slowly injected followed by 5 g intramuscularly every 4 hours as described in Table 27-3. She convulsed no more. (*From Pritchard and co-workers, 1984.*)

trapartum was defined as a decrease in diastolic blood pressure to approach 90 mm Hg but no lower lest placental perfusion be compromised.

Hydralazine so administered has proven remarkably effective. In each instance it has lowered the blood pressure toward normal, and therefore, it has not been necessary to add other antihypertensives because of lack of response to hydralazine. Importantly, cerebral hemorrhage has been avoided.

An example of very severe hypertension in a woman with chronic hypertension complicated by superimposed eclampsia that responded to repeated intravenous injections of hydralazine is cited in Table 27-7. Hydralazine was injected more frequently than recommended in the protocol, and the blood pressure decreased in less than 1 hour from 240/150 mm Hg to 110/80 mm Hg. Ominous fetal heart rate decelerations were evident when the pressure fell to 110/80 mm Hg and persisted until the maternal blood pressure rose somewhat.

Other Antihypertensive Agents. Intravenously administered diazoxide has been championed by some for use in preeclampsia–eclampsia because of its very potent antihypertensive action. Unfortunately, intravenous diazoxide therapy is accompanied by many adverse side effects. As examples: It is very likely to arrest labor. It causes retention of sodium, water, and uric acid. It causes serious hyperglycemia in the mother and newborn infant. It may produce irreversible, and therefore lethal, hypotension when administered with or after other antihypertensive agents. In our experience, as well as that of most obstetricians in academic centers, diazoxide has not been needed, since hydralazine, given as described above, has proven effective. Therefore, we deliberately avoid these serious adverse effects from diazoxide.

Sodium nitroprusside by intravenous infusion is a potent, short-acting antihypertensive agent. Unfortunately, it crosses the placenta and may cause cyanide poisoning in the fetus. Moreover, it has been described to cause worrisome increases in intracranial pressure.

Hypertension Persisting Postpartum

The potential problem of serious compromise of placental perfusion, and, in turn, fetal well-being that can be induced by antihypertensive agents is obviated by delivery. If there is a problem after delivery in controlling severe hypertension and the intravenous hydralazine regimen described above is being used repeatedly early in the puerperium to control persisting severe hypertension, hydralazine is then administered intramuscularly, usually in 10 mg doses at 4 to 6 hour intervals. Rarely are larger doses needed. Once repeated blood pressure readings remain near normal, the hydralazine is stopped. If hypertension of appreciable intensity recurs, oral therapy is given for as long as necessary.

Avoidance of Diuretics and Hyperosmotic Agents

At the time of formulation of this regimen, expansion of the extravascular component of the extracellular fluid compartment, i.e., generalized edema, had long been recognized as a common feature of severe preeclampsia and eclampsia. Most treatment regimens included liberal use of diuretics to try to clear the edema, but most of the diuretic agents that were then available were not very potent. There were also strong suspicions at that time,

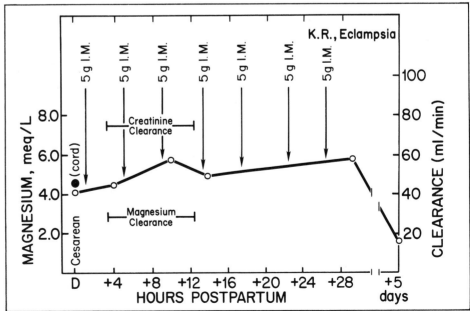

Figure 27-12. B. Maternal magnesium levels during the first 28 hours postpartum and 4 days after magnesium sulfate was discontinued are plotted. Before and the day after delivery the renal clearance of magnesium remained relatively constant at about 35 percent of the somewhat depressed creatinine clearance. The mother recovered fully and the baby thrived. (*From Pritchard and co-workers, 1984.*)

which subsequently have been amply verified, that the maternal blood volume in women with severe preeclampsia and eclampsia typically are constricted appreciably compared to normal pregnancy.

It was reasoned at the outset that potent diuretics could further compromise placental perfusion, since their immediate effects would include further depletion of intravascular volume that most often is already reduced compared to normal pregnancy. Therefore, diuretics were not used to lower blood pressure lest they enhance the intensity of the maternal hypovolemia and hemoconcentration and the adverse effects on the mother and the fetus.

Once delivery is accomplished, in almost all cases of severe preeclampsia and eclampsia, there is a spontaneous diuresis that begins within 24 hours and results in the disappearance of excessive extravascular extracellular fluid over the next 3 to 4 days, as demonstrated in Figure 27-10A, B.

In regard to hyperosmotic agents, the potential exists for an appreciable intravascular influx of fluid in response to their infusion and, in turn, the subsequent escape of intravascular fluid in the form of edema into vital organs, especially the lungs and brain. Moreover, an oncotically active agent that leaks through capillaries into the lungs and brain would promote the accumulation of edema at these sites. Finally, a sustained beneficial effect from their use has not been demonstrated. For all of these reasons, hyperosmotic agents have not been administered, and the use of furosemide or similar agents has been limited to the rare instance in which pulmonary edema was identified or strongly suspected.

Fluid Therapy

Fluid, primarily lactated Ringer's solution containing 5 percent dextrose, has been administered routinely at the rate of 60 ml to no more than 150 ml per hour unless there was unusual fluid loss from vomiting, diarrhea, diaphoresis, or more likely, excessive blood loss at delivery. The presence of oliguria, which is common in cases of severe preeclampsia and eclampsia, coupled with the knowledge that the maternal blood volume is very likely constricted compared to normal pregnancy, makes it tempting to administer intravenous fluids more vigorously. The rationale for controlled, conservative fluid administration is that the typical eclamptic woman already has a considerable excess of extracellular fluid that, for reasons that remain unclear, is inappropriately distributed between the intravascular and extravascular divisions of the extracellular fluid compartment. The infusion of large volumes of fluid could and does enhance the maldistribution of extracellular fluid and thereby increases appreciably the risk of life-threatening edema be it pulmonary, cerebral, or laryngopharyngeal (Gedekah and associates, 1980; Benedetti and Quilligan, 1980; Heller and associates, 1983; Sibai and co-workers, 1981).

The woman with severe preeclampsia or eclampsia, who consequently lacks normal pregnancy hypervolemia,

TABLE 27-7. INTRAVENOUS HYDRALAZINE FOR ACUTE CONTROL OF SEVERE HYPERTENSION

Time	OS, Eclampsia Blood Pressure
1140	240/150
1145	Magnesium sulfate, 4 g IV and 10 g IM
1155	270/130
1156	Hydralazine, 5 mg IV bolus
1200	200/120
1201	Hydralazine, 5 mg IV bolus
1205	230/130
1206	Hydralazine, 10 mg IV bolus
1210	185/120
1220	180/120
1221	Hydralazine, 5 mg IV bolus
1230	150/105
1235	150/105
1250	110/80 —FETAL DISTRESS
1310	130/90
1345	130/100 ⎫ Return to normal
1430	150/105 ⎬ of fetal heart rate
1500	150/90 ⎭

is much less tolerant to blood loss than is the normally pregnant woman. *An appreciable fall in blood pressure very soon after delivery most often means excessive blood loss and not miraculous dissolution of the vasospastic disease.* When oliguria follows delivery, the hematocrit is frequently evaluated to help detect excessive blood loss, which, when identified, is treated by careful blood transfusion.

Until it is understood how to contain more fluid within the intravascular compartment and, at the same time, less fluid outside the intravascular compartment, we remain convinced that, in the absence of marked fluid loss, fluids can be administered safely only in moderation. To date no serious adverse effects have been observed from such a policy. Importantly, dialysis for renal failure has never been required in any of the 245 cases of eclampsia so managed. By way of comparison, in one large European renal dialysis center eclampsia has been identified to be the leading cause of acute renal failure among women (Silke and co-workers, 1980). Moreover, in the great majority of women with eclampsia that we have managed, sufficient follow-up has been achieved to ascertain that either normal renal clearance returned or, in those women with preexisting impaired renal function, subsequent plasma creatinine levels were no higher than before.

Delivery

When this regimen was formulated in the 1950s, the identification of eclampsia immediately caused appropriate concern for the welfare of the mother. Therefore, to avoid risks to the mother from cesarean delivery, steps to effect vaginal delivery were employed even in some circumstances in which it appeared that the fetus might have been better served by cesarean section. It became apparent early on that labor often ensued spontaneously or could be induced successfully even remote from term without subjecting the fetus to greater risk. It also became apparent early on that a magic cure did not immediately follow delivery by any route but that serious morbidity was less common in the puerperium among women delivered vaginally. For these reasons, we have continued to try to effect vaginal delivery and quite often have been successful; labor culminating in vaginal delivery was accomplished in three fourths of pregnancies in which induction was attempted. Moreover, labor was often induced successfully and vaginal delivery accomplished even remote from term, for example, in 16 of the last 20 instances in which the fetuses weighed 1500 g or less.

Although it has been stated that labor is impaired by magnesium sulfate, this claim is not supported by these successes in achieving vaginal delivery in the women with eclampsia so treated nor by observations reported previously (Pritchard, 1955; Stallworth and co-workers, 1981).

Anesthesia

Local or pudendal anesthesia has been used for nearly all vaginal deliveries. General anesthesia, using thiopental, succinylcholine, nitrous oxide and oxygen, has been administered for cesarean delivery. The markedly contracted intravascular compartment with its reduced blood volume is exquisitely sensitive to vasodilatation. Therefore, conduction anesthesia has been avoided in cases of severe preeclampsia and eclampsia because of concern for sudden, severe hypotension induced by splanchnic blockade and, in turn, the immediate danger from pressor agents and subsequent danger from large volumes of aqueous fluid given to try to correct hypotension so induced. Vigorous crystalloid infusion and infusion of oncotically active colloidal solutions have incited very troublesome edema formation, including pulmonary edema, cerebral edema, and pharyngolaryngeal edema.

Meperidine, usually with promethazine, has been given in moderation for discomforts of labor and after cesarean delivery.

Pharmacology and Toxicology of Magnesium Sulfate

Even though magnesium sulfate continues to be very widely used by obstetricians in the United States, probably no drug is so misunderstood and underrated by physicians who do not have personal clinical experience with its efficacy. Magnesium sulfate has been condemned primarily because its mechanism of action in controlling convulsions has not been clearly understood, a problem that also has existed with other anticonvulsant agents, even phenytoin.

Magnesium sulfate USP is $MgSO_4 \cdot 7H_2O$ and not $MgSO_4$. Magnesium sulfate administered as described will practically always arrest eclamptic convulsions and prevent their recurrence. The initial intravenous injection of 4 g is used to establish promptly a therapeutic level that is then maintained by the nearly simultaneous intramuscular administration of 10 g of the compound, followed by 5 g intramuscularly every 4 hours, as long as there is no evidence of potentially dangerous hypermagnesemia. With this dosage schedule, the plasma levels for magnesium that are achieved are therapeutically effective and range from 4 to 7 mEq/L, compared to pretreatment plasma levels of less than 2.0 mEq/L (Chesley and Tepper, 1957; Stone and Pritchard, 1970). Magnesium sulfate injected deeply into the upper outer quadrant of the buttocks, as described above, has not resulted in erratic absorption and, in turn, erratic plasma levels; indeed, the reverse has been true (Fig. 27-12).

Recently, Graham and co-workers (1984) reported on a prospective study in which a comparison between continuous intravenous magnesium sulfate and intramuscular magnesium sulfate was made. There was no significant difference between the mean magnesium levels observed after intramuscular magnesium sulfate and those observed following the intravenous regimen using a maintenance dose of 2 g per hour. However, the intramuscular regimen resulted in serum magnesium levels that were significantly higher than those obtained with a continuous intravenous maintenance does of 1 g per hour (Fig. 27-13). A similar result was reported by Sanders and Hayashi (1983). Both groups concluded that there was no therapeutic advantage to the intravenous route of administration except possibly the avoidance of discomfort at the intramuscular site of in-

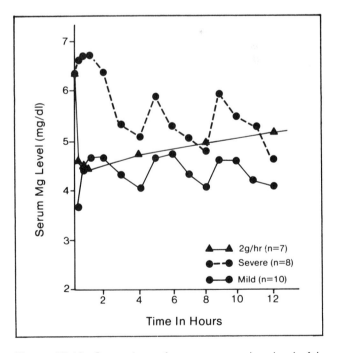

Figure 27-13. Comparison of serum magnesium levels following (1) a 10 g IM loading dose of magnesium sulfate and a 5 g IM maintenance dose every 4 hours (•——•), mild preeclampsia; (2) a 4 g IV loading dose followed by the same regimen as in (1) (•- -•), severe preeclampsia; (3) a 4 g IV loading dose followed by a continuous IV maintenance dose of 2 g per hour (▲——▲). (*From Graham et al.: Am J Obstet Gynecol (in press), 1984.*)

jection. We favor the intramuscular route for reasons of safety as well as the excellent therapeutic results.

The patellar reflex disappears by the time the plasma magnesium level reaches 10 mEq/L, presumably as the consequence of a curariform action. This sign serves to warn of impending magnesium toxicity, since a further increase will lead to respiratory depression.

When the plasma levels rise above 10 mEq/L, respiratory depression develops, and at 12 mEq/L or more, respiratory arrest occurs. Treatment with calcium gluconate intravenously plus the withholding of magnesium sulfate usually will reverse mild to moderate respiratory depression. For severe respiratory depression and arrest prompt endotracheal intubation and ventilation will prove lifesaving. Direct toxic effects on the myocardium from high levels of magnesium have been claimed. However, in humans it appears that a major cause of cardiac dysfunction must be hypoxia, the consequence of respiratory arrest, rather than a direct effect of the magnesium. With appropriate ventilation, cardiac action can be satisfactory even when plasma levels are very high (McCubbin and associates, 1981).

Parenterally injected magnesium is filtered through the glomerulus and variably reabsorbed by the tubule; as the magnesium concentration in plasma increases, more magnesium is filtered and less is reabsorbed. Nonetheless, when glomerular filtration is impaired, so is magnesium clearance. Therefore, an appreciably elevated plasma creatinine level serves to warn of diminished capacity of the kidney to excrete magnesium. A fraction of the injected magnesium is deposited reversibly in surface bone.

The myth is perpetuated that parenterally administered magnesium sulfate is a potent antihypertensive agent. Levine and Coburn (1984) even suggest a mechanism of action to account for an antihypertensive action, namely, the intracellular redistribution of calcium. Many studies in hypertensive human subjects, beginning with those of Winkler and co-workers (1942) in chronically hypertensive subjects and Pritchard (1955) in women with preeclampsia–eclampsia, have identified at most a variable and transient lowering of blood pressure during bolus administration of sizeable doses of the compound!

In monkeys with angiotensin-induced hypertension late in pregnancy, Harbert and co-workers (1969) demonstrated slightly increased uterine blood flow in response to the infusion of magnesium sulfate. At the same time, arterial blood pressure decreased minimally. Altura and associates (1983) observed that when isolated umbilical arteries and veins obtained from normal infants at term were incubated with 0 to 9.6 mmole of magnesium per liter, basal tension of the vessels increased in the absence of magnesium and decreased as the concentration of magnesium increased. They also observed that the absence of magnesium potentiated the contractile response of the vessels to bradykinin, angiotensin II, serotonin, and prostaglandin $F_{2\alpha}$. They thought that their observation might help explain the favorable outcome observed in infants of preeclamptic women who received magnesium sulfate therapy.

Somjen and co-workers (1966) induced in themselves, by intravenous infusion, marked hypermagnesemia, achieving plasma levels to 15 mEq/L. *Predictably, at such high plasma levels, respiratory depression developed that necessitated mechanical ventilation, but depression of the sensorium was not dramatic as long as hypoxia was prevented.*

Borges and Gücer (1978) provided convincing evidence that the magnesium ion exerts an effect on the central nervous system much more specific than generalized depression. They measured the actions of parenterally administered magnesium sulfate on epileptic neural activity induced in awake, undrugged subhuman primates. The infused magnesium sulfate suppressed neuronal burst firing and interictal electroencephalographic spike generation in neuronal populations rendered epileptic by topically applied penicillin G. The degree of suppression increased as the plasma magnesium concentration increased and decreased as the magnesium level fell. Therefore, even though elevated concentrations of magnesium in plasma do decrease acetylcholine release in response to motor nerve impulses, reduce motor end-plate sensitivity to acetylcholine, and decrease the motor end-plate potential, these actions do not account for, nor should they necessarily be implicated in, the explanation of the beneficial effects of magnesium sulfate in controlling the convulsions of eclampsia. Interestingly—indeed, amazingly—Donaldson (1978) and some other neurologists, for reasons that are hard to discern, have erroneously emphasized that magnesium sulfate is a "peripherally" acting anticonvulsant and therefore "bad medicine." They imply that the drug works only in concentrations that cause paralysis and, consequently, the woman with eclampsia so treated is "quiet on the outside but still convulsing on the inside." This conclusion could not have been based on any direct experience with eclampsia and its control with parenterally administered magnesium! At the same time, Donaldson urges other forms of therapy but cites no data whatsoever to support his recommendations. Most other drugs that effectively arrest and prevent eclamptic convulsions do cause appreciable general depression of the central nervous system in both the mother and the newborn infant.

Magnesium ions *in high concentration* will depress myometrial contractility both in vivo and in vitro. With the regimen described above and the plasma levels that have resulted, no evidence of depression of myometrial function has been observed beyond a transient decrease in contraction frequency during and immediately after the initial intravenous loading dose. While the frequency may decrease transiently, the amplitude of the contractions may actually increase (Valenzuela and co-workers, 1983).

Magnesium ions administered parenterally to the mother cross the placenta promptly to achieve equilibrium between mother and fetus. Magnesium sulfate, given as a large single dose intravenously but not with smaller doses, may transiently cause a loss of beat-to-beat variability in the fetal heart rate (Pritchard, 1979).

The newborn infant may be depressed by magnesium only if *severe* hypermagnesemia exists at delivery. The kind of compromises that have been described by Lipsitz and English (1967) to develop at times in the newborn after maternal continuous intravenous therapy with magnesium sulfate have not been observed by us (Stone and Pritchard, 1970) nor by Green and associates (1983).

The dosage schedule and route of administration used by us, coupled with the safeguards observed before each injection, have effectively prevented worrisome adverse effects from hypermagnesemia in newborns at Parkland Memorial Hospital. Indeed, Lipsitz (1971) agreed with our observations after further study in which he found that infants were unlikely to be compromised when the mother had received magnesium sulfate according to the protocol for the treatment of eclampsia used at Parkland Memorial Hospital. The use of magnesium sulfate in PIH, its mechanisms of action, and its possible toxicity in mother and fetus–infant have been described in more detail by Pritchard (1979) and by Cruikshank and associates (1979).

Other Treatment Agents

Although widely used to control convulsions from a variety of causes in nonpregnant individuals, diazepam therapy remains unproven as a substitute for magnesium sulfate. Our experience has been limited to a few women with eclampsia brought to the Obstetrics Emergency Unit after receiving a modest dose of 5 to 10 mg of diazepam elsewhere. Apparently, larger doses of diazepam alone are often required to control eclamptic convulsions. Moreover, Cree and co-workers in 1973 and others more recently have documented in newborns low Apgar scores, apnea persisting several hours after birth, hypotonia, drowsiness, and impaired metabolic response to cooling as the consequence of administration of diazepam to their mothers intrapartum. We have observed one case of respiratory arrest in which diazepam was given repeatedly to a hypertensive woman postpartum to try to arrest convulsions so that a CT scan could be performed. She was then successfully managed with magnesium sulfate given as described above.

Morphine and most sedatives will control convulsions only in doses that render the woman nearly unconscious. Such intense generalized central nervous depression in the mother and her fetus should be avoided. Some other drugs of the great variety that have been used in the treatment of eclampsia and severe preeclampsia are presented in Table 27-3. We have had little personal experience with most of them; for further information, the interested reader is referred to the various reports that are listed.

It should be pointed out that a tendency persists among some medical experts to group together for the purpose of treatment a variety of disease states that appear to have a common functional disturbance. So-called hypertensive encephalopathy is one that from time to time attracts interest and, in turn, incites recommendations for treatment broad in scope, without full appreciation of all the problems created by the disease or evoked by the proposed treatment. Too often, when eclampsia is included under the category of hypertensive encephalopathy, lack of concern for the impact of the recommended therapy on the fetus is apparent. Moreover, it is not unusual for the recommendations to have been based on little or no data (Anonymous, 1979).

The recurrent recognition of thrombocytopenia occasionally and, less often, of other changes in the coagulation mechanism, with or without evidence of abnormal erythrocyte destruction (microangiopathic hemolysis), has led to the recommendation of treatment with heparin, fresh whole blood, fresh frozen plasma, platelets, fibrinogen, and other specific clotting factors as necessary. Merit, if any, from heparin treatment remains to be es-

tablished. In two more recent reports, it was concluded that heparin did not prove effective in ameliorating the clinical course of established preeclampsia (Bonnar and associates, 1976; Howie and co-workers, 1975). These experiences with heparin treatment appear similar to those reported by Butler and associates in 1950. We have never used heparin in these circumstances because of fear of enhancing intracranial hemorrhage and because of an appreciation that correction of the defects occurs promptly after delivery. The outcomes have been satisfactory, as already described. The safety of deliberate anticoagulation with heparin in the presence of severe hypertension is questionable and certainly cannot be recommended until much greater experience attesting to any benefits has been recorded.

Reproduction After Eclampsia

Because of the catastrophic implications of eclampsia, women so affected and their families often are quite concerned over the prognosis for future pregnancies. Moreover, gloomy accounts have repeatedly appeared in the obstetric literature. Hypertension, for example, has been reported to occur in as high as 78 percent of women who previously had eclampsia.

Chesley and co-workers (1962), through meticulous long-term follow-up of women with eclampsia at Margaret Hague Maternity Hospital between the years 1931 and 1952 have provided us with most useful information. For example, of 466 subsequent pregnancies in 189 of the eclamptic women, the fetal salvage was 76 percent, but much of the loss was early abortion. Of the pregnancies that continued to 28 weeks or more, 93 percent resulted in infants who survived.

Of the subsequent pregnancies, 25 percent were complicated by hypertension in the 189 previously eclamptic women observed by Chesley and associates (1964). The hypertension, however, was severe in only 5 percent, while 2 percent were again eclamptic. Our observations on previously eclamptic women are very similar.

Chesley emphasized that many of the recurrences of elevated blood pressure represent nothing more than chronic hypertension. Some women do have normal blood pressures between pregnancies and at follow-up, but, in general, pregnancies following eclampsia are an excellent screening test for latent hypertensive disease. A large percentage of women who develop recurrences of hypertension during subsequent pregnancies ultimately become hypertensive, whereas the prevalence of ultimate hypertension is extremely low in those who are normotensive in later pregnancies.

Chesley and co-workers (1976) traced to 1974 all but 3 of the 270 women who survived eclampsia at the Margaret Hague Maternity Hospital in the period 1931 through 1951. Women who had eclampsia in their first pregnancy carried 28 weeks or more have shown no increase over the expected number of remote deaths. In sharp contrast, women who had eclampsia as multiparas, the majority of whom undoubtedly had underlying chronic vascular disease, have shown three times the expected number of deaths.

Relation of Preeclampsia–Eclampsia to Subsequent Hypertension

Whether preeclampsia and eclampsia actually cause ensuing chronic hypertension has been a subject of debate. One point of view has been that preeclampsia and eclampsia represent an acute vascular disorder in the form of muscle spasm, which, if allowed to continue for several weeks, would result in a permanent structural injury to the vascular wall through hypoxia. This view led some to teach that permanent hypertension might be avoided by delivery of women within 3 weeks after onset of preeclampsia. For some time, Chesley (1978) was of this school, but reappraisal of his data led him to reverse his conclusions. The problem has been confused by the mistaken diagnosis of preeclampsia even in primigravid women who really had chronic renal disease or essential hypertension. Another mistake was that some studies have included a substantial proportion of multiparas, few of whom actually had pure preeclampsia. Contributing to the confusion, nearly 40 percent of women with essential hypertension have significant drops in blood pressure during much of pregnancy. In many of them, as the consequence, normal pressures may be observed from early in gestation. Typically, the blood pressure rises again early in the third trimester, and some edema, with perhaps minimal proteinuria, may occur. Inasmuch as blood pressures before pregnancy were seldom known, the erroneous diagnosis of preeclampsia was likely to have been made.

The results of the long-term follow-up studies of Chesley and associates (1976), who have reexamined women repeatedly for up to 44 years after eclampsia in the first pregnancy, are indicative that the prevalence of hypertension is not increased over that in unselected women matched for age and race. Tillman (1955) accumulated a series of 377 women whose blood pressures were recorded before, during, and at intervals after pregnancy. He could find no indication that normal, preeclamptic, or hypertensive pregnancies had any effect on the blood pressure at follow-up examination and concluded that preeclampsia neither causes residual hypertension nor aggravates preexisting hypertension.

CHRONIC HYPERTENSION

Diagnosis

A diagnosis of chronic hypertension is made in association with pregnancy whenever there is evidence of chronicity of the disorder (p. 528, specific diagnostic criteria). In addition to instances of obvious chronic hypertension, there are instances of repeated pregnancies during which hypertension appears late in pregnancy, but the blood pressure is normal between pregnancies.

Many authors, notably Dieckmann (1952), regarded these recurrent bouts as evidence of latent hypertensive vascular disease. Others concluded that they are repeated attacks of preeclampsia, and still others regarded recurrent hypertension as a separate entity. The results of the long-term follow-up studies of Chesley and co-workers (1976) are supportive of Dieckmann's view (1952).

In most women with chronic hypertensive vascular disease, hypertension is the only demonstrable finding. A few women, however, have secondary alterations that are often grave in relation not only to pregnancy but also to life expectancy. These include hypertensive cardiac disease, arteriosclerotic heart disease, renal disease, and retinal hemorrhages and exudates. The blood pressure, moreover, may vary from levels scarcely above normal to extremes of 300 systolic and 160 or more diastolic.

Hypertensive vascular disease in pregnancy is encountered most frequently in older women. In addition to age, obesity seems to be an important predisposing factor to chronic hypertension. More than 25 percent of pregnant women weighing over 200 pounds have elevated blood pressures. Heredity also seems to play a role in the development of this disorder. Frequently, many members of one family have hypertension.

As already pointed out, the blood pressure often falls by the second trimester of pregnancy, but the decrement is usually temporary, since it is followed in most cases by a rise during the third trimester to levels somewhat above those present in early pregnancy. Commonly, the babies of mothers with chronic hypertension are smaller than expected for their gestational ages. The incidence of abruptio placentae is increased in chronically hypertensive women as well as in women with PIH (Chapter 21, p. 397).

Treatment During Pregnancy

The value of continued administration of antihypertensive agents to pregnant women with chronic hypertension is debated. On the one hand, it may be of benefit to the hypertensive mother to lower her blood pressure. On the other hand, the lower pressure may reduce uteroplacental perfusion and thereby jeopardize the fetus. It is not known at this time whether antihypertensive therapy, as generally prescribed in the absence of pregnancy, is beneficial or deterimental to the pregnancy outcome, and until recently there were few studies that might be used as a clinical guide.

Review of Some Studies. Redman and associates (1976) chose to treat one group of hypertensive women with α-methyldopa and compare the outcome with that of a group of untreated women. They selected patients with blood pressures at or above 140/90 but less than 170/100 at less than 28 weeks gestation. Those women with blood pressures of 170/100 or higher were treated and not included in the control study. A total of 101 women received α-methyldopa, but 107 did not. No di-

TABLE 27-8. PREGNANCY: CHRONIC HYPERTENSION AND SUPERIMPOSED PREECLAMPSIA: METHOD OF TREATMENT AND PERINATAL OUTCOME

Treatment	Number* of Births	Stillbirths	Neonatal Deaths	Uncorrected Perinatal Mortality (deaths/1000)
Redman and associates (1980)†				
Pregnancy: chronic hypertension α-methyldopa and/or hydralazine	184	2	1	16
Superimposed preeclampsia α-methyldopa + other antihypertensive agents	69	6	4	145
Sibai and associates (1983)				
Pregnancy: chronic hypertension No antihypertensive drugs	193	0	1	5
Superimposed preeclampsia α-methyldopa and/or hydralazine	22	2	3	227
Chesley (1978)				
Pregnancy: chronic hypertension‡ (1972–1974) No antihypertensive drugs	593	19§		32
Superimposed preeclampsia ‖ (1960–1974) hydralazine + α-methyldopa	196	42§		214

* The number of births is a larger number than the women cared for because of twin gestations.
† Data extracted from Table 1 from Ounsted and associates (1983) reporting on long term follow-up of children from the original and continuing study of treatment of chronic hypertension in pregnancy by Redman (1980).
‡ Three maternal deaths due to stroke, pulmonary embolus, and aspiration pneumonia.
§ Reported as perinatal deaths.
‖ Two deaths due to stroke and postoperative infection.

uretics were used, and both groups of women underwent early delivery at 37 to 38 weeks gestation. In the control group there was one stillbirth in a pregnancy complicated further by superimposed preeclampsia and one neonatal death likely due to birth asphyxia and trauma. In the treatment group there was one stillbirth in a pregnancy complicated further by superimposed preeclampsia. The average birth weight and laboratory values were essentially the same in both groups. There were four abortions in the control group but none in the treatment group.

A summary of the final results of Redman's carefully conducted study are presented in Table 27-8 and compared to those of Sibai and co-workers (1983) and those of Chesley (1978) in similar women who were managed without antihypertensive medications. All investigators reported that the development of superimposed preeclampsia (pregnancy-aggravated hypertension) was a bad complication. It appears unlikely that treatment with antihypertensive medications will decrease the incidence of this complication (Redman and co-workers, 1976; Redman, 1980).

It is immediately apparent from a review of Table 27-8 that most results were good for pregnant women with chronic hypertension with or without treatment with antihypertensives! The uncorrected perinatal mortality rates were 32, 16, and 5 per 1000, respectively, for Chesley, whose results were obtained from 1972 to 1974,

for Redman whose results were obtained in the late 1970s, and for Sibai whose study was conducted between 1980 and 1982.

The maternal results most often were also satisfactory. The only maternal deaths were those reported by Chesley. A careful analysis of these deaths is therefore warranted. Death from stroke occurred in a woman who was transferred from another hospital. She was in coma and died within 20 minutes of arrival. A second patient died of a pulmonary embolus after a cesarean delivery of a 5000 g infant followed by a stormy postoperative course and a wound evisceration. The final death occurred as the result of aspiration pneumonia that happened during anesthesia for a cesarean delivery.

The use of α-methyldopa during early pregnancy has been questioned because of smaller head circumferences observed in male infants of women who received the drug between 16 and 20 weeks gestation (Redman, 1980). However, the long-term follow-up of the infants in Redman's 1976 and 1980 studies are reassuring. There have been no major adverse effects noted in the infants or children for up to 7½ years of life (Cockburn and associates, 1982; Ounsted and co-workers, 1983).

Despite the good results obtained with α-methyldopa (Redman, 1980) and the comparable results obtained without antihypertensive agents (Sibai and co-workers, 1983; Chesley, 1978), labetalol, a combined α- and β-adrenergic blocker not available in the United

States, and related compounds, are being tested extensively in pregnant women with hypertension in England, Scotland, and Australia (Redman 1982; Walker and associates, 1983; Michael, 1982). The early results (Redman, 1982) of therapy with labetalol are consistent with the view that the agent offers no therapeutic advantage over α-methyldopa.

One other antihypertensive drug must be mentioned but only to condemn its use in pregnancy. Captopril, the angiotensin I converting enzyme inhibitor, has been shown to reduce uteroplacental perfusion and often kill the fetuses of experimental animals (Broughton-Pipkin and associates, 1982; Ferris and Weir, 1983).

At Parkland Memorial Hospital, pregnancy complicated by chronic hypertension has not been treated with antihypertensive agents or diuretics unless (1) blood pressure is above 150/110 or (2) the woman was receiving antihypertensive medications prior to the pregnancy, and her hypertension is well controlled. If the blood pressure increases rapidly and persists above 110 mm Hg diastolic, if significant proteinuria develops, if renal function begins to decrease, or if fetal growth retardation develops, for the reasons that follow, the pregnancy is terminated as recommended above for severe preeclampsia and eclampsia.

PREGNANCY-AGGRAVATED HYPERTENSION

Diagnosis

The common hazard faced by pregnant women with chronic hypertensive vascular disease is the superimposition of preeclampsia. The frequency with which it occurs is difficult to specify precisely, for the incidence varies with the diagnostic criteria employed. If the diagnosis is made only on the basis of (1) significant aggravation of the hypertension (rise of 30 mm Hg systolic and 15 mm Hg diastolic), (2) sustained proteinuria, and (3) gross, generalized edema, the incidence will be relatively low, since delivery is often accomplished before intense superimposed preeclampsia or eclampsia has developed. The incidence reported by the authors listed in Table 27-8 was 25 percent in the Redman series, 10 percent in the Sibai series, and 5.7 percent in the Chesley study. If, however, the diagnosis is made on the basis of a rise in blood pressure and minimal to modest proteinuria, the incidence probably approaches 50 percent.

Pregnancy-aggravated hypertension typically becomes manifest by a sudden rise in blood pressure, which almost always is eventually complicated by substantial proteinuria. In neglected cases especially, extreme hypertension (systolic pressure greater than 200 and diastolic pressure of 130 or more), oliguria, and impaired renal clearance may rapidly ensue; the retina may contain extensive hemorrhages and cottonwool exudates; convulsions and coma are likely. Therefore, in its full-blown form, the resultant syndrome is very similar to

hypertensive encephalopathy. With the development of superimposed preeclampsia or eclampsia, the outlook for both the infant and the mother is grave unless the pregnancy is soon terminated (Table 27-8). The frequency of fetal growth retardation and prematurity is increased appreciably (López-Llera and associates, 1972; Redman, 1980) due to its relatively early onset in pregnancy, as well as the marked severity of the process itself. However, if the infant is liveborn and survives the perinatal period, the long-term prognosis is good (Ounsted and co-workers, 1983).

REFERENCES

Abdul-Karim R, Assali NS: Pressor response to angiotonin in pregnant and nonpregnant women. Am J Obstet Gynecol 82:246, 1961

Altura BM, Altura BT, Carella A: Magnesium deficiency-induced spasms of umbilical vessels: Relation to preeclampsia, hypertension, growth retardation. Science 221:376, 1983

Anonymous: Hypertensive encephalopathy. Br Med J 3:1387, 1979

Assali NS, Douglas RA, Baird WW: Measurement of uterine blood flow and uterine metabolism. Am J Obstet Gynecol 66:248, 1953

Baird D: Combined Textbook of Obstetrics and Gynaecology for Students and Practitioners. Edinburgh and London, E & S Livingstone, Ltd, 1969, p 631

Beer AE: Possible immunologic bases of preeclampsia/eclampsia. Semin Perinatol 2:39, 1978

Benedetti TJ, Quilligan EJ: Cerebral edema in severe pregnancy-induced hypertension. Am J Obstet Gynecol 137:860, 1980

Benedetti TJ, Cotton DB, Read JC, Miller FC: Hemodynamic observations in severe pre-eclampsia with a flow-directed pulmonary artery catheter. Am J Obstet Gynecol 136:465, 1980

Bonnar J, Redman CWG, Denson KW: The role of coagulation and fibrinolysis in pre-eclampsia. In Lindheimer MD, Katz AI, Zuspan FP (eds): Hypertension in Pregnancy. New York, Wiley, 1976

Borges LF, Gücer G: Effect of magnesium on epileptic foci. Epilepsia 19:81, 1978

Brosens IA, Robertson WB, Dixon HG: The role of the spiral arteries in the pathogenesis of preeclampsia. Obstet Gynecol Annu 1:177, 1972

Broughton-Pipkin F, Symonds EM, Turner SR: The effect of Captopril upon mothers and fetuses in the chronically cannulated ewe and in the pregnant rabbit. J Physiol (Br) 323: 415, 1982

Brown RD, Strott CA, Liddle GW: Plasma deoxycorticosterone in normal and abnormal human pregnancy. J Clin Endocrinol Metab 35:736, 1972

Browne FJ: Sensitization of the vascular system in pre-eclamptic toxaemia and eclampsia. Br J Obstet Gynaecol 53:510, 1946

Browne FJ, Dodds GH: Pregnancy in the patient with chronic hypertension. J Obstet Gynaecol Br Emp 49:1, 1942

Browne JCM, Veall N: The maternal placental blood flow in normotensive and hypertensive women. J Obstet Gynaecol Br Emp 60:141, 1953

Browne O: The treatment of eclampsia. Br J Obstet Gynaecol 57:573, 1950

Brunner HR, Gavras H: Vascular damage in hypertension. Hosp Pract 10:97, 1975

Bryant RD, Fleming JG: Veratrum viride in the treatment of eclampsia. Obstet Gynecol 19:372, 1962

Butler BC, Taylor HC, Graff S: The relationship of disorders of the blood-clotting mechanism to toxemia of pregnancy and the value of heparin in therapy. Am J Obstet Gynecol 60:564, 1950

Chesley LC: Hypertensive Disorders of Pregnancy. In Hellman LM, Pritchard JA (eds): Williams Obstetrics, 14th ed. New York, Appleton, 1971, Chap 25

Chesley LC: A short history of eclampsia. Obstet Gynecol 43:599, 1974

Chesley LC: Superimposed preeclampsia or eclampsia. In Chesley LC: Hypertensive Disorders in Pregnancy. New York, Appleton, 1978, p 14, 302, 482

Chesley LC, Tepper I: Plasma levels of magnesium attained in magnesium sulfate therapy for preeclampsia and eclampsia. Surg Clin North Am, April 1957, p 353

Chesley LC, Williams LO: Renal glomerular and tubular function in relation to the hyperuricemia of pre-eclampsia and eclampsia. Am J Obstet Gynecol 50:367, 1945

Chesley LC, Annitto JE, Cosgrove RA: Prognostic significance of recurrent toxemia of pregnancy. Obstet Gynecol 23:874, 1964

Chesley LC, Annitto JE, Cosgrove RA: The familial factor in toxemia of pregnancy. Obstet Gynecol 32:303, 1968

Chesley LC, Annitto JE, Cosgrove RA: Long-term follow-up study of eclamptic women: Sixth periodic report. Am J Obstet Gynecol 124:446, 1976

Chesley LC, Cosgrove RA, Annitto JE: A follow-up study of eclamptic women: Fourth periodic report. Am J Obstet Gynecol 83:1360, 1962

Cockburn J, Moar VA, Ounsted M, Redman CWG: Final report of study on hypertension during pregnancy: The effects of specific treatment on the growth and development of the children. Lancet 1:647, 1982

Combes B, Adams RH: Disorders of the liver in pregnancy. In Assali NS (ed): Pathophysiology of Gestation. New York, Academic, 1972, Vol 1

Cooper DW, Liston WA: Genetic control of severe preeclampsia. J Med Genet 16:409, 1979

Cree JE, Meyer J, Hailey DM: Diazepam in labour: Its metabolism and effect on the clinical condition and thermogenesis of the newborn. Br Med J 4:251, 1973

Cruikshank DP, Pitkin RM, Reynolds WA, Williams GA, Hargis GK: Effects of magnesium sulfate treatment on perinatal calcium metabolism. I. Maternal and fetal responses. Am J Obstet Gynecol 134:243, 1979

Cunningham FG, Cox K, Gant NF: Further observations on the nature of pressor responsivity to angiotensin II in human pregnancy. Obstet Gynecol 146:581, 1975

Cunningham FG, Pritchard JA: How should hypertension during pregnancy be managed? Experience at Parkland Memorial Hospital. Medical Clinics of North America 68:505, 1984

Dewar JB, Morris WIC: Sedation with rectal tribromethanol (Avertin Bromethol) in the management of eclampsia. J Obstet Gynaecol Br Emp 54:417, 1947

DeWolf F, Robertson WB, Brosen I: The ultrastructure of acute atherosis in hypertensive pregnancy. Am J Obstet Gynecol 123:164, 1975

Dieckmann WJ: The Toxemias of Pregnancy, 2d ed. St. Louis, Mosby, 1952

Dieckman WJ, Michel HL: Vascular-renal effects of posterior pituitary extracts in pregnant women. Am J Obstet Gynecol 33:131, 1937

Donaldson JO: Neurology in Pregnancy. Philadelphia, Saunders, 1978

Duenhoelter JH, Jimenez JM, Baumann G: Pregnancy performance in patients under fifteen years of age. Obstet Gynecol 46:49, 1975

Engle WD, Rosenfeld CR: Neutropenia in high-risk neonates. J Pediatr (in press), 1984

Everett RB, Porter JC, MacDonald PC, Gant NF: Relationship of maternal placental blood flow to the placental clearance of maternal plasma dehydroisoandrosterone sulfate through placental estriol formation. Am J Obstet Gynecol 136:435, 1980

Everett RB, Worley RJ, MacDonald PC, Gant NF: Effect of prostaglandin synthetase inhibitors on pressor response to angiotensin II in human pregnancy. J Clin Endocrinol Metab 46:1007, 1978a

Everett RB, Worley RJ, MacDonald PC, Gant NF: Modification of vascular responsiveness to angiotension II in pregnant women by intravenously infused 5α-dihydroprogesterone. Am J Obstet Gynecol 131:352, 1978b

Feeney JG, Scott JS: Pre-eclampsia and changed paternity. Eur J Obstet Gynaecol Reprod Biol 11:35, 1980

Ferris TF: How should hypertension during pregnancy be managed? An internist's apporach. Medical Clinics of North America 68:491, 1984

Ferris TF, Weir EK: Effect of Captopril in uterine blood flow and prostaglandin E synthesis in the pregnant rabbit. J Clin Invest 71:809, 1983

Fisher ER, Pardo V, Paul R, Hayashi TT: Ultrastructural studies in hypertension. IV. Toxemia of pregnancy. Am J Pathol 55:901, 1969

Friedman EA, Neff RK: Pregnancy outcome as related to hypertension, edema, and proteinuria. In Lindheimer MD, Katz AI, Zuspan FP (eds): Hypertension in Pregnancy. New York, Wiley, 1976, p 13

Fritz MA, Stanczyk FZ, Novy MJ: Relationship of uteroplacental blood flow to the placental clearance (PC) of maternal dehydroepiandrosterone (D) through estradiol (E$_2$) formation in the pregnant baboon. Presented at the Society for Gynecologic Investigation, San Francisco, March 21-24, 1984

Gant NF, Chand S, Whalley PJ, MacDonald PC: The nature of pressor responsiveness to angiotension II in human pregnancy. Obstet Gynecol 43:854, 1974a

Gant NF, Madden JD, Siiteri PK, MacDonald PC: The metabolic clearance rate of dehydroisoandrosterone sulfate. III. The effect of thiazide diuretics in normal and future preeclamptic pregnancies. Am J Obstet Gynecol 123:159, 1975

Gant NF, Madden JD, Siiteri PK, MacDonald PC: The metabolic clearance rate of dehydroisoandrosterone sulfate. IV. Acute effect of induced hypertension, hypotension, and natriuresis in normal and hypertensive pregnancies. Am J Obstet Gynecol 124:143, 1976

Gant NF, Daley GL, Chand S, Whalley PJ, MacDonald PC: A study of angiotension II pressor response throughout primigravid pregnancy. J Clin Invest 52:2682, 1973

Gant NF, Jimenez JM, Whalley PJ, Chand S, MacDonald PC: A prospective study of angiotension II pressor responsiveness in pregnancies complicated by chronic essential hypertension. Am J Obstet Gynecol 127:369, 1977

Gant NF, Chand S, Worley RJ, Whalley PJ, Crosby UD, MacDonald PC: A clinical test useful for predicting the development of acute hypertension in pregnancy. Am J Obstet Gynecol 120:1, 1974b

Gedekah RH, Hayashi TT, MacDonald HM: Eclampsia at

Magee-Womens Hospital, 1970–1980. Am J Obstet Gynecol 140:860, 1980

Gilstrap LC, Cunningham FG, Whalley PJ: Management of pregnancy-induced hypertension in the nulliparous patient remote from term. Semin Perinatol 2:73, 1978

Govan ADT: The pathogenesis of eclamptic lesions. Pathol Microbiol (Basel) 24:561, 1961

Graham JM, Sibai BM, McCubbin JH: A comparison of intravenous versus intramuscular MgSO$_4$ in preeclampsia. Am J Obstet Gynecol (in press), 1984

Green KW, Key TC, Coen R, Resnik R: The effects of maternally administered magnesium sulfate on the neonate. Am J Obstet Gynecol 146:29, 1983

Groenendijk R, Trambros JBM, Wallenberg HCS: Hemodynamic measurements in preeclampsia: Preliminary observations. Am J Obstet Gynecol (in press), 1984

Hankins G, Wendel G Jr, Cunningham G, Leveno K: Hemodynamic observation in eclampsia. Presented at Society for Gynecology Investigation, 31st Annual Meeting, San Francisco, March 21–24, 1984 (Abstract)

Hankins GDV, Wendel GW Jr, Whalley PJ Quirk JG Jr: Cardiovascular monitoring in the high-risk pregnancy. Perinatol Neonatol 7:29, 1983

Harbert GM Jr, Cornell GW, Thornton WN Jr: Effect of toxemia therapy on uterine dynamics. Am J Obstet Gynecol 105:94, 1969

Heller PJ, Scheider EP, Marx GF: Pharyngolaryngeal edema as a presenting symptom in preeclampsia. Obstet Gynecol 62:523, 1983

Hertig AT: Vascular pathology in the hypertensive albuminuric toxemias of pregnancy. Clinics 4:602, 1945

Hinselmann H: Die Eklampsie. Bonn, F. Cohen, 1924

Howie PW, Prentice CRM, Forbes CD: Failure of heparin therapy to affect the clinical course of severe preeclampsia. Br J Obstet Gynaecol 82:711, 1975

Hughes EC (ed): Obstetric-Gynecologic Terminology. Philadelphia, Davis, 1972

Ingerslev M, Teilum G: Biopsy studies of the liver in pregnancy. Acta Obstet Gynecol Scand 24:339, 1946

Johnson T, Clayton CG: Diffusion of radioactive sodium in normotensive and preeclamptic pregnancies. Br Med J 1:312, 1957

Karotkin EH, Cashore WJ, Kido M, Redding RA, Douglas W, Stern L, Oh W: The inhibition of pulmonary maturation in the fetal rabbit by maternal treatment with phenobarbital. Am J Obstet Gynecol 124:529, 1976

Kawathekar P, Anusuya SR, Sriniwas P, Lagali S: Diazepam (Calmpose) in eclampsia: A preliminary report of 16 cases. Curr Ther Res 15:845, 1973

Kitzmiller JL, Lang JE, Yelonosky PF, Lucas WE: Hematologic assays in pre-eclampsia. Am J Obstet Gynecol 118:362, 1974

Kraus GW, Marchese JR, Yen SSC: Prophylactic use of hydrochlorothiazide in pregnancy. JAMA 198: 1150, 1966

Landesman R, Douglas RG, Holze E: The bulbar conjunctival vascular bed in the toxemias of pregnancy. Am J Obstet Gynecol 68:170, 1954

Lean TH, Ratnam SS, Sivasamboo R: Use of benzodiazepines in the management of eclampsia. J Obstet Gynaecol Br Commonw 75:856, 1968

Levine B, Coburn JW: Magnesium, the mimic/antagonist of calcium. New Engl J Med 310:1253, 1984

Lichtig C, Luger AM, Spargo BH, Lindheimer MD: Renal immunofluorescence and ultrastructural findings in preeclampsia. Clin Res 23:368A, 1975

Lipsitz PJ: The clinical and biochemical effects of excess magnesium in the newborn. Pediatrics 47:501, 1971

Lipsitz PJ, English IC: Hypermagnesemia in the newborn infant. Pediatrics 40:856, 1967

Llewellyn-Jones D: The treatment of eclampsia. Br J Obstet Gynaecol 68:33, 1961

López-Llera M: Complicated eclampsia. Fifteen years' experience in a referral medical center. Am J Obstet Gynecol 142:28, 1982

López-Llera M, Hernandez-Horta JL, Huttich FC: Retarded fetal growth in eclampsia. J Reprod Med 9:229, 1972

McCall ML: Cerebral circulation and metabolism in toxemia of pregnancy. Observations on the effects of veratrum viride and Apresoline (1-hydrazino-phthalazine). Am J Obstet Gynecol 66:1015, 1953

McCartney CP: Pathological anatomy of acute hypertension of pregnancy. Circulation 30 [Suppl 2]:37, 1964

McCartney CP, Schumacher GFB, Spargo BH: Serum proteins in patients with toxemic glomerular lesion. Am J Obstet Gynecol 111:580, 1971

McCubbin JH, Sibai BM, Abdella TN, Anderson GD: Cardiopulmonary arrest due to acute maternal hypermagnesemia. Lancet 1:1058, 1981

McKay DG: Disseminated Intravascular Coagulation. New York, Harper & Row, 1965

Menon MKK: The evolution of the treatment of eclampsia. J Obstet Gynaecol Br Commonw 68:417, 1961

Menzies D, Prystowsky H: Acute hemorrhagic pancreatitis following chlorothiazide administration in pregnancy. J Florida Med Assoc 54:564, 1967

Metcalfe J, Romney SL, Ramsey LH, Reid DE, Burwell CS: Estimation of uterine blood flow in normal human pregnancy at term. J Clin Invest 34:1632, 1955

Michael CA: The evaluation of labetalol in the treatment of hypertension complicating pregnancy. Br J Clin Pharmacol [Suppl 1] 127:127A, 1982

Minkowitz S, Soloway HB, Hall JE, Yermakov V: Fatal hemorrhagic pancreatitis following chlorothiazide administration in pregnancy. Obstet Gynecol 24:337, 1964

Mojadidi Q, Thompson RJ: Five years' experience with eclampsia. South Med J 66:414, 1973

Morris N, Osborn SB, Wright HP, Hart A: Effective uterine bloodflow during exercise in normal and pre-eclamptic pregnancies. Lancet 2:481, 1956

Naeye RL, Friedman EA: Causes of perinatal death associated with gestational hypertension and proteinuria. Am J Obstet Gynecol 133:8, 1979

Nishimura RN, Koller R: Isolated cortical blindness in pregnancy. West J Med 137:335, 1982

Nochimson DJ, Petrie RH: Glucocorticoid therapy for the induction of pulmonary maturity in severely hypertensive gravid women. Am J Obstet Gynecol 133:449, 1979

Öney T, Kaulhausen H: The value of the angiotensin sensitivity test in the early diagnosis of hypertensive disorders of pregnancy. Am J Obstet Gynecol 142:17, 1982

Ounsted M, Cockburn J, Moar VA, Redman CW: Maternal hypertension with superimposed pre-eclampsia: Effects on child development at 7< years. Br J Obstet Gynaecol 90:644, 1983

Page EW: On the pathogenesis of pre-eclampsia and eclampsia. J Obstet Gynaecol Br Commonw 79:883, 1972

Parker CR, Everett RB, Quirk JG, Whalley PJ, Gant NF, MacDonald PC: Hormone production during pregnancy in the primigravida. II. Plasma levels of deoxycorticosterone (DOC) throughout pregnancy in normal women and women who developed pregnancy-induced hypertension (PIH). Am J Obstet Gynecol 138:626, 1980

Perkins RP, Mattox JH: Evidence against the theory of preeclampsia as a disease of absent immunologic tolerance: Studies on pregnancies resulting from artificial insemination. Am J Obstet Gynecol (in press), 1984

Petrucco OM, Thomson NM, Lawrence JR, Weldon MW: Immunofluorescent studies in renal biopsies in pre-eclampsia. Br Med J 1:473, 1974

Phelan JP, Yurth DA: Severe preeclampsia. I. Peripartum hemodynamic observations. Am J Obstet Gynecol 144:17, 1982

Pritchard JA: The use of the magnesium ion in the management of eclamptogenic toxemias. Surg Gynecol Obstet 100:131, 1955

Pritchard JA: Management of severe preeclampsia and eclampsia. Semin Perinatol 2:83, 1978

Pritchard JA: The use of magnesium sulfate in preeclampsia–eclampsia. J Reprod Med 23:107, 1979

Pritchard JA, Cunningham FG, Mason RA: Coagulation changes in eclampsia: Their frequency and pathogenesis. Am J Obstet Gynecol 124:855, 1976

Pritchard JA, Cunningham FG, Pritchard SA: The Parkland Memorial Hospital protocol for treatment of eclampsia: Evaluation of 245 cases. Am J Obstet Gynecol 148:951, 1984

Pritchard JA, Ratnoff OD, Weismann R Jr: Hemostatic defects and increased red cell destruction in preeclampsia and eclampsia. Obstet Gynecol 4:159, 1954

Pritchard JA, Weisman R Jr, Ratnoff OD, Vosburgh G: Intravascular hemolysis, thrombocytopenia and other hematologic abnormalities associated with severe toxemia of pregnancy. N Engl J Med 250:87, 1954

Raab W, Schroeder G, Wagner R, Gigee W: Vascular reactivity and electrolytes in normal and toxemic pregnancy. J Clin Endocrinol 16:1196, 1956

Redman CWG: Treatment of hypertension in pregnancy. Kidney Int 18:267, 1980

Redman CWG: Controlled trials of treatment of hypertension during pregnancy. Obstet Gynecol Surv 37:523, 1982

Redman CWG, Beilin LJ, Bonnar J, Ounsted MK: Fetal outcome in a trial of antihypertensive treatment in pregnancy. Lancet 2:753, 1976

Robertson AL, Khairallah PA: Effects of angiotensin II and some analogues on vascular permeability in the rabbit. Circ Res 31:923, 1972

Robertson EG: The natural history of oedema during pregnancy. J Obstet Gynaecol Br Commonw 78:520, 1971

Rodriguez SU, Leikin SL, Hiller MC: Neonatal thrombocytopenia associated with antepartum administration of thiazide drugs. N Engl J Med 270:881, 1964

Rosenbaum M, Maltby G: Cerebral dysrhythmia in relation to eclampsia. Arch Neurol Psychiatr 49:204, 1943

Rote NS, Lau RJ, Harrison M, Scott JR: Immunologic mechanisms of maternal and fetal thrombocytopenia in pregnancy-induced hypertension (PIH). Presented at the Society for Gynecologic Investigation, March 21-24, 1984

Ruvinsky ED, Douvas SG, Roberts WE, Martin JN, Rhodes PG, Harris JB, Morrison JC: Maternal administration of dexamethasone in severe pregnancy-induced hypertension. Am J Obstet Gynecol (submitted), 1984

Sanders R, Hayashi R: Intravenous versus intramuscular magnesium sulfate for preeclampsia. Society for Gynecologic Investigation, 30th Annual Meeting, Washington, DC, March 17–20, 1983 (Abstract No 25)

Semchyshyn S, Zuspan F, Cordero L: Cardiovascular response and complications of glucocorticoid therapy in hypertensive pregnancies. Am J Obstet Gynecol 145:530, 1983

Shears BH: Combination of chlorpromazine, promethazine, and pethidine in treatment of eclampsia. Br Med J 2:75, 1957

Sheehan HL: Pathological lesions in the hypertensive toxaemias of pregnancy. In Hammond J, Browne FJ, Wolstenholme GEW (eds): Toxaemias of Pregnancy, Human and Veterinary. Philadelphia, Blakiston, 1950

Shoemaker ES, Gant NF, Madden JD, MacDonald PC: The effect of thiazide diuretics on placental function. Tex Med 69:109, 1973

Sibai BM, Abdella TN, Anderson GD: Pregnancy outcome in 211 patients with mild chronic hypertension. Obstet Gynecol 61:571, 1983

Sibai BM, McCubbin JH, Anderson GD, Lipshitz J, Dilts PV Jr: Eclampsia I. Observations from 67 recent cases. Obstet Gynecol 58:609, 1981

Silke B, Carmody M, O'Dwyer WF: Acute renal failure in pregnancy. In Bonnar J, MacGillivray I, Symonds EM (eds): Pregnancy Hypertension. Baltimore, University Park Press, 1980, p 511

Sims EAH: Pre-eclampsia and related complications of pregnancy. Am J Obstet Gynecol 107:154, 1970

Somjen G, Hilmy M, Stephen CR: Failure to anesthetize human subjects by intravenous administration of magnesium sulfate. J Pharmacol Exp Ther 154:652, 1966

Spargo B, McCartney CP, Winemiller R: Glomerular capillary endotheliosis in toxemia of pregnancy. Arch Pathol 68:593, 1959

Stahnke E: Über das Verhalten der Blutplättchen bei Eklampsie. Zentralbl Gynaekol 46:391, 1922

Stallworth JC, Yeh S-Y, Petrie RH: The effect of magnesium sulfate on fetal heart rate variability and uterine activity. Am J Obstet Gynecol 140:702, 1981

Stone SR, Pritchard JA: Effect of maternally administered magnesium sulfate on the neonate. Obstet Gynecol 35:574, 1970

Talledo OE, Chesley LC, Zuspan FP: Renin-angiotensin system in normal and toxemic pregnancies. III. Differential sensitivity to angiotensin II and norepinephrine in toxemia of pregnancy. Am J Obstet Gynecol 100:218, 1968

Tillman AJB: The effect of normal and toxemic pregnancy on blood pressure. Am J Obstet Gynecol 70:589, 1955

Valenzuela G, Hayashi R, Johns A: Effects of magnesium sulfate upon uterine contractility in humans. Magnesium 2:120, 1983

Vassalli P, Morris RH, McCluskey RT: The pathogenic role of fibrin deposition in the glomerular lesions of toxemia of pregnancy. J Exp Med 118:467, 1963

Volhard F: Die Doppelseitigen Haematogenen Nierenerkrankungen. Berlin, Springer, 1918

Walker JJ, Bonduelle M, Greer I, Calder AA: Antihypertensive therapy in pregnancy. Lancet 1:932, 1983

Weir RJ, Fraser R, Lever AF, Morton JJ, Brown JJ, Kraszewski A, McIlevine GM, Robertson JIS, Tree M: Plasma renin, renin substrate, angiotensin II, and aldosterone in hypertensive disease of pregnancy. Lancet 1:291, 1973

Weis EB Jr, Bruns PD, Taylor ES: A comparative study of the disappearance of radioactive sodium from human uterine muscle in normal and abnormal pregnancy. Am J Obstet Gynecol 76:340, 1958

Wellen I: Specific "toxemia," essential hypertension, and glomerulonephritis associated with pregnancy. Am J Obstet Gynecol 39:16, 1940

Winkel CA, Milewich L, Parker CR Jr, Gant NF, Simpson ER, MacDonald PC: Conversion of plasma progesterone to deoxycorticosterone in men, nonpregnant and pregnant women, and adrenalectomized subjects: Evidence for steroid 21-hydroxylase activity in non-adrenal tissues. J Clin Invest 66:803, 1980

Winkel CA, Casey ML, Guerami A, Rawlins SC, Cox K, MacDonald SC, Parker CR: Ratio of plasma deoxycorticosterone (DOC) levels to plasma progesterone (P) levels in pregnant women who did not develop pregnancy-induced hypertension (PIH). Society for Gynecologic Investigation, 30th Annual Meeting, Washington, DC, March 17–20, 1983 (Abstract No 341)

Winkler AW, Smith PK, Hoff HE: Intravenous magnesium sulfate in the treatment of nephritic convulsions in adults. J Clin Invest, 21:207, 1942

Worley RJ, Everett RB, MacDonald PC, Gant NF: Placental clearance of dehydroisoandrosterone sulfate and pregnancy outcome in three categories of hospitalized patients with pregnancy-induced hypertension. Society for Gynecologic Investigation, 22nd Annual Meeting, March, 1975 (Abstract No 40)

Zeek PM, Assali NS: Vascular changes in decidua associated with eclamptogenic toxemia of pregnancy. Am J Clin Pathol 20:1099, 1950

Zlatnik FJ, Burmeister LF: Dietary protein and preeclampsia. Am J Obstet Gynecol 147:345, 1983

Zuspan FP, Ward MC: Treatment of eclampsia. South Med J 57:954, 1964

Medical and Surgical Illnesses During Pregnancy and the Puerperium

Essentially all diseases that affect a woman when non-pregnant may be contracted during pregnancy. Moreover, the presence of most diseases does not prevent conception.

For most systemic illnesses, the physiologic and anatomic changes inherent in normal pregnancy influence the symptoms, signs, and laboratory values to a considerable degree. Consequently, the physician who is not aware of these changes induced by normal pregnancy may not be able to recognize a disease or may diagnose incorrectly some other disease, to the jeopardy of the mother and her fetus. Throughout this chapter, emphasis is placed on the effect of interaction between the disease and the pregnancy as well as on the problems in diagnosis and treatment imposed by the gestational state. In practically all instances, the following questions are pertinent:

1. Is pregnancy likely to make the disease more serious—if so, how?
2. Does the disease jeopardize the pregnancy—if so, how and to what degree?
3. Should the pregnancy be terminated because of either gross risk to the mother or likelihood of grave damage to the fetus?
4. Should the pregnancy be allowed to continue under a very carefully defined regimen of therapy?
5. If the disease exists before pregnancy, is pregnancy contraindicated—if so, what steps should be taken to protect the woman from pregnancy?

HEMATOLOGIC DISORDERS

Pregnancy normally induces appreciable changes that complicate diagnosis of hematologic disease and assessment of response to treatment. This is true especially for anemia.

ANEMIA AND OTHER DISEASES OF THE BLOOD

Definition of Anemia

A precise definition of anemia in women is complicated by the normal differences in the concentrations of hemoglobin between women and men, between white women and black women, between women who live at high altitudes and those who live near sea level, between women who are pregnant and those who are not, and between pregnant women who receive iron supplements and those who do not. On the basis of data presented in Table 28-1, it can be said that anemia probably exists in women residing at lower altitudes if the hemoglobin is much below 12.0 g/dl in the nonpregnant state or is less than 10.0 g/dl during pregnancy or the immediate puerperium. However, early in pregnancy and again near term, the hemoglobin level of most healthy iron sufficient women is usually 11.0 g/dl or higher.

After delivery, in the absence of excessive blood loss, the hemoglobin level typically fluctuates to a modest degree around the predelivery value for a few days and then rises to a somewhat higher level. The rate and magnitude of increase in the puerperium are to a considerable degree the result of the amount of hemoglobin added to the intravascular compartment during pregnancy and the amount shed during and after delivery.

TABLE 28-1. HEMOGLOBIN CONCENTRATION IN HEALTHY WOMEN WITH PROVEN IRON STORES

Hemoglobin (g/dl)	Stage of Pregnancy		
	Nonpregnant	Midpregnancy	Late Pregnancy
Mean	13.7	11.5	12.3
<12.0 Percent	1	72	36
<11.0 Percent	0	29	6
<10.0 Percent	0	4	1
Lowest	11.7	9.7	9.8

(*From Scott, Pritchard (1967); Pritchard, Scott (1970).*)

Extensive hematologic measurements have been made in healthy nonpregnant women, none of whom were iron deficient, since each had histochemically proven iron stores; nor were any of them deficient in metabolically active forms of folic acid, since marrow erythropoiesis remained normoblastic. The hemoglobin concentration of 85 healthy iron sufficient nonpregnant women averaged 13.7 g/dl and ranged from 12.0 to 15.0 g for ±2 standard deviations from the mean. In healthy iron sufficient women who were 16 to 22 weeks pregnant, the mean hemoglobin was only 11.5 g/dl, and in 3 of the 81 evaluated it was 9.7 or 9.8 g/dl. The hemoglobin level at or very near term averaged 12.3 g/dl; in only 7 out of 95 was the hemoglobin less than 11.0 g/dl, with the lowest value 9.8 g/dl. These data are summarized in Table 28-1.

The modest fall in hemoglobin levels observed during pregnancy in healthy women not deficient in iron or folate is caused by relatively greater expansion of the volume of plasma compared to the increase in hemoglobin mass and volume of erythrocytes. The disproportion beween the rates at which plasma and erythrocytes are added to the maternal circulation normally is greatest during the second trimester. Late in pregnancy, plasma expansion essentially ceases while hemoglobin mass continues to increase (Chapter 9, p. 191).

Frequency

Although anemia is somewhat more common among indigent pregnant women, it is by no means restricted to them. The frequency of anemia during pregnancy varies considerably, depending primarily upon whether supplemental iron is taken during pregnancy. For example, at Parkland Memorial Hospital the hemoglobin levels at the time of delivery among women who took iron supplements averaged 12.4 g/dl, whereas the average was only 11.3 g/dl among those who received no iron. Moreover, in none of the group receiving iron supplements was the hemoglobin less than 10.0 g/dl, but it was below this level in 16 percent of the group who received no supplements (Chapter 13, p. 252). More recently, and confirming many previous observations, Taylor and associates (1982) in the United Kingdom identified hemoglo-

bin levels to average at term 12.7 g/dl among women who received during pregnancy supplemental iron, compared to 11.2 g/dl for those who did not.

Etiology of Anemia

A classification based primarily on etiology and including most of the common causes of anemia in pregnant women follows:

Causes of Anemia During Pregnancy

A. Acquired
 1. Iron deficiency anemia
 2. Anemia caused by acute blood loss
 3. Anemia caused by inflammation or malignancy
 4. Megaloblastic anemia
 5. Acquired hemolytic anemia
 6. Aplastic or hypoplastic anemia
B. Hereditary
 1. Thalassemias
 2. Sickle cell hemoglobinopathies
 3. Other hemoglobinopathies
 4. Hereditary hemolytic anemias without hemoglobinopathy

Although laboratory error as a cause of apparent anemia has not been included in this table, the results from clinical laboratories may sometimes be grossly inaccurate. A common source of laboratory error during pregnancy stems from the rapid sedimentation rate of erythrocytes, induced by the hyperfibrinogenemia of normal pregnancy. If the specimen of blood is not effectively mixed *immediately* before sampling, the results are likely to be inaccurate.

The observed differences between hemoglobin concentrations in pregnant and nonpregnant women, coupled with the well-recognized phenomenon of hypervolemia induced by normal pregnancy, have led to the use of the term *physiologic anemia*. This poor term for describing a normal process is confusing and should probably be discarded, since there is no anemia during normal pregnancy if anemia is defined as a decrease in hemoglobin mass.

Screening for Anemia

A limited but practical hematologic evaluation may be carried out quickly at the time of the mother's visit to the clinic or office. The equipment and reagents required are simple and inexpensive. A few milliliters of venous blood are anticoagulated with Versenate (EDTA). A centrifuge for performing microhematocrit measurements and a hematocrit reading device are employed to detect anemia. For normocytic, normochromic red cells, the hematocrit is almost exactly three times the hemoglobin concentration.

The plasma in the hematocrit tube is examined for icterus, and the thickness of the buffy coat is noted. If icterus is observed, studies to detect hemolytic disease or hepatic dysfunction are initiated. For black patients, a sickle cell preparation is made using isotonic sodium metabisulfite solution or Sickledex; if the result is positive, hemoglobin electrophoresis is indicated. Whenever the hematocrit approaches 30 or less or when there is icterus or when sickling is demonstrated, a blood smear with Wright stain is used to evaluate the blood cells morphologically. These rather simple studies not only detect anemia but also provide important etiologic clues.

IRON DEFICIENCY ANEMIA

The two most common causes of anemia during pregnancy and the puerperium are iron deficiency and acute blood loss. Not infrequently the two are intimately related, since excessive blood loss with its concomitant loss of hemoglobin iron and exhaustion of iron stores in one pregnancy can be an important cause of iron deficiency anemia in the next pregnancy.

As discussed elsewhere (Chapter 9, p. 192; Chapter 13, p. 252) the iron requirements of pregnancy are considerable, but the majority of women have small stores of iron. In a typical gestation with a single fetus, the maternal need for iron induced by pregnancy averages close to 800 mg, of which about 300 mg go to the fetus and placenta, whereas about 500 mg, *if available,* are used to expand the maternal hemoglobin mass. Approximately 200 mg more are shed through the gut, urine, and skin. This amount of iron—1000 mg—exceeds considerably the iron stores of most women. Unless the difference between the amount of stored iron available to the mother and the iron requirements of normal pregnancy is compensated for by absorption of iron from the gastrointestinal tract, iron deficiency anemia develops.

With the rather rapid expansion of the blood volume during the second trimester, the lack of iron often manifests itself by an appreciable drop in the maternal hemoglobin concentration. Although the rate of expansion of the blood volume is not so great in the third trimester, the need for iron remains high because augmentation of the maternal hemoglobin mass continues and considerable iron is now transported across the placenta from mother to fetus. Since the amount of iron diverted to the fetus from an iron deficient mother is not much different from the amount normally transferred, the newborn infant of a severely anemic mother does not suffer from iron deficiency anemia (Murray and co-workers, 1978). Iron stores in the infant are influenced much more by when and how the cord is clamped rather than by the iron stores of the mother.

Identification

Classic morphologic evidence of iron deficiency anemia—erythrocyte hypochromia and microcytosis—is much less likely to be as prominent in the pregnant woman as in the nonpregnant woman with the same hemoglobin concentration. Less severe iron deficiency anemia during pregnancy, i.e., a hemoglobin concentration

of 9 g/dl or so, is usually not accompanied by obvious morphologic changes in the circulating erythrocytes. However, with this degree of anemia from iron deficiency, the serum ferritin levels are usually lower than normal, and there is no stainable iron in the bone marrow. The serum iron-binding capacity is elevated but is in itself of little diagnostic value, since it is also elevated during normal pregnancy in the absence of iron deficiency. Moderate normoblastic hyperplasia of the bone marrow is also found to be similar to that in normal pregnancy. *The anemia is the consequence primarily of the expansion of the plasma volume without normal expansion of maternal hemoglobin mass.*

The initial evaluation of a pregnant woman with moderate anemia should include measurements of hemoglobin, hematocrit, and red cell indices, careful examination of a well-prepared smear of the peripheral blood, a sickle cell preparation if the patient is black, and perhaps measurement of the serum iron concentration, serum ferritin level, or both. Examination of the bone marrow at this point is seldom done, although the demonstration of hemosiderin rules out iron deficiency. The diagnosis of iron deficiency in moderately anemic pregnant women is usually presumptive; it is based largely on the exclusion of other causes of anemia and eventually a response to iron therapy.

When the pregnant woman with moderate iron deficiency anemia receives adequate iron therapy, hematologic response can be detected first in a blood smear. Newly formed erythrocytes that are normal or slightly larger than normal in size and polychromatophilic or basophilic when treated with Wright stain soon appear in the peripheral blood. Examination of a blood smear is simpler than a reticulocyte count and probably provides for a more accurate index of response in the moderately anemic pregnant woman. The rate of increase of the concentration of hemoglobin or of the hematocrit varies considerably but is usually slower than in nonpregnant women. The reason is related largely to the differences in blood volumes. During the latter half of pregnancy the newly formed hemoglobin is added to the characteristically much larger volume of blood. Moreover, during the treatment period the blood volume expands variably depending upon the time in pregnancy. Therefore, the production of an appreciable amount of hemoglobin by the pregnant woman whose plasma volume is expanding simultaneously and rapidly may not result in a rapid increase in hemoglobin concentration, as demonstrated in Figure 28-1. There is no good evidence, however, that pregnancy per se depresses erythropoiesis and hemoglobin generation to any degree.

In severe iron deficiency anemia during pregnancy, the erythrocytes undergo the classic morphologic changes of hypochromia and microcytosis, and the diagnosis is usually made from the red cell indices and confirmed by examination of a well-prepared smear of the peripheral blood. In our now extensive experience, spoon nails, changes in the appearance of the tongue (other than paleness), and other stigmata of the Plummer-

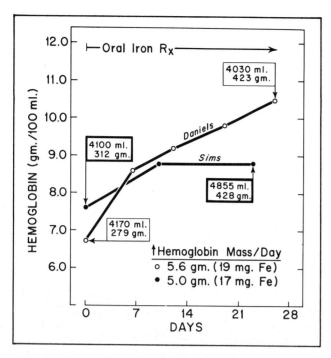

Figure 28-1. Two pregnant women with iron deficiency anemia, when treated with the same simple iron compound, responded by increasing their hemoglobin mass at similar rates but not their hemoglobin levels. The excellent response in Sims treated late in the second trimester was masked by a simultaneous increase in blood volume of nearly 20 percent. The blood volume did not increase in Daniels who was treated late in the third trimester.

Vinson syndrome are rarely found even when the pregnant woman has severe iron deficiency anemia.

Treatment

There has been some divergence of opinion regarding the best way to treat iron deficiency anemia during pregnancy and the puerperium. The use of an effective parenteral iron medication guarantees that the expectant mother receives the iron. Oral preparations are preferred, however, if she understands the importance of taking the medication regularly. If she will not or, much less likely, cannot take the oral doses of iron, parenteral therapy is an alternative. Whatever treatment is employed, the objectives are correction of the severe deficit in hemoglobin mass and eventually restitution of iron stores. Both of these objectives can be accomplished with orally administered, simple iron compounds (ferrous sulfate, fumarate, or gluconate) that provide a daily dose of about 200 mg of *iron*. To replenish iron stores, oral therapy should be continued for 3 months or so after the anemia has been corrected (Pritchard and Mason, 1964).

In our extensive experience with simple iron compounds that provide about 200 mg of iron per day, it makes little

difference in response when the iron is taken. The most important factor is convenience to the patient so that she will take the medication! Unfortunately, she often receives conflicting advice from physicians, nurses, nutritionists, and others concerning when and with or without what items of diet she must take her iron pills. There is no need to prescribe ascorbic acid or fruit juices or to withhold food to enhance iron absorption when ingested as prescribed above, nor is there any advantage from so-called delayed-release or sustained-release medication. Both the treatment regimen and the iron medication should be simple!

Iron preparations that provided significant amounts of iron when administered parenterally have been plagued by adverse reactions that are frequent and, at times, severe. Moreover, the rate of hemoglobin synthesis in response to currently available parenterally administered iron preparations is little, if any, faster than with oral iron taken in the dosage described above. An example of similarity in response during pregnancy is presented in Table 28-21.

The distributor of iron–dextran injection USP (Imferon) in the United States has again emphasized that this preparation "be restricted for use in patients whose medical need is clearly established," and that "the daily dose is recommended to be no more than 2 ml given intramuscularly or intravenously." If iron–dextran is used but after the first few injections of iron–dextran there is no evidence of hematologic response, it is important that the injections be stopped and the cause of the anemia be reevaluated. Hopefully, the total dose infusion technique, which from the outset was obviously unsound therapeutically, has now been abandoned by obstetricians. It is true that storage iron can be created rapidly by injections of iron–dextran, but storage iron so created is much less readily available for hemoglobin synthesis than is storage iron created by oral administration.

Folic acid may, and probably should, be given along with the iron as a safeguard against folate deficiency, although in our experience the response of pregnant women with iron deficiency anemia treated with iron and folic acid is usually not appreciably better than when iron is given alone (Fig. 28-2). There is no good evidence that the addition of cobalt, copper, molybdenum, or ascorbic acid to the iron tablet is advantageous. Ascorbic acid does enhance iron absorption somewhat, so that, theoretically, less iron need be ingested to achieve a comparable level of absorption. However, there is no advantage to reducing the amount of iron ingested, since any adverse gastrointestinal effects from oral iron relate primarily to the amount of iron absorbed rather than to the amount ingested. *Iron preparations that contain significant amounts of iron but are totally free of any adverse effects are likely to be very poorly absorbed and consequently ineffective.*

Transfusions of red cells or whole blood are seldom indicated for the treatment of iron deficiency anemia unless hypovolemia from blood loss coexists or an operative procedure must be performed on a severely anemic

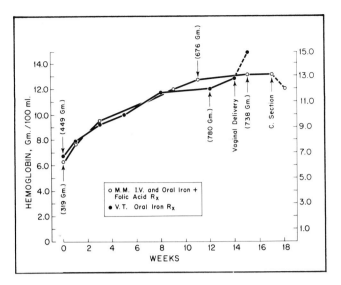

Figure 28-2. Excellent and nearly identical hematologic responses in two pregnant women with severe iron deficiency anemia. The response in one to oral iron alone (65 mg of iron three times a day) was as rapid as it was in the other, who received oral iron in the same dosage plus intravenous iron in excess and folic acid 3 mg per day.

woman. Whereas hypovolemia may be a prominent initial feature of anemia caused by acute blood loss, severe anemia from either failure of production of erythrocytes or their accelerated destruction may lead to cardiac insufficiency and pathologic hypervolemia.

In case of severe anemia and hypervolemia, the administration of packed red cells and any accompanying electrolyte solution must be done with meticulous care to prevent severe circulatory overloading, pulmonary edema, and even death. Exchange transfusion is an effective way to raise the hemoglobin concentration of severely anemic women without inducing or intensifying circulatory overload. Alternatively, the intravenous administration of furosemide shortly before slowly transfusing packed erythrocytes is of value in reducing plasma volume and thereby allowing the intravascular compartment to accommodate the added erythrocytes without causing circulatory overload.

ACUTE BLOOD LOSS ANEMIA

Anemia resulting from recent hemorrhage is more likely to be evident during the puerperium. Both abruptio placentae and placenta previa are likely to cause serious blood loss and anemia before as well as after delivery. Earlier in pregnancy, anemia caused by acute loss of blood is common in instances of abortion, tubal pregnancy, and hydatidiform mole.

Treatment

Acute hemorrhage may have no immediate effect on the hemoglobin concentration even though the hemorrhage leads to hypovolemia so severe as to cause overt collapse. Massive hemorrhage demands immediate blood replacement with whole blood in amounts that restore and maintain adequate perfusion of vital organs (Chapter 21, p. 391 for details of management). Even though the amount of blood replaced commonly does not repair completely the hemoglobin deficit created by the hemorrhage, in general, once dangerous hypovolemia has been overcome and hemostasis has been achieved, the residual anemia should be treated with iron. The moderately anemic woman (hemoglobin greater than 7.0 g/dl) whose condition is stable, who no longer faces the likelihood of further serious hemorrhage, who can ambulate without adverse symptoms, and who is not febrile is usually better treated with iron than with blood transfusions.

ANEMIA WITH CHRONIC DISEASE

A large variety of disorders—chronic infections and neoplasms especially—may produce moderate and sometimes severe anemia, usually with normocytic or slightly microcytic erythrocytes (Lee, 1983). Typically, bone marrow cytology is not markedly altered. The serum iron concentration is decreased, and the serum iron-binding capacity, although lower than in normal pregnancy, is not necessarily much below the normal nonpregnant range. The anemia appears to result, at least in part, from alterations in reticuloendothelial function and iron metabolism. Iron released from the patient's senescent erythrocytes is retained rather than being returned promptly to the plasma to be reutilized by the bone marrow for production of hemoglobin. The fate of iron administered in therapeutic doses is similar. The life span of the erythrocyte, furthermore, is usually slightly shortened. The anemia, therefore, results from decreased erythropoiesis coupled with slightly increased destruction.

Renal disease, suppuration, granulomatous infections, malignant conditions, and rheumatoid arthritis may also cause anemia, presumably by these same mechanisms. At least some cases of so-called *refractory anemia of pregnancy* probably are the consequence of one of these diseases that has gone unrecognized. The anemia of infection, renal disease, and malignancy is refractory in the sense that it is not corrected by treatment with iron, folic acid, vitamin B_{12}, or any other known hematinic agent. Nonetheless, prophylaxis with iron and folic acid usually is desirable to offset any deficiency induced by pregnancy.

It has been our experience that women with acute pyelonephritis and high fever, but not with asymptomatic bacteriuria or mild clinical disease, often develop overt anemia. The genesis of the anemia appears to be increased red cell destruction, coupled with impairment of production that may persist for some weeks (Cunningham and co-workers, unpublished).

MEGALOBLASTIC ANEMIA

The prevalence of megaloblastic anemia during pregnancy varies considerably throughout the world. In the United States, overt anemia with frankly megaloblastic erythropoiesis demonstrable in the bone marrow is a rare complication of pregnancy, but in some other parts of the world it has been found much more frequently.

Folic Acid Deficiency

In the United States, megaloblastic anemia beginning during pregnancy almost always results from folic acid deficiency. It is usually found in pregnant women who consume neither fresh vegetables, especially of the uncooked green leafy variety, nor foods with a high content of animal protein. Women with megaloblastic anemia may have developed troublesome nausea, vomiting, and anorexia during pregnancy. As the folate deficiency and anemia increases, the anorexia often becomes more intense, thus aggravating the dietary deficiency. In some instances of megaloblastic anemia, ethanol ingestion is either the cause or contributes appreciably to its development.

Identification. Deficiency of metabolically active forms of folic acid induces many biochemical and hematologic changes. The sequence of changes from folate deficiency is probably unaltered by pregnancy. In the peripheral blood, the earliest biochemical evidence is low folic acid activity in plasma. The earliest morphologic evidence of folic acid deficiency usually is hypersegmentation of some of the neutrophils during pregnancy. As anemia develops, the newly formed erythrocytes, now being produced in reduced numbers, are macrocytic, even when there has been previous iron deficiency with microcytosis. With preexisting iron deficiency, the more recently formed macrocytic erythrocytes would not be detected from the measurement of the mean corpuscular volume of the erythrocytes. Careful examination of a well-prepared smear of the peripheral blood, however, will usually reveal some macrocytes. As the anemia becomes more intense, an occasional nucleated erythrocyte appears in the peripheral blood. If smears of the buffy coat from peripheral blood are made in order to concentrate the nucleated erythrocytes, several such cells with the distinct features of megaloblasts are usually demonstrable. At the same time, examination of the bone marrow discloses megaloblastic erythropoiesis. As the maternal folate deficiency and, in turn, the anemia become severe, thrombocytopenia, leukopenia, or both may also develop.

Herbert and co-workers (1962) estimated that in normal nonpregnant women the daily folate requirements expressed as folic acid are in the range of 50 to 100 μg per day. During pregnancy, however, the requirements for metabolically active forms of folic acid are increased. The fetus and placenta extract folate from maternal circulation so effectively that the fetus is not anemic even when the mother is severely anemic from folate deficiency. Cases have been recorded in which the newborn hemoglobin levels were 18.0 g or more per dl, while the maternal values were as low as 3.6 g/dl (Pritchard and co-workers, 1970).

Treatment. The treatment of megaloblastic anemia induced by pregnancy should include folic acid, a nutritious diet, and usually iron. As little as 1 mg of folic acid administered orally once a day produces a striking hematologic response. By 4 to 7 days after the beginning of treatment, the reticulocyte count is appreciably increased, and leukopenia and thrombocytopenia are promptly corrected. Sometimes the rate of increase in hemoglobin concentration or hematocrit is disappointing, especially when compared with the usual exuberant reticulocytosis that starts soon after therapy has been initiated. Severe megaloblastic anemia during pregnancy is accompanied frequently by an appreciably smaller blood volume than that of a normal pregnancy, but soon after folic acid therapy has been started the blood volume usually increases considerably. Therefore, even though hemoglobin is being rapidly added to the circulation, the hemoglobin concentration does not precisely reflect the total amount of additional hemoglobin because of the simultaneous expansion of the blood volume.

Women who develop megaloblastic anemia during pregnancy commonly are also deficient in total body iron. Paradoxically, ineffective erythropoiesis resulting from the folate deficiency and, in turn, a decreased amount of iron being incorporated into hemoglobin, induces a considerable elevation of the plasma iron and even some accumulation of storage iron. However, with the onset of effective erythropoiesis, the concentration of iron in the plasma falls precipitously, and any stored iron is rapidly exhausted. Iron may then become the limiting factor in production of hemoglobin.

Megaloblastic anemia recurs rather often in subsequent pregnancies, very likely because of persistence of dietary inadequacies and perhaps in part because of a peculiarity in absorption or utilization of folic acid. Congenital folate malabsorption has been identified rarely (Poncz and associates, 1981).

A great deal of attention has been devoted to the frequency of maternal folate deficiency and megaloblastic anemia in pregnancy and the puerperium, the possible role of folate deficiency in various forms of reproductive failure, and the value of prophylactic administration of folic acid throughout pregnancy, as discussed in some detail in Chapter 13 (p. 255). A good case can be made for supplemental folic acid in circumstances where folate requirements are unusually excessive, for example, in multifetal pregnancy or overt hemolytic anemia. Whether to administer folic acid routinely to all pregnant women in the United States is debatable. If, however, prenatal vitamin supplements are prescribed, folic acid should be included, since there is more evidence that the pregnant woman might suffer from a deficiency of that vitamin than of the several others that are almost always included.

Pernicious Anemia

Megaloblastic anemia caused by lack of vitamin B_{12} during pregnancy is quite rare. *Addisonian pernicious anemia,* in which there is failure to absorb vitamin B_{12} because of lack of intrinsic factor, is extremely uncommon in women of reproductive age. Moreover, unless women with this disease are treated with vitamin B_{12}, infertility may be a complication (Ball and Giles, 1964). There is little reason to withhold folic acid during pregnancy simply out of fear of jeopardizing the neurologic integrity of women who might be pregnant and simultaneously have unrecognized, and therefore untreated, addisonian pernicious anemia.

Breast-fed infants of mothers who suffer vitamin B_{12} deficiency, either as a consequence of lack of intrinsic factor or because of chronic ingestion of a strict vegetarian diet, may develop megaloblastic anemia during infancy (Chapter 13, p. 255).

ACQUIRED HEMOLYTIC ANEMIAS

A variety of acquired hemolytic anemias may complicate pregnancy. Pregnancy, on occasion, may actually incite hemolysis, as described subsequently.

Acquired Hemolytic Anemias

Women with autoimmune acquired hemolytic anemia sometimes demonstrate marked acceleration of the rate of hemolysis during pregnancy. Prednisone and similar compounds seem to be nearly as effective as in the nonpregnant state. Thrombocytopenia, if present, may also be favorably affected by corticosteroid therapy. Pregnancy is not a contraindication to the use of these steroids, but, since the underlying disease is often chronic and progressive, repeated pregnancies are not advisable in women with acquired hemolytic anemia caused by autoimmune disease.

With autoimmune hemolytic anemia, typically both the direct and indirect antiglobulin (Coombs) test is positive. The autoimmune hemolytic anemia and the positive antiglobulin tests may be the consequence of either IgM or IgG antierythrocyte antibodies. IgM antibodies readily agglutinate red cells suspended in saline, whereas IgG antibodies do not and therefore have been referred to as "incomplete antibodies." The antiglobulin test, appropriately performed, does identify IgG antibodies.

IgM antibodies do not cross the placenta, and therefore the fetal red cells are not affected. However, IgG antibodies, especially subclasses IgG_1 and IgG_3, do cross the placenta. The most common example of the adverse fetal effects from maternally produced IgG antibodies is maternal Rh isoimmunization, with hemolytic disease in the fetus and neonate. Whenever IgG antibodies

against red cells are detected in the mother, the fetus should be considered at risk of serious hemolytic disease, and appropriate steps should be taken to gauge its intensity (Chapter 38, p. 775).

Transfusion of red cells into the mother with severe autoimmune hemolytic disease is complicated by the presence of circulating antierythrocyte antibodies. Warming the donor cells to body temperature decreases their destruction by cold agglutinins.

A case of acquired hemolytic anemia with multiple problems cared for recently at Parkland Memorial Hospital is summarized below:

R.A., a 29-year-old gravida 6 para 5, was first seen at Parkland Memorial Hospital in early labor with twin fetuses at 35 to 36 weeks gestation. She also complained of jaundice, pruritus, and malaise of 3 weeks duration. Her hematocrit was 15, MCV 121 fl, reticulocytes 13%, platelets 219,000/mm^3 and serum bilirubin 5.4 mg/dl (3.5 mg direct reacting). Direct and indirect Coombs tests were positive; a warm IgG autoantibody was identified. It was also learned that 8 and 9 months before, or about the time of conception, she had been hospitalized elsewhere because of acquired hemolytic anemia with a hematocrit of 9 on one occasion and 13 on the other; she was transfused with several units of packed red cells, and treatment with prednisone was initiated.

Before red cell transfusion could be accomplished, spontaneous vaginal delivery of twin A was followed by assisted breech delivery of twin B. Their size was appropriate for gestational age. Five minute Apgar scores were 9 for both. Separate placentas were delivered. Blood loss at delivery was not excessive.

There was no clinical or laboratory evidence of hemolytic disease in either twin, although the potential for such existed since IgG antibody was identified in maternal serum. In fact, the central hematocrit of the second twin soon after birth was 70! Exchange transfusion with plasma was performed to lower the hematocrit, and the newborn period remained stormy; necrotizing enterocolitis necessitated left hemicolectomy and colostomy. The infant survived. The first-born twin thrived.

Even though the mother's hematocrit remained at 14, red cell transfusion was withheld because of difficulty in crossmatching and blood loss had not been excessive; she could ambulate without much difficulty. Bone marrow aspirate served to identify marked erythroid hyperplasia with prominent megaloblastic changes and no storage iron. It was hoped that therapy with prednisone (100 mg per day), folic acid (2 mg per day), and iron (200 mg per day), coupled with the termination of the twin gestation without excessive blood loss, would result in rapid hematologic improvement. The reticulocyte count rose promptly to 20 percent and then to as high as 31 percent.

Nine days postpartum she experienced sudden, severe pleuritic pain in the left chest which radiated to the left shoulder and arm. She had difficulty breathing. While breathing room air, arterial Po_2 was 80 mm Hg. Chest roentgenograms and lung scans demonstrated no abnormality. However, two distinct infarcts in the enlarged spleen were detected by technetium scanning ($^{99m}Tc=SC$). Since the hematocrit was only 16 and breathing was shallow, a unit of packed red cells was slowly infused without problems. The signs and symptoms of splenic infarction cleared, the hematocrit rose to 29, and tubal sterilization was performed.

Six months later, severe hemolytic anemia recurred when she stopped taking prednisone. Since then she has maintained an adequate hematocrit on 5 mg of prednisone twice a day.

Pregnancy-Induced Hemolytic Anemia

Unexplained hemolytic anemia in pregnancy is a rare but apparently distinct entity in which severe hemolysis develops early in pregnancy and resolves within few months after delivery. It is characterized by total absence of evidence of an immune mechanism or of any intracorpuscular or extracorpuscular defects (Starksen and co-workers, 1983). The fetus–infant may also demonstrate transient hemolysis. Corticosteroid treatment of the mother is effective. We have observed one such case during several pregnancies. In each instance, intense severe hemolytic anemia was controlled by prednisone until after delivery. The children appear to be normal.

Paroxysmal Nocturnal Hemoglobinuria

This is a rare, acquired hemolytic anemia of insidious onset and chronic course. The hemoglobinuria is not necessarily nocturnal. Hemolysis is the consequence of a defect in the red cell membrane that makes the erythrocyte unusually susceptible to lysis in vivo by complement and in vitro by acid treatment. Platelets and granulocytes are also more sensitive to lysis by complement and appear to share the cell membrane defect. The defect already exists in newly formed cells rather than its being acquired after entering the circulation.

Paroxysmal nocturnal hemoglobinuria is not familial. The disease may range from mild to lethal. Serious complications include marrow aplasia, infections, and thromboses. Except possibly for marrow transplantation, no definitive treatment exists. Heparin therapy, in general, has been disappointing. Corticosteroids may sometimes be of value. Transfusions should be limited to compatible, washed red cells. Iron loss from hemoglobinuria can be high.

There are few case reports of pregnancy complicated by paroxysmal nocturnal hemoglobinuria. Greene and co-workers (1983) and Hurd and associates (1982) have reviewed such cases and added two more. In the case of Hurd and associates, severe anemia was further complicated by skin lesions characteristic of purpura fulminans. Heparin proved of no benefit. Cesarean section was performed primarily because of maternal thrombocytopenia and demonstration of maternal platelet antibody, which caused concern for the status of platelets in the fetus. However, the infant's platelet count at birth was normal. After a stormy postpartum course that included a splenectomy, the mother survived. The pregnant woman cared for by Greene and co-workers (1983) was not so fortunate. She and her fetus succumbed.

Drug-Induced Hemolytic Anemia

Such an anemia is rarely encountered during pregnancy. Infrequently, the hemolysis results from an antibody that, in the presence of a drug such as quinine acting as a hapten, may cause lysis of erythrocytes. Especially in black women, drug-induced hemolysis may much more often be related to an inherited specific enzymatic defect of the erythrocytes, namely, severe *deficiency of glucose-6-phosphate dehydrogenase* (G6PD). There are many variants of this enzyme. The erythrocytes of about 2 percent of black women are markedly deficient in enzyme activity. In this, the homozygous state, both X chromosomes are affected. The heterozygous state, with one deficient and one normal X chromosome, occurs in 10 to 15 percent of black women and results in a modest deficiency of enzyme activity. Several oxidant drugs may induce hemolysis in homozygous women especially.

Since young erythrocytes contain more G6PD activity than do older erythrocytes, in the absence of bone marrow depression the anemia ultimately becomes stabilized and is corrected soon after the drug is discontinued.

Other Acquired Hemolytic Anemias

Overt intravascular hemolysis (visible hemoglobinemia) complicates *preeclampsia–eclampsia* very infrequently (Pritchard and co-workers, 1976). The precise cause of the fragmentation (microangiopathic) hemolysis is unknown (Chapter 27, p. 535). The most fulminant acquired hemolytic anemia encountered during pregnancy is caused by exotoxin of *Clostridium perfringens* and may prove fatal (Chapter 24, p. 488).

APLASTIC ANEMIA

Although rarely encountered during pregnancy, aplastic or hypoplastic anemia is a grave complication. The diagnosis is readily made when anemia, usually with thrombocytopenia and leukopenia, and markedly hypocellular bone marrow are demonstrated. Aplastic anemia may be congenital or acquired. Acquired forms may be induced by drugs and other chemicals, infection, irradiation, leukemia, and immunologic disorders. The basic functional defect appears to be a marked decrease in committed marrow stem cells. In most cases, apalastic anemia and pregnancy appear to have been a chance association. In a few women, however, aplastic anemia has been first identified during pregnancy and then has improved or even resolved when the pregnancy terminated, only to recur with a subsequent pregnancy.

None of the erythropoietic agents that produce remission in other anemias is effective. Corticosteroids such as prednisone are possibly of value, as are large doses of testosterone or other androgenic steroids for treating aplastic anemia. Not all of the effects from the administration of large doses of testosterone or other potent androgens during pregnancy are known. The woman almost certainly would become virilized. The female fetus would probably develop the stigmata of androgen excess (pseudohermaphroditism) depending upon the compound, the dose, and the capacity of the placenta to aromatize the androgen. Liver toxicity has been a common complication of therapy with large doses of androgens.

The treatment for severe aplastic anemia that is most likely to be effective is bone marrow transplantation. This typically requires immunosuppressive therapy for some months after infusion of marrow obtained from a histocompatible donor. Unfortunately, previous blood transfusions enhance considerably the risk of marrow graft rejection. Acute and chronic graft-versus-host disease is a serious complication following marrow transfusion. Antithymocyte globulin is probably the best available adjunctive therapy for patients who do not have a suitable marrow donor (Bayever and co-workers, 1983).

The two great risks to the woman with aplastic anemia during pregnancy are hemorrhage and infection. A continuous search for infection should be made, and if it is found, specific antibiotic therapy should be started promptly. Transfusion of granulocytes should be limited to times of actual infection. Red cell transfusions are likely to be required for symptomatic anemia. If the platelet count is very low, platelet transfusions may be needed to control hemorrhage. However, even when thrombocytopenia is intense, the risk of severe hemorrhage can be minimized by vaginal delivery, performed so as to avoid lacerations and an extensive episiotomy, plus stimulation of the myometrium to contract effectively and thereby minimize bleeding from the placental implantation site.

We have managed throughout pregnancy and the puerperium two patients with severe aplastic anemia characterized by intense pancytopenia. The mothers were transfused to maintain the maternal hemoglobin concentration between 4 and 7 g/dl, and they received large doses of prednisone throughout most of pregnancy. The pregnancies were terminated by vaginal delivery of healthy infants, one of whom has been followed personally by one of us for 21 years. He continues to appear quite healthy.

Experience with pregnancy following marrow transplantation or the use of antithymocyte globulin is limited. A few successful pregnancies after allogenic marrow transplantation have been cited by Deeg and associates (1983). An extensive review of aplastic anemia has been provided by Camitta and associates (1982).

SICKLE CELL HEMOGLOBINOPATHIES

Sickle cell anemia (SS disease), sickle cell–hemoglobin C disease (SC disease), and sickle cell–β-thalassemia disease (S-thalassemia disease) are the most common of the sickle cell hemoglobinopathies. Maternal morbidity and mortality, abortion, and perinatal mortality are appreci-

ably but not uniformly increased with all of these diseases. Therefore, the problems associated with each of the hemoglobinopathies and their management are considered separately.

Sickle Cell Anemia

The inheritance of the gene for the production of sickle, or S, hemoglobin from each parent results in sickle cell anemia (SS disease). In most communities, 1 of every 12 black individuals has the sickle cell trait, which results from inheritance of one gene for the production of S hemoglobin and one for normal hemoglobin A (Schneider and co-workers, 1976). The theoretical incidence of sickle cell anemia among blacks is 1 out of every 576 ($\frac{1}{12} \times \frac{1}{12} \times \frac{1}{4} = 576$), but the disease is usually not this common among pregnant black women. A high death rate especially during early childhood and lower parity among women with SS disease accounts for this.

Pregnancy is a serious burden to the woman with SS disease, for the anemia often becomes more intense, attacks of pain—so-called pain crises—usually become more frequent, and infections and pulmonary dysfunction are more common. In previous decades, at least, maternal mortality has been markedly elevated and nearly one half of pregnancies have terminated in abortion, stillbirth, or neonatal death (Table 28-2).

Adequate care of women with sickle cell anemia or other sickle cell hemoglobinopathies in pregnancy necessitates close observation with careful evaluation of all symptoms, physical findings, and laboratory data. One rather common danger is that the symptomatic woman may categorically be considered to be suffering from a "sickle cell crisis." As a result, ectopic pregnancy, placental abruption, pyelonephritis, and other serious obstetric problems that cause pain or anemia or both may be overlooked. The term sickle cell crisis, if used at all, should be applied only after all other possible causes of pain or reduction in hemoglobin concentration have been excluded.

In our experience, in the absence of infection or nutritional deficiency, the hemoglobin concentration does not fall much below 7 g/dl, a level at or above which pregnant women with sickle cell anemia usually have no

TABLE 28-2. PREGNANCY OUTCOMES REPORTED SINCE 1956 FOR 231 WOMEN WITH SICKLE CELL ANEMIA PREGNANT 511 TIMES AND NOT TRANSFUSED PROPHYLACTICALLY

Maternal Deaths	Spontaneous Abortions	Perinatal Deaths
4,620 per 100,000 births	19.8%	214 per 1000 births

(*Data provided by Milner et al.: Am J Obstet Gynecol 138:239, 1980; Carache et al.: Obstet Gynecol 55:407, 1980.*)

symptoms attributable to low levels of hemoglobin. Since these women maintain their hemoglobin concentration by intense erythropoiesis to compensate for the markedly shortened life span of the erythrocytes, any factor that impairs erythropoiesis or increases destruction of erythrocytes or both aggravates the anemia. The folic acid requirements during pregnancy complicated by sickle cell anemia are considerable. Since the dietary intake of folic acid may be inadequate, especially during episodes of anorexia induced or enhanced by pain, supplementary folic acid is usually indicated; the ingestion of 1 mg per day is adequate.

Labor with SS disease should be managed essentially the same way as for cardiac disease. The woman should be kept comfortable but not oversedated. In all cases, compatible blood should be readily available. If a difficult vaginal delivery or cesarean section is contemplated, the hemoglobin concentration should be raised toward 10 g/dl by careful administration of packed erythrocytes. Exchange transfusion, as described below, may be more beneficial. With any form of transfusion therapy, care must be taken to prevent circulatory overload with heart failure and pulmonary edema. Oxygen therapy should be instituted during times of increased oxygen need.

Intense sequestration of sickled erythrocytes may occur acutely, especially late in pregnancy, during labor and delivery, and early in the puerperium. Dangerous anemia can rapidly appear as a consequence and is accompanied by an increase in the size of the liver and spleen, unless the spleen has been destroyed previously by infarction and fibrosis. The acute sequestration is usually accompanied by severe bone pain. Whenever the hemoglobin spontaneously dropped below 6.0 g/dl or decreased at a rate of 2 g or more per 24 hours, Hendrickse and Watson-Williams (1966) recommended exchange transfusion with donor red cells known to contain only hemoglobin A. It is our impression that such a decrease can result from increased red cell destruction and simultaneously marked inhibition of red cell production.

Hendrickse and Watson-Williams (1966) and some others have also advocated heparin therapy in women with sickle cell anemia who developed severe bone pain during late pregnancy or the puerperium. However, the benefits to be derived from heparin in this circumstance have not been established. Dextran infusion was originally claimed to reduce bone pain and marrow infarction, but a well-controlled study subsequently failed to demonstrate any benefit over that provided by hydration with aqueous glucose solution (Barnes and co-workers, 1965). Liberal hydration appears to be of value prophylactically, reducing the frequency and intensity of attacks of pain.

For severe pain, use of potent analgesics, such as meperidine administered parenterally, is certainly indicated. In our experience, the risk of addiction under these circumstances is remarkably low. Red cell transfusions administered after the onset of severe pain, again

in our experience, have no dramatic effect on the intensity or the duration of the attack of pain, whereas prophylactic red cell transfusions before the pain developed have almost eliminated such pain crises (p. 571).

Because of the chronic debility from sickle cell anemia, the additional complications caused by pregnancy, and the predictably shortened life span of women with sickle cell anemia, sterilization or a least a very effective means of contraception is indicated, even for women of low parity. Oral contraceptives in the form of estrogen-progestin combinations probably are contraindicated in women with SS disease, since erythrocyte sequestration and vascular occlusion inherent in the disease might be intensified. Infection as the consequence of an intrauterine device would likely prove much more dangerous than in an otherwise healthy woman.

Sickle Cell–Hemoglobin C Disease

Although about 1 out of 12 American blacks possesses the gene for production of hemoglobin S, only about 1 in 40 has the gene for hemoglobin C. Therefore, the probability of this genetic combination in a black couple is about 1 in 500, and the probability of their child's inheriting the gene for hemoglobin S and an allelic gene for hemoglobin C is 1 in 4. As the consequence of these genetic frequencies, about 1 out of every 2000 ($\frac{1}{12} \times \frac{1}{40} \times \frac{1}{4}$) pregnant black women can be expected to have sickle cell–hemoglobin C, or SC, disease, barring any significant mortality either before or during the years of reproductivity or an appreciable reduction in fertility, pathologic or voluntary.

In nonpregnant women, morbidity from the sickle cell–hemoglobin C disease is appreciably lower than from sickle cell anemia, and life span is longer. During pregnancy and the puerperium, however, maternal morbidity and mortality are increased considerably. Attacks of severe bone pain and episodes of serious pulmonary dysfunction are much more likely during these times. The pulmonary dysfunction appears to be related commonly to embolization of necrotic bone marrow, both fat and cellular components.

In an 18-year anterospective study at Parkland Memorial Hospital, the maternal mortality rate for a relatively large series of pregnancies in women with sickle cell–hemoglobin C disease was close to 2 percent, and one out of eight pregnancies resulted in abortion, stillbirth, or neonatal death. Thus, the perinatal mortality rate was somewhat greater than that of the general population but not nearly as great as with sickle cell anemia (Pritchard and co-workers, 1973). However, high maternal mortality was a serious problem, a tragic feature that has been observed by others (Table 28-3).

As in other pregnancies complicated by overt hemolytic anemia, the need for metabolically active forms of folic acid in women with sickle cell–hemoglobin C disease is increased, especially when anorexia is present. Iron deficiency can occur during pregnancy, unless the

TABLE 28-3. PREGNANCY OUTCOMES REPORTED SINCE 1956 FOR 211 WOMEN WITH SICKLE CELL–HEMOGLOBIN C DISEASE PREGNANT 605 TIMES AND NOT TRANSFUSED PROPHYLACTICALLY

Maternal Deaths	Spontaneous Abortions	Perinatal Deaths
2,514 per 100,000 births	14.6%	77 per 1000 births

(*Data provided by Milner et al.: Am J Obstet Gynecol 138:239, 1980; Carache et al.: Obstet Gynecol 55:407, 1980.*)

mother has received transfusions previously. Therefore, supplementation not only with folic acid but also with iron is likely to be of benefit unless red cell transfusions have been used previously or are contemplated. Whenever the hemoglobin concentration drops below 8.0 g/dl, a thorough search for the cause or causes is essential. The guidelines we used for simple red cell transfusion to correct anemia are similar to those stated above for sickle cell anemia.

To date, maternal morbidity, especially pain and respiratory insufficiency, has been appreciably less in women with sickle cell–hemoglobin C disease who have been transfused prophylactically as described below.

The frequency of morbidity and the relatively high mortality rate during late pregnancy and the puerperium in women with sickle cell–hemoglobin C disease warrant limitation of family size.

Sickle Cell–β-Thalassemia Disease

The inheritance of the gene for hemoglobin S from one parent and the allelic gene for β-thalassemia from the other results in sickle cell–β-thalassemia disease. Our experience with 37 pregnancies implies that the perinatal mortality and morbidity of this disease are similar to those of sickle cell–hemoglobin C disease (Pritchard and colleagues, 1973). The frequencies of maternal morbidity and mortality perhaps are somewhat less, although maternal mortalities have been observed in association with pregnancy (Morrison and associates, 1972). Our recommendations for general prenatal care, labor, and delivery and the restriction on future pregnancies are similar for sickle cell–thalassemia, sickle cell–hemoglobin C disease, and sickle cell anemia.

Prophylactic Transfusion in Pregnancies Complicated by Sickle Hemoglobinopathies

We continue to transfuse prophylactically during pregnancy women with sickle cell anemia, sickle cell–hemoglobin C disease, or sickle cell–β-thalassemia disease:

At the outset, once the diagnoses of pregnancy and a sickle cell hemoglobinopathy were confirmed, recently collected packed red cells that contained no abnormal hemoglobin were transfused in amounts and frequencies sufficient to reduce and maintain the percentage of red cells that contained hemoglobin S to no more than 60 percent and to keep the hematocrit at 25 or higher as described in detail elsewhere (Cunningham and Pritchard, 1979). (Essentially 100 percent of red cells that contain hemoglobin S will sickle when treated for 1 hour with fresh, isotonic sodium metabisulfite solution sealed between a glass slide and coverslip. An alternative to differential counting of red cells so treated is to separate electrophoretically the S hemoglobin and determine the percentage using a densitometer.)

When the hematocrit was low, as is commonly the case with sickle cell anemia, most often simple transfusions of packed red cells were carefully administered after stimulating a brisk diuresis by giving furosemide, 50 mg, intravenously. When the hematocrit was higher, as it commonly is with SC or S-thalassemia disease, exchange transfusion was commonly employed (Cunningham and Pritchard, 1979). More recently, prophylactic transfusion has not been initiated in women with SC disease or S-thalassemia disease until near the end of the second trimester, since the mothers seldom developed serious debility before that time.

Among the more than 60 cases of sickle hemoglobinopathy so managed, maternal mortality has been zero and maternal morbidity from the sickle hemoglobinopathy has been minimal. The degree of relief from chronically debilitating sickle cell anemia that was provided one woman by transfusion with normal cells during pregnancy is apparent in Figure 28-3.

When maternal morbidity and perinatal mortality for pregnancies in which women were transfused prophylactically were compared to those cared for by us without prophylactic transfusions, a dramatic difference in favor of transfusion prophylaxis was evident (Cunningham and co-workers, 1983). Pregnancy wastage with prophylactic transfusions was limited to one spontaneous abortion very soon after initiation of transfusion therapy and one stillbirth. The stillbirth was associated with fulminant preeclampsia and heart failure in a woman with sickle cell anemia.

Even though there was, at times, worrisome evidence of a compromised intrauterine environment in the form of fetal growth retardation, meconium staining of amnionic fluid, and during labor ominous decelerations of the fetal heart rate, perinatal mortality was remarkably low when compared to previous experiences.

Morbidity from the transfusions has proved troublesome, especially from complications such as alloimmunization and hepatitis. Further transfusion can be anticipated to enhance these complications and to create new ones, especially iron overload and its sequelae. Therefore, we have concluded tentatively that during one pregnancy the mother with sickle cell hemoglobinopathy and her fetus are likely to benefit from prophylactic transfusions of normal donor red cells administered according to the protocol described. Most of the more recently published data concerned with pregnancy wastage and maternal morbidity and mortality as the consequence of a sickle hemoglobinopathy with and without prophylactic transfusion during pregnancy would appear

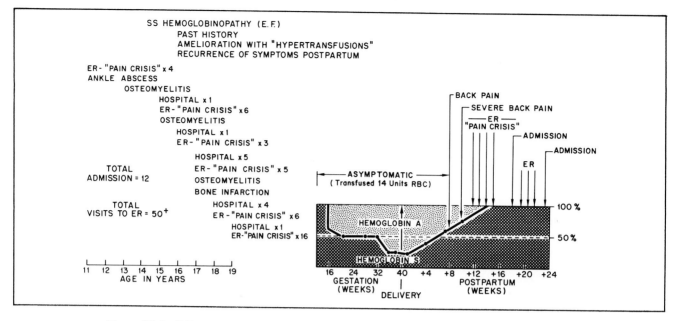

Figure 28-3. E.F., sickle cell anemia. Debility before her first pregnancy is summarized on the left. To the right, the reduction in hemoglobin S level as the consequence of tranfusion of 14 units of packed red cells, and the recurrence of severe pain 9 weeks after delivery are emphasized (ER = Emergency Room). (*From Cunningham, Pritchard. Am J Obstet Gynecol 135:994, 1979.*)

to support this conclusion, even though some individuals who have provided apparently supportive data have concluded otherwise (J. Miller and associates, 1981).

Serious consideration should be given to a number of techniques that can be applied to reduce the adverse effects of transfusions. These include use of red cells that are (1) fresh from the donor, (2) compatible for troublesome minor blood groups, (3) obtained from volunteer donors to reduce the risk of hepatitis, (4) washed to reduce reactions, and (5) predominantly young and therefore capable of surviving longer in the recipient. Young red cells are readily provided by a donor who undergoes frequent phlebotomy and takes iron. Younger donor erythrocytes can be separated to a degree from older red cells by centrifugation, which takes advantage of the lower density of young red cells.

The following biophysical and physiologic changes induced in blood by substituting normal red cells for red cells of sickle cell anemia are of interest: When subjected to reduced oxygen tension, the viscosity of blood containing mixtures of normal red cells and those of sickle cell anemia decreases remarkably, especially as the percentage of normal cells reaches and exceeds the percentage of hemoglobin S-containing cells (Murphy and co-workers, 1976). This phenomenon in vivo would likely affect the microcirculation in a beneficial way. Moreover, D. Miller and associates (1980) have studied exercise performance in subjects with sickle cell anemia before and after exchange transfusion and identified appreciable improvement in work performance following replacement of 50 percent of the abnormal

cells by normal red cells even though the degree of anemia remained essentially unchanged.

Sickle Cell Trait

The inheritance of the gene for the production of S hemoglobin from one parent and for A hemoglobin from the other results in sickle cell trait. In this circumstance, the amount of S hemoglobin produced is distinctly less than the amount of A hemoglobin. The frequency of red cell sickling among black individuals is about 1 in 12 or 8.5 percent. Erythrocytes in smears of blood from women with sickle cell trait usually appear normal unless the blood has previously been markedly depleted of oxygen to produce sickled forms.

Extensive studies of the effect, or lack of effect, of sickle cell trait on pregnancy have been reported (Whalley and associates, 1964; Pritchard and associates, 1973; Tuck and co-workers, 1983). Sickle cell trait did not influence unfavorably the frequency of abortion, perinatal mortality, low birth weight, or pregnancy-induced hypertension. Infection of the urinary tract, however, was about twice as common in the group with sickle cell trait, and further investigations disclosed that twice as many pregnant women with sickle cell trait had asymptomatic bacteriuria as did black women whose erythrocytes did not sickle.

Sickle cell trait should not be considered a deterrent to pregnancy on the basis of increased risks to the mother. Identification and elimination of bacteriuria should avoid the increased risk of pyelonephritis. However, the probability for a debilitating sickle cell hemoglobinopathy in her offspring is one in four whenever the father carries one gene for the production of an abnormal hemoglobin or for β-thalassemia.

Hemoglobin C, C-Thalassemia Diseases, and C-Trait

About 2.5 percent of the black population possesses the gene for hemoglobin C production. Pregnancy and homozygous hemoglobin C disease or hemoglobin C–β-thalassemia disease appear to be rather benign associations (Cunningham and Pritchard, unpublished; Smith and Krevans, 1959). The anemia is usually mild. If severe, it is likely to be the consequence of folic acid or iron deficiency or some other superimposed cause. Supplementation routinely with folic acid and with iron, unless iron is provided by transfusion, is likely to prove of value in pregnant women with any hemoglobinopathy. In our experience, hemoglobin C trait does not predispose to pathologic pregnancies.

Hemoglobin E

Substitution of a single specific amino acid in both β-globin chains gives rise to hemoglobin E. This hemoglobin has become prevalent in the United States since the arrival of a large number of Southeast Asians. Hurst and co-workers (1983), for example, identified homozygous hemoglobin E, hemoglobin E plus α-thalassemia or β-thalassemia, or hemoglobin E trait in 36 percent of Cambodian children and 25 percent of Laotians, but in only 1 percent of Vietnamese; α- and β-thalassemia traits were prevalent in all groups.

The homozygous state for hemoglobin E is characterized by mild anemia even though red cell microcytosis is marked and targeting is common. Pregnancies in women homozygous for hemoglobin E do not appear to be at increased risk as the consequence of this clinically mild hemoglobinopathy. It is not clear at this time whether sickle cell–hemoglobin E disease is as ominous during pregnancy as is sickle cell–hemoglobin C disease.

Anemia from iron deficiency as the consequence of gastrointestinal parasites, repeated pregnancies, or both, has coexisted with the hemoglobin E hemoglobinopathy. We are providing supplements of folic acid as well as iron for pregnant women identified to have homozygous hemoglobin E or hemoglobin E–thalassemia diseases.

Hemoglobinopathy in Newborn

The hemolytic anemia characteristic of these hemoglobinopathies is not operational in utero or at birth, since most of the hemoglobin in the red blood cells is fetal (F) hemoglobin. After birth, as more and more newly synthesized red cells contain more and more abnormal hemoglobin, the disease becomes clinically apparent.

Newborn infants with sickle cell anemia, sickle cell–hemoglobin C disease, and homozygous hemoglobin C disease can be accurately identified at birth by electrophoresis performed on hemoglobin obtained from uncontaminted cord blood using cellulose acetate support medium and buffer at pH 8.4 plus citrate agar gel and buffer at pH 6.0 (Nussbaum and co-workers, 1984).

Genetic Counseling

Identification of the more common hemoglobinopathies and their trait forms involves relatively simple laboratory procedures, and the genetic aspects of these diseases are straightforward. Therefore, genetic counseling can be readily provided. One out of every four children, on the average, will be afflicted with the disease whenever both parents have a trait form, as pointed out above. If one parent has the hemoglobinopathy and the other only the trait form, one half of their children can be expected to inherit the hemoglobinopathy and the other half the trait form. If both parents have a hemoglobinopathy, so will all their children.

Remarkable technical advances have been made for identifying the fetus who is genetically destined to develop sickle cell disease, especially sickle cell anemia. Earlier procedures required the collection of fetal red cells by fetoscope or placental aspiration; the capabilities of these red cells for synthesizing abnormal globin β-chains were then measured in vitro. Unfortunately, fetal loss as the consequence of obtaining fetal blood has been 3 to 5 percent. It was next demonstrated that amniocytes cultured from amnionic fluid could be treated with a restriction endonuclease enzyme that would cleave DNA into fragments that, at first by linkage analysis and subsequently by direct analysis of the fragments, would serve to identify prenatally most or all fetuses who were destined to develop sickle cell anemia. An assay has been developed that is so sensitive that restriction endonuclease enzyme MstII can be applied immediately to cells obtained from 10 to 20 ml of amnionic fluid without prior culture, thereby avoiding the delay that had been imposed by need for cell culture (Chang and Kan, 1982; Orkin and co-workers, 1982).

Hemoglobin C cannot be identified using the enzyme MstII, but hemoglobin C and most instances of β-thalassemia can be identified by analysis of DNA polymorphism or by identifying in vitro the kinds of globin chains synthesized by fetal red cells obtained from the fetus or placenta. The usefulness of DNA polymorphisms in circumstances where the inheritance of these diseases cannot be determined directly is borne out by the experiences of Boehm and associates (1983).

A sample of chorionic villus obtained by aspiration biopsy using a cannula passed transcervically with the guidance of real time sonography during the first trimester has been used to identify the embryo or fetus genetically predisposed to sickle cell anemia or β-thalassemia. DNA extracted from the trophoblast without prior culture was treated with an appropriate restriction enzyme (Old and associates, 1982; Ward and associates, 1983). The extent of jeopardy from biopsy of trophoblast and the precision of diagnosis are not yet known.

HEREDITARY SPHEROCYTOSIS

Hereditary spherocytosis is characterized clinically by varying degrees of anemia and jaundice as the consequence of hemolysis of microspherocytic red cells. Hereditary spherocytosis is usually considered to be transmitted as an autosomal dominant trait with a variable degree of penetrance of the gene, or, possibly, multiple closely linked genes are essential for clinically apparent gene expression. Severe, recessively inherited spherocytosis has been described (Agre and co-workers, 1982).

Hemolysis and, in turn, severe anemia are dependent upon an intact spleen, which is usually enlarged. Splenectomy, while not correcting the red cell microspherocytosis or the increased osmotic fragility, does greatly reduce hemolysis and, in turn, the anemia and jaundice. So-called crises, characterized by severe anemia from accelerated red cell destruction or more likely failure of production, or both, may occur in the woman with a functioning spleen. A previously normal pregnancy does not rule out the sudden development of severe anemia in a subsequent pregnancy (Ventura, 1982). Folic acid supplementation avoids the risk of megaloblastic erythropoiesis and impaired red cell production.

The newborn infant who has inherited hereditary spherocytosis may or may not demonstrate hyperbilirubinemia and anemia during the neonatal period. We have observed the hemoglobin level to fall to as low as 5.0 g/dl by 5 weeks of age in the daughter of a woman with hereditary spherocytosis who became symptomatic during pregnancy.

THALASSEMIAS

The genetically determined hematologic disorders that are classified as thalassemias are characterized by impaired rate of production of one or more of the peptide chains that are normal components of globin. The various forms of thalassemias are classified according to the globin chain that is deficient in amount compared to its partner chain. The two major forms of thalassemias involve either impaired production of α-peptide chains causing α-thalassemia, or of β-chains to cause β-thalassemia.

α-Thalassemias

Four clinical syndromes, the consequence of impaired α-globin chain synthesis, have been identified. For each syndrome a close correlation has been established between clinical severity and the degree of impairment of synthesis of α-globin chains. In most populations the α-globin chain gene loci are duplicated on chromosome 16, and thus the normal genotype for diploid cells can be expressed as $\alpha\alpha/\alpha\alpha$. There are two α-thalassemia genotypes: α-thalassemia-1 is characterized by the deletion of both loci from one chromosome $(-/-)$, whereas α-thalassemia-2 is characterized by the loss of a single locus $(-/\alpha)$.

The deletion of all of the α-globin chain genes $(--/--)$ characterizes homozygous α-thalassemia or *hemoglobin Bart's disease*. Deletion of three of the four genes $(--/-+)$, i.e., there is only one functional α-gene per diploid genome, typifies *hemoglobin H disease*. α-Thalassemia minor is the consequence of deletion of any two of the four α-globin chain genes $(-+/-+$ or $--/++)$, while the deletion of a single α-globin chain gene $(-+/++)$ is responsible for the silent carrier state.

In the homozygous form of α-thalassemia no α-globin chains are produced. The hemoglobin in the fetus consists chiefly of hemoglobin Bart's, the globin of which is made up of four γ-chains rather than the two α and two γ-chains that characterize normal hemoglobin F. Hemoglobin Bart's has an appreciably increased affinity for oxygen. The fetus dies in utero or very soon after birth and demonstrates the typical clinical features of nonimmune hydrops fetalis (Chapter 38, p. 779).

The deletion of three genes is compatible with extrauterine life; the condition is referred to as hemoglobin H disease. The abnormal red cells at birth contain a mixture of hemoglobin Bart's, hemoglobin H (4 β-globin chains), and hemoglobin A. Hemoglobin H disease is characterized by a hemolytic anemia of varying severity and is usually accentuated during pregnancy. The neonate appears well at birth, but as early infancy passes he develops a hemolytic anemia. Most, if not all, of the 20 to 40 percent of hemoglobin Bart's present at birth is replaced by hemoglobin H postnatally.

A deletion of two genes results in α-thalassemia minor, which is characterized by minimal to moderate hypochromic microcytic anemia. Because there is no associated clinical abnormality with α-thalassemia minor, it is often unrecognized. Red cells are hypochromic and microcytic; the hemoglobin concentration is normal to slightly depressed. Women with α-thalassemia minor appear to tolerate pregnancy quite well.

No abnormality is evident in the individual with a single gene deletion.

The relative frequency of α-thalassemia minor, hemoglobin H disease, and hemoglobin Bart's disease varies remarkably among racial groups. All of these variants are encountered in Orientals. However, in individuals of African descent, even though α-thalassemia minor occurs in about 2 percent, hemoglobin H disease is extremely rare, and hemoglobin Bart's disease is unreported. The reason for the discrepancy is that in Orientals with α-thalassemia minor, both gene deletions are typically from the same chromosome $(--/++)$, whereas in blacks with α-thalassemia minor, one gene is deleted from each chromosome $(-+/-+)$. The α-thalassemia syndromes appear sporadically in other racial and ethnic groups.

The simultaneous inheritance of α-thalassemia and sickle cell anemia appears to provide appreciable protection against the ravages so common otherwise in individuals afflicted with SS disease.

β-Thalassemias

Similar to the α-thalassemias, the β-thalassemias are the consequence of impaired globin chain synthesis. The specific defect is impaired production of β-globin chains rather than α-globin chains. The defect accounting for the defective production is not clear but appears to be not the loss of a specific gene or genes but rather a reduction in messenger RNA that codes for β-globin chains. A variety of β-thalassemias has been described.

A deficiency in globin chain synthesis has two important consequences: (1) There is a decrease in the rate of hemoglobin production, and (2) when there is globin chain imbalance, precipitation of the excess globin chain damages the cell membrane, which leads to intense hemolysis. These basic defects lead to the panorama of pathology that characterizes homozygous β-thalassemia (β-thalassemia major, Cooley's anemia). With β-thalassemia minor, a heterozygous state, hypochromia, microcytosis, and slight to moderate anemia exist without the intense hemolysis that characterizes the homozygous state.

In the typical case of β-thalassemia major, the infant appears healthy at birth, but as the hemoglobin F level falls, he becomes severely anemic and fails to thrive. Those females who do survive beyond childhood are often sterile.

With β-thalassemia minor, A$_2$ hemoglobin (comprised of two α and two δ-globin chains) is increased (> 3.5 percent), and hemoglobin F (two α and two γ-globin chains) may be somewhat elevated (> 2.0 percent). The red cells are hypochromic and microcytic, but the anemia is mild.

During pregnancy the hemoglobin concentration in women with β-thalassemia minor is typically 8 to 10 g/dl late in the second trimester, with an increase to between 9 and 11 g/dl near term, as compared with a hemoglobin level of 10 to 12 g/dl in the nonpregnant state (Alger and colleagues, 1979; Freedman, 1969; Pritchard 1962a). There is augmentation of erythropoiesis during pregnancy similar to that of normal women.

There is no specific therapy for β-thalassemia minor during pregnancy. Most often, the outcome for the mother and fetus is satisfactory (Pritchard, 1962a; Smith and associates, 1975; Cooley and Kitay, 1984). Blood transfusions are very seldom indicated except if there is hemorrhage. Iron and folic acid prophylactically, in daily doses of 30 to 60 mg of iron and 1 mg of folic acid, may be of value. Any disease that depresses the function of the bone marrow or increases destruction of erythrocytes naturally intensifies the anemia. Infections, therefore,

should be promptly identified and adequately treated. The modest anemia, when not correctly diagnosed, has led to overzealous treatment especially with parenteral iron and at times with blood transfusions. The potential exists, of course, for the fetus to have inherited the serious problem of β-thalassemia major or sickle cell–β-thalassemia. Techniques for identifying these entities in utero have been discussed (p. 573).

The term β-thalassemia intermedia has been applied to the clinical condition of individuals whose disease was nowhere near as intense as with β-thalassemia major but obviously was more severe than that of β-thalassemia minor. Weatherall and co-workers (1981) have identified in some such individuals, at least, the loss of a single α-globin gene that appeared to have favorably modified homozygous β-thalassemia from a severe transfusion-dependent state into the much milder thalassemia intermedia.

THROMBOCYTOPENIAS

Thrombocytopenia may appear clinically to be idiopathic or, more often, to be associated with one of the following disorders: aplastic anemia, acquired hemolytic anemia, eclampsia or severe preeclampsia, consumptive coagulopathy related to placental abruption or similar hypofibrinogenemic states, lupus erythematosus. megaloblastic anemia caused by severe folate deficiency, drugs, infections, allergies, or excessive irradiation.

Immune (Idiopathic) Thrombocytopenia

The entity long referred to as idiopathic thrombocytopenic purpura is the consequence of an immune process in which antibodies against platelets are the culprits. Antibody-coated platelets are destroyed prematurely by macrophages, especially in the spleen. The mechanism of production of antibodies against platelets is not known. It is usually considered to be an autoantibody but has not been proven to be one. Familial occurrence is virtually unknown.

Splenectomy performed on women with symptomatic immune thrombocytopenia frequently results in significant improvement as the consequence of decreased removal of platelets by the spleen and reduced antibody production. Corticosteroid therapy often proves beneficial by increasing the platelet count and perhaps decreasing capillary fragility. Immunosuppressive drugs have also been used with some success in cases refractory to corticosteroids and splenectomy.

Pregnancy is especially challenging to women with immune thrombocytopenia and to their fetuses and newborn infants. Pregnancy appears to increase the risk of relapse in women previously in remission and to make the condition worse in women with active disease. It is not unusual for women who have been in clinical remission for several years to relapse during pregnancy. The reason or reasons for the deleterious effects of pregnancy

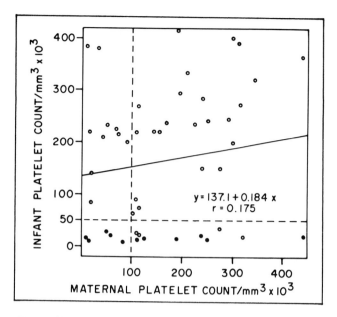

Figure 28-4. Pregnancies complicated by immune thrombocytopenic purpura. Lack of a strong correlation between maternal and newborn infant platelet counts is apparent. (*From Scott et al.: Am J Obstet Gynecol 145:932, 1983.*)

are not known, but hyperestrogenemia has been suspected.

There is no strong contraindication to the use of corticosteroids, such as prednisone, during pregnancy. Large doses may be required for improvement, and most likely treatment will have to be continued for the rest of the pregnancy. When corticosteroid therapy fails to achieve adequate amelioration, splenectomy, if not already accomplished, can be performed. Late in pregnancy the procedure is technically more difficult because of encroachment of the large uterus into the operative field. Cesarean section may be necessary to improve exposure. At the same time, the fetus who may be severely thrombocytopenic avoids the risk of trauma from labor and vaginal delivery.

IgG antibodies are formed in immune thrombocytopenia. IgG antibodies can cross the placenta and cause thrombocytopenia in the fetus and neonate. The severely thrombocytopenic fetus is at increased risk of serious hemorrhage, especially intracranial hemorrhage, as the consequence of labor and delivery.

Considerable attention has been given to the problem of identifying the fetus with potentially dangerous thrombocytopenia. It is evident in Figure 28-4 that there is not a strong correlation between the platelet count in the fetus and in the mother who now has or previously had autoimmune thrombocytopenic purpura. Unfortunately, the conclusion of Karpatkan and associates (1981) that the administration of corticosteroids to the mother assures a platelet count in the fetus–infant adequate for hemostasis during labor and delivery is incorrect. It cannot be substantiated by either the findings

demonstrated by the infant shown in Figure 28-5 and described below or by observations of Cines and associates (1982), Kelton and associates (1982), and Scott and co-workers (1983).

Cines and associates, investigating the relationship, if any, between the levels of maternal IgG circulating platelet antibody, platelet-associated antibody, and the fetal platelet count, reported that monitoring circulating platelet antibody, but not platelet-associated antibody, may help identify a fetus with severe thrombocytopenia. However, Kelton and associates (1982) reported that measurement of platelet-associated antibody could be used to predict thrombocytopenia in the fetus. Scott and co-workers (1983) found neither to be of special value and concluded that no antepartum maternal clinical characteristic or laboratory test tried so far would accurately predict the fetal platelet count. They urge the use, intrapartum, of platelet counts made on blood obtained from the fetal scalp once the cervix is 2 to 3 cm dilated and the membranes are ruptured. (The technique for scalp sampling is described in Chapter 14, p. 288.) Whenever the platelet count in scalp blood was identified to be less than 50,000/mm³, they performed immediate cesarean section. Unfortunately, cesarean section without labor does not provide absolute assurance that the fetus–infant will not hemorrhage as the consequence of severe thrombocytopenia, as exemplified by the infant in Figure 28-5 and described below:

> The multiparous mother was troubled intermittently for several years by thrombocytopenia even though she had undergone splenectomy as a youth. A previous infant bled profusely following circumcision and then was documented to be severely thrombocytopenic. The mother again became severely thrombocytopenic during her last pregnancy. The thrombocytopenia responded well to prednisone, and her platelet count was 130,000 at the time of delivery. Because of the possibility that the fetus might be thrombocytopenic and her desire for sterilization, it was elected to effect delivery by cesarean section. This was accomplished with no serious problems for the mother. However, the infant demonstrated large, expanding cephalohematomas over the occipital bone and both parietal bones, the region of the infant's head that was touched by the operator's hand to lift the head through the uterine and abdominal incisions. The platelet count was 17,000 in cord blood and dropped promptly to as low as 3000 per mm³. Treatment consisted of corticosteroids, platelet transfusions, and exchange transfusions in desperate attempts to remove platelet antibody. The infant survived the hemorrhage and the treatment.

For the mother with an adequate stable platelet count and not taking corticosteroids, cesarean section is unlikely to be of any more risk than it is for the normal woman. The administration of larger doses of steroids increases the risks somewhat of poor wound healing and infection.

The obstetrician faces the dilemma that in delivery what may be best for the fetus–infant is likely to be bad for the mother if the mother has severe thrombocyto-

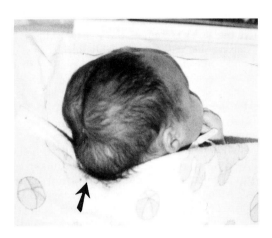

Figure 28-5. Newborn infant with extensive cephalohematomas, especially over the occipital bone (*arrow*). The mother had chronic idiopathic (immune) thrombocytopenic purpura, which was treated with prednisone. Her platelet count at the time of cesarean section was 115,000 per mm^3; the infant's count was as low as 3000 per mm^3.

penia at the time of the operation. Unfortunately, the mother with severe thrombocytopenia who undergoes cesarean section is at appreciably increased risk of serious morbidity and even mortality. It can be anticipated with cesarean section that blood loss commonly will be severe. Moreover, troublesome hematomas prone to infection are common. Platelet transfusions most often prove ineffective, since donor platelets are attacked by antibody and rapidly cleared from the circulation. On the other hand, blood loss at and after vaginal delivery is unlikely to be massive when delivery is so managed as to avoid lacerations, to minimize episiotomy size, and to maximize myometrial contraction and retraction.

In some instances where other accepted treatment modalities had failed to correct dangerous thrombocytopenia, yet life-threatening hemorrhage had developed or extensive surgery needed to be performed, high-dose intravenous polyvalent immunoglobulin therapy has been cited by some as being beneficial. The responses noted have varied from a marked increase in the platelet count within a few days after initiating treatment, with the increase persisting after treatment was stopped, to little or no change in platelet count (Bierling and co-workers, 1982; Carroll and associates, 1983; Fehr and associates, 1982). Blanchette and co-workers (1983) cite evidence that supports reticuloendothelial blockade as the mechanism by which intravenous IgG therapy can increase the platelet count.

The efficacy, if any, of high-dose gamma globulin for correcting severe thrombocytopenia during pregnancy is not known. It is possible that the risk from thrombocytopenia to the fetus–infant, as well as to the mother,

could be reduced appreciably by the administration of this material to the mother with, in turn, placental transfer of IgG to the fetus.

Recently, danazol, a synthetic weak androgen, has been reported to be effective in some cases of idiopathic thrombocytopenic purpura in which splenectomy was ineffective, corticosteroids were ineffective or caused troublesome adverse effects, and vinca alkaloids or colchicine were of no benefit (Ahn and co-workers, 1983). Virilization of the female fetus has been observed when danazol was administered to the mother during pregnancy (Rosa, 1984).

Effective contraception for women with immune thrombocytopenia is desirable. Tubal sterilization meticulously performed at the time of cesarean section should not increase blood loss appreciably. When tubal sterilization is done postpartum or remote from pregnancy, the risk of morbidity relates to the platelet count. Since autoimmune thrombocytopenia is most common in women of reproductive age and often intensifies during pregnancy, estrogen has been implicated in its pathogenesis. Even so, such guilt by association would not appear to negate the advantages of the highly effective contraception and reduced menstrual blood loss that can be achieved with estrogen plus progestin oral contraceptives. An intrauterine device in the presence of thrombocytopenia is likely to enhance appreciably bleeding from the uterus.

Isoimmune thrombocytopenia in the fetus and newborn infant is considered in Chapter 38 (p. 783).

Thrombotic Thrombocytopenic Purpura

This rare entity is characterized by the pentad of thrombocytopenia, fever, neurologic abnormalities, renal impairment, and hemolytic anemia. The classic histologic lesions of thrombotic thrombocytopenic purpura are thrombi consisting mostly of platelets and some fibrin. Throughout the body short segments of arterioles and capillaries are variably occluded by hyaline material that consists mostly of platelet thrombi plus small amounts of fibrin. These characteristic lesions can be identified in biopsy material, for example, from the gingiva.

Neither the precise pathogenesis of the disease nor the mechanisms by which cure is now often achieved are understood at this time. One hypothesis is that a missing plasma factor, which somehow inhibits platelet aggregation, is infused into the patient while an abnormal circulating platelet aggregating factor is removed. As with many vascular phenomena, abnormal production and destruction of prostacyclin and thromboxanes have also been implicated.

The transfusion of platelets appears to make the disease much worse (Harkness and co-workers, 1981). The use of exchange transfusion, transfusion with normal plasma, and plasmapheresis, usually in combination, have improved remarkably the outcome of this once rapidly and highly fatal disease. Frequently, along with these modalities, antiplatelet agents, especially aspirin, and dipyridamole, or dextran 70, have been used in cases with a favorable outcome. Fatality rates have dropped from about 90 percent to about 10 percent.

Only a few dozen cases of thrombotic thrombocytopenic purpura complicating pregnancy appear to have been described (Atlas and associates, 1982). Until recently, at least, most of the mothers, fetuses, and infants died.

Eclampsia complicated further by thrombocytopenia, overt intravascular hemolysis causing hemoglobinemia, and hemoglobinuria has been confused with thrombotic thrombocytopenic purpura. The eclampsia syndrome just described is not characterized by diffuse thrombus formation as is thrombotic thrombocytopenic purpura (Pritchard and associates, 1954; Thiagarajah and co-workers, 1981). Most important, prompt delivery with supportive care appropriate for eclampsia, as described in Chapter 27 (p. 547), results in the remarkably rapid disappearance of evidence of hemolysis and severe thrombocytopenia followed by complete recovery.

It is not evident whether pregnancy worsens the prognosis for thrombotic thrombocytopenic purpura nor if termination of the pregnancy improves the prognosis. Unless the diagnosis is thrombotic thrombocytopenic purpura unequivocally, rather than severe preeclampsia or eclampsia, the response to prompt termination of the pregnancy should be evaluated before resorting to exchange transfusion, plasmapheresis, and antiplatelet drug therapy. Even though Haesslein and associates (1983) imply that maternal mortality is high for severe preeclampsia complicated by hemolysis and thrombocytopenia and therefore recommend plasmapheresis, in our experience, as stated above, prompt delivery with appropriate supportive care is followed by gratifying amelioration of all these stigmata.

INHERITED COAGULATION DEFECTS

Obstetric hemorrhage, a common event, is rarely the consequence of an inherited defect in the coagulation mechanism.

Hemophilia A

This disease, which is characterized by a marked deficiency of small component antihemophilic factor (factor VIII:C), is rare among women as compared to men. With few exceptions, the homozygous state, i.e., the inheritance of two abnormal X chromosomes, is the requisite for classic hemophilia A in women, whereas one affected X chromosome, the hemizygous state, is responsible for the disease in men. In a few instances hemophilia A appears to have developed in women spontaneously, presumably as the consequence of a newly mutant gene.

The degree of risk of serious hemorrhage is influenced markedly by the level of circulating factor VIII:C. If the level is at or very close to zero, the risk is major; if the level is higher, the risk is reduced. Factor VIII:C activity increases appreciably during normal pregnancy, and some increase is likely in hemophiliacs who can synthesize some factor VIII:C. The obstetrician can reduce the risk of grave hemorrhage at and after delivery by avoiding abdominal incisions and vaginal lacerations, minimizing episiotomy, and maximizing myometrial contraction and retraction.

Vaginal delivery of a fetus who inherited hemophilia A usually has not resulted in birth of an infant who has bled seriously during the antepartum or intrapartum periods. After delivery the risk of hemorrhage in the neonate increases, especially if circumcision is attempted. Why labor and vaginal delivery do not commonly incite serious bleeding in the fetus and neonate is not clear. Maternal factor VIII:C does not cross the placenta.

Whenever the mother has hemophilia A, so will all of her sons, and all of her daughters will be carriers. If she is but a carrier, one half of her sons will inherit the disease, and one half of her daughters will be carriers.

Prenatal diagnosis of hemophilia A is possible near midpregnancy if a small amount of fetal plasma can be obtained. Some contamination with amnionic fluid is acceptable, since antigenically active factor VIII (factor VIII:ag) is markedly reduced in affected male fetuses. The identification of fetal sex alone serves to identify those at risk of inheriting hemophilia A, namely, male fetuses.

Factor VIII Inhibitor. Rarely, antibodies directed against factor VIII are acquired and may lead to life-threatening hemorrhage. This phenomenon has been identified in women during the puerperium. The prominent clinical feature was severe, protracted, repetitive hemorrhage from the reproductive tract starting a week or so after an apparently uncomplicated delivery. (Reece and associates, 1982). In the laboratory, the activated partial thromboplastin time was markedly prolonged. Treatment employed has included many transfusions of whole blood and plasma, huge doses of cryoprecipitate, large volumes of an admixture of activated coagulation factors (Autoplex), immunosuppressive therapy, and attempts at various surgical procedures, especially curettage and hysterectomy.

Hemophilia B

The genetic and clinical features of severe deficiency of factor IX (Christmas disease, hemophilia B) are quite similar to those of hemophilia A. The homozygous state, essential for severe disease in women, is rare. Pregnancy, with a favorable outcome from vaginal delivery and not requiring replacement therapy even though factor IX actively remained quite low, has been described in detail by Rust and associates (1975). The male newborn infant appeared to tolerate labor and vaginal delivery without hemorrhage.

Von Willebrand's Disease

The larger component of factor VIII complex, namely, factor VIII-related Willebrand factor or factor VIIIR:WF, is essential for adhesion of platelets to subendothelial collagen and formation of a primary hemostatic plug at the site of blood vessel injury. The factor, synthesized under control of autosomal genes by endothelium and megakaryocytes, is present in platelets as well as plasma.

Clinically, von Willebrand's disease is actually a relatively heterogeneous group of functional disorders involving aberrations of factor VIII complex and platelet dysfunctions. Von Willebrand's disease appears to be inherited by at least three different genetic mechanisms: (1) as an incompletely dominant autosomal trait, (2) as an autosomal recessive, and (3) as an X-linked recessive. The possibility of von Willebrand's disease is usually considered most often in women with bleeding suggestive of a chronic disorder of coagulation. The classic autosomal dominant form is usually symptomatic in the heterozygous state. A less common but clinically more severe autosomal recessive form is manifest when inherited from both parents, each of whom demonstrates little or no disease. Von Willebrand's disease is characterized clinically by easy bruising, mucosal hemorrhage, and excessive bleeding with trauma, including surgery. Its laboratory features are a prolonged bleeding time, prolonged partial thromboplastin time, decreased factor VIII (immunologic activity as well as coagulation-promoting activity), and inability of platelets in plasma from an affected person to react to a variety of stimuli. Von Willebrand's disease is probably a heterogeneous syndrome with various underlying molecular defects (Zimmerman and co-workers, 1979).

Noller and associates (1973) summarized 17 cases of pregnancy complicated by von Willebrand's disease, including 4 of their own. The hemostatic defects may improve during pregnancy. If factor VIII activity is very low, the administration of factor VIII-rich cryoprecipitate is recommended. Most persons with von Willebrand's disease are heterozygous and have only a mild bleeding disorder. When both parents have the disorder, their offspring may, if homozygous, develop a serious bleeding disorder. Fetoscopy has been used to obtain fetal blood that served to identify the fetus as not having severe von Willebrand's disease (Hoyer and colleagues, 1979).

Other Inherited Coagulation Factor Deficiencies

Factor XI deficiency is probably the consequence of an autosomal trait that is manifested as severe disease in the homozygous individuals but as a minor defect in the heterozygote. This deficiency state is most prevalent in persons of Jewish extraction. It is rarely encountered in pregnancy.

Inherited abnormalities of fibrinogen usually involve the formation of a functionally defective fibrinogen, usually referred to as *dysfibrinogenemia. Familial hypofibrinogenemia* has been described very infrequently. Our experiences suggest, at least, that familial hypofibrinogenemia represents a heterozygous autosomal dominant state, with 50 percent of the affected mother's offspring affected. Typically thrombin-clottable protein has ranged from 80 to 110 mg/dl when nonpregnant and then increased by 40 or 50 percent as in normal pregnancy. Those pregnancy complications that give rise to acquired hypofibrinogenemia were common in our cases but most likely only because the existence of such conditions provided the initial impetus for our studies.

Reports of pregnancy experiences for women with congenital afibrinogenemia are rare. The potential for grave problems undoubtedly exists.

OTHER HEMATOLOGIC DISORDERS

Leukemia

In recent years some startling outcomes have been observed for women with leukemia who conceived. Most of the cytotoxic drugs used in treatment cross the placenta, and therefore it was predicted generally that these agents would severely affect the fetus. To date this does not appear to be the case, at least when the drugs are administered only during the second and third trimesters. Several cases of congenital leukemia in infants of nonleukemic mothers have been recorded, although no case of transmission of leukemia to the fetus has been authenticated. Levine and Collea (1979) have considered the problem of pregnancy complicated by chronic granulocytic leukemia, and Lilleyman and associates (1977) and Pizzuto and associates (1980) have done the same for acute leukemia.

Hodgkin's Disease

There are no convincing data to indicate that pregnancy adversely affects the disease. Holmes and Holmes (1978) have analyzed pregnancy outcomes when either the expectant mother or the father had the disease and found the great majority of the outcomes for the 93 pregnancies to be satisfactory. More recently, Jacobs and associates (1981) reported their experiences. Neither chemotherapy during the second and third trimesters nor irradiation to the mediastinum and neck of the mother appeared to affect adversely the fetus or neonate.

Chapman and associates (1979) observed ovarian failure rather commonly to accompany therapy for Hogdkin's disease. Twenty-five of forty-one women were identified clinically and by endocrinologic studies to have ovarian failure. Horning and co-workers (1981) have evaluated the reproductive potential of a relatively large number of women of reproductive age after treatment for Hodgkin's disease. In several instances, signs and symptoms of ovarian failure that developed soon after pelvic irradiation receded and a successful pregnancy outcome followed. No birth defects nor developmental abnormalities were evident in the 24 infants born subsequently.

Polycythemia

Polycythemia during pregnancy is usually secondary and related to hypoxia, most often from congenital cardiac disease or a pulmonary disorder. If the polycythemia is severe, the probability of a successful outcome for the pregnancy is remote.

Polycythemia vera and pregnancy rarely coexist. Ruch and Klein (1964) described a case in which the hematocrit reading in the nonpregnant state was as high as 63. During each of two pregnancies, however, the hematocrit ranged from a low of about 35 during the second trimester to about 44 at term. Fetal loss seems to be high in women with polycythemia vera.

Koeffler and Goldwasser (1981) have reported that measurement of serum erythropoietin by radioimmunoassay can differentiate polycythemia vera (low values) from secondary polycythemia (high values). No experiences during pregnancy were noted, however.

DISEASES OF THE URINARY TRACT

A few diseases of the urinary tract may be associated with pregnancy by chance and be little affected by it. Much more often, pregnancy predisposes to the development or exacerbation of disease. An example of the former is pyelonephritis and of the latter is lupus nephritis. The remarkable changes, anatomic and functional, that are induced in the urinary tract by normal pregnancy are considered elsewhere, especially in Chapter 9 (p. 197).

URINARY TRACT INFECTIONS

Although a urinary infection may involve only the bladder and thus represent true cystitis, infection of the renal calyces and pelvis is invariably accompanied by involvement of the renal parenchyma, a condition better described as pyelonephritis than pyelitis.

During pregnancy, active multiplication of bacteria within the bladder is identified most often when there has been recent instrumentation of the urinary tract or there is persistent asymptomatic bacteriuria. Since bacteria are normally found in the outer portion of the urethra, single catheterization or the use of an indwelling catheter is likely to introduce bacteria into the bladder, where during pregnancy and early puerperium the organisms usually encounter conditions ideal for multiplication. As was shown by Brumfitt and associates (1961), routine bladder catheterization before delivery initiates infection in approximately 9 percent of puerperal women. It follows that the number of puerperal infections can be reduced appreciably by avoiding routine catheterization of the bladder at the time of delivery.

Approximately 5 percent of pregnant women already have bacteriuria at the time of the first prenatal visit. However, prevalence varies considerably, being highest among socioeconomically deprived women of high parity, women who have had previous clinically apparent urinary tract infections, and women whose red cells sickle, including those with sickle cell trait. Approximately 25 percent of women with *untreated asymptomatic bacteriuria* subsequently develop *symptomatic infection* of the urinary tract—cystitis or pyelonephritis—during the course of pregnancy.

Cystitis and Urethritis

Typically, cystitis is characterized by dysuria, particularly at the end of urination, as well as urgency and frequency. There are few associated systemic findings. Usually, there is an abnormal number of leukocytes, as well as bacteria, in the urine. Erythrocytes are also commonly found in the urinary sediment, and occasionally even gross hematuria is seen. Although uncomplicated cystitis occurs, the upper urinary tract may soon be involved in an ascending infection.

Frequency, urgency, dysuria, and pyuria without bacteriuria may also be the consequence of urethritis caused by *Chlamydia trachomatis,* a rather common pathogen of the genitourinary tract.

Acute Pyelonephritis

This disease is the direct result of bacterial infection that may extend upward from the bladder through the blood vessels and lymphatics. The weight of clinical evidence indicates that the ascending route of infection is very much more common.

Acute pyelonephritis is one of the most frequent medical complications of pregnancy. The reported incidence of acute pyelonephritis complicating pregnancy and the puerperium approximates 2 percent and most often appears in the latter part of pregnancy or in the early puerperium (Gilstrap and co-workers, 1981). The disease, when unilateral, is more frequently right sided.

The onset of signs and symptoms of the disease is usually rather abrupt. The woman who has previously been well or has complained of slight bladder irritation or hematuria suddenly develops fever, shaking chills, and aching pain in one or both lumbar regions. There may be anorexia, nausea, and vomiting. The body temperature most often is elevated but, during the course of the disease, may vary remarkably with hyperthermia to as high as 40° C or more and hypothermia to as low as 34° C. Tenderness can usually be elicited by firm palpation in one or both costovertebral angles. The urinary sediment contains many leukocytes, frequently in clumps, and in the sediment are numerous bacteria, usually gram-negative. *Escherichia coli* is the microorganism cultured commonly from the urine. Culture of the blood may demonstrate the same organism.

Pain in one or both lumbar regions and the characteristic urinary findings, as well as fever and costovertebral tenderness, should make the diagnosis clear. The condition may be mistaken, however, for labor, appendicitis, placental abruption, or infarction of a myoma and, in the puerperium, for infection of the uterus and adjacent structures.

Several factors predispose the bacteriuric pregnant woman to acute pyelonephritis. As a result of compression of the ureter at the pelvic brim by the enlarging uterus and by the enlarged ovarian vein, coupled with hormonal effects, there is a progressive dilatation of the renal calyces, pelves, and ureters, accompanied by a decrease in tone and peristaltic action (Chapter 9, p. 198). These changes cause stasis, a factor known to increase susceptibility to renal infection.

In the early puerperium, bladder sensitivity to intravesical fluid tension is often decreased as the consequence of anesthesia, especially epidural or spinal, and after the anesthesia dissipates, from the overriding pelvic discomfort caused by a large episiotomy, lacerations, or hematomas. Moreover, starting immediately after delivery, oxytocin is commonly infused for an hour or so at rates that cause antidiuresis simultaneously with an appreciable volume of fluid. When the oxytocin is stopped, there is likely to be a surge of urine, which rapidly distends the bladder. Marked overdistention of the bladder, coupled with catheterization to provide relief, commonly leads to urinary tract infection!

Asymptomatic Bacteriuria

The term "asymptomatic bacteriuria" is used to indicate persisting, actively multiplying bacteria within the urinary tract without symptoms of a urinary infection. The reported prevalence of bacteriuria during pregnancy varies from 2 to as great as 12 percent, depending on parity, race, and socioeconomic status of the women surveyed. The highest incidence has been reported in black multiparas with sickle cell trait, and the lowest incidence has been found in white, socioeconomically more privileged women of low parity.

In women who demonstrate asymptomatic bacte-

riuria, the bacteriuria is typically present at the time of the first prenatal visit; after an initial negative culture of the urine, fewer than 1.5 percent acquire a urinary infection in the subsequent months until delivery (Whalley, 1967). The diagnosis of asymptomatic bacteriuria requires the demonstration of significant numbers of bacteria in the urine. In most instances, this can be accomplished by culturing clean-voided midstream specimens of urine without resorting to catheterization. A clean-voided specimen of urine containing more than 100,000 organisms of the same species per ml of urine is most often evidence of infection. Smaller numbers of bacteria usually represent contamination of the specimen during collection, although with a higher rate of urine formation, a lesser number of organisms of the same species is likely to represent infection rather than contamination.

Twenty to forty percent of women with asymptomatic bacteriuria during pregnancy subsequently develop an acute symptomatic urinary infection during that pregnancy. However, eradication of bacteriuria with antimicrobial agents has been shown to be effective in the prevention of nearly all clinically evident infections.

Bacteriuria has been thought by some investigators frequently to cause premature labor and, in turn, increased neonatal morbidity and mortality. In an early study by Kass (1962, 1965), the incidence of premature births, defined as a birth weight of 2500 g or less, among 95 women with bacteriuria who received only placebos during pregnancy, was 27 percent, whereas among 84 women with bacteriuria who were treated with antimicrobial agents, the rate was only 7 percent. The corresponding rates of perinatal death were 14 percent and zero, respectively. Kincaid-Smith and Bullen (1965) also reported a relatively high proportion of infants of low birth weight among untreated bacteriuric women, but these investigators were unable to reduce this proportion significantly with antimicrobial therapy (21.5 percent compared to 17.3 percent). They concluded that bacteriuria in pregnancy is commonly a manifestation of underlying chronic renal disease, which accounts for the higher incidence of infants of low birth weight and of perinatal loss. Several other investigators have been unable to corroborate the alleged relation between bacteriuria and low birth weight (Table 28-4). From the evidence currently available, it is concluded that, al-

TABLE 28-4. INCIDENCE OF LOW BIRTH WEIGHT WITH AND WITHOUT BACTERIURIA DURING PREGNANCY

Author	Bacteriuric Patients[a]	Nonbacteriuric Patients[a]
Little (1966)	141 (9)	4735 (8)
Norden, Kilpatrick (1965)	114 (15)	109 (13)
Sleigh et al. (1964)	100 (7)	100 (7)
Whalley (1967)	176 (15)	176 (12)
Wilson et al. (1966)	230 (11)	6216 (10)

[a] Numbers in parentheses indicate percent.

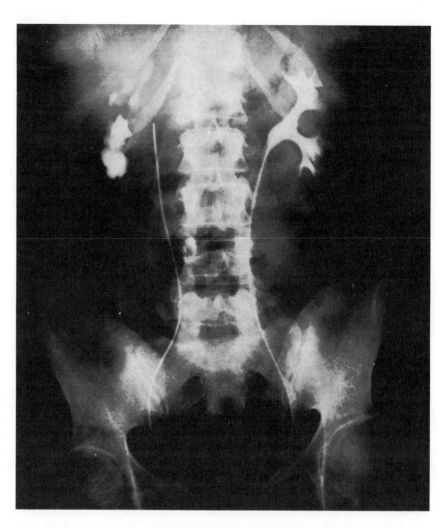

Figure 28-6. Retrograde pyelogram obtained 3 months postpartum, showing marked destruction of the right calyceal system from long-standing asymptomatic infection. The patient, a multipara, had asymptomatic bacteriuria during pregnancy. There was no history of infection of the urinary tract. (*Courtesy of Dr. P. J. Whalley.*)

though there may be a relation between bacteriuria and low birth weight, bacteriuria is not a prominent factor in the genesis of low birth weight or prematurity.

Even though bacteriuria plays a prominent role in the cause of acute pyelonephritis during pregnancy, the majority of women with bacteriuria remain asymptomatic throughout pregnancy. Some of these women certainly have bacteriuria limited to the bladder without involvement of the kidney, but several studies clearly demonstrate that others have potentially serious renal disease. Postpartum urologic investigation of patients shown to have bacteriuria during pregnancy have substantiated that, in many, bacteriuria persists after delivery. Moreover, in a significant number of these women, there is pyelographic evidence of chronic infection, obstructive lesions, or congenital abnormalities of the urinary tract (Kincaid-Smith and Bullen, 1965; Whalley and associates, 1965, 1967).

Routine screening of obstetric clinic patients is advised to detect bacteriuria and, when positive cultures are obtained, to eradicate the infection. Women who do not respond to treatment or who subsequently demonstrate reinfection should be evaluated urologically after the puerperium (Fig. 28-6).

Chronic Pyelonephritis

In contrast to acute pyelonephritis, chronic pyelonephritis may be associated with few or no symptoms referable to the urinary tract. In advanced cases, the major symptoms are those of renal insufficiency. There may or more often may not be a history of prior symptomatic infection of the urinary tract. The pathogenesis of this disease is therefore obscure. As in all chronic progressive renal diseases, the maternal and fetal prognoses in a particular case depend on the extent of renal destruction. Women with hypertension or renal insufficiency have a poor prognosis, whereas those with adequate renal function without hypertension may go through pregnancy without serious complications. Regardless of the extent of renal destruction, chronic pyelonephritis complicated by pregnancy is associated with an increased risk of superimposed acute pyelonephritis, which, in turn, may lead to further deterioration of renal function.

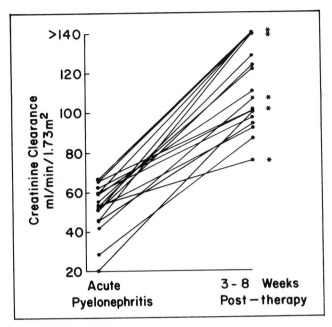

Figure 28-7. Endogenous creatinine clearance values in 18 pregnant women during and 3 to 8 weeks after an attack of acute pyelonephritis; asterisk indicates patients reevaluated while still pregnant. (*From Whalley and co-workers, 1975.*)

Management of Infections of the Urinary Tract

A variety of drugs are now available for the treatment of urinary infections. Ideally, the choice of a particular antimicrobial agent should be based upon studies of the sensitivity of the infecting microorganism. In practice, however, most bacteria causing urinary tract infections in pregnancy are sensitive to the short-acting sulfonamides, nitrofurantoin (Macrodantin), and somewhat less often to ampicillin. Since sensitivity is predictable, treatment can be initiated with one of these three agents and changed, if necessary, when the laboratory results are available.

Treatment of Asymptomatic Bacteriuria. Women with asymptomatic bacteriuria or symptoms confined to the lower urinary tract may be treated without being hospitalized. Treatment for 10 days with Macrodantin, 100 mg once a day, or with sulfisoxazole (Gantrisin), 1 g four times a day, has proved effective in the great majority of cases so treated at Parkland Memorial Hospital. Harris and co-workers (1982) have evaluated single-dose treatment of asymptomatic bacteriuria during pregnancy. In 75 to 80 percent of cases a single dose of sulfisoxazole (2 g), Macrodantin (200 mg), or ampicillin (2 g) plus probenimid (1 g) eradicated the bacteria. Subsequent recurrence rates were 5 percent or less.

Treatment of Acute Pyelonephritis. It is best for pregnant women with systemic manifestations of acute pyelonephritis to be hospitalized during the initiation of

treatment and until clinical improvement is observed. During the first few days of therapy, patients with acute pyelonephritis should be watched carefully to detect signs or symptoms suggesting bacterial shock. Although this serious complication is quite uncommon, its gravity demands early recognition and prompt therapy. Urinary output should therefore be recorded carefully and frequently, the blood pressure measured often, and the body temperature observed closely in all patients with acute pyelonephritis. High fever should be treated usually with a cooling blanket. A marked fall in body temperature is ominous in that it may precede or coincide with worrisome hypotension. The levels of creatinine in plasma should be ascertained early in the course of therapy. It has not been generally appreciated that acute pyelonephritis in pregnancy may in some yet unexplained way cause a considerable reduction in glomerular filtration rate (Fig. 28-7). Fortunately, the impaired renal function is reversed by effective treatment of the infection (Whalley and co-workers, 1975). More recently, respiratory dysfunction similar, at least, to what has been generally termed adult respiratory distress syndrome has been described in some pregnant women seriously ill with acute pyelonephritis (Cunningham and associates, 1984). The investigators postulate that endotoxin caused alveolar-capillary injury that led to the respiratory failure.

Drug Toxicity. Antimicrobial agents used to treat infections of the urinary tract during pregnancy may, in certain circumstances, produce undesirable side effects, both maternal and fetal. Sulfonamides given the mother before delivery will have crossed the placenta and, in the presence of hyperbilirubinemia in the newborn, may possibly increase the danger of kernicterus. Sulfonamides cross the placenta and compete with unconjugated bilirubin for binding by albumin, and as a result there is an increase in unbound, free bilirubin. The sulfonamides, furthermore, may compete with bilirubin for glucuronyl transferase, which is required for conversion of toxic free bilirubin to more benign conjugated pigment.

Nitrofurantoin may lead to hemolytic anemia in women whose erythrocytes are markedly deficient in glucose-6-phosphate dehydrogenase. Perhaps 2 percent of black women are homozygous for the X chromosome-linked enzyme deficiency and therefore are potential candidates for drug-induced hemolysis. Fortunately, hemolysis in the mother or newborn infant has developed rarely in our extensive experience.

Tetracycline administered in the last trimester of pregnancy may lead to subsequent discoloration of the child's deciduous teeth. Therapy with large doses of tetracycline may precipitate a syndrome of fatty liver, jaundice, azotemia, and pancreatitis in pregnant women with impaired renal excretory function (Whalley and colleagues, 1964).

Chloramphenicol may rarely produce serious and even fatal blood dyscrasias, such as aplastic anemia and thrombocytopenia. Streptomycin, kanamycin, and gentamicin may be both ototoxic and nephrotoxic. Ampicillin appears to be effective in about 80 percent of cases of pyelonephritis due to *E. coli* but ineffective against *Enterobacter aerogenes.* In seriously ill pregnant women a combination of ampicillin and gentamicin provides effective treatment until bacterial sensitivities are available.

Most urinary infections respond rapidly to adequate antimicrobial therapy. Clinical symptoms for the most part disappear during the first 2 days of therapy. Even though the symptoms promptly abate, therapy should be continued for at least 10 days. Cultures of urine usually demonstrate no growth after the first 24 hours of therapy if the microorganism is sensitive to the chosen drug. Repeat urine culture of the woman who promptly responds clinically should be performed a week to 10 days after completion of antibacterial therapy.

Since the changes in the urinary tract induced by pregnancy persist, reinfection is always possible. If subsequent cultures of the urine are positive remote from the time of therapy, prolonged treatment is usually indicated using a drug to which the organism appears sensitive.

Prognosis

The prognosis for women with infections of the urinary tract in pregnancy is variable. Pyelonephritis during pregnancy must not be considered cured even though the symptoms subside completely and spontaneously unless the urine remains sterile. The responsibilities are not discharged until the physician is certain that the urine is free from organisms remote from the time of antibacterial therapy. Absence of pyuria is not in itself adequate evidence of cure. All patients who develop repeated infections of the urinary tract should be evaluated urologically after the pregnancy-induced changes in the urinary tract have subsided.

Renal Tuberculosis

Tuberculosis of the kidney is a serious, but rare, complication of pregnancy. Renal tuberculosis is believed by some to pursue a rapidly unfavorable course, particularly during the later months of pregnancy. Therefore, the question of the advisability of allowing the pregnancy to continue in any case of proved renal tuberculosis is raised. A decision regarding termination of pregnancy should be based upon the individual findings in each case, however.

Whether the patient who has undergone nephrectomy for tuberculosis should be allowed to become pregnant is another question. The consensus is that pregnancy should be interdicted for about 2 years until absence of infection and good function have been demonstrated in the remaining kidney.

URINARY CALCULI

Renal and ureteral lithiases are very uncommon complications of pregnancy. Since in many pregnant women there are some of the cardinal prerequisites for the formation of stones—namely, urinary stasis and infection—

the incidence might be expected to be higher were it not for counteracting factors, one of which is undoubtedly the relatively short duration of pregnancy.

Women who have formed renal stones previously are generally at risk of doing so again. Coe and associates (1978), however, could find no evidence in such women that pregnancy increased that risk. Moreover, stone disease did not appear to have any prejudicial effect on pregnancy except for an increased frequency of urinary tract infections. These investigators concluded that a woman with nephrolithiasis need not forego pregnancy as long as renal function is adequate. The calculi during pregnancy seldom cause severe symptomatic obstruction.

Radiopaque stones may be identified by carefully performed roentgenography with or without contrast media. Sonography may help confirm a suspected renal stone. Treatment depends on the symptoms and the duration of pregnancy. Commonly the stone passes spontaneously (Strong and associates, 1978). If the symptoms persist and are severe, surgical removal may be mandatory regardless of other considerations. During the latter half of pregnancy, the blood vessels supplying the kidney and ureter are remarkably enlarged; moreover, proper exposure of the lower ureter without emptying the uterus is often impossible.

Lattanzi and Cook (1980) have described 11 cases of urinary calculi complicating pregnancy and reviewed much of the previous literature. When calculi are discovered, the possibility of hyperparathyroidism should be considered.

GLOMERULONEPHRITIS

Acute Glomerulonephritis

Acute glomerulonephritis rarely develops during pregnancy. In reviewing the literature, Nadler and co-workers (1969) were able to find reports of only 19 women with acute glomerulonephritis occurring between weeks 8 and 37 of pregnancy, and in only 3 of them was the diagnosis verified by biopsy. The diagnosis during pregnancy is made easier if there is a history of a streptococcal infection a few weeks before and supporting evidence is provided by red cell casts in urine and an elevated antistreptolysin titer. Acute glomerulonephritis appearing during the last trimester of pregnancy especially may sometimes be clinically indistinguishable from preeclampsia. Renal biopsy may be of value in some circumstances to try to exclude preeclampsia and identify the type of glomerular disease (Madaio and Harrington, 1983).

In general, the treatment of glomerulonephritis is the same in the pregnant as in the nonpregnant woman. There are insufficient data available to predict fetal or maternal prognosis. Some investigators have noted a high fetal loss from abortion, immaturity, or stillbirth; others have documented otherwise uneventful pregnancies. Since the clinical syndrome usually subsides within 2 weeks, a course of expectant observation is warranted. In nonpregnant women the mortality rate is less than 5 percent, with death usually the result of heart failure or unrelenting renal failure. Some patients never completely recover, lapsing gradually into chronic glomerulonephritis. Women with a history of acute glomerulonephritis that has subsequently healed may undergo additional pregnancies without any appreciable increase in the incidence of complications, according to Felding's survey (1964, 1968).

Singson and associates (1980) have described a case of biopsy-proven acute glomerulonephritis with onset at 6 months gestation and characterized by oliguria, azotemia, elevated C-reactive protein, and antistreptolysin titer, with recovery, including renal function, after about 3 weeks. A healthy infant was delivered at term. Eighteen years later the mother's renal function remained normal.

Chronic Glomerulonephritis

Chronic glomerulonephritis is characterized by the progressive renal destruction, eventually producing the so-called end-stage kidney. In most cases, the cause is unknown, although a few patients appear to develop the disease after a bout of acute glomerulonephritis that failed to heal.

The disease may present in one of six ways:

1. Some patients may remain asymptomatic for years, with proteinuria or an abnormal urinary sediment or both as the only indications of the disease.
2. It may be discovered in some women during the course of evaluation for chronic hypertension.
3. The disease may first become manifest as the nephrotic syndrome.
4. It may present in an acute form similar to acute glomerulonephritis.
5. Renal failure may be the first manifestation.
6. The symptoms and signs of preeclampsia-eclampsia may precede the discovery of chronic glomerulonephritis.

Katz and associates (1980) have reviewed 89 pregnancy experiences in women with chronic renal disease, the exact diagnosis of which was established by renal biopsy. In none of the 38 women with diffuse or focal glomerulonephritis was there evidence before pregnancy of appreciable impairment of renal clearance; plasma creatinine levels were 1.2 mg/dl or less, and blood urea nitrogen levels were 17 mg/dl or less. Nonetheless, of 59 pregnancies in these 38 women with diffuse or focal glomerulonephritis, there were 10 perinatal deaths, 14 infants delivered preterm, and 15 were small for

gestational age. Superimposed preeclampsia was common and severe abruptio placentae developed in 3 instances.

Except for an increased risk of superimposed preeclampsia, women with relatively normal renal function and no hypertension nonpregnant are more likely, but not guaranteed, to have a relatively benign pregnancy. Because of the likelihood of progression of the disease, however, the ultimate maternal prognosis is guarded. Conversely, in women with extreme hypertension or azotemia, the outcome is very likely to be poor for them and for the pregnancy.

Because of the varying rates of renal destruction, it is difficult to evaluate the influence of pregnancy on the progress of the disease. Pregnancy in the absence of superimposed preeclampsia or severe abruptio placentae does not appear to accelerate appreciably deterioration in renal function. In the absence of complications, affected kidneys may show the same pattern of response to pregnancy as do normal kidneys, with some increase in both glomerular filtration and renal plasma flow (Werkö and Bucht, 1956).

Nephrosis

The nephrotic syndrome, or nephrosis, is a disorder of multiple causes, characterized by massive proteinuria (in excess of 5 g per day), hypoalbuminemia, and hypercholesterolemia, usually with hyperlipidemia and edema. Diseases known to be associated with nephrotic syndrome include chronic glomerulonephritis, lupus erythematosus, diabetes mellitus, amyloidosis, syphilis, and thrombosis of the renal vein. In addition, the syndrome may result from poisoning by heavy metals, therapy with some drugs, and allergies to poison ivy or bee and wasp venom.

When the nephrotic syndrome complicates pregnancy, the maternal and fetal prognoses and the treatment depend on the underlying cause of the disease and the extent of renal insufficiency. For example, we have identified two cases of maternal syphilis complicated by nephrosis during the antepartum period. After antibiotic therapy, the nephrosis cleared and pregnancy outcomes were satisfactory. Whenever possible, the specific cause should be ascertained and renal function assessed. In this regard, when the cause is not apparent, percutaneous renal biopsy may be of value. Serial studies of renal function in two of our patients with nephrotic syndrome associated with membranous glomerulonephritis served to demonstrate the usual augmentation of renal function that characterizes pregnancy. Neither woman became hypertensive. A review of additional reported cases of nephrosis indicates that the majority of patients who are not hypertensive and do not have severe renal insufficiency may undergo a successful pregnancy, particularly since the advent of adrenocorticosteroid therapy (Studd and Blainey, 1969; Weisman and colleagues, 1973). In certain cases, however, in which there is evidence of renal insufficiency or moderate to severe hypertension or both, the prognosis for mother and fetus is poor, and interruption of the pregnancy may be indicated, especially if renal function is deteriorating.

ACUTE RENAL FAILURE

In more recent years, acute renal failure associated with pregnancy has become less common from some causes, especially induced abortion and transfusion of incompatible blood. It has certainly not been eliminated, however, as borne out by the experiences of Grünfeld and associates (1980), which are summarized in Table 28-5. Eight of the 57 women died; 19 of the 57 had cortical necrosis. The most common causes of acute renal failure were abruptio placentae and eclampsia.

Identification of the existence of acute renal failure and, in turn, its cause or causes is important. Appropriate therapy initiated promptly will minimize the intensity and duration of functional impairment. Oligura is an important sign of acutely impaired renal function. Unfortunately, potent diuretics, such as furosemide, can increase urine flow without correcting, but rather intensifying, the cause of oliguria. Moreover, their use may negate the value of various urinary indices that might be used to try to differentiate prerenal from intrarenal or postrenal causes of acute renal failure. A high urine:plasma creatinine ratio (> 30) is strongly suggestive, at least, of prerenal azotemia, as is an elevated urine:plasma osmolality ratio (> 1.5). With prerenal azotemia, most filtered sodium is reabsorbed so that the urinary concentration typically is low (< 20 mEq/L). Quite commonly in obstetric cases both prerenal and intrarenal factors are operative. For example, with severe abruptio placentae, severe hypovolemia is common from massive concealed hemorrhage. Moreover, in severe cases of pla-cental abruption, vascular disease, acute or chronic, is frequent. Finally, intense consumptive coagulopathy commonly triggered by the abruption could serve to impede the intrarenal microcirculation.

Acute Tubular Necrosis

The disease is largely preventable (in our experience, at least), by the following means: (1) prompt and vigorous replacement of blood in instances of massive hemorrhage, as in abruptio placentae, placenta previa, rupture of the uterus, and postpartum uterine atony, following the guidelines described in Chapter 21 (p. 393), (2) termination of pregnancies complicated by severe preeclampsia and eclampsia, with careful blood replacement if loss is excessive, (3) close observation for early signs of septic shock, especially in women with septic abortion (Table 24-2), amnionitis, sepsis from other pelvic infections, or pyelonephritis, (4) avoidance of potent diuretics to treat oliguria before initiating appropriate efforts to assure adequate cardiac output for perfusion of the kidney, and (5) avoidance of vasoconstrictors to treat hypotension unless pathologic vasodilatation is unequivocally the cause of the hypotension.

When azotemia is evident and severe oliguria persists, hemodialysis should be initiated before deterioration of general well-being has become marked. Early dialysis appears quite beneficial for lowering mortality and may enhance the extent of recovery of renal function. Acute tubular necrosis is not chronically progressive. In fact, after healing has taken place, renal function usually returns to normal or near normal. Future pregnancies are, therefore, not necessarily contraindicated.

Renal Cortical Necrosis

Compared to acute tubular necrosis, bilateral necrosis of the renal cortex is uncommon. However, when cortical necrosis has developed, according to most published reports, it often has been associated with pregnancy. For example, among 38 cases studied by Kleinknecht and coworkers (1973), 26 were obstetric in origin. Most of the reported cases in pregnant women have followed such complications as abruptio placentae, preeclampsia–eclampsia, or bacterial shock. Histologically, the lesion appears to result from thrombosis of segments of the renal vascular system. The lesion may be focal, patchy, confluent, or gross. Clinically, the disease follows the course of acute renal failure, with oliguria or anuria, uremia, and generally death within 2 to 3 weeks unless dialysis is initiated. Differentiation from acute tubular necrosis during the early phase is possible only by renal biopsy. The prognosis depends on the extent of the necrosis, since recovery is a function of the amount of renal tissue spared. When the lesion is confluent, the mortality rate approaches 100 percent unless chronic dialysis or renal transplantation is applied.

TABLE 28-5. MAIN CAUSE AND COURSE OF ACUTE RENAL FAILURE IN 57 PREGNANT WOMEN

Main Cause	No. of Cases	Cortical Necrosis	Died
Abruptio placentae	13	7	2
Eclampsia	11	1	0
Preeclampsia	1	0	0
Prolonged fetal death	6	5	2
Uterine hemorrhage	4	2	0
Pyelonephritis, acute	3	0	0
Other infections	5	0	0
Amnionic fluid embolism	1	1	1
Ectopic pregnancy	1	0	1
Miscellaneous, "unrelated"	7	0	0
Postpartum, "idiopathic"	5	3	2
Totals	57	19	8

(*From Grünfeld and associates, 1980.*)

Obstructive Renal Failure

Rarely, the compression of the ureters by a very large pregnant uterus is greatly exaggerated, causing ureteral obstruction and, in turn, severe oliguria and azotemia. O'Shaughnessy and co-workers (1980), as well as others, have described this phenomenon as the consequence of a markedly overdistended gravid uterus. Homans and associates (1981) described a case in which massive hydramnios was associated with renal failure in a woman with a single left kidney. When placed in the right lateral recumbent position, diuresis was prompt and the plasma creatinine dropped from 6.0 mg/dl to 2.0 mg/dl over the 60 hour period during which she maintained that posture.

We have observed this phenomenon in one woman with gross hydramnios (9.4 liters) and an anencephalic fetus. Amniocentesis and removal of some of the amnionic fluid was followed promptly by a diuresis and a lowering of the plasma creatinine concentration. In another instance, progressive oliguria and azotemia were identified early in the third trimester in a woman who, as a child, had been subjected to reimplantation of both ureters into the bladder to try to prevent reflux. Ureteral catheters were teased through the markedly narrowed ureteral lumens and provided significant relief from the obstructions.

Postpartum Acute Renal Failure

Wagoner and associates (1968) and Robson and associates (1968) described what they believed to be a new syndrome of acute irreversible renal failure occurring within the first 6 weeks postpartum. Pregnancy and delivery appeared to have been normal in the 7 cases reported, and none of the known causes of renal failure was present. The pathologic changes identified by renal biopsy were necrosis and endothelial proliferation in glomeruli, plus necrosis, thrombosis, and intimal thickening of the arterioles. No vascular abnormalities were demonstrated in the other visceral organs in the 4 cases in which autopsy was performed. Morphologic changes in the erythrocytes consistent with microangiopathic hemolysis and thrombocytopenia were present in the majority of cases. Other authors have described the same or a similar condition under the name *postpartum hemolytic uremic syndrome*.

According to Nissenson and co-workers (1979), 80 percent of affected women have died and only 5 percent have recovered, including a case described by them in which maintenance hemodialysis had been used for over a year.

Postpartum acute renal failure with the characteristic features of hemolytic uremic syndrome has been identified rarely among the large number of women cared for on the Obstetric Service at Parkland Memorial Hospital. Its frequency has not been greater than in the general hospital population. The question persists concerning the role, if any, of pregnancy and puerperium in the genesis of the hemolytic uremic syndrome. Our experiences support the thesis that it is coincidental and thus represents another example of idiopathic sporadic hemolytic uremic syndrome. It is possible that some pregnancy-related event may contribute to its development, such as bacterial sepsis, viral infections, and possibly some drugs, for example, ergot alkaloids. Currently popular and attractive is the concept of faulty intravascular prostacyclin, or prostaglandin I_2, formation in these cases of hemolytic syndrome.

Treatment of apparent hemolytic uremic syndrome has been controversial. Early enthusiasm for heparin was followed by concern over its efficacy and safety, especially in hypertensive, thrombocytopenic individuals. Antiplatelet function agents have been tried, and, more recently, plasma infusion, plasmapheresis, and exchange transfusions have been used commonly as they have in the possibly related phenomenon of thrombotic thrombocytopenic purpura. Treatment postpartum by repeated plasma exchange transfusions and hemodialysis with a favorable outcome has been reported (Spencer and co-workers, 1982). This observation led the authors to suggest that plasma exchange is the preferred treatment.

We continue to observe a case of postpartum hemolytic uremic syndrome managed more than a decade ago with good recovery in which therapy was limited to hemodialysis transiently plus packed red cell transfusions to correct the severe but transient hemolytic anemia (Table 28-6). Quite recently, another case of hemolytic uremic syndrome was treated postpartum with hemodialysis, plasmapheresis, corticosteroids, antiplatelet function agents, and red cells. This treatment was followed by complete recovery over a few months.

PREGNANCY AFTER TRANSPLANTATION

Murray and associates in 1963 reported two successful pregnancies in a woman who had had a kidney transplanted from her identical twin sister. Since that time, many pregnancies have been reported in women who previously had received a kidney from immunologically nonidentical donors.

At the Second European Meeting on Renal Disease (Milan, Italy), analyses were provided for 1068 pregnancies in 717 transplant recipients. Eighty percent of the women had received cadaver kidneys. The incidence of spontaneous abortion was 13 percent, or about the same as in the general population; however, therapeutic abortion was performed on 28 percent of the pregnancies. Of the pregnancies that continued beyond the first trimester, 90 percent culminated in a successful outcome.

Beginning early in pregnancy, glomerular filtration usually increased. Preeclampsia developed in 30 percent of women, and signs of kidney rejection were observed in 9 percent. Unfortunately, without renal biopsy, rejection

TABLE 28-6. POSTPARTUM HEMOLYTIC UREMIC SYNDROME (?) WITH RECOVERY[a]

	Hematocrit	Platelets	Plasma Creatinine	
5/1	Abruptio placentae, hemorrhage, oliguria			
5/3	Transferred to Parkland Memorial Hospital			
5/4	19	46,000	8.0	Hemodialysis
	2 units RBC			
5/5	21	28,000		Hemodialysis
	1 unit RBC			
5/8	18	88,000		Hemodialysis
	2 units RBC			
5/9	26	103,000		
5/10	28	159,000		Hemodialysis
5/11	28	169,000		
5/12	24	206,000		Hemodialysis
5/15	23	290,000		Hemodialysis
5/17	23	354,000		Hemodialysis
5/19	24	525,000		Hemodialysis
5/23	23	627,000		Diuresing
5/30	27	494,000	8.1	Home
6/13	27		4.5	
7/6	28		2.6	
9/14	35		1.8	
10/17			1.6	
+10 Years			1.2	

[a] 42-year-old para 5, severe abruptio placentae, microangiopathic hemolytic anemia, thrombocytopenia, and uremia

may be difficult to distinguish from acute pyelonephritis, recurrent glomerulopathy, and severe preeclampsia. Serious infections, most likely related to immunosuppressive therapy, complicated some pregnancies.

One half of the 618 infants who were successfully delivered were born preterm. Respiratory distress was common among the preterm infants but seldom was fatal. Malformations were identified in 2 percent; no specific type predominated. The newborns, as well as the mothers, were at increased risk of infection because of maternal immunosuppressive therapy.

From these experiences, criteria for not discouraging pregnancy have emerged that emphasize good general health without severe hypertension for 2 years after transplantation and no evidence of graft reaction or persisting proteinuria. Even so, the effects of pregnancy are unpredictable and not necessarily related to previous rejection episodes, lack of problems in previous pregnancies, or HLA types. Prednisone intake should be maintained at 15 mg a day or less and azathioprine at 2 mg/kg or less. We and others have observed azathioprine hepatic toxicity, with severe jaundice developing during pregnancy (Ware and co-workers, 1979). A reduction in dosage is likely to improve hepatic function.

Concern persists over the possibility of late effects in the offspring subjected to immunosuppressive therapy in utero, such as malignancy, germ cell dysfunction, and malformation in the offspring's offspring.

Observations based on many of the pregnancies cited above have been provided in detail by Davison and Lindheimer (1982).

Penn and co-workers (1980) described their extensive experiences with renal transplant and pregnancy. Fifty-six pregnancies in 37 women have culminated in 44 live births, including one set of twins; 3 more women were undelivered at the time of the report. Of 8 abortions, 1 was spontaneous and 7 were therapeutically performed because of impaired renal function, hypertension, or both; and 1 was a stillbirth (from maternal carbon monoxide poisoning). Twenty of the 44 infants were born before 37 weeks gestational age; only 6 of the infants were small for gestational age. Four infants had congenital anomalies, 4 developed respiratory distress, 2 had adrenocortical insufficiency, 2 developed septicemia, and 1 newborn convulsed from an unknown cause. One infant with sepsis died at 10 days of age.

Two of the mothers died 30 and 50 months after pregnancy. Both women refused to continue the immunosuppressive medications and died from graft rejection and uremia. Two others died of overwhelming sepsis 9 months after a third pregnancy and 82 months after a second pregnancy, respectively.

Fifty-eight of 60 babies sired by fathers who had undergone renal transplant were normal. One infant was born with meningomyelocele, hip dislocation, and talipes equinovarus. The other infant with congenital anomalies, including microcephaly and polycystic kidneys, died at birth.

Hemodialysis During Pregnancy

Most often, failing renal function is accompanied by infertility. With chronic hemodialysis, however, fertility may be restored (Perez and colleagues, 1978). A few women have subsequently become pregnant and have been so managed throughout the pregnancy. Liveborn infants with and without evidence of severe growth retardation have been described. Kobayashi and co-workers (1981) summarized several reported cases in which hemodialysis was used during pregnancy. They pointed out that pregnancy does not necessarily need to be terminated because the woman requires hemodialysis. In general, the prognosis must be assumed to be poor.

OTHER DISEASES OF THE URINARY SYSTEM

Polycystic Kidney Disease

An in-depth study of the apparent effects of polycystic kidney disease on pregnancy and vice versa has been provided by Milutinovic and co-workers (1983). Of 137 women at risk of having inherited the autosomal dominant gene, 55 percent demonstrated multiple renal cysts; 45 percent did not. Fertility, spontaneous abortion, stillbirth, and symptomatic urinary tract infection were comparable. Hypertension was more common both when pregnant and nonpregnant in those with polycystic disease, but no evidence was obtained of an adverse effect from pregnancy on the disease. Katz and associates (1979) have recorded a pregnancy in which the growth-retarded infant who was deliberately delivered remote from term survived, even though the mother was uremic from advanced polycystic kidney disease. Polycystic kidney disease is transmitted as an autosomal dominant trait.

Pregnancy After Unilateral Nephrectomy

Because the excretory capacity of two kidneys is much in excess of ordinary needs, and because the surviving kidney usually undergoes hypertrophy with increased excretory capacity, women with one normal kidney most often have no difficulty in pregnancy. If the remaining kidney is chronically infected, however, further damage may result from the stasis induced by pregnancy, with the likelihood of more intense infection. Accordingly, before advising a woman with one kidney about the risk of future pregnancy, a thorough functional evaluation of the remaining organ is essential. Should it be found impaired, childbearing may be risky. Even asymptomatic women should be carefully monitored to make certain that the single kidney is functioning satisfactorily.

Orthostatic Proteinuria

Proteinuria is detectable in urine formed while ambulatory but not when recumbent. No other evidence of renal disease is apparent. The estimate of 5 percent in pregnant women appears too high in our experience. The pregnant woman with orthostatic proteinuria should be evaluated for bacteriuria, abnormal urinary sediment, reduced glomerular filtration rate, and hypertension. In the absence of these abnormalities, the prognosis for pregnancy is good.

Intermittent proteinuria may be the consequence of a suburethral diverticulum that empties its proteinaceous contents into the voided urine from time to time, especially during examination of the anterior vaginal wall.

DISEASE OF THE HEART AND GREAT VESSELS

Heart disease is estimated to occur in approximately 1 percent of pregnancies. Rheumatic heart disease formerly accounted for the great majority of cases, but this has changed remarkably as new cases of rheumatic fever have almost disappeared in this country (Land and Bisno, 1983). Streptococci that are now prevalent appear to have low rheumatogenic potential as well as low nephritogenicity.

At the same time, better medical management, together with a number of newer surgical techniques, has enabled more girls with congenital heart disease to reach the childbearing age in reasonably good health and to conceive. Cardiac disease from hypertension contributes a few cases of organic heart disease in pregnancy, whereas other varieties, such as coronary, thyroid, syphilitic, and kyphoscoliotic cardiac disease, cor pulmonale, various forms of heart block, and isolated myocarditis, are even less common.

Heart disease may be a very serious complication of pregnancy leading to maternal death, but in the great majority of instances it need not be so.

PROGNOSIS

The likelihood of a favorable outcome for the mother with heart disease and her child-to-be depends upon (1) the functional capacity of her heart, (2) the likelihood of other complications that increase further the cardiac load during pregnancy and the puerperium, (3) the quality of medical care provided, and (4) the psychologic and socioeconomic capabilities of the expectant mother, her family, and the community. The last item may assume great importance, since a favorable outcome for the pregnancy is often achieved even in instances of markedly impaired cardiac function if the mother, her family, and the community will accept the need for, and provide an environment suitable for, a very sedentary life. For some women, these requirements may amount to hospitalization with essentially complete bed rest throughout pregnancy and early puerperium.

The prognosis and recommended treatment of cardiac disease have been influenced inappropriately in some instances by certain physiologic measurements, the imprecise or incorrect interpretation of which led the authors to conclude that a maternal hemodynamic burden peaked some weeks before term, following which the risk of cardiac failure dropped dramatically. Considerable emphasis has been placed, for example, on an apparent reduction in cardiac output after the 32nd week of pregnancy (Chapter 9, p. 195). The misconception that cardiac decompensation would seldom occur after this time is not supported by clinical observation. The decrease in maternal blood volume during the last weeks of pregnancy reported by some has been similarly considered to bring about a decrease in cardiac work. Most reported measurements, however, fail to identify a decrease in blood volume of any appreciable magnitude during the last several weeks. It is important that the physician understand that cardiac failure can develop during the last few weeks of the antepartum period, during labor, and during the puerperium. Indeed, of 542 women whose pregnancies were complicated by heart disease reported by Etheridge and Pepperell (1977), 10 died, with 8 of the deaths occurring during the puerperium.

DIAGNOSIS

As discussed at some length in Chapter 9 (p. 194), many of the physiologic changes of normal pregnancy tend to make the diagnosis of heart disease more difficult than it is in the nonpregnant state. For example, in normal pregnancy systolic heart murmurs that are functional are quite common. Moreover, as the uterus enlarges and the diaphragm is elevated, the heart is elevated and rotated so that the apex is moved laterally while the heart is somewhat closer to the anterior chest wall. Cardiac filling is increased, furthermore, accounting for the increase in stroke volume during much of pregnancy. Respiratory effort in normal pregnancy is accentuated, at times suggesting dyspnea. Presumably, this change is brought about in large part by a stimulatory effect of progesterone on the respiratory center. Edema, a further source of confusion, is often prevalent, especially in the lower extremities during the latter half of pregnancy. Therefore, systolic murmurs and edema, as well as changes that suggest cardiac enlargement and dyspnea, are commonplace in normal pregnancy. It becomes obvi-

ous that the physician must be quite careful not to diagnose heart disease during pregnancy when none exists but not fail to detect and treat appropriately heart disease when it does exist.

Burwell and Metcalfe (1958) list the following criteria, any one of which confirms the diagnosis of heart disease in pregnancy: (1) a diastolic, presystolic, or continuous heart murmur, (2) unequivocal cardiac enlargement, (3) a loud, harsh systolic murmur, especially if associated with a thrill, and (4) severe arrhythmia. Pregnant women who fulfill none of these criteria rarely have serious heart disease. While failure to detect clinically significant heart disease is inappropriate, faint suspicion of dysfunction should not lead to diagnostic efforts so intense that procedural costs become great or that seeds of anxiety are firmly planted in the mind of the patient.

Classification of Patients

There is no clinically applicable test for accurately measuring functional capacity of the heart. A helpful classification has been provided by the New York Heart Association, which is based on the woman's past and present disability and is uninfluenced by the presence or absence of physical signs:

- Class I. Uncompromised: Patients with cardiac disease and *no limitation of physical activity.* Patients in this class do not have symptoms of cardiac insufficiency, nor do they experience anginal pain.
- Class II. Slightly compromised: Patients with cardiac disease and *slight limitation of physical activity.* These patients are comfortable at rest, but if ordinary physical activity is undertaken, discomfort results in the form of excessive fatigue, palpitation, dyspnea, or anginal pain.
- Class III. Markedly compromised: Patients with cardiac disease and *marked limitation of physical activity.* These patients are comfortable at rest, but less than ordinary activity causes discomfort in the form of excessive fatigue, palpitation, dyspnea, or anginal pain.
- Class IV. Patients with cardiac disease and *inability to perform any physical activity without discomfort:* Symptoms of cardiac insufficiency or of the anginal syndrome may occur even at rest, and if any physical activity is undertaken, discomfort is increased.

GENERAL MANAGEMENT

The treatment of heart disease in pregnancy is dictated by the functional capacity of the heart. In all pregnant women, but especially in those with cardiac disease, excessive weight gain, *abnormal* retention of fluid, and anemia should be prevented. Increased bodily bulk increases the cardiac work, and anemia with its compensatory rise in cardiac output also predisposes to cardiac failure. The development of pregnancy-induced hypertension is hazardous, for in this circumstance cardiac output can be maintained only by an increase in cardiac work commensurate with the increase in blood pressure. At the same time, hypotension is undesirable, especially in women with septal defects or patent ductus arteriosus that allow shunting of blood from the right to the left heart chambers and from pulmonary artery to aorta.

Management of Classes I and II

With rare exceptions, women in class I and most in class II may be allowed to go through pregnancy. Throughout pregnancy and the puerperium, special attention should be directed toward both prevention and early recognition of heart failure. As emphasized by Sugrue and associates (1981), a more favorable functional classification at the outset should not engender any relaxation in vigilance of management. In 39 percent of their patients who developed frank cardiac failure the functional classification had been class I early in pregnancy!

A specific routine that assures adequate rest should be outlined for each patient. The recommendations of Hamilton and Thomson (1941) are still pertinent: The pregnant woman must rest in bed 10 hours each night and, in addition, must lie down for half an hour after each meal. Light housework and walking about on the level may be permitted. The patient should do no heavy work. Items rich in sodium should be avoided. Weight gain should not exceed the 24 pounds or so that are accounted for by the physiologic changes induced by normal pregnancy. In essence, the pregnant woman must learn to spare herself all unnecessary effort and must rest as much as possible.

Not infrequently, infection has proved to be an important factor in precipitating cardiac failure. Each woman should receive instructions to avoid contact with others who have respiratory infections, including the common cold, and to report at once any evidence of an infection. Pneumococcal and influenza vaccines are probably worthwhile.

The onset of congestive heart failure is often gradual and may be detected if attention is continually directed to certain particular signs. The first warning sign of cardiac failure is likely to be persistent rales at the base of the lungs, frequently with a cough. To be significant, the rales must still be audible after the patient has taken two or three deep breaths, for the rales that are sometimes heard in normal pregnant women disappear after one or two deep inspirations. A sudden diminution in the woman's ability to carry out her household duties, increasing dyspnea on exertion, attacks of smothering with cough, and hemoptysis are other signals warning of serious heart failure, as are progressive edema and tachycardia.

Measurements appropriately made of the vital capacity at each visit are of value, for a sudden decrease may denote cardiac failure. Although the program outlined for the early detection of cardiac failure may seem scarcely applicable to patients in class I or class II, since they seldom decompensate during pregnancy, the interests of the mother and the fetus dictate that all cases of cardiac disease in pregnancy be regarded as at risk of possible decompensation.

Hospitalization before delivery of women with classes I and II cardiac disease has become common practice. Delivery should be accomplished vaginally unless other obstetric complications require cesarean section. In spite of the physical effort inherent in labor and vaginal delivery, less morbidity and mortality have been recorded when delivery has been so accomplished.

Relief from pain and apprehension without undue depression of the infant or the mother is especially important during labor and delivery of women with cardiac disease. For the multiparous woman with a soft, effaced, somewhat dilated cervix, in whom little soft tissue resistance is offered by the vagina and perineum, analgesics in moderate doses usually provide satisfactory pain relief. For women, especially nulliparas, in whom cervical dilatation, descent of the presenting part, and delivery will probably require greater force over a longer time, continuous epidural anesthesia often proves valuable for reducing pain and apprehension. The major danger of conduction anesthesia is maternal hypotension. Hypotension may be fatal in women with cardiac shunts, in whom flow may be reversed, with blood passing from the right to the left side of the heart or the aorta, thereby bypassing the lungs. Continuous conduction anesthesia is considered further in Chapter 18.

For cesarean section, the combination of thiopental, succinylcholine, nitrous oxide, and 50 percent oxygen, with an endotracheal airway placed after previously neutralizing gastric juice, has also proved satisfactory.

During labor, the mother should be kept in a semirecumbent position. Measurements of the pulse and respiratory rates should be made at least four times every hour during the first stage of labor and every 10 minutes during the second stage. Increase in the pulse rate much above 100 per minute or in the respiratory rate above 24, particularly when associated with dyspnea, are signs of cardiac embarrassment that may progress to overt cardiac failure. With any evidence of cardiac embarrassment, intensive medical management must be instituted immediately. Only in the presence of the completely dilated cervix and an engaged presenting part may these changes be taken as indication for delivery. With the cervix only partially dilated and the mother showing obvious evidence of cardiac embarrassment, there is no method of delivery that will not first intensify rather than relieve heart failure.

Immediate medical treatment usually calls for the use of morphine, oxygen, a rapidly acting digitalis preparation, a potent diuretic, and the Fowler position. Morphine should be given intravenously and titrated so as to allay apprehension and also provide relief from pain. It will serve not only to allay apprehension and reduce the elevated respiratory rate, but in the second stage of labor it will reduce the voluntary muscular activity associated with uterine contractions. In the presence of pulmonary edema, oxygen may best be given in the form of intermittent positive-pressure breathing to promote adequate oxygenation and to reduce edema. Digitalis in the form of a rapidly acting glycoside should be given intravenously. Care must be exercised to avoid toxicity, especially in the woman who is depleted of potassium as the consequence of previous diuretic therapy.

Furosemide, given intravenously in a dose of 50 to 100 mg, should not only stimulate diuresis but also relax the capacitance system which, in turn, will reduce venous return to the heart, lower intrapulmonary and left atrial blood pressures, and thereby reduce pulmonary congestion. If the woman is hypertensive, antihypertensive agents should be administered to reduce cardiac afterload. If hypotensive, the cause must be identified. If coincidental hemorrhage is the cause, as for example, severe abruptio placentae with concealed hemorrhage, careful blood replacement and arrest of the hemorrhage are important to a successful outcome. Successful therapy should reflect in a satisfactory hematocrit and a reasonable urinary output.

If the hypotension is the consequence of a severely impaired myocardium, treatment is more difficult, and if there is no improvement after employing the modalities just outlined, invasive hemodynamic monitoring with a functional Swan-Ganz catheter and serial cardiac output measurements may prove important in decision making involving further therapy.

Signs of cardiac embarrassment developing after complete dilatation of the cervix and engagement of the vertex are indications for prompt forceps delivery unless easy spontaneous birth is expected within a few minutes.

Women who have shown little or no evidence of cardiac distress during pregnancy, labor, or delivery sometimes decompensate after delivery. Therefore, it is important that the same meticulous care provided during the antepartum and intrapartum periods be continued into the puerperium. Postpartum hemorrhage, puerperal infection, and puerperal thromboembolism are much more serious complications of pregnancy in the woman with heart disease. If there was no evidence of cardiac embarrassment during labor, delivery, and the early puerperium, breast-feeding is usually not contraindicated. In general, if tubal sterilization is to be performed, it should be delayed until it is obvious that the mother is afebrile, not anemic, and has demonstrated that she can ambulate without evidence of distress. Women who do not undergo tubal sterilization should be given detailed contraceptive advice, as should all puerperal women.

Management of Class III

Women whose cardiac function is so seriously diminished as to fall in class III present difficult problems that demand expert medical judgment and care. The impor-

tant question is whether they should become pregnant. The rational answer is no, but many women will risk much for a baby. They and their families must understand the risk and be willing and able to cooperate to the fullest extent.

The study of Bunim and Appel (1950) demonstrated that about one third of class III cardiac patients will decompensate during pregnancy, unless preventive measures are taken. When such a woman is seen in the first trimester, a question of therapeutic abortion inevitably arises. Her desire for a child may be a determining factor, but class III cardiac disease is an urgent indication for therapeutic abortion unless the mother can be hospitalized for the duration of the pregnancy.

The experience of Gorenberg and Chesley (1958) at the Margaret Hague Maternity Hospital led them to conclude that any woman with heart disease seen early in gestation can be carried through pregnancy successfully if she and her family are willing to abide by certain strict rules. Their recommended regimen included bed rest in the hospital for the duration of the pregnancy in any patient with class III disease. The application of this basic principle, together with good medical and obstetric care to well over 1000 patients in the cardiac clinic, reduced the maternal death rate to not much more than that of the general obstetric population. The extreme importance of rigid adherence to their rules is demonstrated clearly by the fact that cardiac disease was the leading cause of maternal death at the hospital, but those who died were not women attending their cardiac clinic.

The method of delivery is vaginal, as in classes I and II, with cesarean section limited to obstetric indications. Any pregnant woman with a history of previous cardiac failure that was not associated with acute rheumatic carditis or whose cardiac lesion causing the failure has not been corrected surgically is best managed as class III, regardless of the current functional classification.

Even though the woman has recently been in failure or is in failure at the time of labor, vaginal delivery, in general, is safer than cesarean section. These very sick women withstand major surgical procedures poorly; their severe heart disease is a contraindication rather than an indication for cesarean section.

Whereas it is well established that the woman with cardiac disease who receives appropriate care rarely dies during pregnancy or the puerperium, the possibility has been raised that pregnancy causes obscure deleterious effects that ultimately shorten her life span. In other words, it is suggested that pregnancy in some way might accelerate the rate of deterioration of cardiac function. The comprehensive studies by Chesley (1980) of a large number of pregnant women observed over a long period did not demonstrate, or even suggest, that pregnancy has a deleterious remote effect on the course of rheumatic heart disease.

Hospitalization for many months for the woman

who has other children or who perhaps is unmarried and does not desire the pregnancy is a great price, psychologically as well as financially, for her, her family, and, in many instances, the community to pay. Moreover, the life expectancy of the woman with serious cardiac disease is likely to be appreciably shortened. Sometimes, therefore, the child will be motherless at a young age. Thus, even though therapeutic abortion is not mandatory to save the life of the mother when prolonged hospitalization and competent medical care can be provided, if these conditions are not available or are not acceptable to the woman, therapeutic abortion and sterilization, or at least effective contraception, are indicated. Therapeutic abortion demands the application of all of the safeguards discussed previously for safely accomplishing delivery, including vigorous treatment to correct cardiac decompensation before the procedure.

Management of Class IV

The treatment of women with class IV heart disease is essentially that of cardiac failure in pregnancy, labor, and the puerperium. In the presence of cardiac failure, delivery by any known method carries a high maternal mortality rate. Accordingly, the treatment of heart failure in pregnancy is primarily medical rather than obstetric. The prime objective is to correct the decompensation, for only then will delivery be safe.

Effects on Fetus and Newborn

In general, any disease complicated by severe maternal hypoxia is likely to lead to abortion, premature delivery, and intrauterine death. A relation of chronic hypoxia and the polycythemia it causes to the outcome of pregnancy has been demonstrated in studies on women with cyanotic heart disease. Whittemore and colleagues (1980) identified fetal wastage to be 36 percent in pregnancies of women with hypoxic congenital heart disease. When hypoxia is so intense as to stimulate a rise in the hematocrit reading above 65 percent, pregnancy wastage is virtually 100 percent.

Surgical Repair

For some years, to try to improve maternal cardiac function, several kinds of operations have been performed on the heart and large vessels, including open heart surgery with cardiopulmonary bypass.

Heart Valves. A number of women of reproductive age have had a cardiac valvar prosthesis implanted to replace a severely damaged mitral or aortic valve. More recent reports of subsequent pregnancy outcomes in these circumstances include those of Chen and associates (1982) and O'Neill and co-workers (1982). In fact, preg-

nancies with successful outcomes have followed replacement of all three heart valves by prostheses (Nagorney and Field, 1981). Moreover, cardiac bypass and valve replacement procedures have been successfully accomplished during pregnancy (Levy and associates, 1980; Martin and associates, 1981).

The likelihood that a young woman undergoing valve replacement might wish to procreate subsequently has led to the insertion by some of a tissue (typically porcine) valve. Unfortunately, such valves are not proving to be durable; moreover, thromboembolism can occur without anticoagulation (Oakley, 1983).

Continuous anticoagulant therapy is recommended to prevent emboli. If the woman is not pregnant, warfarin is satisfactory, but this drug crosses the placenta and may cause anomalous development, as well as hemorrhage and death in the fetus and newborn. Warfarin during the first trimester is teratogenic. Heparin is the anticoagulant of choice antepartum. It does not cross the placenta. The pregnant woman can usually be instructed to inject heparin satisfactorily into the subcutaneous tissue (Bonnar, 1979). Just before delivery, the heparin is stopped. If delivery occurs while the anticoagulant is still effective and extensive bleeding is encountered, protamine sulfate should be given. Anticoagulant therapy with warfarin or heparin may be restarted the day after vaginal delivery, usually with no problems.

Ueland and associates (1981) have cited data reported by others that heparin given antepartum was accompanied by high perinatal mortality, but they pointed out emphatically that many of the deaths were in pregnancies in serious jeopardy from severe preeclampsia for which heparin was given experimentally! However, chronically administered heparin can affect the pregnancy adversely. As well as the potential danger of hemorrhage, there is the further risk of serious bone demineralization (Howell and associates, 1983; De Swiet and co-workers, 1983).

It is not surprising that severe complications can arise during pregnancy when the mother has a prosthetic valve. Such complications include thrombosis and thromboembolism, hemorrhage, deterioration in cardiac function, and even maternal death. Spontaneous abortions, low birth weight infants, and possibly fetal malformations occur more often than in the general obstetric population. Therefore, sterilization frequently has merit. Because of their possibly thrombogenic action, oral contraceptives containing estrogen and a progestin are usually contraindicated.

Mitral Valvotomy. El-Maraghy and associates (1983) have recorded their experiences in 42 pregnant women with serious disability from mitral stenosis who underwent valvotomy during pregnancy. The 42 mothers and 41 of the fetuses survived; 1 spontaneous abortion occurred 2 days after surgery. Subsequent to surgery, 3 of the 42 women remained in class III.

Patent Ductus Arteriosus

Some patients with patent ductus arteriosus develop pulmonary hypertension and, particularly if the systemic blood pressure falls, may have a reversal of blood flow from the pulmonary artery to the aorta with consequent cyanosis. Sudden drops in blood pressure at delivery, as with conduction anesthesia or hemorrhage, may lead to fatal collapse. Therefore, hypotension should be avoided whenever possible and treated vigorously if it occurs. Burwell and Metcalfe (1958) suggested that the ductus should not be ligated during pregnancy. In our own experience, however, the operation has proved to be relatively simple, and cardiac function improved dramatically.

Cyanotic Heart Disease. If the hematocrit is very high, spontaneous abortion occurs most of the time. With somewhat lesser degrees of polycythemia there is a lesser but still increased incidence of abortion and underweight infants. Whereas uncorrected cyanotic heart disease carries a high risk for both the mother and the fetus, when surgical correction prior to pregnancy is satisfactory, fetal environment is improved remarkably and maternal risks decrease dramatically. Singh and associates (1982), on the basis of 40 pregnancies in 27 patients with surgically corrected *tetralogy of Fallot,* state that a woman with no major residual defects after surgery may be reassured that pregnancy will be well tolerated and delivery can be accomplished in the normal manner.

The prognosis for a pregnancy complicated by *Eisenmenger's syndrome* is poor, as it is with *pulmonary hypertension* from any cause. Both maternal and perinatal mortality rates for Eisenmenger's syndrome have been identified to be about 30 percent (Gleicher and colleagues, 1979).

Coronary Thrombosis and Ischemic Heart Disease

These are rare complications of pregnancy. The treatment is similar to that for the nonpregnant patient. The advisability of a woman undertaking a pregnancy after a myocardial infarction is not clear. Since the underlying vascular disease is usually progressive and since it frequently is associated with hypertension, pregnancy in general appears to be contraindicated. Cortis and Gensini (1977) have advised coronary angiography, and if severe involvement is detected, pregnancy should be discouraged.

Myocardial infarction can occur during pregnancy. Fortunately, it is rare. Hankins and co-workers (1984) have described two cases of myocardial infarction during pregnancy with favorable outcomes for both mothers and infants. They have presented in detail their management techniques, which included labor and vaginal delivery under very close hemodynamic monitoring. They also have provided an extensive review of the literature.

In their two patients, infarction was evident in one at 5 weeks gestation and in the other at 36 weeks gestation. The 39-year-old primigravida at 36 weeks gestation suffered a cardiac arrest for which electroshock was applied twice. In the other woman late in pregnancy angina became severe with any exertion. She was hospitalized for 6 weeks before delivery and treated frequently with nitrates.

In both instances vaginal delivery was planned for under carefully controlled conditions at or very near term. Spontaneous labor developed in one at 39 weeks, 3 weeks after myocardial infarction; in the other it was induced with oxytocin at 38 weeks.

Epidural or epidural plus caudal analgesia was used to minimize both the discomfort of labor and vigorous expulsive efforts that might otherwise have characterized the second stage of labor. Rapid infusion of fluid just before commencing the epidural analgesia was avoided.

Throughout labor, delivery, and the early puerperium maternal hemodynamic function was carefully monitored, including pressure measurements made through an appropriately placed Swan-Ganz catheter, blood pressure measurements through an arterial line, continuous EKG recording, and cardiac outputs determined repeatedly by the thermal dilution technique. Intrauterine pressures were continuously monitored, as was the fetal heart rate.

The 39-year-old primigravida was delivered with low forceps; the other woman delivered spontaneously.

Cardiac outputs were demonstrated to increase 7 to 10 percent during the first stage of labor, 21 to 23 percent during the second stage, and 35 percent during delivery. During the first stage of labor, central venous and pulmonary capillary wedge pressures averaged 10 mm Hg beween uterine contractions but transiently reached levels as high as 25 mm Hg during a contraction.

One year later, both mothers were alive and the infants were thriving.

Postpartal and Peripartal Cardiomyopathy

A cardiomyopathy that develops before, during, or after delivery has been considered by some to be caused somehow by the pregnancy, although the exact etiology is unknown (Burch, 1977). Typically in this country, the woman is black, multiparous, and older. If the mother survives the episode of cardiac decompensation, she may make a complete recovery. The disease has been reported to recur occasionally in a subsequent pregnancy and, at times, remote from pregnancy. Even though the belief prevails that this is a unique syndrome induced in some way by pregnancy and characterized by congestive heart failure with cardiomegaly, pulmonary congestion, and electrocardiographic evidence of nonspecific myocardial damage, it is far from clear whether postpartum heart disease is a distinct clinical entity. Unless the cardiomegaly and other evidence of failure clear promptly and completely, future pregnancies should be avoided.

An extensive review by Veille (1984) serves to emphasize the confusion that surrounds the presumed but certainly not proven syndrome of peripartal cardiomyopathy.

Bacterial Endocarditis

Bacterial endocarditis, acute or subacute, may be encountered during pregnancy and the puerperium. It has contributed appreciably to the relatively few maternal deaths at Parkland Memorial Hospital in recent years. Most often the pregnant women were taking illicit drugs intravenously, then developed bacterial endocarditis, and died from valvar incompetence or emboli to the brain. Surgical intervention with various prosthetic valve replacements of the destroyed valves along with antibiotic therapy and meticulous supportive care may prevent a fatal outcome. Cavalieri and associates (1982) have described a case in which a ruptured, abscessed aortic valve was replaced early in the puerperium. The mother was discharged after 6 weeks of antibiotic therapy. Pastorek and associates (1983) have described in some detail their management of three cases treated antepartum.

Antibiotic Prophylaxis. To minimize the risk of bacterial endocarditis and infective arteritis, women with endocardial damage, valvar prostheses, or mitral valve prolapse or with abnormalities associated with the aorta, such as patent ductus arteriosus or coarctation of the aorta, have often received antibiotics prophylactically around the time of delivery. Even though the evidence that a significant number of cases of bacterial endocarditis have been so prevented is scant to absent, the cost of prophylaxis is not great. If prophylaxis is to be effective, administration should begin during labor and be continued for 48 hours or so after delivery. Aqueous penicillin G (2 million units) plus gentamicin or tobramycin (1.5 mg/kg) every 8 hours intravenously has been recommended by McAnulty and associates (1981). Apparent failures of prophylaxis reported by Durack and associates (1983) include one instance of saline abortion.

For individuals with a history of rheumatic fever or rheumatic heart disease benzathine penicillin G (1.2 million units) intramuscularly each month is recommended.

OTHER DEVELOPMENTAL ABNORMALITIES

Mitral Valve Prolapse

This condition has been suspected to occur in upward to 10 percent of women. In our experience it has not been deleterious to pregnancy, although it may have contributed to pulmonary edema in some women in whom suspected premature labor was treated with β-mimetic agents (Chapter 37, p. 753). Mitral valve prolapse is considered, by some at least, to be a significant risk factor for bacterial endocarditis (Clemens and associates, 1982).

Marfan's Syndrome

This syndrome is characterized by a generalized weakness of connective tissue that can result in dangerous cardiovascular complications. It is considered further on p. 622.

Coarctation of the Aorta

This is a relatively rare lesion. The collateral circulation arising above the level of the coarctation expands, often to a striking extent, to cause localized erosion of the margins of the ribs by the hypertrophied intercostal arteries. The typical findings on physical examination are hypertension in the upper extremities but normal or reduced arterial blood pressures in the lower extremities.

The major complications of coarctation of the aorta are congestive heart failure when there has been long-standing severe hypertension, bacterial endocarditis, and rupture of the aorta. The aortic ruptures are more likely to occur late in pregnancy or early in the puerperium and may be associated with changes in the media that are histologically similar to those characterizing Erdheim's idiopathic medial cystic necrosis.

Congestive heart failure demands vigorous efforts to improve cardiac function and usually warrants interruption of the pregnancy. It has been recommended by some that resection of the coarctation be undertaken during pregnancy to protect against the possibility of dissecting aneurysm and rupture of the aorta. The operation, however, is not without significant risk, especially to the fetus, because all the collaterals must be clamped for variable periods of time during the procedure, possibly leading to serious fetal hypoxia.

Some authorities have recommended that the woman with coarctation of the aorta be delivered by cesarean section lest the transient elevation of arterial blood pressure that commonly accompanies labor lead to rupture of either the aorta or a coexisting cerebral aneurysm. The available evidence, however, suggests that cesarean section should be limited to obstetric indications.

Kyphoscoliotic Heart Disease

During pregnancy especially, severe degrees of kyphoscoliosis commonly cause serious cardiopulmonary problems, sometimes referred to as *kyphoscoliotic heart disease.* In these circumstances, some regions of the lungs in the markedly deformed thoracic cage may be quite emphysematous, while others are atelectatic, with both lesions contributing to an inadequate ventilatory capacity. In these circumstances, *cor pulmonale* is a frequent complication.

The increased oxygen demands and the cardiac work imposed by pregnancy and delivery must be taken into account in reaching a decision whether to allow the pregnancy to continue or to perform a therapeutic abortion. If pulmonary function studies indicate that the vital capacity is not reduced appreciably, the outcome most often is favorable. In women with marked degrees of kyphoscoliosis and markedly impaired pulmonary function, therapeutic abortion is indicated.

Frequently the bony pelvis is so distorted that cesarean section is necessary. The supine position during delivery may result in serious hypotension. The commonly used analgesics, such as meperidine (Demerol), should be used carefully, since respiratory depression is very poorly tolerated. During and after delivery, meticulous care should be directed toward the prevention of further atelectasis, which could lead rapidly to severe hypoxia and death. Intermittent positive-pressure breathing using appropriate concentrations of oxygen with mucolytic agents is of value. Sterilization is often indicated. Kopenhager (1977) has provided an analysis of the obstetric and medical complications of 50 women with kyphoscoliosis.

Arrhythmias

Cardiac arrhythmias occur during pregnancy, but their frequency and intensity are unlikely to be any worse at that time. Bradyarrhythmias, including complete heart block, are compatible with a successful pregnancy outcome.

Tachyarrhythmias are more common. Supraventricular tachycardias and fibrillation can be treated with digoxin or similar preparation. While such alkaloids cross the placenta, they do not appear to harm the fetus. Cardioversion is not contraindicated by pregnancy per se.

Supraventricular tachycardia in association with Wolff-Parkinson-White syndrome has been identified by Gleicher and associates (1981) to have complicated three pregnancies. Propranolol proved effective when used in two instances.

DISEASES OF THE RESPIRATORY SYSTEM

Pregnancy induces a number of changes in the respiratory system. Enlargement of the uterus causes the diaphragm to rise, the transverse thoracic diameter to increase, the vertical chest diameter to decrease, and the residual volume of air in the lungs to be reduced. In response to the modest hyperventilation that occurs normally in pregnancy, the tidal volume is increased somewhat and the plasma carbon dioxide is lowered slightly. Of importance, during the latter part of pregnancy, oxygen consumption is increased 15 to 25 percent above that of normal nonpregnant women (Chapter 9, p. 196).

Pneumonia

Pneumonitis causing an appreciable loss of ventilatory capacity is tolerated less well by women during pregnancy. This generalization seems to hold true irrespective of whether the cause of the pneumonia is bacterial, viral, or chemical. Moreover, as has been emphasized in the discussions of heart disease and of diabetes, hypoxia and acidosis are poorly tolerated by the fetus. Therefore, it is important to the pregnant woman and her fetus that pneumonia be diagnosed as soon as possible and that she be promptly hospitalized so that the disease can be most effectively treated.

There are a few recent reports that deal specifically with pneumonia complicating pregnancy. Benedetti and associates (1982) summarized their experiences with 39 cases caused by a variety of organisms, but most often *Streptococcus pneumoniae*. They utilized prompt hospitalization, antibiotics, measurement of arterial Po$_2$, and, when low, oxygen therapy. All of the mothers survived. One fetus expired whose mother also had sickle cell anemia. These for the most part favorable

outcomes should not serve to minimize the gravity of pneumonia complicating pregnancy but rather to emphasize the value of prompt diagnosis and effective treatment.

Pneumonia caused by *Mycoplasma pneumoniae* is probably fairly common in pregnancy. Unfortunately, it is difficult to diagnose and to treat. A cold agglutinin usually is evident, and eventually complement-fixing antibodies appear. Erythromycin is the antibiotic generally recommended during pregnancy. In the absence of hypoxia, this form of pneumonitis probably does not affect pregnancy adversely.

Aspiration of gastric contents during anesthesia for delivery can cause severe chemical pneumonitis, primarily as the consequence of the necrotizing effects of hydrochloric acid (Mendelson, 1946). Diagnosis and treatment of gastric aspiration are discussed in Chapter 18 (p. 358). The aspiration of gastric contents is not limited to anesthesia for delivery. For example, treatment of eclampsia with large doses of morphine or barbiturates and inebriating the pregnant woman with ethanol to try to arrest labor have sometimes been followed by the aspiration of gastric contents and a bad outcome.

Viral pneumonitis, especially that caused by varicella, can prove devastating to the mother and, in turn, the hypoxic fetus (p. 627), as can influenzal pneumonitis (p. 628).

Thromboembolism and Pulmonary Infarction

Both thromboembolism and pulmonary infarction may be encountered during pregnancy, but they occur more often during the puerperium. Diagnosis and treatment of these serious problems are discussed in Chapter 36.

Asthma

This rather common respiratory illness is encountered relatively often in pregnant women. With active but otherwise uncomplicated asthma, indices of expiratory air flow are reduced while diffusing capacity is normal. A low Pco_2 indicates hyperventilation. An elevated Pco_2 is evidence of CO_2 retention and is ominous.

Pregnancy does not seem to exert any consistent predictable effect on bronchial asthma. In some pregnant women, asthma appears to be less of a problem, in others, it is more, and in still others, it remains about the same. The great majority of women with asthma can be safely carried through pregnancy, labor, and delivery. The pregnant woman in whom signs and symptoms of asthma have previously been mild is at low risk of serious asthmatic attacks during pregnancy. However, the woman who suffers severe attacks when not pregnant is likely to continue to do so when pregnant.

In general, therapeutic regimens that have been beneficial when the patient was not pregnant will continue to be so during pregnancy. This applies both to agents used chronically to minimize bronchospasm and promote clearance of secretions and to those used in vigorous treatment of a severe attack causing hypoxia and hypercapnea. It should be emphasized again that oxygen consumption increases during pregnancy by up to 25 percent and that the fetus tolerates severe hypoxia poorly. Arterial blood gases should be evaluated and oxygen therapy applied when the Po_2 is 70 mm Hg or less. If a favorable response is not soon achieved with oxygen by mask or nasal prongs, mechanical ventilation may be required. At the same time, treatment with α-adrenergic agents such as terbutaline, corticosteroids such as hydrocortisone or methylprednisolone, and, with considerable caution, theophyllines such as aminophylline should be initiated. Hydration without overload is often beneficial. A search for a precipitating or aggravating factor, especially infection, should be undertaken.

The use of medications that contain iodide must be avoided, for iodide is transported across the placenta to the fetus and concentrated in the fetal thyroid. When the mother ingests iodide over a prolonged period of time, the large amount of iodide reaching the fetus may induce a large goiter.

Therapeutic abortion might be indicated in the uncommon woman who, as the consequence of long-standing asthma, has reduced cardiopulmonary function. Since asthma is a chronic disease that in the adult is likely to persist for many years after the pregnancy, sterilization may have merit.

Pulmonary Resection

The effect of pulmonary resection, usually for bronchiectasis or tuberculosis, will depend upon the functional capacity of the remaining pulmonary tissue. In general, if function is equivalent to one normal lung and active pulmonary disease is not present, pregnancy is tolerated without undue risk to the mother and with a good likelihood of delivery of a healthy infant.

Tuberculosis

The considerable influx of women from Southeast Asia, as well as South of the Border, has been accompanied by an increased frequency of tuberculosis in pregnant women, especially in public clinics. Fortunately, the prognosis has improved remarkably for the woman with active pulmonary tuberculosis if the disease is diagnosed and treated. Chemotherapy that has proved to be effective in the absence of pregnancy is also effective during pregnancy. Fortunately, several such drugs do not appear to affect the fetus adversely. Scheinhorn and Angelillo (1977) discovered no increase in birth defects among children whose mothers during pregnancy had been treated with isoniazid, ethambutol, or rifampin. Mild auditory and vestibular abnormalities were identified after streptomycin therapy. When isoniazid is used during pregnancy, supplemental pyridoxine probably should also be administered to minimize the potential for neurotoxicity in the fetus (Atkins, 1982).

Bowes (1975) recommended that all women registering for prenatal care be screened for tuberculosis by appropriate skin testing. If the tine or Mantoux skin test is negative, no further evaluation is needed. If positive, a thorough history is obtained, and a complete physical examination and chest roentgenogram with the abdomen shielded are performed. If both are negative, no treatment is necessary until after delivery, when, generally, isoniazid therapy is carried out for 1 year. However, very few clinics routinely screen all their obstetric patients in this way.

Evaluation of the degree of activity of the pulmonary disease roentgenographically at times may be difficult. As pregnancy advances and the diaphragm rises, the lungs undergo some degree of compression, which may mask the extent of the tuberculous lesion. In fact, this mechanical effect of pregnancy on the lung may conceal actual pulmonary cavitation. Therefore, treatment may have to be undertaken in the pregnant woman on less firm ground than if she were not pregnant.

In the absence of seriously impaired pulmonary function, analgesia and anesthesia for labor and delivery can usually be accomplished with any of the techniques used for normal pregnancy. Tuberculosis is seldom an indication for therapeutic abortion unless there is disseminated tuberculosis or severely compromised cardiopulmonary function. Sterilization is warranted for women who desire no more children. Rifampin, which has been used usually in combination with isoniazid, may impair the efficacy of oral contraceptives.

Congenital tuberculosis is rare even when the mother has widespread disease but does occur and can prove fatal (Myers and co-workers, 1981). The newborn infant is also quite susceptible to tuberculosis. Therefore, the infant should be isolated immediately from the mother suspected of having active disease. Because of the risk of active disease developing in the infant, either isoniazid chemoprophylaxis or BCG vaccination may be beneficial.

Pelvic tuberculosis usually causes intractable sterility. When pregnancy does occur, often it terminates ectopically or in abortion followed at times by activation of the pelvic infection. Although treatment is still controversial, the consensus favors a combination of chemotherapy and surgical extirpation of the pelvic organs. In younger women, however, more conservative therapy may be justified.

Sarcoidosis

This multisystem granulomatous disorder of unknown etiology is rarely identified in pregnant women. The available evidence implies that sarcoidosis seldom affects pregnancy adversely; some authors suggest that pregnancy may actually be beneficial (Dines and Banner, 1967). O'Leary (1968) noted that only women with extensive pulmonary involvement were at risk during pregnancy. We have observed one maternal death in which severe pulmonary sarcoidosis and extensive hilar ade-nopathy were further complicated by placenta previa, extreme obesity, and aspiration of gastric contents.

Pregnancy is not a contraindication to the use of corticosteroids to treat sarcoidosis.

Cystic Fibrosis

This disease is transmitted as an autosomal recessive trait and is estimated to occur in 1 per 1500 white births and 1 per 17,000 black births. Because of improvements in diagnosis and treatment, more girls are surviving to adulthood and conceiving.

Most of the clinical manifestations are caused by abnormal mucus production. Those males who survive to adulthood very often have aspermia. Among females who survive to adulthood, most are infertile because of delay in sexual development and perhaps because of the production of an abnormal cervical mucus.

The pulmonary involvement with cystic fibrosis can prove very deleterious to a pregnancy. Chronic hypoxia and frequent pulmonary infections characterize the pregnancy state. Pancreatic dysfunction can contribute significantly to poor maternal nutrition. Cohen and associates (1980) carried out a survey of cystic fibrosis centers and obtained information on 129 pregnancies. Increased maternal and perinatal mortality were related to severe pulmonary infection.

ENDOCRINE DISORDERS

It is quite evident from the following discussions that a variety of endocrine disorders can complicate pregnancy and vice versa. Diabetes mellitus is made worse by pregnancy, and diabetes increases appreciably the risk of a number of pregnancy complications. With some other conditions, for example, hyperthyroidism, pregnancy often only appears to worsen the endocrinopathy by increasing the concentration of circulating thyroxine but not necessarily the amount of free, or active, hormone.

DIABETES MELLITUS

Before the advent of insulin many women with diabetes were too ill to conceive. For example, Williams (1915), after 13 years as Chief of the Obstetrical Service of the Johns Hopkins Hospital, with a large consulting practice in addition, had encountered only one case of pregnancy complicated by recognized diabetes. The exact cause of the infertility in diabetic women during the preinsulin era is not clear, but amenorrhea was common, the incidence having been placed as high as 50 percent. Of the infrequent patients in whom pregnancy occurred, about one fourth of the mothers and about half of the fetuses and infants died.

Prevalence

The lack of agreement about the minimal requirements for the diagnosis of diabetes mellitus makes it difficult to acquire satisfactory figures for its prevalence. Even so, by diagnostic criteria acceptable to most workers, it is estimated that more than 5 percent of the population now have overt diabetes. The cause or causes for the remarkable increase in recent years are not known, but environmental factors, as well as genetic predisposition, are implicated. Bases for incriminating environmental factors are provided by the following observations: For most young persons with insulin-dependent (type I) diabetes, there is no family history of diabetes. Moreover, the concordance rate for diabetes in monozygous twins, rather than being nearly 100 percent if diabetes were solely genetic in origin, is actually less than 50 percent.

The probability of interaction of environmental factors, especially viral, and of genetic predisposition, is supported by demonstrations of considerable variation in susceptibility to diabetes among different animal strains injected with the same virus. In human population studies, an association has been found between the HLA system and some, but not all, forms of diabetes.

Classification

The National Diabetes Data Group (1979) provided the following scheme for classifying diabetes mellitus, including diabetes apparent only during pregnancy (gestational diabetes):

A. Insulin-dependent type (type I)
B. Noninsulin-dependent type (type II)
    1. Nonobese
    2. Obese
C. Other types (secondary diabetes)
    1. Pancreatic disease
    2. Hormonally induced
    3. Chemically induced
    4. Insulin receptor abnormalities
    5. Certain genetic syndromes
    6. Others
D. Impaired glucose tolerance (subclinical diabetes)
E. Gestational diabetes (pregnancy-induced glucose intolerance)

White (1978) provided an update of her classification of pregnant women with diabetes, which is presented in Table 28-7. Unfortunately, its increasing complexity may have impaired its usefulness.

Diagnosis During Pregnancy

The woman who presents with glucosuria, high plasma glucose levels, ketonemia, and ketonuria is no problem in diagnosis. The woman at the opposite end of the spectrum, with only minimal metabolic derangement caused by diabetes, is difficult to identify. The likelihood of im-paired carbohydrate metabolism and related metabolic stigmata of diabetes is increased appreciably in women who have a strong familial history of diabetes, have given birth to large infants, demonstrate persistent glucosuria, or have unexplained fetal losses.

Reducing substances are commonly found in the urine of pregnant women, but their presence does not necessarily mean diabetes. Often the material is lactose, which should not be a source of needless concern if the urine is tested by a method that is specific for glucose. The commercially available testing substances, Tes-Tape and Clinistix, may be used to identify glucose in the urine while avoiding a positive reaction from lactose. Even when lactosuria is excluded, glycosuria caused by glucose is occasionally identified. Most often, the glucosuria does not reflect hyperglycemia from impaired glucose tolerance but rather the lowered renal threshold for glucose induced by normal pregnancy, as discussed in Chapter 9 (p. 198). Nonetheless, the detection of glucosuria during pregnancy generally warrants further testing.

Fasting Hyperglycemia (Overt Diabetes, White Class B Through T). The criterion for diagnosis of overt diabetes during pregnancy is the identification of fasting hyperglycemia on two or more occasions. Fasting hyperglycemia during pregnancy has been defined by the National Diabetes Data Group (1979) to be a *plasma* level of 105 mg/dl or higher (compared to 140 mg/dl or higher in nonpregnant individuals). The decision to establish a lower value during pregnancy was influenced, in part, by the fact that the plasma glucose level in women is lower during much of normal pregnancy than when nonpregnant.

Abnormal Glucose Tolerance (Class A Diabetes). The diagnosis of class A diabetes requires the use of an oral glucose tolerance test. On the day preceding the glucose tolerance test the woman should not have been fasting but rather should have consumed at least 100 g of carbohydrate. As recommended by the National Diabetes Data Group (1979), after an overnight fast, blood is drawn and then 100 g of glucose in a 50 percent solution is promptly ingested while continuing to otherwise fast. Further venous blood samples are obtained 1, 2, and 3 hours after ingesting the glucose. A diagnosis of class A diabetes is made when two or more plasma glucose levels equal or exceed the following values: fasting—105 mg/dl; 1 hour—190 mg/dl; 2 hours—165 mg/dl; 3 hours—145 mg/dl. If, however, two fasting plasma glucose levels exceed 105 mg/dl, the diabetes is classified as "overt" (at least class B), rather than "chemical" (class A). The values cited above as being critical levels for plasma glucose were derived originally on whole blood by O'Sullivan and Mahan (1964). The concentration of glucose in plasma is typically about 15 percent greater than that in whole blood.

It should be kept in mind that the pregnant woman with a normal fasting level for glucose but an abnormal

TABLE 28-7. CLASSIFICATION OF DIABETES IN PREGNANT WOMEN

A	Chemical diabetes
B	Maturity onset (age over 20 years), duration under 10 years, no vascular lesions
C_1	Age 10 to 19 years at onset
C_2	10 to 19 years duration
D_1	Under age 10 years at onset
D_2	Over 20 years duration
D_3	Benign retinopathy
D_4	Calcified vessels of legs
D_5	Hypertension
E	No longer sought
F	Nephropathy
G	Many failures
H	Cardiomyopathy
R	Proliferating retinopathy
T	Renal transplant

glucose tolerance test early in pregnancy may occasionally develop overt diabetes late in pregnancy. Therefore, the plasma glucose levels while fasting should be checked periodically. Rarely, evidence of diabetes may ameliorate during pregnancy (Sheldon and Coleman, 1974).

The oral glucose tolerance test measures the balance between the absorption of glucose from the intestinal tract, its uptake by tissues, and its excretion in the urine, as well as stimulating the release from the gut of certain hormones that, in turn, augment the release of insulin from β-cells in the islets of Langerhans. In the absence of pregnancy, the oral test is preferred to the intravenous glucose tolerance test because of its greater sensitivity. The oral test during pregnancy suffers from greater variability in the rate of glucose absorption from the gut and, from a very practical standpoint, the likelihood of nausea and vomiting induced by the 100 g of glucose to be ingested rapidly.

Effect of Pregnancy on Diabetes

The diabetogenic properties of pregnancy are borne out by the fact that some women who have no evidence of diabetes when not pregnant develop during pregnancy distinct abnormalities in glucose tolerance and, at times, clinically evident diabetes. Most often these changes are reversible. After delivery, the evidence of either the induction of or a worsening of diabetes usually disappears very rapidly, and the ability of the mother to metabolize carbohydrate returns to the prepregnancy status. As pointed out in Chapter 9 (p. 189), pregnancy per se impairs insulin action. The insulin antagonism during pregnancy is the consequence probably of the actions of *placental lactogen,* which is abundant, and to lesser degrees those of *estrogens* and *progesterone.* Placental *insulinase* may contribute to the diabetogenic effects of pregnancy by accelerating insulin degradation.

During pregnancy, the control of diabetes may be made more difficult by a variety of complications. Nausea and vomiting may lead, on one hand, to insulin shock in women who are receiving insulin and, on the other, to insulin resistance if the starvation is severe enough to cause ketosis. Infection during pregnancy commonly results in insulin resistance and ketoacidosis unless the infection is promptly recognized and both the infection and the diabetes are effectively treated. The vigorous muscular exertion of labor accompanied by the ingestion of little or no carbohydrate may result in troublesome hypoglycemia unless the amount of insulin given is reduced appropriately or an intravenous infusion of glucose is provided.

After delivery, insulin requirements most often decrease at a rapid rate and to a considerable degree. Puerperal infection, however, may obtund this response or perhaps even increase the insulin requirements. Presumably, the rapid decrease in insulin requirements that is usually seen in the absence of other complications stems from the rapid disappearance of placental lactogen, es-

trogens, progesterone, and placental insulinase following delivery of the placenta, while levels of pituitary growth hormone remain low for a few days.

It was thought by some that the fetus ameliorates maternal diabetes by producing insulin, which is transferred in significant amounts across the placenta to the mother. There is no evidence, however, that the fetal pancreas is capable of providing significant amounts of insulin to the mother.

The pregnant woman, even in the absence of diabetes, is more prone to develop metabolic acidosis than when nonpregnant. Presumably, placental lactogen is responsible for this tendency by virtue of its carbohydrate-sparing and lipolytic actions. With diabetes, the likelihood of severe metabolic acidosis is increased appreciably.

Effects of Diabetes on Pregnancy

Diabetes is deleterious to pregnancy in a number of ways. The adverse maternal effects include the following:

1. The likelihood of preeclampsia–eclampsia is increased about fourfold; an increase in preeclampsia–eclampsia is noted even in the absence of demonstrated preexisting vascular disease.
2. Infection occurs more often and is likely to be more severe in women with diabetes.
3. The fetus can be much larger, and fetal size may lead to difficult delivery with injury to the birth canal.
4. Because of the tendency of the fetus to succumb before the onset of spontaneous labor, as well as the possibility of dystocia, the need for cesarean delivery and the maternal risks that are imposed by this operation are increased.
5. Hydramnios is common, and at times the large volume of amnionic fluid, coupled with fetal macrosomia, may cause cardiorespiratory symptoms in the mother.
6. Postpartum hemorrhage is more common than in the general obstetric population.

Maternal diabetes adversely affects the fetus and newborn infant in several ways:

1. In the absence of excellent management of the diabetes and the pregnancy, the perinatal death rate is considerably elevated compared with that of the general population.
2. Morbidity is common in the newborn infant of a mother with diabetes. In some instances, the morbidity is the direct result of birth injury as the consequence of fetal macrosomia with disproportion between the size of the infant and the maternal pelvis. In others, it takes the form of severe respiratory distress and metabolic derangement that includes hypoglycemia and hypocalcemia.

3. Anomalies have been identified more often in the fetuses of women with diabetes.
4. The infant may inherit at least a predisposition to diabetes.

Except for the brain, most organs of the fetus are affected by macrosomia that commonly, but not always, characterizes the fetus of the woman with diabetes (Fig. 28-8). At the same time, body fat is increased. The mechanisms responsible for the extra growth of the fetus are not clear. In several studies, but not all, the degree of fetal macrosomia appeared to correlate well with the degree of maternal hyperglycemia and lack of maternal vascular disease. Both favor the delivery of excessive amounts of glucose across the placenta to the fetus. This stimulates hyperinsulinism in the fetus, and the hyperglycemia plus hyperinsulinism, in concert, enhances glycogen synthesis, lipogenesis, and protein synthesis in the fetus (Hill, 1978). There is abundant experimental evidence to support this concept. Mintz and co-workers (1972) injected the antibiotic streptozotocin into the circulation of the pregnant monkey to destroy the β-cells of the maternal islets of Langerhans. Maternal diabetes so produced was followed by fetal macrosomia. Cheek (1968) injected streptozotocin into the circulation of the monkey fetus to destroy the capacity of the fetus to make insulin, and, conversely, fetal size was reduced appreciably. Moreover, marked fetal growth retardation with very poor development of striate muscle and near absence of adipose tissue has been observed in a newborn infant whose plasma and vestigial pancreas contained no insulin (Hill, 1978).

A fairly common finding at autopsy in the newborn infant of a diabetic mother is hypertrophy and hyperplasia of the islets of Langerhans. Although the changes are not specific, since they are also noted in erythroblastotic infants, they are sufficiently characteristic when found to suggest that the mother had impaired glucose metabolism. This information may be useful in subsequent pregnancies. It has been suggested that maternal hyperglycemia and, in turn, fetal hyperglycemia are responsible for the striking increase in the size, and sometimes the number, of islets.

Management

It is readily apparent from the more recent experiences cited below, as well as other reports, that management based on a full appreciation of the following general principles will provide the best outcome for both the fetus–infant and the diabetic mother:

1. Abnormal carbohydrate metabolism should be detected and defined precisely.
2. Control of maternal glycemia is a very important factor in determining fetal outcome.
3. The pregnant woman with diabetes and her fetus should be cared for throughout her pregnancy by experienced and skilled individuals.
4. The newborn infant of a mother with diabetes should be cared for from the time of birth by experienced and skilled individuals.

Class A Diabetes

Pregnant women without persistent fasting hyperglycemia but with an abnormal oral glucose tolerance test (described above) are treated typically by diet alone and, in the absence of other indications, are delivered at term. In general, for women with gestational diabetes not requiring insulin there is no need to terminate the pregnancy early. In the usual circumstance an acceptable diet is that which is recommended by the American Diabetes Association in amounts that provide about 35 calories per kg each day.

When carefully managed, perinatal mortality for pregnancies of women with class A diabetes is no greater than that for the general obstetric population. Gabbe (1978) cited the figure 16 per 1000 for perinatal mortality. If the diabetes intensifies as pregnancy advances,

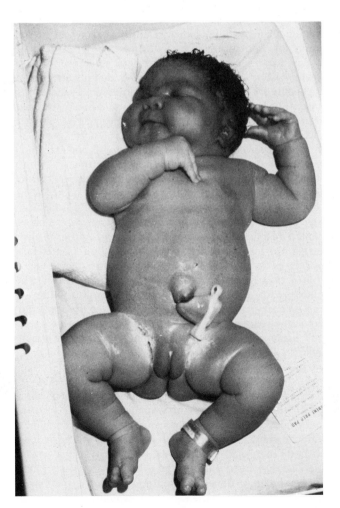

Figure 28-8. Large baby of mildly diabetic mother. Birth weight 6050 g.

however, the prognosis for the fetus–infant worsens. Therefore, throughout the remainder of pregnancy periodic checks for the plasma glucose concentration in the fasting state are essential to detect this event. During pregnancy perhaps 10 to 15 percent of women with class A diabetes will develop overt diabetes.

Overt Diabetes

The likelihood of successful outcomes for the fetus–infant and the overtly diabetic mother relate closely to the degree of control of diabetes that is achieved and the intensity of any maternal cardiovascular or renal disease.

Mortality

In several series of overtly diabetic pregnancies published in recent years, perinatal mortality rates have not been much higher than those for the general population. The perinatal mortality rate reported by Gabbe and associates (1977) was 4.6 percent, by Kitzmiller and co-workers (1978) 3.6 percent, by Leveno and co-workers (1979) 4.5 percent, by Schneider and associates (1980) 3.7 percent, and by Coustan and associates (1980) 4.0 percent. Severe congenital malformations accounted for much of the increase in perinatal mortality over those values observed in the general population. There were no maternal deaths reported in these combined experiences, which amounted to nearly 600 pregnancies.

Management Before Conception

It is now believed by many that the increased frequency of severe malformation in fetuses of diabetic women is the consequence of poorly controlled diabetes preconceptually and early in pregnancy (E. Miller and colleagues, 1981; Cousins, 1983). It is hoped that normalization of maternal plasma glucose during these times will favorably influence development of the embryo and fetus, but this remains to be documented (Ballard and co-workers, 1984).

Prenatal Care

The theme stressed uniformly in all of the more recent reports cited above under Mortality was early diagnosis and meticulous management of the diabetes and of the pregnancy. All emphasized that, ideally, the maternal glucose level should be kept as close to normal as possible and the pregnancy should continue until the fetus is functionally mature unless the intrauterine environment is deteriorating. With evidence of deterioration, the fetus most often is better off being delivered even though premature. Interestingly and importantly, the specific techniques emphasized by the several investigators to provide control of the diabetes and to monitor fetal well-being differed, yet the perinatal outcomes were nearly identical.

The intelligent, well-coached, highly motivated pregnant woman with relatively stable diabetes, who conscientiously follows her appropriate diet, which may have to be ingested in as many as five meals a day, and who either takes multiple forms of insulin two or more times a day, or insulin is infused continuously by pump, has the best chance of achieving the euglycemic state. In actuality, many women who attempt such rigid control commonly run the risk of bouts of hypoglycemia that are dangerous not only to themselves but also to their fetuses. In any event, frequent measurements of plasma glucose, especially preprandially, and adjustment of insulin dosage and of diet on the basis of these measurements will help achieve the goal of avoiding both serious hyperglycemia and hypoglycemia.

Subcutaneous infusion of insulin by a calibrated insulin pump may be used during pregnancy as in the nonpregnant state. The pump has advantages and disadvantages. If distinct advantage to the mother and her fetus from its use can be documented, it will undoubtedly become more popular during pregnancy.

Important to a successful outcome for the fetus is precise knowledge of fetal age. A carefully obtained menstrual history and accurate measurements of uterine height during the second trimester provide useful information. Sonographic confirmation of fetal age often will prove of value. Sonographic evaluation later in pregnancy may serve to document fetal macrosomia, hydramnios, or growth retardation, a complication seen especially when the mother has underlying vascular disease. The value of sonographic examination performed routinely to try to identify fetal malformations early on has not been clearly established.

Effective counseling of the mother is an extremely important function of prenatal care. She must not only be seen often but also be instructed carefully as to how to recognize and deal with problems that arise in the interim. She must be encouraged to report immediately any of a variety of events to the physician who has accepted responsibility for her care. For example, respiratory or urinary infection—rather common occurrences during pregnancy—can rapidly precipitate ketoacidosis that is poorly tolerated by the fetus. The common complication of pregnancy—nausea and vomiting—may, if the mother does not eat appropriately, lead to the characteristic reaction of hyperinsulinism. When more severe and prolonged, the starvation may lead to both serious acidosis and insulin resistance much sooner than if the woman were not pregnant.

The diabetic woman who is pregnant may have to be reeducated about the significance of glucosuria. Similar to the normal pregnant woman, she is likely to develop glucosuria as the consequence of the pregnancy-induced increase in glomerular filtration of the glucose without increased tubular reabsorption. If she were to increase her insulin dosage to a level that avoids glucosuria, she may develop symptomatic hypoglycemia. In general, glucosuria is a signal to evaluate carefully the plasma glucose levels. Frank acetonuria most often means that the insulin dosage should be increased.

Tolbutamide and the other oral hypoglycemic agents should not be used during pregnancy, but instead insulin is given. Tolbutamide in large doses is teratogenic in some species, but there is no evidence that doses used clinically are necessarily teratogenic. Serious hypoglycemia has been observed, however, in the newborn infants of mothers treated with tolbutamide.

For many years, White (1965) administered an estrogen and a progestational agent to diabetic mothers throughout much of pregnancy. Compounds used included estradiol or stilbestrol with either progesterone or ethisterone, or a mixture of estradiol valerate and 17-hydroxyprogesterone caproate. These hormones are no longer used by White (1978). Elimination of these expensive drugs that may be teratogenic certainly has not adversely affected the improved pregnancy salvage witnessed in more recent years.

Timing of Delivery

Ideally, delivery of the overtly diabetic woman is accomplished close to term. At Parkland Memorial Hospital the women are requested to enter the hospital at 34 to 36 weeks gestation and to stay until delivered. Typically the L/S ratio in amnionic fluid is measured at 37 to 38 weeks of gestation, and if 2.0 or greater, delivery is effected. Until that time the fetus is considered not to be in serious jeopardy in utero as long as he is growing and there are no other complications, especially overt maternal hypertension or gross hydramnios. If either severe hypertension or severe hydramnios develops, delivery is carried out even though the L/S ratio is less than 2.0. Of 118 liveborn infants who were delivered according to this regimen, all survived except 1 who suffered from trisomy 18, incompatible with life. Of the 4 stillbirths during the same period, 1 who expired in utero at 34 weeks might have been salvaged if delivery had been performed even earlier (Leveno and co-workers, 1979). Interestingly, an L/S ratio of 2.0 or more as measured in our laboratory has served to exclude severe respiratory distress and its serious sequelae in infants of diabetic mothers receiving insulin. It has become evident, however, from the experiences of others that in some circumstances identification of such a ratio does not always do so, especially in pregnancies complicated by gestational diabetes (Leveno and Whalley, 1982).

Other groups who report very favorable success rates have emphasized other plans of management in an effort to optimize the time selected for delivery. As well as hospitalizing the mothers at 34 weeks, Gabbe and associates (1977) stressed the use, beginning at 30 to 32 weeks, of very frequent measurements of total urinary estriol or, more recently, the concentration of unconjugated plasma estriol (Chapter 7, p. 131) plus the frequent use of the contraction stress test (Chapter 14, p. 281). They believed that they were helped appreciably in their decision making by use of these techniques, whereas the group at Parkland Memorial Hospital did not find the tests to be essential.

Schneider and co-workers (1980) formulated and evaluated a method of management for pregnancies complicated by overt diabetes that emphasized ambulatory care throughout pregnancy until actual delivery. The expectant mother was taught self-measurement of blood glucose using a reflectance meter and, depending upon the results, either the alterations to make in insulin dosage and diet or how to obtain expert advice immediately. They emphasized that an expert especially knowledgeable in obstetrics and diabetes, and who was intimately concerned with the mother's problem, was always available through electronic paging to provide such advice and to direct appropriate action whenever needed. As pointed out above, their low perinatal mortality rate is meritorious.

Estriol Measurement. The daily measurement of 24-hour urinary estriol excretion or of plasma unconjugated estriol concentration to monitor fetal well-being received considerable attention from many workers, including several whose diabetic pregnancy outcomes are cited above. Interestingly, the majority of those cited no longer attempt serial measurements of estriol. Studies have been carried out at several centers to evaluate the benefits that might be achieved from monitoring estriol excretion at very close intervals (daily) during the latter half of the third trimester. As pointed out in Chapter 7 (p. 131), the bulk of evidence indicates that estriol measurements can be grossly misleading, often being abnormally low when the immature fetus is not otherwise compromised (Lavin and co-workers, 1983).

Fetal Heart Reactivity. The contraction stress test and especially the nonstress test (fetal heart reactivity test) have been widely used in diabetic pregnancies, at first on a weekly basis until it became apparent that a week was a long time in the life of a fetus of a diabetic woman, i.e., the fetus could deteriorate remarkably and even die in that period of time. Now advocates are recommending a frequency of nonstress testing that ranges from twice a week to as often as twice a day.

Hemoglobin A_{1c}. Glycosylated hemoglobin A, commonly referred to as hemoglobin A_{1c}, is likely to be elevated in diabetes, and the magnitude of the elevation generally correlates inversely with the degree of long-term control of plasma glucose concentration that has been achieved. Interestingly, Brans and colleagues (1982) found no correlation between maternal hemoglobin A_{1c} levels measured at the time of delivery and either infant birth weight or neonatal hypoglycemia. Conversely, Hahm and associates (1983) have reported that "large birth weight does indicate in a substantial proportion of cases the presence of maternal hyperglycemia reflected by elevated hemoglobin A_{1c} levels during pregnancy." Edidin and Menella (1983), in cases of fetal macrosomia, have also reported elevated glycosylated hemoglobin levels in both maternal and cord blood. It should be emphasized that there are several pitfalls in the analysis of glycosylated proteins, including hemoglobin (Garlick and co-workers, 1983).

Method of Delivery

Cesarean section has been used commonly to avoid traumatic delivery of a large infant at or near term. Moreover, the reduced likelihood of inducing labor safely remote from term has also contributed appreciably to the use of cesarean section to effect delivery of the infant of a diabetic mother. In the several reports cited above with low perinatal mortality, the cesarean section rates were 55 percent in Los Angeles (Gabbe and colleagues, 1977), 70 percent in a midwestern multicenter study (Schneider and co-workers, 1980), 69 percent in Boston (Kitzmiller and associates, 1978), and 81 percent in Dallas (Leveno and associates, 1979).

Induction of labor may be attempted when the following criteria are met: (1) The fetus is not excessively large nor is the pelvis contracted. (2) Parity is not great. (3) The cervix is soft, appreciably effaced, and somewhat dilated. (4) The presenting part is the vertex and is fixed in the pelvis.

It is important to reduce considerably the dose of long-acting insulin given on the day of delivery. Regular insulin should be utilized to meet most or all of the insulin needs of the mother at this time, since the insulin requirements may drop markedly after delivery. During and after either cesarean section or labor and delivery, the mother should be adequately hydrated intravenously as well as supplied with glucose in sufficient dosage to maintain euglycemia. Plasma glucose levels should be checked frequently and regular insulin administered accordingly. The urine, or preferably the plasma, should be checked for ketones. The insulin requirements may fluctuate markedly during the first few days after delivery. Starvation with resistance to insulin must be avoided, and infection must be carefully searched for and promptly treated.

Perinatal Morbidity

Even though perinatal mortality among infants of diabetic mothers has dropped remarkably in many centers in recent years, troublesome morbidity persists. This is clearly evident in the reports just cited. The most serious variety of morbidity is severe *congenital malformations.* Hopefully, normalization of metabolic control before conception and its maintenance during embryogenesis will reduce the frequency and severity of malformations.

Hypoglycemia is commonplace in the newborn infant presumably due, in part at least, to persistent hyperstimulation of the fetal β-islet cells by chronic hyperglycemia. *Hypocalcemia* and *hyperbilirubinemia* are also more common complications of the newborn period. Fortunately, the last three are readily treatable. *Idiopathic respiratory distress* is likely to be somewhat more common among infants of diabetic mothers com-

pared to infants in general of the same gestational age, although Gabbe and associates (1977) and Leveno and colleagues (1979) did not find this to be a major problem.

It is extremely important that the robust appearance of the newly delivered infant not lead to inappropriate care. Although the infant may appear mature on the basis of his size, functionally he may be quite premature and must be so treated.

Contraception

The two most common forms of reversible contraception, estrogen–progestin oral contraceptives and the intrauterine device, may be contraindicated in women who have overt diabetes when nonpregnant. Oral contraceptives are likely to intensify the diabetes. Moreover, the vascular disease that rather often is associated with diabetes may potentiate the variety of hazards from vascular disease that have been described with use of oral contraceptives in the absence of diabetes (Chapter 40, p. 815). The risk of pelvic infection from an intrauterine device is very likely increased in the diabetic woman. Therefore, barrier methods seem the best choice for reversible contraception, followed by sterilization once it is certain that the woman wants no more children.

DISEASES OF THE THYROID

It is difficult at times to differentiate several signs and symptoms of thyroid dysfunction, especially mild to moderate hyperthyroidism, from several of the changes induced by normal pregnancy: (1) Cutaneous blood flow is increased appreciably during pregnancy, and, therefore, some degree of heat intolerance is a common finding in pregnant women especially during warm weather. (2) Modest tachycardia accompanies normal pregnancy. (3) Plasma thyroxine concentration is increased as is thyroid uptake of radioiodine; both are suggestive of hyperthyroidism. However, the free thyroxine concentration is not increased, and the binding in vitro of triiodothyronine by resin is actually decreased, compatible with, but not diagnostic of, hypothyroidism. These diverse changes in thyroxine and triiodothyronine are the consequence of hyperestrogenemia and estrogen-induced increases in binding proteins in plasma, especially thyroid-binding globulin. In some studies, at least, *free* thyroxine and triiodothyronine levels in clinically euthyroid women have been identified actually to be somewhat lower than in healthy nonpregnant women (Franklyn and co-workers, 1983).

Hyperthyroidism

Helpful signs for identifying hyperthyroidism during pregnancy are (1) tachycardia that exceeds the increase caused by normal pregnancy, (2) a high pulse rate while sleeping, (3) an enlarged thyroid gland, (4) exophthalmos, and (5) failure to gain weight normally. In the great majority of cases of hyperthyroidism, the level of thyroxine in plasma is markedly elevated compared with normal values in the nonpregnant state. At the same time, in vitro binding tests fail to demonstrate the appreciably decreased uptake of triiodothyronine that is characteristic of normal pregnancy. Rarely, hyperthyroidism may be associated with normal plasma thyroxine values; instead, the triiodothyronine level is abnormally high (Martin and colleagues, 1976). Measurement of radioiodine uptake by the thyroid is contraindicated during pregnancy. *It is emphasized that careful clinical evaluation, using those signs described above, is most important to a successful pregnancy outcome.*

Treatment may be medical, or medical until such time as the mother is nearly euthyroid, and then surgical. Hyperthyroidism nearly always can be controlled by antithyroid drugs, so that the disease, if treated adequately, need not be a serious threat to the mother.

Medical treatment, however, has the potential for causing fetal complications. Propylthiouracil and similarly acting compounds readily cross the placenta and may induce fetal hypothyroidism and goiter. Therefore, it became common, but unsound, practice to give propylthiouracil in doses that effectively suppressed maternal thyroid activity while the mother received thyroid hormone simultaneously, allegedly to provide hormone to the fetus. Most likely, thyroxine so administered did not cross the placenta to the fetus in significant amounts. Actually, it served only to increase the maternal requirements for propylthiouracil and thereby increase, rather than decrease, the risk to the fetus. Goluboff and co-workers (1974) emphasized that supplemental thyroid hormone may be undesirable because (1) it obscures laboratory indices of propylthiouracil overdosage, (2) it may increase the dosage of propylthiouracil required for control, and (3) it complicates recognition of remission, which sometimes occurs during pregnancy. Moreover, in their experience, supplemental thyroid hormone did not always protect against the development of a goiter in the fetus. However, some physicians persist in administering thyroxine in conjunction with antithyroid drugs (Ramsay and associates, 1983). A regimen employing propylthiouracil without administration of thyroid hormone has always been followed in our clinic with very satisfactory pregnancy outcomes.

The dose of propylthiouracil should be increased until the woman appears clinically to be only minimally thyrotoxic and the level of thyroxine in the blood is reduced to the upper normal range for pregnancy. In case of severe hyperthyroidism, emergency treatment with propranolol and large doses of propylthiouracil are not contraindicated by the pregnancy. Propranolol has also been used for long-term treatment of hyperthyroidism in pregnant women (Bullock and colleagues, 1975; Langer and associates, 1974). However, troublesome adverse effects have been described in newborn infants whose mothers were being treated with propranolol. The adverse effects included fetal distress during labor, low Apgar scores, growth retardation, hypoglycemia, and hyperbilirubinemia (Habib and McCarthy, 1977).

Burrow and associates (1968) have carried out a long-term study of the intellectual and physical development, including thyroid function, of the children born to thyrotoxic mothers treated with propylthiouracil during pregnancy. Although the number of children studied was small, no adverse effects on subsequent growth and development were identified. The prolonged administration of iodide to the mother along with propylthiouracil appears to increase appreciably the likelihood of gross goiter in the fetus. Therefore, iodide, if used, should be used only preceding the time of thyroidectomy and *not* for long-term therapy during pregnancy.

Thyroidectomy may be carried out after the thyrotoxicosis has been brought under control. Opinions differ as to the wisdom of surgical treatment during the first trimester, a time when abortion is relatively common, or during the third trimester, when delivery may occur prematurely. From the beginning of the second trimester until early in the third trimester, however, for the woman who is incapable of adhering to an appropriate plan of medical treatment or for whom drug therapy proves toxic, subtotal thyroidectomy may be the treatment of choice after achieving control medically.

Breast-feeding has been considered by some to be contraindicated when the mother is taking antithyroid drugs, even though the concentrations of antithyroid drugs in breast milk are low and therefore the amount of drug ingested by the infant is quite small.

Women with *Graves disease,* even though they are no longer hyperthyroid, may give birth to infants with manifestations of thyrotoxicosis, including goiter and exophthalmos. Thyroid-stimulating immunoglobulins synthesized by the mother presumably as an autoimmune phenomenon are transferred across the placenta to the fetus and can cause hyperthyroidism in the fetus and newborn infant. The condition is suggested by a maternal history of thyrotoxicosis, identification of appreciable levels of a thyroid-stimulating immunoglobulin in maternal serum, a history of a previously affected fetus–infant, and by persistent fetal tachycardia. Robinson and co-workers (1979) have reported such a case in which the mother was given antithyroid medication to try to treat the fetus plus thyroxine to maintain euthyroidism in the mother. The endpoint used for establishing dosage of the antithyroid medication was the fetal heart rate. The newborn infant may require antithyroid treatment for several weeks until the thyroid-stimulating immunoglobulins are ultimately metabolized.

The infant who was the recipient of thyroid-stimulating immunoglobulins in utero and whose mother was treated until delivery with propylthiouracil may be euthyroid at birth but become hyperthyroid a few days later as propylthiouracil is cleared but the thyrotoxic effect of the immunoglobulin persists.

Thyroid storm can occur during pregnancy and the puerperium. Treatment consists of recognition followed by vigorous therapy simultaneously with large doses of propylthiouracil plus potassium iodide orally (through a nasogastric tube if the patient is unable to swallow), propranolol intravenously, and perhaps a corticosteroid in a large dose intravenously. Supportive care for heart failure, pulmonary edema, and hypoxia is essential.

Hypothyroidism

Overt hypothyroidism is often associated with infertility, and in women who do become pregnant, the likelihood of abortion seems to be increased considerably. In general, hypothyroidism can be diagnosed if the expected rise during pregnancy in the level of circulating thyroxine fails to take place and the level of thyroid-stimulating hormone is elevated. Measurement of serum cholesterol is of little value, since normal pregnancy also induces an increase in the cholesterol concentration.

Effect on Fetus and Infant

In general, the infants of hypothyroid mothers appear healthy, without evidence of thyroid dysfunction (Montoro and co-workers, 1981). The infant of a mother with severe hypothyroidism may be a cretin if the hypothyroidism followed maternal radioactive iodine therapy administered during pregnancy. Any infant whose mother was so treated during pregnancy must be carefully evaluated and probably treated prophylactically for hypothyroidism.

The clinical diagnosis of *congenital hypothyroidism* during the neonatal period is difficult and often missed. If treatment of the affected infant is started early, mental retardation most often can be prevented. According to various reports based on mass screening of newborn infants, the frequency of congenital hypothyroidism so detected is 1 in 4000 to 7000 newborn infants.

Simple colloid goiter in the mother, if unassociated with hypothyroidism, has no influence on pregnancy.

PARATHYROID DISEASE

Hyperparathyroidism

This condition rarely complicates pregnancy, even though the disease is more common in women and has a peak incidence before the menopause. Whalley described four cases cared for at Parkland Memorial Hospital (1963). One case with parathyroid storm, characterized by hypercalcemia and convulsions, was especially interesting. The convulsions, coexistent with chronic pyelonephritis and chronic hypertension, might erroneously have been considered to have been caused by eclampsia.

Tetany has been noted occasionally in the newborn infants of mothers with hyperparathyroidism. At times, neonatal tetany alone has led to a search that identified a maternal parathyroid adenoma. Lowe and associates (1983) and Shangold and colleagues (1982) have reviewed much of the published experiences concerning hyperparathyroidism and pregnancy.

Hypoparathyroidism

This condition is also equally uncommon in pregnancy. Treatment with dihydrotachysterol or large doses of vitamin D (50,000 to 150,000 units per day), together with calcium gluconate or calcium lactate and a diet low in phosphates, usually prevents symptomatic hypocalcemia. The risk to the fetus from large doses of either dihydrotachysterol or vitamin D_2 has not been established. Whether these compounds cause cardiovascular and other anomalies is not clear.

ADRENAL DYSFUNCTION

Addison's Disease

Before 1953, only 50 published cases of Addison's disease in pregnancy had been identified, suggesting that untreated adrenal hypofunction caused sterility (Hunt and McConahey, 1953). With the advent of cortisone and related compounds, pregnancy has become much more common in women with adrenocortical hypofunction.

It is essential during pregnancy and the puerperium to observe the mother quite closely for evidence of either inadequate or excessive steroid replacement. Except at times of stress, replacement therapy need not be greater and sometimes may be less than in the nonpregnant state. There may be little need during pregnancy for compounds with potent mineralocorticoid action. During and after labor and delivery or after a surgical procedure, the amount of steroid replacement should be increased appreciably to approximate the normal response at the time in women with intact adrenals. It is important that shock from causes other than adrenocortical insufficiency be promptly recognized and treated, especially that caused by blood loss or bacterial infection.

Cushing's Syndrome

Pregnancy associated with Cushing's syndrome is rare. The disease has been diagnosed during pregnancy and treated successfully at that time. In one instance, an adrenocortical adenoma was resected (Grimes and colleagues, 1973), and in another, the pituitary-dependent adrenocortical hyperplasia was treated with pituitary irradiation during the pregnancy (Anderson and Walters, 1976); the infants were normal.

Liu and associates (1983) diagnosed Cushing's syndrome in a woman who promptly thereafter conceived before any treatment. The signs of Cushing's syndrome increased appreciably during and after pregnancy. Spontaneous labor and delivery occurred at 32 weeks; *the infant survived respiratory distress.*

Three months postpartum bilateral hyperplastic adrenal glands were excised from the mother with amelioration of the disease.

Primary Aldosteronism

A few cases of primary aldosteronism in association with pregnancy have been reported. In view of the very high levels of aldosterone in normal pregnancies, it is not surprising that there may be amelioration of symptoms as well as of electrolyte disturbances during pregnancy (Biglieri and Slaton, 1967). Although aldosterone is produced in large amounts during much of pregnancy, it is not essential for a successful outcome. Adrenalectomized women may experience normal pregnancies while receiving synthetic adrenocorticoid replacement therapy.

Pheochromocytoma

Pheochromocytoma is a rare complication of pregnancy; both the maternal and the fetal mortality rates have been high. Favorable outcomes have been described more recently for individual patients in whom the diagnosis was made late in pregnancy and the blood pressure was controlled pharmacologically during cesarean section and resection of the tumor (Burgess, 1979; Schenker and Granat, 1982). The diagnosis, localization, and treatment of pheochromocytoma have been well described by Atuk (1983).

DISEASES OF THE PITUITARY

Diabetes Insipidus

The condition is a rare complication of pregnancy. Only two patients have been cared for in the last quarter of a century at Parkland Memorial Hospital, during which there were approximately 170,000 deliveries. As long as the women took vasopressin appropriately for replacement therapy, their pregnancies progressed without serious complication. The specific agent of choice is the synthetic analog of vasopressin, L-deamino-8d-arginine vasopressin.

In a few instances of diabetes insipidus, there appeared to have been an impairment of labor, possibly caused by lack of or reduced amounts of endogenous oxytocin (Hime and Richardson, 1978). Sende and associates (1975) were unable to detect oxytocin by radioimmunoassay in plasma of a pregnant woman with diabetes insipidus before labor, but during labor and puerperium there was a surge of oxytocin. A woman described by Chau and associates (1969) lactated normally, with measured milk ejection pressures comparable to those of normal lactating women.

Diabetes insipidus without anterior pituitary deficiency has been described following massive hemorrhage and prolonged shock from placenta percreta (Collins and co-workers, 1979).

Pituitary Microadenomas

Amenorrhea, galactorrhea, and hyperprolactinemia caused by pituitary microadenomas is amenable to therapy with bromocriptine. A relatively large number of pregnancies have now been observed in women so treated. Jewelewicz and VandeWiele (1980) concluded that the presence of pituitary microadenoma without neurologic or visual symptoms is not a contraindication to ovulation induction and pregnancy. Bromocriptine taken by the mother during pregnancy does not appear to affect the fetus adversely (Turkalj and associates, 1982).

Development of *acromegaly* in a pregnant woman and in turn in her fetus–infant has been described by Fisch and associates (1974). The mother was treated with x-irradiation to the pituitary fossa during the third trimester. The newborn infant suffered from a constellation of skeletal anomalies.

DISEASES OF THE NERVOUS SYSTEM

Pregnancy is not incompatible with most diseases of the nervous system, although the diseases, or their treatment, may adversely affect the pregnancy. Earlier in this century, but not today, eclampsia was a common and very serious disorder involving the nervous system. Eclampsia is considered in Chapter 27.

EPILEPSIES

It is estimated that more than 2 million people in the United States have some form of epilepsy. The new classification of epileptic seizures is provided by Delgado-Escueta and co-workers (1983).

The effect of pregnancy on the frequency of epileptic seizures has been argued for more than 100 years. It would appear that if seizures are well controlled before pregnancy, there is little risk of increased frequency of seizures as the consequence of pregnancy, whereas if seizures are poorly controlled before pregnancy, there is likelihood of even further deterioration during pregnancy (Schmidt and associates, 1983).

Treatment

The therapeutic goal for the treatment of epilepsy during pregnancy is to administer to the mother the least amount of a drug least likely to affect her fetus adversely yet effectively control her convulsions. There is increasing evidence that the use of several of the most effective antiepileptic agents during pregnancy is accompanied by higher frequencies of fetal malformation, as described below.

An increased risk of seizures during pregnancy may be the consequence of several factors: During early pregnancy, nausea and vomiting may interfere with the ingestion and absorption of anticonvulsant medication, increasing the likelihood of seizures. Some women may reduce the dosage of medication or abstain completely because of fear of adverse effects on the fetus and, as a consequence, be seizure prone. During labor, delivery, and the early puerperium, medication may be withheld by the obstetric staff deliberately or inadvertently, similarly increasing the likelihood of convulsions. Phenytoin (diphenylhydantoin), a drug used very commonly during pregnancy, is cleared more rapidly during pregnancy, and, consequently, with a constant dose of medication, plasma levels are likely to be lower during pregnancy than when nonpregnant (Lander and associates, 1977; Kochenour and co-workers, 1980). This should increase the risk of seizures. However, the amount of free (nonprotein bound) drug in plasma increases during pregnancy, and from the standpoint of therapeutic action this should offset to some degree, at least, the lower total concentration of phenytoin (Perucca and associates, 1981). The fall in plasma levels that accompanies pregnancy commonly has been interpreted by many as an indication for frequent measurements of plasma levels and, in turn, adjustment of dosage accordingly, most often by increasing the amount ingested. This approach fails to take into account the enhanced therapeutic effect that results from decreased protein binding of the drug as pregnancy advances. Appropriate plasma levels for women throughout pregnancy have not yet been defined precisely.

Effect of Anticonvulsant on Fetus–Infant

A variety of complications in the offspring of women with epilepsy has been attributed to the anticonvulsant medications, including malformations, low birth weight and prematurity, perinatal mortality, and failure of the neonate to thrive. Hanson and co-workers (1975, 1976) have described a "fetal phenytoin syndrome" that included craniofacial anomalies, distal limb dysmorphosis, and mental deficiency. Eleven percent of infants studied were adversely affected. Use of phenytoin is also accompanied by increased frequencies of cleft lip and cleft palate and of congenital heart lesions. The use of phenobarbital with phenytoin appears to increase the risk of fetal anomalies.

Maternal phenytoin ingestion alone or with phenobarbital has been implicated in the deficiency of four vitamin K-dependent clotting factors (II, VII, IX, and X) in the plasma of the neonate (Mountain and co-workers, 1970). Hemorrhagic disease of the newborn has been described in this circumstance. Hemorrhage can be prevented usually by the prompt parenteral administration of vitamin K to the newborn. However, it might be worthwhile to give the mother vitamin K at least at the onset of labor, if not before, to minimize further the risk of hemorrhage in the fetus and infant. Srinivasan and associates (1982) have described a case of extensive hemorrhage identified several hours after birth and in which, in spite of 1 mg of vitamin K at 1 hour after birth, the prothrombin time was remarkably long. A subcapsular hematoma of the liver that ruptured was identified by liver scan and at laparotomy.

Other anticonvulsants have been implicated in compromise of the fetus and neonate. Trimethadione has proved to be a potent teratogen and should not be used by anyone who is pregnant or is attempting to conceive (Smith, 1977). Carbamazepine (Tegretol), with or without phenobarbital, to control seizures during pregnancy has been linked to small head size in the infant, which persisted at least to age 1½ years (Hiilesmaa and co-workers, 1981). Current clinical data suggest that valproic acid therapy for maternal epilepsy results in an increased frequency of fetal facial, digital, and skeletal malformations, as well as delayed development; several cases of neural tube defects have been identified (Bailey and co-workers, 1983; Robert and Rosa, 1983). Moreover, valproic acid increased the incidence of congenital malformations in animal studies. If the drug is used during the first trimester of pregnancy, measurements of α-fetoprotein and careful sonographic examination of the fetus would appear to be worthwhile.

The possibility still persists that the increased frequency of fetal anomalies and dysmorphism associated with maternal anticonvulsant therapy may be due in part to the epilepsy per se and not be just the consequence of treatment.

Counseling

Consideration should be given to stopping the anticonvulsant medication for the woman who wishes to conceive. If she has not convulsed for a long time on medication and does not do so while off medication before conception, she very likely will have no problem during pregnancy. However, if she does convulse, treatment during pregnancy will be essential. Precautions to protect her and others must be taken during the trial period off medication. The various conditions in which treatment may be stopped with little likelihood of recurrence have been described by Delgado-Escueta and associates (1983).

Several of the anticonvulsant drugs in common use tend to precipitate or aggravate a deficiency of folic acid, and megaloblastic anemia has been described in these circumstances (Chanarin, 1969). At Parkland Memorial Hospital, maternal folate deficiency identified by low plasma folate levels is much more common than in the general obstetric population. Interestingly, no cases of overt megaloblastic anemia have been identified among the pregnant women treated with anticonvulsant drugs even though they did not receive supplemental folic acid (Pritchard and co-workers, 1969). Folic acid has been claimed by some to increase the likelihood of convulsions. However, Hiilesmaa and associates (1983) found no association between the number of seizures during pregnancy and serum folate concentrations. The benefits, if any, to be derived from folic acid supplementation in these circumstances are not clear.

At times, it may be difficult to differentiate between eclampsia and epilepsy in the hypertensive pregnant woman. Magnesium sulfate parenterally administered most often will promptly control the convulsions of epilepsy as well as those of eclampsia (Pritchard and Cunningham, unpublished).

INTRACRANIAL HEMORRHAGE

Among 170 maternal deaths reported by Barnes and Abbott (1959), 36 were caused by cerebral complications. Of these 36 deaths, 17, or about one half, were the result of intracranial hemorrhage.

Hemorrhage within the intracranial cavity is readily recognized using the CT scan. Whether to attempt repair of a potentially accessible vascular lesion during pregnancy is debatable. The advantages achieved by reducing the risk of a subsequent intracranial hemorrhage are obvious. However, the potential for adverse effects on the fetus from maternal hypotension and hypothermia during the surgical procedure is real. Antifibrinolytic agents are commonly used to try to impede clot dissolution and, in turn, perhaps reduce the risk of further hemorrhage. Since fibrinolytic activity is already reduced as the consequence of the pregnancy per se, we have counseled against their use in pregnancy, and thus we avoid the risks associated with their use.

The main obstetric problem concerns the management of pregnancy and delivery in women who survive intracranial hemorrhage. Some, but certainly not all, authorities have favored cesarean section for delivery, and in cases in which the cerebral hemorrhage occurred shortly before or very early in pregnancy, some believe that therapeutic abortion is indicated. On the basis of a review of 142 cases of intracranial aneurysms that ruptured before or during pregnancy, Hunt and co-workers (1974) have concluded that there is little indication for elective cesarean section to replace vaginal delivery. Vaginal delivery following surgical correction of the aneurysm was well tolerated by the patients described by Minielly and co-workers (1979). Barrett and associates (1982) have provided an extensive review of pregnancy-related rupture of arterial aneurysms, including cerebral arterial aneurysms.

OTHER INVOLVEMENT OF THE NERVOUS SYSTEM

Ventriculoperitoneal Shunts

A few instances of pregnancy have been described in women with ventriculoperitoneal shunts for hydrocephalus (Howard and Herrick, 1981; Kleinman and co-work-

ers, 1983). Pregnancy outcomes have been satisfactory. Antibiotic prophylaxis is probably indicated if the peritoneal cavity is entered for cesarean delivery or tubal sterilization.

Maternal Brain Death

A few instances of maternal brain death during pregnancy have been described in which life support systems and parenteral alimentation were utilized for some time while the fetus hopefully achieved sufficient maturity to not only survive but also enjoy good health after birth (Dillon and associates, 1982). The ethical, financial, and legal implications, civil and criminal, that may arise from attempting—or not attempting—such care are profound!

Pseudotumor Cerebri

Idiopathic (benign) intracranial hypertension, or pseudotumor cerebri, is characterized by headache, visual disturbances, and papilledema from increased intracranial pressure in an otherwise healthy individual. Criteria for diagnosis include elevated pressure of cerebrospinal fluid of normal composition and normal CT scan.

Usually, but not always, the disease is self-limited. Corticosteroids usually provide prompt relief. Infrequently, surgical shunting of cerebrospinal fluid is required. Kassam and colleagues (1983) and Koontz and associates (1983) have described several cases during pregnancy and provided a general review.

Trauma to Spinal Cord

Spinal cord lesions caused by trauma or tumor usually do not prevent conception. In women so affected, the pregnancy is likely to be complicated by urinary infections, pressure necrosis of the skin, and autonomic hyperreflexia. Labor often is easy—even precipitous—and comparatively painless. The second stage may be prolonged by an inability to increase intra-abdominal pressure, i.e., bear down. Moreover, trauma causing paraplegia may also cause pelvic deformity and, in turn, fetopelvic disproportion. Young and associates (1983) have described their experiences, especially at parturition.

Multiple Sclerosis

This disease is a rare complication of pregnancy. Pregnancy has been considered by some, but certainly not by all, to precipitate the disease in women who were destined to develop it but at a later time. In most cases, pregnancy appears to have no predictable effect on the course of multiple sclerosis. However, exacerbation during the first few months postpartum is common.

Guillain-Barré Syndrome

Sudo and Weingold (1975) have described 2 instances of pregnancy complicated by the Guillain-Barré syndrome and reviewed 25 others previously reported. Respiratory insufficiency is a most serious problem, as it is in the absence of pregnancy. The fetus does not appear to be affected neurologically.

Ahlberg and Ahlmark (1978) have described a case in which the mother gave birth to twins during respirator ventilation. All survived, although the mother's mechanical paralysis persisted for several more weeks after delivery. Bravo and associates (1982) successfully ventilated a mother for 5 weeks before delivery of a healthy infant.

Myasthenia Gravis

This uncommon disease involving the neuromuscular endplate is most common in women of reproductive age. Long-term therapy has consisted of anticholinesterase drugs, immunosuppression, and thymectomy, alone or in combination. In severely ill women short-term relief may be achieved with plasmapheresis. With occasional exceptions, women with myasthenia gravis go through pregnancy and labor without difficulty; during the second stage of labor the woman may demonstrate impairment of voluntary expulsive efforts.

Acetylcholine receptor antibodies have been detected in most myasthenic patients (Appel and colleagues, 1975). These antibodies, most likely, can be transferred as IgG from the mother to her fetus. If the IgG antibody titers are high, neonatal myasthenia can be anticipated, according to Donaldson and associates (1981).

Transient symptomatic myasthenia gravis occurs in about 10 to 20 percent of the newborn infants of mothers with the disease. The affected infant typically demonstrates a feeble cry, poor suckling, and respiratory distress, which are corrected by parenteral neostigmine. The neonatal myasthenia responds to minute doses of edrophonium or similar drugs and most often subsides completely within 4 to 6 weeks. Without prompt recognition and treatment, including good nursing care, the affected newborn infant may succumb to respiratory insufficiency caused by muscular weakness and the effects of aspiration. The fetus appears to be protected while in utero by a factor that inhibits the interaction between the receptors and antibody to the receptors (Abramsky and co-workers, 1979).

Any drug with a curare-like effect must be used with extreme caution. Such drugs include magnesium sulfate and aminoglycoside antibiotics. Apparently, even the quinine in a gin and tonic may be harmful (Donaldson, 1978).

Huntington's Chorea

The obstetric importance of Huntington's chorea is chiefly eugenic, since this degenerative disease of the cerebral cortex and basal ganglia is inherited as a dominant autosomal trait. To attempt the elimination of this dreaded disease, therapeutic abortion seems justifiable.

Chorea Gravidarum

This is a rare complication of gestation since rheumatic fever has become so rare. Zegart and Schwarz (1968) identified only 1 case in the course of over 100,000 deliveries. Often the woman has previously suffered chorea that sooner or later abated spontaneously, as it is likely to do during or after the pregnancy. Chlorpromazine or haloperidol has been used to treat the disorder (Donaldson, 1982).

Migraine

The effects, if any, of pregnancy on migraine are unpredictable. Ergotamine-containing preparations should probably be avoided during pregnancy, although ergotamine has nowhere near as potent an action on the myometrium as does ergonovine.

Bell's Palsy

This idiopathic paralysis involving the facial nerve may be somewhat more common during pregnancy. Treatment and prognosis are the same as for nonpregnant women.

Psychosis

Pregnancy and the puerperium at times are sufficiently stressful to induce psychosis. The prognosis depends for the most part on the nature of the underlying psychiatric disorder that is almost always present.

Electroshock therapy has been used during pregnancy. However, the risks, if any, to mother and fetus have not been carefully evaluated. Repke and Berger report a case (1984). One pregnant woman was transferred to Parkland Memorial Hospital when she convulsed spontaneously with eclampsia during the course of electroshock therapy. The mother and infant survived.

Lithium carbonate, when used to treat manic-depressive pregnant women, appears to have teratogenic effects that are dose related. Therefore, if used, the smallest effective dose should be administered. The excretion of lithium by the kidney is increased in normal pregnancy but decreased by sodium-depleting diuretics and sodium-poor diets. Lithium toxicity may be the consequence in both mother and fetus. The evidence appears strong for a teratogenic effect, especially on the heart, when lithium is administered during the first trimester (Weinstein and Goldfield, 1975). Källén and Tandberg (1983) identified an increased frequency of low birth weight and prematurity, as well as cardiac anomalies among infants whose manic-depressive mothers were being treated with lithium.

Because of the high frequency of heart disease, especially Ebstein's anomaly, Allan and co-workers (1982) have recommended fetal echocardiography by 20 weeks if the mother had taken lithium during pregnancy. Neonates with goiter, nephrogenic diabetes insipidus, hypothermia, and hypotonia have been identified from pregnancies in which the mothers took lithium. Lithium is concentrated in breast milk; bottlefeeding is probably the better choice in this circumstance.

Treatment with tricyclic antidepressants late in pregnancy appears to cause ill effects in the neonate and probably should be avoided when possible (Østergaard and Pederson, 1982).

DISEASES OF THE LIVER AND GALLBLADDER

Pregnancy normally induces appreciable changes in many of the tests and some physical examinations commonly employed to detect diseases of the liver. The physiologic alterations are considered in Chapter 9 and are (1) serum albumin concentration is decreased about 25 percent, (2) plasma urea nitrogen concentration is lowered, (3) plasma alkaline phosphatase and leucine aminopeptidase activities are increased, (4) excretion of sulfobromophthalein is delayed, and (5) palmar erythema and spider angiomata develop commonly.

Diseases of the liver complicating pregnancy more often than not are coincident with pregnancy. However, there are diseases of the liver that are induced by pregnancy and, unless fatal, disappear following termination of the gestation. The diseases induced by pregnancy are (1) intrahepatic cholestasis of pregnancy with or without icterus gravidarum, (2) hepatocellular damage of varying intensity that is the direct consequence of preeclampsia–eclampsia, (3) acute fatty liver of pregnancy, and (4) hepatic dysfunction associated with hyperemesis gravidarum.

INTRAHEPATIC CHOLESTASIS OF PREGNANCY

This syndrome has also been referred to as *recurrent jaundice of pregnancy, idiopathic cholestasis of pregnancy, cholestatic hepatosis,* and *icterus gravidarum.* This condition is characterized clinically by pruritis, icterus, or both. The major histologic lesion is intrahepatic cholestasis with centrolobular bile staining without inflammatory cells or proliferation of mesenchymal cells. This hepatic derangement has been identified to be especially common among pregnant Scandinavian women and members of a tribe of Indians in Chile (Burroughs and colleagues, 1982; Steven, 1981).

Bile acids are incompletely cleared by the liver and accumulate in plasma. Their levels typically are several-fold greater than in normal pregnancy. The modest hyperbilirubinemia results predominantly from retention of conjugated pigment. Sulfobromophthalein excretion is delayed appreciably, and serum alkaline phosphatase may be elevated above the usual levels for pregnancy. Serum glutamic oxalacetic transaminase activity may be moderately elevated. These changes disappear after delivery but often recur in a subsequent pregnancy or when an oral contraceptive containing estrogen is employed. Its recurrence under these circumstances, coupled with the frequent finding of positive family history, suggests that the disorder is genetically determined.

Ultrasound examination will often serve to exclude an obstruction by gallstones. In the absence of obstruction by gallstones and if the SGOT is not appreciably elevated, thereby excluding viral hepatitis, the likely diagnosis is cholestasis of pregnancy.

Pruritis associated with cholestatic hepatosis is caused by raised plasma levels of bile salts and may be quite troublesome. Cholestyramine has been reported to provide relief. However, Shaw and associates (1982) did not find it to be effective. When cholestyramine is used, absorption of fat-soluble vitamins is impaired. Thus, impaired coagulation as a consequence of vitamin K deficiency may develop late in pregnancy, affecting both the mother and the fetus–neonate, unless supplemental vitamin K is provided.

Reid and associates (1976) reported appreciable pregnancy wastage among women with obstetric cholestasis: (1) there were 5 stillbirths and 1 neonatal death among 56 pregnancies, (2) intrapartum asphyxia was observed in 5 more pregnancies, (3) 18 infants were delivered preterm, and (4) 5 of the mothers suffered postpartum hemorrhage. Johnston and Baskett (1979) observed much lower pregnancy wastage but found an abnormally high incidence of preterm births and postpartum hemorrhage. Shaw and colleagues (1982) recommend delivery once lung maturity has been achieved coupled with close monitoring of fetal well-being.

ACUTE FATTY LIVER OF PREGNANCY

This fortunately rare complication of pregnancy has commonly proved fatal to both mother and fetus (Burroughs and associates, 1982; Hague and co-workers, 1982; Sherlock, 1983; Steven, 1981). The prominent histologic abnormality in acute fatty liver of pregnancy consists of swollen hepatocytes in which the cytoplasm is filled with microvesicular fat with central nuclei and periportal sparing; liver necrosis is not prominent (Fig. 28-9). The

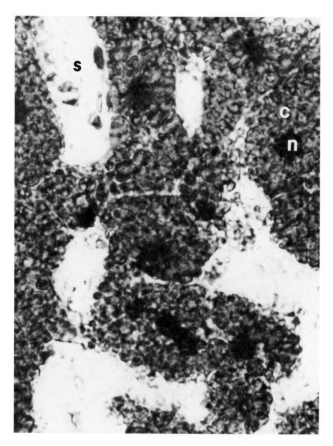

Figure 28-9. Fatty liver of pregnancy. High magnification picture of liver plates and sinusoids (s) showing hepatocyte cytoplasm (c) filled with microvesicular fat globules. Note hepatocyte nucleus (n) remains centrally located in cell despite large amount of fat present. Oil red O fat stain. (*Courtesy of Dr. E. Eigenbrodt.*)

mechanism by which pregnancy incites these changes is not known. Excessive doses of tetracycline, especially in women with impaired renal function, can cause these same histologic changes and clinical picture in nonpregnant individuals as well as pregnant women. The histologic changes in the liver with Reye's syndrome are also very similar to those of acute fatty liver of pregnancy, as are those that are sometimes induced by therapy with sodium valproate.

Acute fatty liver of pregnancy almost always presents during the last trimester of pregnancy. Typically, there is rapid onset of malaise, anorexia, nausea, and vomiting, upper abdominal pain, and progressive jaundice. In some women hypertension, proteinuria, and edema compatible with the diagnosis of preeclampsia have been detected shortly before or coincident with the development of the signs and symptoms of fatty liver of pregnancy.

Fortunately, delivery is likely to achieve, initially, arrest of rapid deterioration in liver function and then relatively rapid recovery, as was the course in the case described here.

The 27-year-old gravida 2, para 2, white woman was transferred to Parkland Memorial Hospital 24 hours after vaginal delivery of an appropriately grown infant of 38 weeks gestational age who survived. About 5 days before delivery, malaise and anorexia were noted, which intensified. Epigastric pain developed and the color of the feces became light. She was admitted in active labor, at which time jaundice was identified. She was not hypertensive at that time but postpartum became so transiently. Vaginal bleeding persisted after delivery, and she was given packed red cells, fresh frozen plasma, and cryoprecipitate at the first hospital.

As shown in Table 28-8, at the time of transfer, coagulation was impaired as the consequence of severe hypofibrinogenemia, pathologic amounts of circulating fibrin degradation products, prolonged prothrombin time, and moderate thrombocytopenia. Vitamin K and fresh frozen plasma were administered without dramatic effect clinically. However, ligation of a previously unrecognized bleeding vaginal artery was followed immediately by an abrupt decrease in vaginal bleeding. By 3 days after delivery, the intensity of the coagulopathy had diminished remarkably. Almost certainly, the coagulopathy resulted from increased consumption of procoagulants (DIC) and probably also from their impaired production by the liver.

Packed red cells were transfused to maintain the hematocrit near 30. Fragmentation (microangiopathic) hemolysis (Fig. 28-10), as well as bleeding from the vagina, was important in the genesis of the anemia that developed postpartum and contributed to the hyperbilirubinemia.

At no time was the SGOT activity elevated to the high levels that would be anticipated if the jaundice were the consequence of viral hepatitis. Liver function, as assessed

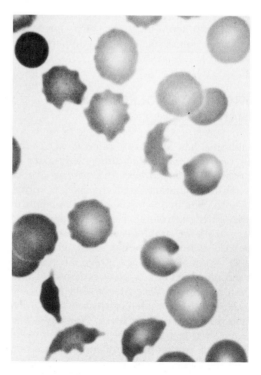

Figure 28-10. Erythrocyte microangiopathy (fragmentation) hemolysis in a case of acute fatty liver of pregnancy. (*Courtesy of Ms. R. Mason.*)

TABLE 28-8. ACUTE FATTY LIVER OF PREGNANCY
Laboratory Studies That Demonstrate Hepatic Dysfunction, Coagulopathy, and Their Repair

Time	Bili-rubin	SGOT	Akalaline Phosphatase	Serum Proteins Total	Albumin	Fibrin-ogen	FSP[a]	Plate-lets	Pro-thrombin	Hema-tocrit
Delivery[b]	8.7	200	358	5.5	—	—	—	73,000	23	40
+1 day[b]	9.6	137	390	4.3	1.9	47	128	111,000	16	30
+3 days[b,c]	11.5	42	—	3.8	2.0	137	8	82,000	15	27
+5 days	10.3	39	264	4.1	2.1	141	8	108,000	13	28
+8 days	7.0	43	276	4.8	2.2	236	8	186,000	—	31
+12 days[d]	4.6	39	283	6.4	3.4	340	8	292,000	13	36
+1 year	0.8	20	130	7.1	4.3	298	2	340,000	12	41

[a] FSP = Fibrin split products (μg/ml of serum).
[b] Transfused with packed RBC and fresh frozen plasma.
[c] Ascites apparent.
[d] 14 kg spontaneous diuresis within 7 days.

by serial measurements of SGOT, alkaline phosphatase, bilirubin, and serum protein concentrations, was improved appreciably by 6 days after delivery. During that time, however, the patient had developed severe ascites; the condition was treated by modest restriction of both sodium and fluids. Her diet during the illness consisted of a general diet with sodium restriction, and she received 150 g of glucose per day intravenously to combat hypoglycemia. She ate little until late in the first week. Diuresis, beginning spontaneously on the seventh day, was vigorous and resulted in a weight loss of 14 kg in less than a week.

Liver biopsy done on the 11th postpartum day confirmed the clinical diagnosis of acute fatty liver of pregnancy (Fig. 28-9). Renal function, which was impaired when she was first hospitalized (plasma creatinine 2.2 mg/dl), began to return to normal by the fifth day after delivery.

One year later, when evaluated for hepatic, renal, and hematologic abnormalities, none persisted.

Delivery is essential for cure. Some authors have recommended cesarean delivery to minimize the time until repair of hepatic function begins. Moreover, immediate delivery is likely to benefit the fetus who is distressed. However, cesarean section in the presence of severe coagulopathy may prove dangerous to the mother, as might an abdominal incision in circumstances in which severe hypoproteinemia and ascites are likely complications of the early puerperium. On the other hand, procrastination in effecting delivery can increase the risk of coma and death from hyperammonemia usually further complicated by hypoglycemia, renal failure, acidosis, and severe hemorrhage.

Interestingly, subsequent pregnancies in an appreciable number of women who had previously suffered severe acute fatty liver of pregnancy have proved to be totally benign.

PREECLAMPSIA–ECLAMPSIA

The liver may be involved in women with preeclampsia and eclampsia. Both the degree of dysfunction and the histologic changes that develop can vary considerably. Typically, upper abdominal pain—epigastric or right upper quadrant—signal potentially dangerous liver involvement. Intrahepatic and subcapsular hemorrhage may develop and become so intense as to rupture the liver and produce extensive, even fatal, hemorrhage. Hepatic dysfunction from preeclampsia and eclampsia is considered in more detail in Chapter 27, p. 537.

HYPEREMESIS GRAVIDARUM

Nausea and vomiting of moderate intensity are especially common complaints from the second to the fourth month of gestation (Chapter 13, p. 260). Fortunately, vomiting sufficiently pernicious to produce weight loss, dehydration, acidosis from starvation, alkalosis from loss of hydrochloric acid in vomitus, and hypokalemia has become quite rare. Hyperemesis may lead to some elevation in SGOT, slight jaundice, and retention of sulfobromophthalein, all of which return to normal with hydration and feeding.

Treatment of pernicious vomiting of pregnancy comprises correction of deficits of fluid and electrolytes and of acidosis or alkalosis. This requires appropriate amounts of sodium, potassium, chloride, lactate or bicarbonate, glucose, and water, which should be administered parenterally until the vomiting has been controlled. *Appropriate steps should be taken to detect other diseases—for example, gastroenteritis, cholecystitis, hepatitis, peptic ulcer, and pyelonephritis.* In many instances, social and psychologic factors contribute to the illness, as in the case of the young unwed mother who continues to live with her parents while they harass her because of her "sin." Commonly, in this circumstance, the woman improves remarkably while hospitalized, only to relapse after discharge. Positive assistance with psychologic and social problems often proves quite beneficial. Only rarely is it necessary to interrupt the pregnancy.

VIRAL HEPATITIS

Almost all forms of liver disease can afflict pregnant women, with the most common being hepatitis. There are at least three distinct forms of viral hepatitis. During the acute phase of the three forms, they often appear to be quite similar. However, long-term complications in the mother and the risks to the fetus and infant are quite different.

The Center for Disease Control has issued guidelines for patients when hospitalized with viral hepatitis. They recommend that feces, secretions, bed pans, and articles in contact with the intestinal tract be handled with glove protected hands. These precautions need not be continued once hepatitis A is excluded. Extra precautions, such as double gloving during delivery, may be wise in case of viral hepatatis B and non A-non B hepatitis. In these instances, instruments in contact with blood should be thoroughly cleaned and appropriately autoclaved.

Viral Hepatitis A

This disease was previously referred to as infectious hepatitis. Individuals who are developing this disease shed the virus in their feces. During the relatively brief period of viremia, their blood is also infectious. This disease is usually spread by ingestion of contaminated blood or water. The incubation period is about 2 to 7 weeks. The signs and symptoms are not very specific, and the infection may go undiagnosed or be considered a flu-like illness unless jaundice is detected. Confirmation of the disease can be made by the appearance of hepatitis A antibody.

The effects of hepatitis A on pregnancy and vice versa are not dramatic in developed countries. However, at least in some underprivileged populations, both perinatal and maternal deaths are increased. Treatment consists of a nutritious diet and sedentary living. We have long followed the policy of hospitalizing all pregnant women with suspected hepatitis until it was clear that they were able to eat and drink and that liver function was not continuing to deteriorate.

There is no evidence that hepatitis A virus is teratogenic. Risk of transmission to the fetus appears to be nil and to the newborn infant quite small. The risk of premature birth appears to be increased somewhat for pregnancies complicated by hepatitis A (Steven, 1981). The pregnant woman who has been recently exposed to hepatitis A may receive gamma globulin prophylactically and benefit from it as she would if she were not pregnant.

Viral Hepatitis B

This disease, once referred to as serum hepatitis, is found worldwide but is endemic in some regions, especially in Asia and in Africa. A variety of immunologic markers have been identified in subjects with acute or chronic disease, in those who have had the disease and now are immune, and in chronic carriers. The hepatitis B virus (Dane particle), core (c) antigen and surface (s) antigen, the antibodies to core and surface antigens, e antigen, and e antibody are all detectable by various techniques.

The viral genome is incorporated into the hepatocyte nucleus, and the viral core of DNA is produced there, while the viral coat is produced in the cytoplasm. These viral components are then assembled and secreted from the cell as infectious virus. The e antigen is very similar to the intact virus and is an indication of the infectious state.

Hepatitis B disease is found most often among drug abusers, homosexuals, health care personnel, and individuals who have been treated often with blood products, for example, hemophiliacs. This form of hepatitis is transmitted usually in infected blood or blood products and in saliva, vaginal secretions, and semen. Thus hepatitis B can be a venereal disease.

The course of hepatitis B infection in the mother does not seem to be altered by pregnancy, at least in developed countries. Prematurity is increased. Treatment is supportive, the same as for hepatitis A.

Transplacental transfer of the virus from the mother to the fetus except at delivery is thought to be rare (Goudeau and co-workers, 1983). Infection of the fetus–infant occurs most often during delivery or subsequent to birth. The infant may possibly obtain the virus through breast-feeding.

Some affected infants are asymptomatic. Some develop fulminant disease and cirrhosis and succumb. Others become chronic carriers and can infect others. The chronic carriers are at appreciable risk of developing fatal hepatoma later in life.

The discovery of the e antigen of hepatitis B virus and its correlation with the number of circulating Dane particles, i.e., virus, led to recognition that vertical transmission of hepatitis B correlates closely with the maternal e antigen status. Mothers with hepatitis B surface antigen and hepatitis B e antigen are very likely to transmit the disease to their infants, whereas those that are negative for e antigen and positive for e antibody do not appear to transmit the infection.

Infection of the newborn infant whose mother harbors the virus usually can be prevented by the administration of hepatitis B immune globulin very soon after birth, followed promptly by hepatitis B vaccine (Beasley and associates, 1983; Wong and co-workers, 1984).

It is probably a good idea to screen pregnant women for hepatitis B surface antigen. Certainly those at high risk should be so tested. If positive, and especially if e antigen is identified in the mother, the offspring should receive immune globulin and vaccine very soon after birth.

Non A-Non B Hepatitis

Most individuals who develop hepatitis after blood or blood products develop the non A-non B form of hepatitis. For example, in one study 18 of 842 cardiac surgery patients developed hepatitis after transfusion; 14 of the cases were attributed to the non A-non B form of hepatitis (Cossart and colleagues, 1982). The disease may be contracted from an infected sexual partner. The injection of some preparations of human normal immunoglobulin has been implicated in the causation of non A-non B hepatitis (Lane, 1983).

Hepatitis from *cytomegalovirus* or *Epstein-Barr virus* can be excluded by checking cytomegaloviral titers and by spot tests for mononucleosis. Hepatitis from *herpesvirus* is rare and usually fatal (Wertheim and coworkers, 1983). Because of its rarity it will seldom be confused with non A-non B hepatitis.

Studies to evaluate immune serum globulin for prophylaxis against non A-non B hepatitis have been somewhat disappointing. Nonetheless, it probably should be given to the newborn of the mother with active disease, since it may prevent acquisition of the disease by the offspring.

Chronic Active Hepatitis

The effect of pregnancy on chronic active hepatitis and vice versa will depend in large part on the intensity of the disease process. The disease has a propensity to progress to cirrhosis, portal hypertension, hepatic failure, and shortened life span. When severe, anovulation is common. Adrenocorticosteroids and immunosuppressants have increased both fertility and survival of women with autoimmune chronic active hepatitis.

Chronic active hepatitis does not necessarily warrant therapeutic abortion. Steven and associates (1979) have concluded that with chronic active hepatitis (1) fertility is reduced but pregnancies that do occur can proceed without serious detriment to the mother if prednisolone treatment is maintained; (2) fetal loss will be increased; and (3) prematurity but not malformations will be common.

CIRRHOSIS OF LIVER

Women with cirrhosis are very likely to be infertile. Cheng (1977) has reviewed the clinical features of pregnancy in women with hepatic cirrhosis and concluded that perinatal loss is high and the maternal prognosis is grave. Esophageal varices were prone to bleed, with fatal hemorrhage as the consequence.

Schreyer and associates (1982) have provided another review of cirrhosis of the liver complicating pregnancy and also confirmed high morbidity and appreciable mortality. They raised the possibility that the high incidence of esophageal hemorrhage and, in turn, the high mortality rate might be decreased by prophylactic portal-systemic shunting but hastened to point out that the procedure and its sequelae are not necessarily benign.

Liver Transplant and Pregnancy

Walcott and associates (1979) described delivery of a normal infant at term after an uncomplicated prenatal course even though the mother had undergone a liver transplant because of necrosis from hepatic venous thrombosis 2 years before. She was being treated continuously with azathioprine and prednisolone, and was not ovulating until treated with clomiphene citrate.

CHOLELITHIASIS AND CHOLECYSTITIS

There is a greater frequency—twice or three times as high—of cholelithiasis in women than in men. Gallbladder kinetics during pregnancy have been investigated by Braverman and associates (1980) using real-time sonography. After the first trimester, both gallbladder volume during fasting and residual volume after contracting in response to a test meal were twice as large as in nonpregnant subjects. Incomplete emptying may result in retention of cholesterol crystals, a prerequisite for cholesterol gallstones. These findings are supportive, at least, of the view that pregnancy increases the risk of gallstones. Presumably, the very high progesterone levels that characterize the second and third trimesters of pregnancy are responsible for the diminished gallbladder activity. Progesterone has been shown to impair the gallbladder response to exogenously administered cholecystokinin in experimental animals.

Acute attacks of gallbladder disease during pregnancy or the puerperium, in general, are managed the same way as for the nonpregnant woman. If cholecystectomy is to be performed, the second trimester is the optimal time, since the risk of spontaneous abortion or delivery of an immature fetus is reduced and the uterus is not yet large enough to impinge on the field of operation. Even so, when surgery is thought to be indicated in the pregnant woman, procrastination should be avoided. Delay can only place the woman and her fetus in greater jeopardy. At times, drainage of the gallbladder is the procedure of choice. Recent surgery does not complicate labor except for the discomfort from the fresh incision.

Hill and associates (1975) described 20 instances of cholecystectomy during pregnancy at the Mayo Clinic. There was one spontaneous abortion at 10 weeks of gestation 42 days after the operation; maternal morbidity was low.

DISEASES OF THE ALIMENTARY TRACT

During normal pregnancy, the alimentary tract undergoes changes—anatomic and functional—that can alter appreciably the criteria for diagnosis and treatment of several diseases to which they are susceptible.

APPENDICITIS

Gestation does not predispose to appendicitis, but because of the general prevalence of the disease, there is an incidence of about 1 in every 2000 pregnancies, as shown in Black's extensive review (1960). Pregnancy often makes diagnosis more difficult. First, anorexia, nausea, and vomiting caused by pregnancy itself are fairly common. Second, as the uterus enlarges, the appendix commonly moves upward and outward toward the flank, so that pain and tenderness may not be prominent in the right lower quadrant (Fig. 28-11). Third, some degree of leukocytosis is the rule during normal pregnancy. Fourth, during pregnancy especially, other diseases may be readily confused with appendicitis, such as pyelonephritis, renal colic caused by a stone or kinking of a ureter, placental abruption, and red, or carneous, degeneration of a myoma.

Appendicitis increases the likelihood of abortion or premature labor, especially if peritonitis develops. The fetal loss rate, therefore, in most series is about 15 per-

cent. As the appendix is pushed progressively higher by the growing uterus, a walling off of the infection becomes increasingly unlikely and appendiceal rupture causes widespread peritonitis. Acute appendicitis in the last trimester, therefore, carries a much graver prognosis. Although antibiotics have reduced the mortality rate from acute appendicitis in pregnancy, the disease remains a serious complication of gestation.

The treatment, regardless of the stage of gestation, is immediate operation (Cunningham and McCubbin, 1975; Gomez and Wood, 1979). *Even though diagnostic errors sometimes lead to the removal of a normal appendix, it is better to operate unnecessarily than to postpone intervention until generalized peritonitis has developed.* The mortality rate of appendicitis today in the obstetric patient is essentially associated with surgical delay.

It is important that during the operation and period of recovery both hypoxia and hypotension be avoided. If they are avoided and generalized peritonitis does not develop, the prognosis is quite good. Seldom, if ever, is cesarean section indicated at the time of appendectomy. Aside from local soreness, a recent abdominal incision should present no problem during labor and vaginal delivery.

Appendicitis during the early puerperium, fortunately, is rare. It may be difficult to diagnose because of

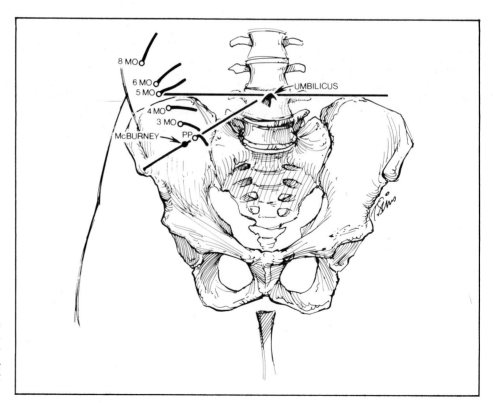

Figure 28-11. Changes in the position of the appendix as pregnancy advances. (MO = calendar month; PP = postpartum). (*Modified from Baer and associates.: JAMA 98:1359, 1932.*)

the frequency with which leukocytosis occurs normally and the frequency of other diseases with similar signs and symptoms. Anorexia with any evidence of peritoneal irritation, such as distention and lack of bowel sounds, should suggest appendicitis.

UPPER ABDOMINAL PAIN

Most obstetricians, but not most internists or gastroenterologists, are aware that upper abdominal pain—epigastric or right upper quadrant—can be an ominous sign of severe preeclampsia and act accordingly. Sonography negative for gallstones, a normal serum amylase value, or absence of free acid in gastric juice does not serve to exclude serious disease but rather supports the diagnosis of severe preeclampsia.

PEPTIC ULCER

An active peptic ulcer is rare during pregnancy, and complications such as perforation or hemorrhage are even rarer. Moreover, women with a symptomatic peptic ulcer most often note considerable improvement during pregnancy.

PANCREATITIS

Pancreatitis during pregnancy is very uncommon. The principles of therapy, in general, are the same as for nonpregnant patients. If the diagnosis is secure, treatment is medical rather than surgical exploration. Two commonly used drugs—tetracycline in large doses and thiazide diuretics—have been implicated in pancreatitis in pregnant women. Corlett and Mishell (1972) and Wilkinson (1973) have reviewed pancreatitis and pregnancy and stress the necessity for prompt medical management.

INTESTINAL OBSTRUCTION

This grave complication of pregnancy results most frequently from pressure of the growing uterus on intestinal adhesions that were caused by previous abdominal operations. The mortality rate can be very high, chiefly because of error in diagnosis, late diagnosis, reluctance to operate on a pregnant woman, and inadequate preparation for surgery.

Kohn and associates (1944) reported a remarkable case in which the same patient was operated upon for *volvulus* four times, three of the operations having been performed in the course of two pregnancies. In a review of the literature, they collected 79 cases of volvulus in pregnancy. In a third of the cases reported by Harer and Harer (1958), emptying the uterus by cesarean section was necessary to obtain proper exposure.

Volvulus, especially of the cecum, has been observed early in the puerperium after cesarean section, as emphasized by Pratt and colleagues (1981).

CHRONIC INFLAMMATORY BOWEL DISEASE

Ulcerative Colitis

In an analysis of one of the largest series of cases reported, Crohn and his associates (1956) found that colitis that had been quiescent at the beginning of gestation was reactivated by pregnancy, usually in the first trimester, in about half the patients. If the colitis was already active at the time of conception, it was materially aggravated in three quarters of the patients. They emphasized also the excessive and prolonged severity of postpartum recurrences.

More recently, Levy and associates (1981) observed in 60 pregnancies among 31 women with ulcerative colitis that the majority experienced no change in the activity of their disease during pregnancy. In one fifth, improvement was noted, while one fifth suffered deterioration. All gave birth to normal children. It was concluded that pregnancy does not usually aggravate the disease nor does the disease adversely affect pregnancy.

When this disease becomes worse in gestation, the etiologic factor may be psychogenic rather than related to any intrinsic effect of pregnancy. The patient's fear that pregnancy will aggravate her disease, for example, may precipitate an exacerbation. Reassurance is therefore an important part of management.

Regional Enteritis

Fieldring and Cooke (1970), in pregnancies complicated by Crohn's disease, found no evidence that pregnancy exerted adverse effects on the course of the disease or increased the mortality rate. Moreover, abortion, prematurity, and stillbirth were not increased. Norton and Patterson (1972) have similarly concluded that pregnancy and regional enteritis do not affect each other adversely. Homan and Thorbjarnarson (1976), however, observed relapse in one fourth of women with Crohn's disease after the pregnancy was completed.

Main and associates (1981) have described a case of Crohn's disease and pregnancy complicated by ileal obstruction for which they were reluctant to attempt surgical resection during the pregnancy. The patient was totally fed intravenously from the 27th week until cesarean section at 36 weeks. A somewhat growth-retarded infant who thrived was delivered. The mother subsequently underwent bowel resection.

Sörökin and Levine (1983) have provided a literature review of pregnancy with inflammatory bowel disease from which they conclude that the fetus is likely to survive despite active disease and that there are few reasons to consider therapeutic abortion.

OBESITY

Marked obesity is a hazard to the pregnant woman and her fetus. For example, Tracy and Miller (1969), in the course of reviewing the pregnancies of 48 women whose weights averaged 284 pounds, noted that nearly two thirds developed some obstetric complication. One of the five mothers diagnosed as having diabetes expired. Over half of the 48 were considered hypertensive, and pyelonephritis developed in five.

In our experience, a large variety of serious complications of pregnancy is more likely to develop in obese women, including hypertension, diabetes, aspiration of gastric contents during anesthesia, wound complications, and thromboembolism. The most extreme case of obesity we have encountered during pregnancy was in a young multipara who early in the third trimester weighed somewhat more than 500 pounds, although she was only 62 inches tall. In spite of a multitude of complications, emotional as well as physical, six pregnancies have produced eight living children.

Management of obesity during pregnancy is a challenge. A program of weight reduction utilizing a diet restricted in calories but providing all essential nutrients has commonly been recommended for obese pregnant women. If such a regimen is to be used, it is mandatory that the quality of the diet be monitored closely and that ketosis not be allowed to develop.

JEJUNOILEAL AND GASTRIC BYPASS

The *small intestinal bypass* operation performed to try to relieve obesity has been followed by pregnancy. Twenty-five children, including three sets of twins and one of triplets, have been born to 16 such women observed by Salmon (1975). Their birth weights averaged 3000 g, or 300 g less than did the children born to women before the bypass operation. Two of the children had serious anomalies.

Eight pregnant women with a jejunoileal bypass have been cared for at Parkland Memorial Hospital. Seven of the pregnancies were benign. All of the women received specifically supplemental iron, folic acid, vitamin B_{12}, plus a commercially available prenatal vitamin–mineral preparation. Seven infants were appropriately grown and in good health. In one woman who had previously undergone a bypass operation, which excluded nearly all of the small intestine and utilized an end-to-end anastomosis, pregnancy created myriad problems: She lost appreciable weight while consuming between 6000 and 9000 calories per day. A slightly growth-retarded infant was delivered by cesarean section, which was necessitated by a prolapsed cord; he subsequently thrived. Postpartum, the mother developed severe hypoproteinemia, hypocalcemia with tetany, hypokalemia, hypomagnesemia, and vitamin K deficiency sufficiently intense to prolong the prothrombin time appreciably. She responded well to vitamin K, calcium gluconate, potassium chloride, and magnesium sulfate (given parenterally) and to a generous high protein diet.

Printen and Scott (1982) have described the experiences during 51 pregnancies of 45 women who underwent *gastric bypass* surgery because of morbid obesity (body weight at least twice that of ideal body weight). Fetal growth retardation was not a problem. Of the 46 infants delivered, 1 had a serious malformation. They concluded that neither the mother nor the developing fetus is endangered unduly by a pregnancy conceived subsequent to the period of rapid postoperative weight loss.

CONNECTIVE TISSUE DISORDERS

The so-called connective tissue or collagen diseases are a group of diseases characterized by disorders of connective tissue especially. A common denominator is immunopathologically mediated organ or system injury as the consequence of a variety of autoantibodies. A review of the pathogenesis and clinical features of several of these disorders has been provided by Kohler and Vaughan (1982).

SYSTEMIC LUPUS ERYTHEMATOSUS

Systemic lupus erythematosus is notoriously variable in presentation, course, and outcome. The American Rheumatism Association has provided the following revised criteria for the identification of systemic lupus erythe-

matosus (Tan and associates, 1982): If any 4 or more of the 11 criteria cited are present, serially or simultaneously, the diagnosis of lupus erythematosus is applicable: (1) malar rash, (2) discoid rash, (3) photosensitivity, (4) oral ulcers, (5) arthritis, (6) serositis, (7) renal disorder, (8) neurologic disorder (seizures), (9) hematologic disorder (hemolysis, leukopenia, thrombocytopenia), (10) immunologic disorder (positive LE preparation, anti-DNA, anti-Sm, false positive serologic tests for syphilis), (11) antinuclear antibody.

It has been estimated that nearly 500,000 individuals in the United States have systemic lupus, the great majority of whom are women. Even so, there are few reports concerned with the interactions of lupus and pregnancy in which a large number of pregnancies provided the basis for the publication. Consequently, it is not surprising that disagreements persist concerning systemic lupus and pregnancy, although opinions expressed in more recent reports seem much less divergent than in the past.

Fine and co-workers (1981) have analyzed their experiences with one or more pregnancies in 39 women with systemic lupus erythematosus to provide answers to the following questions:

1. Does pregnancy alter the natural history of systemic lupus erythematosus? They concluded that pregnancy was not accompanied by an increased prevalence of major systemic *nonrenal* manifestations of lupus unless immunosuppressive therapy was stopped because of pregnancy.
2. Are the effects of systemic lupus on renal function exaggerated by pregnancy? They observed that for those women with no more than minimal renal impairment prepregnancy, renal function remained good in the great majority, deteriorated but recovered postpartum in about 10 percent, and in another 10 percent deteriorated and remained depressed. One such woman who also demonstrated florid extrarenal involvement died soon after hemodialysis was begun. It was difficult to distinguish clinically between preeclampsia and lupus nephritis as the cause of the renal impairment as it was in the case summarized below. Induced abortions were not accompanied by any discernible deleterious effect on renal function.
3. Should pharmacologic treatment of systemic lupus be altered during pregnancy? Their experiences led them to recommend the use of glucocorticoids and azathioprine antepartum in doses no different from those used with nonpregnant patients. Moreover, they concluded that there probably is merit in increasing the dosage during labor and for up to 2 months thereafter to minimize the risk of exacerbation.
4. How does systemic lupus affect the fetus and neonate? Stillbirths were frequent (23 percent), as was prematurity (33 percent) and fetal growth retardation (33 percent). Persistent proteinuria or reduced creatinine clearance was associated with a high prevalence of stillbirths and low birth weights even though the mothers were not overtly azotemic. When both proteinuria and appreciably reduced clearance coexisted, fetal wastage was very high. Talipes equinovarus was the only anomaly detected. Congenital heart block was not described.

Varner and associates (1983) also have reported their experiences with pregnancies in women with systemic lupus erythematosus. One of the 36 mothers died 5 weeks postpartum with poorly controlled vascular disease. Perinatal mortality was increased but was not as great as reported by Fine and co-workers (1981). One

fetus–infant demonstrated heart block. Varner and associates too concluded that women whose disease is in remission and stays in remission can anticipate a favorable pregnancy outcome. They recommend that women on immunosuppressive therapy at the onset of pregnancy remain on therapy, since the risk from therapy is less than the risk from the disease without treatment, a conclusion also reached by Hayslett and Lynn (1980), who analyzed the pregnancy outcomes for a large group of women with lupus nephropathy. It is not clear at this time whether there is any advantage to increasing the dosage at delivery and during the puerperium. It has often been stated that this is the time that activation or exacerbation is most likely to occur, but evidence to support the statement is not striking (Hayslett and Lynn, 1980).

Gimovsky and associates (1984), upon reviewing the pregnancy experiences of a comparable number of women with lupus, have described problems very similar to those reported by Fine, Varner, and their associates and cited above. They also noted maternal diabetes to be a troublesome complication of steroid therapy during pregnancy.

Laboratory Evaluation

Various laboratory procedures have been recommended to try to monitor systemic lupus activity. The sedimentation test is widely used. However, an increase in sedimentation rate is uninterpretable during pregnancy, since there is an appreciable rise induced by normal pregnancy. Serial measurements of C3 and C4 components of complement have been recommended. Falling or low levels are more likely to be associated with active disease, but, unfortunately, higher levels provide no guarantee that significant activation of the disease is not occurring. Varner and co-workers (1983), for example, found no correlation between clinical manifestations of disease and C3 and C4 complement levels in nearly one half of their pregnant patients. Our experiences have been similar.

Frequent hematologic evaluation and measurements of renal and hepatic functions are essential to detect changes in the activity of the disease during pregnancy and the puerperium. Hemolytic anemia is characterized by a lowering of hematocrit, a reticulocytosis, and perhaps hyperbilirubinemia, mostly unconjugated. Thrombocytopenia, leukopenia, or both may develop at any time. Increased serum transaminase activity reflects hepatic involvement, as does a rise in serum bilirubin that is predominantly conjugated. At times azathioprine therapy will induce abnormalities in these tests of hepatic function. Overt and increasing proteinuria that persists is an ominous sign and is even more ominous if accompanied by an abnormal serum creatinine concentration. In general, the prognosis becomes poorer as the number of abnormal findings increases, especially if immunosuppressive therapy provides no amelioration.

Lupus versus Preeclampsia–Eclampsia

It may be difficult, if not impossible, to differentiate clinically lupus nephropathy from severe preeclampsia. Moreover, central nervous system involvement with systemic lupus may culminate in convulsions comparable to those of eclampsia. Thrombocytopenia with or without hemolysis may further confuse the diagnosis. We have elected to manage such problem cases of systemic lupus as if they were the consequences of preeclampsia–eclampsia, utilizing magnesium sulfate, hydralazine intravenously, and delivery as described elsewhere (Chapter 27, p. 547). At the same time immunosuppressive therapy is continued. It should be emphasized that remote from pregnancy the commonest causes of death are malignant hypertension with glomerulonephritis and neurologic catastrophes, such as seizures, strokes, and coma.

Some problems of differential diagnosis of preeclampsia–eclampsia from systemic lupus with vascular, renal, and central nervous system involvement during pregnancy and the puerperium are illustrated by the following case from Parkland Memorial Hospital.

A 21-year-old primigravida was observed throughout most of pregnancy. By term her blood pressure had risen from earlier values of 100/60 mm Hg to 130/80 mm Hg and intrapartum to 140/90. Edema was obvious, but proteinuria was not detected. She convulsed 1 hour after spontaneous delivery of a healthy infant who weighed 3985 g. Transiently, her blood pressure was elevated to 160/108 mm Hg and proteinuria appeared. Hematocrit, platelet count, and plasma creatinine were normal. She was treated with magnesium sulfate parenterally for 24 hours and had no more convulsions. One week later she was discharged normotensive and asymptomatic.

Two weeks after delivery she experienced bizarre neurologic changes, including tremors and transient loss of vision and of consciousness. A CT scan of the brain was normal, but an electroencephalogram was abnormal. The LE preparation was positive, antinuclear antibody titer was 640, and the serologic test for syphilis was positive. While hospitalized she developed a malar (butterfly) rash. The diagnosis was systemic lupus with central nervous system involvement. Did she have eclampsia 2 weeks before? We concluded that she did not; rather she had lupus erythematosus.

Effects on Fetus and Infant

The fetus should be observed closely for adverse effects imposed by a hostile intrauterine environment, especially growth retardation. Evidence of growth retardation warrants prompt delivery unless the fetus is very immature. In that case, further close monitoring should be considered until delivery is effected. Isolated congenital heart block, as a consequence especially of fibrosis in the region between the atrioventricular node and bundle of His, may develop in the fetus. The heart block may be tolerated or may lead to Stokes-Adams attacks or heart failure in the fetus and infant. It may require active treatment with a pacemaker. Heart block may also develop in fetuses whose mothers appear normal but who are destined subsequently to develop clinical lupus erythematosus or some other disease of connective tissue. Mothers of infants with isolated complete heart block should be so evaluated. IgG antibodies to SS-A(Ro) and SS-B(La) have been identified transiently in the serum of neonates with congenital heart block and in many of their mothers (Cobbe, 1983; Vetter and Rashkind, 1983; Lee and Weston, 1984).

Stigmata other than growth retardation and congenital heart block may be found in the newborn. The LE factor has been demonstrated in the circulation of the fetus–infant. Transient discoid lupus has been described. Thrombocytopenia, leukopenia, and hemolytic anemia that cleared subsequently have also been identified (Levy, 1982).

Further Reproduction

If systemic lupus has been induced by a drug, the disease most likely will ameliorate when the drug is stopped. Otherwise, it is a lifelong disease. If the disease has been characterized by prolonged remissions, pregnancy should be undertaken during such a remission.

In general, women with systemic lupus and chronic vascular or renal disease should limit their family size because of the poor prognosis for the fetus and also the mother. Wallace and associates (1981) have made the following observations on 609 patients with systemic lupus erythematosus: The 10-year survival was 87 percent for those without nephritis but only 65 percent for those with nephritis. The most common causes of death were renal disease and sepsis. No appreciable difference between whites and nonwhites was noted.

Tubal sterilization may be advantageous. It is performed with greatest safety when the disease is reasonably quiescent. We have not recommended oral contraceptives for women with systemic lupus, since there is some published evidence that suggests that systemic lupus may be worsened by their use. Moreover, in public hospitals and clinics, at least, it is likely that someone sooner or later will interdict their use and the woman will receive no other contraception and conceive. Intrauterine devices are not recommended by us, especially if the woman is receiving immunosuppressive therapy. The potential for pelvic infection is too great.

Since blood vessel disease, especially of the microvasculature, is common in women with systemic lupus, it is not surprising that vessels so involved during pregnancy can include those of the decidua. This may account for the prevalence of fetal growth retardation and pregnancy wastage associated with maternal systemic lupus.

Lupus Anticoagulant

This prothrombinase complex inhibitor is an IgG immunoglobulin that has been identified in some individuals with systemic lupus and also in others with no apparent evidence of lupus. In vitro the presence of the lupus anticoagulant is characterized by a prolonged kaolin partial thromboplastin time. Paradoxically, in vivo lupus anticoagulant incites thrombosis (Boey and co-workers, 1983).

The lupus anticoagulant in pregnant women has, at times, been associated with decidual vasculopathy, placental infarction, fetal growth retardation, repeated abortion, and recurrent fetal loss (Carreras and co-workers, 1981; DeWolf and co-workers, 1982; Reece and associates, 1984). Evidence suggestive of impairment of prostacyclin formation was obtained in one study. The definition of the role of lupus anticoagulant in pregnancy wastage requires further clarification. Kochenour and associates (1984) have recommended that screening for lupus anticoagulant by measuring the partial thromboplastin time be included in the evaluation of women who suffered recurrent abortion or fetal death. These workers, as well as Lubbe and associates (1984), have administered corticosteroids plus aspirin to try to improve pregnancy outcomes.

RHEUMATOID ARTHRITIS

Although a number of humoral and cellular immunologic abnormalities have been identified, the cause of rheumatoid arthritis, or rheumatoid disease, is unknown. The disease is more common in women than men.

In 1938, Hench reported marked improvement in the inflammatory component of rheumatoid arthritis during pregnancy. The pattern of improvement involved gradual amelioration of the signs and symptoms of the rheumatoid process, as occurs during a spontaneous remission. Apparently on the basis that corticosteroid levels in plasma were considered to be markedly increased in pregnancy, Hench began to treat individuals who had rheumatoid arthritis with cortisone with a favorable effect. Smith and West (1960) demonstrated subsequently that an increased secretion of cortisol did not readily account for all of the remissions rather commonly found in pregnancy.

More recently, Unger and associates (1983) studied a group of women with rheumatoid arthritis for disease activity during pregnancy. In two thirds of them disease activity diminished. In the group in which activity subsided, pregnancy-associated α_2-glycoprotein was considerably higher (mean 1250 mg/L) than in those in whom the disease remained the same or worsened (mean 470 mg/L). Pregnancy-associated glycoprotein is known to have immunosuppressive properties in vitro, and therefore it is tempting to implicate the high level of this protein in the remission of rheumatoid arthritis in pregnancy, as Hench did for cortisol.

Neely and Persellin (1977) similarly identified amelioration of activity of rheumatoid arthritis in 62 percent (35/56) of pregnancies, but in the other 38 percent there was either no change in activity or the arthritis actually became worse. In four women the signs and symptoms of the disease first appeared during pregnancy. Thus in some women the course may occasionally worsen during pregnancy, and sometimes the disease may first appear at that time, as illustrated by the case summarized below.

The drug most commonly used to treat rheumatoid arthritis remote from pregnancy has been aspirin in doses that, if used in pregnancy, might possibly affect the fetus and neonate adversely in one or more of the following ways: impaired hemostasis, prolonged gestation, and premature closure of the ductus arteriosus. Nonetheless, aspirin usually has been the drug of choice during pregnancy. Gold compounds have been used in pregnancy, but there has not been sufficient experience to recommend their use. Prednisolone and similar adrenocorticosteroids have been used, usually without producing serious adverse effects on the pregnancy.

Intense involvement of certain joints may interfere with delivery. For example, severe deformities of the hip may preclude vaginal delivery.

We have observed the clinical onset of rheumatoid arthritis during the first trimester of pregnancy in a 22-year-old nullipara. Treatment with aspirin (600 mg every 4 hours) did not produce relief. Prednisolone, 7.5 mg a day begun at 20 weeks gestation, plus enteric-coated aspirin, three tablets every 4 hours, provided considerable relief. She never was anemic; supplemental iron was provided during pregnancy.

Fetal growth retardation and oligohydramnios became evident during the third trimester. The mother was not hypertensive. The infant when delivered at 35 weeks gestation weighed 1720 g but thrived subsequently. The placenta contained multiple infarcts.

Rheumatoid arthritis requiring vigorous treatment has persisted during the 2 years since delivery. Therapy has consisted primarily of gold by injection and indomethacin. She is contemplating another pregnancy.

DERMATOMYOSITIS

Dermatomyositis (polymyositis) is an uncommon acute, subacute or chronic inflammatory disease of unknown cause involving especially skin and muscle. The disease may manifest itself as a severe generalized myositis with a cutaneous eruption and fever and a fatal outcome within a few days or weeks. It may also assume a chronic form, characterized by the gradual development of paresis with little, if any, cutaneous or systemic involvement.

About 15 percent of adults developing dermatomyositis have an associated malignant tumor. The time of appearance of the two diseases, however, may be separated by several years. Extirpation of the malignant lesion is sometimes followed by a permanent remission of the dermatomyositis. The most common sites of the associated cancer are the breast, lung, stomach, and ovary. The uterus and cervix have also been reported as primary sites.

There are so few reports of dermatomyositis in pregnancy that it is difficult to draw any definite conclusions about the effect of one upon the other. We have observed a case diagnosed and treated with prednisone before pregnancy. During and after the pregnancy the mother actually improved and the infant thrived.

SCLERODERMA

Scleroderma, or progressive systemic sclerosis, occurs mostly in young women of childbearing age, but its rarity prevents an accumulation of extensive data relative to its effect on pregnancy. Scleroderma was formerly considered to have a markedly deleterious effect upon pregnancy. Johnson and associates (1964) were more encouraging in their report of 36 pregnancies in a group of 337 women in whom scleroderma had developed before the age of 45. They concluded that pregnancy had little or no effect on the course of the disease and that scleroderma had a minimal effect on the pregnancy. In our limited experience, however, dysphagia seems to be aggravated by pregnancy. Renal insufficiency and malignant hypertension are common causes of death. Whether preeclampsia enhances their onset and severity is not known. Almost certainly, preexisting vascular–renal disease would increase the risk of preeclampsia–eclampsia. A fatal case of apparent eclampsia in a woman with scleroderma has been reported (Fear, 1968). The fetus also succumbed.

Vaginal delivery may be anticipated unless the changes wrought by scleroderma in the soft tissues produce dystocia, requiring abdominal delivery.

POLYARTERITIS NODOSA

Polyarteritis (periarteritis) nodosa is a rare disease with protean manifestations. The classic variety is a progressive illness characterized clinically by myalgia, neuropathy, gastrointestinal disorders, hypertension, and renal disease. Only a few documented cases of polyarteritis nodosa in association with pregnancy have been reported. The experience is too scant to draw any definitive conclusions about polyarteritis nodosa and pregnancy other than the fact that, generally, the combination is associated with unfavorable maternal outcome (Siegler and Spain, 1965). Typically, the mother died postpartum with hypertension and renal involvement. Burkett and Richards (1982) reported one patient in

whom the disease was considered to be in remission throughout pregnancy and puerperium. Although it was her fourth pregnancy, she developed hypertension (160/110), proteinuria, and edema, which necessitated delivery at 37 weeks gestation. Interestingly, the surviving infant was not growth retarded. The mother continued on antihypertensive therapy but, 18 months later, died of progressive renal failure, uremia, and congestive heart failure.

MARFAN'S SYNDROME

This disorder of connective tissue exhibits a mendelian autosomal pattern of inheritance that may be related to a dominant gene. Both sexes are affected equally, and there appears to be no racial or ethnic basis for the syndrome. There are many mild cases in which the intrinsic lesion of the connective tissue affects neither well-being nor longevity and, consequently, escapes detection. In young adults, the syndrome may be a major cause of *dissecting aortic aneurysm,* which occurs much more commonly in pregnancy, as emphasized by Kitchen (1974).

Although the specific defect is still controversial, there is a degeneration of the elastic lamina in the media of the aorta. The cardiovascular lesion is the most serious abnormality, involving most of the ascending portion of the aorta and predisposing to aortic dilatation or dissecting aneurysm. Early death in Marfan's syndrome is thus ultimately caused either by valvar insufficiency and congestive heart failure or by rupture of a dissecting aneurysm.

Marfan's syndrome alone is not an indication for abdominal delivery, for cesarean section does not protect against excessive stress on the aorta before the onset of labor. The role of cardiovascular surgery in Marfan's disease is poorly defined.

Ehlers-Danlos Syndrome

This genetically transmitted disorder of connective tissue is characterized by a variety of changes in connective tissue, including hyperelasticity of the skin and in the more severe types by a strong tendency for arteries to rupture, causing death. Case reports and literature review have been provided by Snyder and co-workers (1983) and Taylor and associates (1982).

SEXUALLY TRANSMITTED DISEASES

The term *venereal disease* is now defined by law in Texas at least. It includes syphilis, gonorrhea, chancroid, granuloma inguinale, condyloma acuminatum, genital herpes simplex infection, and genital and neonatal chlamydial infections including lymphogranuloma venereum. This list is incomplete since a considerable number of other diseases can be sexually transmitted. Pregnancy

does not make the woman immune to sexually transmitted disease. Moreover, during a single act of sexual intercourse, she may both become pregnant and acquire such a disease.

The following treatment protocols for sexually transmitted diseases attempt to adhere to the intensive, but frequently modified, recommendations provided by the Centers for Disease Control, Venereal Disease Control Division, United States Department of Health and Human Services (1982).

SYPHILIS

An unusually critical time to detect and treat syphilis is during pregnancy, not only to protect the mother and her sexual partner from the numerous complications of syphilis but, especially important, to prevent the extensive pathologic changes that characterize congenital syphilis (Chapter 38, p. 788). Fortunately, of the many congenital infections, syphilis is not only the most readily prevented, it is also the most susceptible to therapy.

Identification

Following an incubation period of 10 to 90 days, primary syphilis appears. When infection is acquired during pregnancy, the primary lesion, or sometimes multiple lesions, involving the genital tract may be of such size or so located as to go unnoticed. In some instances, however, the lesion may be somewhat larger than usual, presumably because of the increased vascularity of the genitalia. The chancre lasts from 1 to 5 weeks and heals spontaneously; a nontender, solitary enlarged nymph node is often present.

Approximately 6 weeks after the appearance of the chancre, secondary syphilis may appear in the form of a highly variable skin rash. The lesions of secondary syphilis are often slight; they may be limited to the genitalia, where they appear usually as elevated areas, or *condylomata lata,* which occasionally cause ulceration of the vulva. Unfortunately, in many women no history of a local sore or rash can be elicited. The first suggestion of the disease is the delivery of an infant that may be either stillborn or liveborn but severely afflicted with congenital syphilis.

A suitable serologic screening test such as the Venereal Disease Research Laboratory (VDRL) slide test must be performed on blood obtained at the time of the first prenatal visit. Testing is required by law. Fortunately, serologic tests for syphilis will almost always be positive by 4 to 6 weeks after contracting the disease. Because such reagin tests lack specificity, a treponemal test such as the Fluorescent Treponemal Antibody Absorption Test is used to confirm a positive result. Especially on women at high risk for syphilis, a second nontreponemal test should be done during the third trimester, and all cord bloods should be tested.

Antibiotic Treatment of Syphilis

Penicillin remains the treatment of choice. The recommendations for treatment provided by the Centers for Disease Control (1982) follow.

I. *Incubating syphilis:* Patients exposed to infectious syphilis within the preceding 3 months, or at high risk based on epidemiologic grounds,

should be treated as for early syphilis outlined below. Where possible, a diagnosis should be established. Women who are culture-positive for gonorrhea with no lesion and a nonreactive serology must also be considered at high risk. The aqueous procaine penicillin G plus probenecid regimen for gonorrhea (described below) is also effective therapy for incubating syphilis. A reagin test for syphilis should be repeated 3 months after the initial therapy.

II. *Treatment for syphilis of less than 1 year's duration*
   A. Benzathine penicillin G: 2.4 million units total, half in each butttock, has the advantage of a single visit treatment.
   B. For patients allergic to penicillin, two alternative regimens are recommended.
      1. Oral erythromycin, 500 mg by mouth, four times a day for 15 days.
      2. Oral tetracycline hydrochloride, 500 mg by mouth, four times a day for 15 days. Tetracycline is not recommended by the Centers for Disease Control during pregnancy.

If during the year following treatment clinical signs recur or persist, a spinal fluid examination should be done and the patient retreated using the regimen described below for syphilis acquired more than 1 year previously. The same retreatment regimen is used if the initial nonspecific antibody titer is greater than 1:8 or fails to decrease to negative or by fourfold within a 12-month period.

III. *Treatment of syphilis of indeterminate length or more than 1 year's duration (except neurosyphilis)*
   A. Benzathine penicillin G: 2.4 million units intramuscularly weekly (1.2 million units in each buttock) for 3 successive weeks, a total of 7.2 million units.
   B. For the patient allergic to penicillin, a spinal fluid examination must be performed prior to therapy. An alternative to penicillin during pregnancy is oral erythromycin, 500 mg, four times a day for 30 days, for a total of 60 g.

IV. *Treatment of neurosyphilis:* If the spinal fluid is positive, treatment must be more intense. Hospitalization is recommended to institute therapy with intravenous crystalline penicillin G therapy, 2 to 4 million units every 4 hours for 10 days, followed by benzathine penicillin G, 2.4 million units intramuscularly each week for three doses.

Alternatively, aqueous procaine penicillin G, 2.4 million units intramuscularly daily, plus probenecid, 500 mg by mouth four times a day, both for 10 days can be given, followed by benzathine penicillin G, 2.4 million units intramuscularly weekly for three doses.

Another alternative—which does not appear to have been adequately evaluated—is benzathine penicillin G, 2.4 million units intramuscularly weekly for three doses.

All patients with positive spinal fluid should have spinal fluid testing at least every 6 months for 3 years.

V. *Treatment of syphilis in pregnancy:* For pregnant patients not allergic to penicillin, treatment is the same as for the corresponding stage of syphilis in nonpregnant patients. For pregnant women who are allergic to penicillin, the only therapy recommended by the Centers for Disease Control is erythromycin in the same form and dosage used in nonpregnant women for the same stage of disease.

The antibiotic of choice in pregnancy is penicillin since it is so very effective. If the pregnant woman is allergic to penicillin, desensitization can be tried, usually with success in our experience, and the disease then treated appropriately with penicillin (Wendel and coworkers 1984). Tetracycline is more likely to be effective than erythromycin in the eradication of the disease in the mother and especially in the fetus. Although tetracycline is generally excluded from use during pregnancy for reasons that are not altogether clear, we agree with Fiumara (1984) that the benefits from its use to treat syphilis during pregnancy outweigh the risk to the fetus. That risk is possibly staining of the deciduous teeth. The permanent teeth are not affected.

The mother who has been treated successfully often remains susceptible to a subsequent syphilitic infection, as does her fetus. Therefore, it is very important during pregnancy to treat her sexual partner, as well as to observe her closely for evidence of reinfection. When reinfection is detected, retreatment is necessary. Women who have been treated for syphilis during pregnancy should have monthly quantitative nontreponemal serologic tests for the remainder of the pregnancy. Women who show a rise in titer of four dilutions or greater should be treated.

VI. *Treatment of congenital syphilis:* Every infant with suspected or proven congenital syphilis should have a cerebrospinal fluid examination prior to treatment and should be followed at monthly intervals until the nontreponemal serologic tests are negative. Symptomatic infants or infants with a positive spinal fluid should be treated with crystalline penicillin G, 50,000 units per kg intramuscularly or intravenously in two divided doses each day for a minimum of 10 days, or with aqueous procaine penicillin G, 50,000 units per kg intramuscularly each day for a minimum of 10 days.

Asymptomatic seropositive infants with a negative cerebrospinal fluid examination can be treated with a single dose of benzathine penicillin G, 50,000 units per kg intramuscularly.

Infants born of mothers treated with erythromycin for syphilis during pregnancy should be managed as though they have congenital syphilis.

GONORRHEA

Infection in women caused by *Neisseria gonorrhoeae* may be limited to the lower genital tract, including the cervix, urethra, and periurethral and Bartholin glands, or it may spread across the endometrium to involve the oviducts and the peritoneum. The organism also enters the bloodstream to cause arthritis uncommonly and endocarditis rarely.

Acute gonococcal salpingitis is not a problem in pregnancy after the third month, when the chorion laeve has fused with the decidua parietalis to obliterate the endometrial cavity between the cervix and oviducts. Rarely, a fallopian tube previously damaged by infection with *N. gonorrhoeae* may become reinfected during pregnancy with other organisms that reach it through the bloodstream or lymphatics.

The greatly increased prevalance of gonorrhea in recent years has not spared pregnant women; many obstetric clinics have noted gonococcal infections of the lower genitourinary tract to be common.

The pregnant woman may have asymptomatic local infection involving singly or, in combination, the lower genital tract, the lower urinary tract, and the rectum. The infection may antedate the pregnancy, or the patient may have acquired the disease at the time of the insemination that resulted in pregnancy, in which case she is likely to develop symptomatic acute salpingitis, or she may have become infected locally after the uterine cavity was obliterated by fusion of chorion to decidua. In any event, either no treatment or inadequate treatment with persistence of the infection allows her to infect her sexual partner, to suffer gonococcal arthritis or other disseminated disease, and to infect her infant at the time of delivery, thereby causing gonorrheal ophthalmia (Chapter 20, p. 383), and to develop an ascending infection of the genital tract after delivery. Consequently, even asymptomatic disease during pregnancy should be identified and eradicated. Ideally, all pregnant women should have endocervical cultures for gonococci made at the time of their first visit and again late in pregnancy if they are at high risk for the infection (Chapter 13, p. 249).

Treatments of Gonorrhea

In recent years there has been an increasing frequency of infections caused by penicillinase-producing *N. gonorrhoeae*. Moreover, a tetracycline-resistant organism may be emerging in some areas at least. Further complicating therapy, chlamydial infections are believed to coexist commonly with gonococcal disease.

Sexual partners exposed to gonorrhea should be examined, cultured, and treated at once, using one of the following regimens. Individuals treated for gonorrhea should be recultured 5 to 7 days after completion of the treatment.

I. *Uncomplicated infection in adults*
A. Aqueous procaine penicillin G, 4.8 million units injected intramuscularly, one half in each of two injection sites, plus 1 g of probenecid by mouth.
B. Ampicillin, 3.5 g, plus probenecid, 1 g, both by mouth. This regimen is not effective against pharyngeal infection.
C. Amoxicillin, 3 g, plus probenecid, 1 g, both by mouth. This regimen is not effective against pharyngeal infection.
D. For pregnant women allergic to penicillin or probenecid, spectinomycin, 2 g intramuscularly, is recommended. (Incubating syphilis is not adequately treated by spectinomycin. Moreover, a penicillin-resistant gonococcus has been identified that is resistant to spectinomycin.)
E. Tetracycline is not recommended for women while actually pregnant. Otherwise, the recommended dose is 500 mg orally four times a day for 7 days.

II. *Coexistent Chlamydial Infection:* The suggested treatment is the addition to the above treatment regimens of *erythromycin,* 500 mg, ingested on an empty stomach four times a day for at least 7 days. However, optimal dosage has not been established.

In the absence of pregnancy, *tetracycline* is currently the drug of choice. (The use of tetracycline to treat serious disease during pregnancy, even for 7 days, is not considered to be a therapeutic atrocity for reasons that hardly justify such strong condemnation!)

III. *Penicillinase-producing gonococci:* Spectinomycin, 2 g intramuscularly, may prove effective. If it is not, either cefoxitin, 2 g intramuscularly, plus probenecid, 1 g orally, or cefoxatime, 1 g intramuscularly, can be used.

IV. *Disseminated gonococcal infections:* There are several acceptable treatment schedules for *arthritis* and *dermatitis,* including the use of aqueous crystalline penicillin intravenously at the outset and either ampicillin or amoxicillin by mouth subsequently for at least 1 week. Tetracycline is recommended in case of penicillin allergy unless the woman is pregnant. Then erythromycin can be used as described above.

For gonococcal *endocarditis* and *meningitis,* long-term, high-dose penicillin intravenously is recommended.

V. *Infants of mothers with gonorrhea:* Aqueous crystalline penicillin, 50,000 units in a single injection, is recommended (20,000 units if premature).

VI. *Gonococcal ophthalmia:* The infant should be isolated until treated for 24 hours with intravenously administered penicillin. Local care of the eyes by an expert is also important. Topical antibiotic preparations are not appropriate. Both parents should be treated for gonorrhea.

CHLAMYDIAL INFECTIONS

Infections caused by *Chlamydia trachomatis* are thought to be the most prevalent of sexually transmitted diseases in the United States. In the pregnant woman, the organism has been linked with an increased risk for the fetus–infant of prematurity, stillbirth, and ophthalmia neonatorum, and with endometritis in the mother postpartum (Martin and co-workers, 1982; Harrison and co-workers, 1983). Chlamydia also appears to be an important agent etiologically in acute salpingo-oophoritis. Unfortunately, culture techniques for *C. trachomatis* are not yet available in many clinics, and where available, they are expensive.

Treatment should be provided for pregnant women who harbor the organism as proven by culture or, if cultures are not available, to those whose sexual partners have nongonococcal urethritis.

Treatment with erythromycin consists of 500 mg orally four times a day on an empty stomach for at least 7 days. Treatment of the male partner at the same time with tetracycline is important.

One serotype of *C. trachomatis* causes lymphogranuloma venereum (lymphopathia venereum). The primary genital infection is transient and seldom recognized. Inguinal adenitis may follow and at times lead to suppuration. Ultimately, the lymphatics of the lower genital tract and the perirectal tissues may be involved in sclerosis and fibrosis, which cause vulvar elephantiasis and especially severe rectal stricture.

Fistula formation involving the rectum, perineum, and vulva may also be quite troublesome. Sometimes attention is first drawn to the disease in pregnant women when rectal examination is attempted. In the absence of pregnancy, tetracycline, 500 mg orally four times a day for at least 2 weeks, is recommended. Otherwise erythromycin, in the same dosage, can be tried, as can sulfamethoxazole, 1 g orally twice a day for at least 2 weeks. Stricture and fistula formation may necessitate surgical intervention.

HERPES SIMPLEX VIRAL INFECTIONS

Virology

Two types of herpesvirus have been distinguished based on immunologic as well as clinical differences. Type I herpes simplex virus is responsible for most nongenital herpetic lesions but infrequently may also involve the genital tract. Type II herpes simplex virus is recovered almost exclusively from the genital tract and probably is transmitted in the great majority of instances, but not necessarily always, by sexual contact (Nerurkar and colleagues, 1983). The incidence of antibody specific for the type II virus approaches 100 percent among prostitutes. In the absence of appropriate antibody, exposure to a sexual partner with herpetic lesions that are shedding virus will in the majority of instances result in clinical disease.

Maternal Disease

The reported prevalence rates for active herpes infection of the genital tract vary considerably. The incubation period is 3 to 6 days for primary infection and 7 to 10 days for secondary infection.

Papules that itch or tingle and then become painful vesicles develop commonly on the vulva and perineum. Inguinal adenopathy sometimes is severe. Transient systemic flu-like symptoms are common. The vulvar and perineal vesicles are easily traumatized and commonly rupture and become secondarily infected. Vulvar lesions are likely to be extremely painful and may cause considerable debility, including urinary retention.

There is no really effective treatment. Acyclovir (Zovirax) used topically perhaps modifies the symptomatology. Severe secondary infection should respond to broad-spectrum antibiotic therapy. For intense discomfort, analgesics and topical anesthetics may provide some relief.

With primary infection of the vulva or perineum, in 2 to 4 weeks all of the signs and symptoms disappear. However, the virus typically retreats to nearby nerve ganglia, from which it can reemerge at any time—*with or without symptoms*—and cause a secondary infection in the mother and possibly a primary systemic infection in the neonate (Wittek and co-workers, 1984). There is not yet highly effective treatment to prevent such recurrences.

The cervix is the most common site of infection of the genital tract. Cervical involvement may take the form of a diffuse inflammation or discrete ulcers. However, involvement of the cervix and vagina is commonly asymptomatic. The virus may be shed from an infected cervix for months. Cervical smears usually, but not always, contain large multinucleate cells with eosinophilic viral inclusion bodies. They may be identified in a smear prepared for cervical cytologic study (Pap smear). Virologic confirmation can be accomplished readily, since the virus in tissue cultures soon induces cytopathic changes. Monoclonal antibodies to herpes simplex virus I and II have been prepared and provide for a rapid diagnostic test to identify both viral types of herpes simplex (Volpi and co-workers, 1983).

When lesions involving the genital tract are present, the virus can be transmitted. The suggestion has been made that when a partner has had genital herpes, condoms should be used subsequently even when he is asymptomatic. Because of the possible association between herpesvirus type II and cervical neoplasia, it has been recommended that women who have herpes undergo cytologic evaluation of the cervix (Pap smear) annually.

Neonatal Disease

Maternal infection appears to be transmitted only rarely across the placenta or an intact chorioamnion to the embryo or fetus. Almost always the fetus becomes infected by virus that was shed from the cervix or lower genital tract and then either invades the uterus following rupture of the membranes or contacts the fetus as he or she descends through the genital tract. The incidence of neonatal herpes simplex viral infection has increased remarkably at least in some, and presumably most, areas of the United States. For example, Sullivan-Bolyai and associates (1983) have reported an increase in King County, Washington, from 2.6 per 100,000 live births in 1969 to 12 per 100,000 in 1981. This increase reflects undoubtedly an increased prevalence of viral infection among adults, including pregnant women.

The infection in the newborn may take one of three forms: (1) disseminated, with involvement of major viscera, (2) localized with involvement confined to the central nervous system, eyes, skin, or mucosa, or (3) asymptomatic. Congenital and neonatal herpes simplex viral infections often prove lethal. Visintine and associates (1978) cite a mortality rate of 60 percent! Serious ocular and central nervous system damage has been identified in at least one half of survivors.

Attempts at treatment of the neonate in general have been disappointing. Therefore, considerable emphasis has been placed upon preventing contact between fetus and virus during delivery.

Delivery

Because of the severity of the disease in the neonate who becomes infected with herpes simplex virus, cesarean delivery is being used widely in instances where herpetic lesions of the genital tract are suspected or a recent culture has identified the virus to be present. For some obstetric services, just the threat of asymptomatic shedding of virus by women previously diagnosed as having genital herpes is considered sufficient grounds for performing cesarean section.

In case of rupture of the membranes, the 4-hour rule has been commonly applied, i.e., if the genital herpes is diagnosed or strongly suspected and the membranes have been ruptured less than 4 hours, cesarean delivery is performed. Otherwise, vaginal delivery is allowed. The validity of the rule is suspect.

The question that persists is: "Should cesarean section be performed on many mothers to try to protect a very few infants from contracting a horrible disease, or should vaginal delivery be accomplished with its safety for the mothers but grave risk for a very few infants?"

We favor cesarean delivery until such time when either the presence of the virus in the genital tract can quickly be tested for and excluded with accuracy or the fetus–infant can be effectively protected from exposure to the virus immunologically or chemotherapeutically.

The infant of a mother known or suspected of having genital herpes should be isolated in the nursery and cultured for herpes. In addition, liver function and spinal fluid should be monitored and the infant kept under close observation for up to 2 weeks.

It has been considered impractical and unnecessary by some neonatologists, but certainly not all, to separate a baby from his or her mother when the mother has herpetic lesions. Instead, she has been urged to wash her hands carefully and avoid any contact between her lesions, her hands, and the baby. Breast-feeding has been allowed under these conditions. It should be pointed out, however, the breast-feeding was implicated in one case of disseminated herpes simplex infection in a newborn infant (Dunkle and colleagues, 1979).

It has been recommended by some authorities (Kibrick, 1980) that parents and personnel with oral herpetic lesions be isolated from newborn infants, although Schriner and associates (1979) found that over 50 percent of 110 neonatal centers questioned did not isolate mothers with oral herpes from their infants.

CHANCROID

The organism *Haemophilus ducreyi* can cause painful nonindurated genital ulcers, or soft chancres, at times accompanied by painful inguinal lymphadenopathy. Chancroid has become rare in the United States but is more common in some developing countries. Prostitutes appear to be an important reservoir of infection (Plummer and associates, 1983). Diagnosis should be confirmed by culture of the organism obtained from the ulcers or in aspirate from the enlarged lymph nodes. Treatment consists of erythromycin, 500 mg orally four times a day for at least 10 days and until the ulcers and nodes have healed. Trimethoprim–sulfamethoxazole, 160 mg/800 mg orally twice a day, has also been recommended.

GRANULOMA INGUINALE

In the pregnant woman the lesions of this now rare disorder tend to be multiple, large, foul-smelling ulcerations of the vulva, lower vagina, perineum, and cervix. The causative organism, *Donovania granulomatis*, at times disseminates to cause remote lesions, especially in bone. Diagnosis depends upon identification of Donovan bodies in large mononuclear cells in Giemsa-stained smears from the lesions. Antibiotic therapy is the same as described for lymphogranuloma venereum, p. 625.

OTHER SEXUALLY TRANSMITTED DISEASES

There is a great variety of infections and infestations that can be acquired as the consequence of sexual intercourse. These include *trichomonal vaginitis* (Chapter 13, p. 263), *monilial vulvovaginitis* (Chapter 13, p. 263), *condylomata acuminata* (Chapter 25, p. 491), *scabies,* and *pediculosis pubis.* Sexual partners at risk of fecal–oral transmission may acquire any of a number of enteric infections.

OTHER TROUBLESOME INFECTIONS DURING PREGNANCY

These infections are considered here because of unique problems that they create during a coexisting pregnancy, for example, chickenpox, or because of historical interest, i.e., smallpox.

VARICELLA

Most individuals have acquired chickenpox during childhood, and, therefore, the disease is uncommon in adults. Unfortunately, when it does occur in adults, it is prone to be much more severe than in children. *This is especiallly so for pregnant women.* Varicella pneumonia, an all too common complication, is likely to prove fatal. Treatment has consisted of oxygenation and control of bacterial superinfection. Acyclovir may be of value in preventing and treating varicella pneumonitis (Hirsch and Schooley, 1983). We have observed severe thrombocytopenia plus prolonged prothrombin and partial thromboplastin times to occur in pregnancies complicated by varicella pneumonia, especially in cases that proved fatal. Because of the remarkably lethal nature of varicella pneumonia during pregnancy, the administration of zoster immune globulin should be considered for non-immune pregnant women exposed to chicken pox.

Development of maternal chickenpox during the first trimester has been implicated very infrequently in congenital malformations as the consequence of transplacental passage and infection of the embryo-fetus (DeNichola and Hanshaw, 1979).

Exposure of the fetus to the virus just before or during delivery, and therefore before he has received antibody from the mother, poses a serious threat to the newborn infant. In some instances the infant will develop disseminated visceral and central nervous system disease, which in the past, at least, was likely to be fatal. Zoster immune globulin should be administered to the neonate whenever the onset of maternal clinical disease occurs during the 4 days before delivery or 2 days postpartum.

An experimental attenuated, live-virus vaccine has been developed and would be of value for susceptible nonpregnant women.

MUMPS

This uncommmon disease during pregnancy probably increases the risk of abortion and premature labor. Pregnancy per se does not appear to increase the frequency or severity of complications associated with mumps. While parotid enlargement is a common feature of mumps, not all parotid enlargement is the consequence of mumps. We have seen overtly enlarged parotid glands as the consequence of *pica* in the form of intense starch eating.

Manson and associates (1960) in 501 cases of mumps found that major fetal anomalies were not much more common than in the general population. Congenital mumps is very rare. Thus, whether or not intrauterine mumps infection endangers the health of the fetus and infant in any way is not clear.

RUBEOLA

Most women are immune to measles as a consequence of previous infection or active immunization. Therefore, it is a rare complication during pregnancy.

An increased frequency of abortion and premature birth has been described if the mother develops measles. If she does so shortly before birth, there is considerable risk of measles developing in the neonate and, in turn, some risk of death, especially in premature infants. Passive immunization can be achieved by administering immune serum globulin intramuscularly. Vaccination should not be attempted during pregnancy, since the vaccine contains live virus.

The teratogenicity of the virus has not been established; the risk if any, is very likely to be small.

INFLUENZA

If pneumonia develops, the prognosis at once becomes serious. Although antibiotics are not effective against the virus of influenza, they are of value in the treatment of a secondary bacterial pneumonia. In the great influenza epidemic of 1918, the disease, particularly the pneumonic type, was a grave complication of pregnancy. Harris (1919), in a statistical study based on 1350 cases, found a

gross maternal mortality rate of 27 percent, which increased to 50 percent when pneumonia developed. The pandemic of so-called Asian influenza that swept the United States and other areas of the world in 1957 also affected pregnant women with particular frequency and severity. In August and September of that year, for instance, 50 percent of the women in the childbearing age who died of influenza in Minnesota were pregnant (Freeman and Barno, 1959). In the same year in that state, the leading cause of maternal death was influenza. In New York City, the incidence of influenza in pregnant women was 50 percent higher than in nonpregnant controls, and the mortality rate was also appreciably higher (Bass and Molloshok, 1960).

No convincing evidence has been derived that Asian influenza causes congenital malformations (Ebert, 1961; Saxen and colleagues, 1960; Walker and McKee, 1959; Wilson and associates, 1959). Vaccination against influenza may be of value for pregnant women, especially when an epidemic is anticipated.

COMMON COLD

The pregnant woman appears to be slightly more susceptible to acute upper respiratory infections than the nonpregnant woman. Cases of pneumonia complicating pregnancy are often preceded by an acute cold. Hemolytic streptococcal puerperal infections may occur in patients who had acute respiratory infections at the time of delivery, and the incidence of hemolytic streptococci in the upper respiratory passages of such patients is much higher than it is in nonpregnant women.

COXSACKIE VIRAL DISEASE

Coxsackie viral infection may be a serious complication of pregnancy, since it can be fatal to the fetus–infant, although causing only symptoms of a minor illness in the mother. Myocarditis and encephalomyelitis are the primary lesions. Whether maternal coxsackie infection ever causes sublethal injuries of the embryo and fetus, thus producing congenital anomalies, is not known.

POLIOMYELITIS

The inactivated poliomyelitis vaccine (Salk) is recommended for adult vaccination, including immunization during pregnancy. With the widespread use of vaccination during childhood, this disease is becoming a rarity in the United States. Siegel and Goldberg (1955), in a carefully controlled study in New York City, demonstrated that pregnant women not only are more susceptible to the disease but also have a higher death rate. The perinatal loss was about 33 percent; rarely, the fetus became infected. Cesarean section was not necessarily required even in the presence of extensive paralysis and diminished expulsive efforts during the second stage of labor.

SCARLET FEVER

Although the causative organism of scarlet fever, *Streptococcus pyogenes,* is sensitive to certain antibiotics, the disease in the early months of pregnancy has a tendency to cause abortion, presumably because of the high fever in the mother. Regardless of antibiotics, rigid isolation must be instituted and maintained in the treatment of a pregnant, parturient, or puerperal patient with scarlet fever. For no obvious reasons, scarlet fever has become very uncommon in recent years.

ERYSIPELAS

Erysipelas is always a very serious disease, but it is particularly dangerous in pregnant women because of the potential hazard of puerperal infection. The hemolytic streptococci associated with erysipelas may become more invasive, causing a septicemia and possibly producing fetal infection and even death. For the protection of other patients, strict isolation of women with erysipelas is absolutely essential. The disease should be actively treated with an appropriate antibiotic agent, which usually frees the patient of hemolytic streptococci in a relatively short time.

TYPHOID FEVER

According to Alimurung and Manahan (1952), pregnancy complicated by typhoid fever in former years resulted in abortion or premature labor in 60 to 80 percent of cases, with a fetal mortality rate of 75 percent and a maternal mortality rate of 15 percent. The more recent experiences of Riggall and co-workers (1974) are much more favorable, however. Chloramphenicol or ampicillin is usually quite effective in arresting the disease. Antityphoid vaccines appear to exert no harmful effects when administered to pregnant women and should be given in an epidemic or when otherwise indicated.

MALARIA

The incidence of abortion and premature labor is increased in malaria, although the likelihood of either relates to the severity of the disease and the promptness with which therapy is instituted. The increased fetal loss may be related to placental and fetal infection with malaria, but the evidence is somewhat contradictory, since parasites rarely cross the placenta to infect the fetus. Covell (1950), who studied this question extensively, cited an incidence of neonatal malaria in Africa of 0.03 percent. According to Jones (1950), parasites have an af-

finity for the decidual vessels and may involve the placenta extensively without affecting the fetus. There is a marked tendency toward recrudescence of the disease during pregnancy and the puerperium, just as after surgical procedures.

Strang and associates (1984) have described a fatal case of falciparum malaria with cerebral involvement and blackwater fever during pregnancy and discuss pathogenesis and treatment.

Pregnancy does not contraindicate the administration of the commonly used antimalarial drugs. Some of the newer antimalarial agents have antifolic acid activity, however, and theoretically may contribute to the development of megaloblastic anemia. In actual practice, this does not appear to be the case. Nonetheless, folic acid supplementation has been recommended (Main and co-workers, 1983; Anonymous, 1983).

Lewis and associates (1973) suggest prophylaxis with chloroquine, 500 mg orally once a week, initiated before entering an epidemic area and continuing until 6 weeks postpartum.

AMEBIASIS

Dysentery caused by *Entamoeba histolytica,* especially with hepatic abscess, may be a serious illness during pregnancy. Therapy is similar to that for the nonpregnant woman.

COCCIDIOIDOMYCOSIS

In the past, disseminated coccidioidomycosis during pregnancy commonly terminated in maternal death. In more recent years, treatment with amphotericin B has been employed successfully in a number of cases (Harris, 1966; McCoy and associates, 1980). The drug must be administered carefully because of the risk of serious toxicity.

HANSEN'S DISEASE

According to Maurus (1978), women with leprosy generally do well in pregnancy. Dapsone and clofazimine appear to be safe for treatment during pregnancy (Farb and associates, 1982).

SMALLPOX

Prior to the thirteenth edition of this book, the first disease discussed in this chapter was smallpox. Now, less than 20 years later, the disease has been declared eradicated throughout the world! Hopefully, medical progress will continue to provide for rapid and extensive replication of this most rewarding medical phenomenon, eradication of serious disease!

DISEASES OF THE INTEGUMENT

Generally, diseases of the skin occur with about the same frequency in pregnant as in nonpregnant women. There are a few dermatoses that appear to be unique to pregnancy.

HERPES GESTATIONIS

A serious but rare dermatologic disease peculiar to pregnancy is herpes gestationis. This blistering disease of pregnancy usually presents as an extremely pruritic widespread eruption (Fig. 28-12). The lesions vary from erythematous and edematous papules to large, tense bullae. Common sites of involvement are the abdomen and the extremities. Morphologic changes also occur in

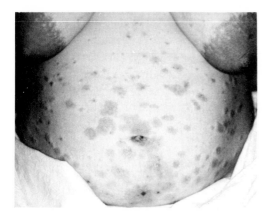

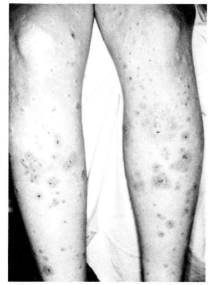

Figure 28-12. Herpes gestationis at 30 weeks gestation. Subsequently, remarkable relief from the intense pruritis, as well as considerable decrease in the intensity of the skin reaction, was provided by glucocorticoid treatment.

the mucosa of the small intestine, similar to those of adult celiac disease, but they do not appear to cause significant malabsorption (Sweiman and Millikan, 1982).

Katz and co-workers (1976) described a herpes gestationis serum factor that is a thermostable IgG class protein. Immunofluorescent techniques applied to a skin biopsy are of value for confirming the diagnosis (Hertz and associates, 1977). IgG and C3 complement are deposited along the basement membrane zone.

Prednisone daily in divided doses usually brings relief promptly and inhibits the formation of new lesions. Pyridoxine has also been used and appears to have been effective in some patients at least. The healed sites are not scarred but are usually hyperpigmented. The process may recur in subsequent pregnancies.

Lesions similar to those of the mother have been observed to develop in her newborn infant and then to clear spontaneously in a few weeks (Chorzelski and colleagues, 1976). C3 complement deposited at the basement membrane of the infant's skin and the herpes gestationis factor in cord serum have been described by Katz and associates (1976). Increased perinatal mortality has been identified.

ACNE

Some women, but certainly not all, note acne to improve during pregnancy. The retinoic acid isotretinoin (Accutane) has been commonly prescribed to treat severe cystic acne. Unfortunately, the use of this drug during the first trimester of pregnancy has been accompanied by a high frequency of abortion and of malformed infants (MMWR, 1984). Therefore pregnant women and women who might become pregnant should not receive this drug.

PAPULAR DERMATITIS OF PREGNANCY

This rare dermatitis is characterized by a pruritic generalized eruption, the lesions of which consist of soft, red to violet to red-brown papules, some of which are centrally crusted. They clear spontaneously soon after pregnancy but can recur in subsequent pregnancies. Corticosteroids taken orally may control this form of pregnancy-induced dermatitis. Perinatal mortality is increased, especially if the mother is not treated with corticosteroids.

ABNORMALITIES OF PIGMENTATION

During pregnancy, increased pigmentation is frequently noted (*chloasma*) and may be particularly marked along the linea alba and about the breasts. In other cases, unsightly, more or less symmetric, brownish splotches appear upon the face. *Melasma gravidarum,* or the mask of pregnancy, involves especially the forehead and cheeks. After the pregnancy, the hyperpigmentation usually disappears or at least recedes appreciably. Oral contraceptives may cause similar changes in pigmentation.

MELANOMA

Some benign nevi become malignant during pregnancy. The resulting melanoma may grow with unusual rapidity and may metastasize widely. The prognosis in pregnant women with melanoma is poor. Despite its rarity, melanoma is the most common tumor reported to metastasize to the placenta and fetus.

ALOPECIA

Postpartum, the numbers of scalp hairs shed may increase considerably. The condition ceases gradually and spontaneously. Fortunately, the mother can be reassured that the phenomenon is temporary, that it is not pathologic, and that she can anticipate full recovery.

MISCELLANEOUS COMPLICATIONS

The following complications are uncommon but can be troublesome during pregnancy.

HIATAL HERNIA

Rigler and Eneboe (1935) performed upper gastrointestinal radiologic examinations on 195 unselected women in the last trimester of pregnancy. Among 116 multiparas, 21, or about 18 percent, had hiatal hernias, and among 79 primigravidas, 4 had hiatal hernias. Ten of these 25 patients were reexamined 1 to 18 months postpartum, and hernias were observed in only 3. Hiatal hernias seen during pregnancy may be produced by intermittent but prolonged increase in intra-abdominal pressure. These hernias are an occasional cause of vomiting, epigastric pain, and even bleeding from ulceration.

Carpal Tunnel Syndrome

The median nerve is vulnerable to compression within the carpal tunnel at the wrist. Typically, the woman awakes with a tingling in one or both hands. The fingers otherwise feel numb and useless. A splint applied to the very slightly flexed wrist and worn during sleep usually provides relief. The signs and symptoms most often regress after delivery.

SYMPHYSEAL SEPARATION

Significant separations or ruptures of the symphysis pubis are associated with clinical symptoms in addition to roentgenologic findings. In general, only separations of more than 1.0 cm are symptomatic. Callahan (1953) reported an incidence of 1 in 2200 deliveries, whereas Waters (1953) cited a frequency of about only 1 in 20,000 at the Margaret Hague Maternity Hospital. The more recent experience at Parkland Memorial Hospital is closer to that of Waters, indicating that the complication is rare in this country today.

The symphysis may separate either during pregnancy or in the course of labor. If it occurs before labor, the separation may develop either spontaneously or after trauma. If the rupture takes place during labor, it is usually the result of a traumatic forceps delivery, but other cases have been attributed to forcible abduction of the patient's thighs during positioning for delivery.

The symptoms are symphyseal pain on motion, such as turning in bed, and tenderness over the symphysis or sacroiliac regions. Roentgenologic examination may reveal a slight separation or a widely gaping defect. Sacroiliac symptoms are noted in about one third of the patients.

Treatment is orthopedic, current opinion favoring simple strapping in most cases. Recovery of function is usually complete, although some separation and motion of the joint may persist. Subsequent vaginal delivery without recurrence of the original symptoms may be anticipated.

BURNS

Although Parkland Memorial Hospital is a major burn center in the United States, we have not seen a large number of pregnant women with severe burns. It has become apparent, however, that pregnant women who suffer chemical pneumonitis from smoke inhalation tolerate the pneumonitis that evolves poorly, as they do most all forms of pneumonitis.

Rayburn and associates (1984) have reviewed their experiences with pregnancies complicated by burns. They confirmed a positive relationship between the extent of the burn, maternal mortality, fetal mortality, and preterm delivery.

Mathews, on the basis of experience with 50 burned pregnant women (1982), has recommended that women in the second or third trimester of pregnancy with burns over 50 percent or more of their body should be delivered immediately, as maternal death is otherwise almost certain and the fetal survival rate is not improved by waiting. He emphasized that, if undelivered, the maternal prognosis is markedly worse than for a nonpregnant woman suffering otherwise comparable burns.

Skin contracture following serious abdominal burns may be painful during a subsequent pregnancy and may even necessitate surgical decompression and split skin autografts (Mathews, 1982). It has been our limited experience that the burn scar during pregnancy undergoes considerable softening and therefore can stretch appreciably.

Loss or distortion of the breast nipples may cause problems in breast-feeding. Daw and Mohandas (1983) describe cases in which breast-feeding was satisfactory from one breast and that the other breast without a nipple created no problems.

BREAST CARCINOMA

A large proportion of breast cancers appear to be estrogen- or progesterone-dependent. Theoretically, they should be more amenable to therapy in the absence of the hyperestrogenemia and hyperprogesteronemia that characterize normal pregnancy. However, so far, proof is lacking that this is actually the case.

Pregnancy does not appear to exert much influence on the course of mammary cancer, and therapeutic abortion does not improve the prognosis for this disease. In the extensive investigations of Westberg (1946), based on 224 women and a control series of 3000 nonpregnant women with mammary cancer, the difference in the survival rates was scarcely significant. Hochman and Schreiber (1953), and others since then, have contended that the 5-year survival rate in cancer of the breast coexisting with pregnancy is primarily dependent on the stage of the disease at the time of diagnosis and that interruption of pregnancy has no bearing on the course. The results to be anticipated will be comparable to the survival rates that can be expected with the same stage of the disease not complicated by pregnancy. Hochman and Schreiber (1953) believed that the increased vascularity of the breast during pregnancy might result in rapid invasion of the lymph nodes and adjacent tissues as well as in more distant hematogenous metastases. Provided that radical mastectomy was promptly performed, however, they maintained the increased vascularity did not affect prognosis.

No strong evidence has been provided that pregnancy after mastectomy for cancer of the breast has an adverse effect on survival (Donegan, 1977; Zinns, 1979).

Several chemotherapeutic agents have been administered for metastatic disease during the second and third trimesters without apparent harm to the fetus–infant.

REFERENCES

Abramowsky CR, Vegas ME, Swinehart G, Gyves MT: Decidual vasculopathy of the placenta in lupus erythematosus. N Engl J Med 303:668, 1980

Abramsky O, Lisak RP, Brenner T, Zeidman A: Significance in neonatal myasthenia gravis of inhibitory effect of amniotic fluid on binding of antibodies to acetylcholine receptor. Lancet 2:1333, 1979

Agre P, Orringer EP, Bennett V: Deficient red-cell spectrin in severe, recessively inherited spherocytosis. N Engl J Med 306:1155, 1982

Ahlberg G, Ahlmark G: The Landry-Guillain-Barré syndrome and pregnancy. Acta Obstet Gynecol Scand 57:377, 1978

Ahn YS, Harrington WJ, Simon SR, Mylvaganam R, Pall LM, So AG: Danazol for the treatment of idiopathic thrombocytopenic purpura. N Engl J Med 308:1396, 1983

Alger LS, Golbus MS, Laros RK Jr: Thalassemia and pregnancy: Results of an antenatal screening program. Am J Obstet Gynecol 134:662, 1979

Alimurung MM, Manahan CP: Typhoid in pregnancy: Report of a case treated with chloramphenicol and ACTH. J Philipp Med Assoc 28:388, 1952

Allan LD, Desai G, Tynan MJ: Prenatal echocardiographic screening for Ebstein's anomaly for mothers on lithium therapy. Lancet 2:875, 1982

Anderson KJ, Walters WAW: Cushing's syndrome and pregnancy. Aust NZ J Obstet Gynaecol 16:225, 1976

Anonymous: Pyrimethamine combinations in pregnancy. Lancet 2:1005, 1983

Appel SH, Almon RR, Levy N: Acetylcholine receptor antibodies in myasthenia gravis. N Engl J Med 293:760, 1975

Atkins JN: Maternal plasma concentration of pyridoxal phosphate during pregnancy: Adequacy of vitamin B_6 supplementation during isoniazid therapy. Am Rev Respir Dis 126:714, 1982

Atlas M, Barkai G, Menczer J, Houlu N, Lieberman P: Thrombotic thrombocytopenic purpura in pregnancy. Br J Obstet Gynaecol 89:476, 1982

Atuk NO: Pheochromocytoma: Diagnosis, localization, and treatment. Hosp Pract, April 1983, p 187

Bailey CJ, Pool RW, Poskitt EME, Harris F: Valproic acid and fetal abnormality. Br Med J 286:190, 1983

Ball EW, Giles C: Folic acid and vitamin B_{12} levels in pregnancy and their relation to megaloblastic anemia. J Clin Pathol 17:165, 1964

Barnes JL, Abbott KH: Cerebral complications incurred during pregnancy and the puerperium. Calif Med 91:237, 1959

Barnes PM, Hendrickse JP deV, Watson-Williams EJ: Low-molecular weight dextran in treatment of bone-pain crises in sickle-cell disease: A double blind trial. Lancet 2:1271, 1965

Barrett JM, Van Hooydonk JE, Boehm FH: Pregnancy-related rupture of arterial aneurysms. Obstet Gynecol Surv 37:557, 1982

Bass MH, Molloshok RE: In Guttmacher AF, Rovinsky JJ (eds): Medical, Surgical and Gynecological Complications of Pregnancy. Baltimore, Williams & Wilkins, 1960, p 526

Bayever E, Champlin R, Ho W, Gale R, Feig S: Results of treatment of aplastic anemia in young patients. Pediatr Res 17 [No 4, Part 2] (Abstract No 852), 1983

Beasley RP, Lee G C-Y, Roan C-H, Hwang L-Y, Lan C-C, Huang FY: Prevention of perinatally transmitted hepatitis B virus infections with hepatitis B immune globulin and hepatitis B vaccine. Lancet 2:1099, 1983

Bellingham F, Mackey R, Winston C: Pregnancy and intestinal

obstruction: A dangerous combination. Med J Aust 2:318, 1949

Benedetti TJ, Valle R, Ledger WJ: Antepartum pneumonia in pregnancy. Am J Obstet Gynecol 144:413, 1982

Bierling P, Farcet JP, Dveradi N, Rochant H, Mondor HH: Gamma globulin for idiopathic thrombocytopenic purpura. N Engl J Med 307:1150, 1982

Biglieri EG, Slaton PE Jr: Pregnancy and primary aldosteronism. J Clin Endocrinol 27:1628, 1967

Black WP: Acute appendicitis in pregnancy. Br Med J 1:1938, 1960

Blanchette V, Hogan V, Hsu E, Luke B, Rock G: Mechanism of action of high-dose intravenous gammaglobulin therapy in childhood immune thrombocytopenic purpura. Pediatr Res 17 [No 4, Part 2] (Abstract No 853) 1983

Blatt J, Mulvihill JJ, Ziegler JL, Young RC, Poplack DC: Pregnancy outcome following cancer chemotherapy. Am J Med 69:828, 1980

Boehm CD, Antonarakis SE, Phillips JA III, Stetten G, Kazazian HH Jr: Prenatal diagnosis using DNA polymorphisms. N Engl J Med 308:1054, 1983

Boey ML, Colaco CB, Gharavi AE, Elkon KB, Loizou S, Hughes GRV: Thrombosis in systemic lupus erythematosus: Striking association with the presence of circulating lupus anticoagulant. Br Med J 287:1021, 1983

Bonnar J: Venous thrombo-embolism and pregnancy. In Stallworthy J, Bourne G (eds): Recent Advances in Obstetrics and Gynecology. New York, Churchill Livingstone, 1979, No 13

Bowes WA Jr: Detection and treatment of tuberculosis. Contemp Ob/Gyn 6:43, 1975

Brans YW, Huff RW, Shannon DL, Hunter MA: Maternal diabetes and neonatal macrosomia. Pediatrics 70:576, 1982

Braverman DZ, Johnson ML, Kern F Jr: Effects of pregnancy and contraceptive steroids on gallbladder function. N Engl J Med 302:362, 1980

Bravo RH, Katz M, Inturisi M, Cohen NH: Obstetric management of Landry-Guillain-Barré syndrome. Am J Obstet Gynecol 142:714, 1982

Brodie MJ, Moore MR, Thompson GG, Goldberg A, Low RAL: Pregnancy and acute porphyria. Br J Obstet Gynaecol 84:726, 1977

Brumfitt W, Davies BI, Rosser E: Urethral catheter as a cause of urinary-tract infection in pregnancy and puerperium. Lancet 2:1059, 1961

Bullock JL, Harris RE, Young R: Treatment of thyrotoxicosis during pregnancy with propranolol. Am J Obstet Gynecol 121:242, 1975

Bunim JJ, Appel SB: A principle for determining prognosis of pregnancy in rheumatic heart disease. JAMA 142:90, 1950

Burch GE: Heart disease and pregnancy. Am Heart J 93:104, 1977

Burgess GE: Alpha blockade and surgical intervention of pheochromocytoma in pregnancy Obstet Gynecol 53:266, 1979

Burkett G, Richardson R: Periarteritis nodosa and pregnancy. Obstet Gynecol 59:252, 1982

Burroughs AK, Seong NH, Dojcinov DM, Scheur PJ, Sherlock SVP: Idiopathic acute fatty liver of pregnancy in 12 patients. Q J Med, New Series LI:481, 1982

Burrow GN, Bartsocas C, Klatskin EH, Grunt JA: Children exposed in utero to propylthiouracil. Am J Dis Child 116:161, 1968

Burwell CS, Metcalfe J: Heart Disease and Pregnancy. Boston, Little, Brown, 1958

Callahan JT: Separation of the symphysis pubis. Am J Obstet Gynecol 66:281, 1953

Camitta BM, Storb R, Thomas ED: Aplastic anemia: Pathogenesis, diagnosis, treatment, and prognosis. N Engl J Med 306:645, 712, 1982

Carache S, Scott J, Niebyl J, Bonds D: Management of sickle cell disease in pregnant patients. Obstet Gynecol 55:407, 1980

Carreras LO, Vermylen J, Spitz B, Van Assche A: "Lupus" anticoagulation and inhibition of prostacyclin formation in patients with repeated abortion, intrauterine growth retardation and intrauterine death. Br J Obstet Gynaecol 88:890, 1981

Carroll RR, Noyes WD, Kitchens CS: High-dose intravenous immunoglobulin therapy in patients with immune thrombocytopenic purpura. JAMA 249:1748, 1983

Cavalieri RL, Watkins L, Abraham RA, Berkay HS, Niebyl JR: Acute bacterial endocarditis with postpartum aortic valve replacement. Obstet Gynecol 59:124, 1982

Chanarin I: The Megaloblastic Anaemias. Oxford and Edinburgh, Blackwell Scientific Publications, 1969

Chang JC, Kan YW: A sensitive new prenatal test for sickle cell anemia. N Engl J Med 307:30, 1982

Chapman RA, Sutcliffe SB, Malpas JS: Cytotoxic-induced ovarian failure in Hodgkin's disease, II. Effects on sexual function. JAMA 242:1882, 1979

Chau SS, Fitzpatrick RJ, Jamieson B: Diabetes insipidus and parturition. Br J Obstet Gynaecol 76:444, 1969

Cheek DB (ed): Human Growth. Philadelphia, Lea & Febiger, 1968

Chen WCC, Chan CS, Lee PK, Wang RYC, Wong VCW: Pregnancy in patients with prosthetic valves: An experience with 45 pregnancies. Q J Med New Series LI:358, 1982

Cheng Y-S: Pregnancy in liver cirrhosis and/or portal hypertension. Am J Obstet Gynecol 128:812, 1977

Chesley LC: Severe rheumatic cardiac disease and pregnancy: The ultimate prognosis. Am J Obstet Gynecol 136:552, 1980

Chorzelski TP, Jablonska S, Beutner EH, Maciejowska EWA, Jarzabek-Chorzelska M: Herpes gestationis with identical lesions in the newborn. Arch Dermatol 112:1129, 1976

Chuang T-Y, Su WPD, Perry JO, Ilstrup DM, Kurland LT: Incidence and trend to herpes progenitalis. May Clin Proc 58:436, 1983

Cines DB, Dusak B, Tomaski A, Mennuti M, Schreiber AD: Immune thrombocytopenic purpura and pregnancy. N Engl J Med 306:826, 1982

Clemens JD, Horwitz RI, Jaffe CC, Feinstein AR, Stanton BF: A controlled evaluation of the risk of bacterial endocarditis in persons with mitral valve prolapse. N Engl J Med 307:776, 1982

Cobbe SM: Congenital complete heart block. Br Med J 286:1769, 1983

Coe FL, Parks JH, Lindheimer MD: Nephrolithiasis during pregnancy. N Engl J Med 298:324, 1978

Cohen LF, DiSant'Agnese PA, Friedlander J: Cystic fibrosis and pregnancy. Lancet 2:842, 1980

Collins ML, O'Brien P, Cline A: Diabetes insipidus following obstetric shock. Obstet Gynecol 53:175, 1979

Committee on Drugs, American Academy of Pediatrics: Psychotropic drugs in pregnancy and lactation. Pediatrics 69:241, 1982

Cooley JR, Kitay DZ: Heterozygous β-thalassemia in pregnancy. J Reprod Med 29:141, 1984

Corlett RC Jr, Mishell DR Jr: Pancreatitis in pregnancy. Am J Obstet Gynecol 113:281, 1972

Cortis BS, Gensini GG: Can the risks of myocardial infarction in pregnancy be reduced? Bull Tex Heart Inst 4:49, 1977

Cossart YE, Kirsch S, Ismay SL: Post-transfusion hepatitis in Australia. Lancet 1:208, 1982

Cousins L: Congenital anomalies among infants of diabetic mothers. Am J Obstet Gynecol 147:333, 1983

Coustan DR, Berkowitz RL, Hobbins JC: Tight metabolic control of overt diabetes in pregnancy. Am J Med 68:845, 1980

Covell G: Congenital malaria. Trop Dis Bull 47:1174, 1950

Crohn BB, Yarnis H, Walter RI, Gabrilov JL, Crohn EB: Ulcerative colitis as affected by pregnancy. NY J Med 56:2651, 1956

Cunningham FG, McCubbin JH: Appendicitis complicating pregnancy. Obstet Gynecol 45:415, 1975

Cunningham FG, Pritchard JA: Prophylactic transfusions of normal red blood cells during pregnancies complicated by sickle cell hemoglobinopathies. Am J Obstet Gynecol 135:994, 1979

Cunningham FG, Pritchard JA, Mason R: Pregnancy and sickle hemoglobinopathy: Results with and without prophylactic transfusions. Obstet Gynecol 62:419, 1983

Cunningham FG, Leveno KJ, Hankins GDV, Whalley PJ: Respiratory insufficiency associated with pyelonephritis during pregnancy. Obstet Gynecol 63:121, 1984

Davison JM, Lindheimer MD: Pregnancy in renal transplant recipients. J Reprod Med 27:613, 1982

Daw E, Mohandas I: Pregnancy in patients after severe abdominal burns. Br J Obstet Gynaecol 90:69, 1983

Deeg HJ, Kennedy MS, Sanders JE, Thomas ED, Storb R: Successful pregnancy after marrow transplantation for severe aplastic anemia and immunosuppression with cyclosporine. JAMA 250:647, 1983

Delgado-Escueta AV, Treiman DM, Walsh GO: The treatable epilepsies. N Engl J Med 308:1508, 1576, 1983

DeNicola LK, Hanshaw JB: Congenital and neonatal varicella. J Pediatr 94:175, 1979

DeSwiet M, Ward PD, Fidler J, Horsman A, Katz D, Letsky E, Peacock M, Wise PH: Prolonged heparin therapy in pregnancy causes bone demineralization. Br J Obstet Gynaecol 90:1129, 1983

DeWolf F, Carreras LO, Moerman P, Vermylen J, Van Assche A, Renaer M: Decidual vasculopathy and extensive placental infarction in a patient with repeated thromboembolic accidents, recurrent fetal loss, and lupus anticoagulant. Am J Obstet Gynecol 142:829, 1982

Dillon WP, Lee RV, Tronolone MJ, Buckwald S, Foote RJ: Life support and maternal death during pregnancy. JAMA 248:1089, 1982

Dines DE, Banner EA: Sarcoidosis during pregnancy. JAMA 200:150, 1967

Donaldson JO: Neurology of Pregnancy. Philadelphia, Saunders, 1978

Donaldson JO: Control of chorea gravidarum with haloperidol. Obstet Gynecol 59:381, 1982

Donaldson JO, Penn AS, Lisak RP, Abramsky O, Brenner T, Schotland DL: Antiacetylcholine receptor antibody in neonatal myasthenia gravis. Am J Dis Child 135:222, 1981

Donegan WL: Breast cancer and pregnancy. Obstet Gynecol 50:244, 1977

Driscoll JJ, Gillespie L: Obstetrical considerations in diabetes in pregnancy. Med Clin North Am 49:1025, 1965

Dunkle LM, Schmidt RR, O'Connor DM: Neonatal herpes simplex infection possibly acquired via maternal breast milk. Pediatrics 63:250, 1979

Durack DT, Kaplan EL, Bisno AL: Apparent failures of endocarditis prophylaxis. JAMA 250:2318, 1983

Ebert JD: First International Conference on Congenital Malformation. Summary and evaluation. J Chron Dis 13:91, 1961

Edidin DV, Menella J: Increased glycosylated hemoglobin in maternal and cord blood of macrosomic infants of diabetic mothers. Pediatr Res 17:288A [Abstract No 1211], 1983

El-Maraghy M, Abou Senna I, El-Tehewy F, Bassiouni M, Ayoub A, El-Sayad H: Mitral valvotomy in pregnancy. Am J Obstet Gynecol 145:708, 1983

Etheridge MJ, Pepperell RJ: Heart disease and pregnancy at the Royal Women's Hospital. Med J Aust 2:277, 1977

Farb H, West DP, Pedvis-Leftick A: Clofazimine in pregnancy complicated by leprosy. Obstet Gynecol 59:122, 1982

Fear RE: Eclampsia superimposed on scleroderma. Obstet Gynecol 31:69, 1968

Fehr J, Hofman V, Kappeler U: Transient reversal of thrombocytopenia by high-dose intravenous gamma globulins. N Engl J Med 306:1254, 1982

Felding C: Obstetric studies in women with renal disease in childhood. Acta Obstet Gynecol Scand 45:141, 1964

Felding C: The obstetric prognosis in chronic renal disease. Acta Obstet Gynecol Scand 47:166, 1968

Fieldring JF, Cooke WT: Pregnancy and Crohn's disease. Br Med J 2:76, 1970

Fine LG and several participants: UCLA Conference: Systemic lupus erythematosus in pregnancy. Ann Intern Med 94:667, 1981

Fisch RO, Prem KA, Feinberg SB, Gehrz RC: Acromegaly in a gravida and her infant. Obstet Gynecol 43:861, 1974

Fiumara NJ: The surgical diagnosis: Ruling out VD. Part 2: Syphilis Infections in Surgery 3:59, 1984

Franklyn JA, Sheppard MC, Ramsden DB: Serum free thyroxine and free triiodothyronine concentrations in pregnancy. Br Med J 287:394, 1983

Freedman WL: Alpha and beta thalassemia and pregnancy. Clin Obstet Gynecol 12:115, 1969

Freeman DW, Barno A: Deaths from Asian influenza associated with pregnancy. Am J Obstet Gynecol 78:1172, 1959

Gabbe SG: Application of scientific rationale to the management of the pregnant diabetic. Semin Perinat 2:361, 1978

Gabbe SG, Mestman JH, Freeman RK, Goebelsmann UT, Lowensohn RI, Nochimson D, Cetrulo C, Quilligan EJ: Management and outcome of diabetes mellitus, classes B-R. Am J Obstet Gynecol 129:723, 1977

Garlick RL, Mazer JS, Higgins PJ, Bunn HF: Characterization of glycosylated hemoglobins. J Clin Invest 71:1062, 1983

Gilstrap LC III, Cunningham FG, Whalley PJ: Acute pyelonephritis in pregnancy: An anterospective study. Obstet Gynecol 57:409, 1981

Gimovsky ML, Montoro M, Paul RH: Pregnancy outcome in women with systemic lupus erythematosus. Obstet Gynecol 63:686, 1984

Gleicher N, Meller J, Sandler RZ, Sullum S: Wolff-Parkinson-White syndrome in pregnancy. Obstet Gynecol 58:748, 1981

Gleicher N, Midwall J, Hochberger D, Jaffin H: Eisenmenger's syndrome and pregnancy. Obstet Gynecol Surv 34:721, 1979

Goluboff LG, Sisson JC, Hamburger JI: Hyperthyroidism associated with pregnancy. Obstet Gynecol 44:107, 1974

Gomez A, Wood M: Acute appendicitis in pregnancy. Am J Surg 137:180, 1979

Gorenberg H, Chesley LC: Rheumatic heart disease in pregnancy: The remote prognosis in patients with "functionally severe" disease. Ann Intern Med 49:278, 1958

Goudeau A, Yvonnet B, Lesage G, Barin F, Denis F, Coursaget P, Chiron JP: Lack of anti-HBc IgM in neonates with HBs Ag carrier mothers argues against transplacental transmission of hepatitis B virus infection. Lancet 2:1103, 1983

Greene MF, Frigoletto FD Jr, Claster S, Rosenthal D: Pregnancy and paroxysmal nocturnal hemoglobinuria: Report of a case and review of the literature. Obstet Gynecol Surv 38:591, 1983

Grimes EM, Fayez JA, Miller GL: Cushing's syndrome and pregnancy. Obstet Gynecol 42:550, 1973

Grünfeld J-P, Ganeval D, Bournérias F: Acute renal failure in pregnancy. Kidney Int 18:179, 1980

Habib A, McCarthy JS: Effects on the neonate of propranolol administered during pregnancy. J Pediatr 91:808, 1977

Haesslein HC, Schneider JM, Caggiano V: Plasmapheresis in the management of severe EPH gestosis complicated by microangiopathic hemolytic/TTP syndrome. Presented at the 3rd Annual Meeting of the Society of Perinatal Obstetricians, San Antonio, Texas, 1983

Hague WM, Duncan SLB, Slater DN: Acute fatty liver of pregnancy. J R Soc Med 76:652, 1983

Hahm S, Kaplan S, Nitowsky HM: Hemoglobin A_{1c} levels in mothers of large birth weight infants. Pediatr Res 17:315A [Abstract No 1370], 1983

Hamilton BE, Thomson KJ: The Heart in Pregnancy and the Childbearing Age. Boston, Little, Brown, 1941

Hankins GDV, Wendel GD, Leveno KJ, Stoneham J: Myocardial infarction during pregnancy. Pathophysiologic considerations. Obstet Gynecol (in press), 1984

Hanson JW, Smith DW: The fetal hydantoins syndrome. J Pediatr 87:285, 1975

Hanson JW, Myrianthopoulos NC, Harvey MAS, Smith DW: Risks to the offspring of women treated with hydantoins during pregnancy. Pediatr Res 10:449, 1976

Harer WB Jr, Harer WB Sr: Volvulus complicating pregnancy and the puerperium: A report of three cases and review of the literature (37 references cited). Obstet Gynecol 12:399, 1958

Harkness DR, Byrnes JJ, Lian E C-Y, Williams WD, Hensley GT: Hazard of platelet transfusion in thrombotic throbocytopenic purpura. JAMA 246:1931, 1981

Harris JW: Influenza occurring in pregnant women. JAMA 72:978, 1919

Harris RE: Coccidioidomycosis complicating pregnancy. Obstet Gynecol 28:401, 1966

Harris RE, Gilstrap LC III, Pretty A: Single-dose antimicrobial therapy for asymptomatic bacteriuria during pregnancy. Obstet Gynecol 59:546, 1982

Harrison HR, Alexander ER, Weinstein L, Lewis M, Nash M, Sim DA: Cervical *Chlamydia trachomatis* and mycoplasmal infections in pregnancy. JAMA 250:1721, 1983

Hayslett JP, Lynn RI: Effect of pregnancy in patients with lupus nephropathy. Kidney Int 18:207, 1980

Hench PG: Ameliorating effect of pregnancy on chronic atrophic (infectious rheumatoid) arthritis, fibrositis and intermittent hydrarthrosis. Proc. Mayo Clin 13:161, 1938

Hendrickse JP deV, Watson-Williams EJ: The influence of hemoglobinopathies on reproduction. Am J Obstet Gynecol 94:739, 1966

Herbert V, Cunneen N, Jaskiel L, Kopff C: Minimal daily adult folate requirement. Arch Intern Med 110:649, 1962

Hertz KC, Crawford PS, Chez RA, Katz SI: Herpes gestationis: An update. Obstet Gynecol 49:733, 1977

Hiilesmaa VK, Teramo K, Granström M-L: Fetal head growth retardation associated with maternal antiepileptic drugs. Lancet 2:165, 1981

Hiilesmaa VK, Teramo K, Granström M-L, Bardy AH: Serum folate concentration during pregnancy in women with epilepsy: Relation to antiepileptic drug concentrations, number of seizures, and fetal outcome. Br Med J 287:577, 1983

Hill DE: Effect of insulin on fetal growth. Semin Perinat 2:319, 1978

Hill LM, Johnson CE, Lee RA; Cholecystectomy in pregnancy. Obstet Gynecol 46:291, 1975

Hime MC, Richardson JA: Diabetes insipidus and pregnancy. Case report, incidence, and review of literature. Obstet Gynecol Survey 33:375, 1978

Hirsch MS, Schooley RT: Treatment of herpesvirus infections. N Engl J Med 309:963, 1983

Hochman A, Schreiber H: Pregnancy and cancer of the breast. Obstet Gynecol 2:268, 1953

Holmes GE, Holmes FF: Pregnancy outcomes of patients treated for Hodgkin's disease: A controlled study. Cancer 41:1317, 1978

Homan WP, Thorbjarnarson B: Crohn disease and pregnancy. Arch Surg 111: 545, 1976

Homans DC, Blake GD, Harrington JT, Cetrulo CL: Acute renal failure caused by ureteral obstruction by a gravid uterus. JAMA 246:1230, 1981

Horning SJ, Hoppe RT, Kaplan HS, Rosenberg SA: Female reproductive potential after treatment for Hodgkin's disease. N Engl J Med 304:1377, 1981

Howard TE, Herrick CN: Pregnancy in patients with ventriculoperitoneal shunts. Am J Obstet Gynecol 141:99, 1981

Howell R, Fidler J, Letsky E: The risks of antenatal subcutaneous heparin prophylaxis: A controlled trial. Br J Obstet Gynaecol 90:1124, 1983

Hoyer LW, Lindsten J, Blomäck M, Hagenfeldt L, Cordesius E, Strömberg P, Gustavii B: Prenatal evaluation of fetus at risk for severe von Willebrand's disease. Lancet 2:191, 1979

Hunt AB, McConahey WM: Pregnancy associated with disease of the adrenal glands. Am J Obstet Gynecol 66:970, 1953

Hunt HB, Schifrin BS, Suzuki K: Ruptured berry aneurysms and pregnancy. Obstet Gynecol 43:827, 1974

Hurd WW, Miodovnik M, Stys SJ: Pregnancy associated with paroxysmal nocturnal hemoglobinuria. Obstet Gynecol 60:742, 1982

Hurst D, Little B, Kleman KM, Emburg SH, Lubin BH: Anemia and hemoglobinopathies in Southeast Asian refugee children. J Pediatr 102:692, 1983

Jacobs C, Donaldson SS, Rosenberg SA, Kaplan HS: Management of the pregnant patient with Hodgkin's disease. Ann Intern Med 95:669, 1981

Jewelewicz R, VandeWeile RL: Clinical course and outcome of pregnancy in twenty-five patients with pituitary microadenomas. Am J Obstet Gynecol 136:339, 1980

Johnson TR, Banner EA, Winkelmann RK: Scleroderma and pregnancy. Obstet Gynecol 23:467, 1964

Johnston WG, Baskett TF: Obstetric cholestasis. Am J Obstet Gynecol 133:299, 1979

Jones BS: Congenital malaria: 3 cases. Br Med J 2:439, 1950

Källén B, Tandberg A: Lithium and pregnancy. A cohort study on manic-depressive women. Acta Psychiatr Scand 68:134, 1983

Karpatkin M, Porges RF, Karpatkin S: Platelet counts in infants of women with autoimmune thrombocytopenia. N Engl J Med 305:936, 1981

Kass EH: Pyelonephritis and bacteriuria. Ann Intern Med 56:46, 1962

Kass EH: Progress in Pyelonephritis. Philadelphia, Davis 1965. (Contains six articles by various authors on bacteriuria in pregnancy.)

Kassam SH, Hadi HA, Fadel HE, Sims W, Joy WM: Benign intracranial hypertension in pregnancy: Current diagnostic and therapeutic approach. Obstet Gynecol Surv 38:314, 1983

Katz AI, Davison JM, Hayslett JP, Singson E, Lindheimer MD:

Pregnancy in women with kidney disease. Kidney Int 18:192, 1980

Katz M, Quagiorello J, Young BK: Severe polycystic kidney disease in pregnancy. Obstet Gynecol 53:119, 1979

Katz SI, Hertz KC, Yaoita H: Immunopathology and characterization of the HG factor. J Clin Invest 57:1434, 1976

Kelton JG, Inwood MJ, Barr RM, Effer SB, Hunter D, Wilson WE, Ginsburg DA, Powers PJ: The prenatal prediction of thrombocytopenia in infants of mothers with clinically diagnosed immune thrombocytopenia. Am J Obstet Gynecol 144:449, 1982

Kibrick S: Herpes simplex infection at term. JAMA 243:157, 1980

Kincaid-Smith P, Bullen M: Bacteriuria in pregnancy. Lancet 1:395, 1965

Kitchen DH: Dissecting aneurysm of the aorta in pregnancy. Br J Obstet Gynaecol 81:410, 1974

Kitzmiller JL, Cloherty JP, Younger MD, Tabatabaii A, Rothchild SB, Sosenkol I, Epstein MF, Singh S, Neff RK: Diabetic pregnancy and perinatal outcome. Am J Obstet Gynecol 131:560, 1978

Kleinknecht D, Grünfeld J-P, Gomez PC, Moreau J-F, Garcia-Torres R: Diagnostic procedures and long-term prognosis in bilateral renal cortical necrosis. Kidney Int 4:390, 1973

Kleinman G, Sutherling W, Martinez M, Tabsh K: Malfunction of ventriculoperitoneal shunts during pregnancy. Obstet Gynecol 61:753, 1983

Kobayashi H, Matsumoto Y, Otsubo O, Ostubo K, Naito T: Successful pregnancy in a patient undergoing chronic hemodialysis. Obstet Gynecol 57:382, 1981

Kochenour NK, Branch DW, Hershgold EJ, Scott JR: The lupus anticoagulant—a recently discovered and treatable cause of recurrent abortion and fetal death. Presented at the Society for Gynecologic Investigation San Francisco, March 21–24, 1984

Kochenour NK, Emery MG, Sawchuk RJ: Phenytoin metabolism in pregnancy. Obstet Gynecol 56:577, 1980

Koeffler HP, Goldwasser E: Erythropoietin radioimmunoassay in evaluating patients with polycythemia. Ann Intern Med 94:44, 1981

Kohler PF, Vaughan J: The autoimmune diseases. JAMA 248:2646, 1982

Kohn SG, Briele HA, Douglass LH: Volvulus complicating pregnancy. Am J Obstet Gynecol 48:398, 1944

Koontz WL, Herbert WNP, Cefalo RC: Pseudotumor cerebri in pregnancy. Obstet Gynecol 62:325, 1983

Kopenhager T: A review of 50 pregnant patients with kyphoscoliosis. Br J Obstet Gynaecol 84:585, 1977

Land MA, Bisno AL: Acute rheumatic fever: A vanishing disease in suburbia. JAMA 249:895, 1983

Lander CM, Edwards VE, Eadie MJ, Tyrer JH: Plasma anticonvulsant concentrations during pregnancy. Neurology 27:128, 1977

Lane RS: Non A-non B hepatitis from intravenous immunoglobulins. Lancet 2:974, 1983

Langer A, Hung CT, McAnulty JA, Harrigan JT, Washington E: Adrenergic blockade: A new approach to hyperthyroidism during pregnancy. Obstet Gynecol 44:181, 1974

Lattanzi DR, Cook WA: Urinary calculi in pregnancy. Obstet Gynecol 56:462, 1980

Lavin JP, Lovelace DR, Miodovnik M, Knowles HC, Barden TP: Clinical experience with 107 diabetic pregnancies. Am J Obstet Gynecol 147:742, 1983

Lee GR: The anemia of chronic disease. Semin Hematol 20:61, 1983

Lee LA, Weston WL: New findings in neonatal lupus syndrome. Am J Dis Child 138:233, 1984

Leveno KJ, Hauth JC, Gilstrap LC III, Whalley PJ: Appraisal of "rigid" blood glucose control during pregnancy in the overtly diabetic woman. Am J Obstet Gynecol 135:793, 1979

Leveno KJ, Whalley PJ: Dilemmas in the management of pregnancy complicated by diabetes. Med Clin North Am 66:1325, 1982

Levine AM, Collea JV: When pregnancy complicates chronic granulocytic leukemia. Contemp Ob/Gyn 13:47, 1979

Levy DL: Fetal-neonatal involvement in maternal autoimmune disease. Obstet Gynecol Surv 37:122, 1982

Levy DL, Warriner RA III, Burgess GE III: Fetal response to cardiopulmonary bypass. Obstet Gynecol 56:112, 1980

Levy N, Roisman I, Teodor I: Ulcerative colitis in pregnancy in Israel. Dis Colon Rectum 24:351, 1981

Lewis R, Lauersen NH, Birnbaum S: Malaria associated with pregnancy. Obstet Gynecol 42:696, 1973

Lilleyman JS, Hill AS, Anderton KJ: Consequences of acute myelogenous leukemia in early pregnancy. Obstet Gynecol Survey 33:393, 1978

Little PJ: The incidence of urinary infection in 5000 pregnant women. Lancet 2:925, 1966

Liu L, Jaffe R, Borowski GD, Rose LI: Exacerbation of Cushing's disease during pregnancy. Am J Obstet Gynecol 145:110, 1983

Lowe DK, Orwoll ES, McClung MR, Cawthon ML, Peterson CG: Hyperparathyroidism and pregnancy. Am J Surg 145:611, 1983

Lubbe WF, Butler WS, Palmer SJ, Liggins GC: Lupus anticoagulant in pregnancy. Brit J Obstet Gynaecol 91:357, 1984

Madaio MP, Harrington JT: The diagnosis of acute glomerulonephritis. N Engl J Med 309:1299, 1983

Main ANH, Shenkin A, Black WP, Russell RI: Intravenous feeding to sustain pregnancy in patient with Crohn's disease. Br Med J 283:1221, 1981

Main EK, Main DM, Krogstad DJ: Treatment of chloroquine-resistant malaria during pregnancy. JAMA 249:3207, 1983

Manson MM, Logan WPD, Loy RM: Rubella and Other Virus Infections during Pregnancy. London, Her Majesty's Stationery Office, 1960

Martin DH, Koutsky L, Eschenbach DA, Daling JR, Alexander ER, Benedetti JK, Holmes KK: Prematurity and perinatal mortality in pregnancies complicated by maternal *Chlamydia trachomatis* infections. JAMA 247:1585, 1982

Martin DH, Montgomery DAD, Harley JMcDG: The occurrence of T₃ thyrotoxicosis in pregnancy. Irish J Med Sci 145:92, 1976

Martin MC, Pernoll ML, Boruszak AN, Jones JW, Lo Cicero J III: Cesarean section while on cardiac bypass. Obstet Gynecol 57:41 [Suppl], 1981

Mathews RN: Obstetric implications of burns in pregnancy. Br J Obstet Gynaecol 89:603, 1982

Mathews RN: Old burns and pregnancy. Br J Obstet Gynaecol 89:610, 1982

Maurus JN: Hansen's disease in pregnancy. Obstet Gynecol 52:22, 1978

McAnulty JH, Metcalfe J, Ueland K: General guidelines in the management of cardiac disease. Clin Obstet Gynecol 24:773, 1981

McCoy MJ, Ellenberg JF, Killam AP: Coccidioidomycosis complicating pregnancy. Am J Obstet Gynecol 137:739, 1980

Mendelson CL: Aspiration of stomach contents into the lungs during obstetric anesthesia. Am J Obstet Gynecol 52:191, 1946

Miller DM, Winslow RM, Klein HG, Wilson KC, Brown FL, Statham NJ: Improved exercise performance after exchange transfusion in subjects with sickle cell anemia. Blood 56:1127, 1980

Miller E, Hare JW, Cloherty JP, Dunn PJ, Gleason RE, Soeldner JS, Kitzmiller JL: Elevated maternal hemoglobin A_{1c} in early pregnancy and major congenital anomalies in infants of diabetic mothers. N Engl J Med 304:1331, 1981

Miller JM Jr, Horger EO III, Key TC, Walker EM Jr: Management of sickle hemoglobinopathies in pregnant patients. Am J Obstet Gynecol 141:237, 1981

Milner PF, Jones BR, Döbler J: Outcome of pregnancy in sickle cell anemia and sickle cell-hemoglobin C disease. Am J Obstet Gynecol 138:239, 1980

Milutinovic J, Fialkow P, Agodoa LY, Phillips LA, Bryant JI: Fertility and pregnancy complications in women with autosomal dominant polycystic kidney disease. Obstet Gynecol 61:566, 1983

Minielly R, Yuzpe AA, Drake CG: Subarachnoid hemorrhage secondary to ruptured cerebral aneurysm in pregnancy. Obstet Gynecol 53:64, 1979

Mintz DH, Chez RA, Hutchinson DL: Subhuman primate pregnancy complicated by streptozotocin-induced diabetes mellitus. J Clin Invest 51:837, 1972

MMWR: Isotretinoin—A new recognized human teratogen. Morbidity Mortality Weekly Report 33:171, 1984

MMWR: Sexually transmitted diseases treatment guidelines 1982. Morbidity Mortality Weekly Report 31:33 [Suppl], 1982

MMWR: Spectinomycin-resistant β-lactamase-producing *Neisseria gonorrheae*—England. Morbidity Mortality Weekly Report 31:495, 1982

Mones JM, Saldana MJ: Nodular regenerative hyperplasia of the liver in a 4-month-old infant. Am J Dis Child 138:79, 1984

Montoro M, Collea JV, Frasier SD: Successful outcome of pregnancy in women with hypothyroidism. Ann Intern Med 94:31, 1981

Montouris GD, Fenichel GM, McLain LW: The pregnant epileptic. Arch Neurol 36:601, 1979

Morrison JC, Fort AT, Wiser WL, Fish SA: The modern management of pregnant sickle cell patients: A preliminary report. South Med J 65:533, 1972

Mountain KR, Hirsh J, Gallers AS: Neonatal coagulation defect due to anticonvulsant drug treatment in pregnancy. Lancet 1:265, 1970

Murphy JR, Wengard M, Brereton W: Rheological studies of Hb SS blood; influence of hematocrit, hypertonicity, separation of cells, deoxygenation, and mixture with normal cells. J Lab Clin Med 87:475, 1976

Murray JE, Reid DE, Harrison JH, Merrill JP: Successful pregnancies after human renal transplantation. N Engl J Med 269:341, 1963

Murray MJ, Murray AB, Murray NJ, Murray MB: The effect of iron status of Nigerian mothers on that of their infants at birth and 6 months, and on the concentration of Fe in breast milk. Br J Nutr 39:627, 1978

Myers JP, Peristein PH, Light IJ, Towbin RB, Dincsoy HP, Dincsoy MY: Tuberculosis in pregnancy with fatal congenital infection. Pediatrics 67:89, 1981

Nadler N, Salinas-Madrigal L, Charles AG, Pollak VE: Acute glomerulonephritis during late pregnancy. Obstet Gynecol 34:277, 1969

Nagorney DM, Field CS: Successful pregnancy 10 years after triple cardiac valve replacement. Obstet Gynecol 57:386, 1981

National Diabetes Data Group: Classification of diabetes mellitus and other categories of glucose intolerance. Diabetes 28:1039, 1979

Neely NT, Persellin RH: Activity of rheumatoid arthritis during pregnancy. Tex Med 73:59, 1977

Nerurkar LS, Jacob AJ, Madden DL, Sever JL: Detection of genital herpes simplex infection in a tissue culture-fluorescent-antibody technique with biotin-avidin. J Clin Microbiol 17:149, 1983

Nerurkar LS, West F, May M, Madden DL, Sever JL: Survival of herpes simplex virus in water specimens collected from hot tubs in spa facilities and on plastic surfaces. JAMA 250:3081, 1983

Nissenson AR, Krumlovsky FA, deGreco F: Postpartum hemolytic uremic syndrome. JAMA 242:173, 1979

Noller KL, Bowie EJW, Kempers RD, Owen CA Jr: Von Willebrand's disease in pregnancy. Obstet Gynecol 41:865, 1973

Norden CW, Kilpatrick WH: In Kass EH (ed): Progress in Pyelonephritis. Philadelphia, Davis, 1965, p 64

Norton RA, Patterson JF: Pregnancy and regional enteritis. Obstet Gynecol 40:711, 1972

Nussbaum RL, Powell C, Graham HL, Caskey CT, Fernbach DJ: Newborn screening for sickling hemoglobinopathies. Houston, 1976 to 1980. Am J Dis Child 138:44, 1984

Oakley C: Pregnancy in patients with prosthetic valves. Br Med J 286:1680, 1983

Old JM, Ward RHT, Karagözlu F, Petrou M, Modell B, Weatherall DJ: First-trimester fetal diagnosis for haemoglobinopathies: Three cases. Lancet 2:1414, 1982

O'Leary JA: A continuing study of sarcoidosis and pregnancy. Am J Obstet Gynecol 101:610, 1968

O'Neill H, Blake S, Sugrue D, MacDonald D: Problems in the management of patients with artificial valves during pregnancy. Br J Obstet Gynaecol 89:940, 1982

Orkin SH, Little PFR, Kazazian HH Jr, Boehm CD: Improved detection of the sickle mutation by DNA analysis. N Engl J Med 307:32, 1982

O'Shaughnessy R, Weprin SA, Zuspan FP: Obstructive renal failure by an overdistended pregnant uterus. Obstet Gynecol 55:247, 1980

Østergaard GZ, Pederson SE: Neonatal effects from maternal clomipramine treatment. Pediatrics 69:233, 1982

O'Sullivan JB, Mahan CM: Criteria for the oral glucose tolerance test in pregnancy. Diabetes 13:278, 1964

Pastorek JG III, Plauche WC, Faro S: Acute bacterial endocarditis. J Reprod Med 28:611, 1983

Penn I, Makowski EL, Harris P: Parenthood following renal transplant. Kidney Int 2:221, 1980

Perez RJ, Lipner H, Abdulla N, Cicotto S, Abrams M: Menstrual dysfunction of patients undergoing chronic hemodialysis. Obstet Gynecol 51:552, 1978

Perucca E, Ruprah M, Richens A: Altered drug binding to serum proteins in pregnant women: therapeutic relevance. J R Soc Med 74:422, 1981

Pizzuto J, Avives A, Noriega L, Niz J, Morales M, Romero F: Treatment of acute leukemia during pregnancy. Cancer Treat Reps 64:679, 1980

Plummer FA, Nsanze H, Karisara P, D'Costa LJ, Dylewski J, Ronald AR: Epidemiology of chancroid and *Haemophylus ducreyi* in Nairobi, Kenya. Lancet 2:1293, 1983

Poncz M, Colman N, Herbert V, Schwartz E, Cohen AR: Therapy of congenital folate malabsorption. J Pediatr 98:76, 1981

Pratt AT, Donaldson RC, Evertson LR, Yon JL Jr: Cecal volvulus in pregnancy. Obstet Gynecol 57:37 [Suppl], 1981

Printen KJ, Scott D: Pregnancy following gastric bypass for the treatment of morbid obesity. Am Surg 48:363, 1982

Pritchard JA: Hereditary hypochromic microcytic anemia in obstetrics and gynecology. Am J Obstet Gynecol 83:1193, 1962a

Pritchard JA, Mason RA: Iron stores of normal adults and replenishment with oral iron therapy. JAMA 190:897, 1964

Pitchard JA, Scott DE: Iron demands in pregnancy. In Hallberg L, Harwerth H-G, Vanotti A (eds): Iron Deficiency Pathogenesis, Clinical Aspects, Therapy. New York, Academic, 1970

Pritchard JA, Scott DE, Whalley PJ: Folic acid requirements in pregnancy-induced megaloblastic anemia. JAMA 208:1163, 1969

Pritchard JA, Scott DE, Whalley PJ, Haling RF Jr: Infants of mothers with megaloblastic anemia due to folate deficiency. JAMA 211:1982, 1970

Pritchard JA, Weisman R Jr, Ratnoff OD, Vosburgh GJ: Intervascular hemolysis, thrombocytopenia, and other hematologic abnormalities associated with severe toxemia of pregnancy. N Engl J Med 250:89, 1954

Pritchard JA, Scott DE, Whalley PJ, Cunningham FG, Mason RA: The effects of maternal sickle cell hemoglobinopathies and sickle cell trait on reproductive performance. Am J Obstet Gynecol 117:662, 1973

Ramsay I, Kaur S, Krassas G: Thyrotoxicosis in pregnancy: Results of treatment by antithyroid drugs combined with T4. Clin Endocrinol 18:73, 1983

Rayburn W, Smith B, Feller I, Varner M, Cruikshank D: Major burns during pregnancy: Effects on fetal well-being. Obstet Gynecol 63:392, 1984

Reece EA, Fox HE, Rapoport F: Factor VIII inhibitor: A cause of severe postpartum hemorrhage. Am J Obstet Gynecol 144:985, 1982

Reece EA, Romero R, Clyne LP, Kriz NS, Hobbins JC: Lupus-like anticoagulant in pregnancy. Lancet I:344, 1984

Reichman RC, Badger GJ, Mertz GJ, Corey L, Richman DD, Connor JD, Redfield D, Savoia MC, Oxman MN, Bryson Y, Tyrrell DL, Portnoy J, Creigh-Kirk T, Keeney RE, Ashikaga T, Dolin R: Treatment of recurrent genital herpes simplex infections with oral acyclovir: A controlled trial. JAMA 251:2103, 1984

Reid R, Ivey KJ, Rencoret RH, Storey B: Fetal complications of obstetric cholestasis. Br Med J 1:870, 1976

Repke JT, Berger NG: Electro-convulsive therapy in pregnancy. Obstet Gynecol 63:39S, 1984

Riggall F, Salkind G, Spellacy W: Typhoid fever complicating pregnancy. Obstet Gynecol 44:117, 1974

Rigler LG, Eneboe JB: Incidence of hiatus hernia in pregnant women and its significance. J Thorac Surg 4:262, 1935

Robert E, Rosa F: Valproate and birth defects. Lancet 2:1142, 1983

Robinson PL, O'Mullane NM, Alderman B: Prenatal treatment of fetal thyrotoxicosis. Br Med J 1:383, 1979

Robson JS, Martin AM, Ruckley VA, MacDonald MK: Irreversible postpartum renal failure. Q J Med 37:423, 1968

Rosa FW: Virilization of the female fetus with maternal danazol exposure. Am J Obstet Gynecol 149:99, 1984

Ruch WA, Klein RL: Polycythemia vera and pregnancy. Obstet Gynecol 23:107, 1964

Rust LA, Goodnight SH, Freeman RK, Johnson CS: Pregnancy and delivery in a woman with hemophilia B. Obstet Gynecol 46:483, 1975

Salmon PA: Pregnancies occurring in patients before and after bypass operation for weight loss. Personal communication, 1975

Saxen L, Hjelt L, Sjostedt JE, Hakosalo J, Hakosalo H: Asian influenza during pregnancy and congenital malformation. Acta Pathol Microbiol Scand 49:114, 1960

Scheinhorn DJ, Angelillo VA: Antituberculosis therapy in pregnancy: Risks to the fetus. West J Med 127:195, 1977

Schenker JG, Granat M: Phaeochromocytoma and pregnancy—An updated appraisal. Aust NZ J Obstet Gynaecol 22:1, 1982

Schmidt D, Canger R, Avanzini G, Battino D, Cusi C, Beck-Mannagetta G, Koch S, Rating D, Janz D: Change of seizure frequency in pregnant epileptic women. J Neurol Neurosurg Psychiatry 46:751, 1983

Schneider JM, Curet LB, Olson RW, Shay G: Ambulatory care of the pregnant diabetic. Obstet Gynecol 56:144, 1980

Schneider RG, Hightower B, Hasty TS, Ryder H, Tomlin G, Atkins R, Brimhall B, Jones RT: Abnormal hemoglobins in a quarter million people. Blood 48:629, 1976

Schreyer P, Caspi E, El-Hindi JM, Eschar J: Cirrhosis—Pregnancy and delivery: A review. Obstet Gynecol Survey 37:304, 1982

Schriner RL, Kleiman MB, Gresham EL: Maternal oral herpes: Isolation policy. Pediatrics 63:247, 1979

Scott DE, Pritchard JA: Iron deficiency in healthy young college women. JAMA 199:147, 1967

Scott JR, Rote NS, Cruikshank DP: Antiplatelet antibodies and platelet counts in pregnancies complicated by autoimmune thrombocytopenic purpura. Am J Obstet Gynecol 145:932, 1983

Sende P, Pantelakis N, Suzuki K, Bashore R: Plasma oxytocin level in pregnancy with diabetes insipidus. Clin Res 23:242A, 1975

Shangold MM, Dor N, Welt SI, Fleischman AR, Crenshaw MC Jr: Hyperparathyroidism and pregnancy: A review. Obstet Gynecol Surv 37:217, 1982

Shaw D, Frohlich J, Wittmann BAK, Willms M: A prospective study of 18 patients with cholestasis of pregnancy. Am J Obstet Gynecol 142:621, 1982

Sheldon J, Coleman T: Remission of diabetes mellitus during pregnancy. Br Med J 1:55, 1974

Sherlock S: Acute fatty liver of pregnancy and microvesicular fat diseases. Gut 24:265, 1983

Siegel M, Goldberg M: Incidence of poliomyelitis in pregnancy. N Engl J Med 253:841, 1955

Siegler AM, Spain DM: Periarteritis nodosa in pregnancy. Clin Obstet Gynecol 8:280, 1965

Singh H, Bolton PJ, Oakley CM: Pregnancy after surgical correction of tetralogy of Fallot. Br Med J 285:168, 1982

Singson E, Fisher KF, Lindheimer MD: Acute poststreptococcal glomerulonephritis in pregnancy: Case report with an 18 year follow-up. Am J Obstet Gynecol 137:857, 1980

Sleigh JD, Robertson JF, Isdale MH: Asymptomatic bacteriuria in pregnancy. J Obstet Gynaecol Br Commonw 71:74, 1964

Smith DW: Teratogenicity of anticonvulsant medications. Am J Dis Child 131:1337, 1977

Smith EW, Krevans JR: Clinical manifestations of hemoglobin C disorders. Bull Johns Hopkins Hosp 104:17, 1959

Smith MB, Whiteside MG, DeGaris CN: An investigation of the complications and outcome of pregnancy in heterozygous beta-thalassaemia. Aust NZ J Obstet Gynecol 15:26, 1975

Smith WD, West HF: Pregnancy and rheumatoid arthritis. Acta Rheumat Scand 6:189, 1960

Snyder RR, Gilstrap LC, Hauth JC: Ehlers-Danlos syndrome and pregnancy. Obstet Gynecol 61:649, 1983

Sórókin JJ, Levine SM: Pregnancy and inflammatory bowel disease: A review of the literature. Obstet Gynecol 62:247, 1983

Spencer CD, Crane FM, Kumar JR, Alving BM: Treatment of postpartum hemolytic uremic syndrome with plasma exchange. JAMA 247:2808, 1982

Srinivasan G, Seeler RA, Tiruvury A, Pildes RS: Maternal anticonvulsant therapy and hemorrhagic disease of the newborn. Obstet Gynecol 59:250, 1982

Starksen NF, Bell WR, Kickler TS: Unexplained hemolytic anemia associated with pregnancy. Am J Obstet Gynecol 146:617, 1983

Steven MM: Progress report: Pregnancy and liver disease. Gut 22:592, 1981

Steven MM, Buckley JD, Mackay IR: Pregnancy in chronic active hepatitis. Q J Med, New Series, 48:519, 1979

Strang A, Lachman E, Pitsoe SB, Marszalek A, Philpott RH: Malaria in pregnancy with fatal complications. Case report. Brit J Obstet Gynaecol 91:399, 1984

Strong DW, Murchison RJ, Lynch DF: The management of ureteral calculi during pregnancy. Surg Gynecol Obstet 146:604, 1978

Studd JWW, Blainey JD: Pregnancy and the nephrotic syndrome. Br Med J 1:276, 1969

Sudo N, Weingold AB: Obstetric aspects of the Guillain-Barré syndrome. Obstet Gynecol 45:39, 1975

Sugrue D, Blake S, MacDonald D: Pregnancy complicated by maternal heart disease at the National Maternity Hospital, Dublin, Ireland, 1969 to 1978. Am J Obstet Gynecol 139:1, 1981

Sullivan-Bolyai J, Hull HF, Wilson C, Corey L: Neonatal herpes simplex virus infection in King County, Washington. JAMA 250:3059, 1983

Tan EM, Cohen AS, Fries JF, Masi AT, McShane DJ, Rothfield NF, Schaller JG, Talal N, Winchester RJ: The 1982 revised criteria for the classification of systemic lupus erythematosus. Arthritis Rheum 25:1271, 1982

Taylor DJ, Mallen C, McDougal N, Lind T: Effect of iron supplementation on serum ferritin levels during and after pregnancy. Br J Obstet Gynaecol 89:1011, 1982

Taylor DJ, Wilcox I, Russell JK: Ehlers-Danlos syndrome during pregnancy: A case report and review of the literature. Obstet Gynecol Surv 36:277, 1982

Thiagarajah S, Harbert GM Jr, Caudle MR, Sturgill BC: Thrombotic thrombocytopenic purpura in pregnancy: A reappraisal. Am J Obstet Gynecol 141:20, 1981

Tracy TA, Miller GL: Obstetric problems of the massively obese. Obstet Gynecol 33:204, 1969

Tuck SM, Studd JWW, White JM: Pregnancy in women with sickle cell trait. Br J Obstet Gynaecol 90:108, 1983

Turkalj I, Braun P, Krupp P: Surveillance of bromocriptine in pregnancy. JAMA 247:1589, 1982

Ueland K, McAnulty JH, Ueland FR, Metcalfe J: Special considerations in the use of cardiovascular drugs. Clin Obstet Gynecol 24:809, 1981

Unger A, Kay A, Griffin AJ, Panayi GS: Disease activity and pregnancy associated α_2-glycoprotein in rheumatoid arthritis. Br Med J 286:750, 1983

Varner MW, Meehan RT, Syrop CH, Strottman MP, Gopelrud CP: Pregnancy in patients with systemic lupus erythematosus. Am J Obstet Gynecol 145:1025, 1983

Veille JC: Peripartum cardiomyopathies: A review. AM J Obstet Gynecol 148:805, 1984

Ventura CS: Hereditary spherocytosis with haemolytic crisis during pregnancy. Aust NZ J Obstet Gynecol 22:50, 1982

Vetter VL, Rashkind WJ: Congenital complete heart block and connective-tissue disorders. N Engl J Med 309:236, 1983

Volpi A, Lakeman AD, Pereira L, Stagno S: Monoclonal antibodies for rapid diagnosis and typing of genital herpes infection during pregnancy. Am J Obstet Gynecol 146:813, 1983

Visintine AM, Nahmias AJ, Josey WE: Genital herpes. Perinatal Care 2:32, 1978

Wagoner RD, Holley KE, Johnson WJ: Accelerated nephro-

sclerosis and postpartum acute renal failure in normotensive patients. Ann Intern Med 69:237, 1968

Walcott WO, Derick DE, Jolley JJ, Snyder DL, Schmid R: Successful pregnancy in a liver transplant patient. Am J Obstet Gynecol 132:340, 1978

Walker WM, McKee AP: Asian influenza in pregnancy: Relationship to fetal anomalies. Obstet Gynecol 13:394, 1959

Wallace DJ, Podell T, Weiner J, Klinenberg JR, Forouzesh S, Dubois EL: Systemic lupus erythematosus—Survival patterns. JAMA 245:934, 1981

Ward RHT, Modell B, Petrou M, Karagölü F, Douratsos E: Method of sampling chorionic villi in first trimester of pregnancy under guidance of real time ultrasound. Br Med J 286:1542, 1983

Ware AJ, Luby JP, Hollinger B, Eigenbrodt EH, Cuthbert JA, Atkins CR, Shorey J, Hull AR, Combs B: Etiology of liver disease in renal transplant patients. Ann Intern Med 91:364, 1979

Waters EG: Discussion of paper by JT Callahan: Separation of symphysis pubis. Am J Obstet Gynecol 66:292, 1953

Weatherall DJ, Pressley L, Wood WG, Higgs DR: Molecular basis for mild forms of homozygous beta-thalassemia. Lancet 1:527, 1981

Weinstein MR, Goldfield MD: Cardiovascular malformations with lithium used during pregnancy. Am J Psychiatr 132:529, 1975

Weisman SA, Simon NA, Herdson PB, Franklin WA: Nephrotic syndrome in pregnancy. Am J Obstet Gynecol 117:867, 1973

Wendel GD, Stark BJ, Jamison RB, Sullivan TJ: Penicillin Allergy and Desensitization in serious maternal/fetal infections. Presented at the Society of Perinatal Obstetricians Feb 2-4, San Antonio, 1984

Werkö L, Bucht H: Glomerular filtration rate and renal blood flow in patients with chronic diffuse glomerulonephritis during pregnancy. Acta Med Scand 153:177, 1956

Wertheim RA, Brooks BJ Jr, Rodriguez FH Jr, Lesesne HR, Jennette JC: Fatal herpetic hepatitis in pregnancy. Obstet Gynecol 62:38 [Suppl], 1983

Westberg SV: Prognosis of breast cancer for pregnant and nursing women. Acta Obstet Gynecol Scand [Suppl 4] 25:1, 1946

Whalley PJ: Bacteriuria of pregnancy. Am J Obstet Gynecol 97:723, 1967

Whalley PJ: Hyperparathyroidism and pregnancy. Am J Obstet Gynecol 86:517, 1963

Whalley PJ, Adams RH, Combes B: Tetracycline toxicity in pregnancy. JAMA 189:357, 1964

Whalley PJ, Cunningham FG, Martin FG: Transient renal dysfunction associated with acute pyelonephritis of pregnancy. Obstet Gynecol 46:174, 1975

Whalley PJ, Martin FG, Peters PC: Significance of asymptomatic bacteriuria detected during pregnancy. JAMA 198:879, 1965

White P: Classification of obstetric diabetes. Am J Obstet Gynecol 130:228, 1978

White P: Pregnancy and diabetes, medical aspects. Med Clin North Am 49:1015, 1965

Whittemore R, Wright MR, Leonard MF, Johnson M: Results of pregnancy in women with congenital heart defects. Pediatr Res 14:452, 1980

Wilkinson EJ: Acute pancreatitis in pregnancy: A review of 98 cases and a report of 8 new cases. Obstet Gynecol Surv 28:281, 1973

Williams JW: The limitations and possibilities of prenatal care. JAMA 64:95, 1915

Wilson MG, Hewitt WL, Monzon OT: Effect of bacteriuria on the fetus. N Engl J Med 274:115, 1966

Wilson MG, Heins HL, Imagawa DT, Adams JM: Teratogenic effects of Asian influenza, JAMA 171:638, 1959

Wong VCW, Ip HMH, Reesink HW, Lelie PN, Reerink-Brongers EE, Yeung CY, Ma HK: Prevention of the HBsAg carrier state in newborn infants of mothers who are chronic carriers of HBsAg and HBeAg by administration of hepatitis-B vaccine and hepatitis-B immunoglobulin. Lancet I:921, 1984

Young BK, Katz M, Klein SA: Pregnancy after spinal cord in-jury: Altered maternal and fetal response in labor. Obstet Gynecol 62:59, 1983

Zegart KN, Schwarz RH: Chorea gravidarum. Obstet Gynecol 32:24, 1968

Zimmerman TS, Abildgaard CF, Meyer D: The factor VIII abnormality in severe von Willebrand's disease. N Engl J Med 301:1307, 1979

Zinns JS: The association of pregnancy and breast cancer. J Reprod Med 22:297, 1979

Zweiman B, Millikan LE: Vesiculobullous skin diseases with prominent immunologic features. JAMA 248:2623, 1982

29

Dystocia Caused by Anomalies of the Expulsive Forces

Dystocia (literally difficult labor) is characterized by abnormally slow progress of labor. It is the consequence of four distinct abnormalities that may exist singly or in combination:

1. Uterine forces that are not sufficiently strong or appropriately coordinated to efface and dilate the cervix.
2. Forces generated by voluntary muscles during the second stage of labor that are inadequate to overcome the normal resistance of the bony birth canal and maternal soft parts.
3. Faulty presentation or abnormal development of the fetus of such a character that the fetus cannot be extruded by the uterine contractions (see Chapter 30).
4. Abnormalities of the birth canal that form an obstacle to the descent of the fetus (see Chapter 31).

Pelvic contraction is often accompanied by uterine dysfunction, and the two together constitute the most common cause of dystocia. Similarly, faulty presentation or unusual fetal size or shape may be accompanied by uterine dysfunction. *As a generalization, uterine dysfunction is common whenever there is disproportion between the presenting part of the fetus and the birth canal.*

UTERINE DYSFUNCTION

As described in Chapter 15 (p. 306), the first stage of labor has commonly, but somewhat artificially, been divided into two distinct phases, the latent phase and the active phase. Typically, the latent phase (*prodromal labor*) will be of several hours duration, during which time the cervix undergoes softening and effacement but only slight dilatation. This phase of cervical change is characterized by uterine contractions of mild intensity, short duration, and variable frequency. The phase of more rapid cervical dilatation, or the active phase, follows. During the active phase, or what has long been

called by both mother and physician simply labor, the cervix dilates more rapidly at 1 to 2 cm per hour and there is descent of the presenting part through the birth canal (Fig. 29-1).

Labor has been further subdivided into three additional divisions or phases, the acceleration phase of active labor, the phase of maximum slope, and the deceleration phase. It must be emphasized that the acceleration and deceleration phases may never be identified during rapid labor. In fact, to anticipate a deceleration phase in labor can result in the delivery of many babies under less than optimal circumstances! Friedman (1980) emphasizes this point when he states that the deceleration phase "is an artifact in the sense that nothing is actually slowing down, but rather, the cervix is now being retracted cephalad around the fetal presenting part, and therefore is no longer being actively dilated by the forces of uterine contraction."

The descent of the presenting part normally begins well before the cervix reaches full dilatation and proceeds until the presenting part reaches the perineum. It should be noted that this pattern is highly variable. The fetal presenting part in a nulliparous women may be at the plus one or even plus two station before the onset of labor, whereas in parous women, descent of the presenting part may not begin until the cervix is nearly fully dilated.

The sigmoid curve for cervical dilatation and the slope of fetal descent, at best, should be considered as *idealized visual aids* to help understand the temporal relationships of cervical dilatation and the descent of the presenting part (Fig. 29-1).

Failure of the cervix to dilate or of the presenting part to descend is cause for appreciable concern. Prolongation of either the first or second stage of labor may result in increased perinatal and maternal morbidity. Any delay in cervical dilatation during the first stage or prolongation of the second stage of labor should alert the obstetrician to possible danger.

Uterine dysfunction in any phase of cervical dilatation is characterized by lack of progress, for one of the prime characteristics of normal labor is its progression. Friedman (1978) defines prolongation of the latent phase

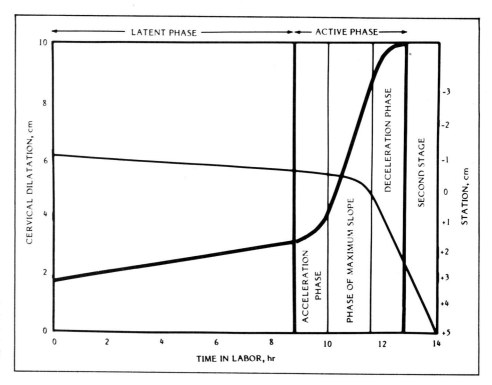

Figure 29-1. Composite of cervical dilatation and fetal descent curves illustrating their interrelationship and their component phases. (*Courtesy of Cohen and Friedman, 1983.*)

as 20 hours in nulliparas and 14 hours in multiparas, and a protracted active phase as cervical dilatation of less than 1.2 cm per hour in nulliparas and 1.5 cm in multiparas (Fig. 29-1; Table 29-1). The diagnosis of uterine dysfunction in the latent phase is difficult and sometimes can be made only in retrospect. One of the most common errors is to treat women for uterine dysfunction who are not yet in active labor.

There have been three significant advances in the treatment of uterine dysfunction: (1) the realization that undue prolongation of labor may contribute to perinatal morbidity and mortality; (2) the use of very dilute intravenous infusion of oxytocin in the treatment of certain types of uterine dysfunction; and (3) the more frequent use of cesarean section to effect delivery rather than difficult midforceps delivery when oxytocin fails or its use is inappropriate (Table 29-2).

Types of Dysfunction

Reynolds and co-workers (1948) emphasized that the uterine contractions of labor are normally characterized by a gradient of myometrial activity, being greatest and lasting longest at the fundus (fundal dominance) and diminishing toward the cervix (see Chapter 15, p. 310). Caldeyro-Barcia and his colleagues in Montevideo (1950) advanced the work of Reynolds by inserting small balloons into the myometrium at various levels. With the balloons attached to strain-gauge transducers, they demonstrated that there was, in addition to a gradient of activity, a time differential in the onset of the contractions in the fundus, midzone, and lower segments of the uterus. Larks (1960) described the exciting stimulus as starting in one cornu and then several milliseconds later in the other, the excitation waves then joining and sweeping over the fundus and down the uterus.

The group in Montevideo (Caldeyro-Barcia, 1950) made another significant contribution to the understanding of uterine dysfunction. By inserting a polyethylene catheter through the abdominal wall into the amnionic fluid, they ascertained that the lower limit of pressure of contractions required to dilate the cervix is 15 mm Hg, a figure in keeping with the findings of Hendricks and co-workers (1959), who reported that a normal spontaneous uterine contraction often exerts a pressure of about 60 mm Hg. From these observations, it is possible to define two types of uterine dysfunction. In one, *hypotonic uterine dysfunction,* there is no basal hypertonus and uterine contractions have a normal gradient pattern (synchronous), but the slight rise in pressure during a contraction is insufficient to dilate the cervix at a satisfactory rate. This type of uterine dysfunction usually occurs during the active phase of labor, after the cervix has dilated to more than 4 cm. In the other, *hypertonic uterine dysfunction,* or *incoordinate uterine dysfunction,* either basal tone is elevated appreciably or the pressure gradient is distorted, perhaps by contraction of the midsegment of the uterus with more force than the fundus or by complete asynchronism of the electrical impulses originating in each cornu, or a combination of abnormalities.

In the hypotonic variety of uterine dysfunction, contractions become less frequent and the uterus is easily indentable even at the acme of a contraction. Contrac-

TABLE 29-1. ABNORMAL LABOR PATTERNS, DIAGNOSTIC CRITERIA, AND METHODS OF TREATMENT

Labor Pattern	Diagnostic Criterion		Preferred Treatment	Exceptional Treatment
	Nulligravidas	*Multiparas*		
Prolongation Disorder				
1. Prolonged latent phase	> 20 hr	> 14 hr	Therapeutic rest	Oxytocin or cesarean sections for urgent problems
Protraction Disorders				
1. Protracted active phase dilatation	< 1.2 cm/hr	< 1.5 cm/hr		
2. Protracted descent	< 1.0 cm/hr	< 2 cm/hr	Expectant and support	Cesarean section for CPD
Arrest Disorders				
1. Prolonged deceleration phase	> 3 hr	> 1 hr	Without CPD*: oxytocin	Rest if exhausted
2. Secondary arrest of dilatation	> 2 hr	> 2 hr		
3. Arrest of descent	> 1 hr	> 1 hr	With CPD: cesarean section	Cesarean section
4. Failure of descent	No decent in deceleration phase or second stage of labor			

* CPD: Cephalopelvic disproportion.
(*Modified from Cohen and Friedman, 1983.*)

tions of the "hypertonic" or incoordinate variety are typically much more painful yet ineffective. As discussed below, hypotonic dysfunction often responds favorably to treatment with oxytocin. The opposite is most often true of the "hypertonic" variety, in which the abnormal pattern of uterine contractions is more likely to become accentuated and the tone of the uterine muscle increased. Exceptions have been documented, however, in which a uterus with basal hypertonus and frequent, incoordinate contractions did convert to orderly physiologic contractions, apparently in response to intravenous oxytocin (Caldeyro-Barcia, 1957). In general, the likelihood of such a response is low and the risk of enhancing the hypertonus is considerable (Cohen and Friedman, 1983).

Etiology

Pelvic contraction and fetal malposition are common causes of uterine dysfunction. That moderate degrees of pelvic contraction and fetal malposition may cause hypotonic uterine dysfunction is of great clinical importance. Overdistention of the uterus, as with twins and with hydramnios, may contribute to the condition. *However, in many—perhaps one half—of instances, the cause of uterine dysfunction is unknown.* The main fault seldom lies within a cervix that is too rigid to dilate. In elderly nulliparas, and in women whose cervices are fibrosed from some cause, however, excessive rigidity of the cervix may be a factor in the production of dystocia.

Complications

Undue procrastination too often leads to an unfortunate outcome whereas intervention too early results in needless cesarean deliveries. Fetal and neonatal deaths are accompaniments of intrauterine infection, which commonly develops in prolonged dysfunctional labor. Although it may be wise for the mother's protection to treat these intrauterine infections with antibiotics, such therapy appears to be of little value in protecting the fetus. Maternal exhaustion may occur if labor is greatly prolonged; however, supportive therapy with adequate

TABLE 29-2. NEONATAL APGAR SCORES BY LABOR PATTERN IN NULLIPARAS AND PERINATAL MORTALITY BY DELIVERY METHOD

Labor Pattern	Percent of Apgar Scores Less than 5		Perinatal Mortality per 1000 by Delivery Method		
	at 1 min	*at 5 min*	*Spontaneous*	*Low Forceps*	*Midforceps*
Normal	12.7	3.2	1.5	2.8	10.8*
Prolongation Disorder	12.9	4.6	0.0	0.0	10.8*
Protraction Disorders	23.7*	3.1	0.0	12.0*	28.5*
Arrest Disorders	25.2*	8.0*	16.1*	24.4*	38.3*

* Statistically significant, p < 0.01.
(*Modified from Cohen and Friedman, 1983.*)

intravenous fluids should be initiated and delivery effected before these complications appear. Difficult labors and deliveries are more likely to leave psychologic scars on the mothers, as emphasized by Jeffcoate (1961), as well as Steer (1950). Both found that difficult labor exerted a definite deleterious effect upon future childbearing. These investigators showed that, although more than two thirds of their patients had further children after spontaneous delivery, only one third did so after midforceps operations.

Treatment of Hypotonic Dysfunction

Two questions must be answered before a plan for treatment can be formulated: (1) Has the woman actually been in active labor? If there has been rhythmic uterine activity of sufficient intensity to produce some discomfort and the cervix has been observed to undergo distinct changes in effacement *and* in dilatation to 3 to 4 cm at least, it is correct to conclude that there has been real, albeit abnormal, labor. (2) Is there cephalopelvic disproportion? Uterine inertia is often a protection against some degree of pelvic contraction or abnormalities of fetal size or presentation. Fortunately, the uterus does not typically persist in spontaneous activity that would lead to its own destruction, that is, rupture. Instead, the usual forces of labor are replaced by hypotonic uterine dysfunction.

Most often, once the diagnosis of active labor followed by hypotonic uterine dysfunction has been made and the head is engaged, or at least well fixed in the pelvis, the membranes, if intact, should be ruptured and ideally an intrauterine pressure catheter and fetal scalp electrode placed. Close observation may be employed for 30 to 60 minutes to see if the amniotomy will improve the quality of labor. Next, a decision must be made whether to stimulate labor with oxytocin or to effect cesarean delivery. The presence of meconium in the amnionic fluid is an ominous sign and makes close monitoring of fetal heart rate and the uterine contraction pattern even more critical.

The choice of whether to augment labor with *hypotonic uterine dysfunction* has been for many years an empiric decision based largely upon clinical judgment as to fetal size, presentation, and position as well as clinical assessment of pelvic size. In practice x-ray pelvimetry usually provides little help (Joyce and associates, 1975; Barton and co-workers, 1982; Anderson, 1983).

Oxytocin Stimulation for Hypotonic Labor

It should be ascertained that the birth canal is most likely adequate for the size of the fetal head and that the fetal head is well-flexed so as to utilize its smallest diameters to negotiate the birth canal (biparietal and suboccipitobregmatic diameters). A contracted pelvis is most unlikely when all of the following criteria are met:

1. The diagonal conjugate is normal.
2. The pelvic sidewalls are nearly parallel.
3. The ischial spines are not prominent.
4. The sacrum is not flat.
5. The subpubic angle is not narrow.
6. The occiput is known to be the presenting part.
7. The fetal head descends through the pelvic inlet with fundal pressure.

If these criteria are not met, the alternatives are cesarean delivery or possibly oxytocin stimulation. If oxytocin is used, it is mandatory that the fetal heart rate and the contraction pattern frequency, intensity, duration and timing in relation to the fetal heart rate be observed closely. If fetal heart action is monitored discontinuously, it is imperative that it be checked *immediately following* contractions rather than waiting a minute or more afterward (see Chapter 14, p. 284).

Technique for Intravenous Oxytocin. Ten units of oxytocin are thoroughly mixed with 1 liter of aqueous solution, usually 5 percent glucose in water or, preferably, a balanced salt solution. More dilute solutions can be prepared by doubling the amount of diluent or halving the amount of oxytocin. Although more dilute solutions have been found effective by numerous authors, the mixture (10 units per liter) is easy to prepare, safe, effective, and likely to cause the least confusion in preparation and administration. Since the oxytocin solution is 10 mU/ml, its rate of flow is easily calculated. Use of a constant infusion pump enhances the precision of the dosage delivered, especially in the lower range, and is recommended.

The needle, *with the flow shut off*, is inserted into an arm vein, or preferably into an already well-functioning intravenous infusion line, and the flow started to deliver no more than 1 mU per minute (Seitchik and Castillo, 1982). For *augmentation* of labor in true hypotonic dysfunction, this amount of oxytocin should not initiate tetanic uterine contractions, although one should be prepared to stop the flow in the event that the uterus is overly sensitive to the drug. The flow can be very gradually increased at not greater than 30-minute intervals to yield no more than 10 mU per minute, according to Seitchik and Castillo (1982, 1983a, 1983b). It is rarely necessary to exceed this rate in the treatment of uterine dysfunction. For the *induction* of labor, if a flow rate of 30 to 40 mU per minute fails to initiate satisfactory uterine contractions, greater rates of infusion are not likely to do so.

The mother should never be left alone while the oxytocin infusion is running. The uterine contractions must be evaluated continually and the flow shut off immediately if they exceed 1 minute in duration or if the fetal heart rate decelerates significantly. When either occurs, immediate discontinuation of the flow nearly always corrects the disturbances, preventing harm to mother and fetus. The oxytocin concentration in plasma rapidly falls since the mean half-life of oxytocin is approximately 3 minutes.

It always must be kept in mind that oxytocin possesses potent antidiuretic action. Whenever 20 mU per minute or more of oxytocin is infused, free water clearance by the kidney decreasees markedly. If aqueous fluids, especially dextrose in water, are infused in appreciable amounts along with the oxytocin, there exists the possibility of water intoxication that may lead to convulsions, coma, and even death (see Chapter 17, p. 346).

At Parkland Memorial Hospital, the following general precautions are exercised with the use of oxytocin to treat hypotonic uterine dysfunction:

1. The woman must have demonstrated true labor, not false or prodromal labor. The only valid evidence of labor is progresssive effacement and dilatation of the cervix. Although the process has come to a standstill, it must have progressed to the extent of at least 3-cm dilatation. One of the most common mistakes in obstetrics is to try to stimulate labor in women who have not been in active labor.

2. There must be no other discernible evidence of mechanical obstruction to safe delivery.

3. Use of oxytocin is generally avoided in cases of abnormal presentations of the fetus and of marked uterine overdistention such as gross hydramnios, a large singleton fetus, or multiple fetuses.

4. Women of high parity (more than 5), in general, are not given oxytocin because their uteri rupture more readiy than those of women of lower parity (Chapter 33, p. 700). For the same reason, oxytocin is usually withheld from women with a previous uterine scar.

5. The condition of the fetus must be good, as evidenced by normal heart rate and lack of heavy contamination of the amnionic fluid with meconium. A dead fetus is, of course, no contraindication to oxytocin unless there is overt fetopelvic disproportion or a transverse lie.

6. The obstetrician must note the time of the first contraction after administration of the drug and be prepared to discontinue its use if a tetanic contraction occurs. It is imperative that hyperstimulation of the uterus be avoided. The frequency, intensity, and duration of contractions, and uterine tone between contractions must not exceed those of normal spontaneous labor.

7. Fetal heart rate and uterine contraction pattern are evaluated frequently. Continous monitoring of the fetal heart and uterine activities is recommended to accomplish this.

Oxytocin is a powerful drug, and it has killed or maimed mothers through rupture of the uterus and even more babies through hypoxia from markedly hypertonic uterine contractions. The intravenous administration of oxytocin, however, as is attested to by many publications, has brought about a distinct advance in both its efficacy and safety. Failure to treat uterine dysfunction exposes the mother to increased hazards from maternal exhaustion, intrapartum infection, and traumatic operative delivery. At the same time, failure to treat uterine dysfunction may expose the fetus to an appreciably

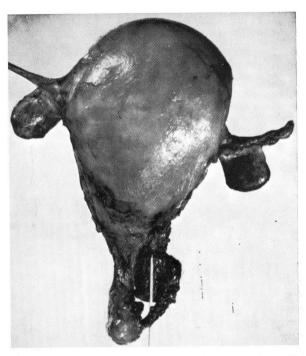

Figure 29-2. Rupture of the lower uterine segment resulting from stimulation by dilute intravenous oxytocin in a 38-year-old multipara.

higher risk of death, whereas the risk from intravenous oxytocin should be negligible when used appropriately. Serious accidents, nevertheless, may accompany its use unless the precautions mentioned here are rigidly observed. The ruptured uterus illustrated in Figure 29-2 should serve as a warning to the physician of the need for these precautions. In this case, oxytocin was administered to a multiparous woman who was 38 years of age. Inasmuch as no other abnormalities were present, it must be assumed that the aging uterine muscle had been previously stretched repeatedly in other labors and could not stand the stress produced by the oxytocin.

One characteristic of intravenous oxytocin is that when successful, it acts promptly, leading to noticeable progress with little delay. For any given rate of infusion the plasma level reaches a plateau after about 30 minutes as the rate of infusion and rate of destruction by oxytocinase achieve equilibrium. Therefore, the drug need not be used for an indefinite period of time to stimulate labor. It should be employed for no more than a few hours (O'Driscoll and co-workers, 1984; Seitchik and Castillo, 1983a, 1983b); if, by then, the cervix has not changed appreciably and if predictably easy vaginal delivery is not imminent, cesarean delivery should be performed. On the other hand, oxytocin should not be used to force cervical dilatation at a rate that exceeds normal (Cohen and Friedman, 1983). Ready resort to cesarean section in cases where oxytocin fails or in which there are contraindications to its use has served to diminish perinatal mortality and morbidity appreciably.

Attempt at Precise Classification of Labor Disorders

In an attempt at precision, Friedman (1978) divided labor disorders into three divisions: prolonged latent phase disorders, protraction disorders, and arrest disorders. The prolonged latent phase is a single entity; the protraction disorders are two in number and consist of two further divisions, a protracted active dilatation phase and protracted descent. The arrest of labor disorders are four in number and consist of prolonged deceleration phase, secondary arrest of dilatation, arrest of descent, and failure of descent. These labor disorders and the diagnostic criteria to establish their diagnoses and treatments are listed in Table 29-1.

The diagnosis of a prolonged latent phase is based upon the passage of excessive time with failure of the cervix to dilate past 3 to 4 cm. Unfortunately, this diagnosis is most often made in retrospect. Also, this disorder of labor is almost impossible to distinguish from false labor. The causes of this form of labor disorder are discussed elsewhere (p. 643), but in summary the most frequent causes are related to the early use of excessive narcotic and/or sedative analgesics and the use of regional epidural anesthetics (Friedman and Sachtleben, 1961). Thus, treatment usually consists of allowing these drugs to be metabolized and cleared from the maternal circulation if sufficient time is available, that is, membranes have not been ruptured for an excessive period of time and the fetal and maternal patients are both in no specific danger. If this is not effective, 85 percent of such patients will respond to an oxytocin infusion.

As simple as these diagnoses and managements may seem, the problem remains that a prolonged latent phase may be due to (1) *injudicious use of anesthetics and/or analgesics,* (2) *false labor,* (3) *hypertonic uterine dysfunction,* or (4) *"unknown" reasons.* Thus, if analgesic or anesthetic causes are not present and if delivery is not mandated for fetal and/or maternal reasons, Friedman (1978) recommends heavily sedating the patient with narcotics. When the patient awakens in 6 to 7 hours she usually will be in progressive labor if the disorder was due to *hypertonic uterine dysfunction* or will not be in labor if she had been in false labor. In those 2 to 3 percent of patients who revert to the same pattern as before the sedation, a diagnosis of *hypertonic uterine dysfunction* is most likely.

The two protraction disorders are closely related and should be considered together. The diagnosis is established when the cervix fails to dilate at the rates listed in Table 29-1 or when the presenting part fails to descend at the rates listed in the same table, but progress continues. The major cause(s) of these disorders is unknown but approximately one third of cases are due to varying degrees of cephalopelvic disproportion.

Treatment of the protraction disorders is not clearly established except in cases where cephalopelvic disproportion can be documented; then delivery by cesarean section is indicated. In other circumstances, Friedman (1978) recommends supportive measures such as hydration and psychologic support but maintains that even with oxytocin stimulation the rate of dilatation of the cervix and the rate of descent of the presenting part cannot be accelerated.

This view of passive support is opposed by O'Driscoll and colleagues (1969, 1970, 1973, 1983, 1984) who actively intervene if cervical dilatation is not achieved at a specific rate. O'Driscoll and co-workers (1983, 1984) discourage the use of intravenous oxytocin in multiparous but not in nulliparous patients as well as the use of midforceps in patients who have experienced either prolongation or arrest patterns of dysfunctional labor. Cohen and Friedman (1983) discourage the use of midforceps in such labors (Table 29-2).

The arrest disorders are considered to be present (Table 29-1) when there is no cervical dilatation for 2 hours, when the deceleration phase is prolonged, or when there is failure of the presenting part to descend for greater than 1 hour or longer. Friedman (1978) maintains that approximately one half of these patients have "insurmountable obstruction" and recommends the judicious use of intravenous oxytocin but cautions that such efforts, while effective in dilating the cervix and ultimately resulting in vaginal delivery, may subject the fetus to substantial risks of hypoxic injury as well as birth trauma. O'Driscoll and associates (1983, 1984) strongly disagree with this approach. They aggressively stimulate such labors in nulliparous patients but not in multiparas. Seitchik and Castillo (1983a, 1983b) take a less aggressive approach than do O'Driscoll and associates.

Buccal Oxytocin. Oxytocin has been administered by placing tablets containing the drug against the buccal mucosa. Since transbuccal absorption is quite variable, either understimulation or overstimulation may occur. This technique has not been used at Parkland Memorial Hospital; rather, the drug is precisely administered intravenously with a calibrated infusion pump. Transbuccal administration of oxytocin to induce or stimulate labor has been disapproved by the Food and Drug Administration.

Prostaglandins

Prostaglandins $F_{2\alpha}$ and E_2 are potent uterotonic agents that are capable of inducing and augmenting labor. The possibility of uterine hypertonus following oral or intravenous administration is worrisome, but it has not been a major problem in two studies of labor induction using prostaglandin E_2 given orally (Cunningham and co-workers, 1976; Hauth and associates, 1977).

Considerable efficacy has been claimed for prostaglandin E_2 suppositories, especially when used to "ripen" the firm, minimally effaced, and little dilated cervix of women in whom labor was to be induced. In the study of Shepherd and associates (1979), a suppository containing 3 mg of prostaglandin E_2 was inserted into the posterior vaginal fornix the evening before induction. If the cervix remained unfavorable, that is, firm, minimally effaced, and little dilated, the next morning a second "ripening" dose was inserted. Labor often followed the first or second suppository. If it did not, and the cervix was now favorable (soft and somewhat effaced and dilated), amniotomy was performed or oxytocin was infused intravenously, or both. The cesarean section rate subsequent to the use of the prostaglandin E_2 suppositories among women with a cervix considered at the outset to be unfavorable was only 2 percent. Only one instance of uterine hypertonus was described. The condition of the fetuses at birth, as judged by Apgar scores, was considered to be satisfactory. Neither prostaglandin $F_{2\alpha}$ nor E_2

has been approved by the Food and Drug Administration for such use in this country.

Treatment of Hypertonic Uterine Dysfunction

Such dysfunction is characterized by uterine pain that appears to be out of proportion to the intensity of contractions and certainly out of proportion to their effectiveness in effacing and dilating the cervix. This type of uterine dysfunction characteristically occurs prior to the cervix reaching a dilatation of 4 cm or more. Because of the relative infrequency of this variety of dysfunctional labor, it has attracted little attention as a clinical entity, and thus its role in perinatal morbidity may be overlooked.

Oxytocin is rarely, if ever, indicated in the presence of uterine hypertonus with a living fetus. Cesarean delivery should be employed if fetal distress is suspected. If the membranes are intact and there is no other evidence of fetopelvic disproportion, administration of morphine or meperidine will relieve pain and rest the mother and may arrest the abnormal uterine activity. When she awakes, hopefully, more effective labor will be evident. As mentioned earlier, it is important that such management does not lead to undue procrastination and unappreciated fetal distress, including the defecation of copious amounts of meconium into the amnionic fluid, and, in turn, serious meconium aspiration by the fetus (see Chapter 38, p. 770). Tocolytic agents, such as ritodrine, have been used, presumably with some success, especially in other countries.

INADEQUATE VOLUNTARY EXPULSIVE FORCE

With achievement of full cervical dilatation the great majority of women cannot resist the urge to "bear down" or "push" each time that the uterus contracts. Typically, the laboring woman inhales deeply, closes her glottis, and contracts her abdominal musculature repetitively with vigor to generate appreciable increases in intraabdominal pressure throughout the time that the uterus is contracting. The combined force created by the contractions of the uterus and of the abdominal musculature propels the fetus down the vagina and, in the case of spontaneous delivery, through the vaginal outlet.

Causes of Inadequate Expulsive Forces

At times, the magnitude of the force created by the contraction of the abdominal musculature is sufficiently compromised to prevent spontaneous vaginal delivery. Conduction anesthesia—lumbar epidural, caudal, or intrathecal—is likely to reduce the reflex urge for the woman to "push," and, at the same time, may impair her ability to contract the abdominal muscles sufficiently to increase intraabdominal pressure. General anesthesia,

with loss of consciousness, certainly imposes these adverse effects, as does *heavy* sedation.

In some instances, the inherent urge to "push" that develops in most women as the cervix becomes fully dilated is overridden by the intensification of pain that is created by bearing down. Rarely, insufficient expulsive efforts may be the consequence of long-standing paralysis of the abdominal musculature, as may occur after poliomyelitis or transection of the spinal cord.

Management

Careful selection of the kind of anesthesia and the timing of its administration are very important if compromise of voluntary expulsive efforts is to be avoided. With rare exception, intrathecal or general anesthesia should not be administered until all conditions for a safe, low forceps delivery have been met, that is, the fetal head is engaged, the sagittal suture is in the anteroposterior position, and the occiput distends the perineum and protrudes somewhat through the vaginal introitus with a contraction. With continuous epidural anesthesia, it may be necessary to allow the paralytic effects to wear off so that the mother in response to coaching can generate intraabdominal pressure sufficient to move the fetal head into position appropriate for low forceps delivery. The alternatives—a possibly difficult midforceps vaginal delivery or cesarean delivery—are unsatisfactory choices in the absence of any evidence of fetal distress.

For the woman who cannot bear down appropriately with each contraction because of great discomfort, analgesia is likely to be of considerable benefit. Perhaps the safest for both fetus and mother is nitrous oxide, mixed with an equal volume of oxygen and provided during the time of each uterine contraction. At the same time, appropriate encouragement and instruction are most likely to be of benefit.

PRECIPITATE LABOR AND DELIVERY

Precipitate, that is, extremely rapid, labor and delivery may result from an abnormally low resistance of the soft parts of the birth canal, from abnormally strong uterine and abdominal contractions, or, *very rarely,* from the absence of painful sensations and thus a lack of awareness of vigorous labor.

Maternal Effects

Precipitate labor and delivery are seldom accompanied by serious maternal complications if the cervix is appreciably effaced and easily dilated, the vagina has been previously stretched, and the perineum is relaxed. However, vigorous uterine contractions combined with a long, firm cervix, and a vagina, vulva, or perineum that resists stretch may lead to rupture of the uterus or troublesome lacerations of the cervix, vagina, vulva, or perineum. It is in these latter circumstances that the rare condition *am-*

nionic fluid embolism is most likely to occur (see Chapter 21, p. 415). *The uterus that contracts with unusual vigor before delivery is likely to be hypotonic after delivery with hemorrhage from the placental implantation site as the consequence* (see Chapter 34, p. 708).

Effects on Fetus and Neonate

Perinatal mortality and morbidity from precipitate labor may be increased appreciably for several reasons. First, the tumultuous uterine contractions, often with negligible intervals of relaxation, prevent appropriate uterine blood flow and oxygenation of the fetal blood. Second, the resistance of the birth canal to expulsion of the head may cause intracranial trauma, although this must be rare. Third, during an unattended birth, the infant may fall to the floor and be injured or may need resuscitation that is not immediately available.

Treatment

Unusually forceful spontaneous uterine contractions are not likely to be modified to a significant degree by the administration of analgesia. Importantly, if tried, the dose should be such that the infant at birth is not further depressed by the maternally administered analgesia. The use of general anesthesia with agents that impair uterine contractibility, such as halothane and ether, is often excessively heroic. Both epinephrine and magnesium sulfate parenterally administered have been claimed to be effective, but the evidence that they are useful is weak. Certainly, any oxytoxic agents being administered should be stopped immediately. Tocolytic agents, such as ritodrine, may prove effective. It is indefensible to lock the mother's legs or hold the baby's head back directly to try to delay delivery. Such maneuvers may damage the infant's brain.

LOCALIZED ABNORMALITIES OF UTERINE ACTION

Pathologic Retraction and Constriction Rings

Very rarely, localized rings or constrictions of the uterus occur in association with prolonged rupture of the membranes and protracted labors. The most common type is the so-called *pathologic retraction ring of Bandl* (Bandl, 1875), an exaggeration of the normal retraction ring described in Chapter 15 (p. 308), and is often, but not always, the result of obstructed labor, with marked stretching and thinning of the lower uterine segment. In such a situation, the ring may be clearly evident as an abdominal indentation and signifies impending rupture of the lower uterine segment (Fig. 30-7). Localized constrictions of the uterus are rarely seen today, since prolonged obstructed labor is no longer compatible with acceptable obstetric practice. They may, however, still

occur occasionally as hourglass constrictions of the uterus following the birth of the first of twins. In such a situation, they can sometimes be relaxed and delivery effected with appropriate general anesthesia, but on occasion prompt cesarean section offers a better prognosis for the second twin (see Chapter 26, p. 522).

Missed Labor

In rare instances, uterine contractions commence at or near term and, after continuing for a variable time, disappear without leading to the birth of the child. The fetus then dies and may be retained in utero for months or years undergoing mummification. This condition is known as missed labor. If uterine contractions disappear without leading to the birth of the child, and especially if the infant dies and is retained, abdominal pregnancy is a much more likely diagnosis than is missed labor. Management of prolonged retention of a fetus dead in utero is discussed in Chapter 21 (p. 412) and of extrauterine (abdominal) pregnancy in Chapter 22 (p. 436).

REFERENCES

Anderson N: X-ray pelvimetry: Helpful or harmful? J Fam Pract 17:405, 1983

Bandl L: Über Ruptur der Gebärmutter. Vienna, 1875

Barton JJ, Garbaciak JA Jr, Ryan GM: The efficacy of x-ray pelvimetry. Am J Obstet Gynecol 143:304, 1982

Caldeyro-Barcia R, Alvarez H, Reynolds SRM: A better understanding of uterine contractility through simultaneous recording with an internal and a seven channel external method. Surg Obstet Gynecol 91:641, 1950

Caldeyro-Barcia R: Oxytocin and pregnant human uterus. Proceedings of the 4th Pan-American Congress on Endocrinology. Buenos Aires, 1957

Cohen W, Friedman EA (eds): Management of Labor. Baltimore, University Park Press, 1983

Cunningham FG, Cox K, Hauth JC, Strong JD, Whalley PJ: Oral prostaglandin E₂ for labor induction in high-risk pregnancy. Am J Obstet Gynecol 125:881, 1976

Friedman EA: Labor: Clinical Evaluation and Management, 2nd ed. New York, Appleton, 1978

Friedman EA: Cervical function in human pregnancy and labor. In Naftolin F, Stubblefield PG (eds): Dilatation of the Uterine Cervix: Connective Tissue Biology and Clinical Management. New York, Raven, 1980

Friedman EA, Sachtleben MR: Dysfunctional labor. I. Prolonged latent phase in the nullipara. Obstet Gynecol 17:135, 1961

Hauth JC, Cunningham FG, Whalley PJ: Early labor initiation with oral PGE₂ after premature rupture of the membranes at term. Obstet Gynecol 49:523, 1977

Hendricks CH, Quilligan EJ, Tyler AB, Tucker GJ: Pressure relationships between intervillous space and amniotic fluid in human term pregnancy. Am J Obstet Gynecol 77:1028, 1959

Jeffcoate TNA: Prolonged labor. Lancet 2:61, 1961

Joyce DN, Giwa-Asagie F, Stevenson GW: Role of pelvimetry in active management of labor. Br Med J 4:505, 1975

Larks SD: Electrohysterography. Springfield, IL, Thomas, 1960

O'Driscoll K, Foley M: Correlation of decrease in perinatal mortality and increase in cesarean section rates. Obstet Gynecol 61:1, 1983

O'Driscoll K, Foley M, MacDonald D: Active management of labor as an alternative to high cesarean section rate for dystocia. Obstet Gynecol 63:485, 1984

O'Driscoll K, Jackson RJ, Gallagher JT: Prevention of prolonged labour. Br Med J 2:477, 1969

O'Driscoll K, Jackson RJ, Gallagher JT: Active management of labour and cephalopelvic disproportion. J Obstet Gynaecol Br Commonw 77:385, 1970

O'Driscoll K, Stronge JM, Minogue M: Active management of labour. Br Med J 3:135, 1973

Reynolds SRM, Heard OO, Bruns P, Hellman LM: A multichannel strain-gauge tokodyanamometer: An instrument for studying patterns of uterine contractions in pregnant women. Bull Johns Hopkins Hosp 82:446, 1948

Seitchik J, Castillo M: Oxytocin augmentation of dysfunctional labor. I. Clinical data. Am J Obstet Gynecol 144:899, 1982

Seitchik J, Castillo M: Oxytocin augmentation of dysfunctional labor. II. Uterine activity data. Am J Obstet Gynecol 145:526, 1983a

Seitchik J, Castillo M: Oxytocin augmentation of dysfunctional labor. III. Multiparous patients. Am J Obstet Gynecol 145:777, 1983b

Shepherd J, Pearce JMF, Sims CD: Induction of labour using prostaglandin E_2 pessaries. Br Med J 2:108, 1979

Steer CM: Effect of type of delivery on future childbearing. Am J Obstet Gynecol 60:395, 1950

30

Dystocia Caused by Abnormalities in Presentation, Position, or Development of the Fetus

BREECH PRESENTATION

Incidence

Breech presentation is common remote from term, as demonstrated in Table 30-1. Most often, however, sometime before the onset of labor the fetus will turn spontaneously to a vertex presentation so that breech presentation persists in only about 3 to 4 percent of singleton deliveries. For example, 3.2 percent of 33,562 infants delivered in recent years at Parkland Memorial Hospital presented as breech.

Etiology

As term approaches, the uterine cavity, for reasons that are not totally clear, most often accommodates the fetus in a longitudinal lie with the vertex presenting. Breeches are much more common at the end of the second trimester of pregnancy than at or near term (Table 30-1). Factors other than prematurity that appear to predispose to breech presentation include uterine relaxation associated with great parity, multiple fetuses, hydramnios, oligohydramnios, hydrocephalus, anencephalus, previous breech delivery, uterine anomalies, and tumors.

Implantation of the placenta in either cornual–fundal region of the uterus has been suspected of predisposing to breech presentation. Fianu and Vaclavinkova (1978) have provided sonographic evidence of a very much higher prevalence of implantation of the placenta in the cornual–fundal region for breech presentations (73 percent) than for vertex presentations (5 percent). The frequency of breech presentation is also increased with placenta previa but only a small minority of cases of breech presentation are associated with placenta previa. No strong positive correlation has been shown between breech presentation and a contracted pelvis in most recent reports.

A live fetus is *not* required for a fetus to change

presentations spontaneously. Recently a woman was admitted to Parkland Memorial Hospital at term with a fetus known to be dead, confirmed by the lack of fetal heart sounds with doppler examination and also by the lack of heart action seen with real-time sonography. The presentation was cephalic at the time of the first oxytocin induction which proved unsuccessful. Three days later, at the time of the second attempt at induction of labor, the fetus was in a breech presentation. Three days later at the time of a third and successful induction of labor, the fetus was again in a vertex presentation!

Significance

If delivery occurs without prior conversion of the breech to a vertex presentation, an *increased* frequency of the following complications can be anticipated: (1) perinatal morbidity and mortality from difficult delivery; (2) low birth weight from prematurity, growth retardation, or both; (3) prolapsed cord; (4) placenta previa; (5) fetal anomalies and developmental abnormalities that appear after the newborn period; (6) uterine anomalies and tumors; (7) multiple fetuses; and (8) operative intervention, especially cesarean section.

Diagnosis

The varying relations between the lower extremities and buttocks of the fetus in breech presentations form the categories of frank breech, complete breech, and incomplete breech presentations (Figs. 12-2-12-4). With a *frank breech* presentation, the lower extremities are flexed at the hips and extended at the knees and thus the feet lie in close proximity to the head. A *complete breech* presentation differs from a frank breech presentation in that one or both knees are flexed rather than both extended. With *incomplete breech* presentation, one or both hips are not flexed and one or both feet or knees lie below the breech, that is, a foot or knee is lowermost in the birth canal. The frank breech appears

651

TABLE 30-1. FETAL PRESENTATION AT VARIOUS GESTATIONAL AGES DETERMINED SONOGRAPHICALLY

Gestation (Weeks Inclusive)	Total (No.)	Cephalic (%)	Breech (%)	Other (%)
21–24	264	54.6	33.3	12.1
25–28	367	61.9	27.8	10.4
29–32	443	78.1	14.0	7.9
33–36	638	88.7	8.8	2.5
37–40	463	91.5	6.7	1.7

(*From Scheer and Nubar: Am J Obstet Gynecol 125:269, 1976.*)

most common when the diagnosis is established radiologically near term.

Abdominal Examination. Typically, the first maneuver identifies the hard, round, readily ballottable fetal head to occupy the fundus of the uterus (Fig. 30-1). The second maneuver indicates the back to be on one side of the abdomen and the small parts on the other. On the third maneuver, if engagement has not occurred, that is, the interotrochanteric diameter of the fetal pelvis has not passed through the pelvic inlet, the breech is movable above the pelvic inlet. After engagement, the fourth maneuver shows the firm breech to be beneath the symphysis. The heart sounds of the fetus are usually heard loudest slightly above the umbilicus whereas with engagement of the fetal head the heart sounds are loudest below the umbilicus.

Vaginal Examination. The diagnosis of a frank breech presentation is confirmed vaginally by palpating its characteristic components. Both ischial tuberosities, the sacrum, and the anus are usually palpable, and after further descent, the external genitalia may be distinguished.

Especially when labor is prolonged, the buttocks may become markedly swollen, rendering differentiation of face and breech very difficult; the anus may be mistaken for the mouth, and the ischial tuberosities for the malar eminences. Careful examination, however, should prevent that error, for the finger encounters muscular resistance with the anus, whereas the firmer, less yielding jaws are felt through the mouth. Furthermore, the finger, upon removal from the anus, is sometimes stained with meconium. The most accurate information, however, is based on the location of the sacrum and its spinous processes, which establishes the diagnosis of position and variety.

In complete breech presentations, the feet may be felt alongside the buttocks, and in footling presentations, one or both feet are inferior to the buttocks (Fig. 30-2). In footling presentations, the foot can readily be identified as right or left on the basis of the relation to the great toe. When the breech has descended farther into the pelvic cavity, the genitalia may be felt; if not markedly edematous, they may permit identification of fetal sex.

X-Ray and Sonographic Examinations. Sonography used to identify a breech presentation usually does not identify the relationship of the lower extremities to the fetal pelvis as well as does x-ray. Fetal anomalies, however, are more likely to be detected with sonography.

Labor

There are fundamental differences between labor and delivery in cephalic and breech presentations as described in Chapter 42. With a cephalic presentation, once the head is delivered, typically the rest of the body follows without difficulty. With a breech, however, successively larger or, in case of the head, very much less compressible parts of the fetus are born.

Spontaneous complete expulsion of the fetus who presents as a breech, as described below, is seldom successfully accomplished. As the rule, either cesarean delivery (see Chapter 43) or vaginal delivery that requires skilled participation by the obstetrician is essential for a favorable outcome (see Chapter 42).

Prognosis

With breech presentation, compared to cephalic presentation, both the mother and the fetus are at greater risk but to nowhere near the same degree.

Maternal. Because of the greater frequency of operative delivery, including cesarean section, there is a higher maternal morbidity and slightly higher mortality for pregnancies complicated by persistent breech presentation (Collea, 1980). Labor usually is not prolonged. Hall and Kohl (1956), in a large series of cases, reported the median duration of labor to be 9.2 hours for nulliparas and 6.1 hours for multiparas.

Fetus-Infant. *The prognosis for the fetus in a breech presentation is considerably worse than when in a vertex presentation.* The major contributors to this perinatal loss are prematurity, congenital anomalies, and birth trauma. Brenner and associates (1974) provided a careful analysis of the characteristics and perils to the fetus from breech presentation. They determined the overall mortality rate for 1016 breech deliveries to be 25.4 percent compared to 2.6 percent for nonbreech deliveries at the University Hospitals of Cleveland. At every stage of gestation, they identified antepartum, intrapartum, and neonatal deaths to be significantly greater among breeches and the average Apgar scores to be lower for those who survived. During the latter half of pregnancy, the birth weight at any gestational age was somewhat less for breech infants than for nonbreech infants. Congenital abnormalities were identified in 6.3 percent of breech deliveries compared to 2.4 percent in nonbreech deliveries.

Tank and associates (1971) examined the character of serious traumatic vaginal delivery. At autopsy, the

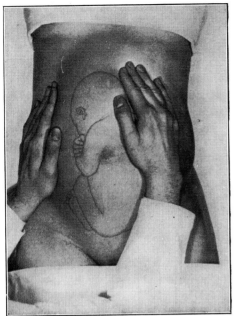

A

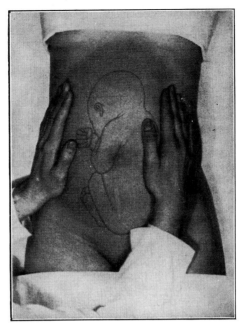

B

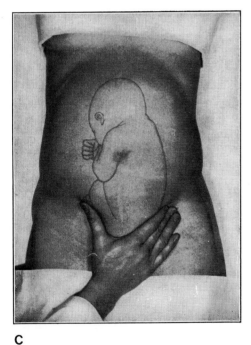

C

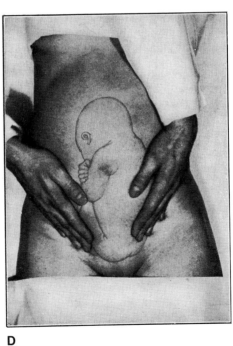

D

Figure 30-1. Palpation in left sacro-anterior position. **A.** First maneuver. **B.** Second maneuver. **C.** Third maneuver. **D.** Fourth maneuver.

organs most frequently found to be injured are, in order of frequency, the brain, spinal cord, liver, adrenal glands, and spleen. It is of interest that, in retrospective analysis of cases of "idiopathic" adrenal calcification, breech delivery was very common. Other sites of injuries from vaginal delivery include the brachial plexus; the pharynx, in the form of tears or pseudodiverticula from the obste-

trician's finger in the mouth as part of the Mauriceau maneuver (see Chapter 42, p. 858, 861); and the bladder, which may be ruptured if distended. Traction may injure the sternomastoid muscle and, if not appropriately treated, lead to torticollis.

Similar results have been reported from the Los Angeles Women's Hospital by Gimovsky and Paul

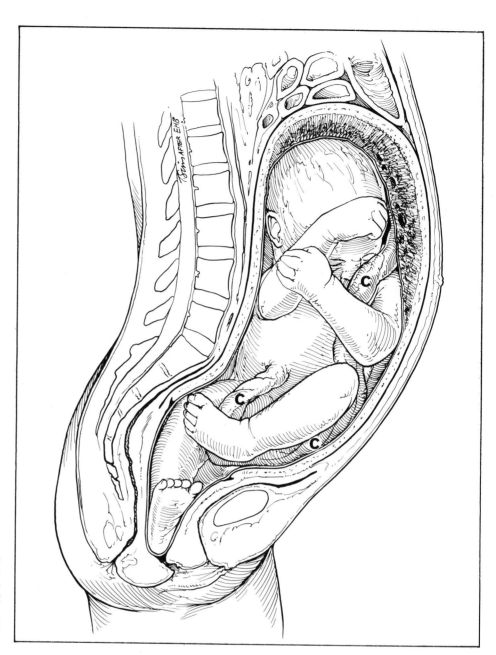

Figure 30-2. Double-footling breech presentation in labor with membranes intact. Note possibility of umbilical cord accident at any instant, especially after rupture of membranes (C = umbilical cord).

(1982). They observed an overall mortality rate for all breech presentations of 8.5 percent compared to a 2.2 percent rate for cephalic presentations. These results were obtained despite a cesarean delivery rate of 74 percent for all breech presentations. Thus, even with liberal use of cesarean section and after exclusion of fetuses who were very premature or had severe congenital anomalies, there still remained a relative twofold risk for the infant delivered as a breech compared to the overall population.

Green and associates (1982) reported a distressing result obtained for breeches managed during 1963–72 at the Royal Victoria Hospital in Montreal compared to the 1978–79 time period. In the decade 1963–72 the ce-

sarean section rate was 22 percent compared to 94 percent for 1978–79. In spite of the significant increase in cesarean section rates, rates of fetal asphyxia remained the same, despite a *trend* toward decreased fetal trauma and death. The authors concluded that cesarean section alone could not guarantee a good infant outcome because the "maneuvers of extracting a breech by cesarean section are similar to that associated with the delivery of a breech via the vaginal route." A similar warning that cesarean section alone cannot assure a better outcome was presented by Calvert (1980), who urged a more liberal use of large uterine incisions for breeches.

Because of the confusing nature of compounding variables in trying to ascertain the safest method of breech delivery for both maternal and fetal patients, several studies have been conducted to contrast outcomes obtained for mature versus premature infants and within such groups to contrast outcomes obtained for different types of breech presentations.

Mature Fetus

Rovinsky and associates (1973), at Mount Sinai Hospital in New York City, looked especially at the risks associated with breech presentation for singleton fetuses who weighed 2500 g or more and were considered to be at or near term. The overall perinatal mortality rate for more than 2000 such infants was 3.17 percent compared to 0.84 percent for infants with a cephalic presentation at or near term. Major congenital anomalies were identified in 2.1 percent of those presenting as breech versus 0.8 percent in those that were vertex. In one third of the perinatal deaths, breech presentation or delivery, or both, were thought to be etiologic factors. Mortality and morbidity rates from trauma were understandably lowest in infants who weighed 2500 to 3000 g and highest among those who weighed 4000 g or more. Morbidity from trauma was progressively higher as the amount of obstetric manipulation required to effect vaginal delivery increased. As might be expected, mortality and morbidity rates from trauma were higher when less experienced obstetricians delivered the breech.

In the Mount Sinai experiences, the incidence of overt prolapse of the cord among frank breeches at term was three times greater (1.7 percent) than for term vertex presentations; for complete and footling breeches, however, cord prolapse was 20 times greater (10.9 percent). Moreover, the incidence of fetal distress of undetermined cause in term breeches was 6.4 percent, or eight times greater than for term vertex presentations. No perinatal deaths were attributable to either breech presentation or delivery among the 425 (19.8 percent) that were delivered by cesarean section.

According to Rovinsky and associates, in retrospect it is likely that the deaths of 17 infants at term who succumbed as the consequence of labor and vaginal delivery, or about 1 percent of all term breech deliveries, would have been prevented by cesarean section. It is also pertinent that Brenner and co-workers (1974) identified in their study the perinatal mortality rate for fetuses of 32 weeks or greater gestational age and alive at the onset of labor to be 3.4 percent for those who were delivered vaginally and 0 percent for those who were delivered by cesarean section.

With careful selection of cases and using cesarean section 58 percent of the time, Lyons and Papsin (1978) achieved zero perinatal mortality for both vaginal and abdominal breech deliveries of infants who weighed over 2500 g. Nonetheless, morbidity was evident in 5.6 percent of those who were delivered vaginally compared to 0.8 percent in those delivered by cesarean section.

Collea and colleagues (1980) reported the results of a *prospective study* designed to identify the optimal method of delivery of the fetus who presented as a frank breech at term. Of those women who were randomly selected as candidates for vaginal delivery, 46 percent were promptly excluded from further consideration because of possible fetopelvic disproportion based on x-ray pelvimetry. Of the 60 infants who eventually delivered vaginally all survived although two sustained injury to the brachial plexus. In this study there were no maternal deaths, but 73 (49.3 percent) of the 148 women who delivered by cesarean section had significant morbidity compared to only 4 (6.7 percent) of the 60 women who delivered vaginally.

Gimovsky and associates (1983) published the preliminary results of a prospective study designed to identify the optimal method of delivery of the fetus who presented as a *nonfrank* breech at term. One hundred five women with nonfrank breech presentations in labor were entered into the study. Seventy (67 percent) were placed in the group to receive a trial of labor and 35 (33 percent) underwent elective cesarean section. Of those placed in the labor group, 31 (44 percent) delivered vaginally and 39 (56 percent) required cesarean section. The largest single reason for a cesarean section being performed in the trial of labor group was inadequate pelvic dimensions observed by x-ray pelvimetry (23 of the 39, or 59 percent). Neonatal morbidity assessed by Apgar scores, cord blood pH, birth injury, and hospital stay was essentially the same for infants delivered vaginally or by cesarean section except for the one infant who died following a vaginal delivery. This infant death was attributed to inadequate resuscitation. Maternal morbidity in terms of fever, blood transfusions, wound infections and length of hospital stay was significantly greater among women delivered by cesarean section. While this report is an interesting preliminary evaluation of vaginal delivery of nonfrank breeches, the 1 death out of 31 patients allowed to deliver vaginally is in essence "one too many." This rate, if maintained, would be equivalent to a fetal death rate of 32 per 1000. The long-term results in this continuing study may, of course, be much more favorable after additional patients are studied.

Premature Fetus

Vaginal delivery as a breech may be much more hazardous to the premature infant than previously thought. Ingemarsson and associates (1978) compared neonatal mortality and the frequency of subsequent developmental abnormalities in 42 premature breech infants delivered by cesarean section versus 48 premature infants who were delivered vaginally. For those delivered vaginally, six (14.6 percent) succumbed and developmental abnormalities were detected at 12 months in 10 (24 percent) of the survivors, compared to two deaths (4.8 percent) and one with developmental abnormalities (2.5 percent) among those who were delivered by cesarean section. In a paired, controlled retrospective study at Parkland Memorial Hospital of low birth weight infants (below 2500 g) who presented as a breech, Duenhoelter and co-workers (1979) identified mortality, as well as morbidity, to be much more common among those infants who were delivered vaginally. Seven of 44 who were delivered vaginally died (15.9 percent), compared to 1 of 44 (2.3 percent) delivered by cesarean section.

Kauppila and associates (1981) reported from Finland that from 1967 to 1976 infant mortality was significantly higher in breech than in cephalic deliveries and that perinatal mortality and neonatal mortality were 1.8-fold and 2.9-fold greater, respectively. The causes of death were primarily intracranial hemorrhage, fetal asphyxia, and prolapsed cord. However, during the last 5 years of the study, even with an increasing cesarean section rate, this policy did not improve the prognosis for 1500- to 2499-g infants. For infants less than 1500 g, there was a higher incidence of cerebral hemorrhage when delivered vaginally, especially if the infant was a footling breech. They concluded that vaginal delivery of infants 1500 g and larger was justified *if proper fetal monitoring and prompt operative capabilities were present for signs of fetal distress.* With added complications such as hypertension, diabetes, fetal growth retardation, and footling breech presentations, primary cesarean section should be undertaken. For infants less than 1500 g, primary cesarean section was recommended. Crowley and Hawkins (1980) reviewed 11 papers published between 1975 and 1979 and reported that with weights between 1000 and 1500 g (28 to 31 weeks gestation) cesarean section seemed to confer an advantage in survival.

The rather universal acceptance of primary cesarean section for infants less than 2000 g recently has been questioned by two groups of investigators. Cox and associates (1982) compared 1973–74 and 1979–80 morbidity and mortality figures for breech infants under 2500 g delivered at Coventry Maternity Hospital. In 1979–80 a neonatal intensive care unit was operating for the first time and the cesarean section rate had increased from 19.9 percent to 42.2 percent. The stillbirth rate had declined from 24.7 percent to 11.1 percent and the neonatal mortality rate (corrected for lethal congenital abnormalities) had decreased from 23.9 percent to 8.7 percent. Infant survival had increased from 66.2 percent to 82.1 percent. However, the long-term survival rates for *normal* babies in the two periods were 63.1 and 64.1 percent, respectively. The 1973–74 period had 1/21.5 handicapped survivors compared to 1/4.6 in 1979–80. The authors concluded that the perinatal mortality rate had decreased but the increased survival rate was accounted for by the survival of handicapped infants. They further speculated that the increased overall survival rate might have been the result of the neonatal intensive care unit rather than the consequence of the increased cesarean section rate. Effer and associates (1983) reported that perinatal mortality decreased by 20 percent from 1976 to 1980 in very low birth weight infants. During the same time the increased cesarean section rate (11.9 to 49.1 percent) was thought to be responsible for the improved outcome. The changes were most marked

in the less than 1000 g weight group. Survival and cesarean section rates for vertex infants of similar birth weights and gestational ages were analyzed for the same years. A similar or greater reduction in mortality rate (85 to 45 percent) was noted in the very low birth weight vertex infants, while the cesarean section rate only increased from 14.2 percent to 22.2 percent. The authors concluded that no clear interpretation of this study was possible but that any hypothesis must include the possibility that the increased cesarean section rate might be incidental and in no way related to the observed improved outcome and that "as yet unidentified perinatal care practices, other than cesarean section, may be more likely to affect outcome in this high-risk group."

An additional and important consideration must be kept in mind when one considers the route for delivery for a premature breech. As mentioned before, congenital anomalies are numerous, as high a frequency as 24 percent in Ingemarsson and associates series (1978).

Prophylaxis

Whenever a breech presentation is recognized during the third trimester, some obstetricians, but not the majority, believe an attempt should be made by *external version* to substitute a vertex presentation (Chapter 42). External version is more readily accomplished in multiparous women with lax abdominal walls than in nulliparous women. Because of possible trauma, anethesia should never be used.

External version, if properly and gently performed, carries little danger, according to Ranney (1973), who reported his experiences with gentle attempts at external cephalic version in 860 instances of either breech presentation or, less often, transverse lie. The initial attempt was successful 781 times. Although many of the 781 fetuses reverted to an abnormal presentation, repeat attempts at conversion were usually successful. The failure rate during the third trimester increased as pregnancy advanced, with a marked rise after the 36th week. During the study, the overall frequency of breech delivery was only 0.6 percent, or about one sixth the expected frequency. No trauma to the fetus was identified. There was no increase in the frequencies of placental abruption or of hemolytic disease in the newborn infants, although these have been reported by others. Ranney believes that successful version relatively early in the third trimester, as well as lowering the risk associated with vaginal delivery, may reduce the likelihood of prematurity, which is more common with breech presentation.

Based on their experiences with 491 pregnancies in which the fetus presented other than cephalic, Ylikorkala and Hartikainen-Sorri (1977) also concluded that a breech presentation any time during the third trimester warrants attempts at external version. These Finnish workers always used ultrasound to confirm the presentation of the fetus and location of the placenta. In some instances they administered spasmolytic, tocolytic, or analgesic drugs but never anesthesia. They were able to convert the presentation of the fetus to that of vertex in three fourths of their attempts with no serious morbidity identified. The incidence of breech presentation decreased to 2.9 percent from the previous value of 4.5 percent. Thus they were unable to lower the incidence of breech delivery to the remarkably low level achieved by Ranney. Moreover, mean duration of pregnancy was no greater after successful external version than in those pregnancies in which attempts were unsuccessful. Similar results, using sonography and tocolytic agents, have been reported recently by Van Dorsten and associates (1981). A follow-up article by Van Dorsten in 1982 details his technique with visual aids to enhance the description of his method (see Chapter 42, p. 864).

Enthusiasm for external cephalic version is not shared by all. Bradley-Watson (1975), for example, seriously questioned the value of attempting external cephalic version. He attributed the following complications to external cephalic version: Antepartum hemorrhage (3 percent); premature labor (1.2 percent); fetal death (0.9 percent); and premature rupture of membranes (0.6 percent). Chapman and associates (1978) described spinal cord transection in utero after an unsuccessful attempt at external cephalic version. Marcus and associates (1975) identified significant fetomaternal hemorrhage in 6 of 100 pregnancies and Gjøde (1980) reported fetomaternal bleeds in 14 of 50 women during the first attempt at external version. Gjøde recommends that immunoprophylaxis with anti–D globulin be given *prior* to attempting external version in pregnant women who are Rh_o (D) negative (see Chapter 38, p. 773).

Problems with Vaginal Delivery

Major problems do arise from vaginal delivery of a fetus in a breech presentation. Delivery of the breech draws the umbilicus and attached cord into the pelvis, which compresses the cord. Therefore, once the breech has passed beyond the vaginal introitus, the abdomen, thorax, arms, and head must be delivered promptly. This entails the delivery of successively less readily compressible parts. With a mature fetus, some degree of molding of the fetal head may be essential for the head to negotiate the birth canal successfully. In this unfortunate circumstance, the alternatives with vaginal delivery are both unsatisfactory: delivery may be delayed many minutes while the aftercoming head accommodates to the maternal pelvis, but hypoxia and acidosis become severe; or delivery is forced, causing trauma from compression, traction, or both, to the brain, spinal cord, skeleton, and abdominal viscera.

With a premature fetus, the disparity between the size of the head and the buttocks is even greater than with a larger fetus. At times, the buttocks and lower extremities of the premature fetus will pass through the cervix and be delivered, and yet the cervix will not be adequately dilated for the head to escape without trauma to the infant. In this circumstance, Dührssen incisions of the cervix may be tried (see Chapter 41, p. 851).

Even so, trauma to the fetus and mother may be appreciable, and hypoxia in the fetus may prove disastrous. The frequency of prolapsed cord is considerable when the fetus is small or the breech is not of the frank variety.

Recommendations for Delivery

A diligent search for any other complication, actual or anticipated, that might further justify delivery by cesarean section has become a feature of many obstetricians' philosophy for managing delivery in breech presentations. To try to minimize infant mortality and morbidity, cesarean section is now commonly used in the following circumstances to deliver all but the very immature fetus whose potential for survival is negligible:

1. Breech presentation and a large fetus.
2. Breech presentation and any degree of contraction or unfavorable shape of the pelvis.
3. Breech presentation and a hyperextended head.
4. Breech presentation not in labor, with maternal or fetal indications for delivery such as pregnancy-induced hypertension or rupture of the membranes for 12 hours or more.
5. Breech presentation and uterine dysfunction.
6. Footling breech presentation.
7. Breech presentation, an apparently healthy but premature fetus of 26 weeks or more gestation, with the mother in either active labor or in need of delivery.
8. Breech presentation and severe fetal growth retardation.
9. Breech presentation and previous perinatal death or children suffering from birth trauma.
10. Breech presentation and a firm request by the mother for sterilization.

Large Fetus. The experiences of Rovinsky and associates (1973) as well as others, have been that morbidity and mortality rates for the fetus at term increase with birth weight. Therefore, the fetus estimated to weigh 3500 g (8 pounds) or more would often benefit from delivery by cesarean section even though the mother's pelvis appears adequate. This allows for underestimation of fetal weight, a relatively common phenomenon when the fetus is large. With the head free in the uterine fundus, sonographic measurements of the biparietal diameter to estimate fetal size, unfortunately, are more likely to be erroneous than with a vertex presentation, as is pointed out in Chapter 31 (p. 678). Nonetheless, the obstetrician could feel much more secure about the estimate of fetal size if there were good agreement between the clinical and sonographic estimates.

Unfavorable Pelvis. In contrast to labor with a cephalic presentation, there is no time for molding of the aftercoming head. Therefore, a moderately contracted pelvis that had not previously caused problems in delivery of

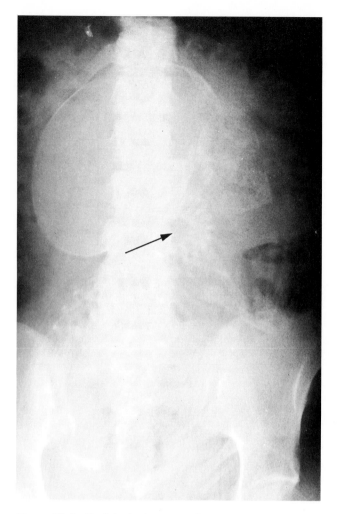

Figure 30-3. Radiologic demonstration of a complete breech presentation with a markedly hyperextended cervical spine (*arrow*) and head. Delivery by cesarean section resulted in a normal newborn infant.

an average size fetus who presented as a vertex might prove dangerous if the fetus were presenting as a breech. Rovinsky and colleagues (1973) urge not only accurate measurements of pelvic dimensions but also precise evaluation of the pelvic architecture rather than reliance on pelvic indexes. Gynecoid (round) and anthropoid (elliptical) pelves are favorable configurations, but platypelloid (anteroposteriorly flat) and android (heart-shaped) pelves are not (see Chapter 11, p. 225). The platypelloid pelvis typically is narrowed anteroposteriorly, which is unfavorable for the aftercoming head. The android pelvis has a narrow forepelvis, which renders the inlet less favorable than the pelvic diameters would suggest.

Hyperextension of Fetal Head. In perhaps 5 percent or less of cases of breech presentation at or near term, a roentgenogram shows the fetal head to be in extreme hyperextension (Fig. 30-3). Most often the cause of the hyperextension is not apparent (Caterini and colleagues, 1975). Vaginal delivery may result in considerable injury to the cervical spinal cord, as reemphasized by Abroms and associates (1973) and Bhagwanani and associates (1973). In general, radiologic evidence of marked hyperextension of the fetal head after labor has been established as an indication for cesarean section.

No Labor or Uterine Dysfunction. Induction of labor in women with a breech presentation is defended by some and condemned by others. Brenner and colleagues (1974) noted no significant differences in mortality rates and Apgar scores between cases with induced labor and those with spontaneous labor. In instances in which oxytocin was used to augment labor, however, infant mortality rates were higher and Apgar scores were lower. Gimovsky and Paul (1982) observed that augmentation of labor was followed by vaginal delivery in two of nine women, both multiparous, but one of the two deliveries resulted in entrapment of the aftercoming head. The general policy at Parkland Memorial Hospital is to resort to cesarean delivery, rather than oxytocin to induce or augment labor, unless the fetus is very immature or has a severe anomaly.

Footling Breech Presentations. The possibility of compression of a prolapsed cord or a cord entangled around the extremities as the breech fills the pelvis, if not before, is a threat to the fetus.

Premature Delivery. If the fetus is premature, the aftercoming head may be trapped by a cervix that is sufficiently effaced and dilated to allow passage of the thorax but not the less compressible head. The consequences of vaginal delivery in this circumstance all too often have been both hypoxia and physical trauma, both of which are especially deleterious to the premature infant. Delivery of the apparently healthy, although premature, fetus by cesarean section reduces the risks of hypoxia, birth trauma, and their sequelae.

Previous Pregnancy Wastage. The compelling desire to minimize any likelihood of trauma to the fetus may lead to the decision to perform cesarean section.

Desire for Sterilization. For the woman with a breech presentation who desires sterilization, the risk of cesarean section to accomplish delivery and sterilization is no greater, and probably less, than the summation of risks from vaginal breech delivery followed by celiotomy for sterilization.

Vaginal Delivery

Vaginal delivery should be relatively safe for a frank breech presentation if (1) the pelvis is in no way contracted when examined by x-ray pelvimetry [a previous cephalic delivery by itself is not proof that the pelvis may not be "contracted" for a breech delivery (Bistoletti, 1981)]; (2) the fetus is judged not to be unusually large (less than 8 pounds) when examined independently by two or more trained examiners or when estimated sonographically; (3) spontaneous labor is demonstrated to effect orderly effacement and dilatation of the cervix and descent of the breech through the birth canal; and (4) individuals skilled in breech delivery, in providing appropriate anesthesia, and in infant resuscitation are in immediate attendance. Even when every attempt is made to fulfill these criteria, the outcome for the infant is not always as good as when cesarean section is performed (Collea and co-workers, 1980; Gimovsky and Paul, 1982).

The physician who might naively champion any childbirth outside of a hospital setting is either not aware of the hazards of breech delivery in such a setting or is totally insensitive to the welfare of the fetus and the mother. The techniques and precautions for vaginal delivery are detailed in Chapter 42.

Cesarean Section

There is little question that perinatal mortality and morbidity from trauma and hypoxia can be reduced by liberal use of cesarean section. Even for fetuses at term (2500 g or more), Rovinsky and associates (1973) concluded from their analyses that cesarean section improved the outcome for the fetus. During the 17-year period studied by them, the use of cesarean section for breech delivery increased dramatically.

This same trend in most training institutions towards delivery by cesarean section of the majority of fetuses that present as a breech means that one important criterion for safe vaginal delivery is becoming more and more difficult to fulfill: most resident training programs within the near future will not provide sufficient opportunity for acquisition of skills essential for successful vaginal breech delivery.

At Parkland Memorial Hospital, cesarean section is used very liberally for breech delivery. In recent years, nearly three fourths of fetuses presenting by the breech have been delivered by cesarean section. This value is remarkably greater than, for example, the cesarean section rate of 10.7 percent reported for breech deliveries in 1956 by Hall and Kohl.

Summary

The fetus in the breech position is likely to benefit from cesarean section carried out early in labor, if not before, but at the expense of an appreciable increase in maternal morbidity and a slight increase in maternal mortality. It is anticipated that the prevailing enthusiasm for offspring of the highest quality but of limited number will continue to stimulate frequent use of cesarean section for breech delivery.

FACE PRESENTATION

In a face presentation, the head is hyperextended so that the occiput is in contact with the fetal back and the chin (mentum) is the presenting part.

Incidence

Cruikshank and White (1973) reported an incidence of 1 in 600, or 0.17 percent; the Obstetrical Statistical Cooperative identified a similar frequency of 0.2 percent. Of 33,562 infants who were delivered at Parkland Memorial Hospital, 0.3 percent presented as a face.

Diagnosis

Although abdominal findings may be suggestive, the clinical diagnosis of face presentation must rest on vaginal examination. On vaginal palpation, the distinctive features of the face are the mouth and nose, the malar bones, and particularly the orbital ridges. It is possible to mistake a breech presentation for a face, since the anus may be mistaken for the mouth and the ischial tuberosities for the malar prominences. The fetal anus is always on a line with the ischial tuberosities, however, whereas the fetal mouth and malar prominences form the corners of a triangle. The roentgenographic demonstration of the hyperextended head with the facial bones at or below the pelvic inlet is quite characteristic (Fig. 30-4).

Etiology

The causes of face presentations are numerous, generally stemming from any factor that favors extension or prevents flexion of the head. Extended positions of the head, therefore, occur more frequently when the pelvis is contracted or the fetus is very large. In a series of 141 face presentations studied by Hellman and co-workers (1950), the incidence of inlet contraction was 39.4 percent. This high incidence of pelvic contraction, as well as large infants, must be kept in mind when considering the successful management of face presentation.

In multiparous women, the pendulous abdomen is another factor that predisposes to face presentation. It permits the back of the fetus to sag forward or laterally, often in the same direction in which the occiput points, thus promoting extension of the cervical and thoracic spine.

In exceptional instances, marked enlargement of the neck or coils of cord about the neck may cause extension. Anencephalic fetuses naturally present by the face because of faulty development of the cranium.

Mechanism. Face presentations are rarely observed above the pelvic inlet. The brow generally presents and is converted to a face presentation after further extension of the head during descent through the pelvis.

The mechanism of labor in these cases consists of

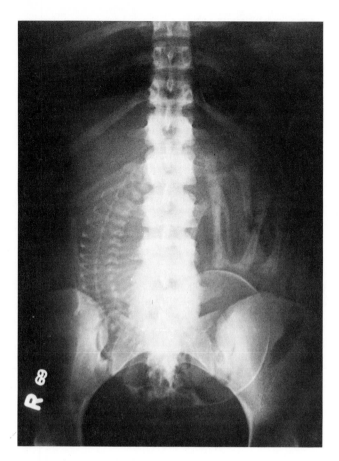

Figure 30-4. Roentgenogram showing face presentation. Note marked hyperextension of head and spine of fetus.

the cardinal movements of descent, internal rotation, and flexion, and the accessory movements of extension and external rotation. Descent is brought about by the same factors as in vertex presentations. Extension results from the relation of the fetal body to the deflected head, which is converted into a two-armed lever, the longer arm of which extends from the occipital condyles to the occiput. When resistance is then encountered, the occiput must be pushed toward the back of the fetus while the chin descends (Fig. 30-5).

The object of internal rotation of the face is to bring the chin under the symphysis pubis. Unless the head is unusually small, natural delivery cannot otherwise be accomplished. Only in this way can the neck subtend the posterior surface of the symphysis pubis. If the chin rotates directly posteriorly, the relatively short neck cannot span the anterior surface of the sacrum, which measures about 12 cm in length (Fig. 30-5). Hence, the birth of the head is manifestly impossible unless the shoulders enter the pelvis at the same time, an event that is out of the question except when the fetus is markedly premature or macerated. Internal rotation in a face presentation results from the same factors as in vertex presentations.

After anterior-rotation and descent, the chin and mouth appear at the vulva, the undersurface of the chin presses against the symphysis, and the head is delivered by flexion (Fig. 30-6). The nose, eyes, brow (bregma), and occiput then appear in succession over the anterior margin of the perineum. After the birth of the head, the occiput sags backward toward the anus. In a few moments, the chin rotates externally to the side toward which it was originally directed, and the shoulders are born as in vertex presentations.

Edema may sometimes distort the face sufficiently to obliterate the features and lead to erroneous diagnosis of breech presentation (Fig. 30-7). At the same time, the skull undergoes considerable molding, manifested by increase in length of the occipitomental diameter of the head.

Treatment

In the absence of a contracted pelvis and the presence of effective spontaneous labor with no evidence of fetal distress, successful vaginal delivery will usually follow. As pointed out above, face presentations among term-size fetuses occur more commonly when there is some degree of contraction of the pelvic inlet. Therefore, cesarean section often proves to be the best method for their delivery.

Other methods of management of face presentations are rarely, if ever, indicated in modern obstetrics. Outmoded are attempts to convert manually a face to a vertex presentation, manual or forceps rotation of a persistently posterior chin to a mentum anterior position, and internal podalic version and extraction. All are likely to be unduly traumatic to both fetus and mother.

BROW PRESENTATION

With a brow presentation, that portion of the fetal head between the orbital ridge and the anterior fontanel presents at the pelvic inlet. The fetal head thus occupies a position midway between full flexion (occiput) and full extension (mentum or face). Except when the fetal head is small or the pelvis is unusually large, engagement of the fetal head and subsequent delivery cannot take place as long as the brow presentation persists.

Etiology

The causes of persistent brow presentation are essentially the same as those of face presentation. The brow presentation is commonly unstable and converts to a face or an occiput presentation. Cruikshank and White (1973), for example, observed either flexion to an occiput presentation or extension to a face presentation to take place in two thirds of cases in which the presentation was initially that of the brow.

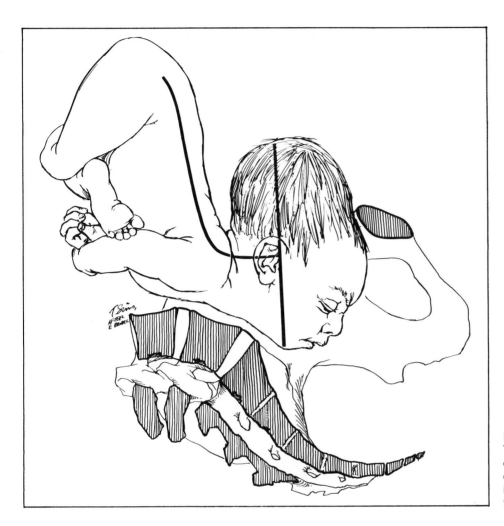

Figure 30-5. Face presentation. The occiput is on the longer end of the head lever. The chin is directly posterior. Vaginal delivery is impossible unless the chin rotates anteriorly.

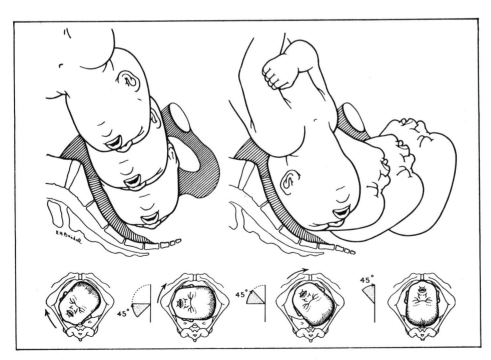

Figure 30-6. Mechanism of labor for right mentoposterior position with subsequent rotation of mentum anterior and delivery.

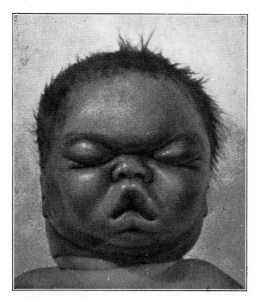

Figure 30-7. Edema in face presentation.

Diagnosis

The presentation may be recognized by abdominal palpation when both the occiput and chin can be easily palpated, but vaginal examination is usually necessary. The frontal sutures, large anterior fontanel, orbital ridges, eyes, and root of the nose can be felt on vaginal examination. Neither mouth nor chin is within reach however (Figs. 30-8, 30-9).

Mechanism

The mechanism of labor varies greatly with the size of the fetus. With a small fetus and a large pelvis, labor is generally easy. With larger fetuses, however, it is usually very difficult, since engagement is impossible until after marked molding that shortens the occipitomental diameter, or, more commonly, either flexion to an occiput presentation or extension to a face presentation.

The considerable molding essential for delivery of the fetus where the brow presentation persists characteristically deforms the head. The caput succedaneum is over the forehead and may be so extensive that identification of the brow by palpation is impossible. In these instances, the forehead is prominent and squared, and the occipitomental diameter is diminished.

Prognosis

In the transient varieties of brow presentation, the prognosis depends upon the ultimate presentation. When the brow presentation persists, the prognosis is poor for vaginal delivery of an uncompromised infant unless the fetus is small or the birth canal is huge.

Treatment

The principles underlying the treatment of brow presentations are much the same as those for a face presentation. If, by chance, spontaneous labor is progressing without any evidence of distress in the closely monitored fetus and without unduly vigorous uterine contractions, no interference is necessary. If labor becomes either unduly vigorous, or, more likely, ineffective, or if fetal distress is suspected, prompt cesarean section is indicated.

SHOULDER PRESENTATION

In this condition, the long axis of the fetus is approximately perpendicular to that of the mother, that is, a *transverse lie*. When the long axis forms an acute angle, an *oblique lie* results. An oblique lie is usually only transitory, however, for either a longitudinal or transverse lie commonly results when labor supervenes. For this reason, the oblique lie is termed *unstable lie* in Great Britain.

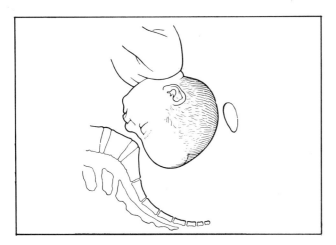

Figure 30-8. Brow posterior presentation.

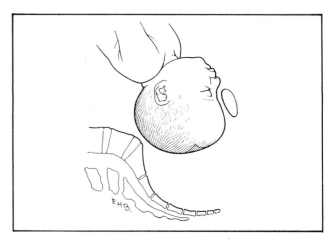

Figure 30-9. Brow anterior presentation.

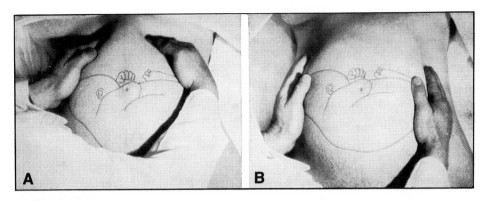

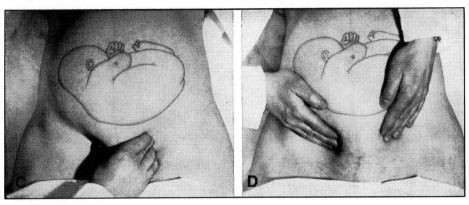

Figure 30-10. Palpation in transverse lie, right acromiodorsoanterior position. **A.** First maneuver. **B.** Second maneuver. **C.** Third maneuver. **D.** Fourth maneuver.

In transverse lies, the shoulder is usually over the pelvic inlet, with the head lying in one iliac fossa and the breech in the other. This condition is referred to as a *shoulder* or an *acromion presentation*. The side of the mother toward which the acromion is directed determines the designation of the lie as right or left acromial. Moreover, since in either position the back may be directed anteriorly or posteriorly, superiorly or inferiorly, it is customary to distinguish varieties as dorsoanterior and dorsoposterior.

Incidence

Transverse lie occurred once in 322 singleton deliveries (0.3 percent) at both the Mayo Clinic and the University of Iowa Hospitals (Johnson, 1964; Cruikshank and White, 1973). At Parkland Memorial Hospital the incidence was 0.4 percent among 33,562 deliveries.

Etiology

The common causes of transverse lie are (1) unusual relaxation of the abdominal wall resulting from great multiparity, (2) prematurity, (3) placenta previa, and (4) contracted pelvis. The incidence of transverse lie increases with parity, occurring approximately ten times more frequently in patients of parity of four or more than in nulliparous women. Relaxation of the abdominal wall with a pendulous abdomen allows the uterus to fall forward, deflecting the long axis of the fetus away from

the axis of the birth canal into an oblique or transverse position. Placenta previa and pelvic contraction act similarly. A transverse or oblique lie occasionally develops in labor from an initial longitudinal position, the head or breech migrating to one of the iliac fossae.

Diagnosis

The diagnosis of a transverse lie is usually readily made, often by inspection alone. The abdomen is unusually wide from side to side, whereas the fundus of the uterus extends scarcely above the umbilicus.

On palpation, with the first maneuver no fetal pole is detected in the fundus. On the second maneuver, a ballottable head is found in one iliac fossa and the breech in the other. The third and fourth maneuvers are negative unless labor is well advanced and the shoulder has become impacted in the pelvis (Figs. 30-10, 30-11). At the same time, the position of the back is readily identified. When the back is anterior, a hard resistance plane extends across the front of the abdomen; when it is posterior, irregular nodulations representing the small parts are felt in the same location (Figs. 30-10, 30-11).

On vaginal examination, in the early stages of labor, the side of the thorax, if it can be reached, may be recognized by the "gridiron" feel of the ribs above the pelvic inlet. When dilatation is further advanced, the scapula and the clavicle are distinguished on opposite sides of the thorax. The position of the axilla indicates the side of the mother toward which the shoulder is

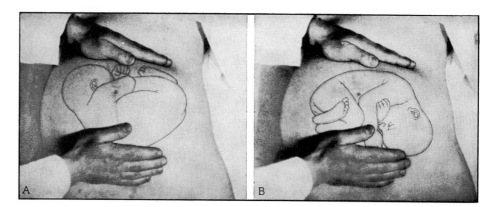

Figure 30-11. Transverse lie, palpation of back in dorsoanterior **(A)** and in dorsoposterior **(B)** positions.

directed. Later in labor, the shoulder becomes tightly wedged in the pelvic canal, and a hand and arm frequently prolapse into the vagina and through the vulva (Figs. 30-12, 30-13).

Course of Labor

The spontaneous birth of a fully developed infant is manifestly impossible in a persistent transverse lie, since expulsion cannot be effected unless both the head and trunk of the fetus enter the pelvis at the same time. At term, therefore, both the fetus and the mother will die unless appropriate measures are instituted.

After the rupture of the membranes, if the mother is left to herself, the fetal shoulder is forced into the pelvis, and the corresponding arm frequently prolapses (Fig. 30-13). After some descent, the shoulder is arrested by the margins of the pelvic inlet, with the head in one iliac fossa and the breech in the other. As labor continues, the shoulder is firmly impacted in the upper part of the pelvis. The uterus than contracts vigorously in an unsuccessful attempt to overcome the obstacle. After a time, a retraction ring rises increasingly higher and becomes more marked. The situation is referred to as neglected transverse lie. If not vigorously and properly treated, the uterus eventually ruptures and the mother, as well as the fetus, die.

If the fetus is quite small and the pelvis large, spontaneous delivery may occur despite persistence of the abnormal lie. In such cases, the fetus is compressed with the head forced against the abdomen. A portion of the thoracic wall below the shoulder thus becomes the most dependent part, appearing at the vulva. The head and thorax then pass through the pelvic cavity at the same time, and the fetus, which is doubled upon itself (*conduplicato corpore*), is expelled. Such a mechanism obviously is possible only in the case of very small infants and occasionally when the second fetus in a twin pregnancy is prematurely born.

Prognosis

Labor with shoulder presentation increases the maternal risk and adds tremendously to the fetal hazard. Most maternal deaths from this complication occur in ne-

glected cases from spontaneous rupture of the uterus or traumatic rupture consequent upon late and ill-advised version and extraction. Even with the best of care, however, the chance of maternal death will be increased slightly for four reasons: (1) the frequent association of transverse lie with placenta previa, (2) the increased likelihood of cord accidents, (3) the almost inevitable necessity of major operative interference, and (4) the likelihood of sepsis after rupture of the membranes and extrusion of the arm through the vagina.

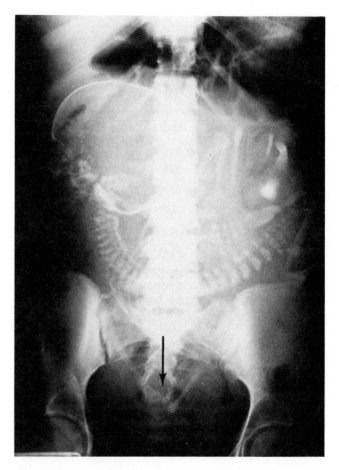

Figure 30-12. Roentgenogram of a transverse lie which illustrates an elbow (*arrow*) at the level of the cervix.

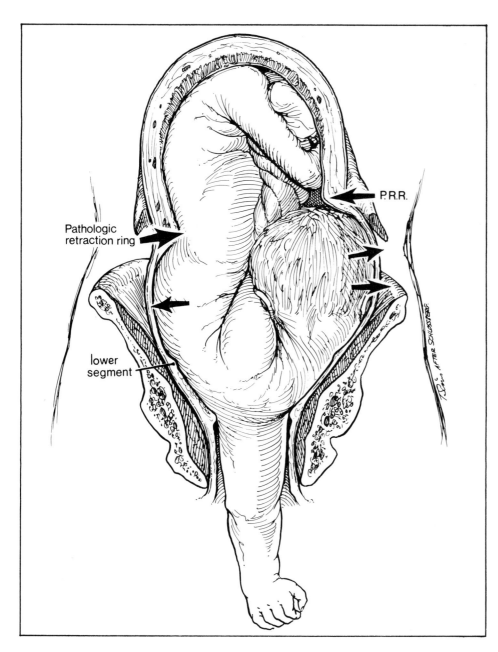

Figure 30-13. Neglected shoulder presentation. A thick muscular band to form a pathologic retraction ring has developed just above the very thin lower uterine segment. The force generated during a uterine contraction is directed centripetally at and above the level of the pathologic retraction ring. This serves to stretch further and possibly to rupture the very thin lower segment below the retraction ring. P.R.R. =pathologic retraction ring.

Management

In general, the onset of active labor in a woman with a transverse lie is an indication for cesarean section. Once labor is well established, attempts at conversion to a longitudinal lie by abdominal manipulation are not likely to be successful. Before labor or early in labor, with the membranes intact, attempts at external version are worthy of a trial in the absence of other obstetric complications that point toward cesarean section. If during early labor the fetal head can be maneuvered by abdominal manipulation into the pelvis, it should be held there during the next several contractions to try to fix the head in the pelvis. The fetal heart rate must be closely checked during this time. If these measures fail in the woman in labor, cesarean section should be performed promptly. Internal podalic version is rarely, if ever, indicated (see Chapter 42, p. 866).

Because neither the feet nor the vertex of the fetus occupies the lower uterine segment, a low transverse incision into the uterus may lead to difficulty in extraction of a fetus entrapped in the body of the uterus above the level of the incision. A vertical incision is therefore generally favored. The treatment of neglected transverse lie entails support in the form of antibiotics, fluid therapy, and transfusion if needed. Delivery may be accomplished abdominally by cesarean section or cesarean section–hysterectomy, as the situation demands (see Chapter 43, p. 871, 879).

If the cervix is fully dilated and the fetus is dead, decapitation by means of a blunt hook and scissors or sickle knife may permit vaginal delivery. However, since destructive procedures may rupture the uterus, cesarean section or cesarean hysterectomy is almost always preferable, even with a dead baby.

COMPOUND PRESENTATION

In compound presentation, an extremity prolapses alongside the presenting part with both entering the pelvis simultaneously (Fig. 30-14).

Incidence

Goplerud and Eastman (1953) identified a hand or arm prolapsed alongside the head once in every 700 deliveries. Much less common was prolapse of one or both lower extremities alongside a vertex presentation or a hand alongside a breech presentation. Weissberg and O'Leary (1973) described compound presentations among infants that weighed 1500 g or more to occur once in 1600 deliveries.

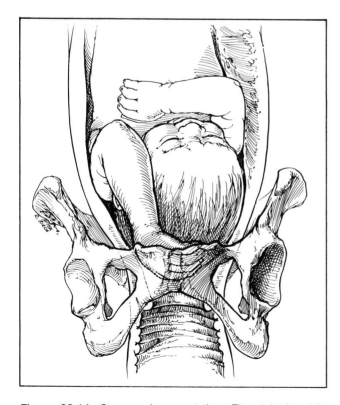

Figure 30-14. Compound presentation. The right hand is lying in front of the vertex. With further labor, the hand and arm may retract from the birth canal and the head descend normally.

Etiology

As expected, the causes of compound presentation are conditions that prevent complete occlusion of the pelvic inlet by the fetal head. In Goplerud and Eastman's series, the incidence of prematurity was twice the expected rate. Often, however, no cause is demonstrable.

Prognosis

Although the reported perinatal loss is above 25 percent, a major portion of the wastage is contributed by prematurity, prolapsed cord, and traumatic obstetric procedures.

Management

In most cases, the prolapsed part should be left alone, since most often it will not interfere with labor. In Goplerud and Eastman's series of 50 cases not associated with prolapse of the cord, 24, or almost one half, had no treatment. Normal delivery ensued in all, with the loss of one infant. If the arm is prolapsed alongside the head, the condition should be observed closely to ascertain whether the arm rises out of the way with descent of the presenting part. If it fails to do so and if it appears to prevent descent of the head, the prolapsed arm should be gently pushed upward and the head simultaneously downward by fundal pressure. Whenever fetal distress is detected, cesarean section is the treatment of choice.

PERSISTENT OCCIPUT POSTERIOR POSITIONS

Most often, occiput posterior positions undergo spontaneous anterior rotation followed by uncomplicated delivery. In 10 percent or less of cases, spontaneous rotation does not occur. Although the precise reasons for failure of spontaneous rotation are not known, transverse narrowing of the midpelvis undoubtedly plays a role.

The conduct of labor and delivery with the occiput posterior need not differ remarkably from that with the occiput anterior. The status of the fetus is monitored by continuous internal electronic techniques or by frequently measuring the fetal heart rate during and especially immediately after a contraction. Progress of labor may be ascertained by checking the rate and extent of cervical dilatation and the descent of the fetal head through the birth canal. In most instances, delivery can usually be accomplished without great difficulty once the head reaches the perineum.

The possibilities for vaginal delivery are (1) await spontaneous delivery, (2) forceps delivery with the occiput directly posterior, (3) forceps rotation of the occiput to the anterior position and delivery, or (4) manual rotation to the anterior position followed by spontaneous or forceps delivery.

Spontaneous Delivery

If the pelvic outlet is roomy and the vaginal outlet and perineum are somewhat relaxed from previous vaginal deliveries, rapid spontaneous delivery will often take place. If the vaginal outlet is resistant to stretch and the perineum is firm, the deceleration portion of the labor curve and/or the second stage of labor may be prolonged appreciably before spontaneous delivery will occur (see Chapter 29, p. 646). During each expulsive effort, with the occiput posterior, the head is driven against the perineum to a much greater degree than when the occiput is anterior. Therefore, forceps delivery after suitable episiotomy often is indicated.

Forceps Delivery as an Occiput Posterior

The need for more traction compared to forceps deliveries from the occiput anterior position can be minimized by making a larger episiotomy. In most instances, a mediolateral incision should be made to avoid lacerations into the anus and rectum. The use of forceps and a large episiotomy warrant more complete anesthesia than may be achieved with pudendal block and local perineal infiltration. The forceps are applied bilaterally along the occipitomental diameter, as described in Chapter 41 (p. 847).

It is important to identify the infrequent case in which the protrusion of fetal scalp through the introitus is the consequence of marked elongation of the fetal head from molding combined with the formation of a large caput. In this circumstance, the head may not even be engaged, that is, the biparietal diameter has not yet passed through the pelvic inlet. Labor characteristically has been long in such a case and, in turn, descent of the head has been slow. Careful palpation above the symphysis discloses the fetal head to be present above the pelvic inlet. Prompt cesarean section is the appropriate method of delivery. It may be necessary at the time of operation to have an associate insert a sterile gloved hand into the vagina to dislodge the head upward.

Forceps Rotation

If the head is engaged, the cervix fully dilated, and the pelvis is adequate, forceps rotation may be attempted if the operator is sufficiently skilled to do so. These circumstances are most likely to prevail when expulsive efforts of the mother during the second stage are ineffective, as, for example, with continuous regional anesthesia. Rotation by the so-called Scanzoni maneuver or with Kielland forceps is described in Chapter 41 (p. 847).

Manual Rotation

The requirements for forceps rotation must be met. When the hand is introduced to locate the posterior ear and thus confirm the posterior position, the occiput often rotates toward the anterior position. The head may be grasped with the fingers over the posterior ear and the thumb over the anterior ear and an attempt made to rotate the occiput to the anterior position (see Chapter 41, p. 847).

Outcome

Phillips and Freeman (1974) have reviewed the extensive experiences with occiput posterior positions at Grady Memorial Hospital, Atlanta, Georgia. Basic management of the persistent occiput posterior position was similar to that for the occiput anterior position, namely, delivery without manual or forceps rotation. Compared to the occiput anterior position, labor was prolonged on the average 1 hour in parous women and 2 hours in nulliparous women. The perinatal mortality rate of 2.2 percent did not differ significantly from the 1.8 percent for the occiput anterior group. No significant rise in Apgar scores of less than 7 was found. Extension of the episiotomy, however, was increased appreciably. Phillips and Freeman (1974) comment that midline episiotomies are not acceptable for occiput posterior deliveries and, instead, adequate mediolateral incisions should be made.

At Parkland Memorial Hospital, either manual rotation to the anterior position followed by forceps delivery, or forceps delivery from the occiput posterior position, is used to effect delivery. When neither can be done with relative ease, cesarean section is performed.

PERSISTENT OCCIPUT TRANSVERSE POSITION

In the absence of an abnormality of the pelvic architecture, the occiput transverse position is most likely a transitory one as the occiput rotates to the anterior position. If hypotonic uterine dysfunction, either spontaneous or the consequence of anesthesia, does not develop, spontaneous rotation is usually soon completed, thus allowing the choice of spontaneous delivery or delivery with outlet forceps.

Delivery

If rotation ceases because of lack of uterine action and in the absence of pelvic contraction, vaginal delivery usually can be readily accomplished in a number of ways: The occiput may be manually rotated anteriorly or posteriorly and forceps delivery carried out from either the anterior or posterior position. Another approach recommended by some is to apply forceps of the Kielland type to the head in the occiput transverse position (see Chapter 41, p. 848), rotate the occiput to the anterior position, and then deliver the head with either the same forceps or with standard outlet forceps. If the failure of spontaneous rotation of the head is caused by hypotonic uterine dysfunction *without cephalopelvic disproportion,* dilute oxytocin may be infused while the fetal heart rate and the uterine contractions are closely monitored.

The genesis of the occiput transverse position is not always so simple, nor is the treatment so benign. With the platypelloid (anteroposteriorly flat configuration) pelvis and the android (heart-shaped) pelvis, there may not be adequate room for rotation of the occiput to either the anterior or the posterior position. With the android pelvis, the head may not even be engaged, yet the scalp may be visible through the vaginal introitus as the consequence of considerable molding and caput formation. This situation, sometimes referred to as *deep transverse arrest,* is fraught with danger to both the fetus and the mother. If forceps are tried for delivery, it is imperative that undue force not be applied but, instead, delivery be accomplished by cesarean section.

FETAL MACROSOMIA

Birth weights rarely exceed 11 pounds (5000 g), although in 1979 the birth of an infant who weighed 16 pounds (7300 g) was widely reported in the United States. Postpartum, delayed glucose metabolism was detected in the mother. She had previously given birth to several infants who weighed 9 and 10 pounds. Certainly one of the largest infants on record weighed 23.75 pounds (10,800 g), as reported by Beach in 1879 (Barnes, 1957).

Several factors, alone or in combination, may be operative in the genesis of macrosomia. These include (1) large size of the parents, especially the mother, (2) multiparity, (3) diabetes in the mother, (4) maternal obesity, (5) prolonged gestation, and (6) previous delivery of an infant weighing more than 4000 g (Houchang and co-workers, 1980).

With large fetuses, dystocia may arise because the head becomes not only larger but harder and less moldable with increasing weight. Moreover, after the head has passed through the pelvic canal, dystocia may be caused by the arrest of even larger shoulders at either the pelvic brim or outlet (Fig. 30-15).

Incidence

It is common practice to designate all newborn infants weighing 4000 g or more as "excessive-sized." The incidence of these infants in more than 104,000 deliveries in the Obstetrical Statistical Cooperative was 5.3 percent, and the incidence of infants weighing 4500 g or more was 0.4 percent. Interestingly, among the often socio-economically deprived, predominantly black population with a relatively low prevalence of diabetes cared for at Parkland Memorial Hospital, the frequency of birth weights of 4000 g or more among 20,000 deliveries was 5.1 percent.

Diagnosis

Inasmuch as the clinical estimation of the size of the fetus may be inaccurate, the diagnosis of excessive size is often not made until after fruitless attempts at delivery. Nevertheless, competent clinical examination should enable experienced examiners to arrive at a fairly accurate estimate. Sonographic evaluation of the dimensions of the head, thorax, and abdomen often enhances appreciably the confidence of the estimate (Wladimiroff and colleagues, 1978).

Serious dystocia may arise when an excessively large head attempts to pass through a normal pelvis, just as when the head of an average size fetus is arrested by a definitely contracted pelvic inlet. At times, the head is delivered without great difficulty but the large shoulder girdle becomes entrapped. Dystocia from a large shoulder girdle is discussed subsequently.

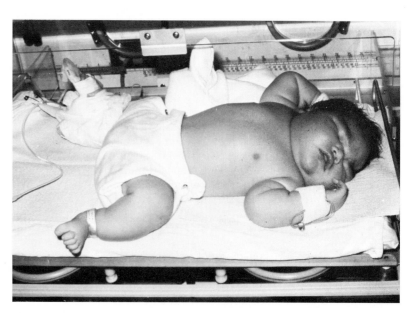

Figure 30-15. This infant weighed 6065 g and was delivered by cesarean section. Delayed glucose metabolism ("gestational diabetes") was detected in the mother.

Prognosis

Since excessive-sized infants are more often born to multiparous mothers and to women with diabetes, both the maternal and fetal risks are increased. In a report on 766 infants who weighed over 4500 g, Sack (1969) cited a perinatal loss of 7.2 percent. More distressing, 16 percent of the infants were severely depressed at birth, 11.4 percent had severe neurologic complications, and 4.5 percent of those who survived the perinatal period were dead before the age of 7 years.

SHOULDER DYSTOCIA

Shoulder dystocia is a serious complication of delivery. The problem is that the head is delivered, causing the cord to be drawn into the pelvis and compressed before it is realized that the shoulders cannot be delivered.

Incidence

Swartz's review (1960) of experiences with shoulder girdle dystocia indicated an incidence of 0.15 percent for all fetuses who weighed more than 2500 g, but an incidence in infants over 4000 g of 1.7 percent. An analysis of experiences at Los Angeles County–University of Southern California Medical Center has served to reemphasize the increased likelihood of shoulder dystocia following a prolonged second stage of labor managed by instrumental vaginal delivery of the head from the midpelvis (Benedetti, Gabbe, 1978). With a prolonged second stage and midpelvic delivery, the incidence of shoulder dystocia was 4.57 percent compared to 0.16 percent in the absence of a prolonged second stage of labor.

Prevention

Elliott and associates (1982) have observed that a transthoracic diameter for an infant of a diabetic mother of 1.4 cm greater than the head circumference served as a predictor of significant fetomaternal disproportion and as such correlated with the possibility of shoulder dystocia. This work was the extension of their previous work with Houchang and associates (1980, 1982), who actually measured newborns over 4000 g. As a result of this study, they reported that a chest minus head circumference difference of 1.6 cm or more or a shoulder minus head circumference of 4.8 cm or more indicated a high likelihood of shoulder dystocia. They recommended that, if such measurements could be obtained in potential candidates for shoulder dystocia, either primary cesarean section be done or, if vaginal delivery were considered, that plans be made to assure the presence of a physician experienced in the delivery of infants with shoulder dystocia plus appropriate anesthesia and pediatric support must be present in order to help minimize the occurrence and sequelae of traumatic deliveries.

Management

There will always be the unexpected case, despite a carefully obtained history that may identify the likelihood of a shoulder dystocia developing and despite the possibility of sonographic evidence being used to identify candidates in whom this complication is likely to occur. Therefore, the practitioner of obstetrics *must* be well versed in the management principles of this occasionally devastating complication.

Reduction in the interval of time from delivery of the head to delivery of the body is of great importance to survival, but overly vigorous traction on the head or neck, or excessive rotation of the body, may cause serious damage to the infant. Infrequently, deliberate fracture of the clavicle may be necessary and lifesaving to the infant. A large mediolateral episiotomy and adequate anesthesia are necessary.

The first step is to clear the infant's mouth and nose. Next, avoiding unnecessary force, the operator sweeps the posterior arm across the chest and delivers it. The shoulder girdle is then rotated into one of the oblique diameters of the pelvis. The anterior shoulder can usually be delivered at this point.

Woods (1943) suggested another method, which utilizes the principle of a screw. The operator applies pressure to the infant's posterior scapula to rotate upward. The posterior shoulder then passes beneath the symphysis in a screwlike motion and is delivered as an anterior shoulder.

Benedetti and Gabbe (1978) recommended that the method suggested by Woods be tried first and if unsuccessful the posterior arm then be delivered. Should both these methods fail, the last measure should be the deliberate fracture of the clavicle of the impacted shoulder. Although this policy may appear excessive, the fracture will heal. Damage to cervical nerve roots may leave permanent sequelae. Prompt, appropriate physiotherapy can often reduce the degree of permanent damage (Chapter 39, p. 795).

HYDROCEPHALUS AS A CAUSE OF DYSTOCIA

Internal hydrocephalus, or excessive accumulation of cerebrospinal fluid in the ventricles of the brain with consequent enlargement of the cranium, occurs in about one in 2000 fetuses and accounts for about 12 percent of all severe malformations found at birth. Associated defects are common, with spina bifida occurring in about one third of cases. Not infrequently, the circumference of the head exceeds 50 cm, and sometimes reaches 80 cm. The volume of fluid is usually between 500 and 1500 ml, but as much as 5 liters may accumulate. Breech presentation is found in about one third of these cases. Whatever the presentation, gross cephalopelvic disproportion is the rule, with serious dystocia as the usual consequence (Figs. 30-16, 30-17).

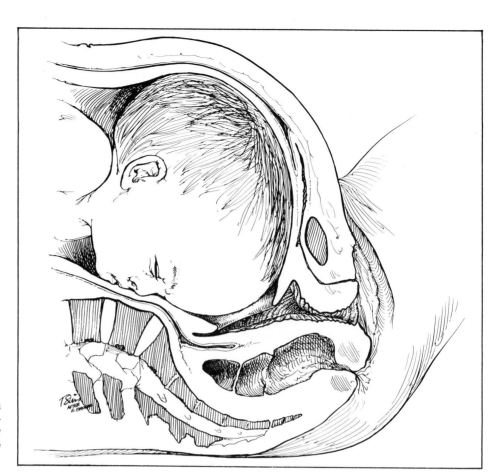

Figure 30-16. Severe dystocia from hydrocephalus, cephalic presentation. Note the disparity between the small size of the face and the rest of the cranium.

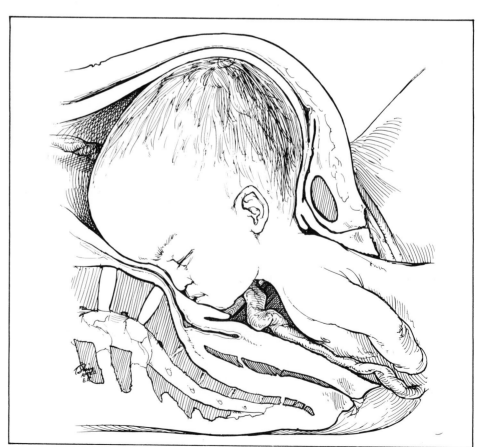

Figure 30-17. Severe dystocia from hydrocephalus, breech presentation. Note the distension of the lower uterine segment.

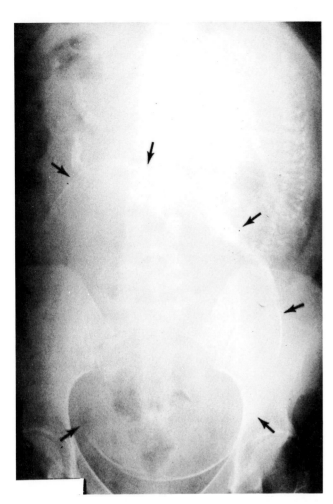

Figure 30-18. Roentgenogram demonstrating huge hydrocephalus, further outlined by arrows; 2300 ml of cerebrospinal fluid was aspirated transvaginally (Figs. 30-20, 30-21).

Diagnosis

Since the treatment of this complication of labor is usually straightforward, early diagnosis is the key to success. In this condition particularly, an empty bladder facilitates both abdominal and vaginal examination. In cephalic presentations, a broad, firm mass above the symphysis is evident from abdominal examination. The thickness of the abdominal wall usually prevents detection of the thin, elastic, hydrocephalic cranium. The high head forces the body of the infant upward, with the result that the fetal heart is often loudest above the umbilicus, a circumstance leading to the suspicion of a breech presentation. Vaginally, the broader dome of the head feels tense, but more careful palpation may disclose very large fontanels, wide suture lines, and an indentable, thin cranium characteristic of hydrocephalus. Roentgenography or sonography provides confirmation by the demonstration of a large, globular head (Figs. 30-18, 30-19).

Hydrocephalus is somewhat more difficult to diagnose radiographically with a breech presentation, since the roentgenographic outline of a normal fetal head often appears enlarged to a degree suggestive of hydrocephalus. This results from the fetal head lying more anterior than with a cephalic presentation and the divergence of x-rays inherent in diagnostic roentgenography. Therefore, in breech presentations hydrocephalus may not have been considered until it is found that the head cannot be extracted. The mistake may be avoided by paying particular attention to the following criteria: (1) the face of the hydrocephalic infant is small in relation to the large head; (2) the hydrocephalic cranium tends to be globular, whereas the normal head is ovoid; and (3) the shadow of the hydrocephalic cranium is often very thin or scarcely visible.

The difficulties inherent in radiologic diagnosis are obviated by the use of sonography to compare the diameter of the lateral ventricles to the biparietal diameter of

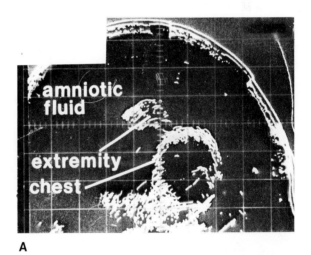

A

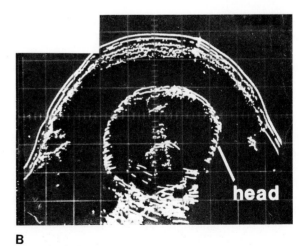

B

Figure 30-19. Sonograms of a fetus with hydrocephalus and associated hydramnios. Visible in **A** are the thorax, an extremity, and an excessive amount of amnionic fluid. In **B**, the head is remarkably enlarged compared to the thorax. (*Courtesy of Dr. R. Santos.*)

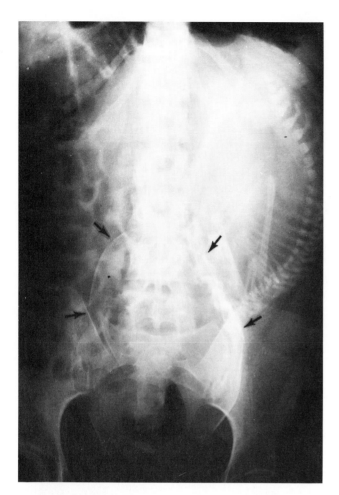

Figure 30-20. Roentgenogram from same case as in Figure 30-18 after 2300 ml of cerebrospinal fluid had been removed.

the head, and to evaluate the thickness of the cerebral cortex, as well as to compare the size of the head to that of the thorax and abdomen. The marked difference between the size of the hydrocephalic head and the thorax is apparent in the sonograms in Figures 30-19A and B.

Prognosis

Rupture of the uterus is a danger and may occur before complete dilatation of the cervix. Hydrocephalus predisposes to rupture not only because of the obvious disproportion but also because the great transverse diameter of the cranium overdistends the lower uterine segment. When fetal hydrocephalus is overlooked, the maternal mortality rate is lamentably high.

Treatment

Most often, the size of the hydrocephalic head must be reduced if the head is to pass through the birth canal. With a cephalic presentation, as soon as the cervix is di-

lated 3 cm or so, the huge ventricles may be tapped transvaginally with a needle. An 8-inch long, 17-gauge needle usually used for intrauterine transfusion has proved quite satisfactory for promptly removing appreciable volumes of cerebrospinal fluid. In the case illustrated in Figures 30-18, 30-20, and 30-21, 2300 ml of cerebrospinal fluid were removed. With cesarean section, it is also desirable at times to remove cerebrospinal fluid just before incising the uterus in order to circumvent dangerous extensions of a low transverse or vertical incision and to avoid deliberately creating a very long vertical incision in the uterus.

With a breech presentation, labor can be allowed to progress and the breech and trunk are delivered. With the head over the inlet and the face toward the mother's back, the needle is inserted transvaginally just below the anterior vaginal wall and into the aftercoming head through the widened suture line. To protect the birth canal from the needle as it is passed toward the head, the more distal part of the needle, including the point, may be covered with a segment of sterile plastic tubing about 6 inches long cut from an intravenous infusion set.

Alternatively, fluid may be withdrawn through a needle inserted transabdominally into the fetal head. After emptying the bladder and cleansing the skin, the needle is inserted in the midline somewhat below the

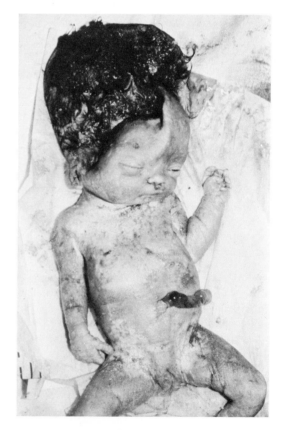

Figure 30-21. Hydrocephalic infant delivered spontaneously after removal of 2300 ml of cerebrospinal fluid.

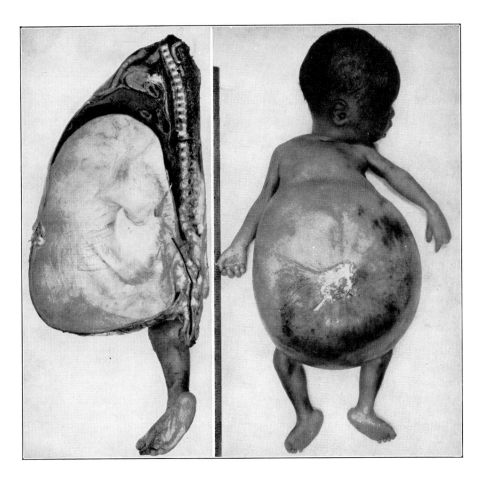

Figure 30-22. Fetus at 28 weeks with immensely distended bladder. Delivery made possible by expression of fluid from bladder through perforation at umbilicus. Median sagittal section shows interior of bladder and compression of organs of abdominal and thoracic cavities. A black thread has been laid in the urethra. (*From Savage: Am J Obstet Gynecol 29:276, 1935.*)

maternal umbilicus and inferior to the top of the fetal skull. The transabdominal approach to remove cerebrospinal fluid can also be used in the event of a cephalic presentation before trying to stimulate labor with oxytocin. The transabdominal approach also has been applied successfully in the breech fetus using ultrasound to guide the needle (Osathanondh, 1980).

Recently, the antepartum identification of fetal hydrocephaly has resulted in the successful "shunt" of the ventricles in such an affected fetus (Clewell, 1982). However, not all attempts have been successful, not only because of mechanical problems, but because many of these fetuses can be expected to have *multiple* abnormalities, many of which are lethal. *This technique is highly experimental at present and should be attempted only in centers capable of screening likely candidates, performing the procedure, and providing adequate neonatal and surgical support for the baby.*

LARGE FETAL ABDOMEN AS A CAUSE OF DYSTOCIA

Enlargement of the fetal abdomen sufficient to cause grave dystocia is usually the result of a *greatly distended bladder* (Fig. 30-22), *ascites, or enlargement of the kidneys or liver.* Occasionally, the abdomen of a

fetus affected with *edema* may attain such proportions that spontaneous delivery is impossible. Enlargement of the fetal abdomen may escape detection until fruitless attempts at delivery have demonstrated an obstruction. An enlarged abdomen and intraabdominal accumulation of fluid can be diagnosed in utero by careful sonographic examination (Figs. 30-23, 30-24).

Treatment

If the abdominal enlargement is not discovered until the fetal head has been delivered, decompression of the fetal abdomen often becomes a necessity. The maternal bladder is emptied and the suprapubic area is cleansed. A large-gauge long needle, as described for hydrocephalus, is inserted through the midline of the maternal abdomen into the fetal abdomen. Fluid in the fetal bladder or peritoneal cavity promptly escapes. The decompression may be aided by use of continuous suction. As the fetal abdomen approaches normal dimensions, the delivery is readily completed. At times, as with severe hydrops fetalis, ascites will be accompanied by such severe edema of the abdominal wall and so great an enlargement of the liver that removal of the peritoneal fluid provides insufficient decompression for easy delivery. Such cases, fortunately, are becoming extremely rare.

If the diagnosis of gross enlargement of the fetal ab-

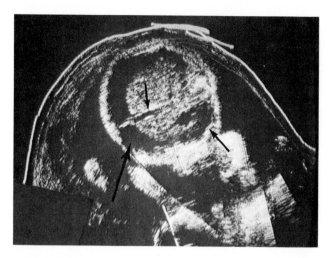

Figure 30-23. Ascites demonstrated sonographically in a transverse scan of the fetal abdomen. The larger lower arrow points to the peritoneal cavity with ascites; the smaller upper arrow overlies the liver and points to the ductus venosus; the smaller arrow to the right is directed toward the stomach. (*Courtesy of Dr. R. Santos.*)

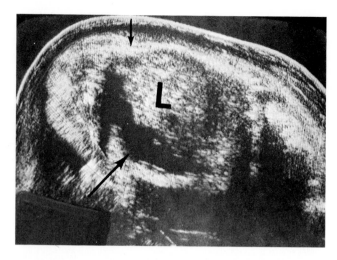

Figure 30-24. A longitudinal scan of the fetal body shown in Figure 30-23. The larger lower arrow is directed toward the peritoneal cavity distended with fluid; the upper smaller arrow points to the spinal column; L = liver. (*Courtesy of Dr. R. Santos.*)

domen is made before delivery, the decision must be made whether or not to perform a cesarean section. In general, the prognosis is very poor for the fetus with abdominal enlargement so marked as to cause dystocia, irrespective of route of delivery.

INCOMPLETE TWINNING CAUSING DYSTOCIA

The embryologic bases of incomplete twinning is considered in Chapter 26. For practical purposes, three groups of double monsters may be distinguished: (1) incomplete double formations at the upper or lower half of the body (diprosopus dipagus); (2) twins that are united at the upper or lower end of the body (craniopagus, ischiopagus, or pygopagus); and (3) double monsters united at the trunk (thoracopagus and dicephalus).

Although twins may be known, conjoining is not always identified until difficulty is encountered in attempting delivery. Since such pregnancies seldom go to term, conjoined twins may not exceed greatly the size of a normal fetus. Also, the connection between the halves is sometimes sufficiently flexible to allow vaginal delivery. Harper and co-workers (1980) recently reported a 300-year review of the obstetric, morphopathologic, neonatal, and surgical problems associated with xiphopagus conjoined twins!

REFERENCES

Abroms IF, Bresnan MJ, Zuckerman JE, Fischer EG, Strand R: Cervical cord injuries secondary to hyperextension of the head in breech presentations. Obstet Gynecol 41:369, 1973

Barnes AC: An obstetric record from The Medical Record. Obstet Gynecol 9:237, 1957

Benedetti TJ, Gabbe SG: Shoulder dystocia. A complication of fetal macrosomia and prolonged second stage of labor with mid-pelvic delivery. Obstet Gynecol 52:526, 1978

Bhagwanani SG, Price HV, Laurence KM, Ginz B: Risks and prevention of cervical cord injury in the management of breech presentation with hyperextension of the fetal head. Am J Obstet Gynecol 115:1159, 1973

Bistoletti P, Nisell H, Palme C, Lagercrantz H: Term breech delivery: Early and late complications. Acta Obstet Gynecol Scand 60:165, 1981

Bradley-Watson PJ: The decreasing value of external cephalic version in modern obstetric practice. Am J Obstet Gynecol 123:237, 1975

Brenner WE, Bruce RD, Hendricks CH: The characteristics and perils of breech presentation. Am J Obstet Gynecol 118:700, 1974

Calvert JP: Intrinsic hazard of breech presentation. Br Med J 281:1319, 1980

Caterini H, Langer A, Sama JC, Devanesan M, Pelosi MA: Fetal risk in hyperextension of the fetal head in breech presentation. Am J Obstet Gynecol 123:632, 1975

Chapman GP, Weller RO, Normand ICS, Gibbens D: Spinal cord transection in utero. Br Med J 2:398, 1978

Clewell WH, Johnson ML, Meier PR, Newkirk JB, Zide SL, Hendee RW, Bowes WA Jr, Hecht F, O'Keeffe D, Henry GP, Shikes RH: A surgical approach to the treatment of fetal hydrocephalus. N Engl J Med 306:1320, 1982

Collea JV, Chein C, Quilligan EJ: The randomized management of term frank breech presentation: A study of 208 cases. Am J Obstet Gynecol 137:235, 1980

Cox C, Kendall AC, Hommers M: Changed prognosis of breech-presenting low birthweight infants. Br J Obstet Gynaecol 89:881, 1982

Crowley P, Hawkins DF: Premature breech delivery: The cesarean section debate. J Obstet Gynaecol 1:2, 1980

Cruikshank DP, White CA: Obstetric malpresentations: Twenty years' experience. Am J Obstet Gynecol 116:1097, 1973

Duenhoelter JH, Wells CE, Reisch JS, Santos-Ramos R, Jimenez JM: A paired controlled study of vaginal and abdominal delivery of the low birthweight breech fetus. Obstet Gynecol 54:310, 1979

Effer SB, Saigal S, Rand C, Hunter DJS, Stoskopf B, Harper AC, Nimrod C, Milner R: Effect of delivery method on outcomes in the very low-birth weight breech infant: Is the improved survival related to cesarean section or other perinatal care maneuvers? Am J Obstet Gynecol 145:123, 1983

Elliott JP, Garite TJ, Freeman RK, McQuown DS, Patel JM: Ultrasonic prediction of fetal macrosomia in diabetic patients. Obstet Gynecol 60:159, 1982

Fianu S, Vaclavinkova V: The site of placental attachment as a factor in the aetiology of breech presentation. Acta Obstet Gynecol Scand 57:371, 1978

Gimovsky ML, Paul RH: Singleton breech presentation in labor. Am J Obstet Gynecol 143:733, 1982

Gimovsky ML, Wallace RL, Schifrin BS, Paul RH: Randomized management of the nonfrank breech presentation at term: A preliminary report. Am J Obstet Gynecol 146:34, 1983

Gjøde P, Rasmussen, Jørgensen J: Fetomaternal bleeding during attempts at external version. Br J Obstet Gynaecol 87:571, 1980

Goplerud J, Eastman NJ: Compound presentation: Survey of 65 cases. Obstet Gynecol 1:59, 1953

Green JE, McLean F, Smith LP, Usher R: Has an increased cesarean section rate for term breech delivery reduced the incidence of birth asphyxia, trauma, and death? Am J Obstet Gynecol 142:643, 1982

Hall JE, Kohl SG: Breech presentation: A study of 1456 cases. Am J Obstet Gynecol 72:977, 1956

Harper RG, Kenigsberg K, Sia CG, Horn D, Stern D, Bongiovi V: Xiphopagus conjoined twins: A 300-year review of the obstetric, morphopathologic, neonatal, and surgical parameters. Am J Obstet Gynecol 137:617, 1980

Hellman LM, Epperson JWW, Connally F: Face and brow presentation: The experience of the Johns Hopkins Hospital, 1896 to 1948. Am J Obstet Gynecol 59:831, 1950

Houchang D, Dorchester W, Thorosian A, Freeman RK: Macrosomia—maternal, fetal, and neonatal implications. Obstet Gynecol 55:420, 1980

Houchang D, Komatsu G, Dorchester W, Freeman RK, Bosu SK: Large-for-gestational age neonates: Anthropometric reasons for shoulder dystocia. Obstet Gynecol 60:417, 1982

Ingemarsson I, Westgren M, Svenningsen NW: Long-term follow-up of preterm infants in breech presentation delivered by cesarean section. Lancet 2:172, 1978

Johnson CE: Transverse presentation of the fetus. JAMA 187:642, 1964

Kauppila O, Grönroos M, Avo P, Aittoniemi P, Kuoppala M: Management of low birth weight breech delivery: Should cesarean section be routine? Obstet Gynecol 57:289, 1981

Lyons ER, Papsin FR: Cesarean section in the management of breech presentation. Am J Obstet Gynecol 130:558, 1978

Marcus RG, Crewe-Brown H, Krawitz S, Katz J: Feto-maternal haemorrhage following successful and unsuccessful attempts at external cephalic version. Br J Obstet Gynaecol 82:578, 1975

Osathanondh R, Birnholz JC, Altman AM, Driscoll SG: Ultrasonically guided transabdominal encephalocentesis. J Reprod Med 25:125, 1980

Phillips RD, Freeman M: The management of the persistent occiput posterior position: A review of 552 consecutive cases. Obstet Gynecol 43:171, 1974

Ranney B: The gentle art of external cephalic version. Am J Obstet Gynecol 116:239, 1973

Rovinksy JJ, Miller JA, Kaplan S: Management of breech presentation at term. Am J Obstet Gynecol 115:497, 1973

Sack RA: The large infant: A study of maternal, obstetric and newborn characteristics; including a long-term pediatric follow-up. Am J Obstet Gynecol 104:195, 1969

Swartz DP: Shoulder girdle dystocia in vertex delivery; clinical study and review. Obstet Gynecol 15:194, 1960

Tank ES, Davis R, Holt JF, Morley GW: Mechanism of trauma during breech delivery. Obstet Gynecol 38:761, 1971

Van Dorsten JP, Schifrin BS, Wallace RL: Randomized control trial of external cephalic version with tocolysis in late pregnancy. Am J Obstet Gynecol 141:417, 1981

Van Dorsten JP: Safe and effective external cephalic version with tocolysis. Contemp Ob/ Gyn 19:44, 1982

Weissberg SM, O'Leary JA: Compound presentation of the fetus. Obstet Gynecol 41:60, 1973

Wladimiroff JW, Bloemsma CA, Wallenburg HCS: Ultrasonic diagnosis of the large-for-dates infant. Obstet Gynecol 52:285, 1978

Woods CE: A principle of physics is applicable to shoulder delivery. Am J Obstet Gynecol 45:796, 1943

Ylikorkala O, Hartikainen-Sorri A: Value of external version in fetal malpresentation in combination with use of ultrasound. Acta Obstet Gynecol Scand 56:63, 1977

31
Dystocia Caused by Pelvic Contraction

Any contraction of the pelvic diameters that diminishes the capacity of the pelvis can create dystocia during labor. Pelvic contractions may be classified as follows:

1. Contraction of the pelvic inlet
2. Contraction of the midpelvis
3. Contraction of the pelvic outlet
4. Combinations of inlet, midpelvis, and outlet contraction

CONTRACTED PELVIC INLET

Definition

The pelvic inlet is usually considered to be contracted if its shortest *anteroposterior diameter is less than 10.0 cm or if the greatest transverse diameter is less than 12.0 cm.* The anteroposterior diameter of the pelvic inlet is commonly approximated by measuring manually the diagonal conjugate, which is about 1.5 cm greater. Therefore, inlet contraction is also usually defined as a *diagonal conjugate of less than 11.5 cm.* (The errors inherent in the use of this measurement are discussed in Chapter 11, p. 228.)

Using clinical and, at times, x-ray pelvimetry (Chapter 11, p. 226), it is important to identify the shortest anteroposterior diameter through which the fetal head must pass. Occasionally, the body of the first sacral vertebra is displaced forward so that the shortest distance may actually be between this false, or abnormal, sacral promontory and the symphysis pubis.

The biparietal diameter of the fetal head at term has been identified by sonography before delivery to *average* from 9.5 to as much as 9.8 cm in different clinic populations; therefore, it might prove difficult or even impossible for some fetuses to pass through an inlet with an anteroposterior diameter of less than 10 cm. Mengert (1948) and Kaltreider (1952), employing x-ray pelvimetry, demonstrated that the incidence of difficult deliveries is increased to a similar degree when either the anteroposterior diameter is decreased below 10 cm or the transverse diameter of the inlet is decreased below 12 cm. When both diameters are contracted, the incidence of obstetric difficulty is much greater than when only one diameter is contracted. The configuration of the

pelvic inlet is also an important determinant of the adequacy of any pelvis, independent of actual measurements of the anteroposterior and transverse diameters and of calculated "areas" (see Fig. 11-9 and Caldwell–Moloy Classification, p. 225).

A small woman is likely to have a small pelvis, but at the same time, she is more likely to have a small infant. Thoms (1937), in a study of 362 primigravid women, found the average weight of the offspring to be significantly lower (278 g) in women with small pelves than in those with medium or large pelves. In veterinary obstetrics, it has been frequently observed that in most species maternal size rather than paternal size is the important determinant of fetal size.

Size of Fetal Head

Manual, radiologic, and ultrasonic techniques are used with varying degrees of success to identify the size of the fetal head relative to that of the pelvic inlet.

Clinical Estimation. Impression of the fetal head into the pelvis, as described by Müller (1880), may provide useful information. In an occiput presentation, the obstetrician grasps the brow and the suboccipital region through the abdominal wall with his fingers and makes firm pressure downward in the axis of the pelvic inlet. Pressure on the fundus by an assistant at the same time is usually helpful. The effect of the forces on the descent of the head can be evaluated by palpation with a sterile gloved hand in the vagina. If no disproportion exists, the head readily enters the pelvis and vaginal delivery can be predicted. Inability to push the head into the pelvis, however, does not necessarily indicate that vaginal delivery is impossible. A clear demonstration of a flexed fetal head that overrides the symphysis pubis is indicative of disproportion.

Radiologic Estimation. In general, measurements of the diameters of the fetal head by roentgenographic techniques have been disappointing. The precision of roentgenocephalometry is much less than for x-ray pelvimetry.

Sonographic Measurements. Measurement of the fetal biparietal diameter by ultrasonic means allows precise

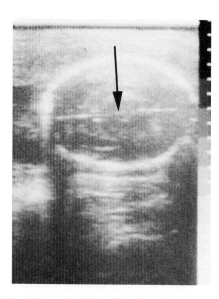

Figure 31-1. Ultrasonic transverse scan of the fetal head (B-mode cephalometry). The arrow is perpendicular to the linear midline structures of the head. The biparietal diameter is significantly smaller than the occipitofrontal diameter. This dolichocephalic or so-called breech head may also develop from crowding in multifetal gestations and from oligohydramnios. (*Courtesy of Dr. R. Santos.*)

measurement more often than does x-ray. The freely floating fetal head, as in breech presentations, may, unfortunately, move sufficiently during sonographic examination to invalidate the measurement. Additionally, the head of the fetus in the breech presentation may be elongated in the occipitofrontal diameter (dolichocephaly) (Kasby, 1982).

This dolichocephalic, or so-called breech head (Fig. 31-1), may also be observed in multifetal gestations and in cases of oligohydramnios (Berkowitz and Hobbins, 1982). Such an observation may lead the sonographer to underestimate fetal weight and gestational age. When a dolichocephalic head is observed, a head circumference measurement will result in a more accurate estimation of fetal size.

Presentation and Position of the Fetus

A contracted pelvic inlet plays an important part in the production of abnormal presentations. In normal nulliparous women, the presenting part commonly descends into the pelvic cavity before the onset of labor at term. When the pelvic inlet is considerably contracted, however, descent usually does not occur until after the onset of labor. if it occurs at all. Vertex presentations still predominate, but since the head floats freely over the pelvic inlet or rests more laterally in one of the iliac fossae, very slight influences may cause the fetus to assume other presentations. For example, *face and shoulder presentations occur three times more frequently in women with contracted pelves, and prolapse of the cord* and of the extremities occurs four to six times more frequently.

Course of Labor

When the pelvic deformity is sufficiently pronounced to prevent the head from readily entering the inlet, the course of labor is prolonged and, often, effective spontaneous labor is never achieved.

Abnormalities in Dilatation of the Cervix

Normally, dilatation of the cervix is facilitated by the hydrostatic action of the unruptured membranes or, after their rupture, by the direct application of the presenting part against the cervix. In contracted pelves, however, when the head is arrested in the pelvic inlet the entire force exerted by the uterus acts directly upon the portion of membranes that overlie the dilating cervix. Consequently, early spontaneous rupture of the membranes is more likely to result.

After rupture of the membranes, the absence of pressure by the fetal head against the cervix and lower uterine segment predisposes to less effective uterine contractions. Hence, further dilatation of the cervix may proceed very slowly or not at all. Cibils and Hendricks (1965) have shown that the mechanical adaptation of the passenger to the bony passage plays an important part in determining the efficiency of uterine contractions. The better the adaptation, the more efficient are the contractions. Since adaptation is poor in the presence of a contracted pelvis, prolongation of labor often results. *With degrees of pelvic contractions incompatible with vaginal delivery, the cervix seldom dilates satisfactorily. Thus, the behavior of the cervix has a prognostic value in regard to the outcome of labor in women with inlet contraction.*

Danger of Uterine Rupture

Abnormal thinning of the lower uterine segment creates a serious danger during a prolonged labor. When the disproportion between the head and the pelvis is so pronounced that engagement and descent do not occur, the lower uterine segment becomes increasingly stretched, and the danger of its rupture becomes imminent. In such cases, a *pathologic retraction ring* may develop and can be felt as a transverse or oblique ridge extending across the uterus somewhere between the symphysis and the umbilicus. Whenever this condition is noted, prompt delivery is urgently indicated. Unless cesarean section is employed to terminate labor, there is the great danger of rupture of the uterus, as well as serious compromise of fetal well-being.

Production of Fistulas

When the presenting part is firmly wedged into the pelvic inlet but does not advance for a considerable time, portions of the birth canal lying between it and the pel-

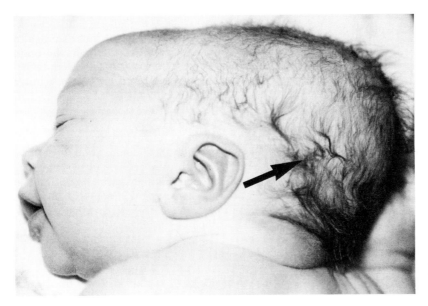

Figure 31-2. Considerable molding of the head and caput formation in a very recently delivered infant. The arrow is directed toward the appreciable scalp edema that overlies the occiput, i.e., caput succedaneum.

vic wall may be subjected to excessive pressure. As the circulation is impaired, the resulting necrosis may become manifest several days after delivery by the appearance of vesicovaginal, vesicocervical, or rectovaginal fistulas. Formerly, when operative delivery was deferred as long as possible, such complications were frequent, but today they are rarely seen, except in neglected cases. In general, pressure necrosis follows a very prolonged second stage of labor.

Intrapartum Infection

Infection is another serious danger to which the mother and the fetus are exposed in labors complicated by prolonged rupture of the membranes. The danger of infection is increased by repeated vaginal examinations and other intravaginal and intrauterine manipulations. If the amnionic fluid becomes infected, fever may or may not develop during labor.

Effects on the Fetus

Prolonged labor in itself is deleterious to the fetus. In women with labors of more than 20 hours or in women with a second stage of labor of more than 3 hours, Hellman and Prystowsky (1952) found, in general, a significant increase in perinatal mortality rates. If the pelvis is contracted and there is associated early rupture of membranes and intrauterine infection, the risk to the infant, as well as the mother, is compounded. Intrapartum infection is not only a serious complication for the mother but also an important cause of fetal and neonatal death, as bacteria in amnionic fluid can make their way through the amnion and invade the walls of the chorionic vessels, thus giving rise to fetal bacteremia. Pneumonia, caused by aspiration of infected amnionic fluid by the fetus, is another serious consequence.

Changes in Scalp and Skull

A large *caput succedaneum* frequently develops on the most dependent part of the head during labor if the pelvis is contracted. The caput succedaneum (Fig. 31-2) may assume considerable proportions and lead to serious diagnostic errors. The caput may reach almost to the pelvic floor while the head is still not engaged, that is, the biparietal diameter has not passed through the pelvic inlet. An inexperienced physician may make premature and unwise attempts at forceps delivery. Typically, the large caput disappears within a few days after birth.

Molding of the Fetal Head. Under the pressure of strong uterine contractions, the bones of the skull overlap one another at the major sutures, a process referred to as *molding* (Figs. 31-2, 39-1). As a rule, the median margin of the parietal bone that is in contact with the sacral promontory is overlapped by that of its fellow; the same result occurs with the frontal bones. The occipital bone, however, is pushed under the parietal bones. These changes are frequently accomplished without obvious detriment to the child, although when the distortion is marked it may lead to tentorial tears and, when blood vessels are torn, to fatal intracranial hemorrhage. Such *molding* of the fetal head may produce a diminution of 0.5 cm or so in the biparietal diameter without cerebral injury, but when greater degrees of molding occur, the likelihood of intracranial injury increases.

Coincident with the molding of the head, the parietal bone, which was in contact with the promontory, may show signs of having been subjected to marked pressure, sometimes becoming very much flattened. Accommodation is more readily accomplished when the bones of the head are imperfectly ossified. This important process may provide one explanation for the differences in the course of labor in two apparently similar cases in which the pelvis and the head present identical

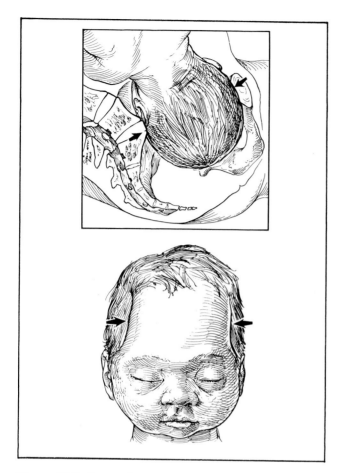

Figure 31-3. Depression of the skull (*arrows*) caused by labor with contracted pelvic inlet.

measurements. In one case, the head is softer and more readily molded, and spontaneous delivery results. In the other, the more resistant head retains its original shape and operative interference is required for its delivery.

Characteristic pressure marks may form upon the scalp, covering the portion of the head that passes over the promontory of the sacrum. From their location, it is frequently possible to ascertain the movements that the head has undergone in passing through the pelvic inlet. Much more rarely, similar marks appear on the portion of the head that has been in contact with the symphysis pubis. Such marks usually disappear a few days after birth, although in exceptional instances severe pressure may lead to necrosis of the scalp.

Fractures of the skull are occasionally encountered, usually following forcible attempts at delivery, though sometimes they may occur with spontaneous delivery. The fractures are of two varieties, appearing either as a shallow groove or as a spoon-shaped depression just posterior to the coronal suture (Fig. 31-3). The former is relatively common but since it involves only the external plate of the bone, it is not very dangerous. The latter, however, if not operated upon, may lead to the death of

the infant, because it extends through the entire thickness of the skull and gives rise upon its inner surface to projections that exert injurious pressure upon the brain and may cause hemorrhage. Accordingly, as soon as feasible after delivery, it is advisable to elevate or remove the depressed portion of the skull.

Prolapse of the Cord

A serious complication for the fetus is prolapse of the cord, the occurrence of which is facilitated by imperfect adaptation between the presenting part and the pelvic inlet. Unless prompt delivery is accomplished, fetal death results from compression of the cord between the presenting part and the margin of the pelvic inlet.

Prognosis

The prognosis for successful vaginal delivery of a term-sized fetus in cases of severe inlet contraction with an anteroposterior diameter of less than 9 cm can be stated as nearly hopeless. For the borderline group in which the anteroposterior diameter is only slightly below 10 cm, the prognosis for successful vaginal delivery is influenced significantly by a number of variables, including the following:

1. The presentation is of extreme importance. All presentations but the occiput are unfavorable.
2. The size of the fetus is of obvious importance. Unfortunately, in spite of the many advances in sonography, estimates of fetal size at term, especially the head, are often imprecise.
3. Not only the diameters of the pelvic inlet but also its configuration plays an important role. With an android configuration (Fig. 11-9), for any given anteroposterior diameter of the inlet, there is less available space, especially in the forepelvis.
4. The frequency and intensity of spontaneous uterine contractions are informative. Uterine dysfunction, typically infrequent contractions of low intensity, is common with significant disproportion. The uterus is not inclined to self-destruct.
5. The behavior of the cervix in labor has great prognostic significance. In general, orderly spontaneous progression to full dilatation indicates that vaginal delivery is most likely to be successful.
6. Extreme asynclitism is unfavorable, as is appreciable molding of the head without engagement.
7. Knowledge of the outcome of previous labor and delivery at term is helpful.
8. Finally, the prognosis for successful vaginal delivery is altered by coincidental conditions that impair uteroplacental perfusion, for example, severe preeclampsia. In such circumstances, uterine contractions sufficient to dilate the cervix and propel the fetus through the birth canal are much more likely to compromise further an already de-

creased placental perfusion to such a degree that the fetus is distressed.

Treatment

The management of inlet contraction is determined principally by the prognosis for safe vaginal delivery. If, on the basis of the criteria reviewed, a delivery that is safe for both mother and child cannot be anticipated, cesarean section should be done. Today it is so rare to employ craniotomy that even dead fetuses are often delivered by cesarean section in cases of contraction of the pelvis. In a minority of instances, the prognosis can be reached before the onset of labor, and cesarean section can be done electively at an appointed time. A carefully managed trial of labor, however, is desirable in most instances. Women with inlet contraction are particularly likely to have both weak uterine contractions during the first stage of labor and a need for vigorous voluntary expulsive efforts during the second stage. Therefore, in general, the use of conduction anesthesia should be avoided. The course of labor should be monitored closely and the prognosis established as soon as reasonably possible. Although signs of impending uterine rupture should always be looked for if the contractions are strong, the danger of this accident occurring is remote in primigravid women. With greater parity, however, the likelihood of rupture of the uterus increases. Finally, the administration of oxytocin in the presence of any form of pelvic contraction, unless the fetal head has unequivocally passed the point of obstruction, can be catastrophic for both the fetus and the mother.

CONTRACTION OF MIDPELVIS

Definition

The so-called plane of the obstetric midpelvis extends from the inferior margin of the symphysis pubis, through the ischial spines, and touches the sacrum near the junction of the fourth and fifth vertebrae. A transverse line theoretically connecting the ischial spines divides the midpelvis into a fore portion and hind portion. The former is bounded anteriorly by the lower border of the symphysis pubis and laterally by the ischiopubic rami. The hind portion is bounded posteriorly by the sacrum and laterally by the sacrospinous ligament, forming the lower limits of the sacrosciatic notch. Average midpelvis measurements are as follows: transverse (interspinous), 10.5 cm; anteroposterior (from the lower border of the symphysis pubis to the junction of the fourth and fifth sacral vertebrae), 11.5 cm; and posterior sagittal (from the midpoint of the interspinous line to the same point on the sacrum), 5 cm. Although the definition of midpelvic contractions has not been established with the same precision possible for inlet contractions, the midpelvis should be considered contracted when the sum of the interischial spinous and posterior sagittal diameters of the midpelvis (normally, 10.5 plus 5 cm, or 15.5 cm) falls to 13.5 or below. There is reason to suspect that midpelvic contraction exists whenever the interischial spinous diameter is less than 10 cm. When it is smaller than 9 cm, the midpelvis is contracted. The preceding definition of midpelvic contraction does not, of course, imply that dystocia will necessarily occur in such a pelvis, but simply that it may develop, depending also upon the size and shape of the forepelvis, and the size of the fetal head, as well as the degree of midpelvic contraction.

Identification

Although there is no precise manual method of ascertaining midpelvic contraction, a suggestion of midpelvic contraction can sometimes be obtained by ascertaining on vaginal examination that the spines are prominent, that the pelvic side walls converge, or that the sacrosciatic notch is narrow. Eller and Mengert (1947), moreover, pointed out that the relationship between the intertuberous and interspinous diameters of the ischium is sufficiently constant that narrowing of the interspinous diameter can be anticipated when the intertuberous diameter is narrow. A normal intertuberous diameter, however, does not always exclude a narrow interspinous diameter.

Prognosis

Midpelvic contraction is probably more common than inlet contraction and is frequently a cause of transverse arrest of the fetal head and, potentially, of difficult midforceps operations.

Treatment

In the management of labor complicated by midpelvic contraction, the main injunction is to allow the natural forces of labor to push the biparietal diameter beyond the potential interspinous obstruction. Forceps operations may be very difficult when applied to a head, the greatest diameter of which has not yet passed a contracted midpelvis. This difficulty may be explained on two grounds: (1) pulling on the head with forceps destroys flexion, whereas pressure from above increases it and (2) although the forceps blades occupy a space of only a few millimeters, this diminishes further the available space. Only when the head has been allowed to descend to such an extent that the perineum is bulging and the vertex is actually visible is it reasonably certain that the head has passed the obstruction. It is then usually safe to apply forceps. Strong suprafundal pressure should not be used to try to force the head past the obstruction.

The use of forceps to effect delivery in midpelvic contraction, usually undiagnosed, has been responsible for much of the stigma attached to the midforceps operation. Midforceps delivery is, therefore, contraindicated in any case of midpelvic contraction in which the bi-

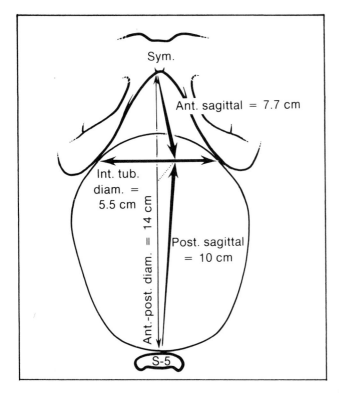

Figure 31-4. Diagram of pelvic outlet of case shown in Figure 31-5. Even though the intertuberous diameter is quite narrow (5.5 cm), vaginal delivery is possible because of the long (10 cm) posterior sagittal diameter. (Int. tub. diam. = intertuberous diameter; Sym. = symphysis pubis; S-5 = fifth sacral vertebra).

parietal diameter of the fetal head has not passed beyond the level of contraction. Otherwise, the perinatal mortality and morbidity rates associated with the operation are prohibitive.

The vacuum extractor (see Chapter 41, p. 850) has been reported by some to be of advantage in some cases of midpelvic contraction *after the cervix has become fully dilated.* Traction need not cause deflection of the fetal head, nor does the vacuum extractor occupy space, as do forceps. Oxytocin, of course, has no place in the treatment of dystocia caused by midpelvic contraction.

CONTRACTION OF THE PELVIC OUTLET

Definition

Contraction of the pelvic outlet is usually defined as diminution of the interischial tuberous diameter to 8 cm or less. The pelvic outlet may be likened roughly to two triangles (Figs. 31-4, 31-6). The interischial tuberous diameter constitutes the base of both. The sides of the anterior triangle are the pubic rami, and its apex the inferior posterior surface of the symphysis pubis. The

posterior triangle has no bony sides but is limited at its **apex** by the tip of the last sacral vertebra (not the tip of **the coccyx**).

Prognosis

It is apparent in Figure 31-4 that diminution in the intertuberous diameter with consequent narrowing of the anterior triangle must inevitably force the fetal head posteriorly. Whether delivery can take place, therefore, **depends** partly on the size of the posterior triangle or, **more** specifically, the interischial tuberous diameter and **the** posterior sagittal diameter of the outlet, as demonstrated in Figures 31-4 through 31-7. A contracted outlet may cause dystocia not so much by itself as through the often associated midpelvic contraction. *Outlet contraction without concomitant midplane contraction is rare.*

Even when the disproportion between the size of the fetal head and the pelvic outlet is not sufficiently great to give rise to serious dystocia, it may play an important part in the production of perineal tears. With increasing narrowing of the pubic arch, the occiput cannot emerge directly beneath the symphysis pubis but is forced increasingly farther down upon the ischiopubic rami. In extreme cases, the head must rotate around a line joining the ischial tuberosities. The perineum, consequently, must become increasingly distended and thus exposed to great danger of disruption. An extensive mediolateral episiotomy is usually indicated.

In view of potential significance of outlet contractions, palpation of the pubic arch and clinical estimation of the intertuberous diameter should be part of the pelvic examination of the pregnant woman.

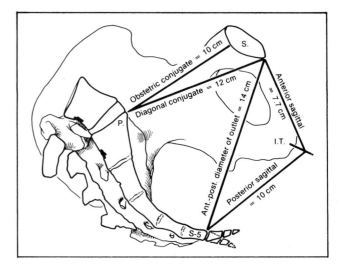

Figure 31-5. Diagram of the lateral view of the same pelvis depicted in Figure 31-4. The long (10 cm) posterior sagittal diameter may allow the fetal head to negotiate the narrow (5.5 cm) intertuberous diameter (I.T. = ischial tuberosity; S. = symphysis pubis; P. = sacral promontory).

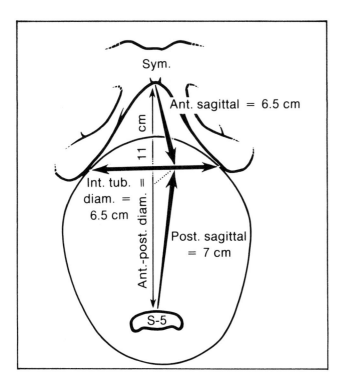

Figure 31-6. Diagram of pelvic outlet in which the intertuberous diameter is narrow (6.5 cm) *and* the posterior sagittal diameter is quite short (7 cm), precluding vaginal delivery of most term-size fetuses (Int. tub. diam. = intertuberous diameter; Sym. = symphysis pubis; S-5 = fifth sacral vertebra).

GENERALLY CONTRACTED PELVIS

Prognosis

Since the contraction involves all portions of the pelvic canal, labor is not rapidly completed after the fetal head has passed the pelvic inlet. The prolongation of labor is caused not only by the resistance offered by the pelvis but also in many instances by the faulty spontaneous uterine contractions that frequently accompany diminution in the size of the pelvis and a fetus of average or larger size.

PELVIC FRACTURES AND PREGNANCY

Speer and Peltier (1972) reviewed their experiences and those of others with pelvic fractures and pregnancy. As expected, trauma from automobile collisions was the common cause of fracture. With bilateral fractures of the pubic rami, compromise of the capacity of the birth canal by callus formation or malunion was very common. The experiences at Parkland Memorial Hospital are that a history of previous fracture of the pelvis warrants careful review of previous x-rays and possibly an additional radiologic evaluation of the pelvis later in pregnancy, unless cesarean section is to be performed for some other reason.

RARE PELVIC CONTRACTIONS*

Kyphotic Pelvis

Kyphosis, or humpback, when involving the lower portion of the vertebral column, is usually associated with a characteristically funnel-shaped distortion. The effect exerted upon the pelvis by kyphosis differs according to its location. When the gibbus, or hump, is situated in the thoracic region, there is usually a compensatory pronounced lordosis beneath it, so that the pelvis itself is but little changed. When situated at the junction of the thoracic and lumbar portions of the vertical column, however, its effect upon the pelvis becomes manifest. It is further accentuated when the kyphosis is lower down and is most marked when it is at the lumbrosacral junction. If the vertebral defect is in the lumbosacral region, the upper arm of the gibbus may overlie the inlet.

Diagnosis. The diagnosis is usually obvious, for the external deformity is readily visible and should at once suggest the possibility of a funnel pelvis. On palpation of the pubic arch, transverse narrowing of the pelvic outlet is observed, whereas by internal examination the lengthening of the obstetric conjugate is found. In lumbosacral kyphosis, there is no longer a promontory, and the bodies of the lower lumbar vertebrae overhang the superior strait. In this type of deformity, therefore, particular attention should be devoted to the length of the "pseudoconjugate," the distance from the upper margin of the symphysis pubis to the nearest portion of the vertebral column. Occasionally, the condition may be mistaken for spondylolisthesis.

Effect upon Labor. The mechanical conditions favor abnormal positions of the fetus. Generally when the distance between the ischial tuberosities is less than 8 cm, labor becomes difficult or impossible, according to the degree of

---

* *Illustrations of several rare pelvic contractions appear in earlier editions of this textbook.*

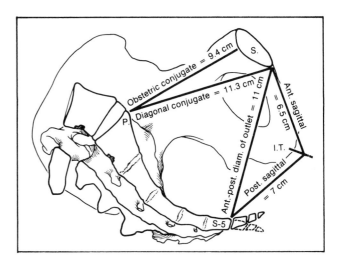

Figure 31-7. Diagram of lateral view of the pelvis from the same case depicted in Figure 31-6. Note the short (7 cm) posterior sagittal diameter (I.T. = ischial tuberosity; S. = symphysis pubis; S-5 = fifth sacral vertebra; P. = sacral promontory).

transverse contraction of the outlet. In such cases, the dystocia is more pronounced than in typical funnel pelves presenting identical measurements, because the anterior displacement of the tip of the sacrum is inevitably associated with shortening of the posterior sagittal diameter.

Effect upon the Heart. In 50 fatal cases of kyphoscoliosis associated with pregnancy that were collected by Jensen (1938), at least 31 were caused by heart failure, far more than resulted from pelvic dystocia. Because of the collapse of the vertebral column, the volume of the thoracic cage in thoracic kyphoscoliosis is diminished, with consequent pressure exerted on the lungs and heart. As a result, the vital capacity is decreased to one half the normal value, as shown by the studies of Chapman and co-workers (1939). This reduction applies to both the absolute and relative vital capacities. In five patients with thoracic kyphoscoliosis studied by them, the vital capacity was from 35 to 53 percent of the total pulmonary volume, whereas in the normal women studied, the fraction was 57 to 69 percent of the total. The ratio of residual air to vital capacity was 1.3 in kyphoscoliotic patients and 0.6 in the normal subjects. In other words, in these deformed women, the usual mechanism of respiration is altered by the greater limitation of costal movement. The ribs move only ineffectively, and breathing is accomplished largely by movements of the diaphragm. Partial collapse and infection are but natural results of these poorly aerated lungs.

Prognosis and Treatment. The kyphoscoliotic patient is severely handicapped in childbearing. If the condition is entirely thoracic, cardiac complications are a threat; if the condition is entirely lumbar, midpelvic contraction is common, and if the condition is lower down, contraction may be extreme. When the gibbus is thoracolumbar, both heart and pelvis may be sources of difficulty.

The prognosis here, as in all other types of contracted pelves, depends not only upon the dimensions of the pelvis but upon the progress of labor. If labor is prolonged with dimensions below the critical levels, delivery is best accomplished by cesarean section.

Kyphorachitic Pelvis

Kyphosis is nearly always of carious origin, but when caused by rachitis it is usually associated with scoliosis. In the rare cases of pure rachitis kyphosis, however, the pelvic changes are slight, for the effect of the kyphosis is counterbalanced to a great extent by that of the rachitis, the former leading to an elongation and the latter to a shortening of the conjugata vera. The kyphosis tends to narrow, and the rachitis to widen, the pelvic outlet. Thus it may happen that a woman presenting a markedly deformed vertebral column of this character may have a practically normal pelvis. The two processes, however, do not always counteract each other, and as a rule, when the kyphosis is high up, the pelvic changes are predominantly rachitic.

Scoliotic Pelvis

With scoliosis involving the upper portion of the vertebral column, there is usually a compensatory corresponding curvature in the opposite direction lower down, thus giving rise to a double, or S-shaped, curve. In such cases, the body weight is transmitted to the sacrum in the usual manner, so that the pelvis is not involved. When the scoliosis is lower down and involves the lumbar region, however, the sacrum takes part in the compensatory process and assumes an abnormal position, leading to slight asymmetry of the pelvis.

Kyphoscoliotic Pelvis

In this type of deformity, the distortion of the pelvis varies according to whether the kyphosis or the scoliosis is predominant. When the extent of the two deformities is approximately equal, however, the kyphotic changes in the pelvis predominate, although the influence of the scoliosis tends to counteract, to a certain extent, the transverse narrowing of the inferior strait.

Kyphoscoliorachitic Pelvis

Kyphosis resulting from rachitis is nearly always complicated by scoliosis, which usually predominates in the production of the pelvic deformity, because the kyphosis and the rachitis tend to counteract each other in their effect on the pelvis. The resulting pelvis, therefore, does not differ materially from that observed in scoliorachitis except that the tendency to anteroposterior flattening is partially counteracted by the action of the kyphotic vertebral column. Because of the scoliosis, the oblique deformity of the pelvic inlet is usually quite marked. Generally, however, this type of pelvis is more favorable, from an obstetric standpoint, than that resulting from scoliorachitis alone.

Extremely Rare Pelvic Contractions

In the past century and a half, descriptions of the seven following extremely rare contracted pelves have appeared in the obstetric literature. A busy obstetrician or even a large obstetric service in this country may in many years encounter none of them. Osteomalacia, for example, although seen in the Far East, is virtually absent from this country. (For details, see *Williams Obstetrics,* 10th ed., 1950.)

1. Robert pelvis
2. Split pelvis
3. Litzmann pelvis
4. Assimilation pelvis
5. Naegele pelvis
6. Osteomalacic pelvis
7. Spondylolisthetic pelvis

Pelvic Anomalies Resulting from Abnormal Forces Exerted by Femurs

Normally, when a woman stands erect, the upward and inward force exerted by the femurs is of equal intensity on either side and is transmitted to the pelvis through the acetabula. In walking or running, the entire body weight is transmitted alternately first to one and then to the other leg. In a person suffering from disease affecting one leg, the sound extremity must bear more than its share of the body weight; consequently, the upward and inward force exerted by the femur is generally greater upon that side of the pelvis. To these mechanical factors are attributed the changes in shape that accompany certain forms of lameness, provided the lesion appeared early in life.

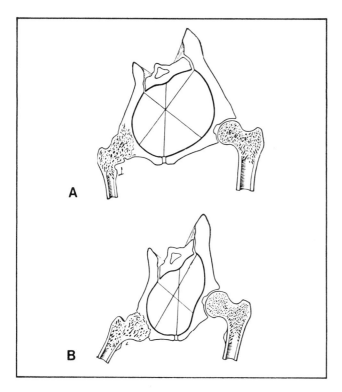

Figure 31-8. Coxalgic pelvis before **A.** and after **B.** the subject has walked.

Pelvic Deformities Caused by Unilateral Lameness

Coxitis occurring in early life nearly always gives rise to an obliquely contracted pelvis. If the disease appeared before the subject learned to walk, or if the child was obliged to keep to bed for a prolonged period, there may have been imperfect development of the pelvis. Added to the generally contracted type are the mechanical effects and atrophic changes resulting from the unilateral disease (Fig. 31-8). They are manifested by imperfect development of the diseased side of the pelvis. The affected innominate bone is smaller than its fellow, and the iliopectineal line forming the arc of a circle has a smaller radius than that of the other side. At the same time, the sacral alae are more poorly developed on the affected side. The entire bone is somewhat rotated about its vertical axis, so that its anterior surface looks toward the normal side.

Oblique contraction of the pelvis may also develop when *unilateral luxation* of the femur occurs in early life, although it is usually less pronounced than that following coxitis. In such circumstances, the head of the bone is displaced backward and upward upon the outer surface of the ilium, where a new articular surface may occasionally be formed. The affected leg becomes considerably shortened, and a disproportionate share of the body weight is transmitted through the normal leg, forcing the healthy side of the pelvis upward, inward, and backward, and resulting in the same oblique contraction seen in coxalgia.

In unilateral poliomyelitis, as well as in those cases in which disease at the knee or ankle or amputation early in life has caused shortening of one leg, unless the patient has had the benefit of proper orthopedic treatment, similar changes occur in the pelvis, though they rarely assume the extreme obliquity that characterizes the coxalgic variety.

Diagnosis. A limp at once suggests an obliquely contracted pelvis. When the condition has been present since childhood, a pelvic deformity on the side corresponding to the unaffected leg is likely.

More accurate information can be obtained by careful examination of the unclothed patient, when the posture of the involved leg as well as the relative positions of the posterior or superior spines and the crests of the ilia may be ascertained. At the same time, the presence or absence of compensatory scoliosis may be noted in such cases.

Effect upon Labor. The effect of this type of pelvis upon labor varies with the extent and position of the deformity. If the affected side is so contracted as to prevent its being occupied by a portion of the presenting part, for all practical purposes a generally contracted pelvis exists. Engagement, if it can occur at all, will take place more readily when the biparietal diameter of the head is aligned with the long oblique diameter of the superior strait. All obstacles to labor have not yet been overcome, however, even after descent has occurred, since in many cases the inward projection of the ischium may lead to abnormalities in rotation. Generally, these pelves are not excessively contracted.

Coxarthrolisthetic Pelvis

Very exceptionally, as the result of localized softening near the acetabulum, the base of one or both acetabula yields to the pressure exerted by the head of the femur, projecting into the pelvic cavity and leading to a unilateral or bilateral transverse contraction. Eppinger (1903) designated such pelves as coxarthrolisthetic and attributed their production to delayed and deficient ossification of the base of the acetabulum. Breus and Kolisko (1912) stated that the deformity is usually related to gonorrheal coxitis, rather than to arthritis deformans or tuberculosis, as was formerly believed. Chiari (1911), however, described a specimen that he believed to have resulted from tabetic arthritis. Benda (1927) collected cases of this rare condition reported up to 1926 and critically considered their mode of production.

Pelvic Deformities Resulting from Bilateral Lameness

Children occasionally are born with *luxation of both femurs,* the heads of the bones lying, as a rule, upon the outer surfaces of the iliac bones, above and posterior to their usual location. In some cases, the acetabula are entirely absent, but more frequently they are rudimentary; new but imperfect substitutes then form higher up. The condition does not usually interfere seriously with learning to walk at the usual age, though the gait is more or less wobbly.

Because the upward and inward force exerted by the femurs is not applied in its usual direction through the acetabula, the pelvis becomes excessively wide and more or less flattened anteroposteriorly. The transverse widening is particularly marked at the inferior strait, while the flattening, as a rule, is not very pronounced. This pelvis, therefore, rarely offers any serious obstacle to labor and delivery.

Atypical Deformities of the Pelvis

The pelvis may rarely be deformed by bone outgrowths at various points and even less frequently by tumors. *Exotoses* are most frequently found on the posterior surface of the symphysis, in front of the sacroiliac joints, and on the anterior surface of the sacrum, although occasionally these may be formed along the course of the iliopectineal line.

Kilian (1854) indicated that such structures may form sharp, knifelike projections. He designated the condition *acanthopelyx* or *pelvis spinosa*. Such formations are rarely sufficiently large to present any obstacle to delivery but because of their peculiar structure may cause considerable injury to the maternal soft parts.

Tumors of various kinds may arise from the walls of the false or true pelvis, so obstructing its cavity as to render labor impossible. Fibromas, osteomas, chondromas, carcinomas, and sarcomas of the pelvis have been described. These sometimes grow large and occasionally become cystic. Chondromas are the most common variety.

Dwarf Pelvis

According to Breus and Kolisko (1900), several varieties of dwarfs must be distinguished: the "true," the hypoplastic, the chondrodystrophic, the cretin, and the rachitic dwarf.

True Dwarf Pelvis (Pelvis Nana). This extremely rare variety of pelvis is generally contracted and tends toward the infantile type, but its most characteristic feature is the persistence of cartilage at all the epiphyses.

Hypoplastic Dwarf Pelvis. According to Breus and Kolisko (1904), this variety of pelvis is found in very small adults and is simply a normal pelvis in miniature. It differs significantly from that of the true dwarf in that it is completely ossified.

Chondrodystrophic Dwarf Pelvis. This variety of pelvis is characterized by an extreme anteroposterior flattening, which at first appears to resemble that of a rachitic pelvis. On closer examination, however, the flattening is seen to result from the imperfect development of the portion of the iliac bone entering into the formation of the iliopectineal line. As a result, the sacral articulation is brought much nearer the pubic bone than usual. In six pelves of this type described by Breus and Kolisko, the conjugata vera varied from 4 to 7 cm, whereas the transverse diameter of the superior strait was only slightly shortened, varying from 11 to 12 cm.

Cretin Dwarf Pelvis. This generally contracted pelvis is formed of imperfectly developed bones. Unlike that of the true dwarf, it does not present infantile characteristics, but signs of a steady though imperfect growth throughout early life are seen. Unossified cartilage may be present focally in young subjects, but it disappears with advancing age and is never found in all the epiphyses as in the true dwarf pelvis.

Rachitic Dwarf Pelvis. True rachitic dwarfs are rare and possess generally contracted rachitic pelves, which do not differ, except by their small size, from other rachitic pelves.

REFERENCES*

Benda R: Contribution to the etiology and pathogenesis of coxitic protrusion of the acetabulum. Arch Gynaek 129:186, 1927

Berkowitz RL, Hobbins JC: How head shape affects BPD. Contemp Ob/Gyn 19:35, 1982

Breus C, Kolisko A: Die pathologischen Beckenformen. Leipzig and Vienna, 1900, Vol. III:I. Teil Spondylolisthesis, pp 17–59; Kyphosen-Becken, pp 163–307; Skoliosen-Becken, pp 355–359

Breus C, Kolisko A: Die pathologischen Beckenformen. Leipzig and Vienna, 1904, Vol. I: Spaltbeken, pp 107–139; Assimilations-becken, pp 169–256; Zwegbecken, pp 259–366

Breus C, Kolisko A: Rachitis-Becken, Die pathologischen Beckenformen. Leipzig and Vienna, 1904, Vol I, part 2, p 435

Breus C, Kolisko A: Coxitis-Becken, Die pathologischen Beckenformen. Leipzig and Vienna, 1912, Vol III, pp 474–593

Chapman EM, Dill DB, Graybiel A: Decrease in functional capacity of lungs and heart resulting from deformities of the chest: Pulmonocardiac failure. Medicine 18:167, 1939

Chiari H: Spondylolisthesis. Bull Johns Hopkins Hosp 22:41, 1911

Cibils LA, Hendricks CH: Normal labor in vertex presentation. Am J Obstet Gynecol 91:385, 1965

Eller WC, Mengert WF: Recognition of mid-pelvic contraction. Am J Obstet Gynecol 53:252, 1947

Eppinger: Pelvis-Chrobak (Coxarthrolisthesis-Becken). Beitrage, Geb Gyn Vienna 2:173, 1903

Hellman LM, Prystowsky H: Duration of the second stage of labor. Am J Obstet Gynecol 63:1223, 1952

Jensen J: The Heart in Pregnancy. St. Louis, Mosby, 1938, pp 333–341

Kaltreider DF: Criteria of midplane contraction. Am J Obstet Gynecol 63:392, 1952

Kasby CB, Poll V: The breech head and its ultrasound significance. Br J Obstet Gynaecol 89:106, 1982

Kilian HS: Das Stachelbecken (Acanthopelyx). Mannheim, Schilderungen neuer Beckenforman, 1854

Litzmann CCT: Die Formen des Beckens, nebst einem Anhang uber Osteomalacie. Berlin, 1861

Mengert WF: Estimation of pelvic capacity. JAMA 138:169, 1948

Müller: On the frequency and etiology of general pelvic contraction. Arch Gynaek 16:155, 1880

Naegele FC: Das schragverengte Becken. Mainz, 1839

Robert F: Beschreibung eines im hochsten Grade querverengten Beckens. Karlsruhe und Freiburg, 1842

Speer DP, Peltier LF: Pelvic fractures and pregnancy. J Trauma 12:474, 1972

Thoms H: The obstetrical significance of pelvic variations: A study of 450 primiparous women. Br Med J 2:210, 1937

---

* In this chapter, several historical references are included. Further information may be found in earlier editions of this textbook.

32
Dystocia from Other Abnormalities of the Reproductive Tract

VULVAR ABNORMALITIES

Complete *atresia of the vulva* or the lower portion of the vagina is usually congenital and, unless corrected by operative measures, precludes conception. More frequently, vulvar atresia is incomplete, resulting from adhesions or scars following injury or infection. The defect may present a considerable obstacle to delivery, but the resistance is usually overcome eventually by the continued pressure exerted by the fetal head, commonly at the cost of deep perineal tears.

Whenever the vulvovaginal outlet is small, rigid, and inelastic, dystocia and extensive lacerations are likely unless prevented by adequate episiotomy. Because of various factors, the vulva may become extremely edematous, but dystocia rarely results from edema alone. Thrombi and hematomas about the vulva, although more common during the puerperium, occasionally form late in pregnancy before or during labor and may give rise to difficulty (see Chapter 36, pp. 738). Inflammatory lesions or tumors near the vulva may have a similar effect. Rarely, *condylomata acuminata* may be so extensive as to make vaginal delivery undesirable (see Chapter 25, p. 491), although it can usually be accomplished without extensive lacerations or hemorrhage. The danger of infection is increased, however. *Bartholin cysts* rarely become large enough to contribute to dystocia.

ABNORMALITIES OF THE VAGINA

Complete *vaginal atresia* is nearly always congenital and, unless corrected operatively, forms an effective bar to pregnancy. Incomplete atresia is either a manifestation of faulty development or results from postnatal accidents.

Occasionally, the vagina is divided by a *longitudinal septum,* which may be complete, extending from the vulva to the cervix, or more often incomplete, limited to either the upper or lower portion of the canal. Since such conditions are frequently associated with other abnormalities in development of the genital tract, their de-

tection should always prompt careful examination to ascertain whether there is a coexistent uterine and/or renal deformity (see Chapter 25, p. 495). A complete longitudinal septum usually does not cause dystocia, since the half of the vagina through which the fetus descends gradually dilates satisfactorily. An incomplete septum, however, occasionally interferes with descent of the head or breech, over which the septum may become stretched as a band of varying thickness. Such structures are usually torn through spontaneously but occasionally are sufficiently resistant that either they must be divided or cesarean section must be performed.

Occasionally, the vagina may be obstructed by an *annular stricture* or band of congenital origin. These are unlikely to interfere seriously with delivery, however, since they usually soften as pregnancy advances and yield before the oncoming head, requiring incision in only extreme cases.

Sometimes the upper portion of the vagina is separated from the rest of the canal by a *transverse septum* with a small opening. Such a stricture is occasionally mistaken for the upper limit of the vaginal vault and, at the time of labor, the opening in the septum is erroneously considered to be an undilated external os. On careful examination, however, the obstetrician can pass a finger through the opening and feel the cervix or on rectal examination can palpate the cervix through the anterior rectal wall above the level of the vaginal septum. After the external os has become completely dilated, the head impinges upon the septum and causes it to bulge downward. If the septum does not yield, slight pressure upon its opening will usually lead to further dilatation, but cruciate incisions may be required occasionally to permit delivery.

Atresia can result from scarring, the consequence of injury or inflammation. Following an infection in which much of the lining of the vagina sloughs, the vaginal lumen during healing may be almost entirely obliterated. Atresia may result from the corrosive action of abortifacients inserted into the vagina. Injuries that lead to extensive scarring, for example, the trauma that may ensue during rape of a child by an adult male, may also cause vaginal atresia.

The effects of atresia vary greatly. In most cases, because of the softening of the tissues incident to pregnancy, the obstruction is gradually overcome by the pressure exerted by the presenting part; less often, manual or hydrostatic dilatation or incisions may become necessary. If, however, the structure is so resistant that spontaneous dilatation appears improbable, cesarean section should be performed at the onset of labor.

A *Gartner duct cyst* may protrude into the vagina and even through the introitus and possibly be confused with a cystocele. A *cystocele* may be managed successfully by emptying the bladder, using a catheter and upward manual pressure on the prolapsed anterior vaginal wall. A Gartner duct cyst may or may not slip above the presenting part. If not, the cyst may be aspirated aseptically.

Among the rare causes of serious dystocia are *neoplasms,* such as *fibroma, carcinoma,* or *sarcoma,* arising from the vaginal walls or adjacent structures.

Tetanic contraction of the levator ani, rarely, may seriously interfere with descent of the head. In that condition, analogous to vaginismus in nonpregnant women, a thick, ringlike structure completely encircles and markedly constricts the vagina about midway between the cervix and the vulva. Ordinarily, the obstruction yields under anesthesia.

ABNORMALITIES OF THE CERVIX

Atresia and Stenosis

Complete atresia of the cervix is incompatible with conception. In pregnancy, therefore, complete *cervical atresia* could only occur after conception.

Cicatrical *stenosis of the cervix* may follow extensive cauterization or difficult labor associated with infection and considerable destruction of tissue. For example, of the ten cases of severe cervical dystocia following treatment of the cervix reported by Gibbs and Moore (1968), previous conization was responsible in six. Cryotherapy is less likely to produce stenosis. Rarely, cervical stenosis is caused by extensive infiltration by carcinoma or syphilitic ulceration and induration. Occasionally, it has resulted from corrosives, such as potassium permanganate tablets, used in an attempt to produce abortion. Amputation of the cervix, with suturing to effect hemostasis and promote reepithelialization, may lead to stenosis, although cervical incompetence is much more likely.

Ordinarily, because of the softening of the tissues during pregnancy, the stenosis gradually yields during labor. In rare instances, however, the stenosis may be so pronounced that dilatation appears improbable, and cesarean section should be employed to effect delivery.

In cases of *conglutination* of the cervical os, the cervical canal at the time of labor undergoes complete obliteration through effacement while the cervical os remains extremely small. Thus the presenting part is separated from the vagina by only a thin layer of cervical tissue. Ordinarily, complete dilatation promptly follows pressure with the fingertip, although in rare instances manual dilatation or cruciate incisions may be required.

Carcinoma of the Cervix

Dystocia may be a consequence of extensive infiltration of the cervix by carcinoma since dilatation is likely to be inadequate even when uterine contractions remain forceful. With less involvement, the cervix will usually dilate. The effects of carcinoma of the cervix upon pregnancy and vice versa, as well as appropriate treatment, are discussed in Chapter 25 (p. 493).

UTERINE DISPLACEMENTS

Anteflexion

Marked anteflexion of the enlarging pregnant uterus is usually associated with diastasis recti and a pendulous abdomen (see Chapter 25, p. 499). When the abnormal position of the uterus prevents the proper transmission of the force of the contractions to the cervix, cervical dilatation, as well as engagement of the presenting part, is impeded. Marked improvement may follow maintenance of the uterus in an approximately normal position by means of a properly fitting abdominal binder.

Retroflexion

As stated in Chapter 25 (p. 499), persistent retroflexion of the pregnant uterus is usually incompatible with advanced pregnancy. If spontaneous or artificial reposition does not occur, the woman either aborts or develops symptoms caused by incarceration of the uterus before the end of the fourth month. In very exceptional instances, however, pregnancy may proceed, in which event the adherent fundus remains applied to the floor of the pelvis, with the anterior wall stretching to accommodate the product of conception. In this condition, known as *sacculation,* the head of the fetus may occupy the displaced fundus, with the cervix drawn up so high that the external os lies above the upper margin of the symphysis pubis. Consequently, during labor the contractions tend to force the infant through the most dependent portion of the uterus, with the cervix dilating only partially. Spontaneous delivery is thus impossible and rupture of the uterus may occur. For these reasons, cesarean section affords the best method of delivery and at the same time facilitates possible repositioning of the uterus.

Previous Operative Correction. Fortunately, operative correction of the retroverted uterus has fallen into disrepute. The one indication may be to bring the retroflexed uterus into the anterior position as part of an operation for extensive pelvic endometriosis. Uterine suspension accomplished by shortening the round ligaments does not adversely affect subsequent labor. If, as part of the operation, the bladder is advanced on the anterior wall of the uterus, urinary frequency, as well as bladder discomfort, may be troublesome during pregnancy.

Pregnancy is contraindicated following the Watkins interposition operation, an operation once performed by some to try to correct a cystocele. Pregnancy after fixation of the fundus of the uterus to the anterior abdominal wall to try to correct either uterine prolapse or uterine retroversion may be complicated by considerable discomfort as the pregnant uterus enlarges. Hopefully, both the Watkins interposition operation and fixation of the uterus to the abdominal wall have been eliminated from contemporary gynecologic surgery.

OTHER PELVIC TUMORS

Uterine Myomas

A myoma may be located immediately beneath the endometrial or decidual surface of the uterine cavity (*submucous myoma*), immediately beneath the uterine serosa (*subserous myoma*), or be confined to the myometrium (*intramural myoma*). An intramural myoma, as it grows, may develop a significant subserous or submucous component, or both. Submucous and subserous myomas may, at times, be attached to the uterus by only a stalk (*pedunculated myoma*).

Similar to the changes that occur in the amount of normal myometrium, myomas increase in size appreciably as pregnancy advances and involute remarkably after delivery. Of the three varieties, submucous myomas of prominent size before conception are most likely to exert deleterious effects on the pregnancy. Implantation of the zygote in endometrium overlying a submucous myoma is seldom successful. Even when implantation occurs, subsequent growth and differentiation of a zygote implanted near a submucous myoma often leads to faulty placental implantation and abortion. Rarely, with a submucous myoma, pregnancy may progress to term, with the myoma then prolapsing through the cervix sometime before, during, or after delivery of the fetus or placenta.

As in the nonpregnant state, pedunculated subserous myomas may undergo torsion with necrosis to the extent that the myoma is detached from the uterus. At times, a subserous myoma may become parasitic, and much or all of its blood is supplied through highly vascularized omentum.

Myomas during pregnancy or the puerperium occasionally undergo "red," or "carneous," degeneration that, in actuality, is *hemorrhagic infarction*. The symptoms and signs of red degeneration are focal pain, with tenderness on palpation and sometimes low-grade fever. Moderate leukocytosis is common. On occasion, the parietal peritoneum overlying the infarcted myoma becomes inflamed and a peritoneal "rub" develops. Red degeneration is difficult to differentiate at times from appendicitis, placental abruption, ureteral stone, or pyelonephritis. Treatment consists of analgesia such as codeine. Most often, the signs and symptoms abate within a few days.

Myomas may become infected during the course of puerperal metritis or septic abortion, and are especially likely to do so if the myoma is located immediately adjacent to the placental implantation site or if an instrument such as a sound or curet perforates the myoma. If the myoma is infarcted, the risk of infection is increased and the likelihood of cure of the infection, except by hysterectomy, is reduced.

Prognosis. When compared to the number of women with uterine myomas who conceive, all these complications are quite infrequent. Most often myomas cause little difficulty except perhaps to make the uterus larger than expected from the menstrual history. Dysfunctional labor, entrapment of the placenta above a submucous myoma, and excessive bleeding from the placental implantation site after delivery have all been cited as worrisome complications. On the basis of our experiences at Parkland Memorial Hospital with a large population of black women, in whom myomas are common, the complications just mentioned are very infrequent. Concern has been expressed at times about the huge size that might have to be achieved by the myomatous pregnant uterus and its contents. This is no more of a problem than exists when twins or hydramnios is a factor.

Myomas in the cervix or in the lower uterine segment may obstruct labor. Sonograms from such a case and a picture of the uterus are shown in Figures 32-1A, B, and C. Myomas that lie within or contiguous to the birth canal earlier in pregnancy may be carried upward as the uterus enlarges, with relief of obstruction to vaginal delivery. Even though relief was not so provided in the cases demonstrated in Figures 32-1 and 32-2, a decision regarding the method of delivery should usually not be made before the onset of labor.

Myomectomy. This procedure should be limited to those tumors with discrete pedicles that can be easily clamped and ligated. Otherwise, myomas should not be dissected from the uterus, during pregnancy or delivery, for bleeding may be profuse and at times the uterus may have to be sacrificed. Typically, the myomas will undergo remarkable involution after delivery. In myomas resected during pregnancy or the puerperium there are often bizarre changes in the nuclei of the smooth muscle cells, changes that may be confused with sarcoma.

When myomectomy results in a defect through or immediately adjacent to the endometrium, subsequent pregnancies should be delivered by cesarean section, preferably before active labor has begun.

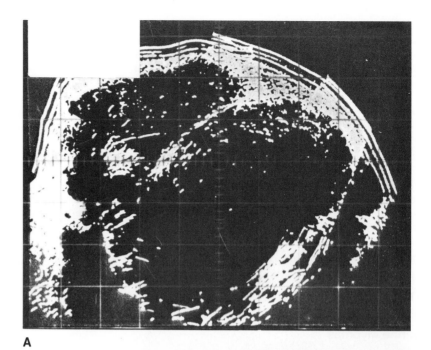

A

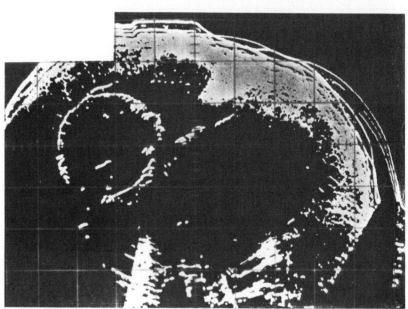

B

Figure 32-1. **A.** Transverse B-scan sonogram of lower abdomen demonstrating a large nearly homogeneous mass which is the myoma shown in Figure 32-1C. (*Courtesy of Dr. R. Santos.*) **B.** Same case as shown in Figure 32-1A. Transverse B-scan sonogram of upper abdomen demonstrating the fetus.

Benign Ovarian Tumors

Ovarian tumors may be serious complications of pregnancy, may undergo torsion, and may pose insuperable obstacles to vaginal delivery. Moreover, even after spontaneous labor and delivery, they may give rise to disturbances during the puerperium.

Although all varieties of ovarian tumors may complicate pregnancy and labor, the most common are cystic (Fig. 32-3). Beischer and associates (1971) noted that of 164 ovarian tumors diagnosed during pregnancy, one

fourth were cystic teratomas, and one fourth were mucinous cystadenomas. Four of the 164 (2.4 percent) were malignant. The most frequent and next most serious complication of ovarian cysts during pregnancy is torsion. The incidence of the accident was 12 percent in Booth's series (1963). Torsion is most common in the first trimester. The cyst may rupture and extrude its contents into the peritoneal cavity as the consequence of torsion, or during spontaneous labor, or during surgical removal. This event is not likely to be as devastating with serous cystomas as with dermoid cysts. Rupture of

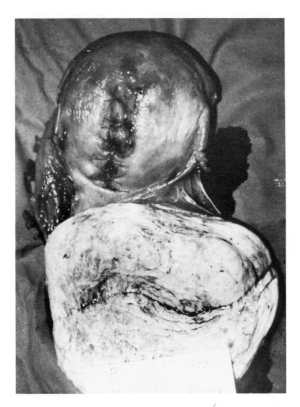

Figure 32-1. C. Same case as shown in Figures 32-1A and 32-1B. Cesarean hysterectomy specimen. The upper mass is the body of the uterus that was just emptied by cesarean section. The lower mass is a huge myoma arising low in the uterus and now incised. The infant weighed 3250 g and the uterus with myoma weighed 2900 g. Red degeneration was not found. Delivery 2 years before had also been by cesarean section.

the latter may be followed by serious, even fatal, granulomatous peritonitis. When the tumor blocks the pelvis, it may lead to rupture of the uterus or the tumor may be forced into the vagina, the rectum, or the intervening rectovaginal septum. It seems surprising that spontaneous rupture of an ovarian cystoma is not more common.

An ovarian tumor complicating pregnancy is often entirely unsuspected. Careful examination of all pregnant women would eliminate a large proportion, but not all, of these errors. If an ovarian tumor does not occupy the pelvis, diagnosis through physical examination is especially difficult, since the abdominal enlargement may be attributed to a pregnancy more advanced than indicated by menstrual data, to multiple fetuses, or to hydramnios, and the true condition may not be recognized until after labor. Usually sonography can provide accurate differentiation between uterine enlargement and an extrauterine cystic mass. A dramatic instance is presented in Figure 32-4.

It must be kept in mind that early in pregnancy an ovary may be somewhat enlarged, creating suspicion of

neoplasm. Enlarged ovaries less than 6 cm in diameter are usually increased in size as the consequence of corpus luteum formation.

In view of the increased incidence of abortion during early pregnancy, the safest time to perform laparotomy is during the fourth month of gestation, provided the operation can be postponed until that time. When the diagnosis is not made until late in pregnancy, it is usually advisable, except in the case of known or suspected malignant tumors, to delay laparotomy until fetal viability has been achieved. If the ovarian cyst is not impacted, it is preferable usually to permit spontaneous labor and remove the tumor later in the puerperium. If the tumor is impacted in the pelvis, cesarean section should be performed, followed by removal of the tumor if it can be mobilized from behind the uterus.

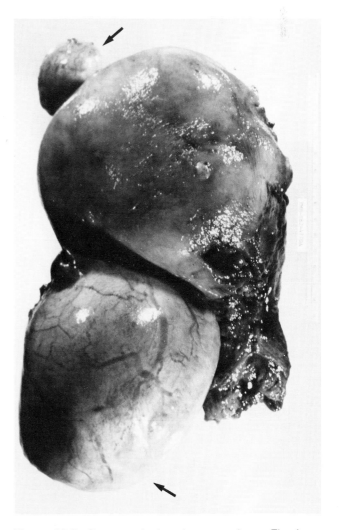

Figure 32-2. Cesarean hysterectomy specimen. The large pedunculated myoma (*lower arrow*) filled the birth canal almost completely and prevented vaginal delivery of near-term large twins. A small myoma (*upper arrow*) protrudes from the fundus. A vertical incision was made in the lower uterine segment for the delivery.

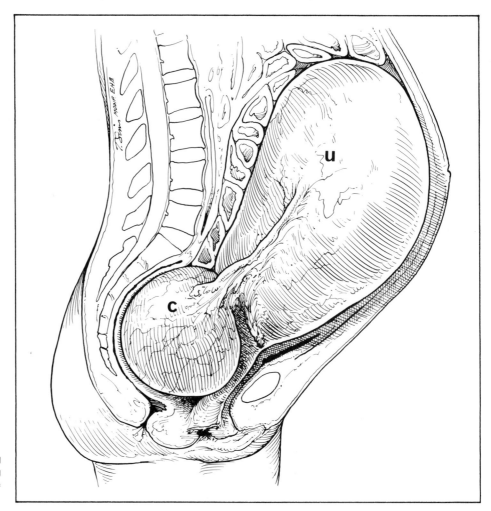

Figure 32-3. Ovarian cyst filling most of true pelvis and causing dystocia. C = ovarian cyst; U = pregnant uterus.

Carcinoma of the Ovary

Malignant ovarian neoplasms are rare in pregnancy. Only 41 cases were found in a literature survey by Valenti (1960), who, along with Amico (1957), believed that the natural course of the disease is uninfluenced by pregnancy. If the tumor is discovered at the time of laparotomy or if the disease is widespread, the treatment should be the same as in the nonpregnant patient. In some circumstances, it is justifiable to remove the tumor and allow the pregnancy to continue when a few more weeks would assure viability of the delivered infant. Even then, delivery should usually be by cesarean section, with decision regarding further surgery and chemotherapy based on the results of clinical and histologic examination.

Pelvic Masses of Other Origins

Labor may be obstructed by pelvic masses of various origins sufficiently large to render delivery difficult or even impossible. A *distended bladder,* with or without a cystocele, may obstruct delivery, as demonstrated in Figure 32-5. However, a less severely distended bladder apparently often does not delay the normal progress of labor (Read, 1980; Kerr-Wilson, 1983). A large *cystocele* or *rectocele,* though occasionally offering slight resistance to labor, can generally be replaced during delivery. Tumors of the bladder may impede passage of the fetus, though rarely seriously enough to require operative delivery. *Pelvic ectopic kidney* is a rare complication of pregnancy. However, a *transplanted kidney* is usually placed in the pelvis. Such a kidney may block the birth canal and sustain injury during passage of the fetus. Most women with an ectopic kidney will deliver vaginally without hazard, but if the kidney is entirely intrapelvic, as is often the case with transplanted kidneys, abdominal delivery is safer.

In rare instances, an enlarged spleen may prolapse into the pelvic cavity and obstruct labor. Echinococcal cysts have been found in the pelvis. An old extrauterine gestation may obstruct the pelvic canal, interfering with the delivery of a subsequent intrauterine fetus. An *enterocele* rarely gives rise to dystocia. The herniated intestine can usually be replaced and the obstacle temporarily overcome, but when reduction is impossible,

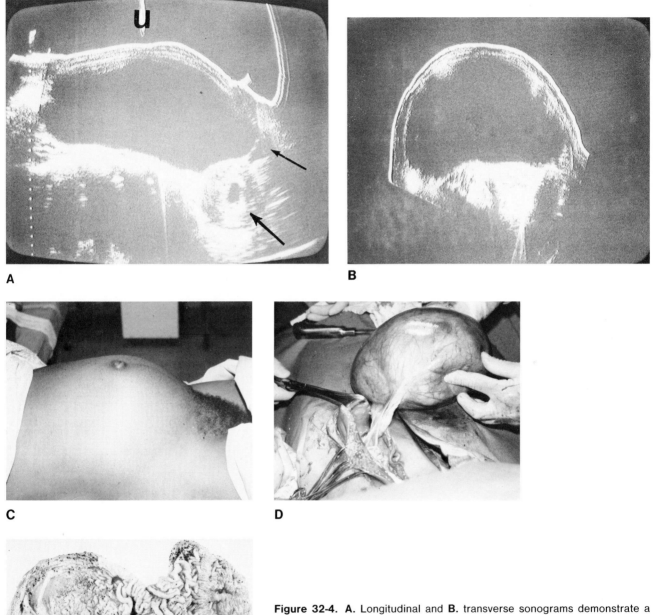

Figure 32-4. A. Longitudinal and **B.** transverse sonograms demonstrate a huge cystic mass above the bladder (*smaller arrow*) and early pregnant uterus (*larger arrow*). The transverse scan was made at the level of the umbilicus (u). **C.** The configuration of the abdomen was suggestive of advanced gestation rather than the correct gestational age of 8 weeks. **D.** A 3500 g ovarian cyst that arose from the tip of the left ovary and incorporated most of the oviduct was readily excised, along with the left tube and ovary, once the incision was extended to near the xiphoid. The external surface of the cyst was free of tumor excrescences. **E.** The cyst was unilocular as evident in the sonograms. (*Courtesy of Dr. R. Santos.*)

694

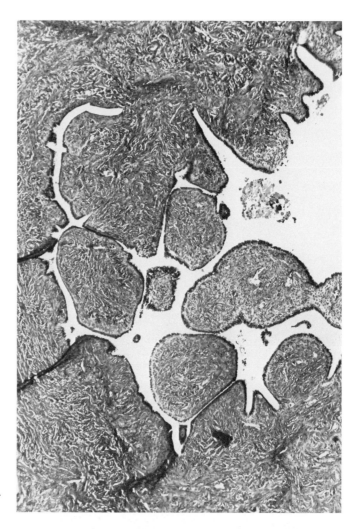

Figure 32-4. F. The histologic diagnosis was serous cystadenofibroma.

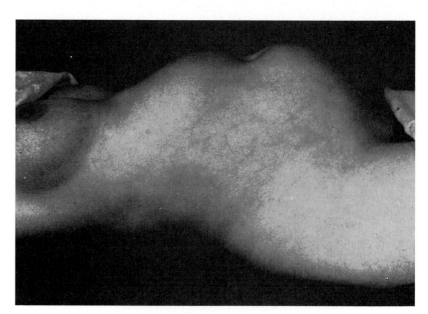

Figure 32-5. Dystocia caused by distension of the bladder. This woman was sent to the hospital after 3 days of ineffectual labor at home. The cervix was thought to have been completely dilated for 24 hours. After catheterization of the greatly distended bladder, which yielded over 1000 ml of urine, the baby's head descended at once and delivery was accomplished easily.

cesarean section is safer than forcing the fetus over a large irreducible hernia. Tumors or inflammation arising from the lower part of the rectum or pelvic connective tissue also may give rise to dystocia.

REFERENCES

Amico JC: Pregnancy complicated by primary carcinoma in the ovary. Am J Obstet Gynecol 74:920, 1957

Beischer NA, Buttery BW, Fortune DW, Macafee CAJ: Growth and malignancy of ovarian tumours in pregnancy. Aust N Z J Obstet Gynaecol 11:208, 1971

Booth RT: Ovarian tumors in pregnancy. Obstet Gynecol 21:189, 1963

Gibbs CE, Moore SF: The scarred cervix in pregnancy and labor. Gen Pract 37:85, 1968

Kerr-Wilson RHJ, Parham GP, Orr JW Jr: The effect of a full bladder on labor. Obstet Gynecol 62:319, 1983

Read JA, Miller FC, Yeh S-Y, Platt LD: Urinary bladder distension: Effect on labor and uterine activity. Obstet Gynecol 56:565, 1980

Valenti C: On carcinoma of the ovary in pregnancy. Minerva Ginecol 9:4, 1960

33
Injuries to the Birth Canal

INJURIES TO THE PELVIC FLOOR AND VAGINA

Perineal Lacerations

All except the most superficial perineal lacerations are accompanied by varying degrees of injury to the lower portion of the vagina. Such tears may reach sufficient depth to involve the rectal sphincter and may extend to varying depths through the walls of the vagina. Bilateral lacerations into the vagina are usually unequal in length and separated by a tongue-shaped portion of vaginal mucosa (see Figs. 17-17 through 17-19). Their repair should form part of every operation for the restoration of a lacerated perineum. Suturing of just the external integuments without approximation of underlying perineal and vaginal fascia and muscle will lead to relaxation of the vaginal outlet and may contribute to rectocele and cystocele formation, as well as uterine prolapse.

Vaginal Lacerations

Isolated lacerations involving the middle or upper third of the vagina but unassociated with lacerations of the perineum or cervix are less commonly observed. Vaginal lacerations in this location are usually longitudinal, resulting from injuries sustained during a forceps operation, although occasionally they accompany spontaneous delivery. Such lacerations frequently extend deep into the underlying tissues and may give rise to copious hemorrhage, which, however, is usually readily controlled by appropriate suturing. They may be overlooked unless thorough inspection of the upper vagina is performed or at least careful attention is paid to bleeding from the genital tract in the presence of a firmly contracted uterus. *Bleeding while the uterus is firmly contracted is strong evidence of genital tract laceration, retained placental fragments, or both.*

Lacerations of the anterior vaginal wall in close proximity to the urethra are relatively common. If superficial and not bleeding, repair is not indicated; otherwise, in order to achieve hemostasis, closure is required. If such lacerations are extensive, difficulty in voiding can be anticipated and an indwelling catheter placed.

Injuries to Levator Ani

Injuries to the levator ani as a result of overdistention of the birth canal may result in separation of muscle fibers or in the diminution in their tonicity sufficient to interfere with the function of the pelvic diaphragm. In such cases, the woman may develop pelvic relaxation. If these injuries involve the pubococcygeus muscle, urinary incontinence may supervene. The likelihood of such injuries is minimized by appropriate episiotomy.

INJURIES TO THE CERVIX

Etiology

Traumatic lesions of the upper third of the vagina are uncommon by themselves but are often associated with extensions of deep cervical tears. In rare instances, however, the cervix may be entirely or partially avulsed from the vagina, with colporrhexis in the anterior, posterior, or lateral fornices. Such lesions usually follow difficult forceps deliveries performed through an incompletely dilated cervix with the forceps blades applied over the cervix. The cervical tears may extend to involve the lower uterine segment and uterine artery and its major branches, and even through the peritoneum. Fortunately, such extensive traumatic lesions are rare in modern obstetric practice. They may be totally unsuspected, but much more often they become manifest by excessive external hemorrhage or by the formation of a retroperitoneal hematoma. These extensive tears of the vaginal vault should be carefully explored. If there is the slightest question of perforation of the peritoneum, or of retroperitoneal or intraperitoneal hemorrhage, laparotomy should be performed. In the presence of damage of this severity, intrauterine exploration for possible rupture is, of course, also mandatory. Formerly, treatment of these lacerations by packing was recommended, *often with poor outcome;* however, surgical repair is much more satisfactory. Effective anesthesia, vigorous blood replacement, and capable assistance are mandatory for a satisfactory outcome.

Cervical lacerations up to 2 cm must be regarded as inevitable in childbirth. Such tears, however, heal rapidly and are rarely the source of any difficulty. In healing, they cause a significant change in the shape of the external os from round before cervical effacement and dilatation to appreciably elongated laterally after delivery and recovery from effacement and dilatation.

Occasionally, during labor the edematous anterior lip of the cervix may be caught and compressed between the head and the symphysis pubis. If ischemia is severe, the cervical lip may undergo necrosis and separation. In still rarer instances, the entire vaginal portion may be avulsed from the rest of the cervix. Such *annular* or *circular detachment of the cervix* probably occurs only in neglected labors or in pregnant women receiving excessive doses of oxytocin.

In all traumatic lesions involving the cervix, there is usually no appreciable bleeding until after birth of the infant, when hemorrhage may then be profuse. Slight cervical tears heal spontaneously. Extensive lacerations have a similar tendency, but perfect union rarely results. As the consequence of such tears, eversion of the cervix with exposure of the delicate mucus-producing endocervical glands is frequently the cause of persistent leukorrhea. If the leukorrhea persists after the puerperium, treatment with cautery or cryotherapy is usually beneficial. If a Papanicolaou smear has not been obtained during pregnancy, it should be obtained and the results reviewed before treatment is initiated.

Diagnosis

A deep cervical tear should always be suspected in cases of profuse hemorrhage during and after the third stage of labor, particularly if the uterus is firmly contracted. For a definitive diagnosis to be made, however, a thorough examination is necessary. Because of the flabbiness of the cervix immediately after delivery, digital examination alone is often unsatisfactory. The extent of the injury can be fully appreciated only after adequate exposure and visual inspection of the cervix.

In view of the frequency with which deep tears follow major operative procedures, the cervix should be inspected routinely at the conclusion of the third stage after all difficult deliveries, even if there is no bleeding. Annular detachment of the vaginal portion of the cervix should be suspected whenever an irregular mass of tissue with a circular central opening is cast off before or after birth of the infant.

Treatment

Deep cervical tears should be repaired immediately. Treatment varies with the extent of the lesion. When the laceration is limited to the cervix, or even when it extends somewhat into the vaginal fornix, satisfactory results are obtained by suturing the cervix after bringing it into view at the vulva. Visualization is best accomplished when an *assistant* makes firm downward pressure on the uterus while the operator exerts traction on the lips of the cervix with fenestrated ovum or sponge forceps. The

vaginal walls are held apart with retractors manipulated with the aid of the assistant (Fig. 33-1). Since the hemorrhage usually comes from the upper angle of the wound, it is advisable to apply the first suture at the angle and suture outward. Interrupted chromic catgut sutures should be employed, since they do not have to be removed. The physician must remember that overzealous suturing to try to restore the normal appearance of the cervix may lead to stenosis during involution of the uterus.

RUPTURE OF THE UTERUS

Frequency

It is apparent from the tabulations provided by Schrinsky and Benson (1978) that the incidence of rupture of the uterus varies appreciably among institutions, ranging from 1 in 100 deliveries to 1 in 11,000. Although the frequency of uterine rupture from all causes has probably not decreased remarkably during the past several decades, the etiology of rupture has changed appreciably and the outcome has improved significantly.

Etiology

Currently, the most common cause of rupture is previous cesarean section and the next most common is probably stimulation of labor with oxytocin. Generally, the previously untraumatized, spontaneously laboring uterus will not persist in contracting so vigorously as to destroy itself.

An extensive classification of the etiology of rupture of the gravid uterus is presented below:

1. Uterine injury before current pregnancy
   A. Surgery involving myometrium
      Cesarean section or hysterotomy
      Repaired previous uterine rupture
      Myomectomy incision close to or through endometrium
      Deep cornual resection to remove interstitial oviduct
      Excision of uterine septum (metroplasty)
   B. Coincidental trauma to uterus
      Instrumented abortion (sounds, curets, or other devices)
      Sharp or blunt trauma (accidents, knives, bullets)
      Silent rupture during previous pregnancy
2. Uterine injury during current pregnancy
   A. Before delivery
      Persistent, intense, spontaneous contractions
      Oxytocin or prostaglandin administration
      Hypertonic solution injected intra-amnionically
      Perforation by monitor catheter
      External trauma, sharp or blunt

Marked uterine overdistention (multiple fetuses, hydramnios)
B. During delivery
   Internal podalic version
   Difficult forceps delivery
   Breech extraction
   Fetal anomaly overdistending lower segment
   Vigorous fundal pressure attempting delivery
   Difficult manual removal of placenta
3. Uterine defects not necessarily related to trauma
  A. Congenital
    Pregnancy in incompletely developed uterus or uterine horn
  B. Acquired
    Placenta increta or percreta
    Invasive mole or choriocarcinoma
    Adenomyosis
    Sacculation of adherent retroverted uterus

Definitions

It is customary to distinguish between *complete* and *incomplete* rupture of the uterus, depending on whether the laceration communicates directly with the peritoneal cavity or is separated from it by the visceral peritoneum over the uterus or that of the broad ligament. An incomplete rupture may, of course, become complete at any instant.

It is important to differentiate between *rupture of a cesarean section scar* and *dehiscence of a cesarean section scar.* Rupture refers, at the minimum, to separation of the old uterine incision throughout most of its length, with rupture of the fetal membranes so that the uterine cavity and the peritoneal cavity communicate. In these circumstances, all or part of the fetus is usually extruded into the peritoneal cavity. In addition, there is usually bleeding, often massive, from the edges of the scar or

from an extension of the rent into previously uninvolved uterus. By contrast, with dehiscence of a cesarean section scar, the fetal membranes are not ruptured and therefore the fetus is not extruded into the peritoneal cavity. Typically, with dehiscence the separation does not involve all of the previous uterine scar, and bleeding is absent or minimal. Dehiscence occurs gradually, whereas ruptures are very likely to be symptomatic and, at times, fatal. With labor or intrauterine manipulations, a dehiscence may become a rupture.

Comparison of Classical and Lower-Segment Cesarean Section Scars

The behavior of a classical scar, that is, a uterine incision through the body of the pregnant uterus rather than the lower uterine segment, in any subsequent pregnancy differs from that of a scar confined to the lower uterine segment. First, the probability of rupture of a classical scar is several times greater than that of a lower segment scar. Second, if a classical scar does rupture, the accident takes place before labor in about one third of the cases. Rupture not infrequently takes place several weeks before term, before a cesarean section is ordinarily scheduled. In fact, Lazarus (1978) described disruption of a previous classical cesarean section scar at 12 weeks gestation with marked hemorrhage and hypovolemia. Therefore, delivery by subsequent cesarean section cannot prevent such ruptures. Lower-segment scars *that are confined to the noncontractile portion of the uterus rarely,* if ever, rupture before labor, and only very infrequently do so during labor.

The statistics available are insufficient to permit a precise calculation of the maternal mortality rate that attends rupture of a cesarean section scar. It is probably less than 1 percent, but the perinatal mortality rate may be as high as 50 percent.

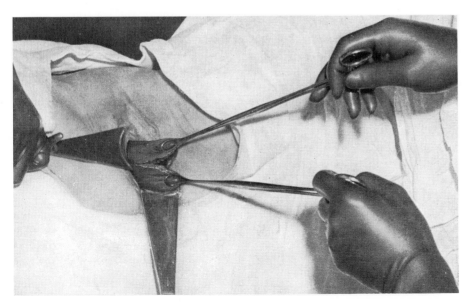

Figure 33-1. Cervical laceration exposed for repair.

Dehiscence of a lower-segment cesarean section scar is much more frequent than actual rupture, especially if the previous uterine incision was transverse. It is remarkable that these separated scars, covered only by the peritoneum, in many instances appear to cause no difficulty in labor or subsequently.

RUPTURE OF A CESAREAN SECTION SCAR

Experiences at Parkland Memorial Hospital

The experience at this institution has been that antepartum and during early labor, separation of the low transverse uterine incision is almost always limited to dehiscence without an appreciable increase in maternal or perinatal morbidity. Separation of a vertical scar, however, is more likely to result in severe hemorrhage, with an increased perinatal morbidity and mortality.

In one sample of 354 cases, in the great majority of which the previous uterine incision was of the low transverse variety, 211, or 60 percent, were considered to be in labor at the time of repeat cesarean section. There were two instances of uterine dehiscence and one of rupture of the scar. One dehiscence involved a previous low transverse uterine incision. The dehiscence was extended to effect delivery of the healthy infant and then the

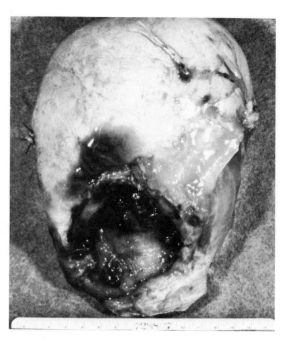

Figure 33-3. Rupture of uterus identified immediately after vaginal delivery; the previous delivery was by cesarean section with a vertical uterine incision.

uterus was closed without much difficulty, using two layers of continuous chromic catgut. In the second case, the dehiscence of the lower vertical incision was not repaired. Instead, cesarean hysterectomy was performed to comply with the woman's request for sterilization. In one case of uterine rupture, a defect believed to be uterine was felt suprapubically during a uterine contraction. With her last two cesarean sections, a vertical uterine incision was made that apparently included some of the upper segment. At laparotomy, the separated vertical scar was covered by a hematoma of about 400 ml that was entrapped beneath the serosa and overlying adherent omentum. Blood had also infiltrated throughout the left broad ligament to the lateral wall of the pelvis. An infant who weighed 2950 g, with an Apgar score of 8 at 5 minutes, was delivered through the ruptured scar. Hysterectomy was performed with some difficulty because of dense adhesions (Fig. 33-2).

Another woman, in whom the cervix was fully dilated and the occiput at +2 station when she was admitted the Labor–Delivery Unit, was promptly delivered using forceps, although she had previously undergone cesarean section. Immediate exploration of the uterus was conducted, as should be done in every case of previous cesarean section. Extensive separation of the vertical cesarean section scar with appreciable hemorrhage was identified and the uterus was removed (Fig. 33-3). Both mother and infant survived.

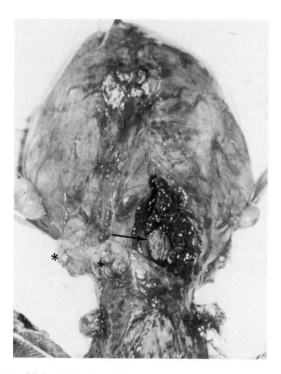

Figure 33-2. Ruptured vertical cesarean section scar (*arrow*) identified at time of repeat cesarean section early in labor; asterisks indicate some of the sites of densely adherent omentum.

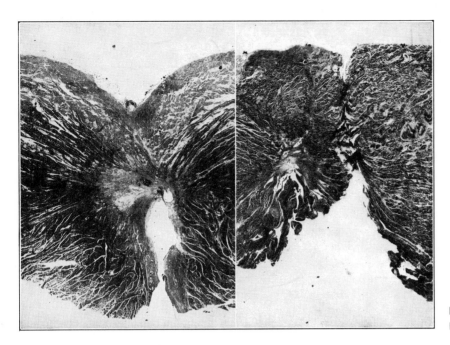

Figure 33-4. Photomicrographs of two poorly healed cesarean section scars.

Healing of the Cesarean Section Scar

Little information on this subject has been garnered from studies of cesarean section scars. Williams (1921) believed that the uterus heals by regeneration of the muscular fibers and not by scar tissue formation. He based his conclusion on the findings of histologic examination of the site of the incision and on two principal observations: First, upon inspection of the unopened uterus at the time of repeated cesarean sections one usually finds no trace of the former incision or, at most, an almost invisible linear scar. Second, when the uterus is removed, often no scar is visible after fixation, or only a shallow vertical furrow in the external and internal surfaces of the anterior uterine wall is seen, with no trace of scar tissue between them. Schwarz and co-workers (1938), however, concluded that healing occurs mainly by the proliferation of fibroblasts. They studied the site of the incision in the human uterus some days after cesarean section, as well as in the uteri of guinea pigs, rabbits, and dogs, and they observed that as the scar shrinks, the proliferation of connective tissue becomes less obvious. Their conclusions appear to be justified by their histologic studies, particularly in cases of adequate approximation of the myometrial edges. If the cut surfaces are closely apposed, the proliferation of connective tissue is minimal, and the normal relation of smooth muscle to connective tissue is gradually reestablished, accounting for the occasional absence of even a trace of a former incision. Even when the healing is so poor that marked thinning has resulted, the remaining tissue is often entirely muscular (Fig. 33-4). The fundamental weakness appears to stem from failure to approximate the inner margins of the incision or from formation of a hematoma or abscess in the immediate vicinity.

RUPTURE OF THE UNSCARRED UTERUS

Traumatic Rupture

Although the uterus is surprisingly resistant to blunt trauma, pregnant women sustaining blunt trauma to the abdomen should be watched carefully for signs of a ruptured uterus. The experiences at Parkland Memorial Hospital, however, have been that rupture of the spleen or traumatic placental abruption, although rare, are relatively more common. Wounds that penetrate the abdomen are much more likely to involve the large pregnant uterus.

Unfortunately, administration of oxytocin in the first or second stage of labor has been a rather common cause of traumatic rupture, especially in women of high parity (Awais and Lebherz, 1970). In the past, traumatic rupture during delivery was most often produced by internal podalic version and extraction. Other causes of traumatic rupture include difficult forceps delivery, breech extraction (Figs. 33-5, 33-6), and unusual fetal enlargement, such as hydrocephalus. The occurrence of a ruptured uterus caused by strong fundal pressure to try to accomplish vaginal delivery is particularly reprehensible.

Spontaneous Rupture of Uterus

This catastrophe is more likely to occur in women of high parity. For this reason, oxytocin should rarely be given to undelivered women of high parity. Similarly, in

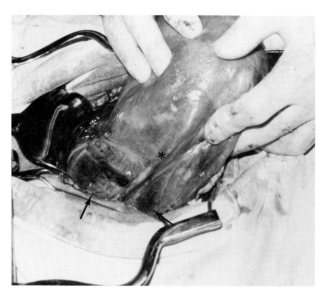

Figure 33-5. A. Rupture of uterus with breech delivery; extensive bleeding beneath uterine serosa and bladder, and in left broad ligament (*arrow*). Asterisk identifies left round ligament.

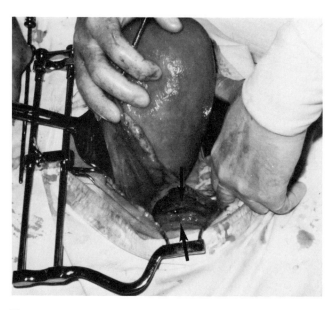

Figure 33-5. B. The broad ligament has been opened and the ureter (*upper arrow*) identified medial to the iliac vessels (*lower arrow*).

women of high parity, a trial of labor in the presence of cephalopelvic disproportion, or abnormal presentation such as a brow, may prove dangerous not only to the fetus but also to the mother.

Pathologic Anatomy

The role in uterine rupture of excessive stretching of the lower uterine segment with the development of a pathologic retraction ring is stressed in Chapter 29 (p. 648). Rupture of the previously intact uterus at the time of labor most often involves the thinned-out lower uterine segment. The rent, when it is in the immediate vicinity of the cervix, frequently extends transversely or obliquely. Usually, the tear is longitudinal, when it occurs in the portion of the uterus adjacent to the broad ligament (Fig. 33-6). Although developing primarily in the lower uterine segment, it is not unusual for the laceration to extend farther upward into the body of the uterus or downward through the cervix into the vagina. At times, the bladder may also be lacerated. After complete rupture, the uterine contents escape into the peritoneal cavity, unless the presenting part is firmly engaged, when only a portion of the fetus may be extruded from the uterus.

Incomplete ruptures frequently extend into the broad ligament. In such circumstances, the hemorrhage tends to be less rapid than in complete ruptures, the blood accumulating between the leaves of the broad ligament, with the formation of a large retroperitoneal hematoma that may involve sufficient blood loss to cause death. More frequently, fatal exsanguination supervenes after secondary rupture of the hematoma relieves the

tamponading effect of the intact broad ligament. With incomplete rupture, the products of conception may remain within the uterus or assume a position between the leaves of the broad ligament.

Apparent spontaneous rupture of the uterus at times follows manipulations that may very well have caused unappreciated injury to the uterus. Three cases of rupture at Parkland Memorial Hospital fall in this category. In one, the previous pregnancy had terminated in an induced septic abortion. During the next pregnancy, at laparotomy following rupture of the uterus, omentum was adherent to the fundus at the site of uterine rupture, strongly suggesting that previous perforation of the uterus had occurred. In the second case, vigorous curettage had followed delivery of a hydatidiform mole and histologically myometrial fragments were identified in the curettings. In this woman's next pregnancy, the uterus ruptured early in labor, the left uterine artery was severed, and rapid exsanguination followed. In the third case, an intrauterine device had been removed by use of a laparoscope with considerable difficulty from the uterine fundus. In the next pregnancy a rent developed in the fundus early in labor, with expulsion of the fetus and placenta, causing fetal death. Taylor and Cummings (1979) described spontaneous rupture of the uterus of a primigravid woman before the onset of labor. The uterine fundus had been traumatized previously by a trocar inserted for laparoscopy.

Instances of uterine rupture have been observed in which hemorrhage was slight. The rupture did not involve large arteries and the emptied uterus contracted well after expulsion of the fetus and placenta into the peritoneal cavity. In very rare cases, the fetus may be

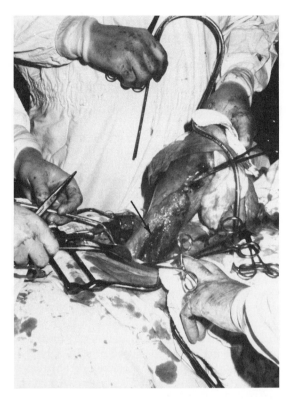

Figure 33-5. C. Extent of rupture (*arrow*) of lateral wall of uterus is now apparent.

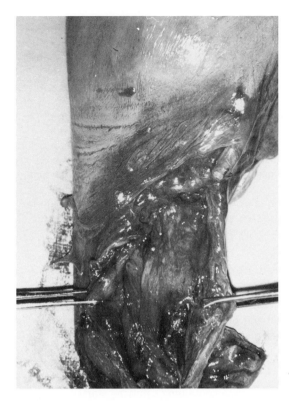

Figure 33-6. Close-up view of resected uterus to show site of rupture observed in Figure 33-5.

extruded into the peritoneal cavity while the placenta remains functional within the uterus and the gestation continues as a *uteroabdominal pregnancy* (Badawy, 1962).

Clinical Course

Prior to circulatory collapse from hemorrhage, the symptoms and physical findings may appear bizarre unless the possibility of rupture of the uterus is kept in mind. As an example, a woman was transferred to Parkland Memorial Hospital near term with the diagnosis of pulmonary embolism. She stated that she had been treated for such following a previous pregnancy. She complained of pain on inspiration and shortness of breath, as well as abdominal pain thought to be labor. The symptoms directed to the chest were not the consequence of an embolus, however, but rather of hemoperitoneum from a ruptured uterus, with blood irritating the diaphragm and causing the pain referred to the chest (see Chapter 22, p. 428).

If the accident occurs during labor, the woman, usually after a period of premonitory signs, at the acme of a uterine contraction suddenly complains of a sharp, shooting pain in the abdomen and may cry out that "something ripped" or "something tore" inside her. Immediately after these symptoms and signs have appeared, there is cessation of uterine contractions, and

the woman, until that point in intense agony, suddenly experiences much relief. At the same time, there may be external hemorrhage, although it is often slight.

Since women who are in labor or who are being delivered are usually given analgesics, pain and tenderness may not be immediately evident, and the condition becomes manifest by the systemic effects of the hypovolemia.

If the fetus is partly or totally extrauterine, abdominal palpation or vaginal examination is helpful in identifying the presenting part, which has moved away from the pelvic inlet. A firm, rounded body, the contracted uterus, may, at times, be felt alongside the fetus. Often fetal parts are more easily palpated than usual. On vaginal examination, it is sometimes possible to palpate a tear in the uterine wall through which the fingers can be passed into the peritoneal cavity, where the viscera may be felt. *Failure to detect the tear by no means proves its absence.* In suspected cases, it is imperative that thorough examination be performed by an experienced examiner before the suspicion is abandoned. At times, either abdominal paracentesis in the flank or culdocentesis is indicated to identify hemoperitoneum. (After delivery, culdocentesis can be performed through the posterior fornix into the cul-de-sac. The posterior lip of the cervix is grasped and a long 15-gauge needle is inserted beneath it through the fornix while the cervix is lifted anteriorly.)

Prognosis

The chances for fetal survival are dismal; the mortality rates found in various studies ranged between 50 and 75 percent. However, if the fetus is alive at the time of the accident, the only chance of continued survival is afforded by immediate delivery, most often by laparotomy. Otherwise, hypoxia from both the separation of the placenta and maternal hypovolemia is inevitable. If untreated, most of the women die from hemorrhage or less often later from infection, although spontaneous recovery has been noted in exceptional cases. Prompt diagnosis, immediate operation, the availability of large amounts of blood, and antibiotic therapy have improved greatly the prognosis for women with rupture of the pregnant uterus.

Immediate Treatment

The life of the woman will depend most often on the speed and efficiency with which hypovolemia can be corrected and hemorrhage controlled. Whenever rupture of the uterus is diagnosed, it is mandatory that the following functions be carried out, immediately and simultaneously: (1) two effective intravenous infusion systems must be established, and lactated Ringer solution or similar electrolyte-containing solutions started; (2) compatible, or at least type-specific, whole blood, must be obtained in large quantities (3 liters to start), and it must be infused vigorously as soon as possible; and (3) a surgical team, including an anesthesiologist must be assembled. The hypovolemia may not be correctable until arterial bleeding has been brought under control surgically. Therefore, delay in operating is contraindicated. Instead, blood must be infused vigorously and the laparotomy begun. In desperate cases, compression applied to the aorta may help to reduce the bleeding. Oxytocin administered intravenously may incite contraction of the myometrium and, in turn, vessel constriction, thereby reducing the bleeding. Clamping the ovarian vessels immediately adjacent to the uterus will help to conserve blood. Techniques for monitoring the adequacy of the circulation, blood and blood-fraction replacement therapy, and the recognition and treatment of coagulation defects are considered in detail in Chapter 21.

Hysterectomy Versus Repair

Hysterectomy is usually required, but in highly selected cases suture of the wound may be performed.

As part of the overall problem of rupture of the uterus, Mokgokong and Marivate (1976), based on a review of 335 cases treated in Durban, South Africa, considered the merits of hysterectomy compared to suture of the laceration. Maternal mortality was 7 percent and fetal mortality was 80 percent. Three fourths of the cases involved women with previously unscarred uteri.

Common specific causes of rupture of the previously unscarred uterus were cephalopelvic disproportion, fetal malpresentation, obstetric instrumentation, oxytocin stimulation, and internal podalic version. The uterine tears were usually longitudinal and lateral, often involving the uterine artery or its major branches. They concluded that total hysterectomy, especially with longitudinal tears, is the surgical procedure of choice, although transverse lower segment lacerations may be dealt with adequately by repair of the rent. The frequency of subsequent successful pregnancies following repair of the rent was not provided.

Sheth (1968) reported the findings in a series of 66 cases in which repair of a uterine rupture was elected rather than hysterectomy. In 25 instances, the repair was accompanied by tubal sterilization. Thirteen of the 41 mothers who did not have tubal sterilization had a total of 21 subsequent pregnancies, but uterine rupture recurred in 4 instances.

In the presence of a large hematoma in the broad ligament, identification and ligation of the uterine vessels can be extremely difficult. In general, efforts to control hemorrhage by clamping indiscriminately at the site of rupture involving the lower segment should be avoided. To do otherwise often leads to clamping and ligation of the ureter, bladder, or both. With uterine ruptures involving the lower uterine segment, bleeding vessels must be visualized free of surrounding tissue before clamping, or the ureter and bladder must be demonstrated to be remote from the tissue that is clamped. Placement of clamps to control bleeding carries little risk when rupture involves the body of the uterus remote from the ureters and bladder. The broad ligament may be entered and the ascending uterine artery and veins safely clamped. Usually, the ovarian vessels should be promptly clamped adjacent to the uterus.

Ligation of the hypogastric arteries at times reduces the hemorrhage appreciably. The ligation is accomplished by opening the peritoneum over the common iliac artery and dissecting down to the bifurcation of the external iliac and hypogastric arteries. The areolar sheath covering the hypogastric artery is incised longitudinally and a right-angle clamp is carefully passed just beneath the artery. Care must be taken not to perforate contiguous large veins. Suture, usually nonabsorbable, is then inserted into the open clamp, the jaws are locked, the suture is carried around the vessel, and the vessel is securely ligated (Figs. 33-7, 33-8). Pulsations in the external iliac artery, if present before tying the ligature, should be present afterward as well. If not, pulsations must be identified after arterial hypotension has been successfully treated in order to assure that the blood flow through the external iliac vessel has not been compromised by the ligature. An important mechanism of action with hypogastric ligation, apparently, is reduction of pulse pressure in those arteries distal to the ligation. It is of interest that bilateral ligation of the hypogastric arteries per se does not appear to interfere seriously with

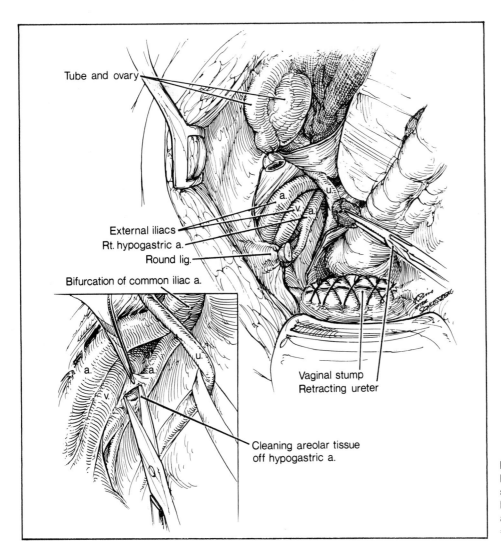

Tube and ovary

External iliacs
Rt. hypogastric a.
Round lig.

Bifurcation of common iliac a.

Vaginal stump
Retracting ureter

Cleaning areolar tissue
off hypogastric a.

Figure 33-7. Ligation of the right hypogastric artery. The areolar sheath covering the artery is being opened (*lower left*) (a. = artery, v. = vein, u. = ureter, lig. = ligament, rt. = right).

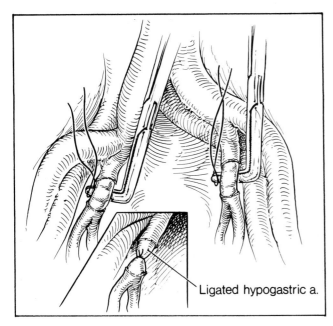

Ligated hypogastric a.

Figure 33-8. Ligation of both hypogastric arteries. After the covering sheath has been opened and the artery has been carefully freed from the immediately adjacent veins, a ligature is carried beneath the artery with a right angle clamp and firmly tied (a. = artery).

subsequent reproduction. Mengert and associates (1969) documented successful pregnancies in five women after bilateral hypogastric artery ligation. In three, the ovarian arteries were also ligated.

GENITAL TRACT FISTULAS FROM PARTURITION

In obstructed labor, the tissues of various parts of the genital tract may be compressed between the fetal head and the bony pelvis. If the pressure is brief, it is without significance, but if it is prolonged, necrosis results, followed in a few days by sloughing and perforation (Chapter 31, p. 678).

In most such cases, the perforation occurs between the vagina and the bladder, giving rise to a vesicovaginal fistula. Less frequently, the anterior lip of the cervix is compressed against the symphysis pubis, and an abnormal communication is eventually established between the cervical canal and the bladder, a vesicocervical fistula. If the woman has no infection, the fistula may heal spontaneously. More often it persists, requiring subsequent repair.

Rarely, the posterior wall of the uterus may be subjected to so much pressure against the promontory of the sacrum that necrosis results, and a fistula communicating with the cul-de-sac develops.

REFERENCES

Awais GM, Lebherz TB: Ruptured uterus, a complication of oxytocin induction and high parity. Obstet Gynecol 36:465, 1970

Badwy AH: Abdominal pregnancy in a previously ruptured uterus. Lancet 1:510, 1962

Lazarus EJ: Early rupture of the gravid uterus. Am J Obstet Gynecol 132:224, 1978

Mengert WJ, Burchell RC, Blumstein RW, Daskal JL: Pregnancy after bilateral ligation of the internal iliac and ovarian arteries. Obstet Gynecol 34:664, 1969

Mokgokong ER, Marivate M: Treatment of the ruptured uterus. Afr Med J 50:1621, 1976

Schrinsky DC, Benson RC: Rupture of the pregnant uterus: A review. Obstet Gynecol Survey 33:217, 1978

Schwarz O, Paddock R, Bortnick AR: The cesarean scar: An experimental study. Am J Obstet Gynecol 36:962, 1938

Sheth SS: Results of treatment of rupture of the uterus by suturing. J Obstet Gynaecol Br Commonw 75:55, 1968

Taylor PJ, Cummings DC: Spontaneous rupture of a primigravid uterus. J Reprod Med 22:169, 1979

Williams JW: A critical analysis of 21 years' experience with cesarean section. Bull Johns Hopkins Hosp 32:173, 1921

34

Abnormalities of the Third Stage of Labor

POSTPARTUM HEMORRHAGE

Definition

Postpartum hemorrhage has most often been defined as loss of blood in excess of 500 ml during the first 24 hours after birth of the infant. Through quantitative measurements of puerperal blood loss, however, the incongruity of this definition has been clearly demonstrated, as blood loss resulting from vaginal delivery is *frequently* somewhat more than 500 ml. Newton (1966), for example, measured the amount of hemoglobin shed by 105 women from the time of vaginal delivery through the next 24 hours and ascertained that the average blood loss was at least 546 ml. If appropriate allowance was made for the maternal blood discarded with the placenta, as well as that not measured because of incomplete recovery of shed hemoglobin, the blood loss during the first 24 hours averaged about 650 ml. Moreover, Pritchard and associates (1962) and DeLeeuw and co-workers (1968) demonstrated that erythrocytes equivalent to approximately 600 ml of blood are lost from the maternal circulation during vaginal delivery and the next several hours. Therefore, a blood loss somewhat in excess of 500 ml by accurate measurement is not necessarily an abnormal event for vaginal delivery. Pritchard and associates noted that about 5 percent of women delivering vaginally lost more than 1000 ml of blood, according to their measurements. These same workers observed that estimated blood loss commonly is only about one half the actual loss. Moreover, based on an estimated blood loss greater than 500 ml, postpartum hemorrhage has been found in many hospitals to occur in about 5 percent of the deliveries. An estimated blood loss in excess of 500 ml in many institutions, therefore, may call attention to mothers who are bleeding excessively and warn the physician that dangerous hemorrhage is imminent. Hemorrhage after the first 24 hours is designated as *late postpartum hemorrhage* and is discussed in the section Hemorrhages During the Puerperium in Chapter 36 (p. 737).

Significance

Postpartum hemorrhage is the most common cause of serious blood loss in obstetrics. As a direct factor in maternal mortality, it is the cause of about one quarter of the deaths from obstetric hemorrhage in the group that includes postpartum hemorrhage, low implanted placentas (placenta previa), placental abruption, ectopic pregnancy, hemorrhage from abortion, and rupture of the uterus.

Immediate Causes

The many factors of importance, singly or in combination, in the genesis of early postpartum hemorrhage are listed below:

1. Trauma to the genital tract
   Large episiotomy
   Lacerations of perineum, vagina, or cervix
   Rupture of uterus
2. Failure of compression of blood vessels at the implantation site
   Hypotonic myometrium
      General anesthesia (especially with halogenated compounds and ether)
      Poorly perfused myometrium (hypotension from hemorrhage or conduction anesthesia)
      Overdistended uterus (large fetus, multiple fetuses, hydramnios)
      After prolonged labor
      After very rapid labor
      After labor from vigorous oxytocin stimulation
      High parity
      Previous hemorrhage from uterine atony
      Uterine infection
   Retention of placental tissue
      Abnormally adherent (placenta accreta, increta, and percreta)
      No abnormality of adherence (succenturiate lobe)

3. Coagulation defects
   Aquired   ⎫ Intensified hemorrhage from
   Congenital   ⎭ all of the above causes

Of all these, the two most common causes of immediate postpartum hemorrhage are hypotonic myometrium (*uterine atony*) and lacerations of the vagina and cervix. Retention of part or all of the placenta, a less common cause, may produce either immediate or delayed hemorrhage, or both. It is uncommon for an episiotomy alone to cause severe postpartum hemorrhage, although blood so lost averages about 200 ml and, at times, is much more (Odell and Seski, 1947).

Predisposing Causes

In the majority of cases, postpartum hemorrhage can be predicted well in advance of delivery. Examples in which trauma is likely to lead to postpartum hemorrhage include delivery of a large infant, midforceps delivery, forceps rotation, delivery through an incompletely dilated cervix, Dührssen incisions of the cervix, any intrauterine manipulation, and vaginal delivery after cesarean section or other uterine incisions. Uterine atony causing hemorrhage can be anticipated whenever an anesthetic agent is used that will relax the uterus. Halothane and ether are prominent examples. The overdistended uterus is very likely to be hypotonic after delivery. Thus the woman with a large fetus, multiple fetuses, or hydramnios is prone to hemorrhage from uterine atony. Blood loss with delivery of twins, for example, averages nearly 1000 ml, or nearly twice that associated with delivery of a singleton, and may be much greater (Pritchard, 1965). The woman whose labor is characterized by uterine activity that is either remarkably vigorous or barely effective is also likely to bleed excessively from uterine atony after delivery. Similarly, labor either initiated or augmented with oxytocin is more likely to be followed by postdelivery uterine atony and hemorrhage. The woman of high parity is at increased risk of hemorrhage from uterine atony. The risk is even greater if she previously has suffered a post partum hemorrhage. Commonly, mismanagement of the third stage of labor involves an attempt to hasten delivery of the placenta short of manual removal. *Constant kneading and squeezing of the uterus that is already contracted are likely to impede the physiologic mechanism of placental detachment, with incomplete placenta separation and increased blood loss as the consequence.*

Clinical Characteristics

Postpartum hemorrhage before delivery of the placenta is called third-stage hemorrhage. Contrary to general opinion, whether bleeding occurs before or after delivery of the placenta or at both times, there may be no sudden massive hemorrhage but rather a steady bleeding that at any given instant appears to be moderate but persists until serious hypovolemia develops. Especially with hemorrhage after delivery of the placenta, the constant seepage may, over a period of a few hours, lead to enormous loss of blood. The effects of hemorrhage depend to a considerable degree upon the nonpregnant blood volume, the magnitude of pregnancy-induced hypervolemia, and the degree of anemia at the time of delivery. A treacherous feature of postpartum hemorrhage is the failure of the pulse and blood pressure to undergo more than moderate alterations until large amounts of blood have been lost, as emphasized in Chapter 21 (p. 391). The normotensive woman may actually become somewhat hypertensive in response to hemorrhage, at least initially. Moreover, the already hypertensive woman may be interpreted to be normotensive although remarkably hypovolemic. Tragically, the hypovolemia may not be recognized until very late.

In instances in which the fundus has not been adequately monitored after delivery, the blood may not escape vaginally but may collect instead within the uterus. The uterine cavity may thus become distended by 1000 ml or more of blood while an incompetent attendant fails to identify the large uterus or, having done so, erroneously massages a roll of abdominal fat. The care of the postpartum uterus must not, therefore, be left to an inexperienced person.

Diagnosis

Except possibly when an intrauterine and intravaginal accumulation of blood is not recognized, the diagnosis of postpartum hemorrhage should be obvious. The differentiation between bleeding from uterine atony and from lacerations is tentatively made on the condition of the uterus. If bleeding persists despite a firm, well-contracted uterus, the cause of the hemorrhage most probably is lacerations. Bright red blood also suggests lacerations. To ascertain the role of lacerations as a cause of bleeding, careful inspection of the vagina, cervix, and uterus is essential. Sometimes bleeding may occur from both atony and trauma, especially after major operative delivery. In general, inspection of the cervix and vagina should be performed after every delivery to prevent hemorrhage from cervical or vaginal lacerations. Anesthesia should be adequate to prevent discomfort to the mother during such an examination and there should have been no contamination of the lower genital tract or adjacent perineum. Examination of the uterine cavity, the cervix, and all of the vagina is essential after breech extraction, after internal podalic version, upon completion of a vaginal delivery in a woman who previously underwent cesarean section. The same is true when unusual bleeding occurs during the second stage of labor and immediately after birth of the infant.

Prognosis

It should be possible to save the life of almost every woman with postpartum hemorrhage, even though hysterectomy may be required to do so in some instances. To obtain this objective, however, requires assiduous attention to all women immediately postpartum, an effective blood bank, and alert action by an experienced obstetric team. Although death from postpartum hemorrhage is rare in current obstetric practice in modern hospitals, it is common under less favorable conditions.

There are other hazards imposed by postpartum hemorrhage, not the least of which are transfusion reactions, including renal failure, hepatitis, and the possibility of developing the acquired immune deficiency syndrome (AIDS).

Sheehan Syndrome

Severe intrapartum or early postpartum hemorrhage, furthermore, is on rare occasions followed by Sheehan syndrome, which, in the classic case, is characterized by failure in lactation, amenorrhea, atrophy of the breasts, loss of pubic and axillary hair, superinvolution of the uterus, hypothyroidism, and adrenal cortical insufficiency. The exact pathogenesis of Sheehan syndrome is not well understood since such endocrine abnormalities in most women who hemorrhage severely are not evident. In some but not all instances of Sheehan syndrome, varying degrees of necrosis of the anterior pituitary gland with impaired secretion of one or more of its trophic hormones account for the endocrine abnormalities. The anterior pituitary of some women who develop hypopituitarism after puerperal hemorrhage does respond to various releasing hormones, however, which implies, at least, impaired hypothalamic function rather than pituitary necrosis. Moreover, confirmatory histologic evidence of hypothalamic involvement has been provided by Whitehead (1963), who, in some cases, identified specific atrophic changes in the hypothalamic nuclei. Lactation after delivery usually, but not always, excludes extensive pituitary necrosis.

The incidence of Sheehan syndrome was originally estimated to be 1 per 10,000 deliveries (Sheehan and Murdoch, 1938), and it appears to be equally rare today in the continental United States, although 100 cases were identified in two decades in one hospital in Puerto Rico (Haddock and colleagues, 1972). Perhaps the application of the many tests of hypothalamic and pituitary function now available will identify milder forms of the syndrome to be much more prevalent (Grimes and Brooks, 1980). A schema of sequential stimulation tests for Sheehan syndrome has been provided by DiZerega and co-workers (1978).

Diabetes Insipidus. Severe hemorrhage at and immediately after delivery has been implicated in the development of diabetes insipidus without apparent anterior pituitary deficiency. The lesion is rare; in fact, Collins and associates (1979) claim to have reported the first case.

Management of Third-Stage Bleeding

Some bleeding is inevitable during the third stage of every labor as the result of transient partial separation of the placenta. As the placenta separates, the blood from the implantation site may escape into the vagina immediately ("Duncan mechanism") or it may be concealed behind the placenta and membranes ("Schultze mechanism") until the placenta is delivered.

In the presence of any external hemorrhage during the third stage, the uterus should be massaged if it is not firmly contracted. If the signs of placental separation have appeared (see Chapter 17, p. 342), expression of the placenta should be attempted by manual pressure on the fundus of the uterus. Descent of the placenta is indicated by the cord becoming slack. If bleeding continues, manual removal of the placenta is mandatory.

Technique of Manual Removal

When this operation is required, aseptic surgical technique should be employed. A sterile glove that covers the forearm to the elbow is recommended. After grasping the fundus of the uterus through the abdominal wall with one hand, the other hand with the long glove is introduced into the vagina and passed into the uterus, along the umbilical cord. As soon as the placenta is reached, its margin is located and the ulnar border of the hand insinuated between it and the uterine wall (Fig. 34-1). Then with the back of the hand in contact with the uterus, the placenta is peeled off its uterine attachment by a motion similar to that employed in separating the leaves of a book. After its complete separation, the placenta should be grasped with the entire hand, which is then gradually withdrawn. Membranes are removed at the same time by carefully teasing them from the decidua, using ring forceps to grasp them as necessary. Some prefer to wipe out the uterine cavity with a sponge. If this is done, it is imperative that a sponge not be left in the uterus or vagina.

Management after Delivery of Placenta

Irrespective of the method of delivery of the placenta, the fundus should always be palpated afterwards to make certain that the uterus is well contracted. If it is not firm, vigorous fundal massage is indicated. In some institutions 0.2 mg of ergonovine (Ergotrate) or methylergonovine (Methergine) is routinely administered either intravenously or intramuscularly. More commonly, because hypertension occasionally develops following administration of these compounds, they are given only

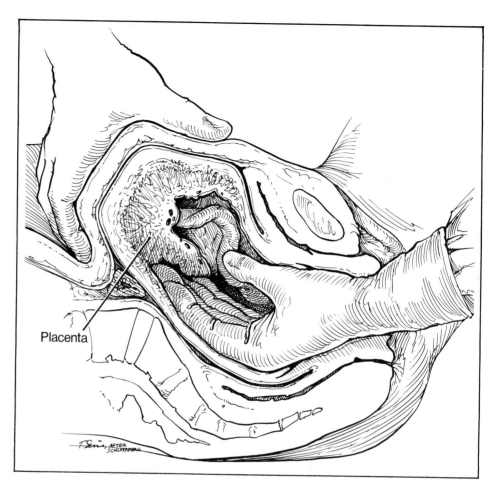

Figure 34-1. Manual removal of placenta. The fingers are alternately abducted, adducted, and advanced until the placenta is completely detached.

Placenta

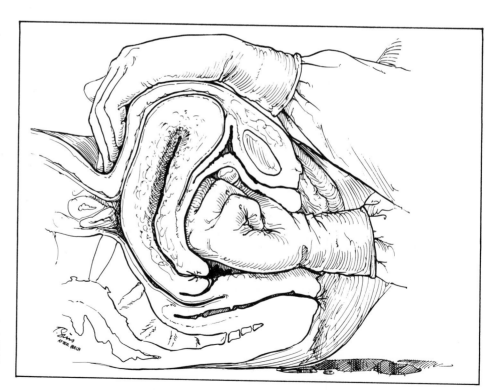

Figure 34-2. Bimanual compression of the uterus and massage with the abdominal hand usually will effectively control hemorrhage from uterine atony.

if there is excessive bleeding not controlled by an intravenous infusion of oxytocin and uterine massage. Most often 20 units of oxytocin in 1000 ml of lacatated Ringer solution or normal saline proves effective when administered intravenously at approximately 10 ml per minute simultaneously with effective massage of the uterus (see Chapter 17, p. 345). If such therapy does not prove effective, ergonovine (Ergotrate) or methylergonovine (Methergine), 0.2 mg administered intravenously, may stimulate the uterus to contract and retract sufficiently to control hemorrhage from the placental implantation site.

If bleeding persists despite these procedures, no time should be lost in haphazard efforts to control hemorrhage, but the following plan of management should be initiated immediately:

1. Employ bimanual uterine compression (Fig. 34-2). (This procedure will control most hemorrhage.)
2. Obtain help!
3. Begin transfusion of blood. The blood group of every obstetric patient should be known before labor, and cross-matched blood should be available for those in whom hemorrhage is anticipated. In an emergency, type-specific but uncross-matched whole blood can be used.
4. Explore the uterine cavity manually for retained placental fragments or lacerations.
5. Thoroughly inspect the cervix and vagina after adequate exposure.
6. Add a second intravenous route using a large bore intravenous catheter so that oxytocin can continue to be given at the same time as blood is being received.
7. Adequacy of cardiac output and arterial filling can be evaluated by monitoring urine output. Put a Foley catheter in the patient's bladder (see Obstetric Hemorrhage, Chapter 21, p. 392).

The technique of bimanual compression (Fig. 34-2) consists simply of massage of the posterior aspect of the uterus with the abdominal hand and massage through the vagina of the anterior uterine aspect with the other fist, the knuckles of which contact the uterine wall. Packing the uterus was an alternative procedure that formerly enjoyed greater popularity. *The late-pregnant uterus cannot be satisfactorily packed immediately after delivery because it dilates under the packing, with further concealed hemorrhage that may be fatal.*

Blood transfusion should be initiated immediately in any case of postpartum hemorrhage in which abdominal massage of the uterus and oxytocic agents fail to control the bleeding. With transfusion and simultaneous manual compression of the uterus and oxytocin infused intravenously, additional measures are rarely required. If the operator's hand tires, an associate can relieve.

Prostaglandins have been used in attempts to control hemorrhage after delivery of the placenta. Takagi and co-work-

ers (1976) found that intravenously and intramuscularly injected prostaglandin $F_{2\alpha}$ was of little value in controlling uterine blood loss at delivery and adverse systemic effects were common; however, they reported excellent results by direct injection into the myometrium of 1 mg of prostaglandin $F_{2\alpha}$. A similar result using intramyometrially injected prostaglandin $F_{2\alpha}$ was reported by Jacobs and Arias (1980). Corson and Bolognese (1977) described a case in which uterine atony following cesarean section appeared to respond to repeated intramuscular doses of prostaglandin $F_{2\alpha}$ after intravenously administered oxytocin and ergonovine were ineffective. More recently, vaginal prostaglandin E_2 suppositories have been reported to be effective in treating persistent uterine atony (Hertz and associates, 1980) as well as intramuscular injection of 0.25 mg of (15-S)-15-methyl prostaglandin $F_{2\alpha}$-tromethamine (Prostin 15/M—Upjohn Company, Kalamazoo, Michigan) (Toppozada and associates, 1981; Hayashi and co-workers, 1981). The direct intramyometrial injection of this compound also has been reported to be effective in arresting postpartum hemorrhage due to uterine atony (Bruce and co-workers, 1982).

The unusual therapeutic failures following the use of (15-S)-15-methyl prostaglandin $F_{2\alpha}$-tromethamine have been associated with uterine infections and delay before attempting its use. Minor side effects of nausea, vomiting, diarrhea, and hyperthermia have been observed following the use of this compound and hypertensive episodes have been troublesome.

Magil (1984) presents the generally favorable experiences of several obstetricians who have tried postaglandin derivatives in an attempt to control postpartum hemorrhage.

It must be emphasized that the use of these prostaglandin compounds, for the purpose of arresting postpartum hemorrhage due to uterine atony has not yet been approved by the Food and Drug Administration and there are few series reported at present. However, with proper informed consent, the use of these compounds as a last resort prior to hypogastric artery ligation, hysterectomy, or both seems justified.

Hemorrhage from Retained Placental Fragments

Immediate postpartum hemorrhage is seldom caused by retained small placental fragments, but a remaining piece of placenta is a common cause of bleeding late in the puerperium. Inspection of the placenta after delivery must be routine. If a portion of placenta is missing, the uterus should be explored and the placental fragment removed, particularly in the face of continuing postpartum bleeding. Retention of a succenturiate lobe (see Figs. 6-15, 6-16) is an occasional cause of postpartum hemorrhage. The late bleeding that may result from a placental polyp is discussed in Chapter 36 (p. 737).

Hemorrhage from Lacerations

If rupture of the uterus is identified, laparotomy, and, most often, hysterectomy, is mandatory for a favorable outcome (see Chapter 33, p. 704). Lacerations of the cervix and the vaginal vault sometimes cause profuse bleeding. Any time that bleeding persists in the presence of a firmly contracted intact uterus, hemorrhage from

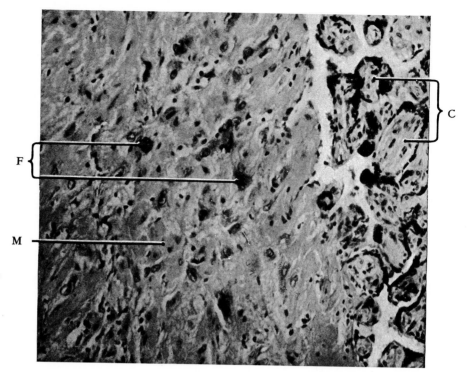

Figure 34-3. Photomicrograph of uterine wall in a case of placenta accreta. Notice the absence of decidua with chorionic villi in contact with the myometrium (C = chorionic villi, M = myometrium, F = trophoblastic giant cells).

lacerations of the cervix or vagina should be suspected. In any case of protracted hemorrhage, moreover, even though the obstetrician is certain that uterine atony is the cause, inspection of the cervix and vagina is a necessary precaution to avoid overlooking a serious laceration. Proper exposure of the cervix and upper vagina to repair such lacerations usually requires an associate. Two retractors are inserted into the vagina, the walls of which are separated widely. Ring forceps are then placed on the anterior and posterior lips of the cervix, which is carefully inspected, especially laterally. Lacerations that are bleeding should be promptly repaired. Either interrupted single sutures or figure-of-eight sutures are employed, with the highest one placed slightly above the apex of the tear, because bleeding from cervical lacerations usually arises from a vessel at this point (see Chapter 33, p. 697).

Hysterectomy

If rupture of the uterus is identified, hysterectomy is lifesaving in most instances (see Chapter 33, p. 704). With an apparently intact uterus, and when other measures to combat postpartum hemorrhage fail, the question of hysterectomy arises. If performed without initiating blood replacement in a woman who is profoundly hypovolemic, hysterectomy may hasten death. On the other hand, hysterectomy should not be delayed unduly. Vigorous transfusion therapy should be initiated and surgery promptly begun. This approach will prevent deaths in cases in which all other measures to arrest hemorrhage fail. A technique is described in Chapter 43 (p. 880).

ABNORMALLY ADHERENT PLACENTA

In most instances, the placenta separates spontaneously from its implantation site during the first few minutes after delivery of the infant. The precise reason for delay in detachment beyond this time is not always obvious, but quite often it seems to be due to inadequate uterine contraction and retraction. Very infrequently, the placenta is unusually adherent to the implantation site, with scanty or absent decidua, so that the physiologic line of cleavage through the spongy layer of decidua is lacking. As a consequence, one or more cotyledons of the placenta are firmly bound to the defective decidua basalis or even to the myometrium. When the placenta is densely anchored in this fashion, the condition is called placenta accreta.

Definitions

The term *placenta accreta* is used to describe any implantation of the placenta in which there is abnormally firm adherence to the uterine wall. As the consequence of partial or total absence of the decidua basalis and imperfect development of the fibrinoid layer (*Nitabuch layer*), the placental villi are attached to the myometrium (*placenta accreta*) (see Fig. 34-3), actually invade the myometrium (*placenta increta*), or even penetrate through the myometrium (*placenta percreta*) (Fig. 34-4). The abnormal adherence may involve all of the cotyledons (total placenta accreta), a few to several cotyledons (partial placenta accreta), or a single cotyledon (focal placenta accreta).

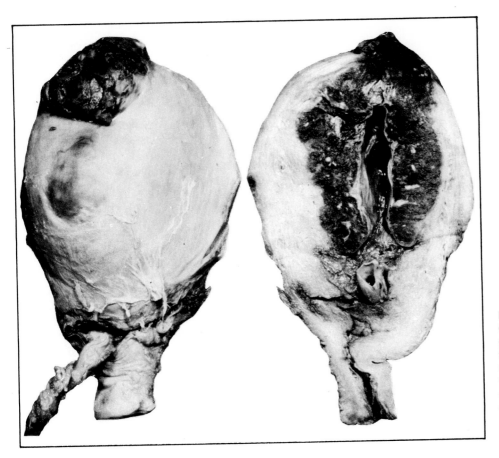

Figure 34-4. Placenta percreta. On the left, the placenta is fungating through the fundus above the old classical cesarean section scar. In the opened specimen on the right, the variable penetration of the fundus by the placenta is evident. (*From Morrison: Obstetrics and Gynecology Annual. New York, Appleton, 1978, p 113.*)

Significance

An abnormally adherent placenta, although an uncommon condition, assumes considerable significance clinically because of morbidity and, at times, mortality from severe hemorrhage, uterine perforation, and infection. The true frequencies of placenta accreta, increta, and percreta are unknown. Breen and associates (1977), for example, reviewed reports of this condition published since 1891. The incidence varied from 1 in 540 deliveries to 1 in 70,000 deliveries, with an average incidence of approximately 1 in 7000. Read and co-workers (1980) reported an incidence of 1 per 2562 deliveries and concluded that the clinical picture today "is one of higher reported incidence, lower parity, greater incidence of associated placenta previa ..." and decreasing maternal and perinatal mortality.

Etiologic Factors

Abnormal adherence of the placenta is found most often in circumstances where decidual formation was likely to have been defective, for example, implantations in the lower uterine segment, or over a previous cesarean section scar or other previous incisions into the uterine cavity, or after uterine curettage. Fox (1972), in his review of 622 reported cases of placenta accreta collected between 1945 and 1969, noted the following characteristics:

(1) placenta previa was identified in one third of affected pregnancies; (2) one fourth of the women had been delivered previously by cesarean section; (3) nearly one fourth of the women had previously undergone curettage; and (4) one fourth of them were gravida six or more. A similar result was observed by Read and co-workers for patients studied in the 1970s. However, the overall incidence and parity had decreased, likely due to limiting family size.

Clinical Course

Antepartum hemorrhage is common, but in the great majority of cases the antepartum bleeding is the consequence of a coexisting placenta previa. Invasion of the myometrium by placental villi at the site of a previous cesarean section scar may lead to rupture of the uterus during labor or even before (Berchuck and Sokol, 1983). Labor is most likely to be normal, however, in the absence of placenta previa or an involved uterine scar.

The problems associated with delivery of the placenta and subsequent developments will vary appreciably, depending upon the site of implantation, the depth of penetration into the myometrium, and the number of cotyledons involved. It is very likely that the focal placenta accreta with implantation in the upper segment of the uterus occurs much more often than is recognized.

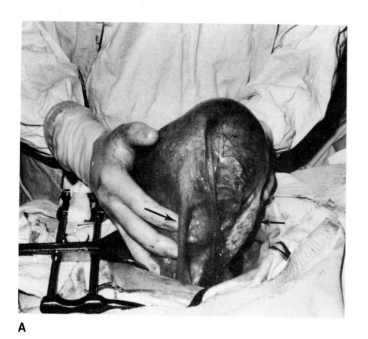

A

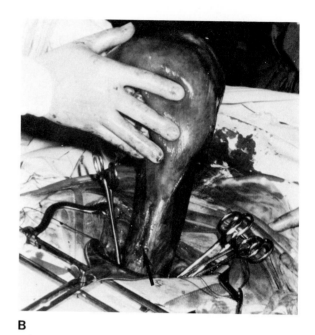

B

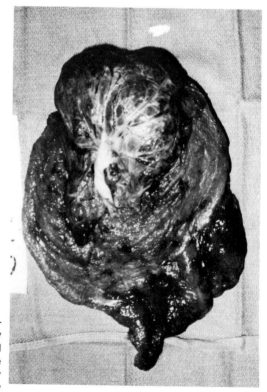

Figure 34-5. A. Hysterectomy for placenta accreta. The uterine fundus contains the adherent placenta. Arrows point to round ligament (*left*) and ovary (*right*) separated by the oviduct. **B.** The infundibulopelvic ligaments, broad ligaments, and cardinal ligaments have been resected. The incision in the lower segment (*arrow*) is used to palpate the margin of the cervix to identify where to enter the vagina. **C.** The uterus has been opened anteriorly to show the adherent placenta (placenta accreta).

C

The involved cotyledon is either pulled off the myometrium with perhaps somewhat excessive bleeding from that part of the implantation site, or the cotyledon is torn from the placenta and adheres to the implantation site with increased bleeding, immediately or later. This is probably the mechanism of formation of many so-called placental polyps (see Chapter 23, p. 443, and Fig. 36-2).

With more extensive involvement, however, hemorrhage becomes profuse as delivery of the placenta is attempted. Successful treatment depends upon immediate blood replacement therapy, as described under Obstetric Hemorrhage in Chapter 21 (p. 393), and nearly always prompt hysterectomy.

With total involvement of the placenta (total placenta accreta), there may be very little or no bleeding from the uterus, at least until manual removal of the placenta is attempted. At times, traction on the umbilical cord will invert the uterus as described below. Moreover, usual attempts at manual removal of the placenta will not succeed, since a cleavage plane between the maternal surface of the placenta and the uterine wall cannot be developed. The safest treatment in this circumstance is prompt hysterectomy. Such a case is illustrated in Figures 34-5A–C.

The possibility exists that the diagnosis of placenta increta might be diagnosed antepartum. Tabsh and co-workers (1982) described a case of placenta previa in which they were also able to identify placenta increta from *the lack of the usual subplacental sonolucent space*. These investigators hypothesize that the presence of this normal subplacental sonolucent area represents the decidual basalis and the underlying myometrial tissue. The absence of this sonolucent area is consistent with the presence of a placenta increta. Pasto and associates (1983) confirmed that the *absence* of a subplacental sonolucent or "hypoechoic retroplacental zone" is consistent with the presence of placenta increta.

> Placenta percreta is more likely to be life threatening than is placenta accreta or placenta increta, and can cause intra-abdominal antepartum hemorrhage (Cario and colleagues, 1983) or intrapartum hemorrhage, as exemplified by a case reported by Collins and associates (1978). During repeat cesarean section, severe hemorrhage began as the uterine serosa adjacent to the bladder was incised. The placenta had perforated the lower segment of the uterus and actually grown into the bladder. Removal of the placenta resulted in a 7-cm hole in the bladder. The massive hemorrhage was combatted with 11 liters of blood. The infant was anemic from blood loss consequent to incision of the placenta to effect delivery. The mother promptly developed diabetes insipidus without evidence of anterior pituitary dysfunction.

In the 622 published cases reviewed by Fox (1972), the most common form of "conservative" management was manual removal of as much placenta as possible and then packing of the uterus. ONE FOURTH OF THE WOMEN DIED, that is, four times as many as when

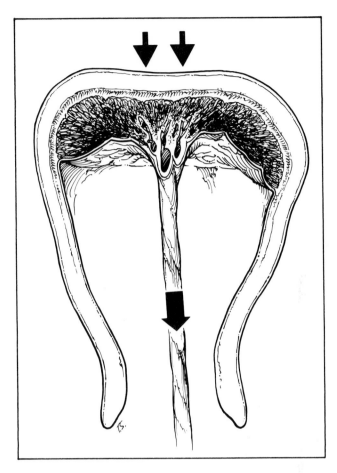

Figure 34-6. Most likely site of placental implantation in cases of uterine inversion. With traction on the cord and the placenta still attached, the likelihood of inversion is obvious.

treatment consisted of immediate hysterectomy. He noted that "conservative" treatment of placenta accreta in at least four instances was followed by an apparently normal pregnancy.

INVERSION OF THE UTERUS

Etiology

Complete inversion of the uterus after delivery of the infant is almost always the consequence of strong traction on an umbilical cord that is attached to a placenta implanted in the fundus of the uterus (Fig. 34-6). Contributing to uterine inversion are a tough cord that does not readily break away from the placenta, combined with fundal pressure and a relaxed uterus, including the lower segment and cervix. Placenta accreta may be implicated although uterine inversion can occur without the placenta being so firmly adherent. At times, the inversion may be incomplete (Fig. 34-7).

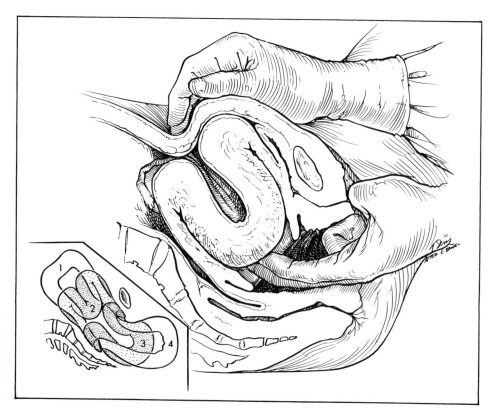

Figure 34-7. Incomplete inversion of the uterus. The diagnosis is made by abdominal palpation of the craterlike depression and vaginal palpation of the fundal wall in the lower segment and cervix. Shown in the insert are progressive degrees of inversion.

The exact frequency of this complication is not known. Kitchin and co-workers (1975) reported an incidence of 1 in 2284 deliveries. Platt and Druzin (1981) reported 28 cases in 60,052 deliveries, for an incidence of 1 in 2148 deliveries. These same investigators suggested that parenteral magnesium sulfate, which was administered to patients with pregnancy-induced hypertension, might have played a role in the etiology of this complication. Pritchard (1982) suggested that the inexperience of personnel performing the deliveries appeared to be a more important factor!

Clinical Course

Inversion of the uterus associated with the third stage of labor is often followed by circulatory collapse. Without prompt treatment, the woman may die (Fig. 34-8). It has been stated that shock tends to be disproportionate to blood loss (Greenhill and Friedman, 1974). Careful evaluation of the effects from transfusion of large volumes of blood in such cases does not support this concept, but, instead, makes it very apparent that blood loss in such circumstances was often massive but greatly underestimated. It is not unusual for even the woman who has received several units of blood because of hypotension to become anemic subsequently when isovolemic. Such outcomes are difficult to reconcile with the concept of shock out of proportion to blood loss (Watson and associates, 1980; Platt and Druzin, 1981).

Treatment

Delay in treatment increases the mortality rate appreciably. It is imperative that a number of steps be taken immediately and simultaneously:

1. Assistance, including an anesthesiologist, is summoned immediately.
2. The freshly inverted uterus with placenta already separated from it may often be replaced simply by immediately pushing on the fundus with the palm of the hand and fingers in the direction of the long axis of the vagina.
3. Preferably two intravenous infusion systems are made operational, and lactated Ringer solution and especially whole blood are given to refill the intravascular compartment and support cardiac output.
4. If attached, the placenta is not removed until the infusion systems are operational, fluids are being given, and anesthesia, perferably halothane, has been administered. Recently, Grossman (1981) reported that 2 g of magnesium sulfate administered intravenously resulted in enough uterine relaxation to enable the physician to restore the uterus to its normal position. To remove the placenta before this time increases the hemorrhage. In the meantime, the inverted uterus, if prolapsed beyond the vagina, is replaced within the vagina.

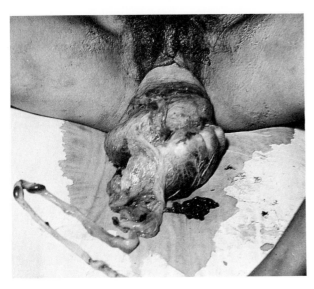

Figure 34-8. A fatal case of inverted uterus following delivery at home. The placenta was firmly adherent to its implantation site in the fundus (placenta accreta).

5. After removing the placenta, the palm of the hand is placed on the center of the fundus with the fingers extended to identify the margins of the cervix. Pressure is then applied with the hand so as to push the fundus upward through the cervix.

6. Oxytocin is NOT given until after the uterus is restored to its normal configuration.

As soon as the uterus is restored to its normal configuration, the anesthetic agent used to provide relaxation is stopped and simultaneously oxytocin is started to contract the uterus while the operator maintains the fundus in normal relationship. Initially, bimanual compression, as illustrated in Figure 34-2, will aid in the control of further hemorrhage until uterine tone is recovered. After the uterus is well contracted, the operator continues to monitor the uterus transvaginally for any evidence of subsequent inversion, although this occurrence is quite unlikely.

Surgical Intervention

Most often, the inverted uterus can be restored to its normal position by the techniques described above. For example, Kitchin and associates (1975) identified 11 "spontaneous" puerperal inversions among 25,000 deliveries, and in each instance the uterus was promptly replaced vaginally without significant morbidity other than hemorrhage from the uterus while in the inverted state. If the uterus cannot be reinverted by vaginal manipulation because of a dense constriction ring, as illustrated in Figure 34-9, laparotomy is imperative. The fundus may

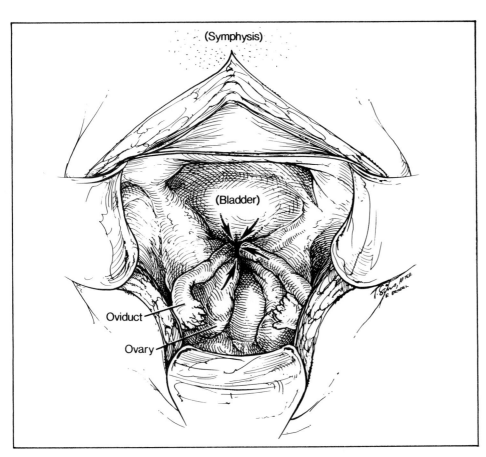

Figure 34-9. Completely inverted uterus viewed from above.

then be simultaneously pushed upward from below and pulled from above. A traction suture well placed in the inverted fundus may be of aid. If the constriction ring still prohibits reposition, it is carefully incised posteriorly to expose the fundus. A graphic outline of this surgical technique has been reported recently (vanVugt and associates, 1981). After replacement of the fundus, the anesthetic agent used to relax the myometrium is stopped, oxytocin infusion is begun, and the uterine incision is repaired. The adjacent viscera are carefully examined for trauma.

REFERENCES

Berchuck A, Sokol RJ: Previous cesarean section, placenta increta, and uterine rupture in second-trimester abortion. Am J Obstet Gynecol 145:766, 1983

Breen JL, Neubecker R, Gregori CA, Franklin JE Jr: Placenta accreta, increta, and percreta. A survey of 40 cases. Obstet Gynecol 49:43, 1977

Bruce SL, Paul RH, Van Dorsten JP: Control of postpartum uterine atony by intramyometrial prostaglandin. Obstet Gynecol 59:47S, 1982

Cario GM, Adler AD, Morris N: Placenta percreta presenting as intra-abdominal antepartum hemorrhage. Case report. Br J Obstet Gynaecol 90:491, 1983

Collins ML, O'Brien P, Tabrah N: Placenta previa percreta with bladder invasion. JAMA 240:1749, 1978

Corson SL, Bolognese RJ: Postpartum uterine atony treated with prostaglandins. Am J Obstet Gynecol 129:918, 1977

DeLeeuw NKM, Lowenstein L, Tucker EC, Dayal S: Correlation of red cell loss at delivery with changes in red cell mass. Am J Obstet Gynecol 84:1271, 1968

DiZerega G, Kletzky OA, Mishell DR Jr: Diagnosis of Sheehan's syndrome using a sequential stimulation test. Am J Obstet Gynecol 132:348, 1978

Fox H: Placenta accreta, 1945–1969. Obstet Gynecol Survey 27:475, 1972

Greenhill JP, Friedman EA: Biological Principles and Modern Practice of Obstetrics. Philadelphia, Saunders, 1974, p 687

Grimes HG, Brooks MH: Pregnancy in Sheehan's syndrome. Report of a case and review. Obstet Gynecol Survey 35:481, 1980

Grossman RA: Magnesium sulfate for uterine inversion. J Reprod Med 26:261, 1981

Haddock L, Vega LA, Aguilo F, Rodriguez O: Adrenocortical, thyroidal and human growth hormone reserve in Sheehan's syndrome. Johns Hopkins Med J 131:80, 1972

Hayashi RH, Castillo MS, Noah ML: Management of severe postpartum hemorrhage due to uterine atony using an analogue of prostaglandin $F_{2\alpha}$. Obstet Gynecol 58:426, 1981

Hertz RH, Sokol RJ, Dierker LJ: Treatment of postpartum uterine atony with prostaglandin E_2 vaginal suppositories. Obstet Gynecol 56:129, 1980

Jacobs MM, Arias F: Intramyometrial prostaglandin $F_{2\alpha}$ in the treatment of severe postpartum hemorrhage. Obstet Gynecol 55:665, 1980

Kitchin JD III, Thiagarajah S, May HV Jr, Thornton WN Jr: Puerperal inversion of the uterus. Am J Obstet Gynecol 123:51, 1975

Magil M: $PGF_{2\alpha}$ for postpartum hemorrhage—How well does it work? Contemp Ob/Gyn p 111, March, 1984

Newton M: Postpartum hemorrhage. Am J Obstet Gynecol 94:711, 1966

Odell LD, Seski A: Episiotomy blood loss. Am J Obstet Gynecol 54:51, 1947

Pasto ME, Kurtz AB, Rifkin MD, Cole-Beuglet C, Wapner RJ, Goldberg BB: Ultrasonographic findings in placenta increta. J Ultrasound Med 2:155, 1983

Platt LD, Druzin ML: Acute puerperal inversion of the uterus. Am J Obstet Gynecol 141:187, 1981

Pritchard JA: Magnesium sulfate and uterine inversion. Am J Obstet Gynecol 143:725, 1982

Pritchard JA: Changes in the blood volume during pregnancy and delivery. Anesthesiology 26:393, 1965

Pritchard JA, Baldwin RM, Dickey JC, Wiggins KM: Blood volume changes in pregnancy and the puerperium: II. Red blood cell loss and changes in apparent blood volume during and following vaginal delivery, cesarean section, and cesarean section plus total hysterectomy. Am J Obstet Gynecol 84:1271, 1962

Read JA, Cotton DB, Miller FC: Placenta accreta: Changing clinical aspects and outcome. Obstet Gynecol 56:31, 1980

Sheehan HL, Murdoch R: Postpartum necrosis of the anterior pituitary: Pathological and clinical aspects. Br J Obstet Gynaecol 45:456, 1938

Tabsh KMA, Brinkman CR III, King W: Ultrasound diagnosis of placenta increta. J Clin Ultrasound 10:288, 1982

Takagi S, Yoshida T, Togo Y, Tochigi H, Abe M, Sakata H, Fujii TK, Takahashi H, Tochigi B: The effects of intramyometrial injection of prostaglandin $F_{2\alpha}$ on severe post-partum hemorrhage. Prostaglandins 12:565, 1976

Toppozada M, El-Bossaty M, El-Rahman HA, El-Din AHS: Control of intractable atonic postpartum hemorrhage by 15-methyl prostaglandin $F_{2\alpha}$. Obstet Gynecol 58:327, 1981.

van Vugt PJH, Baudoin P, Blom VM, van Duersen TBM: Inversio uteri puerperalis. Acta Obstet Gynecol Scand 60:353, 1981

Watson P, Besch N, Bowes WA Jr: Management of acute and subacute puerperal inversion of the uterus. Obstet Gynecol 55:12, 1980

Whitehead R: The hypothalamus in post-partum hypopituitarism. J Pathol Bact 86:55, 1963

Definition

Puerperal infection is infection of the genital tract after delivery. Previously used but less satisfactory synonyms are puerperal fever, puerperal sepsis, and childbed fever.

Puerperal Morbidity

Since most elevations of temperature in the puerperium are caused by puerperal infection, the incidence of fever after childbirth is a reliable index of the incidence of the disease. For this reason, it has been customary to group all puerperal fevers under the general term "puerperal morbidity" and to estimate the frequency of puerperal infection on this basis. Several definitions of puerperal morbidity have been established on the basis of the degree of pyrexia reached. The Joint Committee on Maternal Welfare has defined puerperal morbidity as a "temperature of 38.0° C (100.4° F) or higher, the temperature to occur on any two of the first 10 days postpartum, exclusive of the first 24 hours, and to be taken by mouth by a standard technique at least 4 times daily." This is probably the most commonly employed standard in the United States. This definition may suggest that all fevers in the puerperium are the consequence of infection involving the reproductive tract. Elevations in temperature may, however, be the result of other causes, such as pyelonephritis, upper respiratory infection, breast engorgement, or even thrombophlebitis. Unfortunately, the practical difficulties of differentiating other causes of fever from infection of the reproductive tract are appreciable.

History

Puerperal infection is referred to in the works of Hippocrates and Galen. In the 17th century, Willis (1659) wrote on the subject of *febris puerperarum,* although the English term *puerperal fever* was probably first employed by Strother in 1716.

The ancients regarded the affection to be the result of retention of the lochia, and for centuries this explanation was universally accepted. In the early part of the 17th century, metritis was thought to be the essential cause; the theory of "milk metastasis" of Puzos (1686) followed next. Until Semmelweis (1861) proved the identity of puerperal sepsis

with wound infection and until Pasteur cultivated the streptococcus and Lister (1867) demonstrated the value of antiseptic methods, many theories were suggested concerning the origin and nature of childbed fever. They are comprehensively discussed in the monographs of Eisenmann (1837), Burtenshaw (1904), and Peckham (1935).

Although John Leake (1772) first made the suggestion of the contagious nature of puerperal infection, it remained for Alexander Hamilton to make the earliest positive statement on this subject in 1781. Alexander Gordon of Aberdeen clearly stated in a treatise on epidemic puerperal fever in 1795 the idea of the infectious and contagious nature of the disease, antedating the papers of Holmes (1855) and Semmelweis (1861) by a half-century. Charles White (1773) of Manchester believed puerperal fever to be an absorption fever dependent on stagnation of the lochia. He advised the semirecumbent posture to facilitate drainage and insisted on rigorous cleanliness and ventilation of the lying-in room and complete isolation of infected patients. Although many other British observers had vague ideas upon the subject, it was not until the middle of the 19th century that such views were strongly urged. In 1843, Oliver Wendell Holmes read a paper before the Boston Society for Medical Improvement, entitled *The Contagiousness of Puerperal Fever,* in which he clearly showed that at least the epidemic forms of the infection could always be traced to the lack of proper precautions on the part of the physician or nurse. Four years later, Semmelweis, then an assistant in the Vienna Lying-In Hospital, began a careful inquiry into the causes of the frightful mortality rate attending labor in that institution as compared with the relatively small number of women succumbing to puerperal infection when delivered in their own homes. As a result of his investigations, he concluded that the morbid process was essentially a wound infection caused by the introduction of septic material by the examining finger. Acting upon this idea, he issued stringent orders that the physicians, students, and midwives disinfect their hands with chlorine water, the forerunner of Dakin's solution, before examining parturient women. In spite of immediate, surprising result, the mortality rate falling from over 10 to 1 percent, both his work and that of Holmes were scoffed at by many of the most prominent men of the time, and his discovery remained unappreciated until the influence of Lister's teachings and the development of bacteriology had brought about a revolution in the treatment of wounds.

719

PREDISPOSING CAUSES

In general, the longer the amnionic sac has been ruptured before delivery, the greater the number of vaginal examinations, the more extensive the intrauterine manipulation for delivery of the fetus and placenta, and the greater the size and number of incisions and lacerations, the greater is the likelihood of serious postpartum infection. The impression is widely held that puerperal infection is much more common in women from lower socioeconomic populations than in women who are private patients. The reasons for such a difference need to be diligently investigated.

Several factors operative during pregnancy or delivery have been implicated in the genesis of puerperal infection.

Antepartum Factors

Although the evidence is mostly indirect, anemia, poor nutrition, and sexual intercourse have long been considered to predispose to puerperal sepsis. In spite of lack of strong direct evidence to implicate these three factors in the genesis of puerperal infection, anemia and poor nutrition should be prevented or appropriately corrected, and sexual intercourse should probably be avoided near term.

> *Anemia.* The evidence is far from decisive that anemia per se increases the likelihood of infection (Buckley, 1975; Lukens, 1975). The results obtained in animal experiments and in vitro studies are consistent with the view that iron deficiency anemia does not predispose to infection. In fact, transferrin appears to have significant antibacterial action, and transferrin is increased in iron deficiency anemia. Moreover, growth of a variety of pathogenic bacteria in vitro is inhibited by lack of iron. Finally, impairment of wound healing has not been seen in animals previously made iron deficient.
>
> *Nutrition.* The role of nutrition in the genesis of infection also is not clear, although cell-mediated immunity has been reported more likely to be impaired in malnourished animals. Lymphocyte responses to antigens in vitro are depressed in iron deficiency anemia as well as in kwashiorkor, according to Joynson and associates (1972). Kulapongs and co-workers (1974), however, found no such defect in studies of children with severe iron deficiency anemia.
>
> *Sexual Intercourse.* An increase in puerperal infection resulting from sexual intercourse has not been clearly demonstrated. If, however, the membranes were ruptured at the time of coitus or were to rupture very soon after coitus, the infection rate most likely would be increased. Premature labor has been reported to be more frequent in women who have intercourse late in gestation, and the etiology may possibly be the consequence of infection (Naeye, 1979).

Intrapartum Factors

During the intrapartum period, three factors have been implicated in the genesis of puerperal infection. They are iatrogenic introduction of pathogenic bacteria into the upper genital tract, trauma that devitalizes tissue, and hemorrhage. There is no doubt that the first two are of considerable importance. It is very unlikely that any vaginal manipulation can be carried out with absolute asepsis. Therefore, every intravaginal and intrauterine examination must be carefully considered in terms of benefits to be achieved versus the risks of bacterial contamination. It is not as clear whether hemorrhage per se is of great significance. The trauma that led to hemorrhage and the manipulations associated with control of the hemorrhage and repair of the traumatized structures, however, certainly predispose to infection, as do the hematomas that often form in these circumstances.

Bacterial Contamination. Those who care for the mother may carry infection to the parturient uterus in two ways. First, although the hands are covered with sterile gloves, bacteria already present on the pudenda and in the vagina may be carried into the uterine cavity during the course of examination, insertion of fetal monitoring devices, or operative manipulation. Second, the gloves or instruments may be contaminated by virulent organisms as the result of droplet infection. The nose and mouth of all attendants in the delivery room should therefore be covered, and all persons with a respiratory infection should be excluded. Because the nasopharynx is the most common course of extraneous bacteria brought to the birth canal, all obstetric personnel in the delivery room must wear masks that cover the nose and mouth.

Trauma. Lacerations provide portals of entry for pathogenic bacteria, and devitalized tissue serves as an excellent culture medium.

Blood Loss. Hematomas easily become infected and therefore enhance the likelihood of troublesome sepsis. Whether blood loss per se in the absence of trauma, reparative manipulations, or hematoma formation predisposes significantly to infection is not clear.

PATHOLOGY

After completion of the third stage of labor, the site of placental attachment is raw and elevated, dark red, and about 4 cm in diameter. Its surface is made nodular by the numerous veins that are normally occluded by thrombi. This site is an excellent culture medium for bacteria and a most likely portal of entry for pathogenic organisms. At this time the entire decidua is peculiarly susceptible to bacterial invasion. It is less than 2 mm in thickness, is infiltrated with blood, and presents numerous small openings. Because the cervix rarely escapes some degree of laceration in labor, it is another ready site for bacterial invasion. Vulvar, vaginal, and perineal wounds provide additional portals of entry.

The lesions of puerperal infection, therefore, are basically wound infections. The inflammatory process may remain localized in these wounds or may extend through the blood or lymphatics to tissues far beyond the initial lesion.

Lesions of the Perineum, Vulva, Vagina, and Cervix

A common puerperal lesion of the external genitalia is a localized infection of a repaired laceration or episiotomy wound. The apposing wound edges may become red, brawny, and swollen. The sutures often then cut through the edematous tissues, allowing the necrotic edges of the wound to gape, with the result that frank pus or sanguinopurulent material exudes from the wound. In this manner, complete breakdown of the site may occur. After traumatic or operative delivery, wounds and contusions of the vulva are common. In extreme cases, the entire vulva may become edematous, ulcerated, and covered with exudate.

Lacerations of the vagina are common after operative delivery and may become infected directly or by extension from the perineum. The mucosa becomes swollen and hyperemic and may then become necrotic and slough. Extension may occur by infiltration, resulting in lymphangitis, but more likely the infection remains local.

Cervical infection is probably rather common, since lacerations are frequent and the cervix normally harbors potentially pathogenic organisms. Moreover, since deep lacerations of the cervix often extend directly into the tissue at the base of the broad ligament, infection of such wounds may form the starting point for lymphangitis, parametritis, and bacteremia.

Metritis (Endometritis)

The most common form of puerperal infection involves primarily the endometrium, or more exactly the decidua, and adjacent myometrium. During the first few hours to a few days after delivery, the bacteria successfully invade the decidua that remains, usually at the placental site. If the infection is successfully confined near the surface, the necrotic infected mucosa is shed within a few days.

The appearance of the infected decidua varies widely. In some cases, the necrotic mucosa sloughs, the debris is abundant, and the discharge is foul, profuse, bloody, and sometimes frothy. In others, the discharge is scant. Involution of the uterus may be retarded. Microscopic sections may show a superficial layer of necrotic material containing bacteria and a thick zone of leukocytic infiltration. The term *metritis* is more descriptive than endometritis, because the inflammatory response is almost certain to include to some degree the underlying myometrium.

Thrombophlebitis and Pyemia

One mode of extension of puerperal infection is along the veins, with resultant thrombophlebitis (Fig. 35-1). Halban and Köhler (1919), in autopsies of 163 women who died from puerperal infection before the era of antibiotics, found 82 instances of thrombophlebitis. In 36, it was the only mode of extension identified, whereas in 46, there was obvious coexisting lymphatic involvement. A similar but slightly lower figure (35 percent) was quoted by Collins and co-workers (1951) for the 1937 to 1946 period, which included the early use of antibiotics. Thrombophlebitis results because the exposed placental site is a mass of thrombosed veins and because *Peptostreptococcus, Bacteroides,* and other anaerobic bacteria that frequently inhabit the vagina can thrive in the anaerobic medium provided by venous thrombi.

The ovarian veins may be involved in pelvic thrombophlebitis, since they drain the upper part of the uterus, which most often includes the veins of the placental site (Fig. 35-1). The process is usually unilateral on the right (Munsick and Gillanders, 1981), but extension of the process into the left ovarian vein may reach the junction of the ovarian vein and the renal vein, with involvement of that vessel and consequent renal complications. If the right ovarian vein is affected, the thrombosis may extend well into the inferior vena cava. At times, thrombosis of uterine veins extends to reach the common iliac veins.

Thrombosis of the infected vein may serve to limit the advance of the infection, and the thrombus may undergo organization. In other cases, the thrombus may suppurate, while the surrounding venous wall becomes edematous and necrotic. Very infrequently, large emboli may reach the pulmonary artery and cause sudden death. More often, small septic emboli reach the terminal branches of the pulmonary vessels and may produce, in turn, cor pulmonale. At the same time, bacterial products released into the circulation may cause bacterial shock (Chapter 24, p. 484). Pleurisy, pneumonia, pulmonary infracts, and abscesses may develop in this setting.

Peritonitis

Puerperal infection may extend by way of the lymphatics of the uterine wall to reach either the peritoneum (Fig. 35-2) or the loose tissue between the leaves of the broad ligaments (Fig. 35-3), causing in the former instance peritonitis and in the latter parametritis (pelvic cellulitis).

Generalized peritonitis is a grave complication of childbearing. Typically, fibrinopurulent exudate binds loops of bowel to one another, and locules of pus may form between the loops. The cul-de-sac, the subdiaphragmatic space, and the folds between the infundibulopelvic and broad ligaments are common sites for abscess formation.

Pelvic Cellulitis (Parametritis)

Infection of the retroperitoneal fibroareolar pelvic connective tissue may occur in three main ways:

1. It may be caused by the lymphatic transmission of organisms from an infected cervical laceration, uterine incision for cesarean section, or a laceration of the uterus. Although lacerations of the perineum or vagina may be a cause of localized cellulitis, the process is usually limited to the paravaginal cellular tissue, rarely extending deeply into the pelvis (Fig. 35-3).

2. It may be caused by direct extension of cervical lacerations into the connective tissue at the base of the broad ligaments. This tissue may be exposed to direct invasion by pathogenic organisms in the vagina. A similar outcome may be seen in cases of induced abortion, when a sharp instrument has created a false passage into the paracervical connective tissue.

3. Pelvic cellulitis may be secondary to pelvic thrombophlebitis, which almost always is accompanied by some degree of cellulitis. If the thrombi become purulent, the venous wall may undergo necrosis, and large numbers of organisms may be discharged into the surrounding connective tissue.

Pelvic cellulitis is more often unilateral but need not be so. The cellulitis may remain limited to the base of the broad ligament, but if the inflammatory reaction is

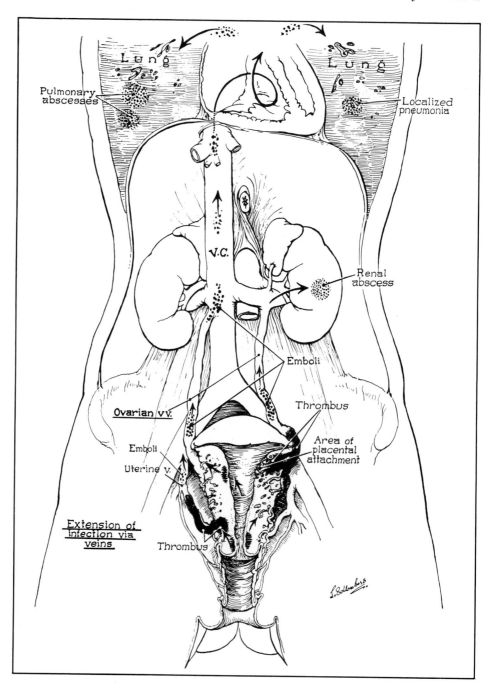

Figure 35-1. Extension of puerperal infection in pelvic thrombophlebitis. V.C. = inferior vena cava.

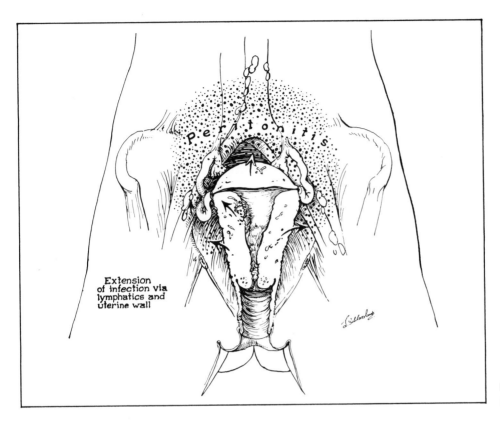

Figure 35-2. Extension of puerperal infection in peritonitis.

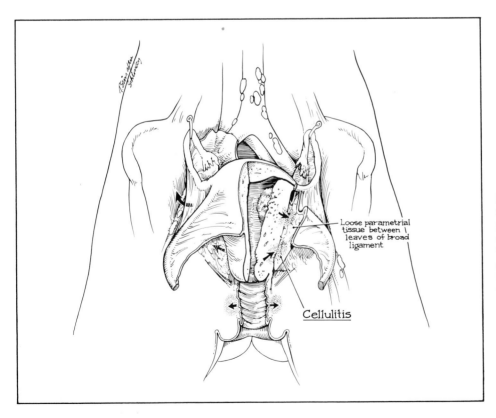

Figure 35-3. Pelvic cellulitis (parametritis) from extension of puerperal infection. Bacteria may enter the parametrial tissue between the leaves of the broad ligament by direct extension or by lymphatic transmission from cervical lacerations or foci of trauma within the uterus, including the site of placental implantation. Bacterial spread may also occur across the wall of an infected vein, the site of thrombophlebitis. Lacerations of the perineum or vagina usually cause only localized cellulitis.

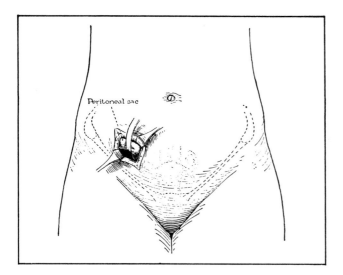

Figure 35-4. Technique for opening localized collection of pus pointing above the inguinal ligament.

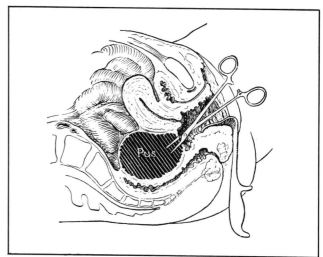

Figure 35-5. Technique for opening collection of localized pus in the cul-de-sac of Douglas (posterior colpotomy).

more intense, the exudate may be forced along natural lines of cleavage. The most common form of extension is directly laterally, along the base of the broad ligament, with a tendency to extend to the lateral pelvic wall. As the mass increases in size, it distends the leaves of the broad ligament and, raising the anterior leaf upward, it may dissect its way forward to reach the abdominal wall just above Poupart's ligament (Fig. 35-4). The uterus is pushed toward the opposite side and fixed. In other cases, high intraligamentous exudates spread from the region of the uterine cornua to the iliac fossae. Retrocervical exudates tend to involve the rectovaginal septum, with the development of a firm mass posterior to the cervix. After cesarean section, involvement of the connective tissue anterior to the cervix results in cellulitis of the space of Retzius with extension upward, beneath the anterior abdominal wall, as high as the umbilicus. Rarely, the process may extend out through the sciatic foramen into the thigh.

Cellulitis in the pelvic connective tissue follows an indolent course but ultimately undergoes either suppuration or, more commonly with appropriate antibiotic therapy, resolution. If suppuration occurs, one outcome is pointing above Poupart's ligament (Fig. 35-4). The skin over the inguinal region becomes edematous, red, and tender; fluctuation is a sign that the abscess is ready for incision. Another outcome is pointing in the posterior cul-de-sac (Fig. 35-5). Either abscess, if not drained, may rupture directly into the peritoneal cavity and cause fulminant putrid peritonitis.

BACTERIOLOGY

Organisms that invade the placental implantation site and incisions, lacerations, and abrasions that are the consequence of labor and delivery may be normal inhab-

itants of the cervix and lower genital tract or may be introduced from exogenous sources. In modern obstetrics, an epidemic of serious puerperal sepsis rarely develops, as virulent bacteria are not usually carried from person to person during labor, delivery, or early in the puerperium. However, such an epidemic resulting from group A β-hemolytic streptococcus has been well documented (Jewett and associates, 1968). Prompt administration of effective antibiotics and identification of the source of the infection prevented deaths and controlled the epidemic.

Common Pathogens

In the great majority of instances of puerperal infection, the bacteria responsible for the infection are those that normally flourish in the bowel and also commonly inhabit the lower genital tract. Gorbach and co-workers (1973) identified in 70 percent of cultures from the external cervix of healthy women one or more potentially pathogenic anaerobic bacteria, as well as aerobic organisms. The anaerobic bacteria included species of *Bacteroides* (57 percent), *Peptostreptococcus* (33 percent), and *Clostridium* (17 percent). Usually multiple species of bacteria were found. The pathogenicity of many of these bacteria is sufficiently great to cause, alone or in combination, extensive cellulitis (parametritis), abscesses, peritonitis, and suppurative thrombophlebitis.

Although the cervix and lower genital tract commonly contain such bacteria, the uterine cavity is sterile before rupture of the amnionic sac. As a consequence of labor and delivery and associated manipulations, the uterus commonly becomes contaminated with anaerobic and aerobic bacteria. For example, Gilstrap and Cunningham (1979) in cultures of amnionic fluid obtained from the uterus at cesarean section performed on laboring women with membranes ruptured more than 6 hours identified the following bacteria: anaerobic and aerobic organisms in 63 percent, anaerobes alone in 30 percent, and aerobes alone in 7 percent. The anaerobic organisms were gram-positive cocci (species of *Peptostreptococcus* and *Peptococcus*) 45 percent, *Bacteroides* species 9 percent, and *Clostridium* species 3 percent. The aerobic organisms were various gram-positive cocci and *Escherichia coli*. An average of 2.5 different organisms per specimen were identified. These observations serve to reemphasize the polymicrobial nature of infections of the genital tract associated with delivery, especially cesarean section. The polymicrobial nature of these infections is further emphasized by the recent reports that genital *Mycoplasma* organisms may possibly play a significant role in the etiology of puerperal metritis (Platt and coworkers, 1980; Andrews and Dann, 1981; Lamey and associates, 1982).

Bacterial Cultures

Precise identification of the bacteria responsible specifically for any given puerperal infection may be quite difficult. Even though satisfactory techniques are used for obtaining and culturing organisms from the uterine cavity, the results are difficult to interpret, since potentially pathogenic bacteria are commonly found in cultures of the uterine cavity during the puerperium without clinical disease. Gibbs and associates (1975), as did Hite and coworkers (1947) 3 decades before, cultured one or more pathogens from swabbings of the uterine cavity in 70 percent or more of clinically healthy puerperal women. Appropriately performed anaerobic and aerobic blood cultures obtained before antibiotic treatment is begun may be more useful to identify the pathogens that actually cause the infection.

CLINICAL COURSE

Lesions of the Perineum, Vulva, Vagina, and Cervix

Local pain and dysuria, with or without urinary retention, are the common symptoms. Provided drainage is good, the reaction in these local conditions is seldom severe, the temperature remaining below 38.5° C (101° F). If, however, purulent material is confined by perineal or vaginal suture, the complication may be signaled by a chill and a sharp rise of fever.

Metritis

The clinical picture of puerperal metritis varies with the extent of the disease. When the infection is strictly confined to the endometrium (dedidua), the cases are mild, with only slight elevation of temperature. More severe cases of metritis may begin with a chill, high fever, and other evidence of a fulminating infection. Postpartum, the temperature begins to rise, often in a sawtooth fash-

ion, to reach levels between 38.5° C and 40° C (101° F and 103° F). The pulse rate typically follows the temperature curve. There is likely to be tenderness over the uterus, and afterpains tend to be bothersome. Even in the early stages there may be changes in the lochia. An offensive odor, long regarded as an important sign of uterine infection, results from invasion of the uterine cavity by anaerobic bacteria. Some infections, however, and notably those with β-hemolytic streptococcus, are frequently associated with scanty, odorless lochia. Indeed, the gravity of a case of metritis may sometimes be in almost inverse proportion to the amount and putridity of the lochia. Leukocytosis may range from 15,000 to 30,000 cells per mm³, but in view of the physiologic leukocytosis of the early puerpertium, these figures are difficult to interpret. The symptoms are variable. Some patients feel well, with no complaints. If the process is localized to the uterus, the temperature falls by lysis, and, even when untreated with antibiotics, by the end of the week the infection is usually over. Localized metritis may be misdiagnosed as a urinary tract infection or be attributed incorrectly to severe breast engorgement or pulmonary atelectasis.

Pelvic Cellulitis

Pelvic cellulitis (parametritis) is the common cause of prolonged, sustained infection in the puerperium. Whenever steady elevations of temperature persist, the condition should be suspected. There is tenderness on one or both sides of the abdomen and tenderness with vaginal examination resulting in movement of the uterus. As the process advances, other findings on vaginal examination may become more characteristic, such as fixation of the uterus by the parametrial exudate or induration in the fornices and the development of a mass in the broad ligament. The exudate may extend upward, and an area of resistance may be felt along the upper border of Poupart's ligament. Not infrequently, it extends posteriorly into the lower part of the broad ligament along the sacrouterine folds and into the cellular tissue surrounding the uterus. In these cases, rectovaginal examination may be very helpful in diagnosis.

Absorption of the exudate occurs in the great majority of patients, but it may require several weeks. During this time, the inflammatory process may become hard, and infrequently the final result may be dense scar tissue in the parametrium. Suppuration of the parametrial mass occurs in the remaining patients. Pointing of the abscess may not occur for weeks after the commencement of the illness. If the abscess can be adequately drained, recovery is usually prompt (Figs. 35-4, 35-5).

Peritonitis

Puerperal peritonitis generally resembles surgical peritonitis except that abdominal rigidity is usually much less prominent. Pain may be severe. Marked bowel distention is a consequence of paralytic ileus. Rarely, in the course of pelvic cellulitis with abscess formation, a large abscess may rupture into the peritoneal cavity and produce catastrophic generalized peritonitis.

Septic Thrombophlebitis

With modern antimicrobial therapy, both the mortality rate and the duration of the disease have been reduced (Cohen and colleagues, 1983). The common cause of death formerly was pulmonary involvement, usually a combination of vascular blockade by septic emboli, infarction, pneumonitis, and abscesses. With prompt, effective antibiotic therapy and, at times in refractory cases, heparin or even ligation of the inferior vena cava and ovarian veins, both the mortality rate and prolonged disease have been reduced appreciably (Duff and Gibbs, 1983; Cohen and colleagues, 1983). Pelvic thrombophlebitis, especially ovarian vein thrombophlebitis, is considered further in Chapter 36, p. 732).

Salpingitis

Most often with postpartum sepsis the fallopian tubes are involved only with perisalpingitis without subsequent tubal occlusion and sterility. Initial attacks of gonorrheal salpingitis during the puerperium are rare.

Toxic-Shock Syndrome

The toxic-shock syndrome is an acute febrile illness that affects multiple organ systems and may result in death. The illness usually is characterized by fever, headache, mental confusion, scarlatiniform rash, subcutaneous edema, nausea, vomiting, watery diarrhea, marked hemoconcentration, oliguria, and renal failure followed by hepatic failure, disseminated intravascular coagulation, and circulatory collapse. During recovery, the rash-covered areas undergo a fine desquamation. *Staphylococcus aureus* has been isolated from a number of lesions, and a *Staphylococcus* endotoxin is suspected to be the causative factor.

Although the syndrome primarily is associated with menstruating women who use tampons, it has been reported in a variety of clinical situations unrelated to menstruation (Reingold and co-workers, 1982). Recently, the disease has been reported to occur in postpartum women (Guerinot and co-workers, 1982; Lauter and Tom, 1982) as well as in a mother and newborn pair (Green and LaPeter, 1982). An excellent review of the problem was provided by Wager (1983).

Ideal therapy for the toxic-shock syndrome remains to be defined. At present, therapy should be parenteral administration of β-lactamase-resistant antibiotics, massive fluid replacement, and other supportive measures as required.

DIFFERENTIAL DIAGNOSIS OF FEVER

Most fevers occurring after childbirth are caused by infection of the genital tract, especially if the preceding labor was attended by extensive vaginal or uterine manipulation, prolonged rupture of the membranes, or intrauterine fetal electronic monitoring. Regardless, every puerperal woman whose temperature rises to 38°C (100.4°F) should be given a complete examination to rule out extrapelvic causes of fever and to establish the diagnosis of puerperal infection by exclusion in the absence of other findings.

The common extragenital causes of fever in the puerperium are *respiratory complications, pyelonephritis, intense breast engorgement, bacterial mastitis, thrombophlebitis, episiotomy infection,* and, in cases of laparotomy, *wound abscess.* Respiratory complications are most often seen within the first 24 hours following delivery. These complications may consist of atelectasis, aspiration pneumonia, or both. Certainly, atelectasis should be prevented with the use of routine coughing and deep breathing on a fixed schedule, usually every 4 hours for at least 24 hours following the administration of an anesthetic agent especially when laparotomy was performed. In instances where aspiration might be suspected, the mother most often will develop a high spiking fever, varying degrees of respiratory wheezing, and, in most instances, obvious signs of oxygen hunger accompanied by varying degrees of cyanosis.

Pyelonephritis is a difficult problem in differential diagnosis. In the typical case, bacteriuria, pyuria, costovertebral angle tenderness, and spiking temperature point clearly to pyelonephritis. However, the clinical picture varies. This is especially true in the puerperal woman, where the first sign of such an infection may be merely an elevation in temperature. Certainly, the costovertebral angle tenderness and nausea and vomiting are late signs to develop. Pyelonephritis should be confirmed by urine culture obtained by catheterization. A significant number of a single species of bacteria should be identified in the urine culture. Empiric therapy should begin immediately pending results of the culture.

Mammary engorgement may occasionally result in a brief temperature rise that rarely exceeds 38.5°C (101°F) during the first few puerperal days. The temperature characteristically lasts no longer than 24 hours. The temperature of true mastitis is usually sustained and associated with mammary signs and symptoms that become overt by 24 hours.

In instances of abdominal wound abscesses, or more rarely, in instances of episiotomy site abscesses, meticulous inspection of either site will usually disclose an abscess when present. Treatment is drainage, culture of the purulent material, and appropriate antibiotic therapy pending the outcome of the culture.

Thrombophlebitis may result in significant temperature elevations in the puerperal woman. The diagnosis is made easy by the observation of a painful, swollen leg, femoral triangle area tenderness, or pain with dorsiflexion of the foot and should be managed with intravenous heparin therapy and appropriate antibiotics (Chapter 36, p. 731).

TREATMENT

Choice of Antibiotics

For many years, the combination of penicillin with a broad-spectrum antibiotic has been used, most often with success, to treat genital tract infections associated with delivery, even though *Bacteroides* species are resistant in vitro, at least, to most of the antibiotic combinations employed. In 1979, diZerega and associates compared the effectiveness of primary treatment of postcesarean section endomyometritis with penicillin plus gentamicin and with gentamicin plus clindamycin, an antibiotic to which *Bacteroides* is usually sensitive. Infection was effectively controlled by the antibiotic regimen in 95 percent of women who received clindamycin plus gentamicin compared to 71 percent of those who received penicillin plus gentamicin. Unfortunately, clindamycin may be toxic in some circumstances. Cunningham and co-workers (1978) observed that metritis and pelvic cellulitis following cesarean section responded satisfactorily to penicillin plus an aminoglycoside about 70 percent of the time and to penicillin plus tetracycline about 85 percent of the time.

For more than 2 decades at Parkland Memorial Hospital, the combination of tetracycline and large doses of penicillin G given intravenously proved to be quite effective for the treatment of the great majority of puerperal infections, as well as septic abortions (Pritchard and Whalley, 1971). However, today, perhaps because of changing bacterial sensitivities to these effective and inexpensive drugs, the most widely used first-line antibiotic is one of the second generation cephalosporins, such as cefoxitin or cefamandole. These agents are administered intravenously every 6 hours. After the patient has become afebrile for 24 hours, an oral cephalosporin is used. This oral antimicrobial therapy is then continued to complete a total of 10 days of antibiotic therapy. With severe infections involving the genital tract, such as those precipitating bacterial shock or producing intense hemolysis, or more often instances where the patient continues to exhibit a febrile course while on a single agent, such as one of the second generation cephalosporins, clindamycin and gentamicin have been added to the cephalosporin already being used. Each of the last two agents, i.e., clindamycin and gentamicin, are administered based upon body weight. In patients in whom there may be impaired renal function, chloramphenicol may be used instead of clindamycin and gentamicin. This is also true in patients in whom there is a significant degree of ileus. Under such conditions, clindamycin may be contraindicated because of its association with pseudomembranous colitis (Kabins and Spira, 1975). However, even in cases of significant ileus, clindamycin may be used in life-threatening instances of anaerobic infection. It is wise to remember that under these instances the bacterium associated with the development of pseudomembranous colitis has been shown to be *Clostridium diffcle,* and under these circumstances it may be judicious to add vibramycin to the treatment regimen to effect eradication of this organism.

Metronidazole (Flagyl) for use in certain life-threatening anaerobic infections may prove to be an additional excellent agent for such infections. Robbie and Sweet (1983) have provided an excellent review of the use of metronidazole and recommend at the present time that this agent not be widely applied for anaerobic infections until its safety has been confirmed. Additionally, these authors emphasize that at the present time, clindamycin or chloramphenicol are adequate for almost all anaerobic infections.

In more recent years, antibiotics have been administered commonly when cesarean delivery has been performed under circumstances that predispose to pelvic infection. Such prophylaxis is considered in Chapter 43 (p. 883).

Lesions of the Perineum, Vulva, and Vagina

These infected external wounds should be treated, like other infected surgical wounds, by establishing drainage. Stitches should be removed and the infected wound opened. Failure to do this may lead not only to infection of the paracervical and paravaginal connective tissue but to a worse ultimate anatomic result. Relief of pain is afforded by effective analgesics. It is advisable to supplement these therapeutic measures with antibiotic therapy during the acute phase of the infection.

Metritis

Mild cases without symptoms, with temperatures under 38° C and no chills, are best handled initially by observation. In this group, it is unnecessary to discontinue breast feeding. In more severe cases, antibiotics are indicated. Breast-feeding is discontinued, not only because it exhausts the mother but also because it is usually futile in the presence of high fever.

Pelvic Cellulitis

Antibiotics must be used. The physician should remain alert for signs of suppuration and abscess formation. The diagnosis of an abscess rests upon detection of a mass, at times by sonography. The mass may be so tender that effective analgesia may be required to perform an adequate examination.

An abscess that forms in the broad ligament and points above Poupart's ligament may be surgically drained extraperitoneally, as illustrated in Figure 35-4. Today, this particular circumstance is rarely encountered. At times, an abscess may form in the posterior cul-de-sac. As the abscess begins to dissect the rectovaginal septum, drainage is established and maintained, as illustrated in Figure 35-5.

Pelvic Thrombophlebitis

Variable degrees of pelvic thrombophlebitis usually accompany parametritis and pelvic cellulitis. Treatment is customarily directed at the pelvic cellulitis rather than at pelvic thrombophlebitis alone. Anticoagulant drugs that are successfully used in femoral thrombophlebitis (Chapter 36, p. 731) may be of less value in these cases, for the primary lesion is extravascular infection rather than thrombosis. Treatment with heparin is certainly indicated in cases of apparent or suspected pulmonary emboli. Ligation of the inferior vena cava and ovarian veins is lifesaving when septic emboli continue to reach the lung in spite of heparinization. In suspected cases of pelvic septic thrombophlebitis *without* embolization, it is not yet clear whether the possible benefits of heparin therapy outweigh the potential dangers of bleeding. Josey and Staggers (1974) believe heparin to be of value in the treatment of such cases, as do others (Munsick and Gillanders, 1981; Cohen and co-workers, 1983; Duff and Gibbs, 1983). The difficulty remains of making this diagnosis without resorting to laparotomy. Computed axial tomography scans can be of diagnostic aid (Fig. 36-1, C, D).

Generalized Peritonitis

It is important to identify the cause of the generalized peritonitis. The treatment of peritonitis as the consequence of an infection that began in the uterus and extended to the peritoneum is medical in most instances. Conversely, peritonitis during the puerperium as the consequence of a lesion of the bowel or its appendages most often should be promptly treated surgically.

Antibiotic therapy should include those agents that are most likely to be effective against *Peptostreptococcus, Peptococcus, Bacteroides, Clostridia,* and aerobic coliform organisms. Clindamycin and gentamicin plus large doses of cephalosporin or penicillin should prove effective in most cases. Chloramphenicol, however, may prove to be less toxic than clindamycin plus gentamicin, as previously discussed (p. 727).

Appropriate fluid and electrolyte therapy is extremely important. With generalized peritonitis, large amounts of fluid are often sequestered in the lumen and the wall of the gastrointestinal tract and, at times, in the peritoneal cavity. Vomiting, diarrhea, and fever also contribute appreciably to loss of fluid and electrolytes. The volumes of fluid and the amounts of electrolytes necessary to replace what is sequestered in the abdomen, aspirated from the gut, and lost through diaphoresis are usually quite large but must not be so massive as to produce circulatory overload.

Most often, paralytic ileus is a prominent feature of the disease process. The gastrointestinal tract should be decompressed by prompt, continuous nasogastric suction. Drugs to stimulate peristalsis are of no value. Oral feeding is withheld throughout the course of treatment until bowel function returns and flatus is expelled.

Procedures to Avoid

Although countless local therapeutic measures have been recommended, such as intrauterine douches, swabbing of the endometrium with antiseptic solutions, continuous irrigation of the uterine cavity, instillations of glycerin, drainage with rubber tubes, and curettage, they all have been abandoned, since each of these measures has been shown to be dangerous as well as futile. In the main, such practices tend to disseminate rather than halt the infection. Surgery is not indicated early in the course of the disease, although abscesses may form at various sites and need to be drained and mechanical intestinal obstruction that has to be relieved may develop.

REFERENCES

Andrews HJ, Dann MJ: *Mycoplasma* and postpartum fever. Lancet 1:43, 1981

Buckley RH: Iron deficiency anemia: Its relationship to infection susceptibility and host defense. J Pediatr 86:993, 1975

Burtenshaw: The fever of the puerperium. New York and Philadelphia Med J, June and July, 1904

Cohen MB, Pernoll ML, Gevirtz CM, Kernstein MD: Septic pelvic thrombophlebitis: An update. Obstet Gynecol 62:83, 1983

Collins CG, McCallum EA, Nelson EW, Weinstein BB, Collins JH: Suppurative pelvic thrombophlebitis: I. Incidence, pathology, etiology. II. Symptomatology and diagnosis. III. Surgical techniques: A study of 70 patients treated by ligation of the inferior vena cava and ovarian veins. Surgery 30:298, 1951

Cunningham FG, Hauth JC, Strong JD, Kappus SS: Infectious morbidity following cesarean section. Comparison of two treatment regimens. Obstet Gynecol 52:656, 1978

diZerega G, Yonekura L, Roy S, Nakamura RM, Ledger WJ: A comparison of clindamycin-gentamycin and penicillin-gentamycin in the treatment of post-cesarean section endomyometritis. Am J Obstet Gynecol 134:238, 1979

Duff P, Gibbs RS: Pelvic vein thrombophlebitis: Diagnostic dilemma and therapeutic challenge. Obstet Gynecol Surv 38:365, 1983

Eisenmann GE: Die Wundfieber und die Kindbettfieber, Erlangen, 1837 Galen: Ars Medicinalis

Gibbs RS, O'Dell TN, MacGregor RR, Schwarz RH, Morton H: Puerperal endometritis: A prospective microbiologic study. Am J Obstet Gynecol 121:919, 1975

Gilstrap LC III, Cunningham FG: The bacterial pathogenesis of infection following cesarean section. Obstet Gynecol 53:545, 1979

Gorbach SL, Menda KB, Thadepalli H, Keith L: Anaerobic microflora of the cervix in healthy women. Am J Obstet Gynecol 117:1053, 1973

Gordon A: A Treatise on Epidemic Puerperal Fever of Aberdeen. London, CG and J Robinson, 1795

Green SL, LaPeter KS: Evidence for postpartum toxic-shock syndrome in a mother-infant pair. Am J Med 72:169, 1982

Guerinot GT, Gitomer SD, Sanko SR: Postpartum patient with toxic shock syndrome. Obstet Gynecol 59:43S, 1982

Halban J, Köhler R: Die pathologische Anatomie des Puerperalprozesses. Vienna and Leipzig, 1919

Hamilton A: A Treatise on Midwifery. London, 1781

Hippocrates: Liber Prior de Muliebrum Morbis

Hite KE, Hesseltine HC, Goldstein L: A study of the bacterial flora of the normal and pathologic vagina and uterus. Am J Obstet Gynecol 53:233, 1947

Holmes OW: Puerperal Fever as a Private Pestilence. Boston, Ticknor & Fields, 1855

Jewett JF, Reid DE, Safon LE, Easterday CL: Childbed fever: A continuing entity. JAMA 206:344, 1968

Josey WE, Staggers SR Jr: Heparin therapy in septic pelvic thrombophlebitis: A study of 46 cases. Am J Obstet Gynecol 120:228, 1974

Joynson DHM, Jacobs A, Walter DM, Dolby AE: Defect of cell-mediated immunity in patients with iron-deficiency anaemia. Lancet 2:1058, 1972

Kabins SA, Spira TJ: Outbreak of clindamycin-associated colitis. Ann Intern Med 83:830, 1975

Kulapongs P, Suskind R, Vithayasai V, Olsen RE: Cell-mediated immunity and phagocytosis and killing function in children with severe iron-deficiency anaemia. Lancet 2:689, 1974

Lamey JR, Eschenbach DA, Mitchell SH, Blumhagen JM, Foy HM, Kenny GE: Isolation of mycoplasmas and bacteria from the blood of postpartum women. Am J Obstet Gynecol 143:104, 1982

Lauter CB, Tom WW: Spiking fever and rash in a postpartum patient. Hosp Pract, Nov 1982

Leake J: Practical Observations on the Child-bed Fever; Also on the Nature and Treatment of Uterine Haemorrhages, Convulsions, and Such Other Acute Disease, As Are Most Fatal to Women During the State of Pregnancy. London, J Walter, 1772

Lister J: On the antiseptic principle in the practice of surgery. Br Med J 2:246, 1867

Lukens JN: Iron deficiency and infection. Am J Dis Child 129:160, 1975

Munsick RA, Gillanders LA: A review of the syndrome of puerperal ovarian vein thrombophlebitis. Obstet Gynecol Surv 36:57, 1981

Naeye RL: Coitus and associated amniotic fluid infections. N Engl J Med 301:1198, 1979

Peckham CH: A brief history of puerperal infection. Bull Int Hist Med 3:187, 1935

Platt R, Lin J-SL, Warren JW, Rosner B, Edelin K, McCormack WM: Infection with *Mycoplasma hominis* in postpartum fever. Lancet 2:1217, 1980

Pritchard JA, Whalley PJ: Abortion complicated by *Clostridium perfringens* infection. Am J Obstet Gynecol 111:484, 1971

Puzos N: Première mémoire sur les depots laiteux, in Traités des accouchements, 1686, p 341

Reingold AL, Shands KN, Dan BB, Broome CV: Toxic-shock syndrome not associated with menstruation. A review of 54 cases. Lancet 2:1, 1982

Robbie MO, Sweet RL: Metronidazole use in obstetrics and gynecology: A review. Am J Obstet Gynecol 145:865, 1983

Semmelweis IP: Die Aetiologie, der Begriff u. die Prophylaxis dis Kindbettfiebers, Pest, Vienna and Leipzig, 1861

Strother: Critical Essay on Fevers. London, 1716

Wager GP: Toxic shock syndrome: A review. Am J Obstet Gynecol 146:93, 1983

White C: Treatise on the management of pregnancy and lying-in women and the means of curing but more especially of preventing the principal disorders to which they are liable. London, EC Dilly, 1773

Willis T: Diatribae duae medico-philosophical . . . de febribus. London, T Raycroft, 1659

36

Other Disorders of the Puerperium

THROMBOEMBOLIC DISEASE

Venous thromboembolic disease is considered under disorders of the puerperium because, in obstetrics, thromboembolism has traditionally been considered primarily as a complication of the puerperium. Deep venous thrombosis and thromboembolism are not limited just to this period, however. In more recent years, there has been a decrease in the frequency of deep venous thrombosis and thromboembolism during the puerperium but perhaps an increase antepartum. Henderson, Lund, and Creasman (1972), for example, described 20 cases that developed antepartum among 29,770 pregnancies, but during the same period, only 16 were identified postpartum.

Undoubtedly, the frequency of venous thromboembolic disease during the puerperium decreased remarkably when early ambulation became widely practiced. Until as late as the 1950s, it had been common practice after delivery to prohibit ambulation for up to 1 week or more. **Stasis is probably the strongest single predisposer to deep vein thrombosis, and, therefore, should be kept to a minimum.** Antecedent events that might possibly predispose to deep vein thrombosis during the antepartum period include the use of oral contraceptives before conception and the greater prevalence of women working during pregnancy at jobs in which they sit for long periods of time.

Venous thrombosis traditionally has been classified as *thrombophlebitis* if an inflammatory response was apparent, or *phlebothrombosis* if such evidence was lacking. The inflammatory response presumably would anchor the clot more firmly and prevent embolism. Unfortunately, contiguous with and proximal to an adherent clot there may form appreciable thrombus that is not adherent and therefore can easily break off to become an embolus. Thrombosis with a significant potential for generating pulmonary emboli may take place in the deep veins of the leg, thigh, and pelvis. A thrombosis that involves only the superficial veins of the leg or thigh is very unlikely to generate a pulmonary embolus.

Superficial Venous Thrombosis

Antepartum or postpartum thrombosis limited strictly to the superficial veins of the saphenous system is treated with analgesia, elastic support, and rest. If it does not soon clear, or if deep venous involvement is suspected, heparin is given intravenously, as described below, until the process clears.

Deep Venous Thrombosis in the Leg

The signs and symptoms with deep venous thrombosis involving the lower extremity vary greatly, depending in large measure on the degree of occlusion and the intensity of the inflammatory response.

Classic puerperal thrombophlebitis involving the lower extremity, sometimes called *phlegmasia alba dolens* or *"milk leg,"* is abrupt in onset, with severe pain and edema of the leg and thigh. The venous thrombosis typically involves much of the deep venous system from the foot to the iliofemoral region. Reflex arterial spasm sometimes causes a pale, cool extremity with diminished pulsations. Seldom is the reaction to deep venous thrombosis this intense, however, There may be appreciable volume of clot yet little reaction in the form of pain, heat, or swelling. Conversely, calf pain, either spontaneous or in response to squeezing, or to stretching the Achilles' tendon (Homan sign), may be caused by a strained muscle or a contusion. The latter can be fairly common during the early puerperium as the consequence of inappropriate contact between the calf and the delivery table leg holders.

In a review, Klotz (1982) outlined in detail the use of doppler and impedance plethysmography techniques that can be used to aid the physician in diagnosing questionable cases. However, despite a variety of diagnostic procedures that have been advocated, probably the only definitive procedure is carefully performed and interpreted *phlebography* (Bonnar, 1979).

Treatment of deep venous thrombosis, in general, consists of heparin intravenously administered as described below, bed rest, and analgesia. Broad-spectrum antibiotic therapy is indicated if there is fever. Most often the pain is soon relieved and the temperature returns to normal. In the great majority of cases, thrombectomy or sympathetic nerve block is not warranted. After the signs and symptoms have completely abated, graded ambulation should be started, with the legs well wrapped in elastic bandages, or, better, well-fitting elastic stockings, and the heparin continued. Recovery to this stage usually takes about 7 to 10 days.

For women who are *postpartum* and suffering their

first attack, who have no obvious chronic vascular disease, and who are observed to be completely asymptomatic while fully ambulatory, anticoagulant therapy may be discontinued. Most often signs and symptoms of deep venous thrombosis do not recur. If, however, symptoms and signs do recur, therapy is promptly restarted but is not stopped when relief is obtained. Instead, prolonged anticoagulant therapy is continued on an outpatient basis. After discharge from the hospital, long-term treatment is maintained either with self-administered, subcutaneously injected heparin, or with warfarin.

During the past several years, considerable controversy has arisen concerning the most effective agent to use in long-term therapy to prevent recurrent thrombophlebitis and thromboembolization. Hull and associates (1979) recommended warfarin as more effective than fixed low-dose heparin for the long-term treatment of venous thrombosis. However, Hull and co-workers (1982a) reported that heparin was as effective as oral warfarin when heparin was administered subcutaneously every 12 hours with the dose adjusted to prolong the partial thromboplastin time to one and one-half times the control value when measured 6 hours after injection. Furthermore, the heparin therapy was associated with a lower risk of bleeding. Subsequently, Hull and colleagues (1982b) reported that by decreasing the dosage of warfarin so that the prothrombin time was not decreased below specified levels, bleeding complications from warfarin could be reduced to the level achieved with heparin and that the effectiveness of the two agents were comparable.

In the absence of pregnancy it seems reasonable to consider warfarin the drug of choice for long-term prophylaxis when appropriate consideration is given to the cost of heparin, the problem of administration, the possibility of heparin-induced thrombocytopenia (Galle and co-workers, 1978; Chong and associates, 1982) and the possibility of osteopenia with fractures (Wise and Hall, 1980; DeSwiet and co-workers, 1983).

Thrombosis, Antepartum. Thrombosis antepartum involving the deep venous system is especially difficult to manage satisfactorily. When deep vein thrombosis involving a leg is not obvious but only suspected antepartum remote from term, it seems reasonable to use doppler and/or impedance plethysmographic techniques to establish or exclude the diagnosis (Klotz, 1982). If these techniques fail, it may be worthwhile to utilize phlebography while shielding the fetus from irradiation to establish or to exclude the diagnosis (Bonnar, 1979). Otherwise, the woman will either have to undergo prolonged anticoagulation with its attendant risks, or run the risk of pulmonary embolism.

Therapy with intravenous heparin usually soon controls active disease, but thrombosis, perhaps with embolization, may recur antepartum, intrapartum, or postpartum unless anticoagulation is continued throughout these periods.

Anticoagulation, Antepartum. Administration of heparin on an outpatient basis can be difficult. All things considered, the best treatment regimen for prophylaxis against recurrence of deep venous thrombosis is self-administered heparin injected subcutaneously in doses of 5000 units two or three times a day (Bonnar, 1979). With so-called low-dose heparin treatment that provides 10,000 to 15,000 units of heparin subcutaneously per day, there is some increase in the risk of recurrent thrombosis and possibly embolism compared to that with larger doses, but a much lower risk of hemorrhage. The regimen described above by Hull and co-workers (1982a) utilizing subcutaneous adjusted dose heparin every 12 hours also appears to be effective and safe. Aspirin and other drugs that impair platelet function increase the risk of hemorrhage, even with "low dose" heparin, and therefore should be avoided.

Warfarin and related compounds that inhibit the synthesis of vitamin K–dependent coagulation factors cross the placenta and thereby also impair the coagulation mechanism of the fetus. Moreover, there is evidence that warfarin may be teratogenic if used early in pregnancy. The administration of warfarin during the first 8 weeks of gestation may result in congenital malformations, which include nasal hypoplasia, ophthalmologic abnormalities, and retarded development (Shaul and Hall, 1977). Whether the malformations are the consequence of microhemorrhages in embryonic cartilage or a more complex teratogenic action is not known. It also must be remembered that a variety of drugs acts to enhance or inhibit the action of warfarin.

Because of the mechanical forces that develop during labor, the fetus is at increased risk of hemorrhage, especially intracranial hemorrhage, at this time. Therefore, if warfarin has been used as an anticoagulant during the antepartum period, the drug should be stopped weeks before the anticipated time of delivery and anticoagulation with heparin initiated.

Pelvic Venous Thrombosis

During the puerperium, thrombi may form transiently in any of the dilated pelvic veins and probably do so relatively often. In general, pelvic venous thrombosis without thrombophlebitis is not likely to incite definitive signs or symptoms unless the thrombosis is extensive or pulmonary embolism occurs.

Ovarian Vein Thrombophlebitis. This lesion is either a very uncommon complication of the puerperium or it resolves spontaneously, at times with the aid of antibiotics that were used to treat pelvic infection.

Munsick and Gillanders (1981) identified the following clinical features from review of cases of ovarian vein thrombophlebitis reported by others and those that they had personally observed: *The cardinal symptom was pain* that developed typically on the second or third postpartum day with or without fever. Pain was present in the lower abdomen, the flank, or both. In some cases, but not all, a tender mass was palpable just beyond the uterine cornu. The thrombophlebitis always involved the right ovarian vein, but in a few instances it involved the left ovarian vein as well. Typical findings at laparotomy were a firm tumefaction of the ovarian vein overlaid by inflamed peritoneum. Peritoneal involvement may have spread to produce perisalpingo-oophoritis and periappendicitis. The thrombus may have extended into the inferior vena cava. If an intra-abdominal lesion that requires surgery, such as appendicitis, can be excluded without performing a laparotomy, treatment for ovarian vein thrombophlebitis recommended by them and others is heparin intravenously and broad-spectrum antibiotics.

Munsick and Gillanders (1981) considered the possible relationship of the direction of blood flow in the ovarian veins to the genesis of ovarian vein thrombophlebitis. From their radioangiographic studies performed during the puerperium, they suspect that in the upright position blood flow from the left ovarian vein is primarily retrograde to the uterus but antegrade from the uterus through the right ovarian vein. With such a flow pattern, bacterial contaminants would more likely ascend the right ovarian vein and provoke intimal damage and thrombophlebitis. They believe that such a mechanism would account for the great preponderance of involvement of the right, rather than the left, ovarian vein.

In one of the very few cases identified in more recent years at Parkland Memorial Hospital laparotomy was performed because of the likelihood of a grave outcome if the suspected diagnosis of right ovarian vein thrombophlebitis proved to be appendicitis, instead. There was extensive inflammation, edema, and induration surrounding the enlarged thrombosed right ovarian vein, the right tube and ovary, and the appendix (Fig. 36-1A, B). The vein was filled with firm clot that extended into the vena cava, and the appendix, right oviduct, and right ovary were resected. The inferior vena cava and uninvolved left ovarian vein were ligated; heparin therapy was started 48 hours after laparotomy; the patient soon recovered.

Even more recently, we have identified an instance of *left* ovarian thrombophlebitis that was clearly visualized by CT scan (Fig. 36-1C, D). Chills and fever spiking as high as 40°C began 36 hours postpartum and persisted for 7 days until intensive broad spectrum antibiotic therapy without heparin was initiated. The woman, who had been remarkably *asymptomatic* except for chills and fever, became afebrile within 48 hours and remained so. It is obvious that much remains to be learned about the diagnosis and treatment of puerperal ovarian vein thrombophlebitis.

Suppurative pelvic thrombophlebitis and *septic emboli* that develop in association with bacterial infection are also discussed in Chapter 35, pp. 722, 726, and 728.

Anticoagulation and Abortion

The treatment of deep venous thrombosis with heparin does not preclude termination of pregnancy by careful curettage (see Chapter 24, p. 478). After all of the products of conception are removed without trauma to the reproductive tract, heparin can be restarted in therapeutic doses at the termination of the procedure without undue risk. If abdominal hysterotomy is to be performed, those precautions presented below for cesarean section are applicable. Experiences are lacking in which hypertonic saline or a prostaglandin has been used as an abortifacient in the presence of effective anticoagulation. The same is true for laparoscopic tubal sterilization. In both circumstances, it is anticipated that serious bleeding might be induced.

Anticoagulation and Delivery

The forces of labor and delivery may induce severe hemorrhage in the fetus if the mother has very recently been treated with warfarin. The effects of warfarin may be reversed by the slow intravenous administration of vitamin K_1 in a dose of 10 mg. The activities of the vitamin K–dependent clotting factors usually increase to safe levels within 8 hours in the mother, but less rapidly in the fetus. Maternal transfusion of plasma or a plasma fraction rich in factors II, VII, IX, and X (Konyne) will correct the deficiency immediately in the mother but, unfortunately, not in the fetus. Hepatitis may be transmitted with this plasma fraction.

Heparin does not cross the placenta. The effects of heparin on blood loss at delivery will depend upon a number of variables, including the following: (1) the dose, route, and time of administration; (2) the magnitude of incisions and lacerations; (3) the intensity of myometrial contraction and retraction once the products of conception have been delivered; and (4) the presence of other coagulation defects. The experiences at Parkland Memorial Hospital have been that measured blood loss is not greatly increased with vaginal delivery if the midline episiotomy is modest in depth, there are no lacerations of the genital tract, and the uterus promptly becomes firmly contracted and remains so after delivery of the placenta. Such ideal circumstances do not always prevail during and after vaginal delivery, however. Mueller and Lebherz (1969), for example, described 10 women with antepartum thrombophlebitis treated with heparin. Three who continued to receive heparin during labor and delivery bled remarkably and developed severe postpartum hemorrhage with large hematomas. Blood replacement of 1500, 2500, and 4500 ml was essential, as was repeated drainage of the hematomas. Therefore, in general, heparin therapy should be stopped during the time of labor and delivery. If the uterus is well contracted and there has been negligible trauma to the lower genital tract, it can soon be restarted. Otherwise, a delay of 2 or 3 days may be prudent. Protamine sulfate administered intravenously most often will promptly and effectively reverse the effect of heparin but, of course,

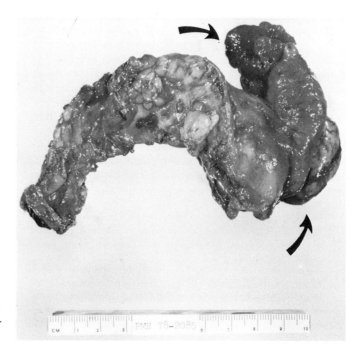

Figure 36-1. Ovarian vein thrombophlebitis. **A.** Resected thrombosed right ovarian vein plus right oviduct (*upper arrow*) and ovary (*lower arrow*).

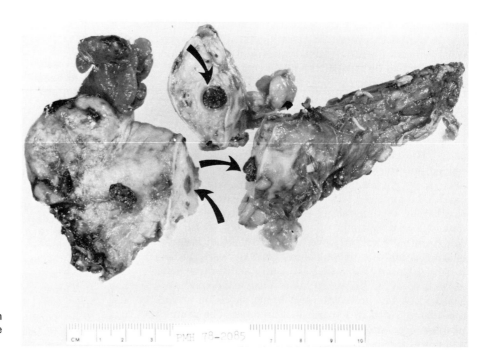

Figure 36-1. B. Same specimen after sectioning to demonstrate the thrombus (*arrows*).

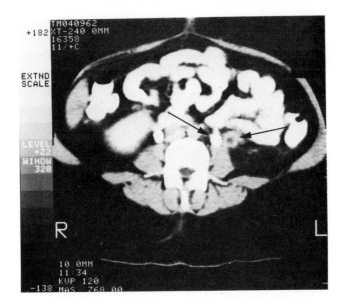

Figure 36-1. C. CT scan in a different woman made at the level of the uterine adnexa. The left ureter (*left arrow*) is filled with contrast material. The left ovarian vein (*right arrow*) appears swollen and inflamed and the lumen is filled with clot. (*Courtesy of Dr. S. Nally.*)

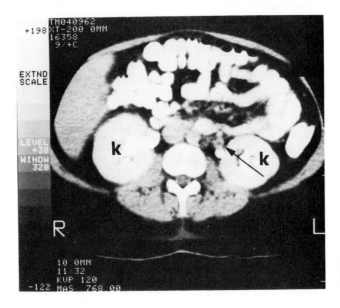

Figure 36-1. D. CT scan of the clotted left ovarian vein (*arrow*) just below the junction of the ovarian and renal veins (k = kidney).

will be of no benefit for hematomas already formed. Protamine sulfate, if used, should not be given in excess of the amount needed to neutralize the heparin. Excess protamine has an anticoagulant effect.

Serious bleeding is likely when heparin in usual therapeutic doses is administered to a woman who has undergone cesarean section within the previous 72 hours. After that, the risk of bleeding decreases with time so that by 1 week in the otherwise uncomplicated case there is slight risk. Again, preexisting defects in the hemostatic mechanism, such as thrombocytopenia, or impaired platelet function as induced by aspirin, enhance the likelihood of hemorrhage with heparin.

The woman who has very recently suffered a pulmonary embolism and who must be delivered by cesarean section presents a grave problem. Cesarean section and ligation of the inferior vena cava above the insertion of the right renal vein and the left ovarian vein near its insertion into the renal vein will usually yield the most favorable outcome. Nearly always in this situation tubal sterilization is also indicated.

Pulmonary Embolism

The greatest danger from venous thrombosis is pulmonary embolism. The reported incidence of pulmonary embolism associated with pregnancy has varied widely, from 1 in 2700 deliveries (Stamm, 1960) to less than 1 in 7000 deliveries (Mengert, 1945).

Chest discomfort, shortness of breath, air hunger, tachypnea, or obvious apprehension are signs and symptoms that should alert the physician to a strong likelihood of pulmonary embolism during the puerperium. Bell and associates (1977) carefully analyzed the clinical findings in a large number of individuals with angiographically identified pulmonary embolism. The most common abnormality was a respiratory rate of greater than 16 per minute. They emphasized that its frequency was so striking that a lower respiratory rate should rule against the diagnosis. Physical examination of the chest may or may not yield findings such as an accentuated pulmonic valve second sound, rales, or friction rub. Right axis deviation may or may not be evident in the electrocardiogram.

Even with massive pulmonary embolism, signs, symptoms, and laboratory data to support the diagnosis of pulmonary embolism may be deceivingly unspecific, as borne out in a cooperative study sponsored by the National Heart and Lung Institute (Wenger and colleagues, 1972). Ninety patients were identified by pulmonary angiography to have massive embolism. Although at least two lobar arteries were obstructed, the classic triad indicative of pulmonary embolism—hemoptysis, pleuritic chest pain, and dyspnea—was noted in only 20 percent of the subjects. Furthermore, there is no definitive laboratory blood test that is diagnostic (Hirsch, 1981).

Great controversy still exists with respect to the safest, least invasive technique that can most accurately diagnose a pulmonary embolus. Some investigators believe that ventilation–perfusion scintigraphy is adequate in the majority of young patients without evidence of underlying cardiopulmonary disease (Viamonte and associates, 1980; Ruckley, 1982; Sassahara and co-workers, 1983). However, these techniques use radioactive agents administered intravenously and they may not provide a definite diagnosis. Hull and associates (1983) reported that ventilation scanning increased the probability of pulmonary embolus in patients with *large perfusion defects and ventilation mismatches* but a ventilation–perfusion match was *not* helpful in ruling out pulmonary embolism. They reported that pulmonary angiography was necessary in most patients with perfusion abnormalities because the diagnosis of pulmonary embolism could not be made or excluded with sufficient accuracy in such patients.

Heparin Dosage

In general, in either category of obstetric patients, therapy with heparin in appropriate doses is effective. Most often, 5000 to 7500 units given intravenously every 4 hours, depending primarily upon the size of the woman, soon accomplishes the therapeutic goals. Heparin can also be given continuously via infusion pump at approximately 1 IU/ml of estimated blood volume over 4 hours (Klotz, 1982).

Attempts to identify by laboratory testing whether the heparin dosage is adequate to inhibit further throm-

bosis, yet not cause serious hemorrhage, have been discouraging unless the laboratory has the capability of measuring heparin in plasma (Bonnar, 1979). Whole blood clotting times have long been used and more recently measurement of the plasma partial thromboplastin time has been recommended (Spaet, 1980). The two tests often correlate poorly. An important test that will aid in detecting hemorrhage, but tends to be forgotten, is the frequent measurement of the hematocrit. Careful clinical evaluation will usually provide the best information concerning adequacy of dosage. Clinical improvement without hemorrhage is the desired goal.

It is important to remember that heparin is being administered whenever blood is to be drawn or medications are ordered to be given parenterally. Serious hemorrhage may occur, especially when arterial blood is drawn for blood gas analyses just before or soon after the administration of heparin.

Therapy with heparin as described may be discontinued in the postpartum woman after 10 days to 2 weeks if the disease process has clearly abated and there is no evidence of underlying chronic venous abnormalities that would predispose to venous thrombosis and no evidence of underlying cardiopulmonary dysfunction. If anticoagulation is to be protracted and a switch to warfarin therapy is the plan, treatment with heparin and warfarin should overlap for 6 days after the prothrombin time has reached the therapeutic level (Wessler and Gitel, 1979; Walsh, 1983).

If the woman is undelivered, there is appreciable risk of recurrence of the venous thrombosis sometime during the subsequent antepartum, intrapartum, and postpartum periods unless an anticoagulant—preferably heparin—is continued. Therefore, anticoagulation should be continued, unless ligation or clipping of the inferior vena cava and left ovarian vein has been carried out, as discussed below.

Venous Ligation

In the very infrequent circumstances where heparin therapy fails to prevent recurrent pulmonary embolism from the pelvis or legs, ligation of the vena cava below the level of the renal veins but above the entry of the right ovarian vein plus ligation of the left ovarian vein below its entry into the left renal vein is usually indicated. Serrated Teflon clips applied to the vena cava may be nearly as effective (Couch and associates, 1975). An intravenously inserted vena caval filter has been used during pregnancy with good results (Scurr and co-workers, 1981). In spite of previous reports suggesting that obstruction of the vena cava causes placental abruption, there are several reports of successful ligation performed antepartum, with favorable outcomes for the mother and usually the fetus (Stone and colleagues, 1968). Caval and ovarian vein ligation for treatment of septic emboli from the pelvis is considered in Chapter 35 (p. 728).

The possibility of pulmonary embolism must always be kept in mind, especially during the puerperium. If the woman develops an embolus during her hospital stay, the diagnosis is more likely to be made and appropriate therapy started. Embolism may occur weeks after delivery, however, with no intervening symptoms. Under these circumstances, it is easy to ascribe the symptoms to some other cause, especially anxiety. A woman readmitted to Parkland Memorial Hospital provides an example:

> A somewhat elderly, multiparous woman was admitted near term with total placental abruption and massive bleeding. Treatment included cesarean section and 15 units of whole blood. Eight days later, after a benign postpartum course, she was discharged. Three weeks after delivery she was awakened during the night by chest pain. In the morning she went to a physician who considered her to be "apprehensive and hyperventilating secondary to grief reaction." Rebreathing into a paper bag and diazepam were prescribed but gave no relief. The same day she came to Parkland Memorial Hospital, where supporting evidence of pulmonary embolism was readily uncovered, including tachypnea, splinting of left side of chest on inspiration, abnormal chest x-ray, pulmonary perfusion defects demonstrated by lung scan in regions free of infiltrate, and, while breathing room air, an arterial blood Po_2 of 62 mm Hg and pH of 7.52. Treatment with heparin intravenously every 4 hours was promptly started. At no time was there clinical evidence of thrombosis in the lower extremities and phlebograms were negative. Presumably the emboli came from the pelvis. She promptly recovered.

In general, whenever there is reasonable suspicion of pulmonary embolus, it is much safer to initiate an effective program of anticoagulation, as outlined in this chapter, rather than risk a second embolus, which may prove fatal.

DISEASES AND ABNORMALITIES OF THE UTERUS

Subinvolution

Subinvolution is an arrest or retardation of involution, the process by which the puerperal uterus is normally restored to its original proportions. Subinvolution is accompanied by prolongation of the period of lochial discharge and sometimes by profuse hemorrhage. It may be followed by prolonged leukorrhea and irregular or excessive uterine bleeding. The diagnosis is established by bimanual examination. The uterus is larger and softer than normal for the particular period of the puerperium. Among the recognized causes of subinvolution are retention of placental fragments and pelvic infection. Since most cases of subinvolution result from local causes, they are usually amenable to early diagnosis and treatment. Ergonovine (Ergotrate) or methyl ergonovine (Methergine), 0.2 mg every 3 to 4 hours for 24 to 48 hours may lead to improvement. Metritis may be best managed by antibiotic therapy.

Postpartum Cervical Erosions

Cervical erosions, or eversions, are a complication of the late postpartum period. Shallow cauterization or cryotherapy can be used to remove persistent exuberant granulations or the delicate exposed endocervical columnar epithelium, without causing stenosis of the endocervix.

Relaxation of the Vaginal Outlet and Prolapse of the Uterus

Extensive lacerations of the perineum during delivery, if not properly repaired, are commonly followed by relaxation of the vaginal outlet. Even when external lacerations are not visible, overstretching or submucosal tears may lead to marked relaxation. The changes in the pelvic supports during parturition predispose, moreover, to prolapse of the uterus and to urinary stress incontinence. These conditions may escape detection unless an examination is made at the end of the puerperium and unless the patients are subjected to long-term follow-up.

In general, operative correction should be postponed until the desired number of children has been achieved, unless, of course, serious disability, notably urinary stress incontinence, results in symptoms sufficient enough for the patient to demand intervention.

HEMORRHAGES DURING THE PUERPERIUM

Occasionally, serious uterine hemorrhage develops in the latter part of the first week, or later in the puerperium. Hemorrhage most often is the result of abnormal involution of the placental site, but it may be caused also by retention of a portion of the placenta. Usually, the retained piece of placenta undergoes necrosis with deposition of fibrin, and may eventually form a so-called *placental polyp* (Fig. 36-2). As the eschar of the polyp detaches from the myometrium, hemorrhage may be brisk.

It has been generally accepted that with late postpartum hemorrhage from the uterus, prompt curettage is necessary. The experiences at Parkland Memorial Hospital, however, have been that curettage subsequent to late puerperal hemorrhage most often did not remove identifiable placental tissue. Hemorrhage was initiated by the separation of the retained products of conception that, in turn, were flushed out by the brisk hemorrhage. Lee and co-workers (1981) support this observation and have presented evidence that the use of sonography can exclude retained placental fragments as the cause of delayed postpartum hemorrhage in the majority of cases. Curettage, rather than reducing hemorrhage, is more likely to traumatize the implantation site and incite more bleeding, at times to such a degree that hysterectomy must be performed. Especially where there is good reason to preserve the uterus for future childbearing, initial treatment may best be directed to control of the

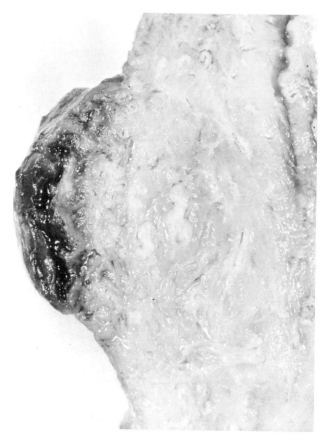

Figure 36-2. Placental polyp. Hysterectomy was performed because of prolonged bleeding which resulted in severe anemia in a woman who wanted no more pregnancies.

bleeding, using intravenous oxytocin, ergonovine, methylergonovine, or prostaglandins (Goldstein and coworkers, 1983; Andrinopoulos and Mendenhall, 1983). If the bleeding subsides, the woman is simply observed; and if the bleeding stops, she is discharged. In general, curettage is carried out only if appreciable bleeding persists or recurs after such management. It is imperative that the physician inform the patient that if a curettage is performed under these conditions, the possibility of a hysterectomy is real. Furthermore, the physician must provide arrangements for adequate blood, appropriate anesthesia, and surgical assistance.

Puerperal Hematomas

Blood may escape into the connective tissue beneath the skin covering the external genitalia or beneath the vaginal mucosa to form vulvar and vaginal hematomas. The condition usually follows injury to a blood vessel without laceration of the superficial tissues, and may occur with spontaneous, as well as operative, delivery. Occasionally, the hemorrhage is delayed, perhaps as a result of sloughing of a vessel that had become necrotic from prolonged pressure.

Less frequently, the torn vessel lies above the pelvic fascia. In that event, the hematoma develops above it. In its early stages, the hematoma forms a rounded swelling that projects into the upper portion of the vaginal canal and may almost occlude its lumen. If the bleeding continues, it dissects retroperitoneally and thus may form a tumor palpable above the Poupart ligament, or it may dissect upward, eventually reaching the lower margin of the diaphragm.

Vulvar Hematomas

Such hematomas, particularly those that develop rapidly, may cause excruciating pain, which is often the first symptom that is noticed (Fig. 36-3). Hematomas of moderate size may be absorbed spontaneously. The tissues overlying the hematoma may give way as a result of necrosis caused by pressure, and profuse hemorrhage may follow. In other cases, the contents of the hematoma may be discharged in the form of large clots.

In the subperitoneal variety, the extravasation of blood beneath the peritoneum may be massive and occasionally fatal. Death may also follow secondary intraperitoneal rupture. Occasionally, rupture into the vagina leads to infection of the hematoma and potentially fatal sepsis.

A vulvar hematoma is readily diagnosed by severe perineal pain and the sudden appearance of a tense, fluctuant, and sensitive tumor of varying size covered by discolored skin. When the mass develops adjacent to the vagina, it may temporarily escape detection, but symptoms of pressure, if not pain, and inability to void should soon lead to a vaginal examination and the discovery of a round, fluctuant tumor encroaching on the lumen. When the hematoma extends upward between the folds of the broad ligament, it may escape detection unless a portion of the tumor can be felt on

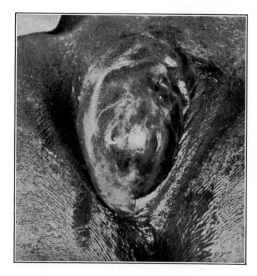

Figure 36-3. Vulvar hematoma bulging into the right vaginal wall.

abdominal palpation or unless evidence of anemia or infection appears.

The prognosis is usually favorable, though bleeding into very large hematomas has led to death.

Treatment. Smaller vulvar hematomas identified after leaving the delivery room may be treated expectantly. If, however, the pain is severe, or if they continue to enlarge, as they often do, the best treatment is prompt incision and evacuation of the blood with ligation of the bleeding points. The cavity can then be obliterated with mattress sutures. *With hematomas of the genital tract, blood loss is nearly always considerably more than the clinical estimate.* Hypovolemia and severe anemia should be prevented by adequate blood replacement. Broad-spectrum antibiotics are of value.

The subperitoneal and supravaginal varieties are more difficult to treat. They can be evacuated by incision of the perineum, but unless there is complete hemostasis, which is difficult to achieve by this route, laparotomy is advisable.

DISEASE OF THE URINARY TRACT

The puerperal bladder is not so sensitive to intravesical fluid tension as in the nonpregnant state. Moreover, it has become commonplace in modern obstetrics to establish an intravenous infusion system during labor in women. After delivery, the infusion system is then used to administer oxytocin during the first hour or so after delivery, if not longer. The oxytocin induces potent antidiuresis until the time the oxytocin is stopped, after which there is a prompt diuresis. The bladder then fills rapidly and may overdistend to a remarkable degree. General anesthesia, and especially conduction anesthesia with the temporarily disturbed neural control of the bladder, are important contributory factors. The woman in this circumstance may, in time, void small volumes of urine ("overflow incontinence"), misleading attendants into believing she is voiding normally. Inspection of the abdomen will disclose the uterine fundus to be much higher than it should be, with an overlying cystic mass, the distended bladder.

As stated above, trauma to the genital tract, especially with large hematoma formation, may cause urinary retention. Therefore, pelvic examination should be performed whenever urinary retention is identified.

The combination of residual urine and bacteriuria introduced by catheterization into a traumatized bladder present the optimal conditions for the development of infection of the urinary tract. The initial symptoms include dysuria, frequency, and urgency. Signs and symptoms of infection will subsequently vary, depending upon whether the infection is localized to the bladder or ascends to involve the upper urinary tract. After urine has been obtained for culture, treatment should consist of appropriate antibiotic or chemotherapeutic agents, as discussed in Chapter 28 (pp. 583).

In cases of overdistension of the bladder, it is usually best to leave an indwelling catheter in place for at least 24 hours so as to empty the bladder completely and prevent prompt recurrence, as well as to allow recovery of normal bladder tone and sensation. When the catheter is removed, it is necessary subsequently to demonstrate ability to void appropriately. If the woman cannot void after 4 hours, she should be catheterized and the volume of urine measured. If there is more than 200 ml of urine, it is apparent that the bladder is not functioning appropriately. The catheter should be left in place and the bladder drained for another day. If less than 200 ml of urine is obtained, the catheter can be removed and the bladder rechecked subsequently as described.

In general, the first time the woman voids spontaneously after removal of an indwelling catheter inserted because of previous inability to void and gross overdistension, she should be immediately catheterized for residual urine. If the volume exceeds 100 ml, constant drainage should be reinstituted and those steps in management just outlined should be resumed. There is evidence that antimicrobial therapy will reduce appreciably the likelihood of bacteriuria developing when bladder catheterization is limited to 4 days or less (Garibaldi and associates, 1974).

DISORDERS OF THE BREAST

Engorgement of the Breasts

For the first 24 to 48 hours after the development of the lacteal secretion, it is not unusual for the breasts to become distended, firm, and nodular. This condition, commonly known as engorged breasts, or "caked breasts," often causes considerable pain and may be accompanied by a transient elevation of temperature. The disorder represents an exaggeration of the normal venous and lymphatic engorgement of the breasts, which is a regular precursor of lactation. It is not the result of overdistension of the lacteal system with milk.

Treatment consists of supporting the breasts with a binder or brassiere, applying an ice bag, and, if necessary, orally administering 60 mg of codeine sulfate or another analgesic. Pumping of the breast or manual expression of milk may be necessary at first (Fig. 36-4), but in a few days the condition is usually alleviated and the infant is able to nurse normally.

Suppression of Lactation

When, for a variety of reasons, the infant is not to be breast-fed, suppression of lactation becomes important. Perhaps the simplest method consists in support with a comfortable binder, application of cold, and mild analgesics for pain. Usually, all signs and symptoms will disappear in a few days if the breasts are not stimulated by pumping. Hormones, particularly estrogens, either alone

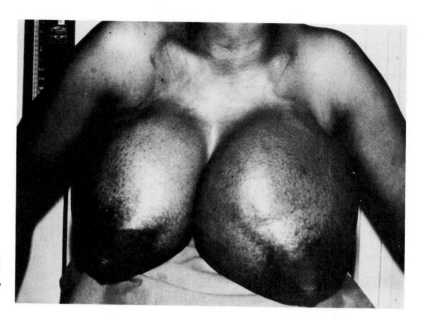

Figure 36-4. Pathologic breast engorgement 3 days after delivery. Pumping of the breasts, uplift support, and analgesia provided relief. (*Courtesy of Dr. J. Duenhoelter.*)

or combined with testosterone, were formerly widely used for this purpose (Harrison, 1979). A single intramuscular injection of 4 ml of long-acting steroid esters in the form of estradiol valerate and testosterone enanthate (Deladumone), administered at the time of delivery, is claimed to be effective.

Several estrogens that have been used to try to suppress lactation have been shown to predispose to venous thrombosis and thromboembolism (Niebyl and colleagues, 1979; Tindall, 1968; Turnbull, 1968). Moreover, their effect of lactation may be one of delay rather than effective suppression. Niebyl and co-workers (1979) challenge their use on the bases of increased risk of thromboembolism and questionable benefit. These agents have not been used at Parkland Memorial Hospital, even though the majority of mothers still do not breast-feed their infants.

Bromocriptine, a dopamine agonist, stimulates the production of prolactin inhibitory factor which, in turn, causes a fall in plasma prolactin and the suppression of lactation. The use of bromocriptine in the puerperium for this purpose has been approved by the Food and Drug Administration, but the recommended duration of treatment is prolonged and the cost of the drug is considerable.

Mastitis

Parenchymatous inflammation of the mammary glands is a rare complication antepartum but is occasionally observed during the puerperium and lactation.

The symptoms of suppurative mastitis seldom appear before the end of the first week of the puerperium and, as a rule, not until the third or fourth week. Marked engorgement usually precedes the inflammation, the first sign of which is chills or actual rigor, soon followed by a rise in temperature and an increase in pulse rate. The breast becomes hard and reddened, and the patient complains of pain. In some cases, the constitutional symptoms attending a mammary abscess are severe. Local manifestations may be so slight as to escape observation, however; such cases are usually mistaken for puerperal infection. In still another group of women, the infection pursues a subacute or almost chronic course. The breast is somewhat harder than usual and more or less painful, but constitutional symptoms are either lacking or very slight. In such circumstances, the first indication of the true diagnosis is often afforded by the detection of fluctuation.

Etiology. By far, the most common offending organism is *Staphylococcus aureus*. The immediate source of the staphylococci that cause this mastitis is nearly always the nursing infant's nose and throat. At the time of nursing, the organism enters the breast through the nipple at the site of a fissure or abrasion, which may be quite small. Whether the bacteria commonly cause mastitis simply by entering the lactiferous ducts of the breast with completely intact integument is not clear. In cases of true mastitis, the offending organism can nearly always be cultured from breast milk. A case of toxic shock has been reported in a woman with a puerperal breast abscess (Dixey and associates, 1982). *Staphylococcus aureus* was cultured from the abscess.

Suppurative mastitis among nursing mothers has at times reached epidemic levels. Such outbreaks most often coincide with the appearance of a new strain of antibiotic-resistant *Staphylococcus* or the reappearance of one previously identified. Typically, the infant becomes infected in the nursery as he comes in contact with nursery personnel who carry the organism. The attendants' hands are the major source of contamination of the newborn. Especially in a crowded, understaffed nursery, it is a simple matter for the personnel inadvertently to transfer staphylococci from one colonized newborn infant to another. The colonization of staphylococci in the infant may be totally asymptomatic or may locally involve the umbilicus or the skin, but occasionally the organisms may cause a life-threatening systemic infection.

Prevention. Safeguards to prevent colonization of the newborn with virulent strains of staphylococci necessitate exclusion from the care of the infant and mother by all personnel with a known or suspected staphylococcal lesion. Also, as a matter of daily routine, close inspection should be made of every infant, with prompt isolation of any who appear to be developing an infection of the cord or of the skin. Frequent use of soap or detergent for handscrubbing by personnel is essential. At the first sign of an outbreak, all personnel should be checked with appropriate cultures and phage-typing of swabbings of the posterior nares to identify carriers of more virulent strains of staphylococci.

At the time of an epidemic, the phenomenon of bacterial interference has been used successfully to prevent colonization of the newborn with a highly virulent strain of *S. aureus* (Light and colleagues, 1967). As each newborn arrives at the nursery, the nares and umbilicus are directly inoculated with a strain of *S. aureus* known to be nonvirulent. This procedure usually blocks subsequent colonization by virulent strains.

Treatment. The advent of antibiotics has markedly improved the prognosis of acute puerperal mastitis. Provided that appropriate antibiotic therapy is started before suppuration begins, the infection can usually be aborted within 48 hours. Before initiating any antibiotic therapy, milk should be expressed from the affected breast onto a swab and promptly cultured. By so doing, the offending organism can be identified and its bacterial sensitivity ascertained. At the same time, the results of such cultures also provide information that is mandatory for a successful program of surveillance of nosocomial infections. The initial choice of antibiotic will undoubtedly be influenced to a considerable degree by the current experiences with staphylococcal infections at the institution in which the woman is receiving care. If, at the time, most staphylococcal infections are caused by organisms sensitive to penicillin, treatment with penicillin G is likely to be curative. If the infection is caused by resistant, penicillinase-producing staphylococci, or if resistant organisms are suspected while awaiting the results of culture, a penicillinase-resistant compound should be used. It is important that treatment not be discontinued too soon. Even though clinical response may be prompt and striking, treatment should be continued for at least 10 days.

Nursing should be discontinued when a diagnosis of suppurative mastitis is made, for it may be quite painful and the milk is infected; moreover, the infant often harbors the organisms and can therefore cause reinfection. Since the infant is almost always colonized by the offending organism, he should be observed very closely for signs of infection. Once established, resistant staphylococcal infections tend to spread and recur among the family for protracted periods of time.

In the case of formation of frank abscesses, drainage, in addition to antibiotic therapy, is essential. The incision should be made radially, extending from near the areolar margin toward the periphery of the gland, to avoid injury to the lactiferous ducts. In early cases, a single incision over the most dependent portion of the area of fluctuation is usually sufficient, but multiple abscesses require several incisions. The operation should be performed under general anesthesia, and a finger should be inserted to break up the walls of the locules. The resulting cavity is loosely packed with gauze, which should be replaced at the end of 24 hours by a smaller pack. If the pus has been thoroughly evacuated, the cavity of the abscess is obliterated and a complete cure is sometimes effected with great rapidity.

Galactocele

Very exceptionally, as the result of the clogging of a duct by inspissated secretion, milk may accumulate in one or more lobes of the breast. The amount is ordinarily limited, but an excess may form a fluctuant mass that may give rise to pressure symptoms. They may resolve spontaneously or require aspiration.

Supernumerary Breasts

One in every few hundred women has one or more accessory breasts (*polymastia*). The supernumerary breasts may be so small as to be mistaken for pigmented moles, or, when without a nipple, for a lipoma. They rarely attain considerable size. They are likely to be situated in pairs on either side of the midline of the thoracic or abdominal walls, usually below the main breasts; they are also found in the axillae, and more rarely on other portions of the body such as the shoulder, flank, groin, or thigh. The number of supernumerary breasts varies greatly. When arranged symmetrically, two or four are most common, although ten have been described.

Polymastia has no obstetric significance, although occasionally the enlargement of supernumerary breasts in the axillae may result in considerable discomfort. Frequently, a tongue of mammary tissue extends out into the axilla from the outer margin of a normal breast, whereas an isolated fragment is sometimes found in the same location. Such structures undergo hypertrophy during pregnancy (Fig. 36-5). When lactation has been established, they may become swollen and painful. Ordinarily, they soon undergo regression and give no further trouble.

Abnormalities of the Nipples

The typical nipple is cylindric, projecting well beyond the general surface of the breast; its exterior is slightly nodular but not fissured. Variations, however, are not

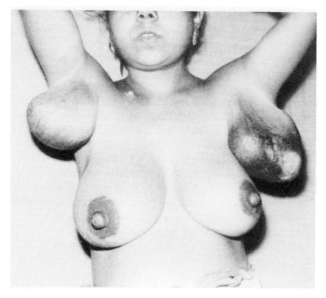

Figure 36-5. Pregnancy with huge bilateral hypertrophic axillary tail of the breasts. (*Courtesy of Dr. P. Bhattacharaya.*)

uncommon, some sufficiently pronounced to interfere seriously with suckling.

In some women, the lactiferous ducts open directly into a depression at the center of the areola. In marked cases of depressed nipple, nursing is out of the question. When the depression is not very deep, the breast may occasionally be made available by use of a breast pump.

More frequently, the nipple, although not depressed, is so greatly inverted that it cannot be used for nursing. In such a case, daily attempts should be made during the last few months of pregnancy to draw the nipple out, using traction with the fingers. Since the maneuver is rarely successful, however, if the nipples cannot be made available by temporary use of an electric pump, suckling must be discontinued.

Nipples that are normal in shape and size may become fissured and therefore particularly susceptible to injury from the child's mouth during suckling. In such cases, the fissures almost invariably render nursing painful, sometimes with a deleterious influence upon the secretory function. Moreover, such lesions provide a convenient portal of entry for pyogenic bacteria. For these reasons, every effort should be made to heal such fissures, particularly by protecting them from further injury with a nipple shield and topical medication. If such measures are of no avail, the child should not be permitted to nurse on the affected side. Instead, the breast should be emptied regularly with a suitable pump until the lesions are completely healed.

Abnormalities of Secretion

There are marked individual variations in the amount of milk secreted, many of which are dependent not upon the general health and appearance of the woman but

upon the development of the glandular portions of the breasts. A woman with large breasts may produce only a small quantity of milk, whereas another with small, flat breasts may produce an abundant supply. Very rarely, there is complete lack of mammary secretion (agalactia). As a rule, it is possible to express a small amount from the nipple on the third or fourth day of the puerperium. Occasionally, the mammary secretion is excessive (polygalactia).

Formerly, persistent lactation or galactorrhea (together with anemorrhea and signs of estrogen deficiency) was referred to as the Chiari–Frommel syndrome. It was believed that this disorder was a pregnancy-induced derangement in the hypothalamic–pituitary control of prolactin and gonadotropin secretion. A similar set of symptoms commencing independent of pregnancy was described by Ahumada (1932) and by Argonz and Del Castillo (1953). With the development of sensitive and accurate radioimmunoassays for prolactin and with the development of polytomography for evaluating the contents of the sella turcica, it has been demonstrated that microadenomas of the pituitary are the most common cause of galactorrhea, amenorrhea, and estrogen deficiency. Thus, the development of this triad should alert the physician to the likelihood of the existence of a microadenoma of the pituitary irrespective of whether the signs and symptoms begin in the puerperal period or remote from pregnancy.

OBSTETRIC PARALYSIS

Pressure on branches of the sacral plexus during labor is demonstrated by complaints of intense neuralgia or cramplike pains extending down one or both legs as soon as the head begins to descend the pelvis. As a rule, the compression is rarely severe enough to give rise to grave lesions. In some instances, however, the pain continues after delivery and is accompanied by paralysis of the muscles supplied by the external popliteal nerve (the flexors of the ankles and the extensors of the toes). Occasionally, the gluteal muscles are affected to a lesser extent. In modern obstetrics, paralysis of this kind is rare. Footdrop results from improper positioning of patients in stirrups or leg holders.

Separation of the symphysis pubis or one of the sacroiliac synchondroses during labor may be followed by pain and marked interference with locomotion (Chapter 28, p. 631).

REFERENCES

Ahumada JC, Del Castillo EB: (Amenorrhea and galactorrhea). Bol Soc Obstet Ginec (Buenos Aires) 11:64, 1932

Andrinopoulos GC, Mendenhall HW: Prostaglandin $F_{2\alpha}$ in the management of delayed postpartum hemorrhage. Am J Obstet Gynecol 146:217, 1983

Argonz J, Del Castillo EB: A syndrome characterized by estrogenic insufficiency, galactorrhea and decreased urinary gonadotropin. J Clin Endocrinol 13:79, 1953

Bhattacharaya P: Pregnancy with huge bilateral hypertrophic axillary tail of the breast. Case report. Br J Obstet Gynaecol 90:874, 1983

Bell WR, Simon TL, DeMets DL: The clinical features of submassive and massive pulmonary emboli. Am J Med 62:355, 1977

Bonnar J: Venous thrombo-embolism and pregnancy. In Stallworthy J, Bourne G (eds): Recent Advances in Obstetrics and Gynaecology. Edinburgh, Churchill-Livingstone, 1979, vol 13, p 173

Chong BH, Pitney WR, Castaldi PA: Heparin-induced thrombocytopenia: Association of thrombotic complications with heparin-dependent IgG antibody that induces thromboxane synthesis and platelet aggregation. Lancet 2:1246, 1982

Couch NP, Baldwin SS, Crane C: Mortality and morbidity rates after inferior vena caval clipping. Surgery 77:106, 1975

DeSwiet M, Ward PD, Fiddler J, Horsman A, Katz D, Letsky E, Peacock M, Wise PH: Prolonged heparin therapy in pregnancy causes bone demineralization. Br J Obstet Gynaecol 90:1129, 1983

Dixey JJ, Swanson DC, Williams TD, Rusin MH, Crook SJ, Midgley J, deSaxe MJ: Toxic-shock syndrome: Four cases in a London Hospital. Br Med J 285:342, 1982

Galle PC, Muss HB, McGrath KM, Stuart JJ, Homesley HD: Thrombocytopenia in two patients treated with low-dose heparin. Obstet Gynecol 52:9S, 1978

Garibaldi RA, Burke JP, Dickman ML, Smith CB: Bacteriuria during indwelling uretheral catheterization. N Engl J Med 291:215, 1974

Goldstein AI, Kent DR, David A: Prostaglandin E$_2$ vaginal suppositories in the treatment of intractable late-onset postpartum hemorrhage. A case report. J Reprod Med 28:425, 1983

Harrison RG: Suppression of lactation. Semin Perinatol 3:287, 1979

Henderson SR, Lund CJ, Creasman WT: Antepartum pulmonary embolism. Am J Obstet Gynecol 112:476, 1972

Hirsh J: Blood tests for the diagnosis of venous and arterial thrombosis. Blood 57:1, 1981

Hull R, Delmore T, Genton E, Hirsh S, Gent M, Sackette D, McLoughlin D, Armstrong P: Warfarin versus low-dose heparin in the long-term treatment of venous thrombosis. N Engl J Med 301:855, 1979

Hull R, Delmore T, Carter C, Hirsh J, Genton E, Gent M, Turpie G, Laughlin D: Adjusted subcutaneous heparin versus warfarin sodium in the long-term treatment of venous thrombosis. N Engl J Med 306:189, 1982a

Hull R, Hirsh J, Jay R, Carter C, England C, Gent M, Turpie AGG, Loughlin D, Dodd P, Thomas M, Taskob G, Ockelford P: Different intensities of oral anticoagulant therapy in the treatment of proximal-vein thrombosis. N Engl J Med 307:1676, 1982b

Hull RD, Hirsh J, Carter CJ, May RM, Dodd PE, Ockelford PA, Coates G, Gill GJ, Turpie G, Doyle DJ, Buller HR, Ras-

kob GE: Pulmonary angiography, ventilation lung scanning, and venography for clinically suspected pulmonary embolism with abnormal perfusion lung scan. Ann Int Med 98:891, 1983

Klotz TA: DVT: Diagnostic advances, therapeutic guidelines. Contemp Ob/Gyn 19:18, 1982

Lee CY, Madrazo B, Drukker BH: Ultrasonic evaluation of the postpartum uterus in the management of postpartum bleeding. Obstet Gynecol 58:227, 1981

Light IJ, Walton RL, Sutherland JM, Shinefield HR, Brackvogel V: Use of bacterial interference to control a staphylococcal nursery outbreak. Am J Dis Child 113:291, 1967

Mengert WF: Venous ligation in obstetrics. Am J Obstet Gynecol 50:467, 1945

Mueller MJ, Lebherz TB: Antepartum thrombophlebitis. Obstet Gynecol 34:867, 1969

Munsick RA, Gillanders LA: A review of the syndrome of puerperal ovarian vein thrombophlebitis with some original observations on ovarian venous blood-flow postpartum. Obstet Gynecol Survey 36:57, 1981

Niebyl JR, Bell WR, Schaaf ME, Blake DA, Dubin NH, King TM: The effect of chlorotrianisene on postpartum lactation suppression on blood coagulation factors. Am J Obstet Gynecol 143:518, 1979

Ruckley CV: Management of pulmonary embolism. Br Med J 285:831, 1982

Sassahara AA, Sharma VRK, Barsamian EM, Schoolman M, Cella G: Pulmonary thromboembolism: Diagnosis and treatment. JAMA 249:2945, 1983

Scurr J, Stannard P, Wright J: Extensive thrombo-embolic disease in pregnancy treated with a Kimray Greenfield vena cava filter. Br J Obstet Gynaecol 88:778, 1981

Shaul WL, Hall JG: Multiple congenital anomalies associated with oral anticoagulants. Am J Obstet Gynecol 127:191, 1977

Spaet TH: Heparin therapy. JAMA 244:1243, 1980

Stamm H: Obstetrical and gynecological mortality due to embolism in Central Europe and Scandinavia. Geburtshilfe Frauenheilkd 20:675, 1960

Stone SR, Whalley PJ, Pritchard JA: Inferior vena cava and ovarian vein ligation during late pregnancy. Obstet Gynecol 32:267, 1968

Tindall VR: Factors influencing puerperal thromboembolism. J Obstet Gynaecol Br Commonw 75:1324, 1968

Turnbull AC: Puerperal thromboembolism and the suppression of lactation. J Obstet Gynaecol Br Commonw 75:1321, 1968

Viamonte M Jr, Koolpe H, Janowitz W, Hildner F: Pulmonary thromboembolism—Update. JAMA 243:2229, 1980

Walsh PN: Oral anticoagulant therapy. Hosp Pract (Jan):101, 1983

Wenger NK, Stein PD, Willis PW III: Massive acute pulmonary embolism: The deceivingly nonspecific manifestations. JAMA 220:843, 1972

Wessler S, Gitel SN: Heparin: New concepts relevant to clinical use. 53:525, 1979

Wise PH, Hall AJ: Heparin-induced osteopenia in pregnancy. Br Med J 281:110, 1980

37

Preterm and Postterm Pregnancies and Fetal Growth Retardation

A fetus or newborn infant whose weight is appreciably below normal is at increased risk of dying or, if he or she survives, at increased risk of being impaired physically or intellectually. The frequency of infants weighing less than 2500 g (5½ pounds) at birth has long served as one indicator of the overall quality of reproductive performance, especially for large populations. It is now fully appreciated, however, that there are two distinct mechanisms responsible for abnormally low birth weight. In one, the rate of growth is normal but for an unduly short period of time; in the other, the fetus fails to maintain a normal rate of growth. Thus, as has been emphasized throughout this book, *a most important factor for the successful management of a pregnancy in which complications develop is precise knowledge of the gestational age of the fetus.* Knowledge of gestational age is certainly essential to any correct decision concerned with the appropriateness of fetal growth. Unfortunately, for a variety of reasons, the gestational age may either be unknown, or worse, be in error. The error may arise as a consequence of the woman's not obtaining prenatal care until very late in pregnancy and therefore long after events important for the identification of fetal age have passed or been forgotten, or the error may evolve from unrecognized delayed ovulation, for example, following menses induced by withdrawal of an oral contraceptive.

Definitions

The fetus or newborn infant is referred to as a *fetus at term* or an *infant at term* during the interval from the 38th through the 42nd week after the onset of a menstrual period that was followed 2 weeks later by ovulation. Of course, the critical date for determining the age of the fetus is the date of ovulation or fertilization, which differ from each other only by minutes to a day or so. *The time of onset of the last menstrual period has assumed clinical importance for determining fetal age only because it is usually known rather precisely, and, when spontaneous and previously regular, it most often is followed by ovulation and fertilization about 2 weeks*

later. Before the 38th week, *preterm* can be applied to categorize the fetus and the pregnancy; at 42 completed weeks and thereafter, *postterm* is appropriate. Importantly, whenever possible, the gestational (menstrual) age should be cited in weeks rather than months or trimesters.

Premature has long been used to designate the fetus or infant before the 38th week of gestational age. In some situations, at least, it might prove more informative not to use "premature" to describe the shortened gestational age of the fetus or infant but rather to use "premature" to describe function. For example, an infant at the time of birth may have achieved a gestational age of only 32 weeks and thus be chronologically premature yet, from the stand-point of pulmonary function, demonstrate no difficulties in adapting to the external environment because pulmonary function was mature. To describe such a fetus or infant as *preterm* with mature pulmonary function rather than premature with mature pulmonary function might provide for greater clarity.

Postterm appropriately describes the fetus or newborn infant whose gestational age has reached 42 weeks or more. *Postdates* has more recently achieved considerable usage, although the word seems to defy precise definition since the dates involved, other than the last menstrual period, are not clear. (Presumably, if the term *postdates* is acceptable, "predates" and "dates" are eligible for incorporation into our medical vocabulary.) It is highly desirable that the actual number of weeks of gestation be stated whenever possible.

A fetus or infant of low birth weight may be the consequence of an abnormally short gestational age but a normal rate of growth (*appropriately grown, preterm fetus or infant*) or of a gestation of normal duration but with an impaired rate of growth (*growth-retarded, term fetus or infant*), or of both a shortened gestation and an impaired rate of growth (*preterm, growth-retarded fetus or infant*). The term "intrauterine growth retardation" seems more cumbersome and much less precise than fetal growth retardation.

The growth-retarded fetus or infant is sometimes

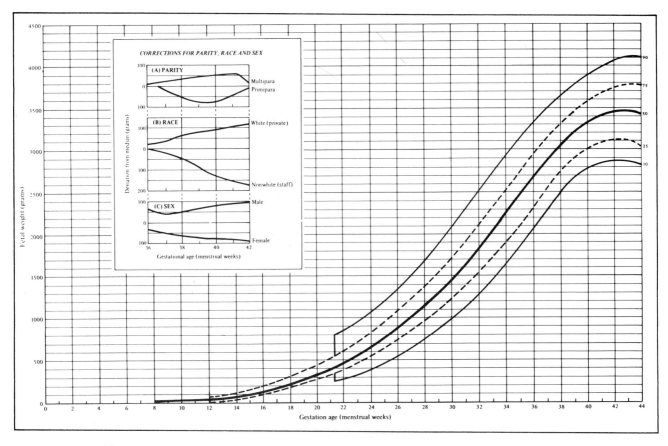

Figure 37-1. Fetal weight. The 10th, 25th, 50th 75th, and 90th percentiles of fetal weight in g throughout pregnancy and correction factors for parity, race (socioeconomic status), and sex are graphed. Data obtained from 31,202 prostaglandin-induced abortions and spontaneous deliveries. (*From Brenner, Hendricks: Am J Obstet Gynecol 126:555, 1976.*)

described as *small for gestational age.* Especially in recent years, "small for gestational age" has been widely used to categorize an infant whose birth weight is clearly below average and usually below the 10th percentile for this gestational age, while an infant whose birth weight is above the 90th percentile has been categorized as *large for gestational age* (Fig. 37-1).

Typically, the fetus continues to grow after 36 weeks gestation but at a slower rate (Fig. 37-2). When gestation is prolonged beyond term, some fetuses—perhaps the majority—continue to grow, and some may achieve a remarkably large size. Those infants who did so have been referred to, at times, as *postmature* as well as postterm. Those fetuses who became undernourished and demonstrated evidence of suffering chronic distress in utero have often been classified as *dysmature.* Unfortunately, some obstetricians and pediatricians use "postmature" to designate all fetuses and infants where the pregnancy is postterm, some apply it only to the large overgrown fetus or infant, while others designate only the undernourished, chronically distressed, newborn infant as postmature. Clarity of terminology must be established if communications between the obstetrician and neona-

tologist are to be effective and serve the best interests of the fetus–infant!

STANDARDS FOR NORMAL FETAL GROWTH AND DEVELOPMENT

By now the practice of equating fetal size with fetal age, which, unfortunately, had been firmly ingrained in obstetric and pediatric practices, should have been abandoned. For normal pregnancies, there is a strong correlation between the two, but at times the infant who is very small at birth may be chronically and functionally quite mature. This phenomenon is likely to be most dramatic when maternal chronic vascular disease complicates pregnancy. Conversely, the infant of normal term size may be dangerously preterm, as in some pregnancies complicated by diabetes. Not merely for nicety of diagnosis but, importantly, for proper care of the infant, the preterm infant whose size is appropriate for his gestational age should be distinguished from the more mature infant who is growth retarded, i.e., small for his gestational age.

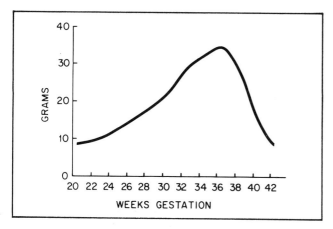

Figure 37-2. Mean daily fetal growth (in g) during previous week of gestation. (*Adapted from Hendricks: Obstet Gynecol 24:357, 1964.*)

Fetal Weights at Various Gestational Ages

It has proven difficult to obtain precise standards for gauging appropriate or inappropriate growth of the human fetus who is remote from term. In order to determine fetal weight directly, obviously the fetus must have been delivered and weighed, but the fetus of known gestational age who is born preterm most often is not the product of a normal pregnancy. For fetuses born preterm, Persson and co-workers (1978) have demonstrated that fetal growth rate, as reflected by the biparietal diameter measured sonographically, typically was somewhat retarded before preterm delivery when compared to that for fetuses who remained in utero to term. The difference increased during the third trimester to reach 3 to 4 mm at 36 weeks. Nonetheless, several investigators are to be congratulated for their laborious efforts to provide needed data, tabulated from birth weights at various gestational ages, even though the data might not be as precise as desired.

There is general agreement that the following factors influence birth weight, at least in term pregnancies:

1. *Sex.* Boys weigh more than girls.
2. *Parity.* Birth weight increases with parity at least through para 2.
3. *Race.* White babies at term weigh more than do black babies.

Ideally, the standardization of birth weight for gestational age would also take into account maternal height and weight, since they also may influence birth weight.

In four different studies in the United States, the mean birth weights identified at 40 weeks gestation were in relatively close agreement for liveborn infants (Brenner and colleagues, 1976; Hoffman and co-workers, 1974; Lubchenco and associates, 1963; Naeye and Dixon, 1978). In these four studies, the mean birth weight at 40 weeks

gestation was 3335 g and ranged from 3280 g to 3400 g. As gestational age decreased, however, the relative differences in mean birth weights increased more markedly, mostly because of the larger weights recorded by Hoffman compared to the other three groups. Fetal weights throughout pregnancy, including the 10th, 25th, 50th, 75th, and 90th percentiles, and correction factors for parity, race, and sex, as determined by Brenner and co-workers (1976), are presented in Figure 37-1. The tabulation provided by Lubchenco and associates appears to be more widely used, although that of Brenner and colleagues may be more appropriate for sea level.

Estimating Gestational Age by Physical Examination

A reasonably precise estimation of gestational age may be quickly performed in the delivery room or nursery by evaluating the infant's development employing the sole creases, size of the breast nodule, scalp hair, earlobe, posture, and for the male infant, testes and scrotum (Fig. 37-3A). A confirmatory neurologic examination can be carried out the day after delivery (Fig. 37-3B).

THE PRETERM INFANT

The problems associated with preterm birth often are deterrents to achievement of the goal that all infants not only will be liveborn and survive but will not suffer physical, intellectual, or emotional impairment as the consequence of a hostile antepartum, intrapartum, or neonatal environment (Pritchard and Whalley, 1974). Any pregnancy in which there is a likelihood that this outcome will not be achieved must be considered high risk.* The great variety of maternal factors that may contribute to preterm birth and to fetal growth retardation are considered throughout this book. Some specific diseases of the newborn infant are discussed in Chapter 38, and birth injuries and malformations are considered in Chapter 39.

Fate of the Preterm Infant

The decrease in the neonatal death rate in the United States from more than 20 per 1000 live births in 1950 to less than 10 per 1000 more recently has been due in large part to the fact that more preterm infants now survive. The availability of remarkably improved neonatal care that in some instances is quite complex has contributed greatly to the reduction in neonatal mortality.

---

* *High-risk pregnancy and fetal distress are two terms commonly used in pregnancy to incite or intensify special concern for the quality of the ultimate product of pregnancy, the newborn infant. Precise definition of fetal distress and of high-risk pregnancy is not simple and will continue to change as the science of perinatology provides new information.*

PATIENT'S NAME _____

▷ **Examination First Hours**

CLINICAL ESTIMATION OF GESTATIONAL AGE
An Approximation Based on Published Data*

PHYSICAL FINDINGS		20	21	22	23	24	25	26	27	28	29	30	31	32	33	34	35	36	37	38	39	40	41	42	43	44	45	46	47	48
		WEEKS GESTATION																												
VERNIX		APPEARS			COVERS BODY, THICK LAYER														ON BACK, SCALP, IN CREASES		SCANT, IN CREASES		NO VERNIX						
BREAST TISSUE AND AREOLA		AREOLA & NIPPLE BARELY VISIBLE NO PALPABLE BREAST TISSUE														AREOLA RAISED		1-2 MM NODULE		3-5 MM	5-6 MM	7-10 MM			7-12 MM			
EAR	FORM	FLAT, SHAPELESS														BEGINNING INCURVING SUPERIOR		INCURVING UPPER 2/3 PINNAE		WELL-DEFINED INCURVING TO LOBE							
	CARTILAGE	PINNA SOFT, STAYS FOLDED														CARTILAGE SCANT RETURNS SLOWLY FROM FOLDING		THIN CARTILAGE SPRINGS BACK FROM FOLDING		PINNA FIRM, REMAINS ERECT FROM HEAD							
SOLE CREASES		SMOOTH SOLES ≥ CREASES														1-2 ANTERIOR CREASES		2-3 ANTERIOR CREASES	CREASES ANTERIOR 2/3 SOLE	CREASES INVOLVING HEEL		DEEPER CREASES OVER ENTIRE SOLE						
SKIN	THICKNESS & APPEARANCE	THIN, TRANSLUCENT SKIN, PLETHORIC, VENULES OVER ABDOMEN EDEMA														SMOOTH THICKER NO EDEMA		PINK		FEW VESSELS	SOME DESQUAMATION PALE PINK	THICK, PALE, DESQUAMATION OVER ENTIRE BODY						
	NAIL PLATES	APPEAR	NAILS TO FINGER TIPS																		NAILS EXTEND WELL BEYOND FINGER TIPS						
HAIR		APPEARS ON HEAD		EYE BROWS & LASHES			FINE, WOOLLY, BUNCHES OUT FROM HEAD								SILKY, SINGLE STRANDS LAYS FLAT				RECEDING HAIRLINE OR LOSS OF BABY HAIR SHORT, FINE UNDERNEATH							
LANUGO		APPEARS	COVERS ENTIRE BODY											VANISHES FROM FACE				PRESENT ON SHOULDERS			NO LANUGO						
GENITALIA	TESTES									TESTES PALPABLE IN INGUINAL CANAL						IN UPPER SCROTUM				IN LOWER SCROTUM							
	SCROTUM									FEW RUGAE						RUGAE, ANTERIOR PORTION		RUGAE COVER		PENDULOUS							
	LABIA & CLITORIS								PROMINENT CLITORIS LABIA MAJORA SMALL WIDELY SEPARATED					LABIA MAJORA LARGER NEARLY COVERED CLITORIS		LABIA MINORA & CLITORIS COVERED										
SKULL FIRMNESS		BONES ARE SOFT							SOFT TO 1" FROM ANTERIOR FONTANELLE					SPONGY AT EDGES OF FONTANELLE CENTER FIRM		BONES HARD SUTURES EASILY DISPLACED		BONES HARD, CANNOT BE DISPLACED							
POSTURE	RESTING	HYPOTONIC LATERAL DECUBITUS				HYPOTONIC			BEGINNING FLEXION THIGH	STRONGER HIP FLEXION	FROG-LIKE	FLEXION ALL LIMBS	HYPERTONIC				VERY HYPERTONIC										
	RECOIL - LEG	NO RECOIL								PARTIAL RECOIL					PROMPT RECOIL												
	ARM	NO RECOIL								BEGIN FLEXION NO RECOIL	PROMPT RECOIL MAY BE INHIBITED		PROMPT RECOIL AFTER 30" INHIBITION														
		20	21	22	23	24	25	26	27	28	29	30	31	32	33	34	35	36	37	38	39	40	41	42	43	44	45	46	47	48

Figure 37-3. A. Clinical estimation of gestational age.

Selection for Neonatal Intensive Care

All hospitals that provide maternity care should ideally possess the facilities and the skilled personnel essential for effective, intensive antepartum, intrapartum, and neonatal care. Lacking a sufficient number of such patients and the financial means for achieving this goal, a system should be developed for identifying high-risk pregnancies and for referral of the mother and her fetus to a regional center. Furthermore, facilities for effecting rapid transport of the newborn infant in need of intensive care to such a center must be made generally available for those hopefully few cases in which delivery occurred before maternal transport could be accomplished.

A rightful concern has arisen from the prediction that, as the survival rate for very young and very small infants improved, there would be a drastic increase in the number of children who would be handicapped in some way. Wright and associates (1972), for example, carefully followed 70 infants who weighed 1500 g or less and compared their courses with normal-sized but otherwise presumably matched controls born between 1952 and 1956 at Chicago Lying-In Hospital. Ten years later, they identified in the study group a remarkable excess of mortality, mental retardation, poor school performance, pyramidal tract disorders, and visual defects. More recent experiences with infants of very low birth weight are much more favorable than those of Wright and associates but are far from ideal.

Survival of the Very Premature Infant

Essentially all neonatal units with adequate facilities and personnel for intensive care of the newborn now are experiencing low neonatal mortality rates for most infants who are born any time during the third trimester (27 or more weeks gestational age) and weigh 1000 g or more but are not malformed. However, as gestational age and birth weight drop below these values, mortality increases

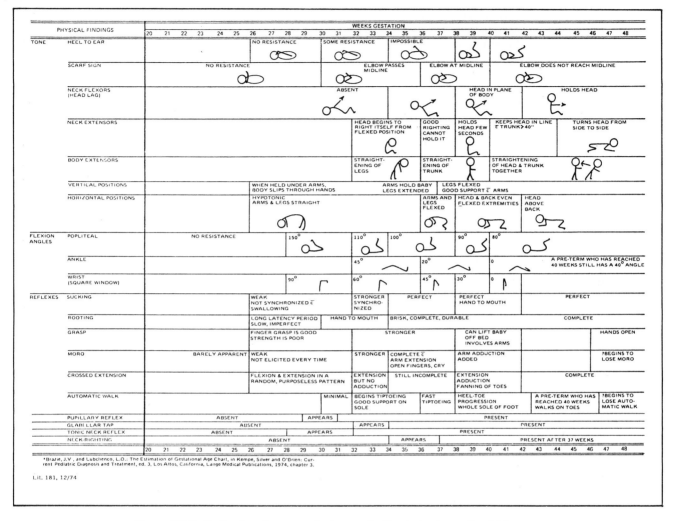

Figure 37-3. B. Confirmatory neurologic examination to be done after 24 hours.

remarkably. For infants as young as 23 weeks gestational age and as small as 600 g, the mortality rate is essentially 100 percent.

Rarely, a quite immature, very, very small infant is born who lives and is acclaimed to be the smallest baby ever to survive. One such infant was reported to weigh 460 g (*Dallas Morning News,* May 30, 1980). Another infant cited in the press weighed 484 g, but his gestational age was stated to be only 22 weeks (5 months). In one instance, the newspaper headline proclaimed appropriately "Thirteen Ounce Baby Beats Big Odds Against Survival." Thus, some infants can survive even though they are so immature that, had they been born without definite signs of life, they typically would have been classified as an abortus!

The fact that some very small infants do survive when provided with prolonged, very expensive intensive care has created serious problems in decision making for the obstetrician who faces the challenge of effecting delivering in such a way as to try to optimize the status of

the fetus–infant at birth in case intensive care is going to be applied, and especially for the neonatologist who must make a judgment as how best to dispense the finite resources for medical care that can be provided by the insurance carrier, the family, government agencies, the hospital, and by himself or herself.

As well as survival, another issue of magnitude is the quality of life that is achieved by immature, very low birth weight infants. It has become apparent that appreciable compromise—physical and intellectual—afflicts too many such children. It is now obvious that three very difficult questions persist regarding care for the very small and immature neonate: "How small is too small?" How handicapped is too handicapped?" "How expensive is too expensive?"

Data such as those provided by Walker and associates (1984) should be considered in answering these questions. They observed that for infants weighing 500 to 599 g, neonatal mortality was 100 percent; for 600 to 699 g, 97 percent; for 700 to 799 g, 76 percent; for 800 to

899 g, 62 percent; and for 900 to 999 g, 40 percent. The average hospital stay ranged from 125 days for the one survivor of 37 infants in the 600 to 699 g birth weight category to 76 days for 39 survivors out of 65 infants in the 900 to 999 g birth weight range. Importantly, among the survivors, the frequency of severe handicaps was 100 percent in the 600 to 699 g birth weight group, 26 percent for the 700 to 799 group, 29 percent for the 800 to 899 g group, and 3 percent for those survivors whose birth weights were 900 to 999 g. They also identified the total costs of hospitalization and comprehensive care expended and calculated the costs per surviving infant. It ranged from $63,442 for survivors in the 900 to 999 g birth weight group to $443,618 for those in the 600 to 699 g weight range.

Even Milligan and co-workers (1984), whose published results have been much better, question the prolonged use of restricted resources at or below 25 weeks gestation. Nonetheless some will argue that the correct answers to these three basic questions are: "The infant is never too small!" "No handicap is too great!" "No expense is too much!" If society decrees these to be the correct answers, more than affirmation is needed; funding must be provided for immediate and, at times, very long-term care!

Interestingly, birth of a very immature infant could have been avoided in many instances by the application of adequate prenatal care—care that was not provided because of lack of funding. The frank statement of Hatwick (1973), made in the course of discussing the economics of obstetric and newborn care, remains true more than a decade later: "While some find the economist's viewpoint repelling, its virtue stems from the fact that it recognizes what none of the other disciplines seem to recognize: Everything has its price! To ignore the cost is to make a decision to use resources in areas which may not be deserving of them." What are the benefits that are likely to be achieved compared to those that would accrue to society from expenditure of the same money in other ways?

PRETERM (PREMATURE) LABOR

Most often, for the reasons presented in Chapter 15 (p. 295) and that follow, it is advantageous to the fetus to remain in utero until term but not unduly long thereafter. At times, however, the fetus is better off being born even though preterm; an example is the severely growth-retarded fetus in a persistently hostile intrauterine environment. Thus, a most important problem in obstetrics and perinatology is how best to identify precisely those circumstances in which the fetus is better off for being born even though he is preterm and may be functionally premature. Conflicting views and recommendations abound at this time, but, appropriately, a great deal of interest currently exists regarding optimal timing of delivery, including the degree of interference that the obstetrician should bring to bear either to prevent or to promote delivery before term.

Causes of Preterm Labor

In the majority of instances, the precise cause or causes of labor before term are not known. Some conditions that predispose to labor before term are listed below:

1. Spontaneous rupture of membranes. Spontaneous labor remote from term commonly is preceded by spontaneous rupture of the membranes. Cause of the rupture is usually unknown. Local infection has been implicated in some cases.
2. Cervical incompetency. No doubt a small percentage of preterm labors and deliveries are the consequence of an incompetent cervix. Remote from term, the incompetent cervix effaces and dilates appreciably, not as the result of increased uterine activity but rather because of an intrinsic weakness in the cervix. Diagnosis and treatment of the incompetent cervix are discussed in Chapter 24, p. 475.
3. Uterine anomalies. Very uncommonly, anomalies of the uterus are identified in cases of preterm labor and delivery. The greater the degree of reduplication of the uterus, for example, the more extensive the septum, and the more complete the separation of the uterus into two distinct horns, the greater the risk of premature labor. Diagnosis and management of this cause of preterm delivery are described in Chapter 25, p. 495.
4. Overdistended uterus. Hydramnios, especially when acute and marked, or the presence of two or more fetuses increases the risk of premature labor, presumably as the consequence of overdistention of the uterus.
5. Anomalies of the products of conception. Malformations of the fetus or of the placenta not only predispose to fetal growth retardation but increase the likelihood of preterm labor as well.
6. Faulty placentation. Abruptio placentae and placentae previa are likely to be associated with preterm labor.
7. Retained intrauterine device. The likelihood of preterm labor is appreciably increased when an intrauterine device persists in a pregnant uterus (Chapter 40, p. 822).
8. Fetal death. Death of the fetus remote from term commonly but not always is followed by spontaneous labor before term is reached.
9. Previous preterm delivery or late abortion. The woman who previously gave birth to a fetus remote from term is more likely to do so again even when no other predisposing factor is identified.

10. Serious maternal disease. Systemic disease in the mother, when it is severe, may cause premature labor and delivery. Serious hypoxia is a feature of some diseases, for example, pneumonia, while high fever characterizes some others, for example, acute pyelonephritis. Neither acute pyelonephritis without marked fever nor asymptomatic bacteriuria has been commonly associated with premature delivery in our experience. Generalized peritonitis is likely to induce labor.
11. Elective induction of labor. Incorrect estimation of gestational age can create undue concern in the mind of the obstetrician over possible adverse effects on the fetus from presumed prolonged gestation, or it leads to considerable pressure from the mother-to-be or her family to intervene. However, induction of labor in some instances has been performed primarily for the convenience of the physician and a preterm infant delivered because of an erroneous estimation of gestational age. The use of oxytocin for *elective* induction of labor has been specifically disapproved by the Food and Drug Administration.
12. Unknown cause. Unfortunately, too many cases have to be so categorized.

Diagnosis of Preterm Labor

Early differentiation between true and false labor is often difficult before the time that the uterus has contracted sufficiently to produce demonstrable effacement and dilatation of the cervix. Unfortunately, by this time, attempts to arrest labor may prove to be ineffective. Successful treatment with available agents so far appears to require early implementation. One result has been the inclusion of a number of cases of false labor that needed no treatment. In turn, the consequence has been confusion and imprecision as to the degree of effectiveness of most of the treatment regimens that have been proposed.

The following features are generally used to identify preterm labor: Uterine contractions are occurring at least once every 10 minutes and last for 30 seconds or more. If labor is soon obvious, treatment may be initiated. If not, uterine function is evaluated further by means of external tocography to record the frequency and duration of contractions. Progressive dilatation of the cervix is, of course, indicative of labor.

Arrest of Preterm Labor

Before an attempt is made to arrest labor, the question must be asked and correctly answered, "Is further intrauterine stay more likely to benefit or harm the fetus?" In the past, the answer has been no more than academic, but highly effective agents for inhibiting labor most

likely will sometime become generally available. Many neonatal deaths continue to be the direct consequence of marked prematurity, and the number of such deaths would undoubtedly be reduced by delaying delivery. Not all fetuses, however, would benefit from further intrauterine stay. This is borne out by an annual stillbirth rate in the United States that now exceeds the neonatal death rate. Some of these stillborn fetuses would have lived if only the fetus had been delivered earlier. For example, retarded fetal growth is confused with prematurity, and the malnourished fetus, to his detriment, is left in a hostile intrauterine environment rather than a more favorable one provided by the nursery. Thus, the problem as to what is best for the fetus—not alone the mother—is not so simple that the obstetrician can automatically attempt to delay delivery in all cases of presumably preterm labor. *The decision is made much easier if the gestational age is precisely known.*

It is not surprising that great interest persists regarding effective treatment regimens for arresting spontaneous labor that develops long before term. Extensive review of pharmacologic attempts to arrest preterm labor was provided by Barden (1977).

Treatment Regimens for Preterm Labor

A number of treatment regimens that have been employed to try to arrest preterm labor are considered below.

Bed Rest. The treatment regimen that has been used most often is simply bed rest, with the mother lying more comfortably on her side. In the relatively few controlled studies of the effect of various treatment modalities, the control group was placed at bed rest and, at times, given a placebo. Satisfactory results in the prevention or arrest of preterm labor may be so obtained. The success is attributable to bed rest and perhaps, in part, to the reassurance of the mother that she is being treated.

Progestational Agents. Historically, with the recognition that parenterally administered progesterone would prolong pregnancy in rabbits, progesterone and subsequently synthetic progestational agents were employed to try to inhibit preterm labor. Most of the evidence to date is not very convincing that such agents are clinically effective, although Johnson and colleagues (1979) reported preterm labor and low birth weight to have occurred less often in mothers who received weekly injections of 17α-hydroxyprogesterone caproate (Delalutin) prophylactically throughout pregnancy. Confirmation of its effectiveness is needed.

Ethanol. The use of intravenously administered ethanol to try to arrest preterm labor became popular following the favorable report by Fuchs and co-workers (1967). Initially, ethanol was thought to block the release of oxytocin from the neurohypophysis. There is now question as to the role, if any, of endogenous oxytocin in human labor (Chapter 15, p. 295). Ethanol may have a direct depressant action on the myometrium. It has become clear that ethanol causes deleterious metabolic derangements, as well as making the fetus–infant and mother drunk. Hopefully, its use has been abandoned.

Magnesium Sulfate.

It has long been recognized that ionic magnesium in a sufficiently high concentration can alter myometrial contractility in vivo as well as in vitro. The role of magnesium presumably is that of an antagonist of calcium.

Steer and Petrie (1977) concluded that intravenously administered magnesium sulfate, 4 g given as a loading dose followed by a continuous infusion of 2 g per hour, will usually arrest labor. The design of their study, however, was far from ideal, and thus the validity of the conclusions that were drawn based on those data are suspect.

Subsequent studies have been reported, some favorable and some not so favorable. Elliott (1983), in a retrospective study, found tocolysis with magnesium sulfate to be "successful, inexpensive, and relatively nontoxic." He reported 87 percent success when the cervix was dilated 2 cm or less and the period of arrest was as short as 48 hours. Spisso and co-workers (1982) were favorably impressed by the efficacy of magnesium sulfate when given intravenously in relatively large dosage to women with intact membranes who had "not begun the active phase of labor." They emphasized that "Treatment during early latent phase labor is the key to successful therapy." (This statement is true undoubtedly for all currently used tocolytic agents.) Miller and associates (1982) compared magnesium sulfate and terbutaline, a β-adrenergic agonist that is considered further subsequently, and on the basis of their small study, reported them to be equally effective for controlling premature labor. They identified less adverse effects from the use of magnesium sulfate. Semchyshyn and associates (1983) failed to stop labor in a woman who was given inadvertently 17.3 g of magnesium sulfate in 45 minutes!

Cotton and associates (1984) compared magnesium sulfate to ritodrine, as well as a placebo. They identified little difference in outcome and therefore concluded, "The fact that delivery occurred in less than 48 hours in nearly one-half of patients under the best of circumstances emphasizes the need for more effective technics for the inhibition of preterm labor."

In any event, the mother must be monitored very closely for evidence of hypermagnesemia that might prove toxic to her and to her fetus–infant, since magnesium promptly crosses the placenta to produce concentrations in fetal plasma comparable to those in the mother. If magnesium intoxication is to be avoided, the patellar reflex should persist and certainly respirations should not be depressed. The pharmacology and toxicology of parenterally administered magnesium are considered in more detail in Chapter 27 (p. 551).

β-Adrenergic Receptor Stimulants.

Earlier in this century, epinephrine in low doses was demonstrated to exert a depressant effect on the myometrium of the pregnant uterus. This observation led to epinephrine's being considered an agent worthy of trial in the emergency treatment of the tetanically contracted uterus. However, its tocolytic effects proved to be rather weak, quite transient, and likely to be accompanied by troublesome cardiovascular effects. Moreover, in larger doses, epinephrine may even enhance myometrial contractility.

In more recent years, a number of compounds capable of reacting predominantly with β-adrenergic receptors have been investigated. Some of these are now used extensively in the practice of obstetrics in other countries. Only one, ritodrine, has been approved so far by the Food and Drug Administration for use in the treatment of preterm labor.

The adrenergic receptors are located on the outer surface of the cell membrane, where a specific agonist can couple with them. Adenylcyclase in the cell membrane of the smooth muscle cell is activated by the coupling of an agonist to the receptor. Adenylcyclase enhances the conversion of adenosine triphosphate to cyclic AMP, which, in turn, initiates a number of reactions that reduce the intracellular concentration of ionized calcium and thereby prevent activation of the contractile proteins, as described in Chapter 15 (p. 305).

There are two classes of β-adrenergic receptors, and these are commonly referred to as β_1 and β_2 adrenergic receptors. The β_1 receptors are dominant in the heart and intestines, while β_2 receptors are dominant in the myometrium, blood vessels, and bronchioles.

A number of compounds generally similar in structure to epinephrine have been evaluated in the search for an ideal one that would provide optimal stimulation of β_2-adrenergic receptors on myometrial cells and thus inhibit uterine contractions but, at the same time, cause little or no adverse effects from stimulation of adrenergic receptors elsewhere. So far no compound has exhibited these utopian properties. Compounds that have been or are being employed to try to arrest labor include the following.

Isoxuprine was one of the first compounds to be extensively evaluated for tocolytic action. It does not appear to be remarkably effective, at least in doses that do not produce potentially dangerous side effects, especially marked tachycardia and hypotension.

Ritodrine has been widely used in recent years. In a multicenter study in the United States, infants whose mothers were considered to be in labor preterm had a lower mortality rate, developed respiratory distress less often, and achieved a gestational age of 36 weeks or a birth weight of 2500 g more often than did infants whose mothers were not so treated (Merkatz and colleagues, 1980). Hesseldahl (1979), however, in a multicenter controlled study in Denmark, did not find any of several ritodrine treatment regimens tested to be more efficacious than "standard treatment," which consisted of bed rest and glucose infusion plus placebo tablets. Hesseldahl, perplexed by the discrepancy between his findings and those reported by some others earlier, did point out that possibly more women who received ritodrine in the Danish study were more predisposed to continue in labor than were those in the "standard treatment" group.

The infusion of ritodrine, and the other β-adrenergic agonists cited now, has resulted in frequent and, at times, serious side effects. In the mother, tachycardia, hypotension, apprehension, chest tightness or actual pain, electrocardiographic S-T segment depression, pulmonary edema, and death have been observed. Maternal metabolic effects include hyperglycemia, hyperinsulinemia (unless diabetic), hypokalemia, and lactic- and keto-acidosis. Perhaps less serious, but, nonetheless, troublesome side effects include emesis, headaches, tremulousness, fever, and hallucinations. The same derangements undoubtedly occur in the fetus. After birth, hypoglycemia, which may become profound, is frequent. If these drugs are used and labor persists, they should be stopped so as to minimize these deleterious effects in the fetus before birth.

A single mechanism has not been identified to explain the development of pulmonary edema. Increased cardiac demands imposed by pregnancy, especially with multiple fetuses, can contribute, as can preexisting cardiac impairment. The fluid load that has been provided to try to help stop labor through hydration can increase pulmonary capillary wedge pressures and thus be a factor in the genesis of pulmonary edema. The simultaneous administration of potent glucocorticoids to try to hasten lung maturation may also contribute, although pulmonary edema has developed in their absence. Caritis and associates (1983) have reported on the pharmacodynamics of ritodrine in women during preterm labor.

Terbutaline has been claimed by some, but certainly not all, to inhibit myometrial contractions effectively even when cervical dilatation is far advanced. Toxicity, especially maternal pulmonary edema, has been evident with its use, as it has with ritodrine.

Salbutamol has been acclaimed by some, similar to terbutaline, to be a very effective agent for arresting labor (Korda and associates, 1974; Liggins and Vaughn, 1973; Rydén, 1977). However, Sims and co-workers (1978) and Reynolds (1978) found salbutamol to be no more effective than ethanol in arresting preterm labor.

Fenoterol structurally is very similar to ritodrine. It is not clear whether fenoterol is any more or less effective or causes more or less adverse reactions than do the other β-mimetic agents currently being used in several countries. Epstein and associates (1979) documented sustained hypoglycemia accompanied by elevated insulin levels in most infants who were delivered within 2 days after the termination of administration of fenoterol to the mother to try to arrest labor. As mentioned above, similar response has been documented for ritodrine and other β-adrenergic agonists.

The use of fenoterol has been extremely popular in West Germany. Kubli (1977) commented that at least 1 million ampules and 6 million tablets of fenoterol have been used annually for a birth rate of about 6 million, yet no evidence has been presented that the use of so much of the compound has been accompanied by any remarkable decrease in the numbers of infants of low birth weight.

Combined Therapy. To try to reduce the adverse effects of ritodrine while effectively arresting premature labor, Ferguson and co-workers (1984) evaluated the response to magnesium sulfate and ritodrine administered together. They were forced to abandon the study because of the frequency and intensity of the maternal side effects that resulted from the use of this combination. Respiratory distress was troublesome, and both symptoms and EKG evidence of myocardial ischemia were common.

Antiprostaglandins. Such agents have been the subject of considerable interest once it was appreciated that prostaglandins are intimately involved in the myometrial contractions that characterize labor (Chapter 15, p. 296). Antiprostaglandin agents may act by inhibiting the synthesis of prostaglandins or by blocking the action of prostaglandins on target organs.

A group of enzymes, collectively called prostaglandin synthetase, are responsible for the conversion of free arachidonic acid to prostaglandin. Several drugs are known to block the prostaglandin synthetase system, including aspirin and other salicylates, indomethacin, naproxen, and meclofenamic acid. Zuckerman and co-workers (1974) and others since 1974 have administered indomethacin to try to inhibit preterm labor and, in general, observed a favorable response.

Extensive investigation in humans of the prostaglandin synthetase inhibitors to try to inhibit labor preterm has been discouraged following recognition that such agents may adversely affect the fetus by inducing major cardiovascular changes, including premature closure of the ductus arteriosus.

Narcotics and Sedatives. Fear of arresting desirable labor by too early administration of narcotics, such as meperidine and morphine, and by sedatives, such as secobarbital and pentobarbital, has long permeated the arena of clinical obstetrics. The evidence is weak, at best, that the fear is justified (Chapter 18, p. 354). Certainly, there is no good evidence that they are very effective in arresting preterm labor. There is good evidence, however, that narcotics and sedatives may dangerously depress the preterm infant when administered to the mother near the time of delivery. Moreover, if they were employed in conjunction with ethanol, maternal depression was likely to be profound. In fact, aspiration pneumonitis, with the death of both mother and fetus, has occurred in this circumstance.

Diazoxide. This very potent antihypertensive agent can also inhibit contractions of the pregnant uterus. Side effects from diazoxide administration include maternal hypotension, tachycardia, increased cardiac output, hyperglycemia, hyperuricemia, and the retention of water, sodium, potassium, chloride, and bicarbonate. It appears likely that these multiple detrimental side effects will outweigh any favorable effect on labor. The drug is not approved for the treatment of threatened preterm labor.

Summary. The benefits to be derived from the use of these various agents that have been employed to try to arrest preterm labor do not appear to be profound. The same cannot be said for complications from their use.

If β-adrenergic agonists are to be used, certain precautions must be taken to avoid misuse. The woman considered to be in premature labor must be carefully evaluated for pregnancy complications that may not be readily apparent but, nonetheless, are ominous. Once it is decided that she is not experiencing uterine contractions as a consequence of or in association with a disease process potentially dangerous to her, to her fetus if left in utero, or to both (examples being placental abruption or intrauterine sepsis), the possibility of underlying maternal disease that would contraindicate their use must be considered. These include any form of heart disease, diabetes, pregnancy-induced or aggravated hypertension, hyperthyroidism, and severe anemias. The status of the fetus must also be considered. Unless the intrauterine environment is normal, he or she may be better off out. This is certainly true for the overtly growth-retarded fetus or when there is intrauterine infection. Finally, if the fetus has achieved reasonable maturity, delivery is more advantageous than are attempts at pharmacologic intervention. At Parkland Memorial Hospital the dividing line of 33 completed weeks of gestational age has proved satisfactory.

RUPTURE OF MEMBRANES BEFORE TERM

Rupture of the membranes remote from term is better referred to as *preterm rupture of the membranes* rather than *premature rupture of the membranes*. "Premature rupture of the membranes" has been applied most commonly to rupture of the membranes at any time before the onset of labor irrespective of whether the duration of gestation at the time of rupture was 24 weeks or 44 weeks.

Rupture of the membranes long before term is an important cause of perinatal morbidity and mortality and of maternal morbidity and even mortality. Most often, the rupture occurs spontaneously and for reasons unknown. At times, unfortunately, the cause is iatrogenic, as the consequence of an ill-timed attempt to induce labor. Techniques for identification of rupture of the membranes are discussed elsewhere (Chapter 17, p. 332).

There is far from unanimity of thought concerning optimal management of pregnancies complicated by rup-

ture of the membranes remote from term. In the majority of cases, labor followed by delivery will ensue within a few days, even when nonintervention is practiced (Wilson and associates, 1982) or tocolysis is attempted. Even so, it appears that for maternity services where the puerperal febrile morbidity rate is low, continued observation without vaginal manipulation may prove to be of greater benefit to the preterm fetus than would steps to effect delivery. *Conversely, in those institutions in which puerperal febrile morbidity is common, the fetus, and the mother as well, may benefit from delivery within 24 hours.* The experiences at Parkland Memorial Hospital provide some verification of the latter attitude. The reason or reasons why infection of the fetus and mother following prolonged rupture of the membranes is so common in many public institutions caring for socioeconomically less affluent women is not clear.

At Parkland Memorial Hospital, pregnancy complicated by rupture of the membranes remote from term has for some time been managed as follows:

1. Perform one sterile speculum examination to identify fluid coming from the cervix or pooled in the vagina. Demonstration of visible fluid or a positive nitrazine test is indicative of ruptures of the membranes. The one sterile examination is concluded with the identification of the extent of cervical effacement and dilatation, confirmation of the presenting part, and exclusion of a prolapsed cord.
2. If the gestational age is 33 completed weeks or less and there are no other maternal or fetal indications for delivery, the pregnancy is allowed to continue without prophylactic antibiotics under very close observation for signs of sepsis.
3. If the gestational age is greater than 33 completed weeks and if labor has not begun spontaneously in 12 hours—a time period that provides for adequate evaluation—it is carefully induced with an intravenous infusion of dilute oxytocin, avoiding hyperstimulation. Breech presentation or transverse lie contraindicates induction. If induction fails, cesarean section is performed. At this and many other institutions, neonatal mortality is now very low for infants born after 33 weeks gestation.
4. Labor and delivery are managed so as to minimize maternal hypotension and fetal hypoxia and acidosis, as well as infection, since these events are known to increase the likelihood of fatal respiratory distress. Unfortunately, simple, expectant management of rupture of the membranes remote from term by no means abolishes perinatal morbidity and mortality (Hankins and associates, 1984).

It has become common practice to give antibiotics prophylactically to the newborn infant born after prolonged (usually 24 hours) rupture of the membranes. If, in the experience of the institution, neonatal infection has proved to be common, antibiotic therapy may well be indicated. At the time of delivery in such circumstances a culture should probably be made of amnionic fluid, gastric aspirate, or a swabbing from the ear of the infant. Not all pediatricians agree on the advantages or the safety of antibiotic prophylaxis.

Accelerated Maturation of Pulmonary Function

The infant who is born long before term is a candidate for the development of severe idiopathic respiratory distress syndrome (Chapter 38, p. 769). The intense hypoxia and acidosis that ensue as the consequence of inadequate alveolar–capillary exchange of oxygen and carbon dioxide may prove fatal. Moreover, some infants who survive severe respiratory distress may suffer lifelong physical or functional impairment (Chapter 38). Since a major factor in the development of the respiratory distress syndrome is inappropriate production of pulmonary surfactant, intense interest persists concerning those phenomena involved in surfactant production (Chapter 8, p. 155).

A variety of clinical events, some well defined and others that are not, predispose to accelerated maturation of surfactant production sufficient to protect against the development of respiratory distress. Gluck (1979) emphasized that surfactant production is likely to be accelerated in pregnancies remote from term complicated by the following conditions:

1. *Maternal:* Chronic renal or cardiovascular disease, long-standing pregnancy-induced hypertension, sickle cell disease, heroin addiction, or hyperthyroidism
2. *Placenta and membranes:* Placental infarction, chronic focal retroplacental hemorrhage, chorioamnionitis, or rupture of membranes
3. *Fetal:* The anemic member of parabiotic twins or the smaller member of nonparabiotic twins

Rupture of the Membranes. Of those conditions listed above, rupture of the membranes remote from term is of exceptional importance. This is true not only because of its frequency but also because of the possibility that delay in delivery may soon be followed by lung maturation, either spontaneous or pharmacologically induced, that would more than offset the risk of infection imposed by delay in delivery. In some reports, but not all, a remarkable decrease in the incidence of respiratory distress has been claimed for the grossly preterm infant who was delivered more than 24 hours after gross rupture of the membranes. Yoon and Harper (1973), for example, in a retrospective study of infants whose birth weights were 1000 g to 2165 g, noted a frequency of respiratory distress of only 3.2 percent if membranes were ruptured more than 24 hours before delivery compared to 21.3 percent if ruptured less than 12 hours, and there are reports by some other investigators that would appear to confirm their observations. However, other reports have provided, at most, only partial confirmation, while more reports have failed to provide any confirmation whatsoever. Interestingly, removal of most of the amnionic fluid does not appear to accelerate pulmonary maturation in the fetal lamb.

Glucocorticoid Therapy. The observations by Liggins and Howie of the effects of glucocorticoids on lung maturation have rightfully received considerable attention (Howie and Liggins, 1977; Liggins and Howie, 1974). On the basis of their previous observations that corticosteroids administered to the ewe accelerated lung maturation in her preterm fetus, they initiated a well-designed study to evaluate the effects of maternally administered betamethasone acetate and phosphate on the prevention of respiratory distress in the subsequently delivered preterm newborn infant. A mixture of 6 mg of each compound was injected intramuscularly at the outset and again 24 hours later. To try to delay birth, ethanol was administered very early in the study, but later salbutamol was used and was considered to be superior. Their results for infants born before 34 weeks of pregnancy demonstrated a significant lowering of the incidence of respiratory distress and of neonatal mortality from hyaline membrane disease if birth was delayed for at least 24 hours and up to 7 days after completion of steroid therapy. Numerous other investigators have made similar observations.

The mechanism by which betamethasone or other corticosteroids reduces the frequency of respiratory distress is not clear. Interestingly, the protective action is likely to be transient. Liggins and Howie (1974) noted that the frequency of respiratory distress increased when the infant was born more than 7 days after treatment with betamethasone compared to that for infants delivered 1 to 7 days after completion of therapy. Moreover, Brown and associates (1979) observed in chronically catheterized fetal lambs that the increase in surfactant that followed dexamethasone administration was transient, with surfactant levels falling to pretreatment values within 8 to 10 days. Therefore, if such compounds are used, retreatment must be considered whenever delivery has not occurred within 7 days of the initial treatment and the risk of early delivery persists.

In contrast to the generally favorable reports just cited, Quirk and co-workers (1979) in a retrospective analysis of 3 years' experiences at Columbia-Presbyterian Medical Center identified no difference in fetal outcomes with and without the use of betamethasone. Of 84 markedly preterm infants whose mothers received betamethasone, 16.4 percent developed the respiratory distress syndrome compared to 14.1 percent of 84 infants whose mothers did not receive the steroid. Seventy-four (88 percent) of the treated group survived compared to 73 (87 percent) of the control group. They attributed the low incidence of respiratory distress in the control population to the avoidance of both compromised labor and traumatic delivery. Most recently, Simpson and Harbert (1984) have similarly reported no difference in respiratory distress with and without the use of glucocorticoids.

The decision whether or not to use potent glucocorticoids to try to minimize the risk of severe respiratory distress in the infant born remote from term is a difficult one. Evidence seems to point to some reduction in the frequency of this serious pulmonary disorder but not to its complete eradication. At the same time, there are risks, immediate and remote, from the use of agents as potent as betamethasone. From the standpoint of the mother, the metabolic derangements that characterize diabetes are likely to be intensified, severe pregnancy-induced hypertension may be worsened, the risk of infection is increased, and wound healing may be impaired, especially so in case of transabdominal delivery. Moreover, the combination of a glucocorticoid to hasten lung maturation and a tocolytic agent to try to delay delivery may incite pulmonary edema. Pulmonary edema has developed during the course of therapy with betamethasone or dexamethasone plus the β-adrenergic stimulators terbutaline or ritodrine, the prostaglandin synthetase inhibitor indomethacin, and magnesium sulfate (Elliott and collegues, 1979; Rogge and co-workers, 1979; Stubblefield, 1978; Tinga and Aarnoudse, 1979).

From the standpoint of the fetus–infant as well as the potential for deterioration in utero as a consequence of the maternal complications just described, there is also increased immediate risk of sepsis from the use of the steroid and delayed delivery. Taeusch and associates (1979) identified serious infection in 13 percent of liveborn infants whose mothers had ruptured membranes and had received dexamethasone; 27 percent of the mothers became infected. By way of comparison, 6 percent of the infants were infected whose mothers had ruptured membranes but did not receive dexamethasone and 12 percent of the mothers became infected. While neonatal deaths due to respiratory distress were decreased in the steroid-treated group compared to the control group, the overall neonatal mortality in both groups was the same because of the increased number of deaths due to sepsis in the steroid-treated group.

The long-term risks to the surviving infant from glucocorticoids so used are not yet known. The adverse effects to experimental animals that have been described following the administration of such steroids around the time of birth are discouraging. For example, in pregnant rats, following betamethasone administration, the fetal death rate was increased, and among survivors growth was impaired so that total body weight and weights of the brain, heart, liver, kidneys, and adrenals were reduced (Mosier and colleagues, 1979). In the rhesus monkey fetus, reduced fetal head circumference has been described (Johnson and co-workers, 1979). However, Liggins (1976, 1982) found no gross difference with regard to intelligence quotient and social adjustment among children at 4 years of age whose mothers had received betamethasone according to the protocol described, and in the preliminary observations made by Brown and associates (1979), no delay in development

was found following antenatal treatment with dexamethasone beyond that seen in infants not so exposed.

At Parkland Memorial Hospital glucocorticoids have not been employed remote from term to try to reduce the risk of respiratory distress for the following reasons:

1. Glucocorticoids have not been approved by the Food and Drug Administration for such use.
2. The long-term effects on the child exposed in utero are not yet known.
3. The incidence of maternal vascular disease at Parkland Memorial Hospital is high.
4. At this institution the likelihood of infection after rupture of the membranes is considerable, while fetal respiratory distress syndrome is uncommon.
5. Mortality from respiratory distress among infants born remote from term is not sufficiently great to warrant the administration of glucocorticoids and attempt to delay delivery for 48 hours or more. During a recent 1-year period, of 85 infants who were delivered at 27 through 32 weeks gestational age, 88 percent survived, as did all of the 85 infants who were 33 or 34 weeks gestational age at birth.

Opinion as to the efficacy of glucocorticoid prophylaxis remains sharply divided in major perinatal centers. However, if there has been a recent trend, it probably has been toward not using them.

MANAGEMENT OF PRETERM LABOR AND DELIVERY

In general, the more immature the fetus, the greater the risks from labor and delivery. This is now well established for breech delivery, which is a common presentation for the preterm fetus (Chapter 30, p. 652), and undoubtedly is true to a degree for all immature fetuses regardless of presentation.

In case of contemplated vaginal delivery, labor, if induced, must not be unduly forceful (Chapter 29, p. 644). Abnormalities of fetal heart rate and uterine contractions should be looked for preferably by continuous electronic monitoring. If the fetal heart is not monitored continuously, it must be evaluated at very close intervals by adequately trained attendants. Tachycardia, especially in the presence of ruptured membranes, is suggestive of sepsis, while periodic decelerations imply cord compression, which is rather common with premature rupture of the membranes and loss of amnionic fluid, or, if late decelerations, placental insufficiency. In either case, if a real attempt is going to be made to salvage the fetus, prompt cesarean section is advisable. It is imperative that the uterine incision be large enough to allow for a nontraumatic exit of the fetus–infant.

Even though fetopelvic disproportion is not a problem, except when there is a transverse lie, the resistance of the cervix and of the lower genital tract to dilatation by the presenting part of the fetus may be formidable, especially if the cervix is long, firm, and little dilated and the mother is nulliparous.

In the absence of a relaxed vaginal outlet, a liberal episiotomy for delivery is advantageous once the fetal head reaches the perineum. Argument persists as to the merits of spontaneous delivery versus forceps delivery to protect the more fragile preterm fetal head. It is doubtful whether use of forceps in most instances produces less trauma. Indeed, to compress and pull on the head of a grossly premature infant is more likely to be traumatic than for him to be pushed out by force applied to the buttocks. The use of outlet forceps of appropriate size may be of aid when conduction anesthesia is used and voluntary expulsive efforts are obtunded. Forceps should not be employed to pull the fetus through a vagina that is resistant to dilatation or over a firm perineum.

At times, conduction anesthesia may be precluded by the maternal disease that led to premature delivery, for example, severe maternal hypertension, hemorrhage, or cyanotic heart disease. For the mother whose discomfort is too unpleasant, a mixture of nitrous oxide, 50 percent, and oxygen, administered during contractions, is likely to provide appreciable analgesia without depressing the fetus. The addition of pudendal or local nerve block provides for delivery (Chapter 18, p. 360).

Importantly, just as the markedly preterm infant is to be afforded special care in the neonatal intensive care unit, the mother and fetus should be very closely observed in the labor and delivery unit. Furthermore, just as especially skilled physicians care for the markedly preterm infant after birth, especially skilled physicians should monitor the labor and personally effect the delivery of the markedly preterm fetus.

A physician proficient in resuscitative techniques who has been fully oriented to the specific problems of the case should be present at delivery. The principles of resuscitation described in Chapter 20 are applicable, including prompt endotracheal intubation and ventilation.

THE GROWTH-RETARDED FETUS

Definition

Generally, a newborn infant is classified as *growth retarded,* or *small for gestational age,* if his birth weight falls below the 10th percentile for his gestational age. Mortality and severe morbidity are not greatly increased among fetuses and infants with lesser degrees of growth retardation and without serious malformations. For any gestational age, however, as weight decreases below the 10th percentile, the risk of fetal death increases remarkably.

Causes of Fetal Growth Retardation

The following conditions predispose to impairment of fetal size:

1. Small mother. For genetic reasons, small women typically have small babies. All that can and need be done to avoid potentially dangerous degrees of growth retardation is to take steps to minimize growth retardation from the other causes listed below. In the case of a small woman, the birth of an infant whose genetically determined weight is somewhat below the average for the whole population is not necessarily an undesirable event. If a fetus were appreciably larger, he or she could experience difficulty in negotiating the typically small pelvis of the small mother.

2. Poor maternal weight gain. When the mother is of average size or smaller, lack of weight gain throughout pregnancy or arrested weight gain during the latter half of pregnancy is more likely to result in a growth-retarded infant. If the mother is large and otherwise healthy, however, below average maternal weight gain in the absence of maternal disease is unlikely to be associated with appreciable fetal growth retardation. Even so, marked restriction of weight gain during pregnancy should not be attempted (Chapter 13, p. 250). In general, calories have to be restricted to less than 1500 per day for some time to cause appreciable growth retardation.

3. Vascular disease. Chronic vascular disease, especially when further complicated by superimposed preeclampsia and proteinuria, commonly causes growth retardation. Pregnancy-induced hypertension occurring late in pregnancy without underlying chronic vascular or renal disease is unlikely to be accompanied by marked fetal growth retardation.

4. Chronic renal disease. Chronic renal disease with appreciably reduced renal clearance is commonly accompanied by retarded fetal growth.

5. Chronic hypoxia. Fetuses of women who reside at high altitude are much more likely to weigh less than those of women who live at a lower altitude. The same is true for fetuses of women with cyanotic heart disease or pulmonary insufficiency.

6. Maternal anemia. A low maternal hemoglobin concentration has been implicated in the genesis of fetal growth retardation. In our experience, however, growth retardation has been common only in the fetuses of women with sickle cell disease or with anemia associated with serious maternal disease.

7. Smoking. Tobacco smoking impairs fetal growth; the more cigarettes smoked, the greater the impairment.

8. Hard drugs. The use of heroin, and almost certainly other hard drugs, during pregnancy impairs fetal growth.

9. Alcoholism. The chronic consumption of appreciable amounts of alcohol by the mother during pregnancy results in growth retardation of the

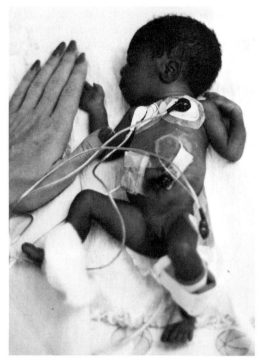

A

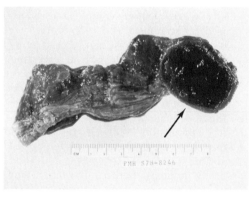

B

Figure 37-4. A. The infant weighed but 650 g when delivered at 29 to 30 weeks gestation. The mother had become severely hypertensive. At delivery by cesarean section there was a subchorial hematoma of many days duration in the placenta (shown in Fig. 37-6B), and the scant amnionic fluid was thick and green. The L/S ratio was 0.64. The infant thrived with no evidence of respiratory distress. **B.** Cross-sectional view of the subchorial hematoma (*arrow*) contained in the placenta of the severely growth-retarded, preterm infant illustrated in Figure 37-4A.

fetus, often accompanied by physical malformation and subsequent intellectual impairment.

10. Abnormalities of placenta and cord. Placental lesions, including chronic focal placental abruption, extensive infarction, or chorioangioma, are likely to cause retarded fetal growth that may be severe (Fig. 37-4A, B). A circumvallate pla-

centa or a placenta previa may impair growth, but usually the fetus is not markedly smaller than normal. Marginal insertion of the umbilical cord and especially velamentous insertion of the cord are more likely to be accompanied by a fetus who is growth retarded.

11. Multiple fetuses. The presence of two or more fetuses is likely to eventuate in appreciable growth retardation of one or both when compared to the normal singleton fetus (Chapter 26, p. 514).

12. Previous birth of a growth-retarded infant. Fetal growth retardation is likely to be repetitive even when no cause is identified. Moreover, the likelihood of fetal growth retardation is somewhat increased among women whose sisters have had a growth-retarded infant.

13. Fetal infections. Cytomegalic inclusion disease, rubella, and probably other chronic infections of the fetus can cause appreciable growth retardation.

14. Fetal malformations. In general, the more severe the malformation, the more likely the fetus is to be small for gestational age. This is especially evident in fetuses with chromosomal abnormalities or with serious cardiovascular malformations.

15. Prolonged pregnancy. The longer pregnancy endures beyond term, the greater the likelihood of the fetus appearing undernourished and chronically distressed. During this time the fetus may not only fail to gain weight but may actually lose weight. Even so, the majority of fetuses probably continue to gain weight.

16. Extrauterine pregnancy. Commonly the fetus who is not housed in the uterus is growth retarded.

Some other factors have been suggested to be important causes of fetal growth retardation although the evidence of a relationship has not necessarily been strong. For example, reduced maternal blood volume has been implicated in fetal growth retardation. The question remains: "Is the fetus growth retarded as the direct and sole consequence of maternal relative hypovolemia, or is the retardation of fetal growth and the retardation of normal pregnancy hypervolemia the consequence of the same basic defect, for example, faulty vascularization of the placental bed?"

As this is being written we are caring for a pregnancy in which maternal blood volume is remarkably less than normal as a consequence of severe megaloblastic anemia, yet the fetus is not growth retarded. Similar observations have been made in this situation, as well as in several cases of eclampsia.

It has also been reported by some that a high maternal hemoglobin concentration is associated with low birth weight, and thus steps ought to be taken to provide for a lower maternal hemoglobin level. Again, failure of the maternal blood volume to expand normally would be reflected in persistence of the normally higher nonpregnant hemoglobin concentration. A low blood volume, in turn, very likely would reflect failure of maternal adaptation, which would simultaneously compromise the fetus.

Diagnosis of Fetal Growth Retardation

Identification through careful history taking of any of the factors listed above that predispose to retarded fetal growth should alert the obstetrician to the possibility of growth retardation in the current pregnancy. Moreover, careful estimation of gestational age and consistently careful evaluation of uterine size during the course of prenatal visits should serve to identify most instances of fetal growth retardation.

Uterine Fundal Height. Belizán and co-workers (1978) correctly identified 86 percent of fetuses whose birth weights fell below the 10th percentile while erroneously suspecting this degree of growth retardation in only 5 percent of pregnancies. Campbell (1983) reported that 85 percent of severely growth-regarded fetuses at 34 weeks gestation were detected by lag in fundal height, compared to 84 percent detected by sonography. Therefore, an appreciation of those circumstances in which fetal growth retardation is more likely to occur, coupled with meticulous clinical mensuration of fundal height and reinforced by sonography, should serve to identify essentially all pregnancies in which a singleton fetus is demonstrating growth retardation. An appropriate technique for measuring uterine fundal height clinically is described in Chapter 13, p. 249).

Sonographic Measurements. To evaluate correctly the results of sonographic measurements, it must be appreciated that the fetus may demonstrate different patterns of growth retardation. In one form, sometimes referred to as *symmetrical growth retardation,* there is retarded growth that is generalized and thus includes the head. With the other pattern, there is *asymmetrical growth retardation,* with the head being spared. With symmetrical growth retardation, the biparietal diameter, the head circumference at the level of the third ventricle, and the abdominal circumference at the level of the umbilical vein or ductus venosus are comparably reduced. Therefore, these findings alone do not serve to differentiate between symmetrical fetal growth retardation and an erroneous gestational age. If, however, gestational age is certain from clinical data or from sonographic measurements made early in pregnancy and microcephaly can be excluded, a small biparietal diameter, head circumference, and abdominal circumference are diagnostic of generalized growth retardation.

Measurement only of the biparietal diameter and head circumference at the level of the third ventricle will not detect asymmetrical growth retardation in which the head is spared. Sonography performed so as to obtain a true cross-sectional view of the fetal abdomen at the level of the umbilical vein or ductus venosus allows the abdominal circumference to be measured rather pre-

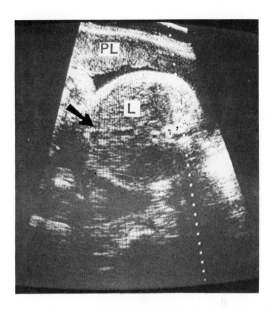

Figure 37-5. Sonographic cross-sectional view of the fetal abdomen at the level of the ductus venosus (*arrow*). L = liver, PL = placenta. (*Courtesy of Dr. R. Santos.*)

cisely (Fig. 37-5). If the head circumference is large compared to the abdominal circumference, and hydrocephalus is excluded (Chapter 30, p. 671), the fetus is asymmetrically growth retarded.

Normally, head circumference is greater than abdominal circumference measured at the level of the umbilical vein or ductus venosus until about 32 weeks gestation, when they become about equal and remain so until about 36 weeks, after which the abdominal circumference normally exceeds head circumference. It is reemphasized that gestational age must be accurate if these measurements are to provide useful information.

Scant amnionic fluid without rupture of the membranes is an ominous sign no matter when it occurs in pregnancy. It is a common finding in cases of severe growth retardation in which the fetus is growth retarded because of maternal factors (Manning and associates, 1981). Clear evidence of oligohydramnios in the presence of any other evidence of growth retardation is usually an indication for delivery even though the fetus is preterm.

Fetal Growth Retardation at or Near Term

Prompt delivery is likely to afford the best outcome for the fetus who is suspected of being severely growth retarded at or near term (Fig. 37-6A, B).

Fetal Growth Retardation Remote from Term

Unfortunately, in many instances of fetal growth retardation remote from term there is no specific treatment that will ameliorate the growth retardation, and, therefore, prompt delivery is often indicated. Possible exceptions are inadequate maternal nutrition, heavy smoking, use of hard drugs, and possibly chronic alcoholism. Ide-

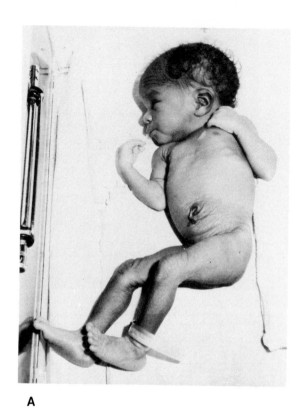

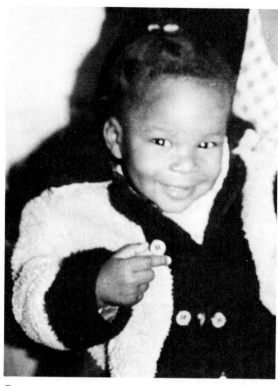

A   B

Figure 37-6. **A.** Severely growth-retarded infant of 38 weeks gestational age but birth weight of only 1800 g. Delivery was by cesarean section. The chronically hypertensive mother had suffered two previous stillbirths. **B.** The same infant at 13 months of age. Physical and intellectual development was normal at that time.

ally, the use of tobacco, hard drugs, and alcohol can be curtailed. In case of maternal undernutrition, the ingestion of a diet adequate quantitatively and qualitatively should favorably influence fetal growth. Very sedentary living that approaches full-time bed rest may also favorably influence fetal growth and, at the same time, possibly reduce the risk of preterm labor.

At times, the overtly growth-retarded fetus is in serious jeopardy irrespective of whether he remains in utero or is delivered. For the fetus who is severely growth retarded but remote from term, the decision to proceed with delivery becomes a matter of trying to ascertain the degree of risk from further stay in utero compared to the risks from preterm delivery. Fortunately, the stress associated with severe fetal growth retardation from causes not intrinsic to the fetus commonly accelerates lung maturation to a sufficient degree that respiratory distress and hyaline membrane disease do not develop. Identification of a lecithin-sphingomyelin (L/S) ratio of 2 or more or identification of phosphatidylglycerol in amnionic fluid is reassuring. However, a lower ratio or no detectable phosphatidylglycerol does not necessarily mean that severe respiratory distress will occur (Chapter 14, p. 274). Generally, delivery of an obviously growth-retarded fetus under the conditions outlined below, rather than procrastination with further fetal deterioration, offers the

chance for survival. By the time in gestation that fetal growth retardation has become severe, the fetus is usually mature enough to survive if (1) he is delivered promptly rather than allowing the risk of further compromise from a longer stay in utero, (2) he is closely monitored during labor to avoid further compromise or delivery is accomplished by cesarean section, and (3) he receives excellent neonatal care beginning immediately after delivery.

The presence of maternal disease that is worsening as a consequence of the pregnancy and thereby threatens the well-being of the mother as well as the fetus should certainly bear on the decision as to whether to deliver the severely growth-retarded fetus or to wait. Almost any maternal disease falls into this category when it is characterized by vascular disease, renal involvement, or both, and superimposed preeclampsia supervenes (Chapter 27, p. 556). With prompt delivery, fetal and neonatal salvage is likely to be improved compared to when delivery is unduly delayed, even though the L/S ratio is less than 2 (Fig. 37-4A). At the same time, with prompt delivery, maternal deterioration is likely to be arrested.

Several observations that have been provided by Creasy (1979) are supportive of the general policy of prompt delivery of the fetus who is believed to be severely growth retarded (below the 10th percentile) even when remote from term. In his experience, as ours, respiratory distress syndrome has been an uncommon complication in the preterm newborn infant who was severely growth retarded. Moreover, when respiratory distress did occur, it seldom proved to be lethal. In the more recent experiences at the University of California at San Francisco, 85 percent of infants *with respiratory distress* who weighed only 1000 to 1250 g at birth survived (Creasy, 1979). Furthermore, from extensive analyses of growth-retarded stillborn infants of various gestational ages, it was apparent that when fetal weight was below the 10th percentile and remained static, additional time in utero did *not* decrease mortality.

Labor and Delivery

Throughout labor, spontaneous or induced, those fetuses who are suspected of being growth retarded should be very closely monitored for evidence of distress, including abnormalities of fetal heart rate and the presence of appreciable amounts of meconium in the amnionic fluid. The likelihood of severe fetal distress during labor is considerably increased, since fetal growth retardation commonly is the result of insufficient placental function as a consequence of either faulty maternal perfusion or ablation of functional placenta or both. These conditions are likely to be aggravated by vigorous labor. Importantly, lack of amnionic fluid predisposes to cord compression and its dangers. The intrauterine environment is likely to prove especially dangerous to the fetus during labor! Consequently, the capabilities for immediate cesarean section should be available. Furthermore, it can be anticipated that the infant at birth may need expert assistance in making a successful transition to air breathing. He is at risk of being born hypoxic and of having aspirated meconium into the lungs, thus compromising chances of successful ventilation. As soon as the head is delivered from the vagina, or from the uterus in case of cesarean section, the mouth, pharynx, and nares should be quickly aspirated by the obstetrician. Moreover, it is essential that care for the newborn immediately after birth be provided by someone who can skillfully clear the airway below the vocal cords of noxious material, especially meconium, and ventilate the infant as needed. The severely growth-retarded newborn infant is unusually susceptible to hypothermia and may also soon develop other metabolic derangements, especially serious hypoglycemia. Polycythemia and blood hyperviscosity occasionally may cause serious difficulty unless effectively treated by limited exchange transfusion with plasma (Jones and Battaglia, 1977).

Subsequent Development of the Growth-Retarded Fetus

Subsequent growth of the individual newborn infant who is growth retarded cannot be reliably predicted from his measurements at birth (Philip, 1978). The infant who is small for gestational age may demonstrate any of a variety of growth patterns during infancy and childhood. Prolonged symmetrical, or generalized, growth retardation in utero is likely to be followed by a slow growth after birth, whereas the asymmetrically growth-retarded fetus is more likely to catch up after birth (Fig. 37-6B). The infant whose length (height) at birth is normal but whose weight is reduced can be expected to grow normally. If length is also compromised, he or she is likely to remain small (Brook, 1983).

The subsequent neurologic and intellectual capabilities of the infant who was growth retarded in utero cannot be predicted precisely. However, Fancourt and associates (1976) found that in children for whom there was sonographic evidence of delayed head growth starting before the third trimester, subsequent neurologic and intellectual development was also delayed.

POSTTERM PREGNANCIES

A postterm pregnancy is one that persists for 42 weeks or more from the onset of a menstrual period that was followed by ovulation about 2 weeks later. Although such a definition would include perhaps 10 percent or even more of pregnancies, some may not be actual postterm pregnancies but rather the result of an error in the estimation of gestational age. Again, the value of precise knowledge of the duration of gestation is evident, for, in general, the longer the truly postterm fetus stays in utero, the greater the risk of a severely compromised fetus and newborn infant.

Causes

Some more rare conditions in which there often is failure of the fetus to be delivered at the usual time include anencephaly, placental sulfatase deficiency, and extrauterine pregnancy. Women who have experienced prolonged gestation with one pregnancy appear to be at increased risk of the same in a subsequent pregnancy. However, until the mechanisms involved in the spontaneous onset and maintenance of normal labor are precisely known, there is little likelihood that the exact cause or causes of prolonged gestation will be identified.

Effects on the Fetus–Infant

The fetus postterm may continue to gain weight in utero and thus be an unusually large infant at birth. The fact that he did grow serves as an indicator of uncompromised placental function and suggests that he should be able to tolerate the rigors of normal labor without distress. However, his continued growth may have created a worrisome degree of fetopelvic disproportion, and as a consequence, labor may not be benign. Moreover, as discussed subsequently, oligohydramnios and cord compression may result in fetal distress, including meconium defecation and aspiration.

At the other extreme, the intrauterine environment may be so hostile to that fetus that further growth in utero is arrested. He or she may appear at birth actually to have lost considerable weight, especially from loss of subcutaneous fat and muscle mass. In the extreme case, the limbs appear long and very thin, there is severe desquamation of the epidermis, and the nails and the amnion are commonly bile-stained. The infant whose gestational age is beyond 42 weeks and who presents this dystrophic appearance has been called "postmature" by some. However, the term "postmature" might best be applied to the postterm fetus who has continued to grow in utero and thus has achieved a size comparable to that of a normal infant who was conceived at the same time but was born at term and thrived after birth. Since "postmature" has been applied in so variable a fashion, perhaps its use ought to be discarded to avoid further confusion. Other commonly used, but not necessarily very precise, descriptions are "postmature and dysmature," "postdates and postmature," and "postterm and dysmature." We favor *postterm* and either *dysmature* or *dystrophic* to describe the obviously undernourished fetus–infant whose gestational age has been prolonged abnormally, i.e., more than 42 weeks.

Importantly, the fetus–infant need not be postterm to have developed the characteristic features of dysmaturity described above, for compromised placental function somewhat earlier in pregnancy may also lead to a similar appearance, as is evident in the dystrophic newborn infant of 38 weeks gestational age illustrated in Figure 37-6A.

Management of Postterm Pregnancy

There remains little doubt that, even in the absence of any recognizable maternal complication, some fetuses who stay in utero much beyond 42 weeks are in progressively greater danger of suffering serious morbidity or even dying in utero or soon after birth. Therefore, it would be advantageous to those fetuses to deliver them by 42 weeks. However, at least five difficult problems persist that serve to discourage a policy of delivering all fetuses whose gestational age is suspected to be at least 42 weeks:

1. Gestational age is not always precisely known, and thus the fetus may actually be less mature than thought.
2. It is very difficult to identify with precision those fetuses who are likely to die or to develop serious morbidity if left in utero.
3. The majority of fetuses fare rather well.
4. Induction of labor is not always successful.
5. Delivery by cesarean section increases appreciably the risk of serious maternal morbidity not only in this pregnancy but to a degree in subsequent ones.

Parkland Management

The general plan of management at Parkland Memorial Hospital of pregnancies believed to be postterm, that is, 42 weeks gestation or more, is as follows:

1. *Postterm and favorable for induction of labor.* If the fetal head is well fixed in the pelvis and well applied to the cervix, and the cervix is soft, somewhat effaced, and 2 cm dilatated or more, induction of labor is attempted with intravenous oxytocin (Chapter 29, p. 644). When so selected, the great majority of women will soon go into labor. If the attempt to induce labor is unsuccessful and the membranes have not ruptured, the woman is allowed to go home if no abnormalities of fetal heart rate were detected by external electronic monitoring and there are no maternal complications, such as hypertension. If by 1 week hence she has not gone into labor, the procedure is repeated.
2. *Postterm but unfavorable for inducing labor.* If at 42 and 43 weeks of gestation, conditions are considered to be unfavorable for inducing labor, no intervention is attempted as long as there are no maternal complications, the fetus is considered by the mother to be active, and amnionic fluid is evident by clinical examination or sonography. Otherwise, an attempt at induction of labor is made with intravenous oxytocin. Management then is the same as described above. Certainly, if still undelivered by 44 weeks gestation, delivery is accomplished promptly. Intravenous oxytocin is infused to try to induce labor. If unsuccessful or contraindicated, cesarean delivery is performed.
3. *Possibly postterm.* In the absence of any identified complication of pregnancy and if amnionic fluid is evident clinically or sonographically, the woman is seen at least weekly and reassured that the risks that accrue from active intervention to effect delivery very likely exceed the potential risks from a possibly prolonged gestation.

In our experience labor at its onset is a particularly dangerous time for the postterm fetus. Therefore, it is important that women whose pregancies are known or suspected to be postterm come to the hospital as soon as they suspect that they are in labor. Upon arrival, while being observed for possible labor, they must be observed very closely for fetal heart rate variations that imply, at least, fetal distress.

Another particularly dangerous time for the postterm fetus is delivery. Aspiration of meconium should be minimized by effective suctioning of the pharynx as soon as the head is delivered but before the thorax is delivered. If meconium is identified, the trachea should be aspirated as soon as possible after delivery by someone skilled in this technique (Chapter 38, p. 770). Immediately thereafter, the infant should be effectively ventilated as needed. At times, the continued growth of the fetus postterm will eventuate in shoulder dystocia following delivery of the head. Therefore, an obstetrician who is experienced in managing this problem should be immediately available to effect delivery (Chapter 30, p. 669).

In general, electronic monitoring of the fetal heart rate and of uterine contractions throughout all of labor is advantageous, especially so whenever personnel appropriately skilled in the detection of fetal distress by auscultation and palpation (Haverkamp and colleagues, 1979) cannot remain continually in attendance.

The question, "When should the membranes be ruptured?" is difficult to answer. Further reduction in amnionic fluid following amniotomy can certainly enhance the possibility of cord compression and perhaps impair placental function. On the other hand, amniotomy is likely to identify the presence of thick meconium that can be dangerous to the fetus if aspirated during labor. Moreover, once the membranes are ruptured, a scalp electrode and intrauterine pressure catheter can then be placed, the use of which usually provides more precise data concerning fetal heart rate and uterine contractions than does external electronic monitoring. Importantly, with internal monitoring the woman is more likely to lie on her side, which should favor placental perfusion, whereas, when balancing external monitoring equipment on her abdomen, she most often is inclined to stay on her back.

Identification of *thick* meconium in amnionic fluid is particularly worrisome. It is evidence of fairly recent fetal distress that may or may not persist. Of great importance, aspiration of meconium may cause severe pulmonary dysfunction and death during the newborn period (Chapter 38, p. 770). The likelihood of successful vaginal delivery of a healthy neonate is reduced appreciably for the nulliparous woman who is in early labor with thick meconium in the amnionic fluid. Strong consideration must be given to prompt cesarean section, especially when cephalopelvic disproportion is suspected or either hypotonic or hypertonic dysfunctional labor is evident.

Other Plans of Management

It has now become common practice in the management of the postterm pregnancy to apply a variety of procedures that have been championed as tests of fetal well-being. Most often these tests have included measurements from one to seven times per week of either the amount of estriol excreted in the urine per 24 hours or its concentrations in plasma, or the evaluation one or more times each week of changes in fetal heart rate either in response to fetal movement (nonstress test) or in response to uterine contractions usually induced with oxytocin (contraction stress test) or both (Chapter 14). As long as these tests remain normal, the fetus is considered to be in little jeopardy from further stay in utero.

The major problems that have arisen with the use of these tests, aside from costs and inconvenience, are frequencies of false positive and false negative results that are unacceptable, at least to some obstetricians. Moreover, careful analyses of published reports concerned with postterm pregnancies provide no convincing

evidence that their use has produced better results than has the preceding plan of management. Unfortunately, as emphasized by Kirschbaum (1979) in the course of discussing the problems associated with prolonged pregnancy, some techniques commonly employed to attempt fetal appraisal were incorporated into clinical practice without vigorous objective proof of value as measured by their predictive strength and the prevention of perinatal morbidity and death. For example, Schneider and co-workers (1978), in their study of postterm pregnancies, found measurements of 24-hour urinary estriol excretion carried out every Monday, Wednesday, and Friday to be of little value in their hands.

Miyazaki and Miyazaki (1981) were disappointed in fetal outcomes in which the nonstress test had been used to try to ascertain fetal well-being. In their relatively small series there were four fetal deaths and one neonatal death following nonstress tests that were interpreted to reassure fetal well-being. Others have reported similar experiences, especially when the interval between testing was as long as a week.

The contraction stress test has been applied to try to identify the suspected postterm fetus who is in jeopardy in utero. Freeman and associates (1981) report excellent outcomes employing this test at weekly intervals and not interfering with the pregnancy as long as the test result remained negative. The experiences of some others have not been so rewarding, however. An example is cited in Figure 37-7. In this case, at 42 plus weeks gestation age, an attempt was made to effect delivery by infusing oxytocin for 8 hours, during which the fetal heart rate was recorded continuously. Throughout the 8-hour period no evidence of ominous decelerations was found, i.e., the contraction stress test was negative. However, effective labor was not established. Three days later the procedure was repeated with the same result. After 3 more days it was repeated for the third time with the same result. Two days later fetal movement ceased. Oxytocin now proved effective for accomplishing labor and delivery. Thick meconium was present in the scant amnionic fluid. Otherwise, careful pathologic examination disclosed no abnormality of the fetus or placenta to account for the death.

Analyses of our experiences with the perplexing problem of appropriate management of prolonged gestation have been made recently by Leveno and associates (1984). Interestingly, the pathophysiology of fetal distress in such cases most likely was oligohydramnios with compromised umbilical cord blood flow, rather than uteroplacental insufficiency.

In summary, lowering perinatal morbidity and mortality associated with the problem of prolonged pregnancy requires precise knowledge of the gestational age of the fetus. Too often, time, effort, and emotion are expended unduly on cases in which gestational age is less than 42 weeks. For the fetus whose gestational age truly exceeds this value, however, the risks are appreciable. Perhaps the most important evidence of impending disaster is scant amnionic fluid. In this circumstance, cord

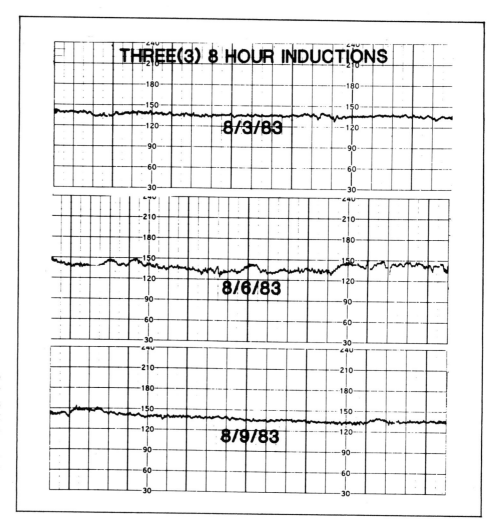

Figure 37-7. Fetal heart rate tracings were made continuously during three 8-hour intravenous oxytocin infusions to try to effect labor in pregnancy at 42 to 43 weeks gestation. Even though there was no evidence of abnormality in fetal heart rate during or after uterine contractions, the fetus died 2 days later. Litigation is pending.

compression can cause fetal distress and too often lead to death. Death may be the direct consequence of hypoxia from the cord compression, or it may be the consequence of abundant meconium shed into a very small volume of amnionic fluid, which is then inhaled as the hypoxic fetus gasps before labor, early in labor, or at delivery and hypoxic death of the neonate.

REFERENCES

Barden TP: Labor. In Pitkin R (ed): Year Book of Obstetrics and Gynecology. Chicago, Year Book, 1977, p 109

Bauer CR, Stern L, Colle E: Prolonged rupture of membranes associated with a decreased incidence of respiratory distress syndrome. Pediatrics 53:7, 1974

Belizán JM, Villar J, Nardin JC, Malamud J, De Vicuña LS: Diagnosis of intrauterine growth retardation by a simple clinical method: Measurement of uterine height. Am J Obstet Gynecol 131:643, 1978

Berkowitz RL, Hobbins JC: A reevaluation of the value of hCS determination in the management of prolonged pregnancy. Obstet Gynecol 49:156, 1977

Brenner WE, Edelman DA, Hendricks CH: A standard of fetal growth for the United States of America. Am J Obstet Gynecol 126:555, 1976

Brook CGD: Consequences of intrauterine growth retardation. Br Med J 286:164, 1983

Brown ER, Nielsen H, Torday JS, Tauesch HW: Reversible induction of surfactant production in fetal lambs treated with glucocorticoids. Pediatr Res 13:491, 1979

Campbell S: Personal communication, 1983

Campbell S, Wilkin D: Ultrasonic measurement of fetal abdomen circumference in the estimation of fetal weight. Br J Obstet Gynaecol 82:689, 1975

Caritis SN, Lin LS, Toig G, Wong LK: Pharmacodynamics of ritodrine in pregnant women during preterm labor. Am J Obstet Gynecol 147:752, 1983

Castrén O, Gummerus M, Saarikoski S: Treatment of imminent premature labour. Acta Obstet Gynecol Scand 54:95, 1975

Cetrulo CL, Freeman R: Bioelectric evaluation in intrauterine growth retardation. Clin Obstet Gynecol 20:979, 1977

Cotton DB, Strasner HT, Hill LM, Schifrin BS, Paul RH: Comparison between magnesium sulfate, terbutaline and a placebo for inhibition of preterm labor: A randomized study, J Reprod Med 29:92, 1984

Creasy RK: Intrauterine growth retardation: Optimal delivery time. Presented at the Seventy-eighth Ross Conference on Pediatric Research (Obstetrical Decisions and Neonatal Outcome), San Diego, May 30, 1979

Dimmick J, Mahmood K, Altshuler G: Antenatal infection: Adequate protection against hyaline membrane disease? Obstet Gynecol 47:57, 1976

Dluholucky S, Babic J, Taufer I: Reduction of incidence and mortality of respiratory distress syndrome by administration of hydrocortisone to mother. Arch Dis Child 51:420, 1976

Eaton CJ: Discussion of paper by Knox GE, Huddleston JF, Flowers CE: Management of prolonged pregnancy: Result of a prospective randomized trial. Am J Obstet Gynecol 134:376, 1979

Elliott JP: Magnesium sulfate as a tocolytic agent. Am J Obstet Gynecol 147:277, 1983

Elliott JP, O'Keeffe DF, Greenberg P, Freeman RK: Pulmonary edema associated with magnesium sulfate and betamethasone administration. Am J Obstet Gynecol 134:717, 1979

Epstein MF, Nicholls E, Stubblefield PG: Neonatal hypoglycemia after beta-sympathomimetic tocolytic therapy. J Pediatr 94:449, 1979

Fancourt R, Campbell S, Harvey D, Norman AP: Follow-up studies of small-for-dates babies. Br Med J 1:1435, 1976

Fedrick J. Anderson ABM: Factors associated with spontaneous pre-term birth. Br J Obstet Gynaecol 83:342, 1976

Ferguson JE III, Hensleigh PA, Kredenster D: Adjunctive use of magnesium sulfate with ritodrine for preterm labor tocolysis. Am J Obstet Gynecol 148:166, 1984

Fitzhardinge PM, Steven EM: The small-for-date infant. 1. Later growth patterns. Pediatrics 49:671, 1972

Freeman, RK, Garite TJ, Modanlou H, Dorchester W, Rommal C, Devaney M: Postdate pregnancy: Utilization of contraction stress testing for primary fetal surveillance. Am J Obstet Gynecol 140:128, 1981

Fuchs, F, Fuchs A-R, Lauersen NH, Zervoudakis IA: Treatment of pre-term labour with ethanol. Dan Med Bull 26:123, 1979

Fuchs F, Fuchs A-R, Poblete V, Resk A: Effect of alcohol on threatened premature labor. Am J Obstet Gynecol 99:627, 1967

Gabert H: Personal communication, 1974

Gluck L: Fetal lung maturity. Presented at the Seventy-Eighth Ross Conference on Pediatric Research, San Diego, May 30, 1979

Graven SN: Ethical dilemmas in current obstetric and newborn care. Report of Sixty-Fifth Ross Conference on Pediatric Research, Columbus, Ohio, Ross Laboratories, 1973

Hankins GDV, Leveno KJ, Whalley PJ, DePalma RT, Williams ML, Nelson S: Maternal, fetal, neonatal, and infant outcomes with expectant management for preterm rupture of the membranes. Presented at the Society of Perinatal Obstetricians, San Antonio, Texas, Feb 2–4, 1984

Hasslein HC, Goodlin RC: Delivery of the tiny newborn. Am J Obstet Gynecol 134:192, 1979

Hatwick RE: Ethical dilemmas in current obstetric and newborn care. Report on Sixty-Fifth Ross Conference on Pediatric Research, Columbus, Ohio, Ross Laboratories, 1973

Haverkamp AD, Orleans M, Langendoerfer S, McFee J, Murphy J, Thompson HE: A controlled trial of the differential effects of intrapartum fetal monitoring. Am J Obstet Gynecol 14:399, 1979

Hemminki E, Starfield B: Prevention and treatment of premature labor by drugs: Review of controlled clinical trials. Br J Obstet Gynecol 85:411, 1978

Hesseldahl H: A Danish multicenter study of ritodrine in the treatment of pre-term labor. Dan Med Bull 26:116, 1979

Hobbins JC, Berkowitz RL, Grannum PAT: Diagnosis and antepartum management of intrauterine growth retardation. J Reprod Med 21:319, 1978

Hoffman HJ, Stark CR, Lunden FE Jr, Ashbrook JD: Analyses of birth weight, gestational age, and fetal viability, U.S. births, 1968. Obstet Gynecol Surv 29:651, 1974

Howie RN, Liggins GC: Clinical trial of antepartum betamethasone therapy for prevention of respiratory distress in preterm infants. Proceedings of Fifth Study Group, Royal College of Obstetricians and Gynecologists, Oct. 1977, p 281

Jimenez J, Tyson J, Santos-Ramos R, Duenhoelter J: Comparison of obstetric and pediatric evaluation of gestational age. Pediatr Res 14:497, 1979

Johnson JWC, Lee PA, Zachary AS, Calhoun S, Migeon CJ: High-risk prematurity-progestin treatment and steroid studies. Obstet Gynecol 54:412, 1979

Johnson JWC, Mitzner W, London WT, Palmer AE, Scott R: Betamethasone and the rhesus fetus. Multisystemic effects. Am J Obstet Gynecol 133:677, 1979

Jones MD Jr, Battaglia FC: Intrauterine growth retardation. Am J Obstet Gynecol 127:540, 1977

Jones MD Jr, Burd LI, Bowes WA Jr, Battaglia FC, Lubchenco LO: Failure of association of premature rupture of membranes with respiratory distress syndrome. N Engl J Med 292:1253, 1975

Jones RAK, Cummins M, Davies PA: Infants of very low birthweight. A 15-year analysis. Lancet 1:1332, 1979

Kirkpatrick SE, Pitlik PT, Hirschklau MJ, Friedman WF: Acute effects of maternal ethanol infusion on fetal cardiac performance. Am J Obstet Gynecol 126:1034, 1976.

Kirschbaum TH: Discussion of paper by Knox GE, Huddleston JF, Flowers CE: Management of prolonged pregnancy: Result of a prospective randomized trial. Am J Obstet Gynecol 134:376, 1979

Knox GE, Huddleston JF, Flowers CE: Management of prolonged pregnancy: Result of a prospective randomized trial. Am J Obstet Gynecol 134:376, 1979

Kopelman AE: The smallest preterm infant. Am J Dis Child 132:461, 1978

Korda AR, Lyneham RC, Jones WR: The treatment of premature labour with intravenously administered salbutamol. Med J Aust 1:744, 1974

Kristoffersen K, Hansen MK: The condition of the foetus and infant in cases treated with ritodrine. Dan Med Bull 26:121, 1979

Kubli F: In Anderson A, et al. (eds): Preterm Labor. London, Royal College of Obstetricians and Gynaecologists, 1977, p 218

Landesman R: Premature labor: Its management and therapy. J Reprod Med 9:95, 106, 1972

Lauersen NH, Merkatz IR, Tejani N, Wilson KH, Roberson A, Mann LI, Fuchs F: Inhibition of premature labor: A multicenter comparison of ritodrine and ethanol. Am J Obstet Gynecol 127:837, 1977

Leveno KJ, Quirk JG, Cunningham FG, Nelson SD, Santos-Ramos R, Toofanian A, DePalma RT: Prolonged pregnancy. I. Observations concerning the causes of fetal distress. Am J Obstet Gynecol (In press) 1984

Levin DL: Effects of inhibition of prostaglandin synthesis on fetal development, oxygenation, and the fetal circulation. Perinatal Seminars (In press), 1984

Liggins GC: The prevention of RDS by maternal betamethasone administration. In Lung Maturation and the Prevention of Hyaline Membrane Disease. Report of the Seventieth Ross Conference on Pediatric Research, Columbus, Ohio, Ross Laboratories, 1976

Liggins GC: Report on children exposed to steroids in utero. Contemp Ob/ Gyn 19:205, 1982

Liggins GC, Howie RN: The prevention of RDS by maternal steroid therapy. In Gluck L (ed): Modern Perinatal Medicine. Chicago, Year Book, 1974

Liggins GC, Vaughn GS: Intravenous infusion of salbutamol in the management of premature labour. J Obstet Gynecol Br Commonw 80:29, 1973

Lubchenco LO: The High Risk Infant. Philadelphia, Saunders, 1976

Lubchenco LO, Hansman C, Dressler M, Boyd E: Intrauterine growth as estimated from liveborn birth weight data at 24 to 42 weeks of gestation. Pediatrics 32:793, 1963

Mann LI, Bhakthavathsalan A, Liu M, Makowski P: Placental transport of alcohol and its effects on maternal and fetal acid-base balance. Am J Obstet Gynecol 122:837, 1975

Manning FA, Hill LM, Platt LD: Qualitative amniotic fluid volume determination by ultrasound: Antepartum detection of intrauterine growth retardation. Am J Obstet Gynecol 139:254, 1981

Mashiach S, Barkai G, Sack J, Stern E, Brish M, Goldman B, Serr DM: The effects of intra-amniotic thyroxine administration on fetal lung maturity in man. J Perinat Med 7:161, 1979

Merkatz IR, Peter JB, Barden TP: Ritodrine hydrochloride: A betamimetic agent developed specifically for use in preterm labor. II. Evidence of efficacy. Obstet Gynecol 56:7, 1980

Miller JM, Keane MWD, Horger EO III: A comparison of magnesium sulfate and terbutaline for the arrest of premature labor. J Reprod Med 27:348, 1982

Milligan JE, Shennan AT, Haskins EM: Perinatal intensive care: Where and how to draw the line. Am J Obstet Gynecol 148:499, 1984

Miyazaki FS, Miyazaki BA: False reactive nonstress tests in postterm pregnancies. Am J Obstet Gynecol 140:269, 1981

Mosier HD Jr, Dearden LC, Tanner SM, Jansons RA, Biggs CS: Disproportionate organ growth in the fetus after betamethasone administration. Pediatr Res 13:486, 1979

Naeye RL, Dixon JB: Distortions in fetal growth standards. Pediatr Res 12:987, 1978

Osler M: Side effects and metabolic changes during treatment with betamimetics (ritodrine). Dan Med Bull 26:119, 1979

Perkins RP: Sudden fetal death in labor. The significance of antecedent monitoring characteristics and clinical circumstances. J Reprod Med 25:309, 1980

Persson P-H, Grennert L, Gennser G: Impact of fetal and maternal factors on the normal growth of the biparietal diameter. Acta Obstet Gynecol Scand [Suppl] 78:21, 1978

Philip AGS: Fetal growth retardation: Femurs, fontanels, and follow-up. Pediatrics 62:446, 1978

Pomerance JJ, Ukrainski CT, Ukra T, Henderson DH, Nash AH, Meredith JL: Cost of living for infants weighing 1000 grams or less at brith. Pediatrics 61:908, 1978

Pritchard JA, Whalley PJ: High risk pregnancy and reproductive outcome. In Gluck (ed): Modern Perinatal Medicine. Chicago, Year Book, 1974

Quirk JG, Raker RK, Petrie RH, Williams AM: The role of glucocorticoids, unstressful labor, and atraumatic delivery in the prevention of respiratory distress syndrome. Am J Obstet Gynecol 1134:768, 1979

Reynolds JW: A comparison of salbutamol and ethanol in the treatment of premature labor. Aust NZ J Obstet Gynaecol 18:107, 1978

Ritchie K, McClure G: Prematurity. Lancet 2:1227, 1979

Rogge P, Young S, Goodlin R: Post-partum pulmonary oedema associated with preventive therapy for premature labor. Lancet 1:1026, 1979

Rydén G: The effect of salbutamol and terbutaline in the management of premature labour. Acta Obstet Gynecol Scand 56:293, 1977

Schifrin BS: The non-stress test. Presented at the Seventy-Eighth Ross Conference on Pediatric Research (Obstetrical Decisions and Neonatal Outcome), San Diego, May 30, 1979

Schneider JM, Olson RW, Curet LB: Screening for fetal and neonatal risk in the postdate pregnancy. Am J Obstet Gynecol 131:473, 1978

Sell E, Harris TR: The influence of ruptured membranes (ROM) on fetal outcome. Pediatr Res 10:432, 1976

Semchyshyn S, Zuspan FP, O'Shaughnessy R: Pulmonary edema associated with the use of hydrocortisone and a tocolytic agent for the management of premature labor. J Reprod Med 28:47, 1983

Simpson GF, Harbert GM Jr: Use of betamethasone in management of preterm gestation with rupture of membranes. Am J Obstet Gynecol (In press), 1984

Sims CD, Chamberlain GVP, Boyd IE, Lewis PJ: A comparison of salbutamol and ethanol in the treatment of preterm labor. Br J Obstet Gynaecol 85:761, 1978

Spellacy WN, Cruz AC, Birk SA, Buhi WC: Treatment of premature labor with ritodrine: A randomized controlled study. Obstet Gynecol 54:220, 1979

Spisso KR, Harbert GM Jr, Thiagarajah S: The use of magnesium sulfate as the primary tocolytic agent to prevent premature delivery. Am J Obstet Gynecol 142:840, 1982

Steer CM, Petrie RH: A comparison of magnesium sulfate and alcohol for the prevention of premature labor. Am J Obstet Gynecol 129:1, 1977

Stewart AL, Turcan DM, Rawlings G, Reynolds EOR: Prognosis for infants weighing 1000 g or less at birth. Arch Dis Child 52:97, 1977

Stubblefield RG: Pulmonary edema occurring after therapy with dexamethasone and terbutaline for premature labor: A case report. Am J Obstet Gynecol 132:341, 1978

Taeusch HW, Frigoletto F, Kitzmiller J, Avery ME, Hehne A, Fromm B, Lawson E, Neff RK: Risks of respiratory distress syndrome after prenatal dexamethasone treatment. Pediatrics 63:64, 1979

Tejani N, Mann LI: Diagnosis and management of the small-for-gestational age fetus. Clin Obstet Gynecol 20:943, 1977

Tinga DJ, Aarnoudse JG: Post-partum pulmonary oedema associated with preventive therapy for premature labour. Lancet 1:1026, 1979

Ulmsten U: Inhibition of myometrial hyperactivity by calcium antagonists. Dan Med Bull 26:125, 1979

Walker D-JB, Feldman A, Vohr B, Oh W: Cost-benefit analysis of neonatal intensive care for infants weighing less than 1000 grams at birth. Pediatrics (in press), 1984

Warshof SL, Gohari P, Berkowitz RL, Hobbins JC: The estimation of fetal weight by computer-assisted analysis. Am J Obstet Gynecol 128:881, 1977

Wilson JC, Levy DL, Wilds PL: Premature rupture of membranes prior to term: Consequences of nonintervention. Obstet Gynecol 60:601, 1982

Wright FH, Blouch RR, Chamberlin A, Ernest T, Halstead WC, Meier P, Poor RY, Naunton RF, Newell FW: A controlled follow-up study of small prematures born from 1952 through 1956. Am J Dis Child 124:507, 1972

Yoon JJ, Harper RG: Observations on the relationship between duration of rupture of the membranes and the development of idiopathic respiratory distress syndrome. Pediatrics 52:161, 1973

Zlatnik FJ, Fuchs F: A controlled study of ethanol in threatened premature labor. Am J Obstet Gynecol 112:610, 1972

Zuckerman H, Reiss U, Robenstin I: Inhibition of human premature labor by indomethacin. Obstet Gynecol 44:787, 1974

Zuelzer WW: Ethical dilemmas in current obstetric and newborn care. Report of the Sixty-Fifth Ross Conference on Pediatric Research. Columbus, Ohio, Ross Laboratories, 1973

38

Other Diseases of the Fetus and Newborn Infant

The fetus and newborn infant are subject to a great variety of diseases, some of which are the direct consequence of maternal disease and have been considered along with the maternal disease, especially in Chapter 28. This chapter provides an introduction to other fetal and neonatal diseases of major clinical importance. Injuries and malformations of the fetus and newborn infant are considered in Chapter 39.

RESPIRATORY DISEASES

To provide prompt blood gas exchange after birth, the infant must rapidly fill his lungs with air while clearing them of fluid, and he must simultaneously increase remarkably the volume of blood that perfuses his lungs. Some of the fluid is usually expressed as the chest is compressed during vaginal delivery; the remainder is absorbed especially through the lymphatics of the lungs. Of great importance is the presence of appropriate surfactant synthesized by the type II pneumonocytes of the lungs to stabilize the air-expanded alveoli by lowering surface tension and thereby preventing lung collapse during expiration.

HYALINE MEMBRANE DISEASE

About two decades ago, the development of idiopathic respiratory distress–hyaline membrane disease was related to deficiency of pulmonary surfactant (Chapter 8, p. 154). If the alveoli cannot be maintained in an expanded state because of inappropriate surfactant action, obvious respiratory distress develops, which is characterized by the formation of hyaline membrane in the distal bronchioles and alveoli, considerable cardiopulmonary shunting of blood, and the likelihood of death from hypoxia and acidosis unless treatment is prompt and appropriate.

Diagnosis

The atelectatic lungs are stiff with very low compliance; thus the work of breathing is increased remarkably. Progressive shunting of blood through nonventilated areas of the lung contributes to the hypoxia and to both metabolic and respiratory acidosis. Clinically, the infants exhibit an increased respiratory rate accompanied by severe retraction during inspiration. Expiration is often accompanied by a whimper and grunt; grunting is very common in the newborn whenever there is uneven expansion of the lungs or lower airway obstruction. Poor peripheral circulation and systemic hypotension may be evident.

Until recently, hyaline membrane disease accounted for one fifth of all neonatal deaths (Farrell and Wood, 1976), but the actual number of deaths from respiratory distress–hyaline membrane disease undoubtedly has decreased since then. Boys are more prone than girls to develop respiratory distress–hyaline membrane disease, and white infants appear to be more often affected than are black infants.

Other forms of respiratory insufficiency may be confused with idiopathic respiratory distress–hyaline membrane disease. These include respiratory insufficiency as a consequence of sepsis, pneumonia, aspiration, pneumothorax, diaphragmatic hernia, and heart failure. Common causes of cardiac decompensation in the early newborn period are patent ductus ateriosus and primary myocardial disease. The chest roentgenogram, coupled with a careful physical examination, is likely to be of considerable aid in differential diagnosis. In case of idiopathic respiratory distress, the chest roentgenogram reveals a diffuse reticulogranular infiltrate throughout the lung fields with an air-filled tracheobronchial tree (air bronchogram).

Pathology

In the fatal case, the atelectatic lungs on gross examination resemble liver. Histologically, many alveoli are collapsed while some are widely dilated. Hyaline membranes of fibrin-rich protein and cellular debris line the dilated alveoli and the terminal bronchioles, and the epithelium underlying the membrane is necrotic.

Treatment

An arterial Po_2 below 40 mm Hg is indicative of a need for effective oxygen therapy. Anaerobically collected blood is required in order to assess Po_2, Pco_2, and pH. The blood may be obtained from a peripheral artery but more easily from a catheter in an umbilical artery, which may also be used for infusion of fluids. The concentration of oxygen administered to these infants should be sufficient to relieve hypoxia and acidosis but not higher. Arterial oxygen tensions of 50 to 70 mm Hg are adequate. Humidification of inspired air also is important in the management of these infants. During recovery, careful blood gas monitoring allows Po_2 to be maintained with progressively lower partial pressure of oxygen. The infant from the time of birth must be kept warm, since chilling increases oxygen consumption.

The use of oxygen-enriched air under pressure to prevent the collapse of unstable alveoli (continuous positive airway pressure) has brought about an appreciable reduction in the mortality rate from the respiratory distress syndrome. In order to be successful, any technique to augment ventilation requires continuous observation by skilled personnel in constant attendance. Successful ventilation usually reduces the high inspired oxygen concentrations that are otherwise required and thereby reduces oxygen toxicity to the lungs and retinas. Disadvantages are that venous return to the heart may be impaired, causing a fall in cardiac output, and there is always the possibility of barotrauma, i.e., rupture of the lung with interstitial emphysema and pneumothorax or pneumomediastinum. These complications are not always the result of overzealous resuscitation and ventilation, however. Vigorous mechanical ventilation is probably an important factor in the genesis of bronchopulmonary dysplasia, as pointed out below.

The establishment of appropriately staffed and equipped neonatal intensive care units has served to reduce dramatically the number of deaths from idiopathic respiratory distress even in very small infants.

Other Complications

Oxygen therapy is not innocuous. Persistent hyperoxia is likely in itself to injure the lung, especially the alveoli and capillaries. If hyperoxemia is produced, the infant is at risk of developing *retrolental fibroplasia* (p. 771). Therefore, the concentration of oxygen administered must be reduced appropriately as the arterial Po_2 rises. Endotracheal tubes after prolonged use cause erosion and serious infection of the upper airway and must be removed as soon as possible. *Bronchopulmonary dysplasia,* or oxygen toxicity lung disease, may develop in infants treated for severe respiratory distress with high

concentrations of oxygen at high pressures. Bronchopulmonary dysplasia is a chronic condition characterized by hypoxia, hypercarbia, and oxygen dependence as a consequence of alveolar and bronchiolar epithelial damage followed by peribronchial and interstitial fibrosis. Pulmonary hypertension is also a frequent complication. In one study the administration of vitamin E during the acute phase of the respiratory distress syndrome appeared to modify the development of bronchopulmonary dysplasia (Ehrenkranz and colleagues, 1978). In a subsequent randomized double-blind study, however, the same investigators were unable to confirm their earlier observations (Ehrenkranz and co-workers, 1979).

Survival

Death from the respiratory distress syndrome formerly was quite common, especially among very small infants. In recent years, fortunately, the mortality rate, even for very small infants, has decreased remarkably. Overt lung disease did persist or reappear following hyaline membrane disease but was not a frequent occurrence in a group of children evaluated by Stahlman and co-workers (1982).

Hopefully, the technique of extracorporeal circulation can be developed sufficiently so it can be used to oxygenate the neonate who is at considerable risk of developing bronchopulmonary dysplasia from prolonged ventilation with highly oxygenated air delivered at increased pressure (Bartlett, 1984).

MECONIUM ASPIRATION

The aspiration of some normal amnionic fluid before birth is most likely a physiologic event (Chapter 8, p. 163). Fetal distress, however, may lead to defecation of meconium into the amnionic fluid and deep, gasping inspiratory efforts by the fetus.

Pathology

Aspiration of meconium is likely to cause both mechanical obstruction of the airways and a chemical pneumonitis. Atelectasis, consolidation, and pneumothorax and pneumomediastinum may prove fatal unless vigorously treated. Yeh and co-workers (1979) emphasized that the initial chest roentgenogram is useful for predicting outcome in infants with meconium aspiration. Consolidation or atelectasis, most commonly associated with aspiration of thick meconium, is indicative of a poor outcome.

Marshall and associates (1978) found no evidence of persistent chronic lung disease among survivors of meconium aspiration whom they followed. However, two of three infants who developed seizures while acutely ill subsequently demonstrated significant psychomotor retardation.

Diagnosis and Management

At Parkland Memorial Hospital, whenever meconium has been identified in amnionic fluid before or during delivery, someone especially skilled in resuscitative techniques is present at the delivery. To prevent further aspiration, the mouth and nares are carefully suctioned by the obstetrician before the shoulders are delivered from the vagina, or as the mouth is visualized through the uterine section at cesarean delivery (Chapter 20, p. 380). As soon as possible after delivery, all meconium-stained fluid that remains above the cords is aspirated and the vocal cords are visualized. Endotracheal intubation and suction are then applied, and as much meconium as possible is aspirated from the trachea. It is essential to perform these procedures swiftly. The stomach is emptied to avoid the possibility of further meconium aspiration. *It is emphasized that ventilation of the lungs must not be delayed unduly while these procedures are carried out.* Subsequent treatment is generally similar to that described for respiratory distress. The value, if any, of corticosteroids, prophylactic antibiotics, and bronchodilators has not been established.

RETROLENTAL FIBROPLASIA

Retrolental fibroplasia had become by 1950 the largest single cause of blindness in this country. After the discovery that the etiology of the disease often was hyperoxemia, its frequency decreased remarkably.

Pathology

The retina of the eye vascularizes centrifugally from the optic nerve starting about the fourth month of gestation and continuing until shortly after birth. During the time of vascularization, the retinal vessels are very sensitive to and thus easily damaged by excess oxygen. The temporal portion of the retina, which is the last to be vascularized, is most vulnerable. Oxygen induces severe vasoconstriction, damage to the endothelium, and obliteration of the affected vessel. When the oxygen level is reduced, there is new vessel formation at the site of previous vasculature damage. The new vessels penetrate the retina and extend intravitreally, where they are prone to leak proteinaceous material or actually burst and leak blood. Adhesions then form that detach the retina.

Prevention

The precise levels of hyperoxemia that can be sustained without causing retrolental fibroplasia are not known. Unfortunately, a cooperative study that was carried out did not provide answers to many difficult but important questions concerning arterial P_{O_2} levels and retrolental fibroplasia (Kinsey and colleagues, 1977). It is felt by many pediatricians that the inhalation of air enriched with oxygen to no more than 40 percent will not cause

retrolental fibroplasia. Some believe, however, that whenever oxygen-enriched air is provided, the blood P_{O_2} must be monitored.

Very small infants born remote from term who develop respiratory distress are most likely to require ventilation with high concentrations of oxygen to maintain life until the respiratory distress clears. During this period, it is important that overzealous treatment does not lead to dangerous hyperoxia and, in turn, retrolental fibroplasia. Frequent measurements of P_{O_2}, therefore, may be necessary first to assure adequate oxygen and then to prevent hyperoxemia as the respiratory distress clears.

Vitamin E has been administered to very low birth weight infants, especially, to try to prevent or minimize the development of retrolental fibroplasia. Hittner and co-workers (1983) are of the opinion that its use has merit and provide a description as to how the vitamin might work.

ANEMIA

Diagnosis

The diagnosis of anemia in the newborn infant is not always a simple process. After 35 weeks of gestation, the mean cord hemoglobin concentration is about 17.0 g/dl; values much below 14.0 g may be regarded as pathologically low. During the first several hours following birth, the hemoglobin value may rise by as much as 20 percent, especially when clamping of the cord was delayed and, as a consequence, an appreciable volume of blood was expressed from the placenta through the cord into the infant. If, however, the placenta was cut or torn, a fetal vessel was perforated or lacerated, or the infant was held well above the level of the placenta for some time before cord-clamping, the hemoglobin concentration is more likely to fall during the hours after delivery.

Fetal to Maternal Hemorrhage

The presence of fetal red cells in the maternal circulation may be identified by use of the acid elution principle first described by Kleihauer, Brown, and Betke, or any of several modifications. Very small volumes of red cells commonly escape from the intravascular compartment of the fetus across the generally intact placental barrier into the maternal intervillous space. Although the bleed is usually small, it may incite maternal isoimmunization, as discussed below. Interestingly, evidence of maternal to fetal bleeding is very much less common (Bernard and co-workers, 1977). Presumably a pressure gradient that is higher on the fetal than on the maternal side persists across the placenta.

Rarely, fetal to maternal hemorrhage may be so severe as to kill the fetus (Fig. 21-5A, B, C). The hypovolemic or severely anemic fetus–infant may be salvaged if the condition is recognized and treatment with blood, red cells, or both is promptly initiated. The fetus who is severely anemic is more likely to demonstrate one or more ominous heart rate patterns (Chapter 14, p. 287). On occasion, the hemorrhage may have been chronic and so severe as to produce evidence of an iron deficiency in the fetus. Maternal iron deficiency, however, even when severe, is not accompanied by anemia in the fetus; the same holds true for maternal megaloblastic anemia due to folate deficiency.

With large fetal to maternal hemorrhage, there is most likely a placental lesion that fostered the leak. Chorioangiomas have been identified. Moreover, we know of two instances of severe fetal to maternal hemorrhage in which the mothers were later found to have choriocarcinoma. While neither placenta was studied, the subsequent recognition of choriocarcinoma in the mothers is suggestive of a placental lesion that was the site of transfer of blood from the fetus to the mother. Abruptio placentae, in our experience, does not appear to lead commonly to severe fetal to maternal hemorrhage.

At Parkland Memorial Hospital, for some time, maternal blood has been investigated for fetal red cells in each instance of stillbirth whenever a cause was not readily apparent. Massive fetal–maternal bleeds have been identified in a small minority of stillbirths. Laube and Schauberger (1982) identified massive fetal to maternal bleeding in 4 of 29 otherwise unexplained antepartum fetal deaths.

Large fetal to maternal hemorrhages may also prove dangerous to the mother. It is possible for up to 400 ml of fetal blood to be transferred from the fetal–placental circulation into the maternal circulation. A transfusion reaction may then develop in the mother whenever A or B antigen is present on fetal red cells but not on the red cells of the mother. Bergin and associates (1978), for example, described many of the characteristic features of a transfusion reaction developing in a mother who was blood type O immediately after delivery of an infant who was blood type B.

HEMOLYSIS FROM MATERNAL Rh$_o$ (D) ISOIMMUNIZATION

Ranking as major contributions to medicine are the delineation of the pathogenesis of most cases of hemolytic disease in the fetus and newborn infant by the observations especially of Levine and associates (1941), the related discovery of the Rh factor by Landsteiner and Wiener (1940), and the development of effective maternal prophylaxis by Freda, Gorman, and Pollack (1963) in the United States and Finn, Clarke, and associates in Great Britain (1961).

Blood Group Factors

Originally, the Rh concept was extremely simple, defined by one antiserum and two blood group factors, namely, Rh positive and Rh negative. The Rh factors, however, have been found to be increasingly complex, and a host

of other red cell antigens have been identified. Although some of them are immunologically and genetically important, fortunately, many are so rare as to be of little clinical significance in the genesis of erythroblastosis fetalis.

Any person who lacks a specific red cell antigen most likely will create an antibody when exposed to that antigen. The antibody may prove harmful to the individual in case of a blood transfusion or to her fetus when she conceives. The vast majority of human beings have at least one such factor inherited from their father and lacking in their mother. In these cases, the mother could be sensitized if enough erythrocytes from the fetus were to reach her circulation and an immune response were to be stimulated by the foreign antigen. In these terms, hemolytic disease is a possibility in nearly every pregnancy. That the disease occurs in very few pregnancies is a result of several circumstances. These include (1) the varying rates of occurrence of the offending red cell antigens, (2) their variable antigenicity, (3) insufficient transplacental crossing of antigen from fetus to mother, (4) the variability of maternal response to the antigen, and (5) lack of transfer of antibody across the placenta from mother to fetus in amounts sufficient to affect the fetus.

The Rh antigens are inherited independent of all other blood group antigens. There is apparently no difference in the distribution of the Rh antigens with regard to sex. There are, however, important racial differences. American Indians and Chinese and other Asiatic peoples are almost all Rh$_o$(D) positive (99 percent). Among black Americans there is a lesser incidence of Rh$_o$(D) negative individuals (7 to 8 percent) than among white Americans (13 percent). Of all racial and ethnic groups studied thus far, the Basques show the highest incidence of Rh$_o$(D) negativity (34 percent).

Rh antigens, other than D, possess low immunogenicity and are typically ignored unless the pregnant woman has already formed an antibody to them, which is detected by an antibody screening test.

At times, hemolysis in the fetus involves other antigen–antibody interactions, especially the ABO system. These are considered subsequently. *All pregnant women should be routinely tested for the presence or absence of Rh$_o$(D) antigen on their erythrocytes and for several irregular antibodies in their serum.*

Mortality

The number of perinatal deaths from Rh$_o$(D) hemolytic disease has dropped dramatically for the following reasons:

1. Pregnant women who are Rh$_o$(D) negative and possess antibody to the Rh$_o$(D) antigen can be readily identified.
2. Hemolysis in the fetus of the sensitized Rh$_o$(D) negative woman can be predicted with considerable accuracy by the identification of abnormally high levels of bilirubin in the amnionic fluid.

3. The fetus who is most likely to be seriously affected can be treated by intraperitoneal transfusions of $Rh_o(D)$ negative red cells or be delivered preterm before he expires in utero or both.
4. Of greatest importance, the appropriate administration to the mother who is $Rh_o(D)$ negative of $Rh_o(D)$ immune globulin during or immediately after pregnancy has eradicated most, but not all, $Rh_o(D)$ isoimmunization among $Rh_o(D)$ negative women.

The favorable impact on reducing perinatal mortality as a consequence of these procedures is exemplified by the experiences in Manitoba. In that Canadian province, the number of perinatal deaths from hemolytic disease decreased from 29 in 1964 to zero in 1974 and 1 in 1975 (Bowman and colleagues, 1977).

Immune Globulin Prophylaxis for the $Rh_o(D)$ Negative, Nonsensitized Mother

Hemolytic disease of the fetus and newborn from $Rh_o(D)$ isoimmunization has become a problem almost totally limited to Rh_o negative women who were sensitized before $Rh_o(D)$ immune globulin* was available. Freda and co-workers (1975) summarized their 10 years of clinical experience with $Rh_o(D)$ immune globulin, confirming their original observations that such immune globulin given to the previously unsensitized Rh_o negative woman within 72 hours of delivery is highly protective, although not absolutely so. There is good evidence to support the practice of giving the immune globulin promptly to previously unsensitized Rh_o negative women who have aborted including ectopic pregnancies and possibly hydatidiform moles, to women who undergo amniocentesis, and to those who bleed vaginally during pregnancy. The observation of Blajchman and co-workers (1974) of detectable fetal–maternal hemorrhage after at least 6 percent of amniocenteses has provided support for a policy that all unsensitized $Rh_o(D)$ negative women suspected of having an $Rh_o(D)$ positive fetus should receive $Rh_o(D)$ immune globulin following such a procedure.

$Rh_o(D)$ negative women who receive blood or some blood fractions are at risk of becoming sensitized. Red cells, of course, can supply massive amounts of foreign antigen if the cells are $Rh_o(D)$ positive and their recipient is $Rh_o(D)$ negative. It is not appreciated by all that platelet transfusions and large volume plasmapheresis can provide sufficient $Rh_o(D)$ antigen to cause sensitization, which could easily have been prevented by an injection of $Rh_o(D)$ antiglobulin. *Freda (1973) emphasized that when in doubt whether or not to give $Rh_o(D)$ immune globulin, the rule of thumb should be to give it.*

While adherence to the above guidelines, including the administration of $Rh_o(D)$ immune globulin to the

apparently nonsensitized mother within the first 72 hours after delivery of an $Rh_o(D)$ positive infant, dramatically decreased the risk of maternal isoimmunization, the problem was not eliminated. For example, Bowman and Pollock (1978) identified 1.8 percent of women to become isoimmunized in spite of adherence to the above recommendations for administering $Rh_o(D)$ immunoglobulin. They and their colleagues deduced that most often the failures were the consequence of spontaneous silent fetal–maternal bleeds that occurred some time before delivery and therefore some time before the administration postpartum of $Rh_o(D)$ immune globulin. To try to avoid isoimmunization from such fetal–maternal bleeds that occurred remote from term, 300 μg of antibody was routinely administered intramuscularly to all nonsensitized, $Rh_o(D)$ negative women at 28 weeks and again at 34 weeks gestation, as well as at the time of amniocentesis or uterine bleeding. If the infant was $Rh_o(D)$ positive, another dose of the immunoglobulin was administered to the mother after delivery. This program was followed by a reduction in the incidence of development of $Rh_o(D)$ isoimmunization during pregnancy from 1.8 percent to 0.07 percent. A single dose at about 28 weeks proved to be almost as effective as did the two doses antepartum; only 2 of 1799 $Rh_o(D)$ negative women showed evidence of $Rh_o(D)$ immunization, despite antenatal prophylaxis (Bowman and Pollock, 1978).

The small amount of antibody—perhaps 15 percent—that crossed the placenta resulted at times in a weakly positive direct Coombs test on cord and infant blood. None of the infants, however, showed evidence of anemia or exaggerated hyperbilirubinemia.

Recommendations. A single intramuscular dose of 300 μg of Rh_o immunoglobulin is administered routinely to all $Rh_o(D)$ negative, *nonimmunized* women at 28 to 32 weeks of gestation and again within 72 hours of the birth of a $Rh_o(D)$ positive infant. A similar dose is also given at the time of amniocentesis and whenever there is uterine bleeding, unless the routine dose at 28 to 32 weeks had been given very recently. If a massive fetal–maternal hemorrhage is recognized, more immune globulin should be given, as described below. One dose of 300 μg will protect the mother against a bleed of up to 15 ml of $Rh_o(D)$ positive red cells. Adoption of these dosage schedules will reduce the incidence of maternal isoimmunization to essentially zero.

Rarely, a woman who is classified as *RhD^u positive* may, when challenged with $Rh_o(D)$ antigen, develop antibodies that can hemolyze $Rh_o(D)$ positive red cells (Lacey and associates, 1983; White and associates, 1983). However, this phenomenon is rare. Whether to provide routinely $Rh_o(D)$ antiglobulin prophylaxis for RhD^u positive women is debated. We do not do so.

Maternal–Fetal Bleed. Rarely, the $Rh_o(D)$ negative woman will have been exposed in utero to $Rh_o(D)$ antigen from her mother and become sensitized as the consequence. For this to occur, the woman's mother must have been $Rh_o(D)$ positive and a maternal–fetal bleed

---

* $Rh_o(D)$ immune globulin is a 7S immune globulin (IgG) extracted by cold alcohol fractionation from plasma containing high titered Rh_o antibody. Each dose provides not less than 300 mg of Rh_o antibody as determined by radioimmunoassay.

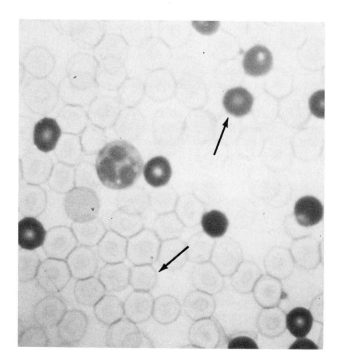

Figure 38-1. Massive fetal to maternal hemorrhage. After acid-elution treatment, fetal red cells rich in hemoglobin F stain darkly (*upper arrow*), whereas maternal red cells with only very small amounts of hemoglobin F (*lower arrow*) stain lightly.

must have occurred sometime before the cord was severed. As with fetal–maternal bleeds, a major blood group (ABO) incompatibility most often appears to offer appreciable protection against Rh_o sensitization. Jennings and Clauss (1978) in a study of 105 Rh_o(D) negative infants born to Rh_o(D) positive mothers identified a maternal–fetal bleed in only 2 instances, or 1.9 percent, a value in very close agreement with that found by Cohen and Zuelzer (1965). Jennings and Clauss (1978) and Bowman (1978), on the basis of their extensive studies, do not believe that Rh_o(D) immune globulin prophylaxis is warranted for Rh_o(D) negative babies born to Rh_o positive mothers.

Large Fetal to Maternal Bleed. In case of larger fetal–maternal hemorrhage, the Rh_o(D) positive erythrocytes may by careful examination be identified, at times, as clumps in the crossmatch of the erythrocytes from maternal blood and the Rh_o(D) immune globulin. The acid-elution technique, however, for identifying erythrocytes that contain appreciable hemoglobin is best used to identify a major bleed and to approximate its magnitude.

When the acid-elution test is performed appropriately, red cells rich in fetal hemoglobin are easy to identify (Fig. 38-1). A careful differential count will serve to approximate closely the percentage of fetal cells in the maternal blood. From this value, multiplied by maternal

hematocrit and by maternal blood volume, an estimate of the volume of fetal red cells in the maternal circulation can be made. (Maternal blood volume, i.e., the apparent volume of distribution of red cells in the intravascular compartment, will average about 5 liters before delivery and 4 liters shortly afterward.) The volume of fetal red cells so calculated, then divided by 15 (volume of red cells effectively inhibited by 300 μg of antibody), provides a reasonable estimate of the number of 300 μg ampules of Rh_o(D) immune globulin required for protection. If the estimate is doubled, almost certainly more than adequate protection would be afforded the mother. In practice, in cases of fetal–maternal hemorrhage, sensitization of the mother can be prevented by injecting sufficient Rh_o(D) immune globulin intramuscularly to provide demonstrable free antibody in the maternal serum.

In a case of massive fetal–maternal hemorrhage successfully treated at Parkland Memorial Hospital, 14 units of Rh_o(D) immune globulin (4200 μg at least) were injected intramuscularly over 48 hours to maintain a clearly demonstrable excess of antibody after delivery of a recently exsanguinated, very large infant. From the differential count of erythrocytes of maternal and fetal origin identified by acid-elution treatment of maternal blood (Fig. 38-1) and measurements of maternal hematocrit and blood volume, at least 150 ml of type O, Rh_o(D) positive fetal erythrocytes were demonstrated to have entered the maternal circulation. The mother did not become sensitized and subsequently gave birth to three unaffected type O, Rh_o(D) positive infants, including a set of twins. She remains free from evidence of Rh_o(D) sensitization.

The Rh_o(D) Negative Sensitized Mother

The mother who is sufficiently immunized to produce enough antibody to cause overt hemolytic disease in the fetus and newborn infant will have demonstrable Rh_o(D) antibody in her serum by the 36th week of gestation. Most often, if appropriate techniques are used, the antibody will be demonstrable much earlier.

According to Freda (1973), if nothing is done to interfere in the pregnancy of a sensitized Rh_o(D) negative woman with an Rh_o(D) positive fetus, the perinatal mortality rate can be anticipated to be about 30 percent. With aggressive management, including diagnostic amniocentesis, intrauterine transfusions in selected cases, and early delivery in most cases, the perinatal mortality rate can be lowered remarkably (Harman and co-workers, 1983).

For optimal outcome, individualization of management should be practiced, aided by the following information:

1. Past obstetric history with emphasis on fetal outcome and how that outcome was achieved
2. Accurate knowledge of fetal age
3. The Rh_o(D) zygosity of the father to identify those pregnancies in which the fetus has about a 50 percent chance of being Rh_o(D) negative

4. Maternal antibody measurements repeated throughout pregnancy
5. Spectrophotometric analyses of amnionic fluid
6. Identification of other pregnancy complications

Antibody Titer. An antibody titer (indirect Coombs test) that goes no higher than 1:16 almost always means that the fetus will not die in utero from hemolytic disease and that with appropriate care after birth he will survive. A titer higher than this indicates the *possibility* of severe hemolytic disease. It is emphasized that the titer in the previously sensitized woman may, during a subsequent pregnancy, rise infrequently to high levels even though her fetus is Rh₀ negative.

Amniocentesis. A suspicious titer, i.e., 1:16 or higher, in most cases warrants appropriately timed amniocentesis and measurements of bilirubin pigment in amnionic fluid. The technique for amniocentesis is described in Chapter 14 (p. 268). If use of intrauterine transfusion is being considered, amniocentesis may be initiated as early as 22 weeks gestation.

The absorbance of the breakdown pigment, mostly bilirubin, in the supernatant of amnionic fluid, when measured in a continuously recording spectrophotometer, is demonstrable as a hump with maximum absorbance at 450 nm wavelength (ΔOD_{450}), as shown in

Figure 38-2. The magnitude of the increase in optical density above baseline at 450 nm most often, but not always, correlates well for any gestational age with the intensity of the hemolytic disease.

Liley (1964) constructed a graph that provided for reasonably precise prediction of the severity of the hemolytic disease (Figure 38-3). His recommendations were as follows:

• If the increase in optical density falls in Zone 1 at 28 to 31 weeks, the fetus will be unaffected or will have mild hemolytic disease. Repeat the amniocentesis in 2 or 3 weeks.
• For Zone 2, the prognosis is less accurate and may require repeated amniocenteses to indicate a trend. In lower Zone 2, the infant's expected hemoglobin at birth will be between 11.0 and 13.9 g, whereas in upper Zone 2, the infant's anticipated hemoglobin will range from 8.0 to 10.9 g. Trends and time of gestation will obviously indicate the necessity for early delivery or intrauterine transfusions.
• Values in Zone 3 indicate a severely affected infant, and fetal death within 1 week to 10 days may be expected. The treatment—early delivery or intrauterine transfusion—will depend on the stage of gestation.

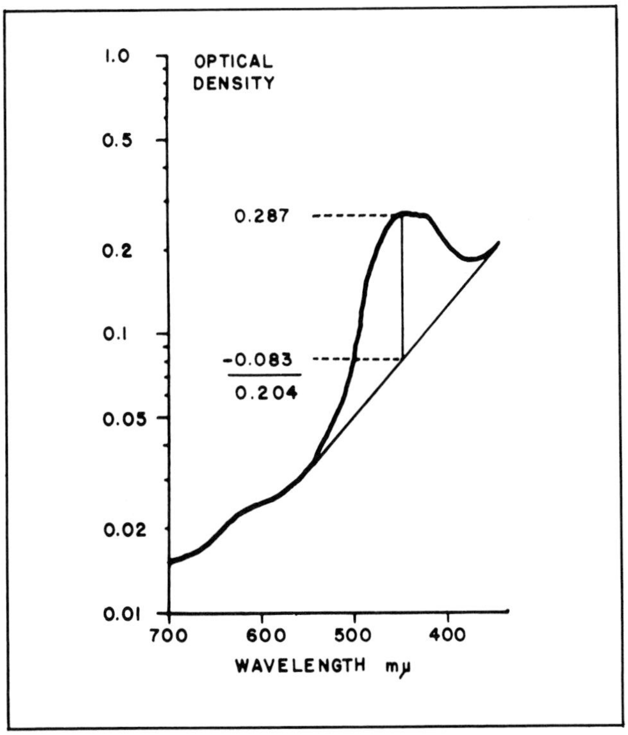

Figure 38-2. Spectral absorption curve of amnionic fluid in hemolytic disease. (*From Liley: In Greenhill (ed): Yearbook of Obstetrics and Gynecology, 1964–1965. Chicago, Year Book, 1964, p 156.*)

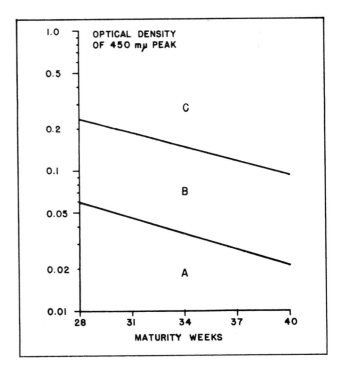

Figure 38-3. Clinical significance of the height of the peak of pigment in the amnionic fluid at different maturities. Zone A, mild or no hemolytic disease; zone B, moderate; zone C, severe. (*From Liley: In Greenhill L. (ed): Year Book of Obstetrics and Gynecology, 1964–1965 series. Year Book, 1964, p. 256.*)

Pathologic Changes in Hemolytic Disease of the Fetus and Newborn

Maternal antibodies gain access to the fetal circulation. In Rh positive infants, such antibodies are both absorbed upon the $Rh_o(D)$ positive erythrocytes and exist in a free form in the infant's serum. The adsorbed antibodies act as hemolysins, leading to an accelerated rate of destruction of the red cells. The earlier this process begins in utero and the greater its intensity, the more severe will be the effect upon the fetus.

Maternal antibodies detectable at birth gradually disappear from the infant's circulation over a period of 1 to 4 months. Their rate of disappearance is influenced to some extent by exchange transfusion. Detection of adsorbed antibodies is best accomplished by the direct Coombs test. If $Rh_o(D)$ red cells coated with $Rh_o(D)$ antibody are typed with an anti-$Rh_o(D)$ saline agglutinin serum, they may be reported incorrectly as $Rh_o(D)$ negative because of the blocking effect produced by the adsorbed antibody. Therefore, erythrocytes reported to be $Rh_o(D)$ negative from an infant whose mother may be isoimmunized must always be checked by the direct Coombs test.

Immune Hydrops. The pathologic changes in the organs of the fetus and newborn infant vary with the severity of the process. The severely affected fetus or infant may show considerable subcutaneous edema as well as effusion into the serous cavities (*hydrops fetalis*). At times, the edema is so severe that the diagnosis can be easily identified in the fetus by use of sonography (Fig. 38-4). In these cases, the *placenta* also is markedly edematous, appreciably enlarged, and boggy, with large, prominent

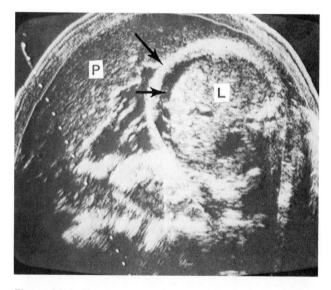

Figure 38-4. Transverse sonogram of a hydropic fetus. Illustrated are fetal ascites (*lower arrow*), edema of fetal abdominal wall (*upper arrow*), liver (L), and large placenta (P). (*Courtesy of Dr. R. Santos.*)

cotyledons and edematous villi. Excessive and prolonged hemolysis serves to stimulate marked erythroid hyperplasia of the bone marrow as well as large areas of *extramedullary hematopoiesis*, particularly in the spleen and liver. Histologic examination of the liver may serve to demonstrate, in addition, fatty degenerative parenchymal changes as well as deposition of hemosiderin and engorgement of the hepatic canaliculi with bile. There may be cardiac enlargement and pulmonary hemorrhages. Heart failure, however, at least at the outset, does not appear to play a major role in the development of ascites. Rather, portal hyptertension and severe hypoalbuminemia are more likely prominent factors in its development. The ascites, and to a lesser degree hepatomegaly and splenomegaly, may be so massive as to lead to severe dystocia as a consequence of the greatly enlarged abdomen. Hydrothorax may be so severe as to compromise respirations after birth.

Fetuses with hydrops fetalis may die in utero from profound anemia and circulatory failure (Fig. 38-5). The liveborn hydropic infant appears pale, edematous, and limp at birth, often requiring resuscitation. The spleen and liver are enlarged, and there may be widespread ecchymoses or scattered petechiae. Dyspnea and circulatory collapse are common. Death may occur within a few hours in spite of transfusions.

Hyperbilirubinemia. Less severely affected infants may appear well at birth, only to become jaundiced within a few hours. Marked hyperbilirubinemia, if untreated, may lead to central nervous system damage, especially to the basal ganglia, which is characterized clinically by lethargy, stiffness of the extremities, retraction of the head, squinting, a high-pitched cry, poor feeding, and convulsions. These signs are indicative of *kernicterus* (p. 780). In such cases, death usually occurs within the first week of life. Surviving infants may be physically helpless, unable to support their heads or sit. Ability to walk is delayed or never acquired. In less severe forms, there may be varying degrees of motor incoordination, whereas some infants demonstrate residual nerve deafness as the only manifestation of neurologic injury.

Anemia, in part resulting from impaired erythropoiesis, may persist for many weeks to months in the infant who had demonstrated hemolytic disease at birth. In the absence of hypoxia, erythrocyte production normally falls after birth, especially in the premature infant. The observations of McIntosh (1975) serve to implicate low production of erythropoietin in this phenomenon.

Fetal Transfusions

The refinement in prognostic precision furnished by the analysis of amnionic fluid led Liley (1963) to try in apparently hopeless cases intrauterine transfusion of blood into the fetal peritoneal cavity. The procedure, in general, should be limited to cases in which, between 23 and

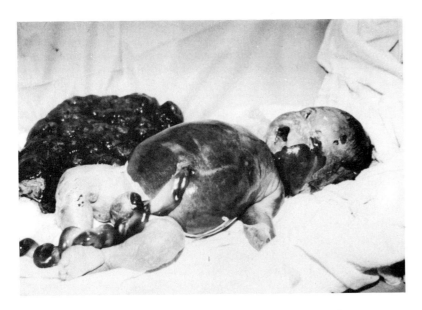

Figure 38-5. Fatal erythroblastosis fetalis. Severely hydropic macerated stillborn infant and characteristically large placenta.

32 weeks, the spectrophotometric tracings and history forecast, in all likelihood, death of the fetus. Thirty-two weeks represents about the earliest gestational age at which the nontransfused affected fetus, if delivered, has a reasonable likelihood of surviving the adverse effects of prematurity, hemolytic disease, and exchange tranfusion. For reasons that are not clear, the preterm infant with hemolytic disease from maternal Rh isoimmunization, unfortunately, is at increased risk of developing severe respiratory distress with hyaline membrane disease. Bowman (1978) has emphasized that, in his hands, mortality following fetal transperitoneal transfusions at 32 weeks gestation and delayed delivery is appreciably lower than with delivery at 32 weeks of an infant who lacks pulmonary maturity.

With intrauterine transfusion the overall survival rate in more recent years probably has been about 50 percent. However, the team in Winnipeg have been much more successful! They have reported recently 100 percent survival of nonhydropic fetuses and 75 percent survival of hydropic fetuses when treated with exchange transfusion, or an overall survival rate of 22 out of 24, or 92 percent (Harman and co-workers, 1983). They emphasized improved fetal evaluation through the use of real-time sonography before, during, and after intrauterine transfusion.

At the Winnipeg Center, 731 intrauterine transfusions have been carried out on 302 fetuses since the first transfusion was attempted in 1964. Mortality has decreased progressively as follows: 1964 to 1968, 55 percent; 1968 to 1972, 34 percent; 1972 to 1976, 34 percent; 1976 to 1980, 29 percent; the recent study cited above, 8 percent. (Importantly, the publicly funded Rh prophylaxis program in Manitoba has lowered the risk of sensitization of mothers in that province from 13 percent to 0.18 percent, and, in turn, has virtually eliminated the need for intrauterine transfusions among pregnant Manitoba residents. This is health care at its best!)

Other Modalities to Try to Minimize Fetal Hemolysis

In an attempt to prevent $Rh_o(D)$ antibody formation, to remove antibody already formed, or to block the action of the antibody on the red cell, a number of techniques have been tried without obvious success. *Plasmapheresis* does not appear to provide benefits that outweigh the risks and the costs. *Promethazine* (Phenergan) in large doses has been cited by some as being beneficial. It is not clear whether its benefits outweigh risks and costs; Charles and Blumenthal (1982) and some others believe this to be so. $Rh_o(D)$ positive *erythrocyte membrane* in enteric-coated capsules has been administered orally to sensitized women throughout pregnancy on the basis that such treatment might induce T suppressor cell formation that would, in turn, reduce antibody response to challenges by the $Rh_o(D)$ antigen. It does not appear to provide any benefit (Gold and co-workers, 1983). Attempts at immunosuppression with corticosteroids once were considered by some to be beneficial but subsequently were proven of no benefit.

Subsequent Child Development. In Bowman's experience (1978) the great majority of fetal transfusion survivors developed normally; 74 of 89 tested when 18 months of age or older were completely normal and 4 were abnormal, while development in 11 appeared to be delayed somewhat, perhaps because of preterm birth.

Delivery Before Term. In many circumstances, delivery somewhat before term is advantageous. Obviously, when it was considered necessary to utilize intrauterine transfusions, delivery, rather than further attempts at intrauterine transfusion, is desirable once sufficient maturity has been achieved to provide an excellent chance of survival.

Sinusoidal fetal heart rate and repetitious *decelera-*

tions have been identified in a number of circumstances, including erythroblastosis fetalis. These changes in the presence of Rh isoimmunization serve to imply, at least, that there is severe fetal anemia. Thus their message is ominous and should stimulate strong consideration for prompt delivery (Visser, 1982).

Whenever a decision is reached to terminate pregnancy before term, facilities adequate for care of premature infants must be available, as well as the necessary equipment for carrying out exchange transfusion. The neonatologist should be advised of the situation well in advance of delivery, so that skilled personnel, blood, and equipment can be immediately available in or adjacent to the delivery room. The need for immediate transfusion is determined by the hemoglobin concentration. Subsequently, the plasma bilirubin concentration is the important determinant.

Method of Delivery. The fetus who is to be delivered remote from term because of evidence of hemolytic disease will sometimes benefit from cesarean section. By so doing, the time of birth is set and the first team of neonatologists and laboratory personnel can be assembled to provide for precise evaluation of the infant at birth and optimal treatment at that critical time, as well as subsequently. Moreover, the likelihood of a difficult, prolonged, or unsatisfactory induction of labor is avoided. In any event, the fetus must be protected from hypoxia, acidosis, and sepsis.

Exchange Transfusion for Hemolytic Disease of the Newborn

Examination of cord blood should be carried out immediately for any pregnancy in which the $Rh_o(D)$ negative mother is known to be sensitized. The cord blood hemoglobin concentration and the direct Coombs test are of considerable importance when the infant is $Rh_o(D)$ positive. If the infant is overtly anemic, it is often best to carry out the initial exchange promptly to correct the anemia, using recently collected packed type O, $Rh_o(D)$ negative red cells.

For infants who are not overtly anemic, exchange transfusion is determined by the rate of increase in bilirubin concentration, the maturity of the infant, and the presence or absence of other complications. Exchange transfusion is not an innocuous procedure. However, if moribund, hydropic, and kernicteric infants are excluded, the mortality rate is 1 percent or less.

Sensitization to Other Blood Group Factors

A variety of other fetal red cell antigens that are lacking in the mother may be involved in the genesis of hemolytic disease in the fetus and infant.

ABO Incompatibility. The major blood group factors A and B have become the most common, but not the most serious, cause of hemolytic disease in the newborn. For example, group O women may from early life have anti-A and anti-B agglutinins, which may be augmented by pregnancy, particularly if the fetus is a secretor. Although about 20 percent of all infants have a major maternal blood group incompatibility, only 5 percent of them show overt signs of hemolytic disease. Moreover, when they do, the disease is usually much milder than that concerned with the Rh_o factor. Black infants are more likely to develop ABO disease than are white infants, according to Kirkman (1977). The disease does not appear to be any more severe, however, in black than in white infants (Peevy and Wiseman, 1978).

Desjardins and co-workers (1979) intensively studied a large number of infants of blood group O mothers to try to identify a relationship between the degree of red cell sensitization by antibody and the cord blood hemoglobin and bilirubin concentrations. They found that when the infant blood type was A or B, the bilirubin was higher and hemoglobin was lower than in cord blood from blood group O infants even when no antibody was identified on the type A or B red cells. They concluded that ABO incompatibility represents a spectrum of hemolytic disease that ranges from those in whom there is little laboratory evidence of red cell sensitization but some evidence of hemolysis to those with severe hemolytic disease in whom red cell sensitization is readily demonstrable.

The usual criteria for diagnosis of hemolysis due to ABO incompatibility include the following: (1) The mother is major blood group O, with anti-A and anti-B in her serum, while the fetus is group A, B, or AB. (2) There is onset of jaundice within the first 24 hours. (3) There are varying degrees of anemia, reticulocytosis, and erythroblastosis. (4) There has been careful exclusion of other causes of hemolysis. Unlike the result in Rh hemolytic disease, the Coombs antiglobulin test in ABO incompatibility may be negative, although it is usually positive.

The principles of management of the newborn infant with Rh disease may be applied to ABO hemolytic disease, particularly with reference to the behavior of hemoglobin and bilirubin. For simple transfusion or exchange transfusion, group O blood is used. Quite dissimilar to Rh hemolytic disease, the incidence of stillbirths among ABO incompatible pregnancies is not elevated. There is seldom justification for early induction of labor on this basis or for performing an amniocentesis except in the rare situation in which the previous infant was hydropic and no other cause was found.

Since there is no adequate method of antenatal diagnosis, careful observation is essential in the neonatal period if cases are to be detected. Although the infants with ABO hemolytic disease most often are less severely affected than are those with Rh hemolytic disease, they are equally incompetent in coping with excess bilirubin and its toxic effects on the central nervous system. Unlike Rh hemolytic disease, ABO disease frequently occurs in infants of primigravidas. It is likely, but not absolutely certain, to recur in subsequent pregnancies. Katz and co-workers (1982) identified a recurrence rate of 87 percent, with 62 percent of the affected infants needing treatment, most often just phototherapy for hyperbilirubinemia.

Other Fetal–Maternal Blood Group Incompatibilities

$Rh_o(D)$ incompatibility and ABO heterospecificity account for approximately 98 percent of all cases of hemolytic disease. However, nearly 400 other antigens have been identified so far on the red cell membrane. For each antigen there is the potential for hemolytic disease in the fetus and infant if the fetus possesses the antigen but the mother does not, the antigen has reached the mother and she has responded with antibody formation, the antibody is of IgG type and can cross the placenta to reach the fetus, and the antibody does so in amounts sufficient to cause hemolysis.

The possibility of hemolytic disease from rarer blood groups may be suspected from the results of the screening test for abnormal antibodies in maternal serum. Listed in Table 38-1 are a number of red cell antigens and their capacity for causing hemolytic disease when the fetus possesses that antigen and the mother is isoimmunized.

Mother as Provider of Rare Type Red Cells. Following isoimmunization of the mother who possesses a rare blood type, the possibility exists of hemolytic disease in the fetus and neonate. This could create a need for red cells devoid of the antigen or antigens to which the mother is isoimmunized. Moreover, the mother herself may require red cells, for example, because of a complication of placental implantation or a problem at delivery. For such circumstances usually she can successfully donate during pregnancy her own red cells, which are then appropriately frozen for subsequent use as demonstrated by the following case:

> G.D., a 17-year-old gravida 2, para 1, lacked immunologic evidence of all Rh antigens except $Rh_o(D)$ and had acquired antibodies during the previous pregnancy and puerperium to these missing antigens. Compatible red cells available in the United States were limited to 2 units frozen in Portland, Oregon. Therefore, repeated phlebotomies, according to the schedule provided in Table 38-2, were performed during the pregnancy, and the red cells were promptly frozen for possible use subsequently. In spite of her small size (57 inches tall and 109 pounds nonpregnant), she tolerated quite well the removal of 6 units (3 liters total) of blood at the rate of 500 ml every 3 to 5 weeks. Iron was provided orally and parenterally along with supplementary folic acid. Oral iron alone, if taken regularly, would have provided sufficient iron (Chapter 28, p. 564).
>
> Repeat cesarean delivery was accomplished without incident. The hemolytic disease in the newborn was treated with exchange transfusions using all of the red cells harvested and stored from the 6 phlebotomies plus the 2 frozen units from Portland (Pritchard and Cunningham, unpublished).

Others have reported on drawing blood from women with rare blood types during pregnancy for possible use at or after delivery. However, the timetables sometimes employed have made little sense. For example, in one instance, while albumin and crystalloid was being infused, 450 ml of blood was collected 10 days and again 3 days before planned delivery (Sandler and associates, 1979). The advantage gained, if any, from such manipulations is not clear, since red cell regeneration during the 10 days and 3 days before would be so slight as to not even cover the red cell loss imposed by collection and storage!

NONIMMUNE HYDROPS FETALIS

Hydrops fetalis, i.e., generalized edema of the fetus and newborn infant, need not have an immunologic basis as it does in cases of Rh-sensitized pregnancies. Anderson and co-workers (1983) found nonimmune hydrops in recent years to be more common than that associated with fetal red cell destruction by antibody of maternal origin. Hutchison and associates (1982) identified nonimmune hydrops to occur once in 3700 pregnancies. Nonimmune hydrops has been identified in utero much more frequently since high-resolution ultrasonography became available.

The formation and the accumulation of serous fluid in body cavities have been attributed to a great variety of causes, many of which were tabulated by Davis (1982) and by Hutchison and associates (1982) and are presented in Table 38-3. We and others (Mueller-Heubach and Mazer, 1983) have observed sonographic evidence of fetal hydrops, especially ascites, remote from term only to have the ascites disappear subsequently and the fetus to be normal at birth. Thus, there appears also to be a category of transient idiopathic hydrops.

Treatment, obviously, should vary considerably dependent upon the cause of the hydrops. However, the cause may be obscure to unknown before delivery. In general, when the hydrops persists and the fetus is mature enough to probably survive, delivery should be accomplished. When hydrops appears to be the consequence of heart failure, digitalization through maternal administration should be considered before delivery is attempted.

HYPERBILIRUBINEMIA

Disposal of Bilirubin

Before birth, unconjugated or free bilirubin is readily transferred across the placenta from the fetal to the maternal circulation (and vice versa, if the maternal plasma level of unconjugated bilirubin is high). Whereas the glucuronide of bilirubin is water soluble and is normally excreted by the liver and when the plasma level is elevated by the kidney, unconjugated bilirubin is not excreted in the urine or to any extent in the bile.

TABLE 38-1. OTHER RED CELL ANTIGENS AND THEIR PROPENSITY TO CAUSE HEMOLYTIC DISEASE IN THE FETUS–INFANT WHOSE MOTHER IS ISOIMMUNIZED

Blood Group System	Antigens Related to Hemolytic Disease	Severity of Hemolytic Disease	Proposed Management
Lewis[a]			
Kell	K	Mild to severe with hydrops fetalis	Amnionic fluid bilirubin studies
	k	Mild only	Expectant
	Ko	Mild only	Expectant
	Kp[a]	Mild only	Expectant
	Kp[b]	Mild only	Expectant
	Js[a]	Mild only	Expectant
	Js[b]	Mild only	Expectant
Duffy	Fy[a]	Mild to severe with hydrops fetalis	Amnionic fluid bilirubin studies
	Fy[b] [b]		
Kidd	Jk[a] [b]	Mild to severe	Amnionic fluid bilirubin studies
	Jk[b]	Mild to severe	Amnionic fluid bilirubin studies
MNSs	M	Mild to severe	Amnionic fluid bilirubin studies
	N[c]	Absent to moderate	Expectant
	S	Mild to severe	Amnionic fluid bilirubin studies
	s	Mild to severe	Amnionic fluid bilirubin studies
	U	Mild to severe	Amnionic fluid bilirubin studies
	Mi[a]	Moderate	Amnionic fluid bilirubin studies
	Mt[a]	Moderate	Amnionic fluid bilirubin studies
	Vw	Mild only	Expectant
Lutheran	Lu[a]	Mild only	Expectant
	Lu[b]	Mild only	Expectant
Diego	Di[a]	Mild to severe	Amnionic fluid bilirubin studies
	Di[b]	Mild only	Expectant
Xg	Xg[a]	Mild only	Expectant
Public Antigens	Yt[a]	Moderate to severe	Amnionic fluid bilirubin studies
	Lan	Mild only	Expectant
	Ge	Mild only	Expectant
	Co[a]	Severe	Amnionic fluid bilirubin studies
Private Antigens	Batty	Mild only	Expectant
	Becker	Mild only	Expectant
	Berrens	Mild only	Expectant
	Biles	Moderate	Amnionic fluid bilirubin studies
	Evans	Mild only	Expectant
	Gonzales	Mild only	Expectant
	Good	Severe	Amnionic fluid bilirubin studies
	Heibel	Moderate	Amnionic fluid bilirubin studies
	Hunt	Mild only	Expectant
	Jobbins	Mild only	Expectant
	Radin	Moderate	Amnionic fluid bilirubin studies
	Rm	Mild only	Expectant
	Ven	Mild only	Expectant
	Wright	Severe	Amnionic fluid bilirubin studies
	Zd	Moderate	Amnionic fluid bilirubin studies

[a] Not a proven cause of hemolytic disease.
[b] Not a cause of hemolytic disease.
[c] A rare cause of hemolytic disease.
(*With slight modification from Weinstein: Obstet Gynecol Surv 31:581, 1976.*)

Glucuronic acid is made available for this reaction by transfer from uridine diphosphoglucuronic acid catalyzed by the microsomal enzyme uridine diphosphoglucuronyl transferase. The conjugated bilirubin is secreted from the hepatocytes through the canalicular apparatus into the biliary tree and then into the small intestine.

Kernicterus

The great concern over hyperbilirubinemia in the newborn infant is its association with *kernicterus*. This complication occurs with greater frequency in premature infants. The yellow staining of the basal ganglia and hip-

TABLE 38-2. G.D., ISOIMMUNIZED AGAINST MOST Rh ANTIGENS EXCEPT Rh₀ (D)
(Gr 2, P 1, 17 Years, 57 Inches, 109 pounds Prepregnant)

Gestation (weeks)	Hemoglobin (g/dl)	Hemato-crit	MCV (mm^3)	Phlebotomy (ml)	Iron–dextran
14	12.0	35		500	500 mg
19		32		500	
24	11.4	34		500	500 mg
28		33		500	500 mg
31	11.1	32	95	500	500 mg
35		34		500	
36	11.1	32	Blood Volume 3826 ml (47% above nonpregnant)		
37	11.5	34	95	Cesarean section	

3060 g boy; Apgar score 9/9; hemolytic anemia; 4 exchange transfusions, subsequently thriving.

pocampus is indicative of profound degeneration in these regions. If the infants survive, they show spasticity, muscular incoordination, and varying degrees of mental retardation. There is a postive correlation between kernicterus and unconjugated bilirubin levels above 18 to 20 mg/dl, although kernicterus may sometimes develop at levels lower than this, especially in very premature infants.

Factors other than the serum bilirubin concentration contribute to the development of kernicterus. Hypoxia and acidosis enhance bilirubin toxicity. Both hypothermia and hypoglycemia predispose the infant to kernicterus by raising the level of nonesterified fatty acids, which compete with bilirubin for the binding sites on albumin and inhibit bilirubin conjugation. Sepsis contributes to kernicterus too, although the mechanism of action is not altogether clear. Sulfonamides and salicylates, such as aspirin, may increase the incidence of kernicterus because they compete with unconjugated bilirubin for protein-binding sites. Sodium benzoate in injectable diazepam, as well as furosemide and gentamicin, also uncouple bilirubin from albumin. Excessive doses of vitamin K analogs may be associated with hyperbilirubinemia. The importance of the serum albumin concentration and the binding sites so provided is obvious.

Breast Milk Jaundice

Breast-feeding can cause nonphysiologic jaundice in the otherwise normal newborn infant. The jaundice has been attributed to the excretion of pregnane-3(alpha), 20(beta)-diol into the breast milk by some mothers. This steroid was reported by Arias and colleagues (1964) to block bilirubin conjugation by inhibiting glucuronyl transferase activity. These observations have not been confirmed, however. Milks that cause hyperbilirubinemia have been described to have an unusually high lipolytic activity and thus can liberate large quantities of fatty acids that could inhibit bilirubin conjugation (Foliot and co-workers, 1976). Another explanation that has been provided is that bilirubin is broken down in the intestine to form free bilirubin, and the free bilirubin can be reabsorbed. However, cow's milk and normal breast milk appear to block the reabsorption of free bilirubin, whereas the milk of mothers with jaundiced offspring does not do so and may even enhance its reabsorption.

With breast milk jaundice, the serum bilirubin level rises from about the fourth day after birth to a maximum by 15 days. If breast-feeding is continued, the high levels persist for another 10 to 14 days and decline slowly over the next several weeks.

No cases of overt bilirubin encephalopathy have been reported due to this phenomenon, according to Maisels (1979), who also points out that there have been no prospective studies of the problem. One obvious solution to severe jaundice as the consequence of ingestion of breast milk is to discontinue breast-feeding and substitute an appropriate formula.

Physiologic Jaundice

By far the most common form of unconjugated nonhemolytic jaundice is so-called physiologic jaundice. In the mature infant, the jaundice increases for 3 to 4 days to achieve serum levels up to 10 mg/dl or so and then falls rapidly. In premature infants, the rise is more prolonged and may be more intense. The mechanisms involved in physiologic jaundice include, when compared to older children and adults, (1) normally increased rate of erythrocyte destruction and, therefore, of bilirubin production, (2) probably a decreased rate of uptake of free bilirubin by hepatic cells because of lower levels of Y and Z anion-binding proteins, (3) decreased rate of conjugation of bilirubin in the liver, and (4) reduced conversion of bilirubin to urobilinogen by bacteria in the intestines, which, in turn, allows a greater fraction of excreted bilirubin to be reabsorbed (enterohepatic circulation). Thus, almost every phase of bilirubin metabolism has been implicated.

Jaundice in the newborn infant should not be ignored as being physiologic in the following circumstances:

1. The infant is visibly jaundiced in the first 24 hours after birth.
2. The total bilirubin concentration in serum is increasing daily by more than 5 mg/dl.
3. The total bilirubin concentration is above 15 mg/dl.
4. Jaundice is visible for more than 1 week in a term infant or 2 weeks in a preterm infant.

Treatment for Hyperbilirubinemia

Exchange transfusion for hyperbilirubinemia is discussed earlier in this chapter. While exchange transfusion is not an innocuous procedure, the mortality rate is less than 1 percent when moribund, hydropic, and kernicteric infants are excluded from analysis.

Phototherapy is now widely used to treat hyperbilirubinemia. In most instances, its use leads to a lower bilirubin level from photooxidation of the compound. Light that penetrates the skin also increases peripheral blood flow, which enhances photodestruction of bilirubin. By some unknown mechanism, light seems to promote excretion of unconjugated bilirubin by the liver. Moreover, intestinal transit may be shortened, thereby reducing reabsorption of bilirubin from the gut. A common situation in which phototherapy is justified, beside that of the infant with hemolytic disease, is the jaundiced infant of low birth weight who appears otherwise well.

As much of the infant's surface as possible should be exposed, and he should be turned every 2 hours. His eyelids should be closed and completely shielded from the light. The infant's temperature must be closely monitored, and dehydration from the heat should be guarded against. Effective photodecomposition requires that the fluorescent bulbs be carefully selected and monitored for appropriate wavelength. The serum bilirubin concentration needs to be monitored for at least 24 hours after phototherapy has been stopped.

Phenobarbital has been shown to induce microsomal enzymes and thereby increase hepatic bilirubin conjugation and excretion. Possible adverse effects from such phenobarbital therapy must be considered, however. For example, phenobarbital inhibits fetal lung development in the rabbit fetus (Karotkin and colleagues, 1976) and brain growth in newborn rats (Diaz and associates, 1977).

HEMORRHAGIC DISEASE OF THE NEWBORN

Hemorrhagic disease of the newborn is a syndrome characterized by spontaneous internal or external bleeding accompanied by hypoprothrombinemia and very low levels of other vitamin K-dependent coagulation factors (V, VII, IX, and X). Bleeding may begin any time after birth but typically is delayed for a day or two. The infant may be mature and healthy in appearance, although

TABLE 38-3. CONDITIONS ASSOCIATED WITH NONIMMUNE HYDROPS FETALIS

Fetal
Hematologic
  Chronic transfusion—fetomaternal
              —twin to twin
  Homozygous α-thalassemia
  G6PD deficiency
  Multiple fetuses with parasitic fetus
Cardiovascular
  Congenital heart disease (septal defects, hypoplastic left heart, pulmonary insufficiency, intracardiac tumor, Ebstein's malformation, subaortic stenosis, tricuspid valvular dysplasia, tetralogy of Fallot)
  Premature closure of foramen ovale
  Tachyarrhythmias—supraventricular tachycardia
              —atrial flutter
  Bradyarrhythmias—heart block
  Fibroelastosis
  Myocarditis
  Hemangioendothelioma
  Arterial calcification
Pulmonary
  Cystic adenomatoid malformation
  Pulmonary lymphangiectasia
  Pulmonary hypoplasia
Renal
  Congenital nephrosis
  Renal dysplasia
  Renal venous thrombosis
  Polycystic kidneys
  Hydronephrosis
Intrauterine Infection
  Cytomegalovirus disease
  Toxoplasmosis
  Syphilis
  Leptospirosis
  Congenital hepatitis or cirrhosis
  Chagas disease
Congenital anomalies
  Chromosomal—trisomy 18
           —trisomy 21
           —Turner syndrome
           —XX/XY mosaicism
  Achondroplasia
  Tuberous sclerosis
  Storage disease
  Sacral teratoma
  Cystic hygromas
  Polycystic ovaries
Miscellaneous
  Meconium peritonitis
  Fetal neuroblastomatosis
  Small bowel volvulus
  Diaphragmatic hernia

Maternal
Diabetes mellitus
Severe preeclampsia-eclampsia

Placental
Umbilical venous thrombosis
Chorionic venous thrombosis
Chorioangioma

Idiopathic

(Adapted from Davis: J Reprod Med 27:594, 1982.)

a greater incidence of the disease has been noted in premature infants.

The prothrombin time and partial thromboplastin time are greatly prolonged. The coagulation changes of vitamin K deficiency, especially if accompanied by a lowered platelet count, might lead to an erroneous diagnosis of disseminated intravascular coagulation, which has a much poorer prognosis (Hathaway and co-workers, 1975). Moreover, the treatment of disseminated intravascular coagulation with anticoagulants, as recommended by some but not all, would intensify hemorrhagic disease of the newborn. In the differential diagnosis, hemophilia, congenital syphilis, sepsis, thrombocytopenic purpura, erythroblastosis, and traumatic intracranial hemorrhage must also be considered.

Plasma vitamin K_1 levels have been measured in normal nonpregnant adults and in pregnant women at term and their infants by Shearer and associates (1982). The levels were somewhat lower in pregnant women than in nonpregnant adults, but the vitamin was undetectable in cord plasma. One mg of vitamin K_1 administered intravenously to mothers shortly before delivery raised their plasma levels remarkably but produced only low levels in the cord plasma. Therefore, the physiologic hypoprothrombinemia in the neonate appears to be the consequence of poor placental transport of vitamin K_1 to the fetus. Subsequently, the chief cause of hemorrhagic disease of the newborn appears to be a dietary deficiency of vitamin K as a consequence of the small amount of the vitamin in breast milk in an infant already depleted at birth. The prothrombin time 24 hours after the start of feedings with cow's milk is comparable to that found 24 hours after vitamin K administration, whereas in infants receiving breast milk, it remains prolonged (Keenan and colleagues, 1971).

Serious reduction of vitamin K-dependent clotting factors during the first week after birth in infants of women with epilepsy treated with anticonvulsant drugs has been described by Mountain and associates (1970).

Prophylaxis. As prophylaxis against hemorrhagic disease of the newborn, the intramuscular injection of 1 mg of vitamin K_1 has proved very efficacious. For treatment of active bleeding, the vitamin is injected intravenously. Abnormalities in clotting are usually corrected over several hours.

The toxic effects of menadione, a synthetic vitamin K, and its derivatives in causing hyperbilirubinemia were the consequence of unnecessarily large doses, particularly to premature infants. Allison's original report (1955) and the deluge of subsequent publications relating the administration of vitamin K to the development of hyperbilirubinemia and kernicterus without exception dealt with excessive doses of the drug. In short, there is no evidence that the small but effective dose of 1 mg of vitamin K_1 (phytonadione) to the infant, or 2.5 to 5 mg given to the mother before delivery, is associated with significant hyperbilirubinemia or its sequelae.

IMMUNE THROMBOCYTOPENIA

Antiplatelet IgG antibody transferred from the mother to the fetus and causing thrombocytopenia in the fetus–neonate can be suspected when the mother has thrombocytopenia from an autoimmune disease, especially *autoimmune (idiopathic) thrombocytopenic purpura.* Avoidance of traumatic delivery and appropriate corticosteroid therapy to try to improve hemostasis are important to a successful outcome (Chapter 28, p. 575). The maternally produced antibody most often is directed against almost all platelets. Transfusion of donor platelets, therefore, is not of much benefit. Corticosteroids given to the infant may be of benefit and, in desperation, exchange transfusion and platelet transfusion may be tried. Blood transfusion may be necessary to help combat hemorrhage.

Isoimmune thrombocytopenia, in which there is maternal isoimmunization against fetal platelet antigens, is another cause of thrombocytopenia in the fetus–neonate. Even though diagnostic tests to type platelet antigens are not commonly available, the diagnosis can most often be made correctly on clinical grounds: (1) The mother has a normal platelet count, and there is no history or evidence on physical examination of a disorder that causes autoimmune thrombocytopenia. (2) The infant has thrombocytopenia without evidence of other disease. In case of active bleeding, treatment, ideally, should include transfusion with platelets compatible with those of the mother. Unfortunately, most of the donor population will have the platelet antigen to which the maternal antibody is directed. However, the mother's platelets are appropriate, since they lack antigen to which the platelet and antibody are directed. Therefore, platelets collected from the mother by plasmapheresis and differential centrifugation are likely to be of greatest benefit to the infant. When one infant has been affected, there is appreciable likelihood that a subsequent one will also be affected. Cesarean section to minimize birth trauma is likely to be advantageous to the affected fetus–infant, yet of little added risk to the mother, since she is not thrombocytopenic.

Thrombocytopenia develops rather often in newborn infants who suffer a variety of illnesses, especially those sick infants who are born remote from term.

POLYCYTHEMIA AND HYPERVISCOSITY

Several conditions predispose to polycythemia and hyperviscosity of the blood in the neonate. These include *transfusion* from the placenta, from a twin, or, much more rarely, from the mother, and *chronic hypoxia* in utero. As the hematocrit reading rises above 65, blood viscosity increases markedly. Signs and symptoms include plethora, cyanosis, and neurologic aberrations. Laboratory findings include hyperbilirubinemia, thrombocytopenia, fragmented erythrocytes, and hypoglycemia, as well as the high hematocrit reading. Treatment consists of prompt recognition and lowering of the hematocrit by partial exchange transfusion with plasma.

SOME INFECTIONS OF THE NEWBORN

The active immunologic capacity of the fetus and neonate is impaired compared to that of older children and adults. Passive immunity is provided by the mother, chiefly in the form of IgG transferred across the placenta. Unfortunately, the degree of passive immunity is much lower in premature infants than in term infants.

Infection, especially in its early stages, may be difficult to diagnose because of the newborn infant's failure to respond in classic fashion. The signs of infection can be vague, nonspecific, and certainly not dramatic until the infant becomes moribund. If infected in utero, he may have had a poor Apgar score for no other apparent reason. The infant may suck poorly, vomit, or develop abdominal distention. He may develop respiratory distress, which is quite similar in many ways to idiopathic respiratory distress–hyaline membrane disease. He may be lethargic or jittery. The response to sepsis may be hypothermia rather than hyperthermia, and the total leukocyte count in blood and the neutrophil count may not be influenced by sepsis, although the band count is likely to be increased.

Bacteria, viruses, fungi, or parasites may cross the placenta from the mother, or they may cross the membranes even though unruptured but, most commonly after rupture of the membranes. The organisms may infect the fetus in utero or during delivery. Thus, premature rupture of the membranes, prolonged labor, and excessive obstetric examinations and manipulations increase appreciably the risk of infection in the newborn infant. Sources of neonatal bacterial infections are as follows:

I. Intrauterine
  A. Transplacental
  B. Ascending amnionitis
    1. Premature rupture of membranes (common)
    2. Intact membranes (rare)
II. Intrapartum
  A. Maternal vaginal and cervical flora
  B. External contamination
III. Postnatal
  A. Transmission from handlers
  B. Equipment containing moisture
  C. Indwelling catheters

Infection at less than 72 hours of age is usually but not always caused by bacteria acquired in utero or during delivery, while infections after that time are most likely to have been acquired after birth.

A major mechanism for inducing infection in the infant subsequent to birth is by transfer of pathogens from those caring for the infant; the handler may harbor the organisms or may passively transfer the organisms from another infected infant. The use of indwelling venous and arterial catheters in the umbilical vessels after delivery demands scrupulous care to prevent infection. Life-support systems that involve moisture easily become contaminated with bacteria and can be the source of a life-threatening infection. It is apparent that the very low birth weight infant who survives the first few days after birth can be at considerable risk of dying later from infection that he or she acquires in the nursery unit (LaGamma and co-workers, 1983).

Any infant who appears ill should be suspected of having an infection. If infection is suspected at vaginal delivery, cultures of a swabbing from the ear or of gastric aspirate may be made; at cesarean section, amnionic fluid can be collected from the sac and promptly cultured. Subsequently, cultures of blood and cerebrospinal fluid are essential for appropriate evaluation of such an infant.

Bacteria Responsible

The bacteria most often responsible for sepsis in the newborn infant in the United States have varied remarkably during the past several decades. For example, in the 1930s and 1940s, group A β-hemolytic streptococci were principally involved. With the widespread use of penicillin, these streptococcal infections were reduced remarkably. Next came the staphylococcus in the 1950s and group B streptococcus in the 1970s.

At similar times elsewhere in the world, other pathogens were likely to have been more prominent than these in causing neonatal sepsis (Siegal and McCracken, 1981).

Staphylococci. In the 1950s, penicillin-resistant staphylococcal disease was observed in epidemic proportions. Reemphasis on handwashing, screening for carriers of unusually virulent staphylococci, and newer antibiotics controlled the epidemics.

Currently recommended procedures to control staphylococcal disease, especially in newborn nurseries, include the following: (1) Close attention is paid to each staff member's technique for handling infants; frequent, careful washing of the hands is important. (2) Routine umbilical care is performed, applying triple dye. (3) A program of continuous epidemiologic surveillance is essential.

Group B Streptococci. Currently, gram-negative organisms are the most common pathogens; however, group B β-hemolytic streptococci also are cause for concern.

It is clear that transmission to the fetus of group B streptococci from a colonized maternal genital tract can occur intrapartum, with the onset of severe sepsis in the infant soon after birth. Up to 40 percent of women during the third trimester of pregnancy harbor group B streptococci in the lower genital tract, and up to 20 percent of newborn infants are colonized. However, very few infants—perhaps 2 to 3 per 1000—develop clinical disease. For those who do demonstrate infection, unfortunately, the mortality rate is very high.

During the 1970s, group B streptococcal infections in the newborn increased remarkably in frequency, but then in many institutions the frequency decreased. The reasons for either the marked increase or the subsequent decrease are not clearly understood.

With the septicemia from group B streptococci that characterizes *early onset disease,* signs of serious illness develop within 48 hours of birth. Typically, membranes have been ruptured for some time before delivery, although rarely the organisms may infect the fetus even though the membranes remain intact. The preterm infant is more likely to develop serious clinical infection. The signs of early onset infection include those of respiratory distress, apnea, and shock. At the outset, therefore, the physician must be astute to differentiate the illness from idiopathic respiratory distress or transient tachypnea of the newborn. Immediate treatment with antibiotics, as well as treatment of the respiratory problems, is mandatory if the infant is to survive. The mortality rate with early onset disease has varied from 30 percent to as high as 90 percent!

Late onset disease usually becomes evident as meningitis a week or more after birth. Whereas the serotype with early onset disease varies from infant to infant, and most often is the same as in the maternal vagina, the serotype in cases of meningitis most often is serotype III. The mortality rate is appreciably less for late onset meningitis than for early onset sepsis.

Neonatal Prophylaxis. Steigman and associates (1978) from a retrospective evaluation reported an absence of early onset group B streptococcal sepsis in 130,000 newborn infants who had received 50,000 units of aqueous penicillin G intramuscularly at birth as prophylaxis against ophthalmia neonatorum. An extensive study (18,738 infants) was then carried out by Siegal and co-workers (1980). Aqueous procaine penicillin G, 50,000 units for infants who weighed 2000 g or more and 25,000 units for those who were smaller, was administered intramuscularly within 1 hour of birth as prophylaxis against ophthalmia neonatorum and also to evaluate its impact on group B streptococcal infections. The incidence of group B streptococcal disease was appreciably less, but not absent, in those who received penicillin. While the incidence of early onset group B streptococcal disease was decreased in the penicillin-treated infants compared to the control group, the incidence of infection caused by penicillin-resistant organisms and mortalities from these organisms appeared to be increased.

Pyati and co-workers (1983) did not identify penicillin prophylaxis to be of major benefit in preventing early onset group B streptococcal disease, in low birth weight neonates at least. The marked variation in the virulence of this organism makes identification of benefits from regimens of treatment and of prophylaxis very difficult to quantify.

Prophylactic administration of penicillin or ampicillin to women who were demonstrated to harbor the organism in the vagina during the third trimester has not proved to be very effective (Siegal and McCracken, 1981). Recurrence was observed commonly. Moreover, an appreciable number of women whose cultures were negative when evaluated in the third trimester were demonstrated subsequently by the time of delivery to harbor the organism.

A nosocomial source of infection has been identified for some cases of group B infections in the newborn infant, again emphasizing that careful attention to hygiene among personnel is essential.

Anaerobic Infections. Infection with anaerobic pathogens also has been recognized more frequently, in part because of better culture techniques and increased awareness of their importance. Anaerobic bacteremia may be self-limited with a favorable prognosis, regardless of antimicrobial therapy, but more often, it is associated with serious perinatal morbidity or mortality.

Epidemic Diarrhea of the Newborn

Outbreaks of epidemic diarrhea of the newborn may occur at any time, and many have been reported. Although it is unlikely that a single pathogen is responsible for all epidemics, certain pathogenic strains of *Escherichia coli* have been isolated in many outbreaks. It is probable that many of the epidemics are caused by these pathogenic colon bacilli and that the organism is brought into the nursery either by infected personnel, with or without symptomatic disease, or by an already infected infant.

The clinical symptoms are diarrhea with loose, watery, greenish stools, lethargy, dehydration, unstable temperature, and anorexia. The mortality rate varies, at times ranging as high as 6 percent in term infants and 35 percent in premature infants. No more infants should be admitted to the nursery, those affected should be isolated, and after the unit is evacuated, rigid cleansing of all equipment and of the nursery itself should be carried out. A stool culture should be obtained from all exposed infants to identify carriers and potentially ill babies.

NECROTIZING ENTEROCOLITIS

This condition commonly presents with the clinical findings of abdominal distention, ileus, and bloody stools and with radiologic evidence of pneumotosis intestinalis (gas in the intestinal wall as the consequence of invasion by gas-forming bacteria) and bowel perforation.

The disease is seen primarily in very small, premature infants but can also occur in larger, more mature neonates. Various causes have been suggested for necrotizing enterocolitis, including perinatal hypotension, perinatal hypoxia, sepsis, umbilical catheters, exchange transfusions, and the feeding of cow's milk and hypertonic solutions. The disease tends to occur in clusters.

Suspicion of developing necrotizing enterocolitis is raised by the presence of abdominal distention or blood in the stools. Usually, further oral feeding is withheld until these conditions clear. Although the prognosis appears to be improving with medical management and at times bowel resection, the etiology is not yet clear. Kliegman and Fanaroff (1984) have provided an extensive review of necrotizing enterocolitis.

RUBELLA

Rubella, or German measles, a disease of minor importance in the absence of pregnancy, has been directly responsible for inestimable pregnancy wastage and, even more serious, for severe malformations in the liveborn infant. The relation between maternal rubella and grave congenital malformations was first recognized by Gregg (1942), an Australian ophthalmologist.

Prevention

Epidemics of rubella have disappeared in the United States, but the disease and its potential for malforming offspring still prevail. Of the cases reported to the Centers for Disease Control in 1982, 62 percent were in people 15 or more years of age. To eradicate the disease completely, the following approach is recommended for immunizing the adult population, particularly women of childbearing age:

1. Raise awareness among health-care providers and the general public of the dangers of rubella infection.
2. See that susceptible women are vaccinated as part of routine medical and gynecologic care.
3. Encourage vaccination of all women visiting family planning clinics.
4. Identify and vaccinate unimmunized women immediately after they undergo childbirth or abortion.
5. Vaccinate susceptible women identified maritally.
6. Require proof of immunity for all hospital personnel who might be exposed to patients with rubella or who might have contact with pregnant women.

Diagnosis

The diagnosis of rubella is at times quite difficult. Not only are the clinical features of other illnesses similar, but subclinical cases with viremia and the capability of infecting the embryo and fetus do occur. Absence of rubella antibody indicates lack of immunity. The presence of antibody denotes an immune response to rubella viremia that may have been acquired anywhere from a few weeks to many years earlier. If maternal rubella antibody is demonstrated at the time of exposure to rubella, the mother can be assured that it is exceedingly unlikely that her fetus will be affected.

The nonimmune person who acquires rubella viremia demonstrates peak antibody titers 1 to 2 weeks after the onset of the rash, or 2 to 3 weeks after the onset of viremia, since the viremia precedes clinically evident disease by about 1 week. The promptness of the antibody response, therefore, may complicate serodiagnosis unless serum is collected initially within a very few days after the onset of the rash. If, for example, the first specimen was obtained 10 days after the rash, detection of antibodies would fail to differentiate between two possibilities: 1, that the very recent disease was actually rubella, or 2, that it was not rubella but the person was already immune to rubella. The demonstration of specific IgM in the pregnant woman indicates a primary infection within the previous month or so. Therefore, specific IgM estimations, if available, are useful for diagnosing recent rubella infection.

There is no known chemotherapeutic or antibiotic agent that will prevent viremia in nonimmune subjects exposed to rubella. The use of gamma globulin for this purpose is *not* recommended.

Effects of Natural Virus

The numerous reports concerned with the frequency of major fetal developmental defects that are thought to be caused by rubella are difficult to interpret because of the lack of precision inherent in the diagnosis of rubella. The frequency of congenital malformations, therefore, is probably higher than some reports have indicated. Rubella during the first month of pregnancy probably causes serious defects in up to 50 percent of the embryos and perhaps even more if those that abort spontaneously are considered. During the second month, the rate appears to be halved to about 25 percent, and during the third month, approximately halved again to about 15 percent.

It is now evident that many infants who are born alive suffer stigmata of continuing intrauterine and neonatal rubella infection. The syndrome of congenital rubella includes one or more of the following abnormalities:

1. Eye lesions, including cataracts, glaucoma, microphthalmia, and various other abnormalities
2. Heart disease, including patent ductus arteriosus, septal defects, and pulmonary artery stenosis
3. Auditory defects
4. Central nervous system defects, including meningoencephalitis
5. Retarded fetal growth
6. Hematologic changes, including thrombocytopenia and anemia
7. Hepatosplenomegaly and jaundice
8. Chronic diffuse interstitial pneumonitis

9. Osseous changes
10. Chromosomal abnormalities

Infants born with congenital rubella may shed the virus for many months and thus be a threat to other infants, as well as to susceptible adults who come in contact with the affected infants.

Infants whose mothers contracted the disease after the first trimester of pregnancy will not necessarily be healthy, as demonstrated by the investigations of Hardy and associates (1969). Their long-term prospective epidemiologic inquiry to assess the impact of the extensive 1964 rubella epidemic in this country revealed 24 instances of serologic evidence of infection by rubella virus after the first trimester. Of the 22 liveborn infants, only 7 could be considered completely normal when followed for periods of up to 4 years. Townsend and colleagues (1975) and Weil and co-workers (1975) have reported progressive panencephalitis beginning in the second decade in children with congenital rubella infection. An unusually high incidence of juvenile diabetes has been identified among individuals who had congenital rubella (Rayfield and Seto, 1978).

It is generally advised that rubella vaccination be avoided shortly before or during pregnancy. The vaccine is an attenuated live virus and can cross the placenta. Fortunately, there is little evidence so far that the vaccine administered to pregnant women induces serious malformations in the embryo or fetus.

TOXOPLASMOSIS

This protozoal infection is caused by *Toxoplasma gondii,* which is transmitted by eating infected raw or undercooked meat or through contact with infected cat feces. It can be acquired congenitally by transfer from the infected mother across the placenta to the fetus.

Maternal immunity appears to protect against intrauterine transmission of the parasite. Therefore, for congenital toxoplasmosis to occur, the mother must have acquired the infection during pregnancy rather than sometime earlier.

Fatigue, muscle pains, and sometimes lymphadenopathy are identified in the infected mother, but most often the maternal infection is subclinical. Infection in pregnancy may lead to abortion or to a liveborn infant with evidence of disease. Virulence of the fetal infection is greatest when maternal infection is acquired early in pregnancy. Most infants born with congenital toxoplasmosis do not manifest signs of clinical illness in the neonatal period. Those who do usually present evidence of generalized disease with low birth weight, hepatosplenomegaly, icterus, and anemia. Some infants will develop primarily neurologic disease with convulsions, intracranial calcifications, and hydrocephaly or microcephaly. Both groups of infants eventually develop chorioretinitis.

Screening blood tests include the Sabin-Feldman dye test, IgM fluorescent antibody test, and indirect fluorescent antibody test.

CYTOMEGALOVIRAL INFECTION

Cytomegalovirus is the most common cause of congenital infection, occurring in 0.5 to 2 percent of births. Perhaps 10 percent of infected infants will be severely and permanently damaged.

Fetal infection results presumably from hematogenous spread of the virus from the mother. Then the virus disseminates widely in the fetus. The disease may induce abortion, or the fetus–infant may suffer from a wide spectrum of serious abnormalities, including microcephaly, hydrocephaly, mental retardation, cerebral palsy, epilepsy, deafness, chorioretinitis, and blindness. Hepatosplenomegaly is common in severe cases. Hemolytic anemia and thrombocytopenia are also prominent in severe cases. The congenital disease may prove fatal.

Infected children shed the virus for protracted periods and can infect those who come in contact with them. Congenital infection can be documented by isolation of the virus from the nasopharynx or the urine. Specific IgM antibody is present in most, but not all, infected infants. The virus may be present in the infected mother's milk. The virus may also be acquired from transfusion of infected blood during the newborn period.

Children who appear normal neurologically at 2 years of age are likely to have escaped all or most of the ravages induced by this virus. There is no known effective treatment. Hopefully, a vaccine will prove preventive. Congenital disease can recur in subsequent pregnancies, although it seldom does so.

TORCH TESTS

In recent years, TORCH (*To*xoplasmosis, *O*ther, *Ru*bella, *C*ytomegalovirus, *H*erpes simplex) testing has become popular in the United States even though on careful analysis the information obtained often has not proven to be of any value and the cost is appreciable. Sever (1981) analyzed thoroughly the results obtained from TORCH package testings and condemned their routine use. The results from a significant number of laboratories were unreliable. Moreover, the presence of antibody did not exclude the presence of the pathogen in case of cytomegalovirus or herpes simplex (Table 38-4). He urged that such tests, when ordered, be selected on an individual basis.

CHLAMYDIA INFECTION

The microbe *Chlamydia trachomatis* has been cultured from the cervix of up to 13 percent of pregnant women (Alexander, 1979; Frommell and co-workers, 1979). Infants delivered vaginally, or after prolonged rupture of

TABLE 38-4. UNNECESSARY TORCH TESTS

Tests for	Unnecessary Use	Basis for Designating as Unnecessary
Toxoplasma	Routine screening of women	Clinical laboratory tests unreliable
	Routine test of paired sera during pregnancy	Outcome data for similarly tested women in US limited
Cytomegalo-virus	Routine screening of women	Reliability of clinical laboratories uncertain
	Routine paired sera during pregnancy	No outcome data on similarly tested women in US
		Recurrent shedding of virus occurs in presence of antibody
		Virus isolation best method for documenting active infection
Herpes simplex	Routine screening of women	Most antibody tests crossreact with HSV-1 and HSV-2; some cross with other herpes viruses
	Documentation of clinical herpes	Recurrent shedding of virus occurs in presence of antibody
		Antibody frequently does not increase with recurrence of infection
		Virus isolation best method for documenting active infection

(From Sever: Contemp Ob/Gyn 18:175, 1981.)

the membranes, from infected women are at some risk of developing conjunctivitis and pneumonia. The pregnant woman with a chlamydial infection can be treated with erythromycin, as can an infected infant.

The absence of elevated IgM in the cord blood of infants whose mothers harbored *Chlamydia* in their cervices is evidence against intrauterine infection; rather it is supportive of the infection being acquired during labor and delivery.

Whether chlamydial infection involving the reproductive tract is responsible for spontaneous abortion or preterm delivery is not clear at this time.

SYPHILIS

In the past, syphilis accounted for nearly one third of all fetal deaths. Indeed, delivery of a macerated fetus was considered diagnostic of syphilis. Today syphilis plays a smaller but certainly a persistent role in the causation of fetal and neonatal death.

Syphilitic lesions in the internal organs comprise essentially interstitial changes in the lungs (pneumonia alba of Virchow), liver (hypertrophic cirrhosis), spleen, and pancreas, and osteochondritis in the long bones. Osteochondritis is most readily recognizable radiologically at the lower end of the femur and the lower ends of the tibia and radius.

Under the influence of syphilitic infection, the placenta becomes larger and paler. Microscopically, the villi appear to have lost their characteristic arborescent appearance and to have become thicker and more club-shaped. There is a marked decrease in the number of blood vessels, which in advanced cases almost entirely

disappear as a result of endarteritis and proliferation of the stromal cells. Spirochetes are sparsely scattered through the placenta even when they are present in large numbers in the fetal organs. They may be demonstrated, however, by examination under the darkfield microscope of scrapings from the intima of the vessels of the fresh cord.

Shown in Figure 38-6A is an infant suffering from congenital lues with a large abdomen due mostly to marked hepatosplenomegaly. His placenta is seen in Figure 38-6B. It weighed more than the infant! Syphilis is discussed further in Chapter 28, p. 623.

DRUG ADDICTION

An unfortunately large number of women use heroin and other hard drugs during pregnancy. These women and their offspring suffer not only from the direct effects of the drug or drugs but are at appreciably increased risk of coincidental infections and varying degrees of malnutrition. Pelosi and co-workers (1975) observed the risks of the following pregnancy complications to be increased two to six times among pregnant women who used heroin: low birth weight (< 2500 g) from prematurity, growth retardation, or both; pregnancy-induced hypertension; late pregnancy bleeding; malpresentation; and puerperal morbidity. Interestingly, accelerated fetal lung maturation, manifested by a high L/S ratio in amnionic fluid and a low incidence of idiopathic respiratory distress in the newborn, is characteristic of pregnancies complicated by maternal heroin addiction.

One half or more of newborn infants of heroin addicts will develop withdrawal symptoms. Without treat-

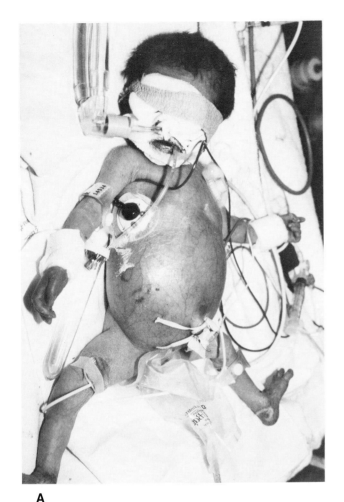

A

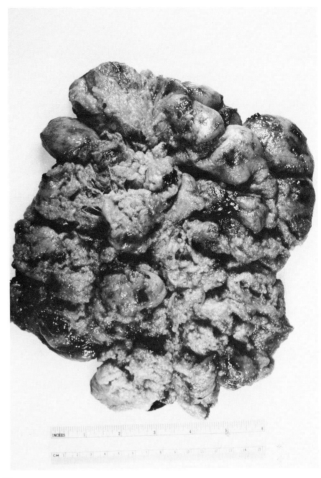

B

Figure 38-6. A. An infant born at 29 weeks gestation and gravely ill with congenital lues. Note the enlarged abdomen caused by marked hepatosplenomegaly plus ascites. (*Courtesy of Dr. G. Wendel.*) **B.** The large syphilitic placenta of the infant in Figure 38-6A. The placenta weighed 1200 g, almost the birth weight of the infant. (*Courtesy of Dr. G. Wendel.*)

ment, an appreciable number of these infants will die. The newborn infant must be closely watched during the first week of life for irritability, convulsions, nasal congestion, vomiting, diarrhea, tachypnea, and fever. Treatment has included paregoric, phenobarbital, chlorpromazine, and diazepam. Therapy is slowly withdrawn but reinstituted if the symptoms recur. Treatment may be required for many days to weeks.

Methadone treatment programs have commonly included pregnant women. Even though the drug is deleterious to the fetus–infant, it is probably less so than heroin. The newborn infant of the methadone-treated mother is also very likely to demonstrate withdrawal symptoms; Newman and co-workers (1975) reported an incidence of 80 percent and Harper and associates (1974) an incidence of 94 percent. Whereas withdrawal symptoms in the infant whose mother is addicted to heroin usually develop within 24 hours of delivery, the infant whose mother has been using methadone may not dem-

onstrate signs of withdrawal for a week or so after birth.

The mother's ability to care for her infant after discharge from the hospital should be assessed by frequent observations, including some in the home setting.

REFERENCES

Akenzua GI, Hui YT, Milner R, Zipursky A: Neutrophil and band counts in the diagnosis of neonatal infections. Pediatrics 54:38, 1974

Alexander ER: Chlamydia: The organism and neonatal infection. Hosp Pract 14:63, 1979

Allison AC: Danger of vitamin K to newborn (Letters to the Editor). Lancet 1:669, 1955

Anderson HM, Hutchison AA, Fortune DW: Non-immune hydrops fetalis: A changing contribution to perinatal mortality. Br J Obstet Gynaecol 90:636, 1983

Arias IM, Gartner LM, Seifter S, Furman M: Prolonged neonatal unconjugated hyperbilirubinemia associated with breast feeding and steroid, pregnane-3(alpha),20(beta)-diol in maternal milk that inhibits glucuronide formation in vitro. J Clin Invest 43:2037, 1964

Bartlett RH: Extracorporeal oxygenation in neonates. Hospital Practice 19:139, 1984

Bergin FT, Cefalo RC, Lewis PE: Self-limited hemolytic transfusion reaction in an ABO-incompatible maternal-fetal unit. Am J Obstet Gynecol 132:116, 1978

Bernard B, Presley M, Caudillo G, Clauss B, Rouault CL, McGregor J, Jennings ER: Maternal-fetal hemorrhage: Incidence and sensitization. Pediatr Res 11:467, 1977

Blajchman MA, Maudsley RF, Uchida I, Zipursky A: Diagnostic amniocentesis and fetal-maternal bleeding. Lancet 1:993, 1974

Bowman JM: The management of Rh-isoimmunization. Obstet Gynecol 52:1, 1978

Bowman JM: Suppression of Rh isoimmunization. A review. Obstet Gynecol 52:385, 1978

Bowman JM, Pollock JM: Antenatal Rh prophylaxis: 28 week gestation service program. Can Med Assoc J 118:622, 1978

Bowman JM, Chown B, Lewis M, Pollock J: Rh isoimmunization, Manitoba, 1963–1975. Can Med Assoc J 116:282, 1977

Charles AG, Blumenthal LS: Promethazine hydrochloride therapy in severe Rh-sensitized pregnancies. Obstet Gynecol 60:627, 1982

Cohen F, Zuelzer WW: The transplacental passage of maternal erythrocytes into the fetus. Am J Obstet Gynecol 93:566, 1965

Davis CL: Diagnosis and management of nonimmune hydrops fetalis. J Reprod Med 27:594, 1982

Desjardins L, Blajchman MA, Chintu C, Gent M, Zipursky A: The spectrum of ABO hemolytic disease of the newborn infant. J Pediatr 95:447, 1979

Diaz J, Schain RJ, Bailey BG: Phenobarbital-induced brain growth retardation in artificially reared rat pups. Biol Neonate 32:77, 1977

Ehrenkranz RA, Ablow RC, Warshaw JB: Prevention of bronchopulmonary dysplasia with vitamin E administration during the acute stages of respiratory distress syndrome. J Pediatr 95:873, 1979

Ehrenkranz RA, Bonta BW, Ablow RC, Warshaw JB: Amelioration of bronchopulmonary dysplasia after vitamin E administration. N Engl J Med 299:564, 1978

Farrell PM, Wood RE: Epidemiology of hyaline membrane disease in the United States: Analysis of national mortality statistics. Pediatrics 58:167, 1976

Finn R, Clarke CA, Donohoe W, McConnell RB, Sheppard PM, Lehane D, Kulke W: Experimental studies on the prevention of Rh haemolytic disease. Br Med J 1:1486, 1961

Foliot A, Ploussard JP, Housset E, Christoforov B: Breast milk jaundice: In vitro inhibition of rat liver bilirubin-uridine diphosphate glucuronyltransferase activity and Z protein-bromosulfonphthalein binding by human breast milk. Pediatr Res 10:594, 1976

Freda V: Hemolytic disease. Clin Obstet Gynecol 16:72, 1973

Freda VJ, Gorman JG, Pollack W: Successful prevention of sensitization to Rh with an experimental anti-Rh gamma$_2$ globulin antibody preparation. Fed Proc 22:374, 1963

Freda VJ, Gorman JG, Pollack W, Bowe E: Prevention of Rh hemolytic disease: Ten years clinical experience with Rh immune globulin. N Engl J Med 292:1014, 1975

Frommell GT, Rothenberg R, Wang S, McIntosh K: Chlamydial infections of mothers and their infants. J Pediatr 95:28, 1979

Gold WR Jr, Queenan JT, Woody J, Sacher RA: Oral desensitization in Rh disease. Am J Obstet Gynecol 146:980, 1983

Gregg NM: Congenital cataract following German measles in the mother. Trans Ophthalmol Soc Aust 3:35, 1942

Hamilton EG: Intrauterine transfusion for Rh disease: A status report. Hosp Pract 13:113, 1978

Hardy JB, McCracken GH, Jr, Gilkeson MR, Sever JL: Adverse fetal outcome following maternal rubella after the first trimester of pregnancy. JAMA 207:2414, 1969

Harman CR, Manning FA, Bowman JM, Lange IR: Severe Rh disease—Poor outcome is not inevitable. Am J Obstet Gynecol 145:823, 1983

Harper RG, Solish GI, Purow HM, Sang E, Panepinto WC: The effect of a methadone treatment program upon pregnant heroin addicts and their newborn infants. Pediatrics 54:300, 1974

Hathaway WE, Mahasandana C, Makowski EL: Cord blood coagulation studies in infants of high-risk pregnant women. Am J Obstet Gynecol 121:51, 1975

Hittner HM, Godio LB, Speer ME, Rudolph AJ, Taylor MM, Blifeld C, Kretzer FL: Retrolental fibroplasia: Further clinical evidence and ultrastructural support for efficacy of vitamin E in the preterm infant. Pediatrics 71:423, 1983

Holt EM, Boyd IE, Dewhurst CH, Murray J, Naylor CH, Smitham JH: Intrauterine transfusion: 101 consecutive cases treated at Queen Charlotte's Maternity Hospital. Br Med J 3:39, 1973

Hutchison AA, Drew JH, Yu VYH, Williams ML, Fortune DW, Beischer NA: Nonimmunologic hydrops fetalis: A review of 61 cases. Obstet Gynecol 59:347, 1982

Jennings ER, Clauss B: Maternal-fetal hemorrhage: Its incidence and sensitizing effects. Am J Obstet Gynecol 131:725, 1978

Karotkin EH, Kido M, Redding R, Cashore WJ, Douglas W, Stern L, Oh W: The inhibition of pulmonary maturation in the fetal rabbit by maternal treatment with phenobarbital. Am J Obstet Gynecol 124:529, 1976

Katz MA, Kanto WP Jr, Korotkein JH: Recurrence rate of ABO hemolytic disease of the newborn. Obstet Gynecol 59:611, 1982

Keenan WJ, Jewitt T, Glueck HI: Role of feeding and vitamin K in hypoprothrombinemia of the newborn. Am J Dis Child 121:271, 1971

Kinsey VE, Arnold HJ, Kalina RE, Stern L, Stahlman M, Odell G, Driscoll J, Elliott J, Payne J, Patz A: PaO$_2$ levels and retrolental fibroplasia: A report of the cooperative study. Pediatrics 60:655, 1977

Kirkman HN Jr: Further evidence for a radical difference in the frequency of ABO hemolytic disease. J Pediatr 90:717, 1977

Kliegman RM, Fanaroff AA: Necrotizing enterocolitis. N Engl J Med 310:1093, 1984

Lacey PA, Caskey CR, Werner DJ, Moulds JJ: Fatal hemolytic disease of a newborn due to anti-D in an Rh-positive Du variant mother. Transfusion 23:91, 1983

LaGamma EF, Drusin LM, Mackles AW, Machalek S, Auld PAM: Neonatal infections. Am J Dis Child 137:838, 1983

Landsteiner K, Wiener AS: An agglutinable factor in human blood recognized by immune sera for rhesus blood. Proc Soc Exp Biol NY 43:223, 1940

Laube DW, Schauberger CW: Fetomaternal bleeding as a cause for "unexplained" fetal death. Obstet Gynecol 60:649, 1982

Levine P, Katzin E, Burnham L: Isoimmunization in pregnancy. JAMA 116:825, 1941

Liley AW: Intrauterine transfusion of foetus in hemolytic disease. Br Med J 2:1107, 1963

Liley AW: Amniocentesis and amniography in hemolytic disease. In Greenhill JP (ed): Yearbook of Obstetrics and Gynecology, 1964–1965 series. Chicago, Year Book, 1964, p 256

Maisels MJ: Neonatal jaundice: III. Breast feeding and jaundice. Perinat Press 3:19, 1979

Marshall R, Tyrala E, McAlister W, Sheehan M: Meconium aspiration syndrome. Neonatal and follow-up study. Am J Obstet Gynecol 131:672, 1978

McIntosh S: Erythropoietin excretion in the premature infant. J Pediatr 86:202, 1975

Mountain K, Hirsh J, Gallus AS: Neonatal coagulation defect and maternal anti-convulsant treatment. Lancet 1:265, 1970

Mueller-Heubach E, Mazer J: Sonographically documented disappearance of fetal ascites. Obstet Gynecol 61:253, 1983

Newman RG, Bashkow S, Calko D: Results of 313 consecutive live births of infants delivered to patients in the New York City methadone maintenance treatment program. Am J Obstet Gynecol 121:233, 1975

Palmer A, Gordon RR: A critical review of intrauterine fetal transfusion. Br J Obstet Gynaecol 83:688, 1976

Peevy KJ, Wiseman HJ: ABO hemolytic disease of the newborn: Evaluation of management and identification of racial and antigenic factors. Pediatrics 61:475, 1978

Pelosi MA, Frattarola M, Apuzzio J, Langer A, Hung CT, Oleske JM, Bai J, Harrigan JT: Pregnancy complicated by heroin addiction. Obstet Gynecol 45:512, 1975

Pyati SP, Pildes RS, Jacobs NM, Ramamurthy RS, Yeh TF, Raval DS, Lilien LD, Amma P, Metzger WI: Penicillin in infants weighing two kilograms or less with early-onset group B streptococcal disease. N Engl J Med 308:1383, 1983

Rayfield EJ, Seto Y: Viruses and the pathogenesis of diabetes mellitus. Diabetes 27:1126, 1978

Renaer M, Van de Putte R, Vermylen C: Massive feto-maternal hemorrhage as a cause of perinatal mortality and morbidity. Eur J Obstet Gynecol Reprod Biol 6:125, 1976

Robertson EG, Brown A, Ellis MI, Walker W: Intrauterine transfusion in the management of severe rhesus isoimmunization. Br J Obstet Gynaecol 83:694, 1976

Sandler SG, Beyth Y, Laufer N, Levene C: Autologous blood transfusions and pregnancy. Obstet Gynecol 53:62 [Suppl], 1979

Sever JL: Is this test necessary? Contemp Ob/Gyn 18:175, 1981

Shearer MJ, Barkhan P, Rahim S, Stimmler L: Plasma vitamin K_1 in mothers and their newborn babies. Lancet 2:460, 1982

Siegal JD, McCracken GH Jr: Sepsis neonatorum. N Engl J Med 304:642, 1981

Siegal JD, McCracken GH Jr, Rosenfeld CR: Effects of a single intramuscular dose of penicillin on neonatal colonization and disease rates due to group B and D streptococci. Presented at 11th International Congress of Chemotherapy—19th Interscience Conference on Antimicrobial Agents and Chemotherapy, Boston, Oct 1979

Siegal JD, McCracken GH Jr, Threlkeld N, Milvenan B, Rosenfeld CR: Single-dose penicillin prophylaxis against neonatal group B streptococcal infections. N Engl J Med 303:769, 1980

Stahlman M, Hedvall G, Lindstrom D, Snell J: Role of hyaline membrane disease in production of later childhood lung abnormalities. Pediatrics 69:572, 1982

Steigman AJ, Bottone EJ, Hanna BA: Control of perinatal group B streptococcal sepsis: Efficacy of single injection of aqueous penicillin at birth. Mt Sinai J Med 45:685, 1978

Taylor WW, Scott DE, Pritchard JA: Fate of compatible adult erythrocytes in the fetal peritoneal cavity. Obstet Gynecol 18:175, 1966

Townsend JJ, Baringer JR, Wolinsky JS, Malamud N, Mednick JP, Pantich HS, Scott RAT, Oshiro LS, Cremer NE: Progressive rubella panencephalitis: Late onset after congenital rubella. N Engl J Med 292:990, 1975

Visser GHA: Antepartum sinusoidal and decelerative heart rate patterns in Rh disease. Am J Obstet Gynecol 143:538, 1982

Weil ML, Itabashi HH, Cremer NE, Oshiro LS, Lennette EH, Carnay L: Chronic progressive panencephalitis due to rubella virus simulating subacute sclerosing panencephalitis. N Engl J Med 292:994, 1975

White CA, Stedman CM, Frank S: Anti-D antibodies in D- and D^u-positive women: A cause of hemolytic disease of the newborns. Am J Obstet Gynecol 145:1069, 1983

Workshop on Bronchopulmonary Dysplasia. J Pediatr 95:815, 1979

Yeh TF, Harris V, Srinvasin G, Lilien L, Pyati S, Pildes RS: Roentgenographic findings in infants with meconium aspiration syndrome. JAMA 242:60, 1979

Zuspan FP (ed): Drug addiction in pregnancy: An invitational symposium. J Reprod Med 20:301, 1978

39

Injuries and Malformations of the Fetus and Newborn Infant

Considered in this chapter are several varieties of birth injuries and malformations. Other birth injuries and malformations are described elsewhere in connection with the specific obstetric complication that led to or contributed to the injury or was created by the malformation. Hydrocephaly, for example, is considered under Dystocia Caused by Abnormalities of the Fetus (Chapter 30, p. 669).

INJURIES

Intracranial Hemorrhages

Hemorrhage within the head of the fetus–infant may be located at any of several sites: subdural, subarachnoid, cortical, white matter, cerebellar, intraventricular, and periventricular. Birth trauma may cause intracranial hemorrhage but is no longer a common cause. The head of the fetus may undergo molding during passage through the birth canal. The skull bones, the dura mater, and the brain itself permit considerable alteration in the shape of the fetal head without untoward results. The dimensions of the head are changed, with lengthening especially of the occipitofrontal diameter of the skull (Fig. 39-1). Bridging veins from the cerebral cortex to the sagittal sinus may tear as a consequence of severe molding and marked overlap of the parietal bones or of difficult forceps delivery. Less common are rupture of the internal cerebral veins, the vein of Galen at its junction with the straight sinus, or the tentorium itself. Compression of the skull can stretch the tentorium cerebelli and may tear the vein of Galen or its tributaries. The common types and locations of intracranial hemorrhages are illustrated in Figure 39-2. Wigglesworth and Pape (1980) have provided lucid descriptions of the pathophysiology of intracranial hemorrhages in the newborn.

Illingworth (1979), an English pediatrician, rightfully contended that obstetricians have been blamed unjustifiably for causing brain damage and other injuries, the genesis of which was not limited just to difficulties during labor and delivery but involved prenatal factors, in-

cluding those that were genetic and social in nature. Nonetheless, the elimination of difficult forceps operations, the use of cesarean section when there was cephalopelvic disproportion, the correct management of breech delivery, and the virtual eradication of internal podalic version and extraction have all contributed significantly to the reduction in the incidence of all birth injuries, including intracranial hemorrhage.

Signs and Symptoms. Commonly, infants suffering intracranial hemorrhage from mechanical injury are born depressed, but their conditions appear to improve until about 12 hours of age. Then drowsiness, apathy, feeble cry, pallor, failure to nurse, dyspnea, cyanosis, vomiting, and convulsions may become evident. Atelectasis, asphyxia, meconium aspiration, and forceps trauma may be associated findings. To help rule out diaphragmatic hernia, congenital heart disease, atelectasis, idiopathic respiratory distress, and pneumonia, prompt roentgenographic examination of the chest is useful. In very recent years, scanning of the neonate's head using sonography and computerized tomography (CT scan) has not only proved of diagnostic value but also has contributed appreciably to an understanding of the etiology of some forms of intracranial hemorrhage and the frequency with which they occur. For example, periventricular and intraventricular hemorrhages are relatively common in infants who were born quite prematurely. Moreover, such hemorrhages occur in the absence of birth trauma. Hadlock and co-workers (1983) and Shankarin and associates (1983) have well described the use of high-resolution real-time ultrasound scanners to identify intracranial hemorrhages.

Treatment. Therapy includes oxygen for the dyspnea and cyanosis and sedation to control convulsions. The blood can be removed from some subdural hematomas by careful needle aspiration. In other instances, surgical intervention may be required. The value of administering clotting factors from plasma to infants with an intracranial hemorrhage is not clear. However, prompt

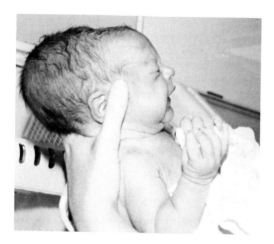

Figure 39-1. Molding of head, newborn child.

intramuscular administration of vitamin K to all newborn infants is indicated (Chapter 38, p. 782).

The surviving infants may subsequently develop functional disturbances, including cerebral palsy and mental deficiency. Certain cases of idiopathic epilepsy may also be caused by intracranial injury sustained at birth.

Cerebral Palsy

Multiple definitions have been proposed for *cerebral palsy*. The term is probably most widely used to identify persons handicapped by motor disorders due to nonprogressive abnormalities of the brain that appeared early in life. Recognized patterns of motor disturbances include the spastic type, the atheoid type, the ataxic type, the atonic type, and mixed forms. Cerebral palsy may result from preterm birth complicated by asphyxia in utero or in the newborn period, from severe hyperbilirubinemia, from cerebellar or cerebral malformations, and from infections acquired in utero, such as cytomegalovirus. Holm (1982) has provided a review of 142 cases of cerebral palsy. One half were the consequence of events that occurred before labor and delivery. No more than 10 percent were considered to be caused by labor and the method of delivery. Whenever possible, the specific brain lesion and its probable cause should be stated, rather than simply applying the term *cerebral palsy*.

Cephalohematoma

A cephalohematoma is usually caused by injury to the periosteum of the skull during labor and delivery (Fig. 39-3), although it may develop in the absence of birth

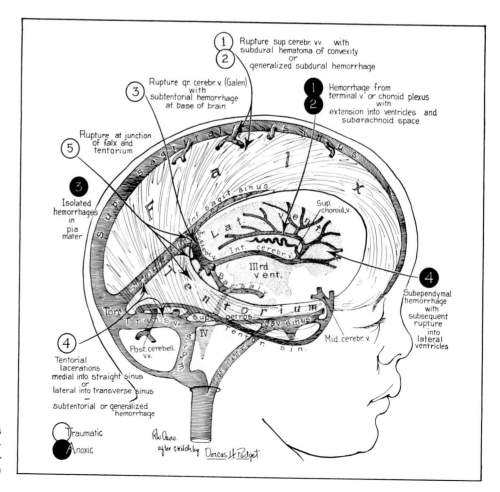

Figure 39-2. The common types and locations of intracranial hemorrhage. (*From Haller et al.: Obstet Gynecol Surv 11:179, 1956.*)

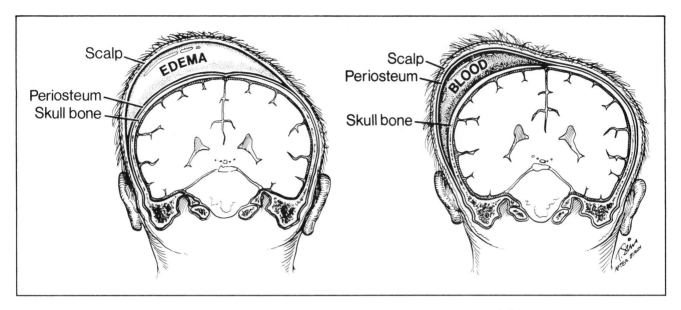

Figure 39-3. Difference between a large caput succedaneum (*left*) and cephalohematoma (*right*). In a caput succedaneum, the effusion overlies the periosteum and consists of edema fluid; in a cephalohematoma, it lies under the periosteum and consists of blood.

trauma when hemotasis is defective. The subperiosteal hemorrhages may develop over one or both parietal bones. The periosteal limitations with definite palpable edges differentiate the cephalohematoma from *caput succedaneum.* The latter lesion consists of a focal swelling of the scalp from edema fluid that overlies the periosteum (Fig. 39-3). Furthermore, a cephalohematoma may not appear for hours after delivery, often growing larger and disappearing only after weeks or even months (Fig 39-4A, B). In contrast, a caput succedaneum is at maximum at birth, grows smaller, and disappears usually within a few hours if small and within a few days even when very large.

Increasing size of the hematoma and other evidence of extensive hemorrhage are indications for additional investigation, including roentgenographic studies of the skull and assessment of coagulation factors, since the infant may have defective blood clotting, as exemplified by the infant with severe thrombocytopenia illustrated in Figure 28-5.

Spinal Injury

Overstretching of the spinal cord and associated hemorrhage may follow excessive traction during a breech delivery, and actual fracture or dislocation of the vertebrae may occur. Complete data on such lesions are lacking, since even the most careful autopsy does not always include thorough examination of the spinal column.

Brachial Plexus Injury

As a result of a difficult delivery and in rare cases after an apparently easy one, the infant is sometimes born with a paralyzed arm. *Duchenne's* or *Erb's paralysis* in-

volves paralysis of the deltoid and infraspinatus muscles, as well as the flexor muscles of the forearm, causing the entire arm to fall limply close to the side of the body with the forearm extended and internally rotated. The function of the fingers is usually retained.

The lesion results from stretching or tearing of the upper roots of the brachial plexus, which is readily subjected to extreme tension as a result of pulling laterally upon the head, sharply flexing it toward one of the shoulders. As traction in this direction is employed frequently to effect delivery of the shoulders in normal vertex presentations, Erb's paralysis may result without the delivery appearing to be difficult. In extracting the shoulders, therefore, care should be taken not to impose excessive lateral flexion of the neck. Most often, in case of cephalic presentations, the afflicted fetus is unusually large, typically weighing 4000 g or more. In breech extractions, particular attention should be devoted to preventing the extension of the arms over the head. Extended arms not only materially delay breech delivery but also increase the risk of paralysis. The prognosis is usually good with prompt, appropriate physiotherapy (Bennett and Harrold, 1976). Occasionally, however, a case may resist all treatment, and the arm may remain permanently paralyzed.

Less frequently, trauma is limited to the lower nerves of the brachial plexus, which leads to paralysis of the hand, or *Klumpke's paralysis.*

Occasionally, the child may be born with *facial paralysis,* a condition that may develop also shortly after birth (Fig. 39-5). It usually occurs in the delivery of an infant in whom the head has been seized obliquely with forceps. It is caused by pressure exerted by the posterior blade of the forceps on the stylomastoid foramen, through which the facial nerve emerges. Very often, fa-

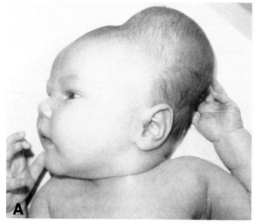

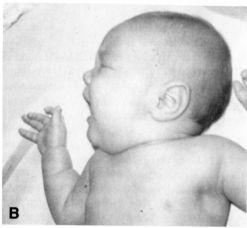

Figure 39-4. A. A very large cephalohematoma photographed 2 weeks after delivery. **B.** The same infant 4 weeks later. (*Courtesy of Dr. William Austin.*)

cial lacerations from the forceps are quite obvious. Not every case of facial paralysis following delivery by forceps should be attributed to the operation, however, since the condition is also encountered after spontaneous delivery. In fact, Hepner (1951) identified facial palsy to be as common following spontaneous delivery as after forceps delivery. Recovery in a few days is the rule (Figs. 39-5, 39-6).

Skeletal Fractures

Fractures of the clavicle and of the humerus are found with about the same frequency. Difficulties encountered in the delivery of the shoulders in cephalic deliveries and extended arms in breech deliveries are the main factors in the production of such fractures. A fractured femur is relatively uncommon and is usually associated with breech delivery. Fractures associated with delivery are often of the greenstick type, although complete fracture with overriding of the bones may occur. Palpation of the clavicles and long bones should be performed on all newborn infants when a fracture is suspected, and any crepitation or unusual irregularity should be investigated

by roentgenography. It is also important to seek evidence of brachial palsy so that treatment for that condition can be instituted.

Fracture of the skull may occur, usually following forcible attempts at delivery, although it may follow spontaneous delivery (Fig. 31-3).

In the roentgenogram in Figure 39-7, a focal but marked depressed fracture of the skull is apparent. Labor was characterized by vigorous uterine contractions, full dilatation of the cervix, and arrest of descent of the head, which was tightly wedged in the pelvis. The fracture was the consequence of compression of the skull against the sacral promontory of the mother or perhaps by pressure from an assistant's hand in the vagina as the head was pushed upward out of the birth canal at cesarean delivery. Surgical decompression was successful.

Muscular Injuries

Injury to the sternocleidomastoid muscle may occur, particularly during a breech delivery. There may be a tear of the muscle or possibly of the fascial sheath, leading to a hematoma and gradual cicatricial contraction. As the neck lengthens in the process of normal growth, the child's head is gradually turned toward the side of the injury, since the damaged muscle is less elastic and does not elongate at the same rate as its normal counterpart on the opposite side, thus producing the deformity of *torticollis*. Roemer (1954) reported that 27 of 44 infants showing this deformity had been delivered by breech or internal podalic version. He postulates that lateral hyperextension sufficient to rupture the sternocleidomastoid may occur as the aftercoming head passes over the sacral promontory.

Congenital Amputations and Constricting Bands

Focal ring constrictions of the extremities and actual loss of a digit or a limb are rare complications. Their genesis is debated. Streeter (1930) and others since have maintained that localized failure of germ plasm usually is responsible for the abnormalities. Torpin (1968), Higginbottom and co-workers (1979), and others more recently have contended that the lesions are the consequence of early rupture of the amnion, which then forms adherent tough bands that constrict and, at times, actually amputate an extremity of the fetus. Occasionally, the amputated part may be found within the uterus. A lesser constriction may result in considerable edema (Baker and Rudolph, 1971).

An unusual fatality from cord vessel occlusion by strings of amnion is demonstrated in Figure 39-8.

Congenital Postural Deformities

Mechanical factors arising from chronically low volumes of amnionic fluid and restrictions imposed by the small size and inappropriate shape of the uterine cavity may mold the growing fetus into distinct patterns of de-

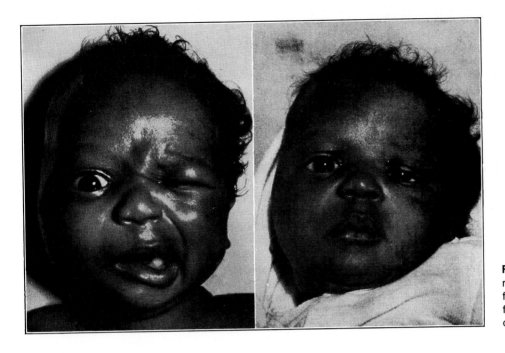

Figure 39-5. (*Left*) Paralysis of right side of face 15 minutes after forceps delivery. (*Right*) Same infant 24 hours later. Recovery was complete in another 24 hours.

formity, including talipes (clubfoot), scoliosis, hip dislocation, limb reduction and body wall deficiency (Miller and co-workers, 1981). Hypoplastic lungs can also result from oligohydramnios.

Coincidental Injuries

Experience at Parkland Memorial Hospital, with a very large trauma service, has been that severe trauma to the fetus inflicted at the time of severe trauma to the mother is less common than might be expected. As the fetus is floating in amnionic fluid, he is likely to be effectively shielded from forces that cause serious injury to maternal structures close by.

Even so, the fetus is not completely immune to trauma from external forces, as emphasized by Buchsbaum (1979) in his book *Trauma In Pregnancy.* Moreover, fetal well-being may be indirectly jeopardized by injuries to the mother that lead to inadequate maternal oxygenation and, in turn, inadequate fetal oxygenation or to maternal cardiac output insufficient for adequate perfusion of vital organs, including the placenta.

It is important that in case of accident the readily measurable vital sign of the fetus, i.e., the fetal heart rate, should be monitored, especially in the third trimester, when the fetus has achieved considerable potential for survival. At times, however, the fetus may expire be-

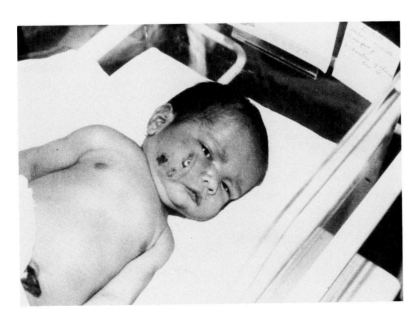

Figure 39-6. Healing abrasions and lacerations from a difficult forceps delivery. Palsy of the right facial nerve has nearly cleared.

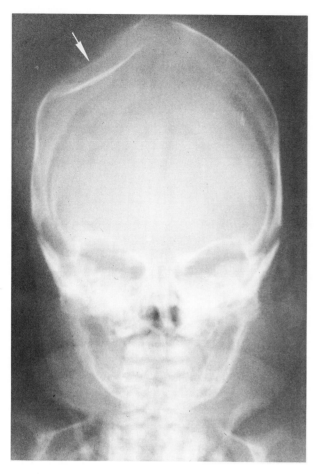

Figure 39-7. Depressed skull fracture evident immediately after birth. Delivery followed vigorous but obstructed labor and dislodgment upward of the fetal head from the birth canal by an assistant's hand in the vagina at the time of cesarean section.

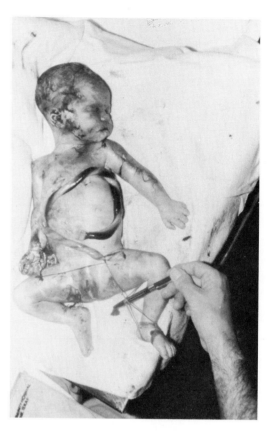

Figure 39-8. Death of a fetus at term from an amnionic band that formed after premature rupture of the amnion. A tough string of rolled amnion was wrapped centrally around the cord and at each end was adherent to the right thigh and the left foot and ankle. Movements of these extremities tightened the amnionic string and constricted the cord. (*Courtesy of Dr. Allan Dutton.*)

fore delivery can be safely accomplished. Such an instance is illustrated in Figures 21-5A and 5B (p. 399). The placenta was partially separated and grossly lacerated as a consequence of the mother's lower abdomen forcibly striking the steering wheel during an auto accident. The cause of fetal death was massive fetomaternal hemorrhage resulting from the gross laceration of the placenta. The fetus was not injured otherwise. The uterus was intact.

An unusual case was described by Buchsbaum and Caruso (1969) in which a pregnant woman was shot in the abdomen (Fig. 39-9). A roentgenogram showed that the bullet was lodged most likely somewhere in the fetus, and at laparotomy an entrance wound was evident in the large pregnant uterus. However, a liveborn, apparently uninjured infant was delivered, and no bullet was present in the uterus or elsewhere in the mother. It was then discovered that the rapidly decelerating bullet had entered the mouth of the fetus and was swallowed; it was subsequently expelled per rectum.

MALFORMATIONS

Frequency

Congenital malformations are the third leading cause of deaths under 1 year of age, with 18 percent of deaths attributed to this underlying cause. Moreover, severe developmental defects are even more common among spontaneously aborted fetuses and stillbirths than among those who are liveborn.

Genetics and Environment

As was emphasized by Fraser (1959), a minority of congenital malformations appear to have a major environmental cause, while a minority of congenital malformations have a major genetic cause. Most malformations probably result from complicated interactions between genetic predisposition and subtle factors in the intrauterine environment.

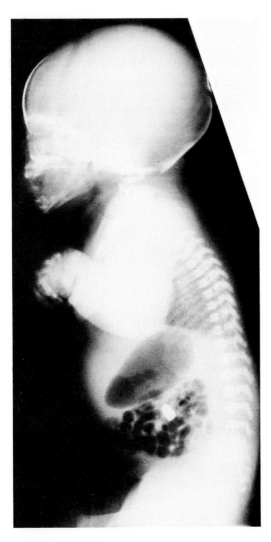

Figure 39-9. A bullet in the stomach of a fetus following a gunshot wound to the mother's abdomen with penetration of the uterus. The fetus swallowed the bullet. (*From Buchsbaum and Caruso: Obstet Gynecol 3:673, 1969.*)

Perhaps the most dramatic example in past years of a major environmental cause of human malformation was maternal rubella during early pregnancy (Chapter 38, p. 786). When contracted during the first 8 to 10 weeks of pregnancy, it causes a variety of malformations in the fetus, including cataracts, cardiac defects, deafness, microcephalus, and mental retardation.

In experimental animals, chiefly rodents, fetal malformations have been produced by withdrawing various vitamins from the maternal diet and adding their chemical analogs, by injecting certain chemicals at particular stages in pregnancy, by the administration of cortisone, by irradiation, by hyperthermia, and by other means. Although in many respects the results of these investigations may not be applicable to man, such research has brought out certain principles underlying induced malformations that bear on the etiology of many human de-

formities. They have been outlined by Wilson (1959) as follows:

1. The susceptibility of an embryo to a teratogen depends upon the developmental stage at which the agent is applied. The real determinant is the degree of differentiation within a susceptible tissue. Generally, all organs and systems seem to have a susceptible period early in the differentiation of the primordia. Susceptibility to teratogenic agents, in general, decreases as organ formation advances and usually becomes negligible after organogenesis is substantially completed.
2. Each teratogenic agent acts on a particular aspect of cellular metabolism. Different teratogenic agents, therefore, tend to produce different effects, although acting at the same period of embryonic development and on the same system. The same agent, moreover, may produce different effects when acting at different stages of embryonic development.
3. The genotype influences to a degree the animal's reaction to a teratogenic agent. In many malformations, therefore, both a genetic predisposition and a teratogenic agent are required to produce an anomaly.
4. An agent capable of causing malformations also causes an increase in embryonic mortality. This concept provides one explanation for early abortions.
5. A teratogenic agent need not be deleterious to the maternal organism. Subclinical maternal rubella, for instance, may lead to congenital malformations.

Kalter and Warkany have provided an update on etiologic factors in congenital malformations (1983) that clearly identifies the progress that has been made in teratology in the past 25 years.

The influence of purely genetic factors in the causation of congenital malformations is demonstrable in experimental animals and human beings. In certain strains of mice, for instance, about 15 percent of newborn young have cleft palate, but none has microphthalmia; in another strain, however, about 8 percent of the young have microphthalmia, but none has cleft palate (Fraser, 1959). These two examples indicate that the genes predispose one variety of embryo to cleft palate and the other to microphthalmia. In human beings, the high frequency of supernumerary digits in black infants compared to white infants, not only in this country but throughout the world, requires a genetic explanation.

Among the several drugs known to be definitely teratogenic in the human being are certain antifolic acid compounds and thalidomide. In addition, some progestational compounds masculinize the female fetus. A great many other drugs are suspect, either because they are teratogenic in animals or because there are clinical im-

TABLE 39-1. MAJOR FINDINGS IN ESTABLISHED CHROMOSOMAL ANOMALIES IN MAN (FREQUENCY PER 1000)

Syndrome	Chromosomal Complement	Sex Chromatin	Newborn Babies	Institution Populations	Signs Recognizable at Birth	Mean Parental Age[a]	
						Maternal	*Paternal*
Turners	45/X	Negative[b]	0.4		Lymphangiectatic edema of hands and feet Webbed neck	27.5	30.3
Klinefelters	47/XXY	Positive	2.0	10–30	None	33.6	37.7
Triple X	47/XXX	Double	0.6	4–7	None	32.5	35.8
YY	47/XYY	Negative	1.4–4[c]	10–30[d]	None		
Downs trisomy 21	47	Depends on sex; ordinarily not abnormal	1.6	100	Mongoloid facies Simian line	36.7	
Translocation	46			Rare	Same		
Trisomy 13–15	47			Rare	Cleft palate Harelip Eye defects Polydactyly		
Trisomy 16–18	47			Rare	Finger flexion Lowset ears Digital arches	32.8	35.2
Cat cry	46 (Deletion B 5)			Rare	Cat cry Moon face		

[a] (*Data from Hamerton (ed.): Chromosomes in Medicine, London, Heinemann Medical Books Ltd., and from Rohde RA, Hodgeman JE, Cleland RS: Pediatrics 33:258, 1964.*)
[b] May be positive with iso-X complement.
[c] (*Ratcliffe and associates: Lancet 1:121, 1970; Sergovich and associates: N Engl J Med 280:851, 1969.*)
[d] (*Court Brown: J Med Genet 5:341, 1968. Refers to penal institutions.*)
(*Data from Maclean and associates: Lancet 1:286, 1964.*)

pressions of prevalence of congenital malformations associated with their use. Evidence from experimental animals can be misleading in support and elucidation of an etiologic relation between drugs and human congenital malformations. For example, on one hand, it was difficult to find an animal that demonstrates the teratogenic effect of thalidomide. On the other hand, some antihistaminic drugs are teratogenic in rodents but not in man (Yerushalmy and Milkovich, 1965). Obviously, pregnant women, for the well-being of their unborn child, should restrict the intake of all but essential drugs, especially during the early months of gestation.

Chromosomal Abnormalities

The incidence of chromosomal abnormalities in liveborn infants has been established by six studies to be between 1 in 50 and 1 in 200, and averages 1 in 178, or 0.56 percent (Boué and Boué, 1978). The frequency among stillbirths and infants who died during the neonatal period was 6 to 7 percent. The incidence of various chromosomal abnormalities among liveborn infants is presented in Table 39-1 and among stillbirths and neonatal deaths in Table 39-2. As pointed out in Chapter 24, chromosomal abnormalities occur in 60 percent or so of early spontaneous abortions.

Whether the involved chromosome is an autosome or a sex chromosome, the pathogenetic mechanism seems to be the same. During meiotic division in the gonad, a chromosome may drop out of the dividing cell (anaphase lagging) and thus be lost. Fertilization of such a gamete results in a zygote with one chromosome too few. In trisomies, one of the explanations of a chromosomal gain is *nondisjunction* or failure of the gamete to split equally at meiotic division. If the cell with the extra chromosome is fertilized, the zygote becomes *trisomic*. These errors of meiotic division produce individuals whose cells are chromosomally equal but abnormal. If,

TABLE 39-2. INCIDENCE OF VARIOUS CHROMOSOMAL ABNORMALITIES AMONG STILLBIRTHS AND NEONATAL DEATHS

Abnormality	Percent
Sex chromosome	1.2
Autosomal trisomies	
Trisomy 21	0.7
Trisomy 18	1.8
Trisomy 13	0.5
Structural anomalies	
Balanced	0.35
Unbalanced	0.5
Others	0.7
Triploidy	0.35
TOTAL	6.1

(*Adapted from Boué, Boué: In Shrimgeout (ed.): Towards the Prevention of Fetal Malformation. Edinburgh, Edinburgh University Press, 1978.*)

however, nondisjunction occurs during mitosis after fertilization, the result is an individual with cells of two or, rarely, more, different chromosomal constitutions, or a chromosomal *mosaic*. In mosaicism, appraisal is more difficult, since the major phenotypic defects may be much less obvious, and karyotypes may be misleading unless many cells are examined.

Down Syndrome (Mongolism). This is the most common chromosomal defect reliably detected by amniocentesis early in the second trimester (Chapter 14, p. 276). Most cases of Down syndrome result from an extra chromosome (trisomy 21). Less common is a chromosomal translocation defect. *Translocation* is the transfer of a segment of one chromosome to a different site on the same chromosome or to a different chromosome. In Down syndrome, such translocations are recognized by study of the karyotype. The important translocations in mongolism are 13–15/21, 21/21, and 21/22. A female carrier with a 13–15/21 translocation has about a 20 percent chance of producing a mongoloid infant. If either parent is a 21/21 carrier, 100 percent of the children will be affected, but if any normal children have been produced or if one of the carrier's parents has the same balanced translocation, the carrier almost certainly has a 21/22 defect. The rate of recurrence of this specific type of translocation is reported to be low. A 21/21 translocation cannot be distinguished from 21/22 except by the birth of a normal child, which rules out the 21/21 translocation.

Down syndrome presents a striking clinical picture often recognizable at birth. The facies of the infants are mongoloid, with narrow, slanting, closely set palpebral fissures. The tongue is thick and fissured, and the palatal arch is often high. Fingers are stubby, and the hands present clearcut dermatoglyphic patterns, particularly a simian line. Mental retardation subsequently becomes apparent.

Whereas in mothers up to the age of 30 the risk of birth of a liveborn infant with Down syndrome is less than 1 in 800, this risk increases to about 1 in 100 by age 40, and to 1 in 32 by age 45 (Table 39-3). The frequency of Down syndrome among conceptuses is higher than this, but a sizable fraction, perhaps twice as many, are expelled from the uterus as abortuses or stillborn infants (Hook, 1978).

Often, but not always, an experienced individual can accurately diagnose Down syndrome from the general appearance of the newborn infant. Ideally, the capability for confirmation by chromosomal analysis should be immediately available for those instances in which other major complications are detected. Using bone marrow aspirate for culture, a karyotype can be obtained in a few hours. Thus, a decision as to the extent of treatment could be made promptly after *informed* consent for such treatment had been obtained from the parents (Francke and colleagues, 1979).

Pregnancy in a woman with Down syndrome is rare but does occur. Bovicelli and associates (1982) have reviewed the pregnancy experiences of 26 affected mothers. No man afflicted with Down syndrome is known definitely to have fathered a child.

TABLE 39-3. RISK OF GIVING BIRTH TO A DOWN SYNDROME INFANT BY MATERNAL AGE

Maternal Age	Frequency of Down Syndrome Infants among Births
30	1/885
31	1/826
32	1/725
33	1/592
34	1/465
35	1/365
36	1/287
37	1/225
38	1/176
39	1/139
40	1/109
41	1/85
42	1/67
43	1/53
44	1/41
45	1/32
46	1/25
47	1/20
48	1/16
49	1/12

(*From Hook, Lindsjo: Am J Hum Genet 30:19, 1978.*)

Effect of Paternal Age. Paternal age does not appear to be an important risk factor for Down syndrome. However, the age of the father does play a role in the development of autosomal dominant genetic diseases. The relative frequency of new autosomal dominant mutations in offspring increases logarithmically with paternal age during the usual period of fatherhood (Friedman, 1981). The absolute frequency of autosomal dominant disease as a consequence of new mutations among children whose fathers are 40 years of age or older is at least 0.3 percent.

Inborn Errors of Metabolism

There are several rare but heritable inborn errors of metabolism, most of which result from the absence of crucial enzymes, with resulting incomplete metabolism of proteins, sugars, or fats. In some cases, there are consequent high levels of toxic metabolites in the blood, causing mental retardation and other defects. These metabolic errors are true congenital defects, which are inherited most often as autosomal recessives (Table 14-1, p. 269).

Phenylketonuria. The inability to metabolize phenylalanine appropriately to tyrosine because of inappropriate phenylalanine hydroxylase activity is an example of an inborn error of metabolism that is inherited in an autosomal recessive manner. It has been reported to occur about once in 10,000 to 15,000 white infants but much less often in black infants. Early diagnosis is important, since the associated mental retardation can often be prevented by a low phenylalanine diet. Optimal early treatment with limitation of phenylalanine consumption will result in normal levels of intelligence (Williamson and associates, 1981). Many states now require that a screening test for phenylketonuria be applied to all newborn infants. Five cases were identified by the Texas Newborn Screening program in the first half of 1983.

Women with phenylketonuria adequately managed during childhood may have poor pregnancy outcomes, including high frequencies of spontaneous abortion, microcephaly, and mental retardation. Women with phenylketonuria who wish to have children should be advised to switch to a diet low in phenylalanine before conception (Tenbrinck and Stroud, 1982). Even then, a normal outcome cannot be guaranteed (Lenke and Levy, 1982).

Teratogenic Agents

Different teratogenic agents produce different effects (Kalter and Warkany, 1983). One that produced devastating effects on the human embryo in the form of phocomelia is thalidomide.

Phocomelia. Phocomelia is a congenital malformation characterized by severe deformities of the long bones. Either the radius is absent or both radius and ulna are defective; in extreme cases, the radius, ulna, and humerus are lacking and the hand buds arise from the shoulders. The legs may be affected in the same manner. In extremely severe cases, both arms and legs are missing. The mental development of the vast majority of the children is normal, and about two thirds of them survive (Taussig, 1962).

In 1961–1962, an outbreak of phocomelia occurred in West Germany, and conclusive evidence indicated that it was attributable to the widespread use by pregnant women of a sedative and tranquilizing drug, thalidomide. In a large proportion of the cases, the drug was administered early in pregnancy for the treatment of nausea and vomiting. The fetus was most vulnerable to the teratogenic action when the drug was ingested by the mother between the 30th and 50th day of pregnancy. It has been estimated that the thalidomide tragedy involved at least 5000 infants and possibly many more.

The most important practical lesson to be drawn from the experience with thalidomide is that no drug should be administered to pregnant women in the absence of a real therapeutic indication. This is especially true for new drugs.

Genetic Predisposition and Environmental Factors

The genotype of the embryo may influence the response to environmental factors that otherwise would not be teratogenic. Possible examples follow:

Anencephaly. Anencephaly is a malformation characterized by cerebral hemispheres that are either rudimentary or absent and absence of the overlying skull (Fig. 39-10). Most often the pituitary gland also is either absent or markedly hypoplastic. The absence of the cranial vault renders the face very prominent and somewhat extended; the eyes often bulge from their sockets, and the tongue hangs from the mouth. About 70 percent of anencephalic fetuses are females.

In addition to the virtual absence of brain tissue in anencephalic fetuses, typically there is extreme diminution in the size of the adrenal glands, the combined weight of which may be well under 1 g in contrast to the usual weight of 5 g for the adrenals in normal term infants. The small size of the gland reflects the absence of fetal, or provisional, cortex; it is commonly believed that the adrenal hypoplasia is secondary to the absence of the pituitary gland.

Nothing definite is known about the cause of anencephaly, but it again appears that both genetic and environmental factors are involved. The possible role of folic acid in the genesis of neural tube defects is considered in Chapter 13 (p. 255). A genetic factor is strongly suggested, of course, by the frequency with which this malformation recurs in subsequent pregnancies. Yen and MacMahon (1968) have pointed out, however, that the relatively small increase (about 5 percent) in sibship risk over the rate in the general population furnishes a strong argument against a single major gene hypothesis. A polygenic predisposition is possible, but the very rare occurrence of concordance in twins is difficult to reconcile with either genetic or, for that matter, environmental causes.

Extreme examples of recurrence in siblings have been reported, in which women have produced four successive anencephalic infants (Horne, 1958). The reported

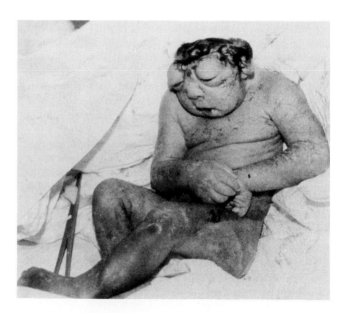

Figure 39-10. Anencephalic monster.

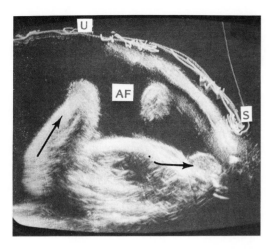

Figure 39-11. Longitudinal sonogram that demonstrates an anencephalic fetus. The right arrow points to the rudimentary head without a calvarium. The left arrow overlies a lower extremity. Hydramnios is evident from the magnitude of the amnionic fluid (AF) between the fetus and the abdominal wall (S = symphysis; U = umbilicus). (*Courtesy of Dr. R. Santos.*)

geographic differences in the incidence of anencephaly, however, have led to the belief that different environmental conditions in these several areas, notably differences in diets, predispose to the anomaly.

Inability to palpate a fetal head abdominally is suggestive of anencephaly, but sonographic or radiologic examination provides for definitive diagnosis (Fig. 39-11). Since accompanying hydramnios occurs in the majority of cases, it too suggests anencephaly or perhaps another malformation. Anencephaly is probably the most common cause of gross hydramnios, which may occasionally be sufficiently massive to require amniocentesis. Because of the diminutive size and abnormal shape of the fetal head, breech and face presentations are the rule.

The most frequent practical question posed by pregnancies complicated by anencephaly is whether to initiate labor as soon as the diagnosis is confirmed. The uterus containing an anencephalic fetus may be somewhat refractory to oxytocin. Late in pregnancy, when severe hydramnios is almost the rule, the slow aspiration of 2 to 3 liters of excess amnionic fluid usually will reduce the risk of abruptio placentae following spontaneous rupture of the membranes with sudden loss of amnionic fluid and marked decomposition of the uterus. Moreover, the myometrium appears to contract more effectively after slow removal of some of the fluid. The insertion into the cervical canal of laminaria tents (Chapter 24, p. 479), followed by the administration of prostaglandin in compounds to terminate the pregnancy by vaginal delivery, has proved ultimately to be effective in cases of anencephaly so managed by Osathanondh and associates (1980).

The duration of anencephalic pregnancies may be remarkably long, especially in the absence of hydramnios, and exceed that reported in any other form of ges-

tation with a living fetus. In the well-authenticated case of Higgins (1954), for example, the duration of pregnancy was 1 year and 24 days after the last menstrual period, with fetal movements perceived until the moment of delivery.

Elevated levels of α-fetoprotein (Chapter 14, p. 277) in amnionic fluid reliably predict the great majority of cases of larger open neural tube defects, including anencephaly. Knowledge of the duration of pregnancy is essential, however, since the level of α-fetoprotein normally varies remarkably with gestational age. Closed or very small open neural tube abnormalities may not be so detected. Lemire and co-workers' book (1978) deals specifically with anencephaly.

Spina Bifida, Meningomyelocele. Spina bifida consists of a hiatus, usually in the lumbosacral vertebrae, through which a meningeal sac may protrude, forming a meningocele (Fig. 39-12). If the sac contains the spinal cord as well, the anomaly is called meningomyelocele. In the presence of complete rachischisis, the spinal cord is represented by a ribbon of spongy, red tissue lying in a deep groove. In these circumstances, the infant dies soon after birth. In other instances, the defect may be very slight, as in *spina bifida occulta*. Associated malformations, particularly hydrocephaly, anencephaly, and clubfoot, are common. If part of the brain protrudes into the

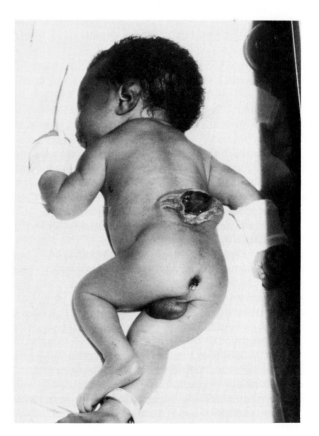

Figure 39-12. Ruptured meningocele.

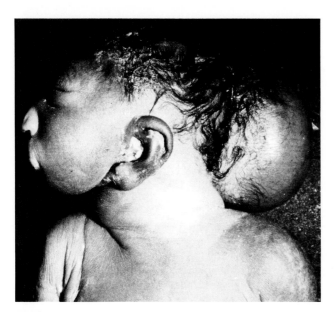

Figure 39-13. A large meningoencephalocele associated with agnathia.

sac, a meningoencephalocele results (Fig. 39-13). In cases of open neural tube defects, α-fetoprotein is likely to be unusually high in both maternal plasma and amnionic fluid (Chapter 14, p. 277).

The incidence of neural tube defects appears to be decreasing in more recent times for unknown reasons (Owens and associates, 1981; Stein and colleagues, 1982).

Hydrocephaly. Because of the clinical importance of hydrocephaly as a cause of dystocia and rupture of the uterus and difficulties in decision making concerning the route of delivery, this malformation is considered also in Chapter 30 (p. 669), together with other fetal causes of dystocia.

The characteristic ultrasonographic finding is dilatation of the lateral ventricles. Associated anomalies, including spina bifida, are fairly common. When hydrocephaly has been identified at or before midpregnancy, pregnancy termination has often been offered.

There are several reports of attempts to relieve the hydrocephalus by transcranial drainage of the cerebrospinal fluid from a ventricle into the amnionic sac, thereby reducing destruction of the cerebral cortex while in utero. Intermittent needle aspiration has been performed through the mother's abdomen, or a shunt has been inserted which, hopefully, would provide a persistent drainage system from ventricle to amnionic sac. The risks versus benefits from such a procedure cannot now be stated. A group of very active investigators has provided the following recommendation: "Prenatal decompression should be performed only if the fetus with isolated ventriculomegaly has evidence of progressive dilatation and decreasing mantle thickness on serial sonograms, is too immature to be delivered for postnatal shunting, and has no other central nervous system ab-

normalities on careful sonography screening" (Occasional Notes, 1982).

A protocol for management of congenital hydrocephalus, including incidence, epidemiology, embryology, pathophysiology, and genetic counseling, has been provided by Vintzileos and associates (1983).

Renal Agenesis. The incidence of complete absence of the kidneys is about 1 in 4000 births (Potter, 1965). The malformation occurs more frequently in male infants and is characteristically accompanied by oligohydramnios. The infant has prominent epicanthal folds, a flattened nose, and large, lowset ears. The skin is loose, and the hands often seem large. A cardiac malformation is common. One third of the infants are stillborn. The longest reported survival is 48 hours, since pulmonary hypoplasia is found in practically all infants. Renal agenesis should be suspected when sonographic evidence is indicative of scant to absent amnionic fluid and neither kidneys nor a filled bladder can be demonstrated. Renal agenesis and the associated changes are commonly referred to as *Potter syndrome.*

Urinary Tract Obstruction. Persistent obstruction of the urine-collecting system of the fetus will destroy the kidneys unless the obstruction is relieved. Therefore, when obstruction of the lower urinary tract has been detected, relief has been attempted in some circumstances by providing drainage from the bladder. Persistent obstruction very likely is always accompanied by oligohydramnios. With normal amounts of amnionic fluid, obstruction most likely is intermittent and probably does not warrant attempts at drainage in utero. The risks versus the benefits from attempts to relieve obstruction in utero remain to be established.

Congenital Heart Disease. Because of the irregularity with which cases of congenital heart disease are reported, the frequency of this malformation cannot be stated precisely, but it is one of the more common abnormalities. The cardiac malformations include such conditions as patent ductus arteriosus, coarction of the aorta, septal defects, pulmonary stenosis, and tetralogy of Fallot. They commonly occur as part of a syndrome, such as Marfan's, Ellis-van Creveld's, and Down and other chromosomal disorders.

Infants with severe congenital heart disease may look and react quite normally at birth, only to deteriorate later. Therefore, one should consider the possibility of a cardiovascular defect in the mature infant who appears normal at birth and then develops tachypnea, cyanosis, marked tachycardia, and hepatomegaly in the early hours or days after birth. Arrhythmias are rare in the newborn.

Clubfeet (Talipes Equinovarus). The extremities are involved in a large number of congenital defects, most of which are rare. Clubfeet, however, are the most common, occurring about once in 1000 births. Since the borderline between the normal and the pathologic is not sharp in this malformation, early orthopedic consultation is essential.

Congenital Dislocation of the Hip. This fairly common malformation is six times more frequent in girls than in boys (Record and McKeown, 1949) and more common in breech than in vertex deliveries. It shows geographic variations, having been noted with unusual frequency in northern Italy, for example. It is rarely seen in black infants. The cause is defective formation of the acetabulum, particularly its upper lip. As a result, the head of the femur may migrate upward and backward. In most cases, the displacement probably does not begin until after birth, developing gradually during the early weeks or months of life. From an obstetric point of view, this fact is worthy of note because it is sometimes alleged that these malformations were overlooked in the neonatal period. Carter (1963), reviewing the genetic aspects of the disease, found concordance in 40 percent of monozygous twins with congenital dislocation of the hip but in only 3 percent of dizygous twins. One percent of subsequent male siblings and 5 percent of later female siblings were affected.

Polydactylism. Supernumerary digits are occasionally seen, especially in black newborns. They usually consist of a small amount of skin and cartilage attached by a fine pedicle to the base of the fourth finger or toe. Simple ligation of the stalk with a silk thread is generally sufficient treatment. If the base is broad and the digit is well developed, however, surgical removal may be required.

Cleft Lip and Cleft Palate. A cleft in the lip, either unilateral or bilateral, may or may not be associated with a cleft in the alveolar arch or a cleft in the palate. It is one of the most frequent congenital deformities, with an incidence of approximately 1.3 per 1000 births. Because of difficulties in feeding, it is advisable to operate upon a cleft lip as soon as the condition of the infant permits. Cleft palate may represent even greater difficulties in feeding, requiring the use of a prosthesis until the age of 2 or 2½ years.

While the risk of the first child of unaffected parents having a cleft lip is about 1 per 1000, or 0.1 percent, the risk of cleft lip in the second child is about 40 times greater, or 4 percent. If both children are affected, the risk of the third child having a cleft lip is 10 percent. If a parent has a cleft lip, the risk of the first child being affected is about 4 percent and when the first child is affected, the risk to the second child is about 10 percent (Habib, 1978). Identification of cleft lip and cleft palate have been made at or before midpregnancy using real-time ultrasonography (Seeds and Cephalo, 1983).

Omphalocele. The large circular defect left as the midgut returns to the abdomen at about 10 weeks gestation is normally closed by the rectus muscles and their inter-connected fascial sheaths. At times, this closure fails to take place. An omphalocele results, consisting of a peritoneal sac covered with amnion and filled with intestines. Rupture of the sac, evisceration, and peritonitis are grave complications. Surgical correction may prove successful. An omphalocele is likely to be associated with elevated levels of α-fetoprotein in maternal serum and amnionic fluid (Chapter 14, p. 277).

Hernia, Umbilical and Inguinal. Umbilical hernias are common, especially in black infants. They are rarely serious, and strangulation of the bowel is almost unknown. Most small umbilical hernias disappear spontaneously within a few months, whereas the larger varieties are generally treated successfully by simple mechanical measures, such as strapping the surrounding skin with a band of adhesive tape. Inguinal hernias may correct themselves spontaneously during the first year of life. Inguinal hernias may undergo incarceration, especially in premature infants.

Imperforate Anus. In this abnormality, because of atresia of the anus, the rectum ends in a blind pouch. Examination of the newborn in the delivery room will usually reveal the condition. More commonly perhaps, it is discovered on the first attempt to record the infant's rectal temperature. Surgical intervention is, of course, imperative.

Sacrococcygeal Teratoma. These tumors are located over and under the coccyx; large ones fill the sacrum and buttocks. Perhaps 25 percent are malignant. An amniogram and a subsequent roentgenogram of a newborn infant with a very large sacrococcygeal tumor are shown in Figures 39-14A and B. The mass ruptured during delivery, with considerable bleeding, and the infant expired. Especially with smaller lesions, resection may be accomplished successfully and the child not be subsequently incapacitated.

Musci and associates (1983) have described an intriguing case in which all of the fetus except the very large teratoma (2120 g when excised the next day) was delivered vaginally; however, the tumor could not be extricated from the birth canal. The infant was intubated and resuscitated until cesarean delivery was undertaken 10 minutes later. The fetus–infant was pushed back through the birth canal into the uterus and then through the uterine incision once again into the external environment. The infant with tumor weighed 5060 g. The "born again" infant underwent excision of the tumor mass 24 hours later and at 3 years of age was described as normal.

GENETIC COUNSELING

Genetic counseling supplies information to families with genetic problems, helping them to make intelligent decisions regarding future childbearing. A malformed child

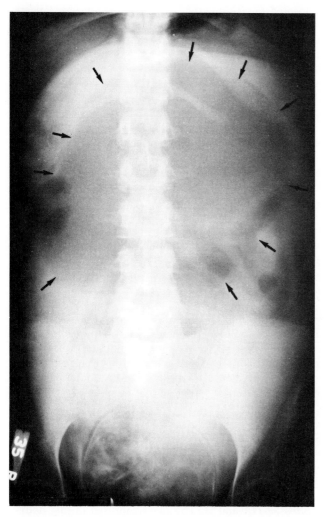

Figure 39-14. A. Amniogram showing a large, relatively radiolucent area corresponding to the location of the sacrococcygeal tumor clearly outlined in the roentgenogram in B.

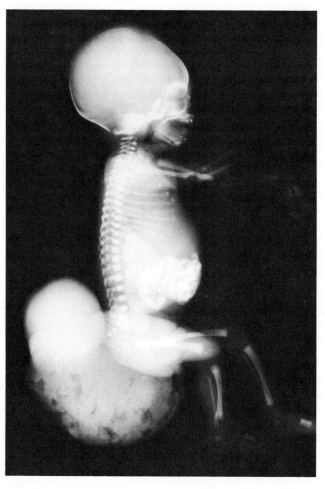

Figure 39-14. B. The large sacrococcygeal tumor contains air at the sites of rupture during labor and delivery. Note the outline of the intestinal tract from contrast material in the amnionic fluid swallowed in utero and concentrated in the intestine.

often precipitates the request for such guidance, although other problems leading to consultation include inheritable disease in the family and maternal age. Human genetic counseling is becoming increasingly complex with the rapid accumulation of new information. Amateurish advice, particularly of the unjustifiably optimistic variety, may produce tragic results.

Forecasting the probability of an inherited disorder is an important step, but it requires a precise medical history. In addition to the routine history obtained on all women who are pregnant (Chapter 13, p. 247), the specific questions listed in Figure 39-15 should be asked to help identify the expectant mother whose fetus is at unusual risk of having or subsequently acquiring a serious disability. The completed record also serves to document that the mother was informed of any unusual risk of the fetus being abnormal or that referral for further genetic counseling was advised.

Upon completion of the history, it is often possible to decide whether the disease follows an easily recognized pattern of inheritance or represents an isolated congenital defect. Most often, further steps to identify the fetus at risk of a serious disorder and to counsel the expectant parents are best handled through a specialized genetics center with established expertise in counseling and quality control of the variety of laboratory procedures that may be employed. The Council on Accreditation and Certification of the American Society of Human Genetics has established standards of accreditation for genetic counselors.

In addition to supplying positive information, appropriate genetic studies and subsequent counseling help to dispel many misapprehensions and ill-founded rumors concerning congenital malformations. It also helps relieve the feeling of guilt after the birth of a defective child.

Techniques for intrauterine diagnosis of fetal defects of genetic origin are considered in Chapter 14 (p. 275).

	Circle Appropriate Answer
1. Will you be age 35 or older when the baby is due?	YES NO

2. Have you or the baby's father or anyone in either of your families ever had:

a. Down syndrome or mongolism?	YES NO
b. Spina bifida or meningomyelocele (open spine)	YES NO
c. Hemophilia (blood won't clot)?	YES NO
d. Muscular dystrophy?	YES NO

3. Have you or the baby's father had a child born dead or alive with a birth defect not listed in Question 2 above?   YES   NO

If Yes, describe: _____

4. Do you or the baby's father have any close relatives who are mentally retarded?   YES   NO

If Yes, list cause if known: _____

5. Do you or the baby's father or close relative in either of your families have any inherited genetic or chromosomal disease or disorder not listed above?   YES   NO

6. Have you, or the spouse of this baby's father in a previous marriage, had three or more spontaneous pregnancy losses?   YES   NO

7. Do you or the baby's father have any close relatives descended from Jewish people who lived in Eastern Europe (Ashkenazic Jews)   YES   NO

If Yes, have either you or the baby's father been screened for Tay-Sachs disease?   YES   NO

If Yes, indicate results and who screened: _____

8. If patient or her spouse is black—
Have you or the baby's father, or any close relative been screened for sickle cell trait and found to be positive?   YES   NO

I have discussed with my doctor the above questions which are answered "Yes" and understand that I am at increased risk for _____ and that it is usually possible to diagnose an affected fetus by testing amniotic fluid at about 16 weeks of pregnancy and I DO NOT want the test.

_____ _____
(PATIENT SIGNATURE)   (DATE)

Patient wants amniocentesis and fetal diagnoses for: _____

Patient referred for further testing or counseling concerning: _____

Figure 39-15. Prenatal diagnosis screening questions. (*From Antenatal Diagnosis, NIH Publication No. 79–193, April, 1979.*)

Evaluation of Malformed Infants Who Die in the Perinatal Period

A *detailed history* of events from before the time of conception through delivery should be obtained. Times of exposure to potential teratogens are especially important. *Photographs* should be made of the face, the body, and all anomalies. A *radiographic skeletal survey* may prove valuable. *Chromosomal analysis* is carried out either on 2 to 3 ml of blood collected aseptically from a large vessel or the heart or on sterile skin, umbilical cord, amnion, or lung. A *complete autopsy* performed on all malformations, both external and internal, should be described in detail. Histologic sections should be made of any tissue that appears abnormal.

MODES OF INHERITANCE

Dominant Inheritance

A mutant gene producing its effects when present on one or both chromosomes of a given pair is referred to as a "dominant gene." A recessive gene produces its effect only when present on both chromosomes. A dominantly inherited disease caused by a single dominant gene is transmitted from one generation to the next in a direct line, so that each affected individual has an affected parent and there are no skipped generations. There is a 50 percent chance that the children of an affected parent married to an unaffected mate will inherit the condition. These affected children will in turn transmit the defect to half of their offspring.

A dominant trait may be sex-linked or autosomal. If the trait is dominant and linked to the X-sex chromosome, all of the daughters of an affected father whose wife is normal will inherit the gene, and none of the sons will be affected. If, however, the mother is heterozygous and affected and the father normal, she will transmit the condition to half of her daughters and half of her sons. If the mother is homozygous and affected, she will transmit the condition to all her children.

Nongenetic factors may mimic inherited determinants in the production of disease, but these phenocopies can often be detected by adequate history, appropriate clinical examination, and studies in the laboratory. Familial recurrence is unlikely with phenocopies.

Penetrance

A dominant gene with phenotypic expression in all individuals who carry the gene is said to be 100 percent penetrant. If not expressed in some individuals even though they have the gene, the gene is not completely penetrant. The degree of penetrance may be quantitatively expressed as the percentage ratio of carriers who show the trait to the total number of individuals who have the gene. A gene that is 80 percent penetrant is expressed in only 80 percent of the people who have that gene. The term *penetrant* is applicable not only to heterozygous dominant genes but also to homozygous genes, whether dominant or recessive.

The same gene may express itself in a variety of ways in different people. This characteristic is known as the *expressivity* of the condition. The expressivity of a gene varies from complete manifestation of the condition to complete absence.

Recessive Inheritance

A child with an inherited disease that requires for its clinical expression the contribution of a duplicate mutant gene from each of its parents, as, for example, sickle cell anemia, is affected by a recessively inherited disease. Almost all inherited enzyme defects are recessive disorders. The parents in these circumstances may be either heterozygous carriers of the mutant gene or homozygous and therefore affected.

If the recessively inherited disease is autosomal, either sex may be similarly affected, and the parents and more remote ancestors are usually unaffected. The probability of a subsequent child's being affected in such a family is 1 in 4. The likelihood that a normal sibling of an affected child is a carrier of the defect is 2 in 3. The carrier child will not produce affected children, however, except by mating with another carrier or an affected individual. If a recessive gene is rare, there is, of course, only a remote chance that unrelated carriers will marry.

In sex-linked recessive inheritance, the affected individuals are nearly always males. The female must have mutations in both her X chromosomes in order to manifest the disease. Red-green color blindness and hemophilia are well-known examples of sex-linked recessive inheritance. The mothers of the affected males are the carriers,

and, as with all sex-linked inheritance, male-to-male transmission does not occur. Positive information in this type of inheritance comes from the maternal side of the family pedigree, whereas the paternal history is of little consequence.

Multifactorial or Polygenic Inheritance

The largest source of genetic variability comes from the combined actions of a number of genes, each with a very small individual effect. The great range of effects so produced is thought to be responsible for the continuous variation seen in the vast majority of differences among normal human beings, as expressed in stature, intelligence, blood pressure, and quite likely in the susceptibility to a number of common diseases.

Many of the more common congenital malformations have a genetic factor in their causation. The increased incidence in relatives, compared with the incidence in the general population, is difficult to explain in terms of any known environmental factors and is much below that found in single-gene transmission. Common congenital malformations with an incidence at birth of at least 1 in 1000, such as cleft lip, pyloric stenosis, talipes equinovarus, congenital dislocations of the hip, spina bifida, anencephalus, and congenital heart defects, are polygenically inherited, with varying degrees of environmental modification.

Empiric Risks

In the majority of cases, a simple pattern of inheritance cannot be demonstrated. In such patients, prognosis is derived from data on empiric risk, based on the pooled experience of many investigators. Such pooled data may be inapplicable to the individual case and occasionally misleading because they include high-risk and low-risk families. The average so obtained may thus either overestimate or underestimate the true risk. In many instances, however, such average data represent the only estimates available. As a rule of thumb, the risk of a significant malformation in any pregnancy is approximately 1 to 1.5 percent. The risk of a second malformed child is about 5 percent, increasing with subsequent malformed children.

Consanguinity

The risks of recurrence of affected offspring is obviously greater for related than for nonrelated parents, and the closer the relationship, the greater is the risk. Even for closely related couples, however, such as first cousins, the chance of having a significantly abnormal child, although twice that expected for children of nonrelatives, has been estimated by Motulsky and Hecht (1964) not to exceed 2 percent. Reed (1963) reported a risk of malformation of about 10 percent in a child resulting from a brother–sister union. Because the likelihood of a normal child resulting from a cousin marriage is greater than that of an affected child, there is no compelling genetic reason to discourage cousin marriage unless there is familial evidence of recessive disease.

REFERENCES

Baker CJ, Rudolph AJ: Congenital ring constrictions and intrauterine amputations. Am J Dis Child 121:393, 1971

Bennett GC, Harrold AJ: Prognosis and early management of birth injuries to the brachial plexus. Br Med J 1:1520, 1976

Boué A, Boué J: Chromosomal abnormalities associated with fetal malformations. In Schrimgeour J (ed): Towards the Prevention of Fetal Malformation. Edinburgh, Edinburgh University Press, 1978

Bovicelli L, Orsini LF, Rizzo N, Montacuti V, Bacchetta M: Reproduction in Down syndrome. Obstet Gynecol 59:13 [Suppl], 1982

Buchsbaum HJ: Trauma in Pregnancy. Philadelphia, Saunders, 1979

Buchsbaum HJ, Caruso PA: Gunshot wound of the pregnant uterus. Obstet Gynecol 3:673, 1969

Buist NRM, Lis EW, Tuerck JM, Murphey WH: Maternal phenylketonuria. Lancet 2:589, 1979

Carter CO: Genetic factors in congenital dislocation of the hip. Proc R Soc Med 56:803, 1963

Francke U, Brown MG, Jones KL: Immediate chromosome diagnosis on bone marrow cells: An aid to management of the malformed newborn infant. J Pediatr 94:289, 1979

Fraser FC: Causes of congenital malformations in human beings. J Chron Dis 10:97, 1959

Friedman JM: Genetic disease in the offspring of older fathers. Obstet Gynecol 57:745, 1981

Habib Z: Genetic counselling and genetics of cleft lip and cleft palate. Obstet Gynecol Surv 33:44, 1978

Hadlock FP, Garcia-Prats JA, Courtney JT, Park SK: Sonographic diagnosis of neonatal intracranial hemorrhage. Perinatol Neonatol Jan 1983

Hepner WR Jr: Facial paresis in newborn infant. Pediatrics 8:494, 1951

Higginbottom MC, Jones KL, Hall BD, Smith DW: The amniotic band disruption complex: Timing of amniotic rupture and variable spectra of consequent defects. J Pediatr 95:544, 1979

Higgins LG: Prolonged pregnancy. Lancet 2:1154, 1954

Holm VA: The causes of cerebral palsy: A contemporary perspective. JAMA 247:1473, 1982

Hook EB: Spontaneous deaths of fetuses with chromosomal abnormalities diagnosed prenatally. N Engl J Med 299:1036, 1978

Horne HW: Anencephaly in four consecutive pregnancies. Fertil Steril 9:67, 1958

Illingworth RS: Why blame the obstetrician? A review. Br Med J 1:797, 1979

Kalter H, Warkany J: Congenital malformations. N Engl J Med 308:424, 491, 1983

Lemire J, Beckwith JB, Warkany J: Anencephaly. New York, Raven Press, 1978

Lenke RR, Levy HL: Maternal phenylketonuria—Results of dietary therapy. Am J Obstet Gynecol 142:548, 1982

Lowe CR: Congenital malformations and the problems of their control. Br Med J 3:151, 1973

Miller ME, Graham JM Jr, Higginbottom MC, Smith DW: Compression-related defects from early amnion rupture: Evidence for mechanical teratogenesis. J Pediatr 98:292, 1981

Miller ME, Graham JM, Jr, Higginbottom MC, Jones KL, Hall BD, Smith DW: The amniotic band disruption complex: Timing of amniotic rupture and variable spectra of consequent defects. J Pediatr 95:544, 1979

Motulsky A, Hecht F: Genetic prognosis and counseling. Am J Obstet Gynecol 90:1227, 1964

Musci MN Jr, Clark MJ, Ayres RE, Finkel MA: Management of dystocia caused by a large sacrococcygeal teratoma. Obstet Gynecol 62:10 [Suppl], 1983

Occasional Notes: Fetal treatment. N Engl J Med 307:1651, 1982

Osathanondh R, Donnenfeld AE, Frigoletto FD, Driscoll SG, Ryan KJ: Induction of labor with anencephalic fetus. Obstet Gynecol 56:655, 1980

Owens JR, McAllister E, Harris F, West L: Nineteen-year incidence of neural tube defects in area under constant surveillance. Lancet 2:1032, 1981

Potter EL: Bilateral absence of ureters and kidneys: a report of 50 cases. Obstet Gynecol 25:3, 1965

Potter EL: Pathology of the Fetus and Infant, 2nd ed. Chicago, Year Book, 1961

Record RG, McKeown T: Congenital malformations of the central nervous system: I. A survey of 930 cases. Br J Soc Med 3:183, 1949

Reed SC: Counseling in Medical Genetics, 2nd ed. Philadelphia, Saunders, 1963

Roemer RJ: Relation of torticollis to breech delivery. Am J Obstet Gynecol 67:1146, 1954

Seeds JW, Cephalo RC: Technique of early sonographic diagnosis of bilateral cleft lip and palate. Obstet Gynecol 62:2 [Suppl], 1983

Shankaran S, Slovis TL: Neurosonography and neonatal intracranial hemorrhage. Perinatol Neonatol, Nov Dec 1983

Smith I, Erdohazi M, MacCartney FJ, Pincott JR, Wolff OH, Brenton DP, Biddle SA, Fairweather DVI, Dobbing J: Fetal damage despite low-phenylalanine diet after conception in a phenylketonic woman. Lancet 1:17, 1979

Starfield B, Holtzman NA: A comparison of effectiveness of screening for phenylketonuria in the United States, United Kingdom and Ireland. N Engl J Med 293:118, 1975

Stein SC, Feldman JG, Friedlander M, Klein RJ: Is myelomeningocele a disappearing disease? Pediatrics 69:511, 1982

Streeter GL: Contrib Embryol 22:1, 1930

Taussig HB: A study of the German outbreak of phocomelia. JAMA 180:1106, 1962

Tenbrinck MS, Stroud HW: Normal infant born to a mother with phenylketonuria. JAMA 247:2139, 1982

Torpin R: Fetal Malformations Caused by Amnion Rupture during Gestation. Springfield, Il, Thomas, 1968

Vintzileos AM, Ingardia CJ, Nochimson DJ: Congenital hydrocephalus: A review and protocol for perinatal management. Obstet Gynecol 62:539, 1983

Wigglesworth JS, Pape KE: Pathophysiology of intracranial hemorrhage in the newborn. J Perinat Med 8:1119, 1980

Williamson ML, Koch R, Azen C, Chang C: Correlates of intelligence test results in treated phenylketonuric children. Pediatrics 68:161, 1981

Wilson JG: Experimental studies on congenital malformations. J Chronic Dis 10:111, 1959

Yen S, MacMahon B: Genetics of anencephaly and spina bifida. Lancet 2:623, 1968

Yerushalmy J, Milkovich L: Evaluation of the teratogenic effect of meclizine in man. Am J Obstet Gynecol 93:553, 1965

40
Family Planning

WHO NEEDS CONTRACEPTION?

The sexually active couple, both of whom are fertile but do not desire pregnancy, needs to use effective contraception. **When no contraception is used by presumably fertile sex partners, about 80 percent of the women will conceive within 1 year.**

Young women who do not want to be pregnant are best advised to use contraception whenever they become sexually active, no matter how young. At least some girls, and perhaps the majority, ovulate before their first menstrual period.

A more difficult question to answer is, "How late in life does a woman remain capable of becoming pregnant?" Results of one study of women in the age range of 40 to 50 imply that ovulation is related more closely to the regularity of menstruation than to the age of the woman (Metcalf, 1979). *When menstruation remained regular, there was evidence of ovulation in almost every cycle.* A recent history of oligomenorrhea or of increasing cycle length was associated with a diminished frequency but not the complete absence of ovulation. Even the presence of hot flashes, amenorrhea, and elevated levels of follicle-stimulating hormone in plasma or urine do not absolutely guarantee against subsequent ovulation (Metcalf and Donald, 1979). Primordial follicles with apparently normal oocytes have been observed in ovaries removed from women over 50 years of age and evidence of ovulation has been witnessed through the laparoscope.

Even so, pregnancies are rare in women over 50, and extremely rare after the age of 52 (Francis, 1970). Therefore, older women are probably best advised as follows: Regular menstrual periods imply recurrent ovulation irrespective of age; however, pregnancy is rare after the age of 50. A woman younger than this who has not menstruated for 2 years is very unlikely to ovulate spontaneously and to conceive, although there are reported instances in which conception occurred more than 2 years after the onset of documented hypergonadotropic, hypoestrogenic amenorrhea (Szlachter and co-workers, 1979).

COMMONLY EMPLOYED CONTRACEPTIVE TECHNIQUES

Methods of contraception of variable effectiveness currently employed include (1) oral steroidal contraceptives, (2) injected steroidal contraceptives, (3) intrauterine devices, (4) physical, chemical, or physicochemical barrier techniques, (5) withdrawal before ejaculation, (6) sexual abstinence around the time of ovulation, (7) breast-feeding, and (8) permanent sterilization.

The results of a national survey of the contraceptive status and most of the methods used by women of reproductive age are presented in Figure 40-1. Estimates of the failure rate with each of these techniques *during the first year of use* are presented in Table 40-1. It is emphasized that failures from patient misuse of the method are included. Effective education, as well as motivation, undoubtedly would have reduced appreciably the failure rate cited in Table 40-1. The results of the Oxford/Family Planning Association contraceptive study provide strong support for this view (Vessey and co-workers, 1982). Their failure rates for more than 17,000 women who have been observed for an average of 9½ years are among the lowest reported. Failure rates for various contraceptive techniques per 100 woman-years of use were as follows: estrogen plus progestin oral contraceptives, 0.16 to 0.32; various intrauterine devices, 0.4 to 2.4; diaphragm, 1.9; and condom, 3.6. Failure rates demonstrated a strong negative association between both the age of the woman and the duration of use, that is, the mature woman who continued to use one technique for a long time typically experienced a very low failure rate.

Abortion, strictly speaking, is not a contraceptive technique, although it serves at times as a less than ideal means for preventing unwanted children (see Chapter 24).

HORMONAL CONTRACEPTIVES

Nearly 9 million women in the United States use one of the variety of hormonal contraceptives available for fer-

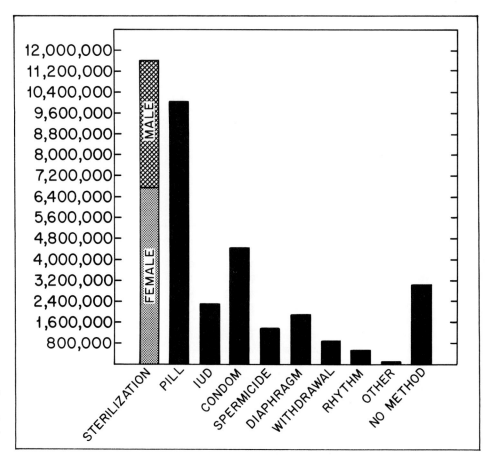

Figure 40-1. Contraceptive methods used in 1982 by women aged 15 to 44 who did not wish to conceive. (*Data from Alan Guttmacher Institute, 1983.*)

tility control. Although hormonal contraceptives represented a dramatic departure from previous traditional methods, they also created a unique therapeutic dilemma. As stated in a report of an advisory committee to the Food and Drug Administration, "Never will so many people have taken such potent drugs voluntarily over such a protracted period for an objective other than for the control of disease." For some women, however, an unwanted pregnancy is in some ways a venereal disease.

ESTROGEN PLUS PROGESTIN CONTRACEPTIVES

The oral contraceptives most often employed now consist of a combination of an estrogen and a progestational agent taken daily for 3 weeks and omitted for 1 week, during which time withdrawal uterine bleeding normally occurs. In the United States the estrogen is ethinyl estradiol or its 3-methyl ether (mestranol), which is promptly metabolized to ethinyl estradiol. A greater variety of compounds with progestational activity is used, including norethindrone, norgestrel, ethynodiol diacetate, and norethynodrel.

Mechanisms of Action

The contraceptive actions of the combined estrogen–progestin steroidal medication are multiple. A most important effect is to prevent ovulation, almost certainly by suppression of hypothalamic releasing factors, which, in turn, leads to inappropriate secretion by the pituitary of follicle-stimulating and luteinizing hormones (Fig. 40-2). Other contraceptive effects induced by the combined steroids include altered maturation of the endometrium, rendering it inappropriate for successful implantation if a

TABLE 40-1. FAILURE RATES DURING FIRST YEAR OF ATTEMPTED USE OF CONTRACEPTION*

Method	Percent
Oral Contraceptives	2.4
Intrauterine Devices	4.6
Condom	9.6
Spermicides	17.9
Diaphragm	18.6
Rhythm	23.7
Other	11.9

*(*From Schirm AL, Trussell J, Menken J, Grady WR: Contraceptive failure in the United States. Family Planning Perspectives 14:2, 1982.*)

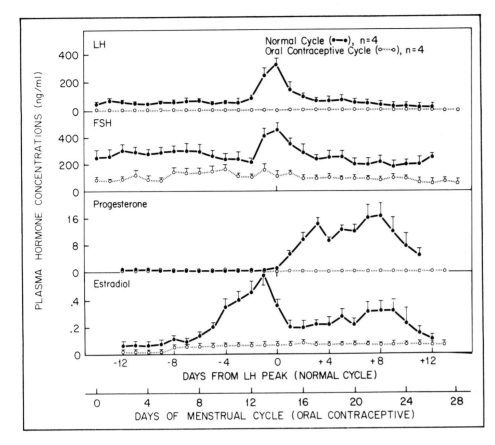

Figure 40-2. Plasma levels of luteinizing hormone (LH), follicle-stimulating hormone (FSH), progesterone, and 17-β estradiol in four ovulatory women and in four women who were ingesting one tablet daily of an oral contraceptive that contained 80 µg of mestranol and 1 mg of norethindrone. Note the suppression of all four hormones in the women taking the oral contraceptives. (*From Carr, Parker, Madden, MacDonald, and Porter: J Clin Endocrinol Metab 49:346, 1979.*)

blastocyst were to develop, and the production of cervical mucus hostile to penetration by sperm. The possible role, if any, of altered tubal and uterine motility induced by the hormones is not clear. As the consequence of these actions, combined estrogen plus progestin oral contraceptives, *if taken daily for 3 weeks out of every 4,* provide virtually absolute protection against conception. An important exception, however, is the period of about a week immediately following initiation of use of an oral contraceptive. Indeed, in the woman with a maturing follicle who is soon to ovulate spontaneously, ovulation may actually be triggered by starting oral contraceptives in this circumstance.

Dosage and Administration

So as to prevent induction of ovulation, as well as to help recognize preexisting early pregnancy, it is generally recommended that women begin the use of oral contraceptives on the fifth day of the menstrual cycle. Many women, however, start their use after delivery or abortion, before the return of spontaneous menses. If their use is initiated at any time other than during or immediately after a normal menstrual cycle, or within 3 weeks of delivery, another means of birth control should be used throughout the first week to avoid the risk of induced ovulation.

To help achieve regular administration of the combined oral contraceptive, and thereby obtain maximum protection, several suppliers offer dispensers that provide sequentially 21 individually wrapped, identically colored tablets that contain hormones, followed by seven inert tablets of another color (Fig. 40-3).

It is important for maximum contraceptive efficiency and for peace of mind that the woman adopt an effective scheme for assuring daily (or nightly) self-administration. One technique is to keep her pill supply and toothbrush close to each other and to swallow a pill at the time of brushing the teeth. If one dose is missed, nothing serious will happen; it may be desirable to double the next dose to minimize breakthrough bleeding and to "stay on schedule." If several doses are missed, another form of effective contraception (a barrier technique) should be used whenever intercourse is contemplated. The pill can be started after withdrawal bleeding. Without any bleeding, the possibility of pregnancy must be considered.

Since oral contraceptives have come into use, the amounts of estrogen and progestational agent contained in each tablet have been reduced considerably. It is now known that effective contraception can be achieved with doses of the steroids that are quite small compared to those originally used. This is of considerable importance, since adverse effects are to a degree dose-related. The

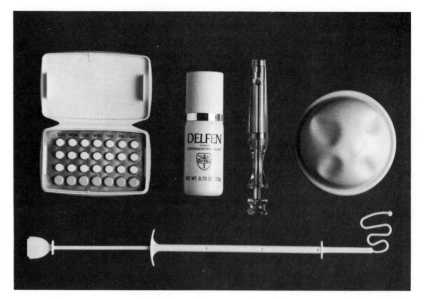

Figure 40-3. Shown left to right are oral contraceptive tablets in a container, a tube of vaginal contraceptive cream plus applicator, a diaphragm, and, below, a Lippes Loop intrauterine device and inserter. Just before insertion, the rod is withdrawn until all of the device is pulled into the inserter tube.

lowest acceptable limit of dosage is set by the ability of the medication to prevent unacceptable breakthrough bleeding from the endometrium (Edelman and associates, 1983). The amount of estrogen most commonly administered daily is 30 to 50 μg of either mestranol or ethinyl estradiol. Oral contraceptive tablets that contain as little as 20 μg of ethinyl estradiol per tablet are commercially available. No tablet sold in the United States contains more than 100 μg. The amount of progestin varies in two ways: (1) Among older, now well-evaluated formulations the progestational activity will vary depending upon the compound used but the daily dosage of the compound ingested throughout the cycle is constant, for example, 1 mg of norethindrone daily. (2) In some more recent preparations the dosage of the progestin varies throughout the cycle, for example, 0.5 mg of norethindrone daily during the first week, 0.75 mg daily the second week, and 1.0 mg daily the third week. This, of course, reduces the amount of progestin administered.

Adverse and Beneficial Effects from Oral Contraceptives

The combined estrogen plus progestin pill taken 3 weeks out of every 4 is the most effective reversible form of contraception available. Failure rates of 0.32 per 100 woman-years or lower have been documented (Vessey and co-workers, 1982). Other beneficial effects include reduced menstrual blood loss; less dysmenorrhea, functional ovarian cysts and salpingitis; less premenstrual complaints; less endometrial and ovarian cancer; reduction in various benign breast diseases and possibly breast cancer; and less rheumatoid arthritis (Andersch and Hahn, 1981; Mishell, 1982; Centers for Disease Control, 1983).

At the outset, concern was rightfully raised for the safety of users of oral contraceptives. Fortunately, no major disasters have occurred, and, in general, the use of oral contraceptives, when appropriately monitored as outlined below, has proved to be safe for the great majority of women.

The possibility of adverse effects from oral contraceptives has received so much attention for so long that the major adverse effect among their users may be the anxiety that has been created by the almost incessant publicity so generated. It would seem that among the data banks of several centers the slightest suggestion of variation in the apparent health status of pill users automatically triggers an outflow of statistical probabilities to word processors for manuscript production, followed soon thereafter by publication and instant dissemination by the lay press, radio, and television. Physicians and public alike are frequently confused by the many and often conflicting reports with which they continue to be bombarded.

Metabolic Changes. A variety of metabolic changes, often qualitatively similar to those of pregnancy, have been identified in women taking oral contraceptives. For example, plasma thyroxine and thyroid binding proteins are elevated appreciably whereas triiodothyronine uptake by resin is lowered. Another change similar to that induced by normal pregnancy is elevation of plasma cortisol concentration with a nearly comparable increase in transcortin. It is extremely important, therefore, that evaluation of results of these laboratory tests and others be considered in light of whether or not the woman is using an estrogen-containing oral contraceptive. The estrogen in a combined estrogen plus progestin pill appears to increase high-density-lipoprotein cholesterol, but some progestins, at least, cause the reverse (Stadel, 1981). The importance of such changes in the genesis of *vascular disease* in users of oral contraceptives is not clear but, nonetheless, is cause for concern.

The contraceptive steroids may intensify preexisting *diabetes* or may prove sufficiently diabetogenic to induce clinically apparent disease in women prone to develop diabetes. However, the risk of the latter appears slight since in the great majority of women the effect on carbohydrate metabolism is slight. Phillips and Duffy (1973), for example, identified serum glucose levels 1 hour after administration of 75 g of glucose orally to average 11 mg/dl more in users of oral contraceptives than in nonusers. As with pregnancy, diabetogenic effects most often appear to be reversible when use of the oral contraceptive is terminated (Wingrave and associates, 1979).

Argument persists as to whether women with diabetes should use oral contraceptives. A general policy established early in the development of the Greater Dallas Family Planning Program operated by the Department of Obstetrics and Gynecology of the University of Texas Southwestern Medical School would preclude their use in this circumstance. The policy is as follows: *No women with systemic chronic disease shall be given an oral contraceptive except in circumstances where it can be verified that the merits from its use undoubtedly outweigh any risks.*

Cholestasis and *cholestatic jaundice* are uncommon complications in users of oral contraceptives; the signs and symptoms clear when the medication is stopped. A somewhat increased risk of surgically identified gallstones and *gallbladder disease* was reported for users of oral contraceptives. However, results of a more recent study by the Royal College of General Practitioners (1982) suggest that oral contraceptives may only accelerate the development of gallbladder disease in women who are susceptible and that there is no overall increased long-term risk. There appears to be no reason to withhold oral contraceptives from women fully recovered from viral hepatitis.

Neoplasia. The possible role of hormonal contraception in the causation of neoplasia is not clear. There are reports that suggest that the risk of malignant and premalignant change in the cervix and breast is increased, or decreased, or unchanged. If there is an increased risk, it most likely is slight (Vessey and co-workers, 1983a, 1983b; Pike and co-workers, 1983; McPherson and associates, 1983; Wiseman, 1983); Food and Drug Administration Advisory Committee, 1984). Oral contraceptive use has been claimed to protect the ovary from malignant change.

Use of estrogen plus progestin contraceptives has been linked circumstantially with the development of *hepatic focal nodular hyperplasia* and actual tumor formation that most often, but not necessarily always, is benign. A prominent feature of the benign tumor nodules is increased vascularity with extensive proliferation of large and small thin-walled blood vessels. Therefore, the lesions, upon rupture, can be complicated by bleeding, hemoperitoneum, and shock, which in 8 of 24 cases cited by Antoniades (1975) proved fatal. The liver may become enlarged to palpation, and by means of sonography, liver scans, and angiography, a space-occupying lesion or lesions can be visualized. If identified before rupture, resection of the lesion, along with stopping the use of oral contraceptives, has been recommended. Some liver lesions appear to have disappeared after merely stopping the use of oral contraceptives. Increased growth and vascularity during pregnancy or the puerperium leading to rupture, and causing death of the mother, have been described (Kent and co-workers, 1978). Fortunately, such liver lesions associated with the use of oral contraceptives are rare.

Nutrition. Aberrations in the levels of several *nutrients* have been described for women who use oral contraceptives and typically are similar to changes induced by normal pregnancy. Lower plasma levels in users compared to nonusers have been described by some investigators, but not all, for ascorbic acid, folic acid, vitamin B_{12}, niacin, riboflavin, and zinc. Moreover, biochemical changes compatible with, but not necessarily proof of, vitamin B_6 deficiency have been documented repeatedly but do not differ from those that accompany normal pregnancy (Theur, 1972; Wynn, 1975).

The possibilities of folate deficiency and of vitamin B_6 deficiency as the consequence of oral contraceptives have received considerable attention. *Folate deficiency* developing from use of oral contraceptives was suggested by Streiff (1970), who described in a few women who were using oral contraceptives severe megaloblastic anemia that responded to pteroylmonoglutamic acid but not to pteroylpolyglutamic acid unless the ingestion of the contraceptive was stopped. He believed that the estrogen of the contraceptive blocked intestinal conjugase (pteroylpolyglutamate hydrolase) and thereby prevented the cleavage of pteroylglutamate to an absorbable active form, a view not supported by the studies of Stephens and co-workers (1972). Shojania and associates (1968) had reported serum folate levels of women who used oral contraceptives to be somewhat lower than those who did not. This triggered a chain reaction of reports that about equally confirmed and denied the findings of Shojania.

The observations of Pritchard and associates (1971) may provide an explanation for the discrepancies. In our initial study, we compared plasma folate levels of socioeconomically somewhat privileged users and nonusers of oral contraceptives who were employed by the hospital or medical school or were wives of employees. No difference in serum folate levels was found. We subsequently carried out similar studies of socioeconomically less privileged women who attended the free family planning clinics. Again we found no difference in plasma folate levels between users and nonusers, but their plasma folate levels were lower than those of the more affluent groups first studied. In other words, less affluent users and nonusers of oral contraceptives had lower folate levels than more affluent users.

Prasad and associates (1978) would appear to have utilized about all of the possible permutations for apparent effects of oral contraceptives on blood folate levels when they reported the following: For nonusers of oral contraceptives blood folate levels were higher in women of upper socioeconomic class. With the use of oral contraceptives by women of upper socioeconomic class blood folate levels were lower than for nonusers in that class. In women of lower socioeconomic class, however, the blood folate levels were no lower in users than in nonusers.

A number of women with overt megaloblastic anemia resulting from folate deficiency during pregnancy have subsequently been followed by us, some of whom used an oral contraceptive beginning shortly after delivery (Scott and Pritchard, 1975). One relapsed remote from pregnancy while using an oral contraceptive, as did one who did not use an oral contraceptive. In both instances, relapse occurred while the women were consuming atrocious diets essentially devoid of any folate. We are therefore of the opinion that use of the typical estrogen–progestin oral contraceptive is rarely by itself a cause of clinically significant folate deficiency. This opinion is not shared by all.

Pyridoxine deficiency in women who use oral contraceptives has been implicated as a cause of mental depression, a phenomenon that is not a frequent complication of oral contraceptive use. Estrogens induce in the liver the rate-limiting enzyme, tryptophan oxygenase, that enhances tryptophan metabolism in a way that suggests pyridoxine deficiency (Wynn, 1975). To abolish these biochemical variations suggestive of pyridoxine deficiency, as much as 20 to 30 mg of pyridoxine, or 10 times the usual intake, need be ingested! Since altered tryptophan metabolism persists in contraceptive users even when other indices of vitamin B_6 nutrition are normal, Leklem and co-workers (1975) believe that oral contraceptives specifically affect tryptophan metabolism by some means other than through vitamin B_6 deficiency.

It has also been suggested that altered tryptophan metabolism, as the consequence of oral contraceptives, may have a diabetogenic effect. For example, tryptophan has been reported to bind to insulin (Larrson-Cohn, 1975). Moreover, Spellacy and associates (1972) claimed that women who were taking oral contraceptives and who experienced deterioration of glucose tolerance showed partial improvement in glucose tolerance after administration of pyridoxine. These observations have not been confirmed (see Chapter 13, p. 255).

The similarity of the changes in tryptophan and pyridoxine metabolism to those of normal pregnancy strongly implies that estrogen–progestin contraceptives do not induce significant pathologic changes as the consequence of pyridoxine deficiency any more than does normal pregnancy.

Combined estrogen–progestin oral contraceptives conserve *iron* by reducing blood loss from menstruation. Nilsson and Sölvell (1967) compared hemoglobin shed by apparently normal women during spontaneous menses with hemoglobin of withdrawal bleeding following estrogen–progestin contraceptives and they noted that the contraceptives reduced the amount of hemoglobin shed by one half. By quantitative measurements, we have demonstrated blood loss from spontaneous menses to decrease from as much as 400 ml per cycle to less than 30 ml when 100 μg of mestranol plus 2 mg of norethindrone was ingested daily by two young women with cyclic menorrhagia of unknown cause. The menorrhagia recurred when the oral contraceptive was stopped. It is apparent, therefore, that women who typically lose more

than the average amount of blood with their periods may benefit from oral contraceptives by becoming iron sufficient. Moreover, women with *dysmenorrhea* from endometriosis or from idiopathic causes are likely to enjoy appreciable relief from pain while using combined oral contraceptives.

At times, while using the combined medication, the amount of blood and endometrium shed is so scant that the woman believes she is amenorrheic and concludes that she is pregnant, especially if she has missed a tablet or two. She then stops taking the medication and, unfortunately, soon thereafter does conceive.

Cardiovascular Effects. Certain vascular phenomena that are induced or enhanced by oral contraceptives, while rare, can be quite serious. In various studies, the risk of *deep vein thrombosis* and *pulmonary embolism* has been estimated to be 3 to 11 times greater in women who used oral contraceptives than in otherwise apparently similar women who did not (Stadel, 1981). Moreover, the use of oral contraceptives during the month before an operative procedure appears to increase the risk of postoperative thromboembolism significantly. Pills that contain less estrogen appear to reduce the risk of venous thrombosis and thromboembolism.

The mechanism by which estrogen–progestin contraceptives enhance the risk of venous thrombosis and thromboembolism is not altogether clear. The development of distinctive vascular intimal and medial lesions with associated occlusive thrombi have been described (Irey and co-workers, 1970). Moreover, platelet aggregation may be accelerated and both plasma antithrombin III activity and endothelial plasminogen activator are likely to be reduced somewhat while using estrogen plus progestin oral contraceptives (Stadel, 1981).

The enhanced risk of thromboembolism appears to decrease rapidly once the oral contraceptive is stopped. The woman who developed thromboembolism while taking estrogen-containing contraceptives, however, appears also to be at increased risk of thromboembolism during pregnancy and the early puerperium (Badaracco and Vessey, 1974).

Arterial thrombosis has also been attributed to the use of estrogen plus progestin contraceptives. The relative risk of a cerebrovascular accident, or *stroke*, seems to be about four times greater than in women who do not use oral contraceptives and appears to be confined largely to women about 35 years old or older (Stadel, 1981).

An association between oral contraceptives and *hypertension* became apparent in the late 1960s, when several reports appeared of the occasional woman who, while using an estrogen–progestin contraceptive, became overtly hypertensive. Usually, but not always, she became normotensive when the medication was stopped. The oral contraceptives, presumably in response chiefly to the estrogen contained, were shown to increase markedly the plasma level of renin substrate and, to a lesser degree, renin to near the levels found in normal preg-

TABLE 40-2. ESTIMATES OF MORTALITY RATES (PER 100,000) ASSOCIATED WITH PREGNANCY AND CHILDBIRTH, FIRST TRIMESTER LEGAL ABORTION, ORAL CONTRACEPTIVES, AND INTRAUTERINE DEVICES

| Age Group (Yr) | Pregnancy and Childbirth | First Trimester Legal Abortion | Oral Contraceptives | | Intrauterine Devices |
			Nonsmokers	Smokers	
15–19	11.1	1.2	1.2	1.4	0.8
20–24	10.0	1.2	1.2	1.4	0.8
25–29	12.5	1.4	1.2	1.4	1.0
30–34	24.9	1.4	1.8	10.4	1.0
35–39	44.0	1.8	3.9	12.8	1.4
40–44	71.4	1.8	6.6	58.4	1.4

(*Adapted from Tietze: Fam Plan Perspect 9:74, 1977.*)

nancy. The great majority of women using oral contraceptives demonstrate these changes, as in pregnancy, yet do not become hypertensive. Fisch and Frank (1977), for example, have evaluated blood pressures of a large number of women who were using oral contraceptives and identified the mean systolic and diastolic blood pressures to be only 5 to 6 and 1 to 2 mm Hg higher, respectively, than in the age-adjusted control group. Not surprisingly, the risk of hypertension attributable to oral contraceptives has been observed to increase with age (Stadel, 1981).

Unfortunately, normotensive women who are destined to become hypertensive in response to oral contraceptives usually cannot be identified in advance. The development of hypertension during pregnancy does not preclude subsequent use of oral contraceptives. Pritchard and Pritchard (1977) evaluated the pressor response to oral contraceptives in young black women who had developed overt pregnancy–induced hypertension but postpartum had diastolic blood pressures of 90 mm Hg or less when oral contraceptives were started. The contraceptive dose provided 50 µg of mestranol and 1 mg of norethindrone daily. Over an average of 1½ years, only 6 percent demonstrated a rise in diastolic pressure above 90 mm Hg, a frequency not remarkably different from that observed in initially normotensive young nulligravid black women who used the same kind of oral contraceptive. Moreover, Fisch and Frank (1977) found no significant association between hypertension from use of oral contraceptives and previous hypertension during pregnancy.

The frequency and intensity of attacks of *migraine* may be enhanced appreciably by estrogen plus progestin contraceptives. Therefore, this method of contraception is likely to be unacceptable to the woman who is prone to such attacks.

Several epidemiologic studies very strongly imply, at least, that use of estrogen plus progestin oral contraceptives increases the risk of *myocardial infarction*. Mann and Inman (1975) noted a significant association, which became stronger with increasing age. Use of oral contraceptives by women who were heavy smokers, were obese, were being treated for hypertension and diabetes, or had type II hyperlipoproteinemia increased the risk of

myocardial infarction remarkably, the effects being synergistic rather than merely additive.

In keeping with the policy of not giving estrogen plus progestin contraceptives to women who demonstrate systemic chronic disease, we do not give them to hypertensive women. Moreover, every woman's blood pressure is rechecked when contraceptive refills are provided 3 months after starting the medication, and every 6 months thereafter. At each visit, usually a nurse or, at times, a physician performs a brief but pertinent interrogation designed to uncover other possibly adverse effects from the use of oral contraceptives. Smoking is discouraged. Physical examination is repeated annually, or more often if an abnormality is suspected. Whenever hypertension is detected, the oral contraceptive is stopped and another form of contraception is substituted.

Lethality of Oral Contraceptives. A number of adverse effects has been identified for users of oral contraceptives. As borne out by the data in Table 40-2, the risk of death from the use of an oral contraceptive is very low if the woman is under 35, has no systemic illness, and does not smoke. The risk of dying as the consequence of using an oral contraceptive is certainly less than that imposed by pregnancy and delivery, even though the risk with the latter is actually quite low. Moreover, serious morbidity, as well as mortality, almost certainly would be minimized by avoiding the use of the estrogen plus progestin pill in those circumstances listed in Table 40-3.

Effects on Reproduction. When the estrogen–progestin contraceptive is discontinued, ovulation usually, but not always, promptly resumes. Similar to the postpartum period, within 3 months after discontinuance at least 90 percent of women who previously ovulated regularly will have done so again. *Post-pill amenorrhea* poses no long-term threat to fertility (Hull and associates, 1981; Linn and colleagues, 1982).

In the rare instance in which *anovulation* persists and is not caused by unrecognized early pregnancy or by premature menopause (in which case there would be high levels of follicle-stimulating hormone in plasma and urine), ovulation may be induced successfully.

Whether very recent use of oral contraceptives be-

TABLE 40-3. SOME IMPORTANT CONTRAINDICATIONS TO USE OF ESTROGEN–PROGESTIN CONTRACEPTIVES

1. Thromboembolism, current or past
2. Cerebrovascular accident, current or past
3. Coronary artery disease
4. Impaired liver function
5. Liver adenoma, current or past
6. Breast cancer
7. Hypertension
8. Diabetes
9. Gallbladder disease
10. Cholestatic jaundice during pregnancy
11. Sickle cell hemoglobinopathy
12. Surgery contemplated within 4 weeks
13. Major surgery on or immobilization of lower extremity
14. Over 40 years of age
15. Smokes heavily

fore a pregnancy or continued use during early unrecognized pregnancy might adversely affect the fetus has been the source of much concern. The more recent report by Linn and co-workers (1983) provides some assurance that they do not. Their study did not show an increased risk of major fetal malformations among users of oral contraceptives (or for users of diaphragm or foam barrier techniques).

Even though an association between *congenital defects* and the use of oral contraceptives during early pregnancy has not been established, the woman who thinks that she may be pregnant might best be advised to stop the oral contraceptive (*but use another contraceptive technique!*) until it can be established whether or not she is pregnant.

Harlap and Eldor (1980) and others have reported a slight increase in both major and minor fetal malformations when the mother had recently used combined oral contraceptives. They also noted a preponderance of male offspring and significantly increased frequency of twinning. Teratogenic effects in pregnancies conceived while taking or soon after taking the pill reported to date have included fetal limb–reduction deformities (Janevich and co-workers, 1974; Nora and Nora, 1975). Rothman and Louik (1978) and Savolainen (1981), however, found little difference for major malformations between infants whose mothers had very recently used oral contraceptives and those whose mothers had not.

Use of contraceptive hormones by nursing mothers tends to reduce the amount of *breast milk;* very small quantities of the hormones are excreted in the milk.

Other Effects. *Cervical mucorrhea* is fairly common in response to the estrogen contained, and the mucus at times may be irritating to the vagina and vulva. *Vaginitis* or *vulvovaginitis,* especially that caused by *Candida,* may develop. Antibiotic therapy in pill users increases the frequency of such an infection.

Hyperpigmentation of the face and forehead (*chloasma*) is more likely to occur in women who demon-

strate such a change during pregnancy. *Acne* may improve or, at times, be aggravated.

Uterine *myomas* may increase in size more rapidly in response to the estrogen of oral contraceptives than they would otherwise but this is not a consistent phenomenon.

Weight gain has been a troublesome complaint from women who use oral contraceptives, although an increase in weight is far from a uniform phenomenon. Some of the weight may be caused by fluid retention, but it is likely to be a consequence of increased dietary intake.

Oral contraceptives often ameliorate the *dysmenorrhea* associated with endometriosis. Their use may even reduce the risk of a woman developing severe endometriosis.

Postpartum Use. Recently pregnant women who do not nurse their children, and especially those who have undergone abortions, may ovulate before 6 to 7 weeks after pregnancy termination (Chapter 19, p. 376; Chapter 24, p. 484). There is an advantage, therefore, to starting oral contraceptives before the traditional "6 weeks postpartum check." On the other hand, increased risks of adverse effects, especially venous thromboembolism, might be anticipated from use of estrogen–progestin contraceptives earlier in the puerperium. So far, in our now extensive experience in which oral contraceptives have been started typically during the third week postpartum, there has been no evidence of increased morbidity.

Cost. Unfortunately, the cost of oral contraceptives has increased remarkably in recent years perhaps as the consequence of extensive and expensive litigation arising from lawsuits filed by some users. Their price cannot accurately reflect the cost of the ingredients.

PROGESTATIONAL AGENTS ALONE

Oral Progestins Alone

The so-called mini-pill, consisting solely of 0.5 mg or less of a progestational agent daily, has not achieved widespread popularity because of a much higher incidence of irregular bleeding and a higher pregnancy rate. The progestational agent alone presumably impairs fertility, without necessarily inhibiting ovulation, by causing formation of cervical mucus that impedes sperm penetration and by altering endometrial maturation sufficiently to thwart successful implantation of a blastocyst.

Injectable Hormonal Contraceptives

The advantages of injected medroxyprogesterone acetate (Depo-Provera) are a contraceptive effectiveness comparable to the combined oral contraceptives, long-lasting action with injections required only two to four times a year, and lactation not likely to be impaired. The mechanisms of action appear to be multiple, and include inhibition of ovulation, increased viscosity of cervical mucus, and an endometrium unfavorable to ovum implantation.

The disadvantages are prolonged amenorrhea, or uterine bleeding, or both, during and after its use, and prolonged anovulation after discontinuation (Cheng and associates, 1974). The risk of venous thrombosis and thromboembolism appears to be increased, as with estrogen plus progestin oral contraceptives (Schwallie, 1974). Obviously, these adverse effects must be explained to the woman and her consent obtained to use such a preparation for contraception. Unfortunately, the woman who may be best served by such a contraceptive agent may not be able to comprehend these potential problems.

Injected medroxyprogesterone acetate (Depo-Provera) has been widely used for contraception in several countries but not in the United States. It has been estimated that one million women throughout the world depend on an injectable progestin for contraception. Food and Drug Administration hearings are held periodically, with great public awareness through television, radio, newspapers, and magazines, but medroxyprogesterone acetate is still not marketed in the United States for contraceptive use, presumably because of the possibility that the compound may cause cancer (Contraceptive Technology Update, 1983). Interestingly, it is approved for use in this country to treat metastatic endometrial cancer. Moreover, studies on a large number of women users have not identified an increased risk of cancer (Liang and co-workers, 1983).

Hormonal implants are being studied currently in several countries. The Norplant system, especially, which provides the progestin levonorgestrel in a silastic container that is implanted subdermally, continues to be evaluated. Some, but not all, ovulatory cycles are prevented by the progestin, which works presumably by altering the endometrium and cervical mucus.

POSTCOITAL CONTRACEPTION

Stilbestrol administered after intercourse to prevent unwanted pregnancy has come to be known as the "morning-after pill." Kuchara (1971) reported no pregnancies in 1000 women who had inadequate contraceptive protection at the time of intercourse but within 3 days began to take stilbestrol, 25 mg twice daily for the next 5 days. The mechanism of action is not fully understood but very likely implantation is interfered with in some way. Nausea and vomiting are common side effects. The possible teratogenic effect of the drug must be kept in mind if pregnancy does occur. Prevention of pregnancy has also been reported using either ethinyl estradiol or conjugated equine estrogens (Premarin) when taken in large doses for several days.

More recently Yuzpe and colleagues (1982) devised

an estrogen plus progestin regimen in which the combination was taken in two doses 12 hours apart starting within 72 hours of exposure. In a multicenter trial involving 692 women the pregnancy rate observed by them was 1.6 percent.

Luteinizing Hormone–Releasing Hormone. The natural hormone agonists and antagonists of luteinizing hormone–releasing hormone (LHRH) are being evaluated for contraceptive properties. Further studies of possible efficacy are awaited.

INTRAUTERINE CONTRACEPTIVE DEVICES

Since early in this century, attempts have been made, sporadic at the outset but very intense in recent years, to design a device that when inserted into the uterus would prevent pregnancy without causing adverse effects. One intriguing but unconfirmed story describes the first successful experience with an intrauterine device to have been the insertion of small stones into the uteri of camels to prevent pregnancy during long caravans.

It is estimated that in the United States 6 to 7 percent of sexually active women of reproductive age use an intrauterine device for contraception (Fig. 40-1). Some of the devices used are demonstrated in Figures 40-3–40-5. The pregnancy rates in larger studies generally vary from 0.5 to 5 per 100 woman-years (Population Reports, 1982).

Theoretical Advantages

Ideally, an intrauterine device would need to be inserted but once, would provide complete protection against pregnancy, would neither be expelled spontaneously nor have to be removed for adverse effects, and, after re-

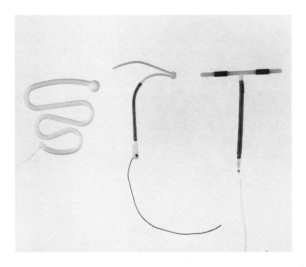

Figure 40-4. Intrauterine contraceptive devices left to right are Lippes Loop (size D), a Cu7, and a Copper T (380 A).

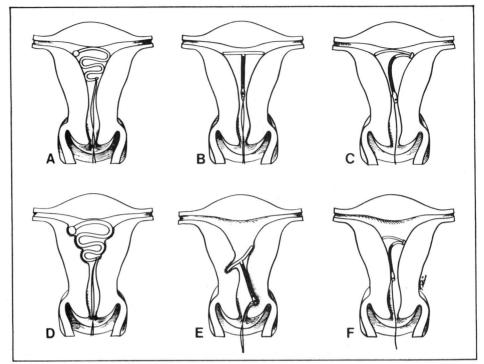

Figure 40-5. Illustrated above are a Lippes Loop (A), Copper T (B), and Cu7 (C), that are of appropriate size and are correctly positioned. Below are a Lippes Loop that is too large (D), a prolapsed Copper T that has perforated the uterine isthmus and cervix (E), and a Cu7 that is too small and has prolapsed into the uterine isthmus and cervical canal (F).

moval to allow a planned pregnancy, would have in no way induced changes detrimental to pregnancy. These objectives have not been fully achieved by any device so far.

Types of Intrauterine Devices

In general, devises are of two varieties: (1) those that appear to be chemically inert, in that they are made of a nonabsorbable material, most often polyethylene impregnated with barium sulfate for radiopacity; and (2) those in which there is more or less continuous elution from the device of a chemically active substance, such as copper or a progestational agent.

Of the chemically inert devices, the *Lippes Loop,* in various sizes, appears to be most popular. Of the chemically active devices, those whose surface is covered with metallic copper are being used extensively. The *Copper T* and *Cu7* devices have been extensively evaluated in this country and elsewhere and have demonstrated desirable qualities. A T-shaped device (*Progestasert*) that releases progesterone, approximately 65 μg a day, through the wall of the vertical shaft of vinyl acetate copolymer has become popular, especially in the circumstance where use of another device had caused excessive bleeding or cramping.

Mechanisms of Action

The mechanisms of action of the chemically inert device have not been defined precisely. Interference with successful implantation of the fertilized ovum in the endometrium seems to be the most prominent contraceptive action. The interference may result from induction of a local inflammatory response that, in turn, leads to lysosomal action on the blastocyst and perhaps phagocytosis of spermatozoa (Population Reports, 1982). Providing support for such a mechanism of action are the observations of Buhler and Papiernik (1983), who described two successive pregnancies in each of four women who had been fitted with intrauterine devices but were chronically taking anti-inflammatory drugs. For the chemically inert devices, contraceptive effectiveness generally increases with size and extent of contact with the endometrium.

Certain metals, especially copper, greatly enhance the contraceptive action of inert devices. For example, one small T-shaped polyethylene device allowed a pregnancy rate of about 18 per 100 woman-years until the addition of fine copper ribbon with a surface area of 200 mm^2. Then the pregnancy rate dropped to about 2 per 100 woman-years. A local, rather than systemic, action from copper must be of major importance, since metallic copper placed in one uterine horn of a rabbit prevents blastocyst implantation there but not in the adjacent horn (Zipper and co-workers, 1971). The experiences of Lippes and co-workers (1978) that insertion of a Copper T or Cu7 device up to 7 days after coitus effectively prevents pregnancy strongly support the concept that the copper-bearing device compromises the blastocyst.

Adverse Effects

A great variety of complications have been described during the use of various intrauterine devices, but, for the most part, the common side effects have not been serious while the serious side effects have not been common. The earliest adverse effects are those associated with insertion. They include clinically apparent or silent *perforation of the uterus,* either while sounding the uterus or during insertion of the device, and *interruption of an unsuspected pregnancy.* The frequency of these complications will depend upon the skill of the operator and the precautions taken to avoid interrupting a pregnancy. Although devices may migrate spontaneously into and through the uterine wall at any time, most perforations occur, or at least begin, at the time of insertion.

Uterine *cramping* and some *bleeding* are likely to develop soon after insertion of an intrauterine device and to persist for variable periods of time. The smaller the device, the less the likelihood of cramping and bleeding but the greater the likelihood of a pregnancy with the device in situ or especially after spontaneous expulsion. Conversely, the larger and more rigid the device, the lower the probability of expulsion and pregnancy but the greater the likelihood of troublesome cramping and bleeding.

Blood loss with menstruation is commonly increased by a factor of about 2 but may be so great as to cause severe iron deficiency anemia (Guttorm, 1971). Therefore, it is wise to make an annual check of the hemoglobin level or hematocrit of women with intrauterine devices as well as any time they complain of heavy menstruation. Antifibrinolytic agents such as epsilon–aminocaproic acid and tranexamic acid have been used by some to reduce excessive uterine bleeding from intrauterine devices, the rationale being that plasminogen activation is inhibited by such agents. Unfortunately, these drugs may prove thrombogenic as well as antifibrinolytic and fatal cerebral thrombosis during the course of such treatment has been reported (Agnelli and associates, 1982).

As an aid for ascertaining appropriate placement in the uterine cavity, most devices have an attached synthetic filament, or tail, which protrudes through the external os and is cut off so that 2 cm or so are visible through the vagina. There has been concern from the outset that the tail might act as a wick and promote invasion of the uterine cavity by pathogenic bacteria. Purrier and co-workers (1979) have identified potentially pathogenic bacteria colonizing the mucus that coated the tails of more than half of intrauterine devices.

Pelvic infections, including septic abortion, have developed following the use of a variety of intrauterine devices. Tuboovarian abscesses, which may be unilateral, have been described by W. Taylor and associates (1973), E. S. Taylor and co-workers (1975), Dawood and Birnbaum (1975), and several others. When infection is suspected, the device should be removed and the woman treated with effective antibiotics. She must be observed closely because there have been deaths from sepsis associated with the use of an intrauterine device. Even so, mortality attributable to such devices is probably lower than that attributed to estrogen plus progestin oral contraceptives or to pregnancy. Nonetheless, because of the risk of salpingitis, pelvic peritonitis, and pelvic abscess,

and, as a consequence, sterility, use of an intrauterine device is usually discouraged for young women of no or very low parity as well as in women who appear to be at increased risk of developing an infection of the pelvic viscera. Vessey and associates (1983) have provided data recently that reinforce their earlier observations that parous women having an intrauterine device removed to try to achieve pregnancy have no prolonged impairment of fertility. They conclude that pelvic infection sufficient to impair fertility must be very uncommon, at least in parous users of such devices.

Actinomyces-like structures identified in Papanicolaou smears and the prolonged use of an intrauterine device have been linked, but the clinical importance of this finding is not clear but worrisome. In most studies an increased prevalence of *Actinomyces israelii* or actinomyces-like organisms was apparent only after several years of use of the device. Furthermore, the organisms were much less frequent when a copper-bearing device was used rather than an inert one, possibly because the former was changed more frequently. Of importance, the percentage of women reporting gynecologic symptoms did not differ significantly between users with and without actinomyces-like organisms on smear (Petitti and associates, 1983). Keebler and co-workers (1983) identified actinomyces in 12.6 percent of device users. Once the smear became positive for actinomyces bodies, all subsequent smears remained positive until the intrauterine device was removed. Authorities agree that, if signs or symptoms of infection develop in women who harbor actinomyces bodies, the device should be removed and antibiotic therapy instituted. However, in the absence of signs or symptoms of pelvic infection there is considerable disagreement as to whether uniform removal of the device or simply close observation is the correct approach.

Locating a Lost Device

When the tail cannot be visualized protruding from the cervical canal, the possibilities of expulsion or of extrauterine location must be considered. In either event, pregnancy is likely to occur. The tail may, however, simply be in the uterine cavity along with a normally positioned device. Often, gentle probing of the uterine cavity using a rod with a terminal hook or with a Randall stone clamp will retrieve the device. The simple assumption that the device had been expelled and that therefore another should be inserted was carried to an extreme in the case demonstrated in Figure 40-6. Adherent to the placenta at delivery were two Dalkon Shields (no longer available!) and one Lippes Loop, each having been inserted because a tail was not visible through the vagina. Almost certainly, each tail was drawn into the uterine cavity by the rapidly growing pregnant uterus. The pregnancy, fortunately, was not otherwise complicated.

When the tail is not visible, sonography has been tried to identify a device that is in the uterine cavity. If a hysteroscope is available, this may also be used in the absence of pregnancy to identify a device in utero.

If not found in the cavity, an extrauterine location may be confirmed by radiographic studies performed in

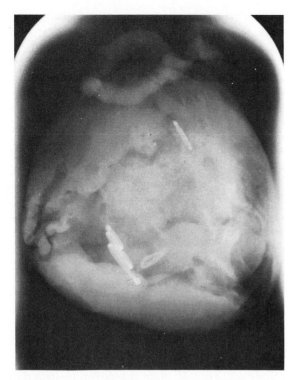

Figure 40-6. A roentgenogram of a term placenta demonstrating two adherent Dalkon Shield intrauterine devices and one Lippes Loop.

the absence of pregnancy with either an opaque probe or another intrauterine device in the uterine cavity, or by filling the uterine cavity with appropriate radiocontrast material (hysterography), as shown in Figure 40-7.

An open device of inert material, such as the Lippes Loop, located outside the uterus may or may not do harm. Perforations of large and small bowel and bowel

fistulas, with attendant morbidity, have developed remote from the time of insertion of the so-called inert devices. Closed devices, such as the Birnberg Bow, can cause *bowel obstruction* and for this reason are no longer used. A copper-bearing device in an extrauterine location is prone to induce an intense local inflammatory reaction and adhere to the inflamed structure. A Copper-T device firmly attached to the appendix is demonstrated in Figure 40-8. Although chemically inert devices have been readily removed from the peritoneal cavity by laparoscopy or through a posterior colpotomy, the copper-bearing device is likely to be too firmly adherent for successful removal by these techniques.

A device may penetrate the uterine wall in varying degrees. At times part of the device may extend into the peritoneal cavity while the remainder is firmly fixed in the myometrium (Fig. 40-9). In this case, at the time of repeat cesarean delivery, part of a Lippes Loop that was inserted 3 years before was found protruding from the fundus posteriorly. Omentum was firmly adherent to the uterus around the protruding loop. Oozing from the tract left after the loop was extracted was controlled with a deep mattress suture.

The intrauterine device can also penetrate into the cervix and actually protrude into the vagina (Fig. 40-5). This is more common with the Cu7 and Copper-T device than with the Lippes Loop. A more likely cause for pregnancy with a device in situ is displacement of the device into the uterine isthmus and cervix (Fig. 40-5), although successful nidation may occur with the device in the fundus of the uterus.

Pregnancy with a Device in Utero

As emphasized in Chapter 13, it is important to identify all pregnant women who might be harboring an intrauterine device, whether it be within the uterine cavity or

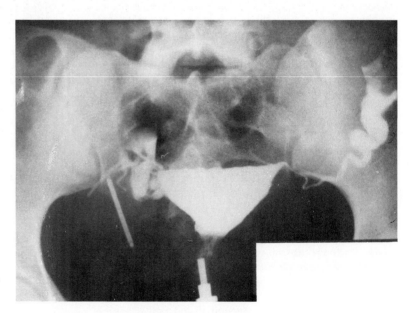

Figure 40-7. Extrauterine location of a Copper T device is confirmed by hysterography.

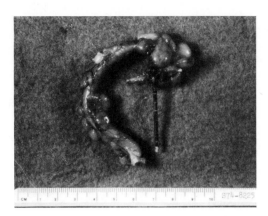

Figure 40-8. Copper T device adherent to appendix.

elsewhere. A device in utero coexisting with a pregnancy is risky to both the fetus and the mother. A device residing beyond the uterus is risky, especially to the mother. Unless removed earlier, appropriate steps must be taken at delivery to identify and assure removal of the device. It is patently obvious that to perform a laparotomy for delivery and not recognize and remove an extrauterine, intra-abdominal device is a serious disservice to the mother!

Fortunately, in some pregnancies the statistical probability of a poor outcome is defied, for example, the favorable outcome for one fetus even though three devices coexisted in utero with her (Fig. 40-6), and the excellent outcome for twin fetuses, who throughout pregnancy were accompanied in utero by an intrauterine device until they were delivered at term (Fig. 40-10).

Nonetheless, when pregnancy is recognized and the tail of the device is visible through the cervix, the device should be removed. This will help reduce subsequent complications in the form of late abortion, sepsis, and prematurity. Tatum and co-workers (1976) observed the abortion rate to be 54 percent with the device left in compared to 25 percent if promptly removed. Moreover, with the device remaining in situ, the frequency of low birth weight, chiefly from prematurity, was 20.3 percent, compared to 4.7 percent if the device was removed early. Vessey and associates (1979) confirmed these observations. If the tail is not visible, attempts to locate and remove the device from the uterus by instrumentation may lead to abortion.

Not only is the likelihood of abortion during the second trimester much increased if an intrauterine device remains in a pregnant uterus, but, very importantly, the abortion is likely to be septic, with the sepsis, at times, being fulminant and killing the mother. Women pregnant with a device in utero and who demonstrate any evidence of uterine infection must have the products of conception and the device removed promptly as well as intensive antibiotic therapy.

An increased incidence of malformation has not been noted with pregnancies complicated by the presence of an intrauterine device.

Extrauterine Pregnancies

Although most intrauterine pregnancies are prevented, the device provides no protection against nidation in other locations. There has been concern that use of an intrauterine device inordinately increases the risk of *ectopic pregnancy,* but Vessey and co-workers (1979) found that the risk remains rather constant with duration of use at 1.2 per 1000 women per year. However, since the device does not prevent extrauterine pregnancy, women already at high risk of an ectopic pregnancy (previous salpingitis, ectopic pregnancy, or tubal surgery) are poor candidates for an intrauterine contraceptive device.

Procedures for Insertion

The Food and Drug Administration requires that before an intrauterine device is inserted physicians must give women who request a device a detailed brochure spelling out the side effects and apparent risks from use of such a device.

Most devices have a special inserter, usually a sterile graduated plastic tube into which the device is withdrawn just before insertion (Fig. 40-3). Timing of insertion of the device influences the ease of placement as well as the pregnancy and expulsion rates. Insertion near the end of a normal menstrual period when the cervix is usually softer and the canal somewhat more dilated may facilitate insertion and at the same time exclude an early pregnancy. However, insertion need not be limited only to this period. For the woman who is reasonably sure that she is not pregnant and she does not want to be pregnant, insertion may be carried out anytime during the menstrual cycle. Even though she

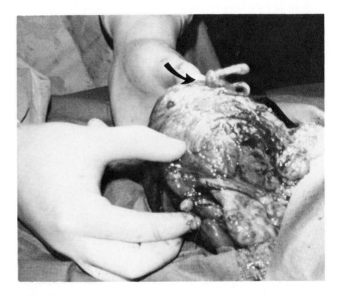

Figure 40-9. Part of a Lippes Loop (*arrow*) covered by adhesions protruding from the uterine fundus posteriorly. Repeat cesarean section has just been performed.

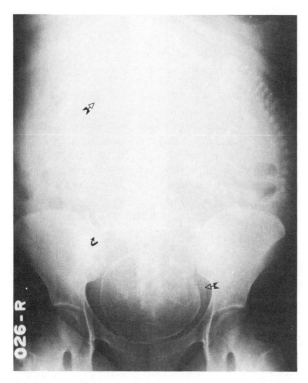

Figure 40-10. Near-term twin fetuses plus a Lippes Loop (*curved arrow*) in utero.

engaged in coitus during the previous week, she is unlikely to conceive if a Copper T or Cu7 device is used (Lippes and associates, 1978).

Insertion at the time of delivery or very soon thereafter is followed by an unsatisfactorily high expulsion rate. The recommendation has been made, therefore, to withhold insertion for at least 8 weeks to reduce expulsion as well as to minimize the risk of perforation. The experience of the Greater Dallas Family Planning Program, however, has been that earlier insertion has not led to perforation or expulsion rates significantly higher than for insertion remote from pregnancy. In the absence of infection, the device may be inserted immediately after early abortion.

A satisfactory technique for insertion and plan for follow-up are outlined below:

1. Obtain a careful gynecologic history. Contraindications to the use of an intrauterine device include the following: Untreated gonorrhea even though asymptomatic, a recent pelvic infection or a history of recurrent pelvic infections, severe dysmenorrhea, cervical stenosis, abnormalities of the uterine cavity, heavy menses, overt anemia, and abnormalities of blood coagulation. The woman who has had a previous ectopic pregnancy should be counseled against the use of an intrauterine device because she is already at considerable risk of another ectopic pregnancy and an intrauterine device does not prevent ectopic pregnancy.
2. Describe the various problems associated with use of an intrauterine device and obtain informed consent.
3. Perform a thorough pelvic examination to identify espe-

cially the position and size of the uterus and adnexa. If abnormalities are found, an intrauterine device often is contraindicated.

4. Visualize the cervix and grasp it with a tenaculum. Use sterile instruments and sterile intrauterine device. Wipe the cervix and the vaginal walls with an antiseptic solution. It is commonly recommended that the uterus first be sounded to help identify the direction and depth of the uterine cavity. Before identifying the depth of the uterine cavity with a sound, the cervical canal and uterine cavity are first straightened by applying gentle traction on the tenaculum. A device of appropriate size is selected based on the length of the uterine cavity. The inserter (Fig. 40-3), with the device contained within its most distal portion, is gently inserted to the fundus of the uterus. After rotating the inserter so that the device is positioned high in the transverse plane of the uterus (Fig. 40-5), the inserter is removed while the device is held in place in the fundus by the plastic rod within the inserter behind the device. Thus, the device is not pushed out of the tube, but rather it is held in place by the rod while the inserter tube is withdrawn.
5. Cut the marker tail 2 cm from the external os, remove the tenaculum, observe for bleeding from the tenaculum puncture sites, and if there is no bleeding, remove the speculum.
6. Provide analgesia with aspirin or codeine to allay cramps. Invite the woman to report promptly any apparent adverse effects.

Expulsion. Loss of the device from the uterus is most common during the first month of use. The recipient should be instructed on how to palpate the strings protruding from the cervix by either sitting on the edge of a chair or squatting down and then advancing the middle finger into the vagina until the cervix is reached. The woman should be checked in 1 month for appropriate placement of the device by identifying the tail protruding appropriately from the cervix. Barrier contraception may be desirable during this time, especially if a device has been expelled previously.

Replacement. The chemically inert device may be left in the uterus indefinitely. The copper-bearing devices will have to be replaced periodically. For the Cu7 and Copper T devices, replacement every 3 years is recommended even though the device may remain effective for 6 to 8 years. The progesterone-bearing intrauterine device, Progestasert, should be replaced annually.

LOCAL BARRIER METHODS

Condoms, vaginal diaphragms, and spermicidal agents placed in the vagina have long been used for contraception with variable success.

Condoms

To date, the condom represents in the United States the only reversible, effective "male method" of contraception except for *coitus interruptus*. Condoms can provide effective contraception. Their failure rate with experienced and strongly motivated couples has been as low as 3 or 4 per 100 couple-years of exposure. Generally, and during the first year of use especially, the failure rate is much higher (Table 40-1). Perhaps the recent availability in the United States of a condom with a spermicidal lubricant (Ramses Extra) will lower the failure rate.

When used properly, condoms provide considerable but not absolute protection against a broad range of sexually transmitted diseases, including gonorrhea, syphilis, herpes, chlamydia and trichomoniasis; they possibly prevent and ameliorate premalignant changes in the cervix (Population Reports, 1982). It is estimated that up to 40 million couples in the world use condoms, with 50 percent of married couples of reproductive age doing so in Japan alone.

Historically, the original condoms were made of intestine and other material, but with the introduction of rubber, the condom became much more effective, less expensive, and more widely available.

The origin of the word "condom" is unknown. It has been stated, probably incorrectly, that it refers to Dr. Condom, a physician who provided King Charles II with a means of preventing more illegitimate offspring. Casanova (1725–1798) is said to have mentioned condoms several times in his exhaustive memoirs.

In Texas, and elsewhere, the earliest father–son discussion of sex and reproduction often was stimulated by the presence of condom-dispensing machines in the men's room of service stations. It is of interest that condoms were widely available at a time when attempts to make other family planning techniques more readily available were discouraged by much of society lest they promote sexual promiscuity or offend someone's religious beliefs. The condoms, or "prophylactics," in the gas stations, allegedly, were provided only to prevent venereal disease.

Intravaginal Contraceptives

Such contraceptive agents are variously marketed as creams, jellies, suppositories, and in aerosol containers (Fig. 40-3) and are widely used in this country, especially by women who find the oral contraceptive or an intrauterine device unacceptable, or who need temporary protection, for example, during the first week after starting oral contraceptives or while nursing.

Most such intravaginal agents can be purchased over-the-counter, that is, a prescription is not needed. Typically, such preparations work by providing a physical barrier to sperm penetration as well as chemical spermicidal action. *To be highly effective, the agents must, shortly before intercourse, be deposited high in the vagina in contact with the cervix.* Their duration of maximal spermicidal effectiveness is usually no more than 1 hour and therefore they must be reinserted into the vagina before intercourse is repeated; douching should be avoided for at least 6 hours after intercourse.

High pregnancy rates are attributable chiefly to inconsistent use rather than to failure of the method during use. If inserted regularly and correctly, use of the

foam preparations for contraception probably results in no more than 5 pregnancies per 100 woman-years of use (Population Reports, 1984).

The spermicides in current use appear to provide some protection against some sexually transmitted disease, including gonorrhea and probably candidiasis and trichomoniasis.

Malformations. Data obtained in one study suggested that the use of vaginal spermicides during the year before conception might be associated with an increased frequency of malformations in offspring. However, a well-defined syndrome of congenital disorders was not identified, and the investigators considered their results to be tentative (Jick and associates, 1981). Importantly, in studies by both Mills and co-workers (1982) and Shapiro and associates (1982) no association was identified between congenital malformations and maternal spermicide exposure before or after the last menstrual period.

Diaphragm Plus Spermicidal Agent

The vaginal diaphragm (Fig. 40-3), consisting of a circular rubber dome of various diameters supported by a circumferentially placed metal spring, has long been used for contraception, in combination with a spermicidal jelly or cream. The spermicidal agent is applied to the superior surface both along the rim and centrally. The device is then placed in the vagina so that the cervix, vaginal fornices, and anterior vaginal wall are effectively partitioned from the rest of the vagina and the penis. At the same time, the centrally placed spermicidal agent is held against the cervix by the diaphragm. When appropriately positioned in the vagina, the rim of the diaphragm is lodged superiorly deep in the posterior vaginal fornix and inferiorly the rim lies in close proximity to the inner surface of the symphysis immediately below the urethra (Fig. 40-11). If the diaphragm is too small, it will not remain in place. If too large, it will be uncomfortable when it is forced into position. A cystocele or uterine prolapse is very likely to result in instability of position and therefore expulsion.

The diaphragm and spermicidal agent can be inserted even hours before intercourse, but if more than 2 hours elapse, additional spermicide should be placed in the upper vagina for maximum protection and be reapplied before subsequent exposure. The diaphragm should be left for at least 6 hours after intercourse before removal.

The so-called toxic-shock syndrome following use of a diaphragm has been described in a few reports (Alcid and associates, 1982). For this reason, it may be worthwhile to remove the diaphragm at the end of 6 hours or so (or the next morning) to minimize this very uncommon event.

The diaphragm requires a high level of motivation for proper use that, when expended, is accompanied by a low pregnancy rate. Vessey and Wiggins (1974) reported a pregnancy rate of only 2.4 per 100 woman-years for already established users of the diaphragm. They right-

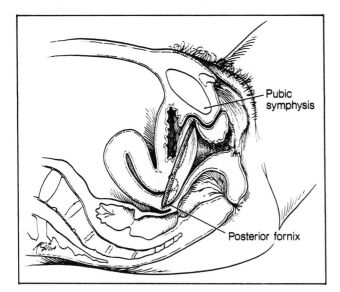

Figure 40-11. A diaphragm in place creates a physical barrier between the vagina and cervix and importantly provides for intimate contact between the contraceptive jelly or cream and the cervix. (The woman is lying supine.)

fully emphasized that established users need not be encouraged to change to a "more modern" method of birth control.

Sponge With or Without a Spermicidal Agent

Contraceptive sponges to be placed in the upper vagina continue to undergo extensive evaluation. One polyurethane sponge soaked with a spermicide has been approved by the Food and Drug Administration and is marketed under the trade name "Today." It has been claimed to be about as effective as other vaginal methods, although studies to date are not really adequate to define precisely its efficacy (Population Reports, 1984).

A sponge of collagen that contains no spermicide is also being evaluated. The key to its effectiveness will be the avidity with which it entraps sperm.

BREAST-FEEDING

Breast-feeding is important to infant health and to child-spacing. For mothers who are fully nursing their infants, ovulation during the first 10 weeks after delivery is very unlikely according to Pérez (1981). However, it is not a very reliable method of family planning for women whose infants are on a 3- to 4-hour, daytime-only feeding schedule and are receiving other food (see Chapter 19, p. 376). Waiting for first menses involves a risk of pregnancy because ovulation may antedate menstruation. Certainly, after the first menses effective contraception is essential unless the woman desires another pregnancy so soon after her last one.

Combined estrogen–progestin contraceptives have been thought by some to reduce somewhat both the rate and the duration of milk production. The benefits from prevention of pregnancy by the use of combined oral contraceptives would appear to outweigh the unsubstantiated risks.

Intrauterine devices have been recommended for the lactating but potentially ovulating, sexually active woman. An increased rate of uterine perforation has been identified in lactating women with an intrauterine device, perhaps as the consequence of vigorous myometrial contractions and involution brought about by the release of oxytocin in response to the stimulation from suckling (Heartwell and Schlesselman, 1983). However, the risk is not so great that intrauterine devices should not be used.

PERIODIC (RHYTHMIC) ABSTINENCE

The pregnancy rate with the various methods for application of periodic abstinence (rhythm methods, "natural" family planning) has been placed at from 5 to 40 per 100 woman-years (Population Reports, 1981).

The human ovum probably is susceptible to successful fertilization only for about 12 to no more than 24 hours after ovulation. Motile sperm have been identified in cervical mucus as many as 7 days after coitus or artificial insemination and in oviducts of women undergoing laparotomy as long as 85 hours after coitus (Ahlgren, 1975). However, it is unlikely that sperm retain the capability for successful fertilization for this long a period.

Ovulation most often occurs about 14 days before the onset of the next menstrual period, but, unfortunately, not necessarily 14 days after the onset of the last menstrual period. Therefore, *calendar rhythm* is not always reliable.

Temperature rhythm relies on *slight* changes in basal body temperature that may occur just before ovulation. The temperature rhythm method is much more likely to be successful if during each menstrual cycle intercourse is avoided until well after the ovulatory temperature rise.

> A bedside clock, the Rite Time, is now marketed. Promotional literature claims that accuracy of the temperature rhythm method is greatly enhanced by the combination of a preprogrammed computer, a digital clock, and a very precise oral thermometer. (Another reason to ask "What time is it?")

Cervical mucus rhythm ("Billings method") depends upon awareness of "dryness" and "wetness" in the vagina as the consequence of changes in the amount and kind of cervical mucus formed at different times in the menstrual cycle. This approach has not achieved popularity.

An extensive review of "natural family planning" has been provided by Klaus (1982).

SURGICAL CONTRACEPTION

Prevalence

Surgical sterilization of one or both sexual partners is the second most popular form of contraception among couples of reproductive age (Fig. 40-1). In 1981, according to the Association for Voluntary Sterilization, nearly 900,000 sterilization procedures were performed in the United States; 52 percent were performed on women.

Until recently, sterilization of women as a technique for effective family planning has been frowned upon by important segments of society, including not only some churches, but also medical groups and a variety of political bodies. For example, until 1969, the American College of Obstetricians and Gynecologists recommended that a woman 30 years of age should have four living children before qualifying for sterilization! Even now, multiple restrictions imposed by the federal government serve to discourage voluntary sterilization among financially underprivileged women by threatening to sever federal funding to the organization that provides the service.

TUBAL STERILIZATION

Over 5,000,000 women underwent tubal sterilization in the United States during the 1970s. Medically speaking, the operation can be performed at any time. Many are done at cesarean section. For women who deliver vaginally the early puerperium is a particularly convenient time. Because the fundus is near the umbilicus and the oviducts are readily accessible directly beneath the abdominal wall for several days after delivery, the operation is technically simple and hospitalization need not be prolonged.

Sterilization immediately following vaginal delivery has some disadvantages. Most often the mother is multiparous and has delivered without receiving anesthesia appropriate for entering the peritoneal cavity. The likelihood of postpartum hemorrhage in multiparous women subsides remarkably during the first 10 hours after delivery. Of particular importance, the status of the newborn infant can be determined much more precisely several hours after birth.

It was recommended previously that puerperal sterilization by partial resection of the oviducts be accomplished before 72 hours postpartum so as to minimize infection from ascending bacterial invasion of the fallopian tubes. However, in several studies no correlation was apparent between time interval and postoperative morbidity. At Parkland Memorial Hospital, the operation is performed in the obstetric surgical suite, most often the morning after delivery, in order to minimize hospital stay.

Types of Tubal Sterilization

The first tubal sterilization reported in the United States more than 100 years ago consisted of ligating the oviducts with a strong silk ligature about 1 inch from their uterine attachment following the woman's second cesarean delivery (Lungren, 1881). Literally, the woman had her tubes tied. Subsequently, it became apparent that an unacceptably high failure rate followed ligation without some form of tubal resection to create discontinuity of the tubal lumen. A variety of techniques are now employed to try to disrupt tubal patency and thereby thwart union of sperm and egg, several of which are considered below.

Irving Procedure. This operation is least likely to fail. Briefly, the procedure, as illustrated in Figure 40-12A, involves severing the oviduct and separating it from the mesosalpinx sufficiently to create a medial segment of tube, the end of which is buried within a tunnel into the myometrium posteriorly, and a short lateral segment of tube, the proximal end of which is then buried within the mesosalpinx. The procedure requires considerably more exposure than do most other techniques and the likelihood of hemorrhage is much greater.

Pomeroy Procedure. Of all the techniques that divide the tube, the simplest, reasonably effective method of performing abdominal sterilization is the so-called Pomeroy procedure (Fig. 40-12B). It has generally been considered important that plain catgut be used to ligate the knuckle of tube, since the rationale of this procedure is based on prompt absorption of the ligature and subsequent separation of the severed tubal ends, which most often become sealed over by fibrosis.

Parkland Procedure. We avoid the initial intimate approximation of the cut ends of the oviduct that is inherent in the Pomeroy procedure (Fig. 40-12C). Through an infraumbilical abdominal wall incision, typically just long enough to allow a small Richardson retractor to be inserted, the oviduct is positively identified by grasping the midportion in a Babcock clamp and confirming by direct observation that indeed fimbriae are present on the distal end of the structure so held. Otherwise, it is easy to confuse the round ligament with the midportion of the oviduct. *Whenever the oviduct is inadvertently dropped, it is mandatory to repeat in toto the identification procedure just described!*

An avascular site (Fig. 40-13A) in the mesosalpinx adjacent to the oviduct is then perforated with a small hemostat and the jaws are opened to separate the oviduct from the adjacent mesosalpinx for about 2.5 cm (Fig. 40-13B). The freed oviduct is ligated proximally and distally (Fig. 40-13C) with 0 chromic suture and the intervening segment of about 2 cm is excised with sharp scissors (Fig. 40-13D). After inspecting for hemostasis, the now discontinuous oviduct is dropped in place and the procedure is repeated on the other side. Both re-

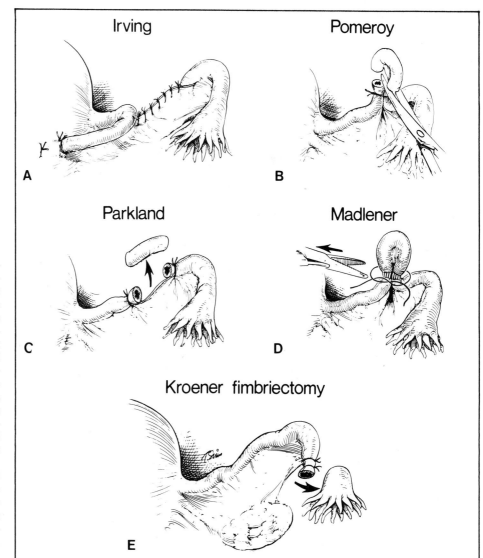

Figure 40-12. Various techniques for tubal sterilization. **A.** Irving procedure: The medial cut end of the oviduct is buried in the myometrium posteriorly and the distal cut end is buried in the mesosalpinx. **B.** Pomeroy procedure: A loop of oviduct is ligated and the knuckle of tube above the ligature is excised. **C.** Parkland procedure: A midsegment of tube is separated from the mesosalpinx at an avascular site, the separated tubal segment is ligated proximally and distally and then excised. **D.** Madlener procedure: A knuckle of oviduct is crushed and then ligated without resection. **E.** Kroener procedure: The tube is ligated across the ampulla and the distal portion of the ampulla, including all of the fimbriae, is resected.

sected segments of oviduct are labeled and submitted for histologic confirmation. Excluding the rare instance in which the operator failed to resect the fallopian tube, which can be confirmed promptly in the surgical pathology laboratory, the subsequent failure rate has been approximately 1 in 400 procedures.

Madlener Procedure. A knuckle of tube is crushed and ligated with nonabsorbable suture but not resected (Fig. 40-12D). This procedure is mentioned only to discourage its use. Early experiences at Parkland Memorial Hospital indicated a failure rate of about 7 percent.

Fimbriectomy. Removal of all of the fimbriae to effect sterilization has been recommended by Kroener (1969) and by others. Kroener doubly ligated the oviduct with silk suture and then excised the fimbriated end (Fig. 40-12C). Although Kroener reported no failures, others

have, and in some instances the rate has been unacceptable. Taylor (1972), for example, observed 6 pregnancies among about 200 women who were subjected to fimbriectomy; when the oviducts were subsequently examined, usually a small amount of fimbrial tissue had been left. Metz (1977) identified 7 failures among 388 women upon whom bilateral fimbriectomy was performed. Catgut suture had been used and the resected surface had been lightly electrocoagulated. In the cases that failed, tuboperitoneal fistulas lined with tubal epithelium were found in the remaining ampullary portion of the tube.

Postoperative Care

After puerperal sterilization, analgesia should be provided for abdominal soreness, which at times is aggravated in multiparous women by uterine "afterbirth pains." Meperidine, 50 to 75 mg intramuscularly, given

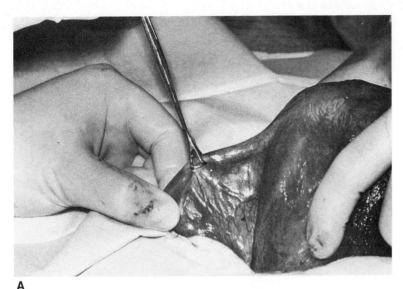

A

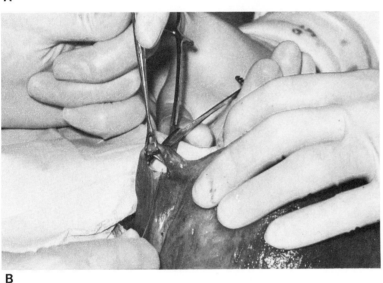

B

Figure 40-13. Sterilization at cesarean section. **A.** An avascular site in the mesosalpinx adjacent to the midportion of the oviduct is looked for. **B.** A small hemostat has been inserted through the avascular site and the jaws of the clamp opened to separate mesosalpinx from tube for about 2.5 cm. A ligature is being inserted.

intermittently as needed during the first 24 hours, provides excellent analgesia. Within 8 hours, most women can ambulate, eat a regular diet, and care for their babies, including breast-feeding. We have found discharge from the hospital the day after the procedure to be satisfactory in most instances.

Nonpuerperal Tubal Sterilization

The techniques, including modifications that have been recommended to accomplish sterilization through tubal occlusion, are almost bewildering in number. Basically, they consist of (1) ligation and resection as described above for puerperal sterilization, (2) the permanent application of a variety of rings or clips to the fallopian tubes, and (3) electrocoagulation of a segment of the oviducts.

Laparotomy to perform sterilization can be a much more formidable procedure once the uterus has completely involuted and returned to the true pelvis. However, much of the difficulty of obtaining exposure is removed if the uterus and adnexa are pushed out of the true pelvis to beneath the abdominal wall above the symphysis using a manipulator previously inserted into the uterus with the handle protruding from the vagina. Utilizing this technique, "mini-laparotomies" are being performed through a 3-cm incision made suprapubically and tubal sterilization effected.

Vaginal tubal sterilization can usually be performed on women who have delivered vaginally once the uterus has involuted and pregnancy-induced hyperemia has subsided. The peritoneal cavity is entered through the posterior vaginal fornix (colpotomy, culdotomy), the oviducts are grasped and drawn into view, and then, most often, either a Pomeroy type resection or fimbriectomy is performed.

Enthusiasm was generated for interval as well as post-abortal sterilizations using *laparoscopy* by an article in *Life* magazine (July 28, 1972) that referred to the technique as "Band-Aid" surgery. Commonly, the woman is cared for in an ambulatory surgical setting. Anesthesia, either general, usually with endotracheal intubation, or local, is induced, and after producing pneumoperitoneum with carbon dioxide, the sterilization procedure is accomplished. Most often the woman can be discharged several hours later.

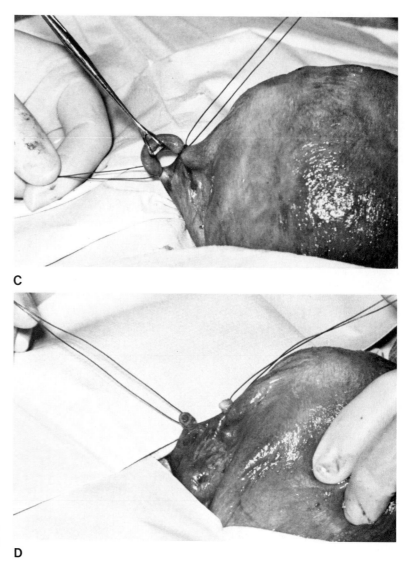

Figure 40-13. C. The segment of oviduct separated from mesosalpinx has been ligated. **D.** The ligated segment of oviduct has been resected.

Hazards from Tubal Sterilization

The principal hazards associated with tubal sterilization are anesthetic complications, inadvertent coagulation of vital structures, the rare occurrence of pulmonary embolism, and failure to produce sterility with an unrecognized and therefore inappropriately treated ectopic pregnancy as the result (see Chapter 22, p. 423). Peterson and co-workers (1982, 1983) have considered all deaths temporally associated with tubal sterilization and estimated the case-fatality frequency to be 8 per 100,000 procedures. When only deaths directly attributable to the procedure per se were considered, the case-fatality rate was at least 4 per 100,000. The leading cause of death, general anesthesia without endotracheal intubation, almost certainly could have been avoided by use of an endotracheal tube or another form of anesthesia.

Results of a multicenter, multinational randomized study of minilaparotomy with tubal ligation plus a midsegment resection procedure compared to laparoscopy with tubal electrocoagulation have been provided by the World Health Organization Task Force on Female Sterilization (1982). Significant complications were identified in 1.5 percent of the former and 0.9 percent of the latter. They concluded, however, that minilaparotomy is the preferred approach for such a service when provided away from a major institution.

DeStefano and co-workers (1983) identified intraoperative or postoperative complications in 1.7 percent of a large number of women who, remote from pregnancy, underwent laparoscopic tubal electrocoagulation for sterilization. Factors identified to increase morbidity were previous abdominal or pelvic surgery, a history of previous pelvic infection, obesity, diabetes, and general rather than local anesthesia. These same factors would, undoubtedly, increase the risk of morbidity with minilaparotomy.

"Post–Tubal Ligation Syndrome." The possibility has been raised of a "post–tubal ligation syndrome" variably characterized by pelvic discomfort, ovarian cyst formation, and especially menorrhagia. That tubal ligation induces any of these changes remains to be established. Kasonde and Bonnar (1976) actually measured menstrual blood loss before and for 6 to 12 months after tubal sterilization and found that the operation made no significant difference in menstrual blood loss. They also noted that women who presented with menorrhagia soon after sterilization usually had had the problem beforehand or had been using oral contraceptives, which reduced blood loss, and then reverted to spontaneous heavier periods when their use was stopped after sterilization. More recently, DeStefano and co-workers (1983) followed 2456 women for 2 years after tubal sterilization surgery and noted that, except for menstrual pain among women who underwent unipolar electrocoagulation procedures, there was no increase in the prevalence of adverse menstrual function. In fact, 50 percent or more of women with adverse menstrual function before sterilization had an improvement over the 2 years following the procedure. Vessey and associates (1983) have compared the frequency of gynecologic and psychiatric disorders among women who had undergone tubal sterilization with the frequencies in women who had not, but their husbands had undergone vasectomy, and found little difference between the two groups.

Some women who had undergone tubal sterilization were reported by Hargrove and Abraham (1981) to have high serum estradiol and low serum progesterone levels compared to normal controls. Ladehoff and co-workers (1980), however, identified no change in ovarian endocrine function following tubal sterilization. Other investigators have failed to identify luteal phase dysfunction after tubal sterilization, except possibly after techniques that can cause obstruction of the uteroovarian artery (Donnez and associates, 1981).

Although complete transection of the oviduct is mandatory, at the same time preservation of blood supply through the adjacent mesosalpinx is desirable to minimize the possibility of "postligation" abnormalities that have been attributed by some to tubal sterilization. The Parkland technique (Fig. 40-12C) should not compromise blood supply to the ovary. Interestingly, El-Minawi and associates (1983), by means of venography, identified uterovaginal and ovarian varicosities commonly after the Pomeroy and some other procedures but not following the Parkland technique.

Restoration of Fertility

Despite the recent enthusiasm for performing "microsurgery" on oviducts previously rendered nonpatent surgically, no woman should undergo tubal sterilization believing that her fertility can be restored by such means. Sterilization reversal is costly, difficult, and uncertain. Restitution of tubal continuity is technically feasible, but the success rate is unknown and probably no more than 50 percent and there is appreciable subsequent risk of tubal pregnancy. If any doubt exists in the mind of the recipient, the sterilization should not be done.

Hysterectomy

For the woman who desires no more children, hysterectomy has many theoretical advantages. The only known potential of the uterus, other than to house products of conception, is to harbor disease. However, in the absence of uterine or other pelvic disease, hysterectomy for sterilization at the time of cesarean section, early in the puerperium, or remote from pregnancy, is difficult to justify (Barclay and associates, 1976; Laros and Work, 1975). Unfortunately, morbidity, mortality, and cost compared to tubal sterilization, usually preclude hysterectomy. With cesarean hysterectomy, blood loss is nearly always greater than with cesarean section plus tubal sterilization, leading to much more frequent use of blood transfusions and its sequelae. Injury to the urinary tract is also appreciably more common.

For reasons that are hard to identify, an increased failure rate for sterilization at the time of cesarean section has been reported by some. However, with the technique for tubal sterilization used at Parkland Memorial Hospital and described above, no difference was identified (Husbands and co-workers, 1970).

Hysteroscopy

Sterilization utilizing *hysteroscopy* to visualize the tubal ostia and somehow obliterate them is a worthy goal and has received considerable attention. To date, the failure rate and other problems limit the clinical utility of this approach.

VASECTOMY

Sterilization of the male has emerged as a popular form of family planning. It has been estimated that one-half million men undergo vasectomy annually in the United States. Through a small incision in the scrotum, the lumen of the vas deferens is disrupted to block the passage of sperm from the testes (Fig. 40-14). The procedure is usually performed in 20 minutes or so on an outpatient basis under local anesthesia. The procedure has less morbidity and mortality and is less expensive than female sterilization. The cost of vasectomy has been estimated to be only about one fifth that of tubal sterilization ($240 compared to $1180).

A disadvantage of vasectomy is that sterility is not immediate. Complete expulsion of sperm stored in the reproductive tract beyond the interrupted vas deferens may take a week to several months. The time appears to depend in part on the frequency of ejaculation. Semen should be checked until two consecutive sperm counts are zero. During this period, another form of contraception must be used. The failure rate for vasectomy is estimated to be about 1 in 100 (Population Reports, 1975).

Restoration of fertility after a successful vasectomy does not always succeed. A review of several reports suggests that odds for success are about 50–50, with somewhat higher success rates following microsurgical

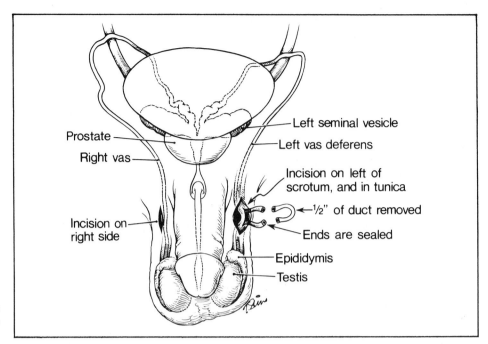

Figure 40-14. Male reproductive system showing the site of vasectomy.

reanastomosis. As with women, the risks of regret after sterilization appear to relate primarily to immaturity at the time of sterilization (Howard, 1982). Three factors that appear to be important in restoration of fertility after previous vasectomy are (1) the application of meticulous microsurgical techniques for reanastomosis, (2) the length of time after vasectomy, since chronic obstruction of the vas and possibly the development of sperm antibodies reduce progressively the capacity for spermatogenesis, and (3) the presence or absence of sperm granulomas.

Long-term storage of semen collected before vasectomy remains an experimental procedure. The cost of storing frozen semen is high, the availability of facilities is limited, and the results remain uncertain (Beck, 1978).

Sperm antibodies can be identified rather often after vasectomy. Concern was raised over the possibility that the immune response may cause systemic changes of a harmful nature. Moreover, in some preliminary studies on previously vasectomized monkeys, atherosclerosis appeared to be increased. However, observations carefully made on a very large number of males who had undergone vasectomy several years before have not identified an increase in cardiovascular disease, circulating immune complexes, or damage to blood vessels of the retina (Linnet and co-workers, 1982; Petitti, 1982; Walker and associates, 1981; Goldacre and colleagues, 1983).

Reversible Systemically Acting Contraceptives for Men

A safe, practical, consistently reliable, and reversible contraceptive for men that does not impair sexual function has not yet been developed.

In China, gossypol, extracted from cottonseed, has been widely used. The compound was discovered after an outbreak of illness and impaired fertility among Chinese farmers exposed to raw cottonseed oil after a change in processing techniques. Gossypol directly affects the testes to inhibit spermatogenesis. Toxic side effects limit its use.

The administration of some analogues of luteinizing hormone–releasing hormone has produced a decline in sperm density, a fall in sperm motility, and a decrease in testosterone production (Linde and co-workers, 1981). The loss of libido makes such a regimen unacceptable.

REFERENCES

Agnelli G, Gresele P, DeCunto M, Nenci GG: Tranexamic acid, intrauterine contraceptive devices and fatal cerebral arterial thrombosis. Br J Obstet Gynaecol 89:681, 1982

Ahlgren M: Sperm transport to and survival in the human fallopian tube. Gynecol Invest 6:206, 1975

Alcid DV, Kothari N, Quinn EP, Geismar L, Glowinsky LZ: Toxic-shock syndrome associated with diaphram use for only nine hours. Lancet 1:1363, 1982

Andersch B, Hahn L: Premenstrual complaints. II. Influence of oral contraceptives. Acta Obstet Gynecol Scand 60:579, 1981

Antoniades K, Campbell WN, Hecksher RH, Kessler WB, McCarthy GE Jr: Liver cell adenoma and oral contraceptives. JAMA 234:628, 1975

Badaracco MA, Vessey MP: Recurrence of venous thromboembolic disease and use of oral contraceptives. Br Med J 1:215, 1974

Barclay DL, Hawks BL, Frueh DM, Power JD, Struble RH: Elective cesarean hysterectomy: A five year comparison with cesarean section. Am J Obstet Gynecol 124:900, 1976

Beck WW Jr: Artificial insemination and preservation of semen. Urol Clin N Am 5:593, 1978

Buhler M, Papiernik E: Successive pregnancies in women fitted with intrauterine devices who take anti-inflammatory drugs. Lancet 1:483, 1983

Centers for Disease Control: Oral contraceptive use and the risk of breast cancer. JAMA 249:1591, 1983

Centers for Disease Control: Oral contraceptive use and the risk of ovarian cancer. JAMA 249:1596, 1983

Centers for Disease Control: Oral contraceptive use and the risk of endometrial cancer. JAMA 249:1600, 1983

Cheng MCE, Lim YC, Ng AYH, Ratnam SS: Six-monthly Depo-Provera injection as a contraceptive agent: Its accceptability in Singapore. Aust NZ J Obstet Gynaecol 14:231, 1974

Contraceptive Technology Update. 4:25 (March), 1983

Dawood MY, Birnbaum SJ: Unilateral tubo-ovarian abscess and intrauterine contraceptive device. Obstet Gynecol 46:429, 1975

DeStefano F, Greenspan JR, Dicker RC, Peterson HB, Strauss LT, Rubin GL: Complications of interval laparoscopic tubal sterilization. Obstet Gynecol 61:153, 1983

Donnez J, Wauters M, Thomas K: Luteal function after tubal sterilization. Obstet Gynecol 57:65, 1981

Edelman DA, Kothenbeutel R, Levinski MJ; Kelly SE: Comparative trials of low-dose combined oral contraceptives. J Reprod Med 28:195, 1983

El-Minawi MF, Masor N, Reda MS: Pelvic venous changes after tubal sterilization. J Reprod Med 28:641, 1983

Fisch IR, Frank J: Oral contraceptives and blood pressure. JAMA 237:2499, 1977

Francis WJA: Reproduction at menarche and menopause in women. J Reprod Fertil (Suppl) 12:89, 1970

Goldacre JM, Holford TR, Vessey MP: Cardiovascular disease and vasectomy. N Engl J Med 308:805, 1983

Guttorm E: Menstrual bleeding with intrauterine contraceptive devices. Acta Obstet Gynecol Scand 50:9, 1971

Hargrove JT, Abraham GE: Endocrine profile of patients with post-tubal ligation syndrome. J Reprod Med 26:359, 1981

Harlap S, Eldor J: Births following oral contraceptive failures. Obstet Gynecol 55:447, 1980

Heartwell SF, Schlesselman S: Risk of uterine perforation among users of intrauterine devices. Obstet Gynecol 61:31, 1983

Howard G: Who asks for vasectomy reversal and why? Br Med J 285:490, 1982

Hull MGR, Savage PE, Bromham DR, Jackson JAM: Normal fertility in women with post-pill amenorrhea. Lancet 1:1329, 1981

Husbands ME Jr, Pritchard JA, Pritchard SA: Failure of tubal sterilization accompanying cesarean section. Am J Obstet Gynecol 107:966, 1970

Irey NS, Nanion WC, Taylor HB: Vascular lesions in women taking oral contraceptives. Arch Pathol 89:1, 1970

Janevich DT, Piper JM, Glebatis DM: Oral contraceptives and congenital limb reduction defects. N Engl J Med 291:697, 1974

Jick H, Walker AM, Rothman KJ, Hunter JR, Holmes LB, Watkins RN, D'Ewart DC, Danford A, Madsen S: Vaginal spermicides and congenital disorders. JAMA 245:1329, 1981

Kasonde JM, Bonnar J: Effect of sterilization on menstrual blood loss. Br J Obstet Gynaecol 83:572, 1976

Keebler C, Chatwani A, Schwartz R: Actinomyces infection associated with intrauterine contraceptive devices. Am J Obstet Gynecol 145:596, 1983

Kent DR, Nissen ED, Nissen SE, Ziehm DJ: Effect of pregnancy on liver tumor associated with oral contraceptives. Obstet Gynecol 51:148, 1978

Klaus H: Natural family planning: A review. Obstet Gynecol Surv 37:128, 1982

Kroener WF Jr: Surgical sterilization by fimbriectomy. Am J Obstet Gynecol 104:247, 1969

Kuchara LK: Postcoital contraception with diethylstilbestrol. JAMA 218:562, 1971

Ladehoff P, Lindholm P, Qvist K, Sørenson T: Gonadotropins and estrogens before and after laparoscopic sterilization. Acta Obstet Gynecol Scand (Suppl) 93:77, 1980

Laros RK Jr, Work BA Jr: Female sterilization. III. Vaginal hysterectomy. Am J Obstet Gynecol 122:693, 1975

Larrson-Cohn U: Oral contraceptives and vitamins : A review. Am J Obstet Gynecol 121:84, 1975

Leklem JE, Brown RR, Rose DP, Linkswiler HM: Vitamin B_6 requirements of women using oral contraceptives. Am J Clin Nutrit 28:535, 1975

Liang AP, Levenson AG, Layde PM, Shelton UD, Hatcher RA, Potts M, Michelson MJ: Risk of breast, uterine corpus, and ovarian cancer in women receiving medroxyprogesterone injections. JAMA 249:2909, 1983

Linde R, Doelle GC, Alexander N, Kirchner F, Vale W, Rivier J, Rabin D: Reversible inhibition of testicular steroidogenesis and spermatogenesis by a potent gonadotropin-releasing hormone agonist in normal men. N Engl J Med 305:663, 1981

Linn S, Schoenbaum SC, Monson RR, Rosner B, Ryan KJ: Delay in conception for former "pill" users. JAMA 247:629, 1982

Linn S, Schoenbaum SC, Monson RR, Rosner B, Stubblefield PG, Ryan KJ: Lack of association between contraceptive usage and congenital malformations in offspring. Am J Obstet Gynecol 147:923, 1983

Linnet L, Møller NPH, Bernth-Perersen P, Ehlers N, Brandslund I, Svehag S-E: No increase in arteriosclerotic retinopathy or activity in tests for circulating immune complexes 5 years after vasectomy. Fertil Steril 37:798, 1982

Lippes J, Tatum HJ, Maulid D, Zielezny M: A continuation of the study of postcoital IUDs. Paper presented at the annual meeting of the Association of Planned Parenthood Physicians, San Diego, October 25, 1978

Lungren SS: A case of cesarean twice. Am J Obstet Dis Women Child 14:78, 1881

Mann JI, Inman WHW: Oral contraceptives and death from myocardial infarction. Br Med J 2:245, 1975

McPherson K, Neil A, Vessey MP, Doll R: Oral contraceptives and breast cancer. Lancet 2:1414, 1983

Metcalf MG: Incidence of ovulatory cycles in women approaching the menopause. J Biosoc Sci 11:39, 1979

Metcalf MG, Donald RA: Fluctuating ovarian function in a perimenopausal woman. Aust NZ Med J 89:45, 1979

Metz KGP: Failures following fimbriectomy. Fertil Steril 28:66, 1977

Mills JL, Harley EE, Reed GF, Berendes HW: Are spermicides teratogenic? JAMA 248:2148, 1982

Mishell DR Jr: Noncontraceptive health benefits of oral contraceptives. Am J Obstet Gynecol 142:809, 1982

Nilsson L, Sölvell L: Clinical studies on oral contraceptives. Acta Obstet Gynecol Scand Suppl 8:46, 1967

Nora AH, Nora JJ: A syndrome of multiple congenital anomalies associated with teratogenic exposure. Arch Environ Health 30:17, 1975

Perez A: Natural family planning: Postpartum period. Int J Fertil 26:219, 1981

Peterson HB, DeStefano F, Greenspan JR, Ory HW: Mortality risk associated with tubal sterilization in United States Hospitals. Am J Obstet Gynecol 143:125, 1982

Peterson HB, DeStefano F, Rubin GL, Greenspan JR, Lee NC, Ory HW: Deaths attributed to tubal sterilization in the United States, 1977 to 1981. Am J Obstet Gynecol 146:131, 1983

Petitti DB: Atherosclerotic disease in men 10 or more years after vasectomy. Presented at the annual meeting of the Association of Planned Parenthood Professionals, Baltimore, November 19, 1982

Petitti DB, Yamamoto D, Morgenstern N: Factors associated with actinomyces-like organisms on Papanicolaou smear in users of intrauterine contraceptive devices. Am J Obstet Gynecol 145:339, 1983

Phillips N, Duffy T: One-hour glucose tolerance in relation to the use of oral contraceptive drugs. Am J Obstet Gynecol 116:91, 1973

Pike MC, Henderson BE, Krailo MD, Duke A, Roy S: Breast cancer in young women and use of oral contraceptives: Possible modifying effect of formulation and age at use. Lancet 2:926, 1983

Population Reports: Periodic abstinence: How well do new approaches work? Series L, No 3, September 1981

Population Reports: Vasectomy—What are the problems? Series D, No 1, January 1975

Population Reports: Update on condoms—Products, protection, promotion. Series H, No 6, September–October 1982

Population Reports: OC's—Update on usage, safety, and side-effects. January 1979, p A-133

Population Reports: IUDs: An appropriate contraception for many women. Series B, No 4, July 1982

Population Reports: Barrier Method—New developments in vaginal contraception. Series H, No 7, January–February, 1984

Prasad AS, Lei KY, Moghissi KS: The effect of oral contraceptives on micronutrients. In Mosely WH (ed): Nutrition and Human Reproduction. New York, Plenum, 1978

Pritchard JA, Pritchard SA: Blood pressure response to estrogen-progestin oral contraceptive after pregnancy-induced hypertension. Am J Obstet Gynecol 129:733, 1977

Pritchard JA, Scott DE, Whalley PJ: Maternal folate deficiency and pregnancy wastage. IV. Effects of folic acid supplements, anticonvulsants, and oral contraceptives. Am J Obstet Gynecol 109:341, 1971

Purrier BGA, Sparks RA, Watt PJ, Elstein M: In vitro study of the possible role of the intrauterine contraceptive device tail in ascending infection of the genital tract. Br J Obstet Gynaecol 86:374, 1979

Rothman KJ, Louik C: Oral contraceptives and birth defects. N Engl J Med 299:522, 1978

Royal College of General Practitioners' Oral Contraceptive Study: Oral contraceptives and gallbladder disease. Lancet 2:957, 1982

Savolainen E, Saksela E, Saxén L: Teratogenic hazards of oral contraceptives analyzed in a national malformation register. Am J Obstet Gynecol 140:521, 1981

Schwallie PC: Experience with Depo-Provera as an injectable contraceptive. J Reprod Med 13:113, 1974

Scott DE, Pritchard JA: Hematologic effects of oral contraceptives after megaloblastic anemia in pregnancy. Gynecol Invest 6:40, 1975

Shapiro S, Slone D, Heinonin OP, Kaufman DW, Rosenberg L, Mitchell AA, Helmrich SP: Birth defects and vaginal spermicides. JAMA 247:2381, 1982

Shojania AM, Hornaday G, Barnes PH: Oral contraceptives and serum-folate levels, Lancet 1:1376, 1968

Spellacy WN, Buhi WC, Birk SA: The effects of vitamin B_6 on carbohydrate metabolism in women taking steroid contraceptives: preliminary report. Contraception 6:265, 1972

Stadel BV: Oral contraceptives and cardiovascular disease. N Engl J Med 305:612, 672, 1981

Stephens MEM, Craft I, Peters TJ, Hoffbrand AV: Oral contraceptives and folate metabolism. Clin Sci 42:405, 1972

Streiff RR: Folate deficiency and oral contraceptives. JAMA 214:105, 1970

Szlachter BN, Nachtigall LE, Epstein J, Young BK, Weiss G: Premature menopause: A reversible entity? Obstet Gynecol 54:396, 1979

Tatum HJ: Copper-bearing intrauterine devices. Clin Obstet Gynecol 17:93, 1974

Tatum HJ, Schmidt FH, Jain AK: Management and outcome of pregnancies associated with Copper-T intrauterine contraceptive device. Am J Obstet Gynecol 126:869, 1976

Taylor TS: Editorial comment. Obstet Gynecol Surv 27:168, 1972

Taylor ES, McMillan JH, Greer BE, Droegemueller W, Thompson HE: The intrauterine device and tubo-ovarian abscess. Am J Obstet Gynecol 123:338, 1975

Taylor WW, Martin FG, Pritchard SA, Pritchard JA: Complications from Majzlin spring intrauterine device. Obstet Gynecol 14:404, 1973

Theur RC: The effect of oral contraceptive agents on vitamin and mineral needs: A review. J Reprod Med 3:13, 1972

Vessey MP: Thromboembolism, cancer, and oral contraceptives. Clin Obstet Gynecol 17:65, 1974

Vessey MP, Wiggins P: Use-effectiveness of the diaphragm in a selected family planning clinic population in the United Kingdom. Contraception 9:15, 1974

Vessey MP, Doll R, Jones K: Oral contraceptives and breast cancer. Lancet 1:941, 1975

Vessey MP, Doll R, Jones K, McPherson K, Yeates D: An epidemiological study of oral contraceptives and breast cancer. Br Med J 1:1757, 1979

Vessey MP, Meisler L, Flavel R, Yeates D: Outcome of pregnancy in women using different methods of contraception. Br J Obstet Gynaecol 86:548, 1979

Vessey MP, Yeates D, Flavel R: Risk of ectopic pregnancy and duration of use of an intrauterine device. Lancet 2:501, 1979

Vessey MP, Lawless M, Yeates D: Efficacy of different contraceptive methods. Lancet 1:841, 1982

Vessey MP, Lawless M, McPherson K, Yeates D: Fertility after stopping use of intrauterine contraceptive device. Br Med J 286:106, 1983

Vessey MP, Huggins G, Lawless M, Yeates D: Tubal sterilization: Findings in a large prospective study. Br J Obstet Gynaecol 90:203, 1983

Vessey MP, McPherson K, Lawless M, Yeates D: Neoplasia of the cervix uteri and contraception: A possible adverse effect of the pill. Lancet 2:930, 1983a

Vessey MP, Baron J, Doll R, McPherson K, Yates D: Oral contraceptives and breast cancer. Final report of an epidemiological study. Br J Cancer 47:455, 1983b

Walker AM, Hunter JR, Watkins RN, Jick H, Danford A, Alhadeff L, Rothman KJ: Vasectomy and non-fatal myocardial infarction. Lancet 1:13, 1981

Wingrave AJ, Kay CR, Vessey MP: Oral contraceptives and diabetes mellitus. Br Med J 1:23, 1979

Wiseman RA: Oral contraceptives and breast cancer rates. Lancet 2:1415, 1983

World Health Organization Task Force on Female Sterilization: Minilaparotomy or laparoscopy for sterilization: A multicenter, multinational randomized study. Am J Obstet Gynecol 143:645, 1982

Wynn V: Vitamins and oral contraceptive use. Lancet 1:561, 1975

Yuzpe AA, Smith RP, Rademaker AE: A multicenter clinical investigation employing ethinyl estradiol combined with *dl*-norgestrel as a postcoital contraceptive agent. Fertil Steril 37:508, 1982

Zipper JA, Tatum JH, Medel M, Pastene L, Rivera M: Contraception through the use of intrauterine metals: I. Copper as an adjunct to the T device. Am J Obstet Gynecol 109:771, 1971

41

Forceps Delivery and Related Techniques

Obstetrics forceps are designed for extraction of the fetus. The intriguing history of the early development and use of these instruments is presented at the end of this chapter.

GENERAL DESIGN

Forceps vary considerably in size and shape but consist basically of two crossing *branches* that are introduced separately into the vagina. Each branch is maneuvered into appropriate relationship with the fetal head and then articulated. Basically, each branch has four components. These are the *blade,* the *shank,* the *lock,* and the *handle.* Each blade has two curves, the *cephalic* and the *pelvic.* The cephalic curve conforms to the shape of the fetal head and the pelvic curve with that of the birth canal. The blades are oval to elliptical in outline and some varieties are fenestrated rather than solid to permit a more firm hold on the fetal head.

The cephalic curve (Fig. 41-1) should be large enough to grasp the fetal head firmly without compression, but not so large that the instrument slips. The pelvic curve (Fig. 41-1) corresponds more or less to the axis of the birth canal but varies considerably among different instruments. The blades are connected to the handles by the shanks, which give the requisite length to the instrument.

The kind of articulation, or *forceps lock,* varies among different instruments. The common method of articulation consists of a socket located on the shank at the junction with the handle and into which fits a socket similarly located on the opposite shank (Figs. 41-1, 41-2). This form of articulation is commonly referred to as the *English lock.* A *sliding lock* is used in some forceps, for example, Kielland forceps (Fig. 41-3) and Barton forceps in which a single U-shaped receptacle mounted midway on the left shank accepts the shank of the right branch. The sliding lock allows the shanks to move forward and backward independently. The components of a quite different type of lock, the *French lock,* are a threaded eye bolt screwed partway into a threaded hole in the left shank and a notch in the right shank that articulates with the eye bolt. After each branch has been applied to the fetal head, the notch is moved over the stem of the eye bolt and the eye bolt is tightened to lock the branches firmly together. With one style, the Tarnier forceps (Fig. 41-4), there is included behind the French lock a hinged bolt with a wing nut mounted on one branch that, after the forceps are locked, is depressed medially into a U-shaped receiver mounted on the opposite shank. As the wing nut is tightened against the receiver, both blades of the forceps are forced against the fetal head. Use of Tarnier forceps was abandoned at Parkland Memorial Hospital long ago for obvious reasons.

DEFINITIONS AND CLASSIFICATION

Forceps operations on a fetus presenting by the vertex are classified as follows, according to the level and position of the head in the birth canal at the time the blades are applied:

Low forceps (outlet forceps) operations are those in which the instrument is applied after the fetal head has reached the perineal floor, the sagittal suture is in the anteroposterior diameter of the outlet, and the scalp is visible at the vaginal introitus.

Midforceps operations are those in which forceps are applied before the criteria for low forceps are met but after engagement of the fetal head has taken place. Clinical evidence of engagement is usually afforded by the descent of the lowermost part of the skull to or below the level of the ischial spines, since the distance between the level of the ischial spines and the pelvic inlet is ordinarily greater than the distance from the biparietal diameter to the leading part of the fetal head (see Chapter 11, p. 227). Especially after vigorous labor, elongation of the fetal head from the combination of a marked degree of molding and caput formation will create the erroneous impression that the head is engaged even though the biparietal diameter has not passed through the pelvic inlet (see Chapter 31, p. 679).

The definition of midforceps as stated includes many levels of the fetal head and, therefore, a range of difficulty. For this reason, Dennen (1964) and some others subdivided midforceps operations as follows: A *midforceps delivery* is one performed when the leading bony portion of the head is at or just below the level of the ischial spines, with the biparietal diameter through the pelvic inlet; the head nearly fills the hollow of the

837

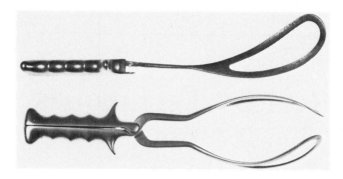

Figure 41-1. Simpson forceps. Note the ample pelvic curve in the single blade above and cephalic curve evident in the articulated blades below. The fenestrated blade and the wide shank in front of the English style lock characterize the Simpson forceps.

sacrum. A *low midforceps delivery* is one performed when the biparietal diameter is at or below the level of the ischial spines and the leading part is within a finger's breadth of the perineum between contractions; the head fills the hollow of the sacrum.

The danger of trauma to the fetus and the mother from a so-called low midforceps delivery will vary remarkably depending upon the circumstances preceding delivery. At times, the fetal head, as the consequence of appropriate uterine contractions and voluntary expulsive efforts of the mother, will descend to lie firmly against the perineum with the sagittal suture anteroposterior; subsequent to anesthesia for delivery, however, the fetal head will recede somewhat from the perineum and the sagittal suture will revert to an oblique position. Forceps delivery with episiotomy in this circumstance is very likely to be a benign procedure. On the other hand, if the fetal head has never reached the perineum and the sagittal suture has never achieved the anteroposterior position, so-called low midforceps delivery may prove traumatic to fetus, mother, or both. Forceps delivery in this latter situation should really be classified as a midforceps delivery.

High forceps operations are those in which forceps are applied before engagement has taken place. High forceps delivery has no place in modern obstetrics.

Incidence

During much of the first half of this century, polarization of opinions over the use of forceps in obstetrics resulted in two very distinct schools of thought. One school vigorously maintains that forceps delivery should be accomplished as soon as the fetal head was engaged and the cervix fully dilated (or, at times, dilatable). The other contends with equal vigor that spontaneous delivery should be awaited. Subsequently, in objective analyses of outcomes it has been demonstrated repeatedly that increased perinatal morbidity and mortality and maternal morbidity result from midforceps delivery (see Chapter 29, Table 29-2). Moreover, for reasons presented sub-

sequently, there may be less perinatal and maternal morbidity with truly low forceps (outlet forceps) delivery and an adequate episiotomy compared to delayed spontaneous delivery without episiotomy. In general, the incidence of low forceps operations compared to spontaneous deliveries in any given institution will depend upon the attitude of the staff, the kinds of analgesia and anesthesia used for labor and delivery, and the parity of the obstetric population.

Functions and Choice of the Forceps

The forceps may be used as a tractor or a rotator, or both. Its most important function is traction, although, particularly in transverse and posterior positions of the occiput, forceps may be employed successfully for rotation. Any properly shaped instrument will give satisfactory results, provided it is used intelligently. For general purposes, either Simpson or Tucker–McLane forceps are quite useful. In some circumstances, more specialized forceps may be preferable, for example, in some cases of *deep transverse arrest.* (When the progress of labor ceases with the fetal head in the transverse position, well down in the pelvis with the occiput below the spines, the situation is referred to as deep transverse arrest.) If there is no cephalopelvic disproportion, transverse arrest may be overcome with oxytocin stimulation, with resulting descent of the head to the perineum and spontaneous anterior rotation. *If, however, there are indications for prompt delivery, as in instances of fetal distress, but easy vaginal delivery with no delay cannot be anticipated, cesarean section should be used.*

Forces Exerted by the Forceps

Obstetricians have long been interested in the forces exerted by the forceps blades on the fetal skull and maternal tissues. If excessive, these forces can be damaging to both the woman and her fetus. From experiments con-

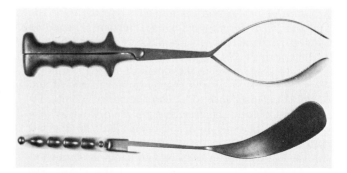

Figure 41-2. Tucker–McLane forceps. The blade is solid and the shank is narrow.

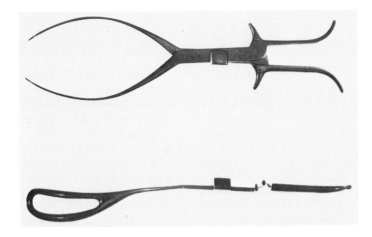

Figure 41-3. Kielland forceps. The characteristic features are the sliding lock, a minimal pelvic curvature, and lightweight.

ducted on women in labor more than a century ago, Joulin (1867) estimated that a pull in excess of 60 kg might damage the fetal skull. These crude studies and subsequent ones have furnished only a gross approximation, for the force produced by the forceps on the fetal skull is a complex function of both pull and compression by the forceps and of friction produced by the maternal tissues.

Indications for the Use of Forceps

The termination of labor by forceps, provided it can be accomplished without trauma, is indicated in any condition threatening the mother or fetus that is likely to be relieved by delivery. Such maternal indications include heart disease, acute pulmonary edema, intrapartum infection, or exhaustion. Fetal indications include prolapse of the umbilical cord, premature separation of the placenta, and abnormalities in fetal heart rate indicative of fetal distress.

Elective Low Forceps

The vast majority of forceps operations performed in this country today are elective low forceps. One reason is that sometimes drug-induced analgesia, and often conduction analgesia and anesthesia, interfere with the woman's voluntary expulsive efforts, in which circumstances low forceps delivery becomes the most reasonable procedure.

The fact that the methods employed to relieve pain frequently necessitate forceps delivery is not an indictment of the procedures, provided the obstetrician adheres strictly to the definition of low forceps. The fetal head must be on the perineal floor with the sagittal suture anteroposterior. In these circumstances, forceps delivery preceded by episiotomy is a simple and safe operation requiring only gentle traction. By allowing the woman in labor ample time, the criteria for low forceps can usually be met despite the effects of analgesia. *However, if the head does not descend and rotate, any forceps operations performed is not a low forceps but rather a midforceps operation.* Although midforceps op-

erations, especially those in which anterior rotation is the only criterion of low forceps not met, may occasionally be easy in expert hands; in general, the head is higher before rotation and more traction is usually required. To maximize safety for both mother and fetus, therefore, forceps should not be used *electively* until the criteria of a low forceps operation, as here defined, are fulfilled.

"Prophylactic" Forceps Delivery

In a minority of nulliparous women, marked resistance of the perineum and the vaginal introitus may sometimes present a serious obstacle to the passage of the fetus, even when the expulsive forces are normal. In such

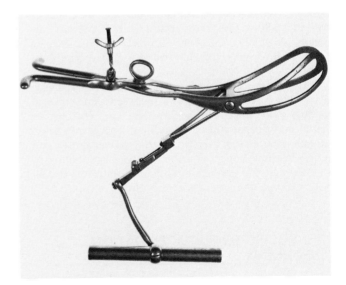

Figure 41-4. Tarnier forceps and axis traction handle. The characteristic features are the French lock, the wing nut (which when dropped in place and tightened can apply excessive pressure against the fetal head), and the traction handle. These forceps have been used to effect vaginal delivery even in the presence of cephalopelvic disproportion. Trauma to fetus and mother, however, was a common result.

cases, an episiotomy and outlet forceps delivery are beneficial to mother and fetus. Prolonged pressure of the fetal head against a rigid perineum sometimes results in injury to the fetal brain. To prevent cerebral injury and to spare the mother the strain of the last minutes of the second stage, DeLee (1920) recommended the "prophylactic forceps operation," more commonly called "elective low forceps," on the grounds that the obstetrician elects to interfere knowing that it is not absolutely necessary, for spontaneous delivery may normally be expected within approximately 15 minutes.

Prophylactic Low Forceps for Small Fetuses. Bishop and associates (1965), after analyzing data from the Collaborative Perinatal Project, suggested that prophylactic low forceps delivery improved neonatal outcome in low-birth-weight infants. There appeared to be improved mental and motor performance at 8 months and improved neurologic function at 1 year of age in low-birth-weight infants delivered by low forceps rather than spontaneously. Dewhurst (1976) and Hobel and associates (1980) recommended this approach in the management of preterm and small fetuses, apparently based upon the report of Bishop.

Recently, the practice of prophylactic forceps for the delivery of small fetuses has been questioned. Haesslein and Goodlin (1979) reported that the incidence of intraventricular hemorrhage in vertex infants 800 to 1350 g was two times as high in neonates delivered electively by low forceps as in infants delivered spontaneously. O'Driscoll and associates (1981) reported that in preterm infants only those delivered by low forceps suffered traumatic intracranial hemorrhage at birth. Fairweather (1981) reported no statistically significant difference in neonatal outcome in neonates (500 to 1500 g) delivered spontaneously and by low forceps. A similar study by Schwartz and co-workers (1983) with a similar conclusion has recently been published.

At present, there appears to be no obvious advantage to low forceps delivery of a small fetus and the real possibility of harm. In such cases, the obstetrician should perform an appropriately large episiotomy in an attempt to increase the size of the vaginal outlet and perineum, thus hopefully ensuring the least trauma to the infant. If the perineum and vaginal introitus are already relaxed, an incision is not necessary.

PREREQUISITES FOR APPLICATION OF FORCEPS

There are at least six prerequisites for the successful application of forceps:

1. *The head must be engaged and preferably deeply engaged.* Application of the blades before engagement, that is, high forceps, is an extremely difficult operation, often entailing brutal trauma to the maternal tissues and death of a large proportion of the babies. Many years ago, when cesarean section was also a highly dangerous operation, high forceps might have had a certain place in operative obstetrics. Delivery by high forceps is rarely employed today, however, and is mentioned here only to be condemned. Even after engagement occurs, the higher the station of the fetal head, the more difficult and traumatic the forceps delivery becomes. Moreover, whenever the blades are applied before the head has reached the perineal floor, it is common to find the head decidedly higher than was believed to be the case from the findings of vaginal examination. This occurs because of extensive caput succedaneum formation and molding. These difficulties of midforceps operation may occur even in the presence of a valid maternal indication for forceps delivery. For instance, it is generally agreed that women with heart disease should be spared, as much as safely possible, the effort of bearing down during the second stage of labor. Such efforts, however, may prove much less harmful than a difficult midforceps delivery. Therefore, forceps should not be used until the station of the head is low enough to ensure a nontraumatic operative procedure. The same generalization applies to forceps for fetal distress when the head is not close to the perineal floor. Granted that the fetal heart rate in such a case may suggest that the infant is hypoxic, it may still be judicious to allow more time for the head to descend rather than superimpose the trauma of a difficult midforceps operation on an already distressed infant. If delivery is mandatory, cesarean section is preferable to a difficult and damaging forceps operation.

2. *The fetus must present either by the vertex or by the face with the chin anterior.* The use of forceps is not applicable, of course, to transverse lies (shoulder presentation), nor is it intended for the breech.

3. *The position of the head must be precisely known so that the forceps can be appropriately applied to the fetal head.* So-called pelvic application can be dangerous.

4. *The cervix must be completely dilated before the application of forceps.* Even a small rim of cervix may offer great resistance when traction is applied, causing extensive cervical lacerations that may reach the lower uterine segment. If prompt delivery becomes imperative before complete dilatation of the cervix, cesarean section is preferable.

5. *Before forceps application, the membranes must be ruptured to permit a firm grasp of the head by the blades of the forceps.*

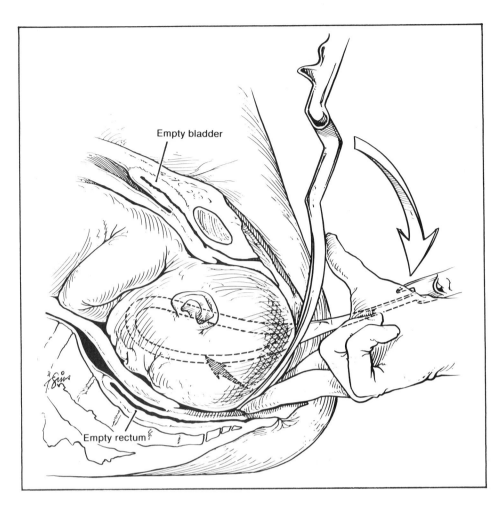

Empty bladder

Empty rectum

Figure 41-5. Occiput anterior and crowning. Application of left blade of Simpson forceps. The right blade is next applied and the blades are articulated.

6. *There should be no disproportion between the size of the head and that of the pelvic inlet, the midpelvis or the outlet.*

TECHNIQUES OF FORCEPS DELIVERY

Preparations for Operation

In the absence of previously instituted adequate continuous conduction anesthesia, a decision as to the type of anesthesia is made based on factors considered especially in Chapter 18. Pudendal block is not likely to provide sufficient anesthesia for forceps delivery. If spinal anesthesia is to be used, the anesthetic agent is introduced before placing the woman in the lithotomy position for delivery. If general anesthesia is to be used, the woman is placed in the lithotomy position, the pudenda are scrubbed and draped, and the obstetrician is ready to perform the forceps delivery before administering the anesthetic.

The woman's buttocks should be brought to the edge of the delivery table, and her legs held in position by appropriate stirrups. She is scrubbed and draped as described in Chapter 17 (p. 338). The bladder should be emptied by catheterization if a midforceps delivery is planned.

Application of Forceps

Forceps are constructed so that their cephalic curve is closely adapted to the sides of the fetal head (Fig. 41-5). The biparietal diameter of the fetal head corresponds to the greatest distance between the appropriately applied blades. Consequently, the head of the fetus is perfectly grasped only when the long axis of the blades corresponds to the occipitomental diameter, with the tips of the blades lying over the cheeks, while the concave margins of the blades are directed toward either the sagittal suture (occiput anterior position) or the face (occiput posterior position). Thus applied, the forceps should not slip, and traction may be applied most advantageously as illustrated in Figure 41-6. When forceps are applied obliquely, however, with one blade over the brow and the other over the opposite mastoid region, the grasp is less secure, and the fetal head is exposed to injurious pressure (Fig. 41-7). With most forceps, if one blade is applied over the brow and the other over the occiput, the instrument cannot be locked (Fig. 41-8), or, if locked, the blades slip off when traction is applied (Fig. 41-9),

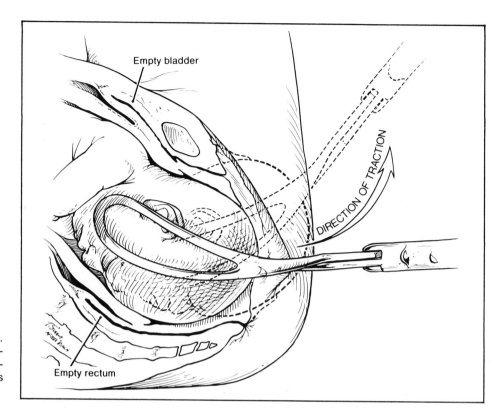

Figure 41-6. Occiput anterior. Delivery by low forceps (Simpson). The direction of gentle traction for delivery of the head is indicated.

causing appreciable trauma. For these reasons, the forceps must be applied directly to the sides of the head along the *occipitomental diameter,* in what is termed the biparietal or bimalar application.

Identification of Position

Precise knowledge of the exact position of the fetal head is essential to a proper cephalic application. With the head low down in the pelvis, diagnosis of position is made by examination of the sagittal suture and the fontanels, but when it is at a higher station, an absolute diagnosis can be made by locating the posterior ear.

The term *pelvic application* is employed when the left blade is applied to the left and right blade to the right side of the woman's pelvis, irrespective of the posi-

tion of the fetal head. It follows that the head is grasped satisfactorily only when the sagittal suture happens to be directed anteroposteriorly. Pelvic application is likely to be injurious to the fetus and should not be practiced.

Low Forceps Delivery

Delivery by low forceps is illustrated in Figures 41-10–41-17. With the head at the low station required in the definition of low forceps, the obstacle to delivery is usually insufficient expulsive forces, appreciable resistance of the perineum, or both. In such circumstances, the sagittal suture occupies the anteroposterior diameter of the pelvic outlet, with the small (posterior) fontanel directed toward either the symphysis pubis or the concavity of the sacrum. In either event, the forceps, if ap-

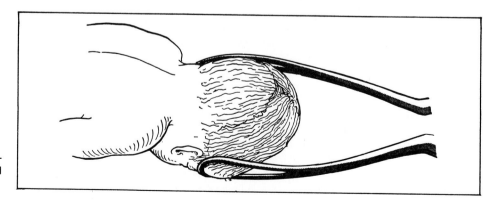

Figure 41-7. INCORRECT application of forceps over brow and mastoid region.

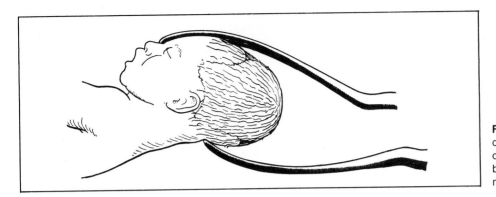

Figure 41-8. INCORRECT application of forceps, one blade over occiput and the other over the brow. Note that the forceps cannot be locked.

plied to the sides of the pelvis, grasps the head ideally. The left blade is introduced into the left side of the pelvis and then the right blade into the right side of the pelvis, as follows: Two fingers of the right hand are introduced inside the left, posterior portion of the vulva and into the vagina beside the fetal head. The handle of the left branch is then grasped between the thumb and two fingers of the left hand, as in holding a pen, and the tip of the blade is gently passed into the vagina between the fetal head and the palmar surface of the fingers of the right hand, which serve as a guide. The handle and branch are held at first almost vertically, but as the blade adapts itself to the fetal head, they are depressed, eventually to a horizontal position. The guiding fingers are then withdrawn, and the handle is left unsupported or held by an assistant. Similarly, two fingers of the left hand are then introduced into the right, posterior portion of the vagina to serve as a guide for the right blade, which is held in the right hand and introduced into the vagina. These guiding fingers are then withdrawn and the horizontally positioned branches are articulated, usually without difficulty. Otherwise, first one and then the other blade should be gently maneuvered until the handles are repositioned to effect easy articulation.

Appropriateness of Application. The application is now checked before any traction is applied. For the occiput anterior position, appropriately applied blades are equidistant from the sagittal suture. In the occiput pos-

terior position the blades are equidistant from the midline of the face and brow. If cervical tissue has been grasped, the forceps should be loosened and, if possible, the incompletely retracted cervix pushed up over the head. Otherwise, the procedure is abandoned and labor is allowed to continue.

Traction with Forceps. When it is certain that the blades are placed satisfactorily and the cervix is not entrapped, gentle, intermittent, horizontal traction is exerted until the perineum begins to bulge. As the vulva is distended by the occiput, the handles are gradually elevated, eventually pointing almost directly upward as the parietal bones emerge. With the fetal head in the occiput anterior position, this maneuver takes advantage of the smallest diameters of the fetal head and brings the suboccipital region beneath the symphysis. As the handles are raised, the head is extended. Episiotomy is rarely performed immediately prior to application of the blades but most often when forceps traction on the head begins to distend the perineum. During upward traction, the four fingers should grasp the upper surface of the handles and shanks, while the thumb exerts the necessary force upon their lower surface, as shown in Figure 41-16.

During the birth of the head, spontaneous delivery should be simulated as closely as possible, employing minimal force. Traction should therefore be intermittent, and the head should be allowed to recede in intervals, as

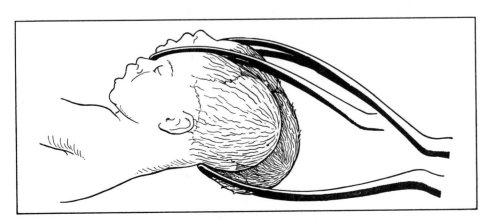

Figure 41-9. Forceps applied INCORRECTLY as in Figure 41-8. Note extension of head and tendency of blades to slip off with traction.

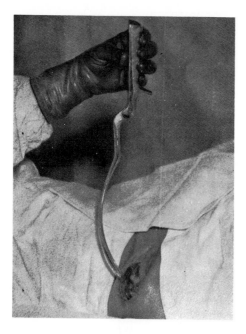

Figure 41-10. The left handle held in the left hand. Simpson forceps.

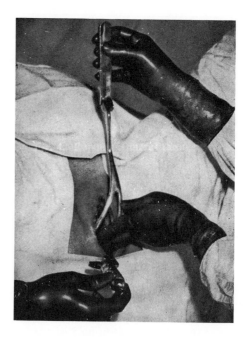

Figure 41-12. Left blade in place; introduction of right blade by right hand.

in spontaneous labor. Except when urgently indicated, as in severe fetal distress, delivery should be sufficiently slow, deliberate, and gentle to prevent undue compression of the fetal head.

After the vulva has been well distended by the head and the brow can be felt through the perineum, the delivery may be completed in several ways. Some obstetri-

cians keep the forceps in place, in the belief that greatest control of the advance of the head is thus maintained. The thickness of the blades may at times add to the distension of the vulva, however, thus increasing the likelihood of laceration or necessitating a large episiotomy. In such cases, the forceps are removed and delivery is completed by the modified Ritgen maneuver (Fig. 41-17),

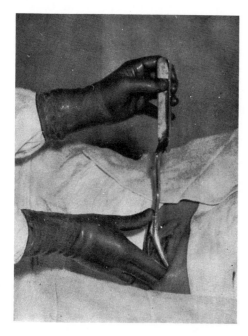

Figure 41-11. Introduction of left blade into left side of pelvis.

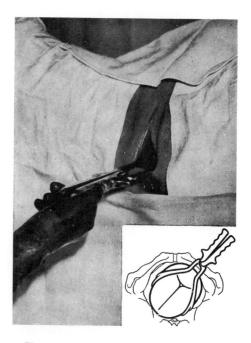

Figure 41-13. Forceps has been locked.

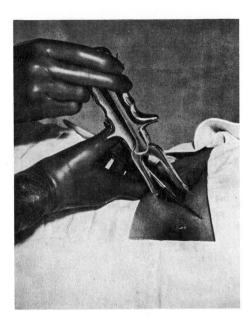

Figure 41-14. Median or mediolateral episiotomy may be performed at this point. Left mediolateral episiotomy shown here.

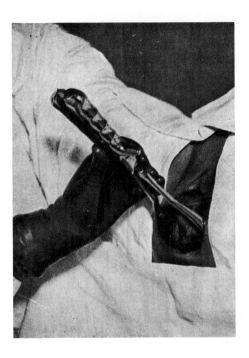

Figure 41-16. Upward traction.

slowly extending the head by using upward pressure upon the chin through the posterior portion of the perineum, while covering the anus with a towel to minimize contamination from the bowel. If the forceps are removed prematurely, the modified Ritgen maneuver may prove to be a tedious and inelegant procedure.

Midforceps Operations

When the head lies above the perineum, the sagittal suture usually occupies an oblique or transverse diameter of the pelvis. In such cases, the forceps should always be applied to the sides of the head. The application is best

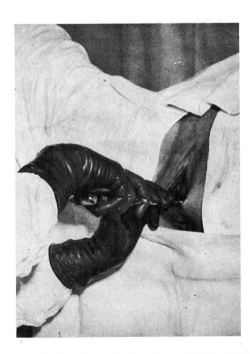

Figure 41-15. Horizontal traction; operator seated.

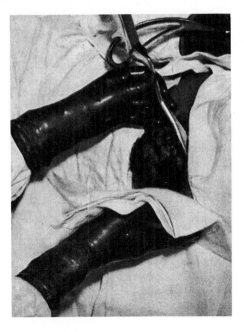

Figure 41-17. Disarticulation of branches of forceps. Beginning modified Ritgen maneuver.

accomplished by introducing two or more fingers into the vagina to a sufficient depth to feel the posterior fetal ear, over which, whether right or left, the first blade should be applied.

Left Occiput Anterior Position

In left occiput anterior positions, the right hand, introduced into the left posterior segment of the vagina, should identify the posteriorly located left ear and at the same time serve as a guide for introduction of the left branch of the forceps, which is held in the left hand and applied over the left ear. The guiding hand is then withdrawn, and the handle is held by an assistant or left unsupported, the blade usually retaining its position without difficulty. Two fingers of the left hand are then introduced into the right posterior portion of the pelvis, but no attempt is yet made to reach the anteriorly located right ear, which lies near the right iliopectineal eminence. The right branch of the forceps, held in the right hand, is then introduced along the left hand as a guide. It must then be applied over the anterior ear of the fetus by gently sweeping the blade anteriorly until it lies directly opposite the blade that was introduced first. Of the two branches, when articulated, one occupies the posterior and the other the anterior extremity of the left oblique diameter.

Right Occiput Anterior Position

In right positions, the blades are introduced similarly but in opposite directions, for in those cases the right ear of the fetus is the posterior ear, over which the first blade must be placed accordingly. After the blades have been applied to the sides of the head, the left handle and shank lie above the right. Consequently, the forceps does not immediately articulate. Locking of the branches is easily effected, however, by rotating the left around the right to bring the lock into proper position.

Occiput Transverse Positions

If the occiput is in a transverse position, the forceps are introduced similarly, with the first blade applied over the posterior ear, and the second rotated anteriorly to a position opposite the first. In this case, one blade lies in front of the sacrum and the other behind the symphysis. The conventional Simpson or Tucker–McLane forceps (Figs. 41-1, 41-2) or the specialized Kielland (Fig. 41-3) or Barton forceps (Fig. 41-18) may be used.

Rotation from Anterior and Transverse Positions

When the occiput is obliquely anterior, it gradually rotates spontaneously to the symphysis pubis as traction is exerted. When it is directed transversely, however, in order to bring it anteriorly a rotary motion of the forceps is required. The direction of rotation, of course, varies with the position of the occiput. Rotation from the left

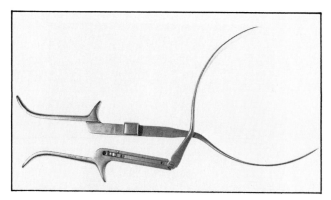

Figure 41-18. Barton forceps. The characteristic features are the sliding lock and one hinged blade.

side toward the midline is required when the occiput is directed toward the left, and in the reverse direction when it is directed toward the right side of the pelvis. Infrequently, particularly when the Barton forceps is used in transverse positions in anteroposteriorly flattened (platypelloid) pelves, rotation should not be attempted until the fetal head has reached or approached the pelvic floor. Premature attempts at anterior rotation under such conditions may result in injury to the fetus and maternal soft parts. Regardless of the original position of the head, delivery is eventually effected by exerting traction downward until the occiput appears at the vulva; the rest of the operation is completed as described.

In exerting traction before the head appears at the vulva, one or both hands may be employed. To avoid excessive force, the operator should sit with his arms flexed and elbows held closely against the thorax, since the obstetrician's body weight must not be applied.

It is reemphasized that the possibility of serious trauma to the mother, and especially the fetus, must be kept in mind whenever midforceps delivery is considered. The remote fetal effects may be subtle. For example, Friedman and associates (1977) reported that the mean IQ scores of 4-year-old children who were delivered by midforceps was somewhat lower than the scores of those who were delivered spontaneously or by low forceps.

Use of Forceps in Obliquely Posterior Positions

Prompt delivery may at times become necessary when the small (occipital) fontanel is directed toward one of the sacroiliac synchondroses, namely, in right occiput posterior and left occiput posterior positions. When interference is required in either instance, the head is often imperfectly flexed (Fig. 41-19A,B). In some cases, when the hand is introduced into the vagina to locate the posterior ear, the occiput rotates spontaneously toward the anterior, indicating that manual rotation of the fetal head might be easily accomplished.

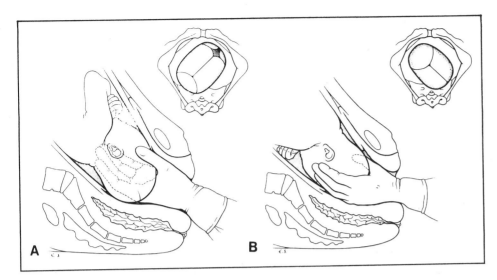

Figure 41-19. A. Manual rotation; left hand in position grasping the head. **B.** Manual rotation accomplished to ROA. Note that with rotation to the ROA position the fetal head may become more flexed. (*Both A and B from Douglas and Stromme: Operative Obstetrics, 3rd ed. New York, Appleton, 1976.*)

Manual Rotation from Posterior Positions

The requirements for forceps must be met. A hand with the palm upwards is inserted into the vagina and the fingers are brought in contact with that side of the fetal head that is to be pushed toward the anterior position while the thumb is placed over the opposite side of the head (Fig. 41-19A,B). With the occiput in a right posterior position, the left hand is used to rotate the occiput anteriorly in a clockwise direction; the right hand is used for the left occiput posterior position. At the beginning of the rotation, it may be helpful to dislodge the head *slightly* upward in the birth canal but the head must not be disengaged. After the occiput has reached the anterior position, labor may be allowed to continue or, more commonly, forceps used to effect delivery. First one blade is applied to that side of the head which is held by the fingers to help maintain the occiput in the anterior position. The other blade is immediately applied and delivery accomplished as described for occiput anterior forceps delivery.

Forceps Delivery as Occiput Posterior

If manual rotation cannot be accomplished easily, application of the blades to the head in the posterior position and delivery from the occiput posterior position is the safest procedure. In many of these cases, the cause of the persistent occiput posterior position and of the difficulty in accomplishing rotation is an anthropoid pelvis, the architecture of which predisposes to posterior delivery and opposes rotation. When the occiput is directly posterior, horizontal traction should be applied until the root of the nose is under the symphysis. The handles should then be slowly elevated until the occiput gradually emerges over the anterior margin of the perineum. Then, by imparting a downward motion to the instrument, the nose, face, and chin successively emerge from the vulva. The extraction is more difficult than when the occiput is anterior, and because of greater distension of

the vulva, perineal lacerations are more common (Fig. 41-20).

Forceps Rotations from Posterior Positions

Tucker–McLane, Simpson, or Kielland forceps may be used to try to rotate the fetal head. The occiput may be rotated 45 degrees to the posterior position or 135 degrees to the anterior (Fig. 41-21). Except in the hands of experts with extensive experience, however, forceps rotation is more likely to result in maternal and fetal injury than is delivery of the head as an occiput posterior. In rotating the occiput anteriorly with forceps, the pelvic curvature, originally directed upward, at the completion of rotation is inverted and directed posteriorly. Attempted delivery with the instrument in that position is likely to cause serious injury to maternal soft parts. To avoid such trauma, it is essential to remove and reapply the instrument as described in the following text.

TYPES OF SPECIAL MANEUVERS

Scanzoni–Smellie Maneuver

The double application for forceps, which was first described by Smellie (1752) and rediscovered by Scanzoni (1853) about a century later, has produced satisfactory results in some hands, but it is rarely necessary and is generally employed in only a small percentage of all obliquely posterior occipital positions. Because the right posterior variety is much more frequent, the steps of the operation in that case are detailed.

In the first application, the blades of the forceps are applied to the sides of the head with the pelvic curve toward the face of the fetus, whereas in the second application the pelvic curve is directed toward the occiput. For the first application, the right hand is passed into the vagina posteriorly and the rear ear is located. The left blade is applied over the ear and held in position by

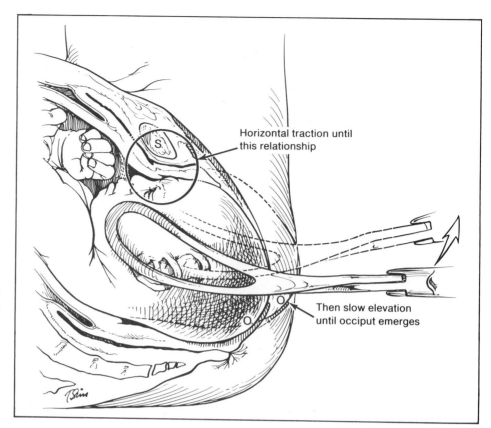

Figure 41-20. Occiput directly posterior. Low forceps (Simpson) delivery as an occiput posterior (O = occiput; S = symphysis). The arrow illustrates the point at which time the head should be flexed after the bregma passes under the symphysis. It is evident that to prevent serious perineal lacerations an extensive episiotomy is most often required.

Horizontal traction until this relationship

Then slow elevation until occiput emerges

an assistant, while the operator's left hand is passed into the right side of the vagina to control the introduction of the right blade, which is then rotated anteriorly until it lies over the left ear and opposite the first blade. The forceps is then locked and the handles elevated to flex the fetal head. Rotation may be facilitated by dislodging the fetal head very slightly upward. *The head must not be disengaged from the pelvis.* To compensate for the pelvic curvature in Tucker–McLane forceps, or others with a pelvic curvature, the handles of the forceps are gently rotated clockwise through an arc that extends well lateral to the circumference of the birth canal (Fig. 41-21). This serves to rotate the fetal head about the occipitomental diameter. With an appropriate initial forceps application, it is often possible to rotate the head completely to the occiput anterior position without undue force.

Once the occiput is rotated anteriorly, it is necessary to remove and reapply the forceps as described for an occiput anterior delivery. The forceps are unlocked and the branch now on the left side of the pelvis (right branch) is removed by gently pulling the handle simultaneously downward and inward. During this maneuver, the other branch is held in position anteriorly by an assistant to help stabilize the occiput in an anterior position. The right branch is now inserted immediately after the remaining branch has been removed. During this time, the occiput will typically rotate back to a right occiput anterior position. After reapplication, some

difficulty may arise in proper articulation, since the handle of the left branch lying above the right cannot be locked, but this can be readily overcome by rotating the handle of the left branch around the right to bring the lock into proper position. In left occiput posterior position, the blades are applied similarly but in the reverse order.

Rotation with Kielland Forceps

Kielland (1916) described a forceps with narrow, somewhat bayonet-shaped blades that he claimed could readily be applied to the sides of the head in the occiput transverse position and surpassed all other models as a rotator (Fig. 41-3). He held that his forceps was particularly useful when the station of the fetal head was high and when the sagittal suture was directed transversely. The Kielland forceps has almost no pelvic curve, but does have a sliding lock and is very light. On each handle is a small knob that indicates the direction of rotation.

There are two methods of applying the anterior blade. In one, *which may prove dangerous,* the anterior blade is introduced first with its cephalic curve directed upward and, after it has entered sufficiently far into the uterine cavity, it is turned through 180 degrees to adapt the cephalic curvature to the head. Kielland advised a more safe "wandering" or "gliding" method of application for the anterior blade when the uterus is tightly

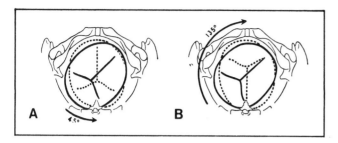

Figure 41-21. Rotation of obliquely posterior occiput to sacrum. **A.** and symphysis pubis, **B.**

contracted about the head and the lower uterine segment is stretched and thin. In such cases, when the pelvis is slightly contracted, it is dangerous to introduce the anterior blade with its cephalic curvature directed upward to be followed by rotation of the blade. In the wandering or gliding method, the anterior blade is introduced at the side of the pelvis over the brow or face to an anterior position, with the handle of the blade held close to the opposite maternal buttock throughout the maneuver. The second blade is introduced posteriorly and the branches are locked. Rotation is then accomplished at the station at which it may be most easily accomplished but not so high as to disengage the head from the pelvis.

Rubin and Coopland (1970) summarized the experiences with Kielland's forceps rotation at Winnipeg General Hospital. Of the 1000 consecutive cases surveyed, almost exactly one half were occiput posterior and the remainder were occiput transverse. Rotation was accomplished successfully in 970. The same forceps were nearly always used for delivery, followed by reapplication when necessary. There were eight perinatal deaths, including four with serious anomalies. Injuries to the infant were considered mostly minor. There were 27 injuries that were not minor, however, including seven fractured skulls.

Rotation with Barton Forceps

A forceps described by Barton and co-workers (1928) is illustrated in Figure 41-18. It differs from the usual types in that the anterior blade is hinged where it joins the shank. This forceps appears to be particularly useful when the sagittal suture occupies the transverse diameter of a platypelloid pelvis with a straight sacrum. For such cases, it has been used with presumably satisfactory results in several clinics in this country. The usual method of employing the Barton forceps involves wandering the hinged blade over the occiput or, less frequently, over the face. The posterior blade is then inserted directly into the hollow of the sacrum and the two branches of the forceps are articulated, adjusting the application, when necessary, by means of the sliding lock. Traction is applied in the transverse diameter of the pelvis with rotation effected at or near the pelvic

floor. Traction and rotation should not be performed simultaneously.

Injury from Forceps Rotation

With any forceps rotation, serious trauma may result to both fetus and mother unless considerable care is exercised. In a scholarly and extensive (108 references) review of midforceps delivery, Richardson, Evans, and Cibils (1983) proposed three prerequisites for the uses of midforceps: (1) midforceps must rationally be needed as an alternate method of delivery to cesarean section; (2) midforceps must be proven to be associated with a lower maternal morbidity rate than cesarean section; and (3) midforceps should improve fetal outcome, or, at the least, not result in fetal harm. With respect to the first requirement, there appears to be little doubt that there is a need for such a method in cases of fetal distress, maternal exhaustion, prolapsed umbilical cord, and cases of secondary labor arrest due to conduction anesthesia.

The issue of maternal morbidity following the use of midforceps procedures compared to cesarean section is not clear-cut. The use of midforceps is not a benign procedure (O'Driscoll and associates, 1981) for either mother or infant; however, neither is cesarean section (see Chapter 43). Infection rates postpartum can be 30 to 90 percent and hospital stays lengthened considerably (Cunningham and associates, 1978). Cesarean sections are associated with significant increases in morbidity and likely mortality when compared to vaginal deliveries; therefore, despite occasional terrible consequences, it must be concluded that midforceps procedures carry less morbidity for the mother than does cesarean section. The same cannot be said for the fetus.

Damage to the fetus with a midforceps application can result in trauma and death immediately or long-term morbidity in the form of cerebral palsy and lowered intelligence. The immediate consequences of midforceps rotations have recently been reviewed by three groups whose reports included control series. Hughey and colleagues (1978) compared 458 midforceps operations to 17 cesarean section deliveries. The cesarean section patients were selected when the cervix was completely dilated and the occiput failed to rotate to the anterior position from transverse or posterior position. Using a "perinatal morbidity index," an unfavorable result of 30 percent was reported for the fetuses delivered by midforceps versus a 0 percent morbidity with cesarean section. Bowes and Bowes (1980) compared the fetal outcome in midforceps deliveries to fetal outcome in patients delivered by cesarean section or by vacuum extraction. Morbid events occurred in 14 of 71 midforceps deliveries (19.7 percent) compared to 2 morbid events in the 37 cesarean sections (5.4 percent) and 3 instances of fetal trauma occurring in 15 vacuum extractions (20 percent). Chiswick and James (1979) have looked carefully at neonatal morbidity and mortality following vaginal delivery with Kielland forceps or cesarean section after attempts at vaginal delivery with these forceps. Birth trauma was evident in 15 percent of infants delivered with forceps. Neonatal mortality, most often from tentorial tears, was 3.5 percent. Factors significantly associated with the use of Kielland forceps were nulliparity, short maternal stature, induction of labor, late engagement of the fetal head, slow dilatation of the cervix, and epidural anesthesia during labor (James and Chiswick, 1979).

Long-term morbidity for the newborn delivered by midforceps in terms of cerebral palsy appears to be increased (Fuldner, 1957; Eastman and co-workers, 1962), but this has not been universally observed (Steer and Boney, 1962). The issue of intelligence following midforceps delivery is unsettled and is likely to remain so because of the multitude of variables affecting intelligence such as gender, mother's education, race, and socioeconomic status. Broman and co-workers (1975), controlling for socioeconomic status, race, and gender but *not* fetal weight, reported that infants delivered by midforceps had slightly higher IQ scores at 4 years of age than children delivered spontaneously. There were no significant differences among the IQ scores by type of delivery. The results published by Friedman and associates (1977) are in contrast to those reported by Broman. Friedman reported significant decreases in IQ for both black and white infants delivered by midforceps.

Application of Forceps in Face Presentations

In face presentations with the chin directed toward the symphysis, the application of forceps is occasionally used to effect vaginal delivery. The blades are applied to the sides of the head along the occipitomental diameter, with the pelvic curve directed toward the neck. Downward traction is exerted until the chin appears under the symphysis. Then, by an upward movement, the face is slowly extracted, the nose, eyes, brow, and occiput appearing in succession over the anterior margin of the perineum (Fig. 41-22). Forceps should not be applied when the chin is directed toward the hollow of the sacrum, since delivery cannot be effected in that position.

Trial Forceps and Failed Forceps

In trial forceps, the operator attempts midforceps delivery with the full knowledge that a certain degree of disproportion at the midpelvis may make the procedure incompatible with safety for the fetus. With an operating room both equipped and staffed for immediate cesarean section, and after a good forceps application has been achieved, firm downward pulls on the instrument are made. If no descent occurs, the procedure is abandoned and cesarean section is performed (Douglass and Kaltreider, 1953).

The term *failed forceps* is applied to a case in which a forceps delivery was anticipated and a vigorous but unsuccessful attempt was made to deliver with forceps. The three fundamental factors responsible for such a failure are disproportion, incomplete cervical dilatation, and malposition of the fetal head. Most but not all such

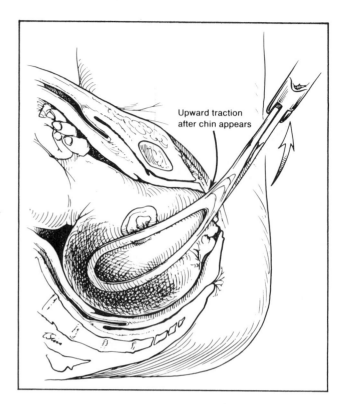

Figure 41-22. Face presentation, mentum (chin) anterior. Delivery with low forceps (Simpson).

cases stem from inexperience and ignorance of obstetric fundamentals. In most areas of the United States, these cases are becoming much less frequent.

> Since incomplete dilatation of the cervix is the cause of many cases of failed forceps, at times the problem can be solved by additional labor. Similarly, if the head does not rotate in occiput posterior positions, the case should be managed according to the principles set forth on page 846). In the presence of overt disproportion, cesarean section is the only recourse if the fetus is alive. The prognosis for the infant is usually poor because of the trauma he has received. The outlook for the mother, however, is usually better, although it varies with the extent of trauma and infection.

VACUUM EXTRACTOR

There have been numerous attempts in the past to attach a tractor by suction to the fetal scalp. The theoretic advantages of the vacuum extractor over forceps include the fact that insertion of space-occupying steel blades within the vagina and positioning the blades precisely over the fetal head, as is required for safe forceps delivery, can be avoided, the fetal head can be rotated without the vacuum extractor impinging upon maternal soft tissues, and there is great reduction in intracranial pressure during traction. All previously described instruments were unsuccessful until Malmström (1954) applied a new principle, namely, traction on a metal cap so designed that the suction creates an artificial caput within the cup that holds firmly and allows adequate traction.

In spite of some early enthusiasm for the instrument in the United States, the vacuum extractor is not used extensively now, partly because of reports of fetal damage, such as lacerations and abrasions of the scalp, cephalohematomas, intracranial hemorrhage, and death of infants. In contrast to the American hesitancy about the instrument, there has been an enthusiastic reception in other parts of the world, although the enthusiasm has waned in at least at some foreign institutions (Patel, 1984).

Craniotomy

The term *craniotomy,* as used in obstetrics, means an operation to collapse the fetal head for the purpose of facilitating its delivery. Widespread prenatal care, more astute management of pelvic contraction, antibiotics, and improvements in cesarean section have rendered craniotomy an exceedingly rare operation in modern obstetrics. As indicated in Chapter 30 (p. 672), cases of hydrocephalus are managed better by needle puncture and drainage than by craniotomy.

Operations Preparatory to Forceps

Hysterostomatomy (Dührssen Incisions). When immediate delivery is desirable before the cervix is fully dilated, multiple radial incisions may be made in the cervix and repaired immediately after delivery. These incisions are usually called Dührssen incisions, after the German obstetrician who described them in 1890. While the complications may be formidable, the technique of the operation is simple: Three incisions, corresponding approximately to the hours of 2, 6, and 10 on the face of a clock, are made with scissors. Delivery is then effected by forceps or breech extraction, depending on the presentation. The operation should never be done unless the cervix is fully effaced and more than 7 cm dilated, lest profuse or even fatal hemorrhage result. The procedure is, of course, contraindicated in placenta previa.

Most obstetricians now consider the operation obsolete. It is included here only because of the rare possibility of its use in fetal distress when the cervix is almost fully dilated or the aftercoming head is trapped by the cervix.

Although the incisions themselves are simple to perform, the procedure involves major potential hazards, and cesarean section is most often preferable. For instance, in cases of uterine dysfunction in which the cervix is not yet fully dilated, the head is usually well above the pelvic floor, and a difficult midforceps operation, with its attendant trauma to mother and fetus, is often required. In such circumstances, severe maternal hemorrhage is common. Moreover, poor anatomic results, such as deep scars and adhesions between the cervix and the vaginal mucosa, are likely to be a result.

Manual Dilatation of the Cervix

In practice, there is no such procedure as "manual dilatation of the cervix." What actually occurs when it is attempted is manual laceration of the cervix. The operation has no place in modern obstetrics.

Symphysiotomy and Pubiotomy

Symphysiotomy is the division of the pubic symphysis with a wire saw or knife to effect an increase in the capacity of a contracted pelvis sufficient to permit the passage of a living child. In pubiotomy, the pubis is severed a few centimeters lateral to the symphysis. Because of interference with subsequent locomotion, bladder injuries, and hemorrhage, and because of the greater safety of cesarean section, these two operations have been abandoned in the United States. Symphysiotomy is still performed in parts of Africa and elsewhere, especially when it may be impossible to follow a patient in a subsequent pregnancy. Since, in these circumstances, a woman delivered by cesarean section for a mildly contracted pelvis might well die with a ruptured uterus in her next pregnancy, symphysiotomy may be indicated in such a case in an attempt to produce sufficient enlargement of the pelvis to allow vaginal delivery. Hartfield (1973) described a technique for subcutaneous symphysiotomy and summarized his experiences.

History of Forceps

Crude forceps are an ancient invention, several varieties having been described by Albucasis, who died in 1112. Since their inner surfaces were provided with teeth to penetrate the head, however, it appears that they were intended for use only on dead fetuses.

The true obstetric forceps was devised in the latter part of the 16th or the beginning of the 17th century by a member of the Chamberlen family. The invention was not made public at the time, but was preserved as a family secret through four generations, not becoming generally known until the early part of the 18th century. Previously, version had been the only method that permitted the operative delivery of an unmutilated child. When that operation was impossible, imperative delivery was accomplished with hooks and crochets, which usually led to the destruction of the child. Thus, before the invention of forceps, the use of instruments was synonymous with the death of the child, and frequently of the mother as well.

William Chamberlen, the founder of the family, was a French physician who fled from France as a Huguenot refugee and landed at Southhampton in 1569. He died in 1596, leaving a large family. Two of his sons, both of whom were named Peter, and designated the elder and younger, respectively, studied medicine and settled in London. They soon became successful practitioners, devoting a large part of their attention to midwifery, in which they became very proficient. They attempted to control the instruction of midwives and, to justify their pretensions, claimed that they could successfully deliver patients when all others failed.

The young Peter died in 1626 and the elder in 1631. The elder left no male children, but the younger was survived by several sons, one of whom, born in 1601, was likewise named Peter. To distinguish him from his father and uncle, he is usually spoken of as Dr. Peter, since the other two did not possess that title. He was well educated, having studied at Cambridge, Heidelberg, and Padua, and on his return to London was elected a Fellow of the Royal College of Physicians. He was most successful in the practice of his profession and counted among his clients many members of the royal family and nobility. Like his father and uncle, he attempted to monopolize control of the midwives, but his

pretensions were set aside by the authorities. These attempts gave rise to much discussion, and many pamphlets
were written about the mortality of women in labor attended by men. He answered them in a pamphlet entitled
"A Voice in Ramah, or the Cry of Women and Children as
Echoed Forth in the Compassions of Peter Chamberlen."
He was a man of considerable ability, combining some of
the virtues of a religious enthusiast with many of the de-
vious qualities of a quack. He died at Woodham Mortimer
Hall, Moldon, Essex, in 1683, the place remaining in the
possession of his family until well into the succeeding century. He was formerly considered the inventor of the forceps, a fact now known to be incorrect.

Dr. Peter Chamberlen left a very large family, and three
of his sons, Hugh, Paul, and John, became physicians who
devoted special attention to the practice of midwifery. Of
them, Hugh (1630–?) was the most important and influen-
tial. Like his father, he was a man of considerable ability
who took a practical interest in politics. Since some of his
views were out of favor, he was forced to leave England for
Paris, where in 1673 he attempted to sell the family's secret
to Mauriceau for 10,000 lires, claiming that with forceps he
could deliver in a very few minutes the most difficult case.
Mauriceau placed at his disposal a rachitic dwarf whom he
had been unable to deliver, and Chamberlen, after several
futile hours of strenuous effort, was obliged to acknowledge
his inability to do so. Notwithstanding his failure, he maintained friendly relations with Mauriceau, whose book he
translated into English. In his preface he refers to the forceps in the following words: "My father, brothers, and my-
self (though none else in Europe as I know) have by God's
blessings and our own industry attained to and long practiced a way to deliver women in this case without prejudice
to them or their infants."

Some years later he went to Holland and sold his secret
to Roger Roonhuysen. Shortly afterward the Medical-
Pharmaceutical College of Amsterdam was given the sole
privilege of licensing physicians to practice in Holland, to
each of whom, under the pledge of secrecy, was sold Chamberlen's invention for a large sum. The practice continued
for a number of years until Vischer and Van de Poll purchased and made public the secret, whereupon it was discovered that the device consisted of only one blade of the
forceps. Whether that was all Chamberlen sold to Roonhuysen, or whether the Medical-Pharmaceutical College
had swindled the purchasers, is not known.

Hugh Chamberlen left a considerable family, and one of
his sons, Hugh (1664–1728), practiced medicine. He was a
highly educated, respected, and philanthropic physician,
who numbered among his clients members of the best families in England. He was an intimate friend of the Duke of
Buckingham, who had a statue erected in Chamberlen's
honor in Westminster Abbey. During the later years of his
life he allowed the family secret to leak out, and the instrument soon came into general use.

For more than 100 years Dr. Peter Chamberlen was considered the inventor of the forceps, but in 1813 Mrs. Kem-
ball, the mother of Mrs. Codd, who was the occupant of
Woodham Mortimer Hall at the time, found in the garret a
trunk containing numerous letters and instruments, among
them four pairs of forceps together with several levers and
fillets. As the drawings indicate (Fig. 41-23), the forceps
were in different stages of development, one pair hardly applicable to the living woman, although the others were
useful instruments. Aveling (1882), who carefully investi-

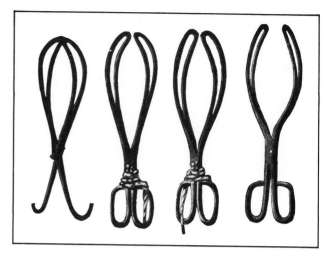

Figure 41-23. Chamberlen forceps.

gated the matter, believes that the three pairs of available
forceps were used, respectively, by the three Peters, and
that in all probability the first was devised by the elder
Peter, son of the original William. The forceps came into
general use in England during the lifetime of Hugh Chamberlen, the younger. The instrument was employed by
Drinkwater, who died in 1728, and was well known to
Chapman and Giffard.

In 1723, Palfyn, a physician of Ghent, exhibited before
the Paris Academy of Medicine a forceps he designated
mains de fer. It was crudely shaped and impossible to articulate. In the discussion following its presentation, De la
Motte stated that it would be impossible to apply it to the
living woman, and added that if by chance anyone should
happen to invent an instrument that could be so used, and
kept it secret for his own profit, he deserved to be exposed
upon a barren rock and have his vitals plucked out by vul-
tures. He had little knowledge at the time he spoke such an
instrument had been in the possession of the Chamberlen
family for nearly 100 years.

The Chamberlen forceps, a short, straight instrument
with only a cephalic curve, is perpetuated in the short forceps of today. It was used, with but little modification, until
the middle of the 18th century, when Levret, in 1747, and
Smellie, in 1751, independently added the pelvic curve and
increased the length of the instrument. Levret's forceps
was longer, with a more decided pelvic curve than that of
Smellie. From these two instruments, the long forceps of
the present day are descended.

As soon as forceps became public property, they were
subjected to various modifications. As early as 1798,
Mulder's atlas included illustrations of nearly 100 varieties.
The modifications attempted in improving the instrument
are pictured in Witkowski's *Obstetrical Arsenal,* illustrating several hundred forceps but representing only a small
fraction of those devised. The monograph of Das contains
excellent historical sketches of the development of the instrument. It is remarkable, however, that little advance was
made over the instruments of Levret and Smellie until
Tarnier, in 1877, clearly enunciated the principle of axis
traction. These forceps were designed to cope with high
stations of the fetal head and contracted pelves. Such
problems today, however, are generally solved by other

means. Episiotomy, furthermore, has eliminated many of the difficulties stemming from the pelvic curve, and severe traction at the fenestra, as in the axis–traction forceps, is therefore unnecessary and probably undesirable (Rhodes, 1958).

Except for two specialized forceps, those of Barton and Kielland, very little that is both new and useful in modern obstetrics has been added to the development of the instrument in over 200 years.

REFERENCES

Aveling JH: The Chamberlens and the Midwifery Forceps. London, Churchill, 1882

Barton LG, Caldwell WE, Studdiford WE: A new obstetrical forceps. Am J Obstet Gynecol 15:16, 1928

Bishop E, Israel L, Briscoe C: Obstetric influences on the premature infants' first year of development: A report from the Collaborative Study of Cerebral Palsy. Obstet Gynecol 26:628, 1965

Bowes WA, Bowes C: Current role of midforceps operations. Clin Obstet Gynecol 23:549, 1980

Broman SH, Nichols PL, Kennedy WA: Preschool IQ: Prenatal and Early Developmental Correlates. Hillside, NJ, Lawrence Earlbaum, 1975

Chiswick ML, James DK: Kielland's forceps: Association with neonatal morbidity and mortality. Br Med J 1:7, 1979

Cunningham FG, Haugh JC, Strong JD, Kappus SS: Infectious morbidity following cesarean sections: Comparison of two treatment regimens. Obstet Gynecol 52:656, 1978

DeLee JB: The prophylactic forceps operation. Am J Obstet Gynecol 1:34, 1920

Dennen EH: Forceps Deliveries, 2d ed. Philadelphia, Davis, 1964

Dewhurst C (ed): Integrated Obstetrics and Gynecology for Postgraduates, 2nd ed. Oxford, Blackwell, 1976, p 440

Douglas RG, Stromme WB: Operative Obstetrics, 3rd ed. New York, Appleton, 1976

Douglass LH, Kaltreider DF: Trial forceps. Am J Obstet Gynecol 65:889, 1953

Dührssen A: On the value of deep cervical incisions and episiotomy in obstetrics. Arch Gynaekol 37:27, 1890

Eastman NJ, Kohl SG, Maisel JE, Kaveler F: The obstetrical background of 753 cases of cerebral palsy. Obstet Gynecol Surv 17:459, 1962

Fairweather D: Obstetric management and follow-up of the very low-birth-weight infant. J Reprod Med 26:387, 1981

Friedman EA, Sachtleben MR, Bresky PA: Dysfunctional labor. XII. Long-term effects on the fetus. 127:779, 1977

Fuldner RV: Labor complication and cerebral palsy. Am J Obstet Gynecol 74:159, 1957

Haesslein H, Goodlin R: Survey of the tiny newborn. Am J Obstet Gynecol 134:192, 1979

Hartfield VJ: Subcutaneous symphysiotomy—Time for a reappraisal? Aust NZ J Obstet Gynaecol 13:147, 1973

Hobel C, Oakes G: Special considerations on the management of preterm labor. Clin Obstet Gynecol 23:147, 1980

Hughey MJ, McElin JW, Lussky R: Forceps operation in perspective. I. Midforceps rotation operations. J Reprod Med 20:253, 1978

James DK, Chiswick ML: Kielland's forceps: Role of antenatal factors in prediction of use. Br Med J 1:10, 1979

Joulin M: Study on the use of force in obstetrics. Arch Gen Med, 6th Series 9:149, 1867

Kielland C: On the application of forceps to the unrotated head, with description of a new model of forceps. Monatsschrift fur Geburtshilfe und Gynealkologie 43:48, 1916

Malmström T: The vacuum extractor, an obstetrical instrument. Acta Obstet Gynecol Scand (Suppl) 4:33, 1954

O'Driscoll K, Meagher D, MacDonald D, Geoghegan F: Traumatic intracranial haemorrhage in firstborn infants and delivery with obstetric forceps. Br J Obstet Gynaecol 88:577, 1981

Patel N: Personal communication, 1984

Richardson DA, Evans MI, Cibils LA: Midforceps delivery: A critical review. Am J Obstet Gynecol 145:621, 1983

Rubin L, Coopland AT: Kielland's Forceps. Can Med Assoc J 103:505, 1970

Scanzoni FW: Lehrbuch der Geburtshülfe, 3rd ed. Vienna, Seidel, 1853, pp 838–840

Schwartz DB, Miodovnik M, Lavin JP Jr: Neonatal outcome among low birth weight infants delivered spontaneously or by low forceps. Obstet Gynecol 62:283, 1983

Smellie W: A Treatise on the Theory and Practice of Midwifery. London, Wilson & Durham, 1752

Steer CM, Boney W: Obstetric factors in cerebral palsy. Am J Obstet Gynecol 83:526, 1962

42

Techniques for Breech Delivery and Version

BREECH PRESENTATION

The indications for vaginal versus cesarean delivery for breech presentations have been considered in Chapter 30 (p. 657). Labor and techniques for vaginal delivery of breech presentation are considered below.

Mechanism of Labor

Unless there is disproportion between the size of the fetus and the pelvis, engagement and descent of the breech in response to labor usually takes place with the bitrochanteric diameter of the breech in one of the oblique diameters of the pelvis. The anterior hip usually descends more rapidly than the posterior hip, and when the resistance of the pelvic floor is met, internal rotation usually occurs, bringing the anterior hip toward the pubic arch and allowing the fetal bitrochanteric diameter to occupy the anteroposterior diameter of the pelvic outlet. Rotation usually takes place through an arc of 45 degrees. If, however, the posterior extremity is prolapsed, it always rotates to the symphysis pubis, ordinarily through an arc of 135 degrees, but occasionally in the opposite direction past the sacrum and the opposite half of the pelvis through an arc of 225 degrees.

After rotation, descent continues until the perineum is distended by the advancing breech, while the anterior hip appears at the vulva and is stemmed against the pubic arch. By lateral flexion of the body, the posterior hip is then forced over the anterior margin of the perineum, which retracts over the buttocks, thus allowing the infant to straighten out when the anterior hip is born. The legs and feet follow the breech and may be born spontaneously, although the aid of the obstetrician is usually required.

After the birth of the breech, there is slight external rotation, with the back turning anteriorly as the shoulders are brought into relation with one of the oblique diameters of the pelvis. The shoulders then descend rapidly and undergo internal rotation, with the bisacromial diameter occupying the anteroposterior diameter of the inferior strait. Immediately following the shoulders,

the head, which is normally sharply flexed upon the thorax, enters the pelvis in one of the oblique diameters and then rotates in such a manner as to bring the posterior portion of the neck under the symphysis pubis. The head is then born in flexion, with the chin, mouth, nose, forehead, bregma (brow), and occiput appearing in succession over the perineum. Usually the breech engages in the transverse diameter of the pelvis, with the sacrum directed anteriorly or posteriorly. The mechanism of labor in the transverse position differs only in that internal rotation occurs through an arc of 90 degrees.

Infrequently, rotation occurs in such a manner that the back of the infant is directed toward the vertebral column instead of toward the abdomen of the mother. Such rotation should be prevented if possible. Although the head may be delivered by allowing the chin and face to pass beneath the symphysis, the slightest traction on the body may cause extension of the head. Extension, if uncorrected, increases the diameters of the head, which must pass through the pelvis.

Vaginal Delivery

There are three general methods of breech delivery through the vagina:

1. *Spontaneous breech delivery:* The infant is expelled entirely spontaneously without any traction or manipulation other than support of the infant. This form of delivery of mature infants is rare.
2. *Partial breech extraction:* The infant is delivered spontaneously as far as the umbilicus, but the remainder of the body is extracted.
3. *Total breech extraction:* The entire body of the infant is extracted by the obstetrician.

Since the technique of breech extraction differs in complete and incomplete breeches on the one hand, and frank breeches on the other, it is necessary to consider these conditions separately. (The varieties of breech presentation are illustrated in Figs. 12-2–12-4.)

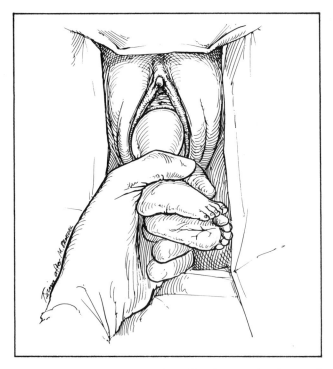

Figure 42-1. Breech extraction. Traction on the feet and ankles.

Timing of Delivery

In general, preparations for breech extraction should be initiated by the time that the buttocks or the feet appear at the vulva. It is essential that the delivery team include (1) an obstetrician skilled in the art of breech extraction, (2) an associate who is also scrubbed and gowned to assist with the delivery, (3) an anesthesiologist who can quickly induce appropriate general anesthesia when needed, (4) an individual trained to resuscitate the infant effectively, including endotracheal intubation, and (5) someone to provide general assistance.

Delivery is easier and, in turn, perinatal morbidity and mortality are lower when the breech of the fetus is allowed to deliver spontaneously. If fetal distress develops before this time, however, a decision must be made whether to perform a total breech extraction or, more likely, a cesarean section. It must be remembered that, for a favorable outcome with any breech delivery, at the very minimum the birth canal must be sufficiently large to allow passage of the fetus without trauma and the cervix must be effaced and fully dilated. If these conditions are lacking, cesarean section nearly always is the more appropriate method of delivery.

Extraction of Complete or Incomplete Breech

During total breech extraction of a complete or incomplete breech presentation, the obstetrician's hand is introduced through the vagina and both feet of the fetus grasped; the ankles are held with the second finger lying between them. The feet are brought with gentle traction through the vulva. If difficulty is experienced in grasping both feet, first one foot should be drawn down the vagina to, but not through, the introitus and then the other foot is so manipulated (Fig. 42-1).

Now both feet are grasped and pulled through the vulva simultaneously. Unless there is considerable relaxation of the perineum, an *episiotomy* is made. The episiotomy is an important adjunct to any type of breech delivery. A mediolateral episiotomy is usually preferred with a term-sized infant because it furnishes greater room and is less likely to extend into the rectum.

As the legs begin to emerge through the vulva, they should be wrapped in a sterile towel to obtain a firmer grasp, for the vernix caseosa renders them slippery and difficult to hold. Many obstetricians prefer the towel to be moistened. The sterile water or normal saline used should be warm but not so hot as to burn the infant. Downward gentle traction is then continued.

As the legs emerge, successively higher portions are grasped, first the calves and later the thighs. When the breech appears at the vulva, gentle traction is applied until the hips are delivered. As the buttocks emerge, the back of the infant usually rotates to the anterior. The thumbs of the operator are then placed over the sacrum and the fingers over the hips, and gentle downward traction is continued until the costal margins, and then the scapulas become visible (Figs. 42-2, 42-3). As traction is exerted and the scapulas become visible, the back of the infant tends to turn spontaneously toward the side of the mother to which it was originally directed (Fig. 42-4). If turning does not occur, however, slight rotation should be added to the traction, with the object of bringing the bisacromial diameter of the fetus into the anteroposterior diameter of the pelvic outlet.

A cardinal rule in successful breech extraction is to employ steady, gentle, downward traction until the lower halves of the scapulas are delivered outside the vulva, making no attempt at delivery of the shoulders and arms until one axilla becomes visible. Frequently, failure to follow this rule will make an otherwise easy procedure difficult. The appearance of one axilla indicates that the time has arrived for delivery of the shoulders. Provided the arms are maintained in flexion, it makes little difference which shoulder is delivered first. Occasionally, while plans are made to deliver one shoulder, the other is born spontaneously.

There are two methods of delivery of the shoulders: (1) With the scapulas visible, the trunk is rotated in such a way that the anterior shoulder and arm appear at the vulva and can easily be released and delivered first. In Figure 42-4, the operator is shown rotating the trunk of the fetus counterclockwise to deliver the right shoulder and arm. The body of the fetus is then rotated in the reverse direction to deliver the other shoulder and arm. (2) If trunk rotation was unsuccessful, the posterior shoulder must be delivered first. The feet are grasped in one hand and drawn upward over the groin of the mother toward

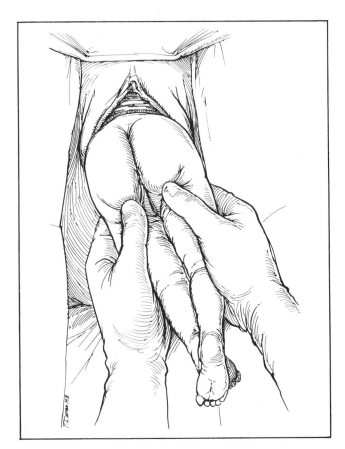

Figure 42-2. Breech extraction. Traction on the thighs. A warm, moist towel is most often applied over the fetal parts to reduce slippage from vernix as traction is applied and to keep the exposed parts warm.

which the ventral surface of the fetus is directed; in this manner, leverage is exerted upon the posterior shoulder, which slides out over the perineal margin, usually followed by the arm and hand (Fig. 42-5). Then, by depressing the body of the fetus, the anterior shoulder emerges beneath the pubic arch, and the arm and hand usually follow spontaneously (Fig. 42-6). Thereafter, the back tends to rotate spontaneously in the direction of the mother's symphysis. If upward rotation fails to occur, it is effected by manual rotation of the body. Delivery of the head may then be accomplished.

Unfortunately, however, the process is not always so simple, and it is sometimes necessary first to free and deliver the arms. These maneuvers are much less frequently required today, presumably because of adherence to the principle of continuing traction without attention to the shoulders until an axilla becomes visible. Attempts to free the arms immediately after the costal margins emerge should be avoided.

Since there is more space available in the posterior and lateral segments of the normal pelvis than elsewhere, the posterior arm should be freed first. Since the corresponding axilla is already visible, upward traction

upon the feet is continued, and two fingers of the obstetrician's other hand are passed along the humerus until the elbow is reached (Fig. 42-5). The fingers are now used to splint the arm, which is swept downward and delivered through the vulva. To deliver the anterior arm, depression of the fetal body of the infant is sometimes all that is required to allow the anterior arm to slip out spontaneously. In other instances, the anterior arm can be swept down over the thorax using two fingers as a splint. Occasionally, however, the body must be seized with the operator's thumbs over the scapulas and rotated to bring the undelivered shoulder near the closest sacrosciatic notch. The legs are then carried upward to bring the ventral surface of the infant to the opposite groin of the mother; subsequently, the arm can be delivered as described previously.

If the arms have become extended over the head, their delivery, although more difficult, can usually be ac-

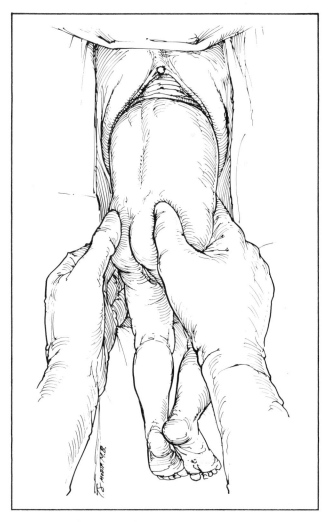

Figure 42-3. Breech extraction. Extraction of the body. The obstetrician's hands are applied over, but not above, the infant's pelvis. Rotation is not attempted until the scapulae are clearly visible.

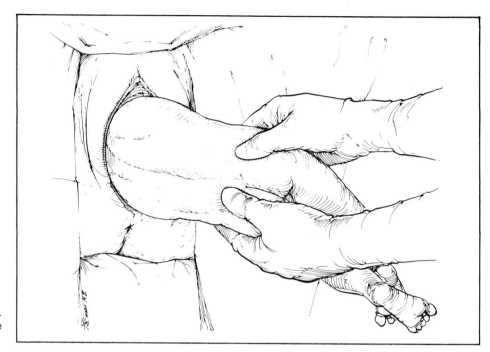

Figure 42-4. Breech extraction. The scapulas are visible and the body is rotating.

complished by the maneuvers just described. In so doing, particular care must be taken to carry the operator's fingers up to the elbow and to use the fingers as a splint, for if the operator's fingers are merely hooked over the fetal arm, the humerus or clavicle is exposed to great danger of fracture. Infrequently, one or both fetal arms is found around the back of the neck (*nuchal arm*), and delivery is still more difficult. If the nuchal arm cannot be freed in the manner described, extraction may be facilitated by rotating the fetus through half a circle in such a direction that the friction exerted by the birth canal will serve to draw the elbow toward the face. Should rotation of the fetus fail to free the nuchal arm, it may be necessary to push the fetus upward in an attempt to release them. If the rotation is still unsuccessful, the nuchal arm is often forcibly extracted by hooking a finger over it. In that event, fracture of the humerus or clavicle is very common. Fortunately, good union almost always follows appropriate treatment.

After the shoulders are born, the head usually occupies an oblique diameter of the pelvis with the chin directed posteriorly. The fetal head may then be extracted either with forceps, as described below and illustrated in Figures 42-7A,B and 42-11–42-16, which is the method preferred by many obstetricians and is described subsequently, or by the so-called *Mauriceau maneuver* (Fig. 42-8).

Employing the Mauriceau maneuver to help flex the head, the operator's index and middle finger of one hand are applied over the maxilla, while the fetal body rests upon the palm of the hand and forearm, which is straddled by the fetal legs. Two fingers of the operator's other hand are then hooked over the fetal neck, and grasping the shoulders, downward traction is applied until the

suboccipital region appears under the symphysis. Moderate suprapubic pressure simultaneously applied by an assistant helps keep the head flexed. The body of the fetus is then elevated toward the mother's abdomen, and the mouth, nose, brow, and eventually the occiput emerge successively over the perineum. Gentle traction should be exerted by the fingers over the shoulders. At the same time, appropriate suprapubic pressure applied by an assistant, as shown in Figure 42-8, is helpful in delivery of the head.

Extraction of Frank Breech

At times, extraction of a frank breech may be accomplished by *moderate* traction exerted by a finger in each groin and facilitated by a generous episiotomy (Fig. 42-9). If moderate traction does not effect delivery of the breech, and cesarean section is not used, vaginal delivery can only be accomplished by *breech decomposition*. This procedure involves intrauterine manipulation to convert the frank breech into a footling breech. The procedure is more readily accomplished if the membranes were ruptured recently but becomes extremely difficult if considerable time has elapsed after the escape of the amnionic fluid and the uterus has become tightly contracted over the fetus.

In many cases, the *Pinard maneuver* aids materially in bringing down the feet. In that procedure, two fingers are carried up along one extremity to the knee to push it away from the midline. Spontaneous flexion usually follows, and the foot of the fetus is felt to impinge upon the back of the hand. The fetal foot may then be readily grasped and brought down (Fig. 42-10). As soon as the buttocks are born, first one leg and then the other are drawn out and extraction is accomplished as described under the section on Extraction of Complete or Incomplete Breech (p. 856).

Forceps to Aftercoming Head

Piper forceps (Figs. 42-7A,B, 42-11–42-16) should be applied when the Mauriceau maneuver cannot be easily accomplished, or they may be applied electively instead of the Mauriceau procedure. The blades of the forceps should not be applied to the aftercoming head until it has been brought into the pelvis by gentle traction, combined with suprapubic pressure, and is engaged (Fig. 42-7). As shown in Figure 42-16, suspension of the body of the fetus in a towel keeps the arms out of the way and prevents excessive abduction of the trunk.

Entrapment of the Aftercoming Head

Occasionally, especially with small preterm fetuses, the incompletely dilated cervix will not allow delivery of the aftercoming head. Prompt action is necessary if a living infant is to be delivered. With gentle traction on the fetal body, the cervix, at times, may be manually slipped over the occiput. If this maneuver is not readily successful, Dührssen incisions can be made in the cervix.

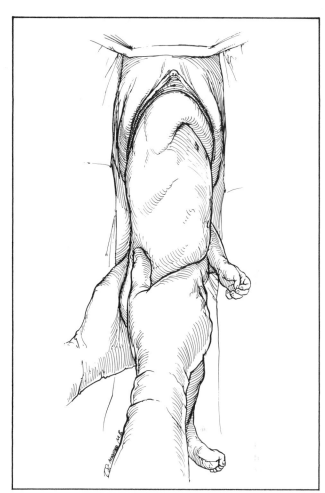

Figure 42-6. Breech extraction. Delivery of the anterior shoulder by downward traction. The anterior arm may then be freed the same way as the posterior arm in Figure 42-5.

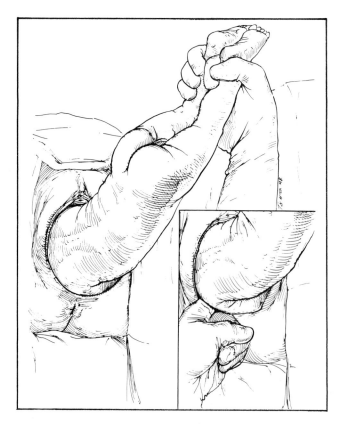

Figure 42-5. Breech extraction. Upward traction to effect delivery of the posterior shoulder, followed by freeing the posterior arm (insert).

This is one of the few indications for this procedure in modern obstetrics (see Chapter 41, p. 851).

Bracht Maneuver

In an effort to stimulate the forces of nature, Bracht (1936) employed a maneuver whereby the breech was allowed to deliver spontaneously to the umbilicus. The baby's body was then held, not pressed, against the mother's symphysis. The force applied in this procedure should be equivalent to that of gravity. The mere maintenance of this position, added to the effects of uterine contractions and moderate suprapubic pressure by an assistant, often suffices to complete delivery spontaneously. The *Bracht maneuver* has been popular in Europe but has not gained wide acceptance in the United States. The procedure was thoroughly reviewed by Plentl and Stone (1953).

Anesthesia for Breech Delivery

It is wise to allow the breech to deliver spontaneously to the umbilicus. Anesthesia for episiotomy and intrava-

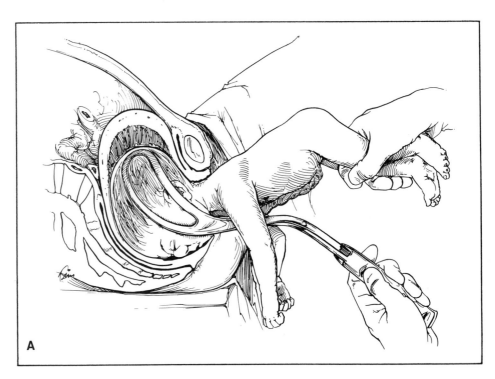

A

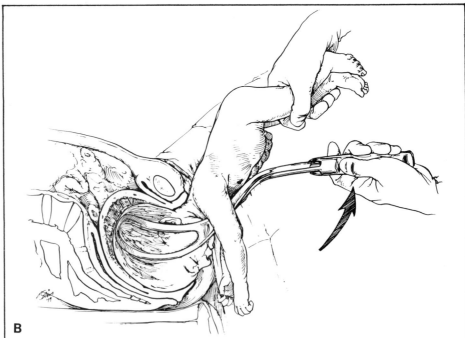

B

Figure 42-7. A. Forceps applied to the aftercoming head. The head has entered the pelvis and forceps have been applied (see Figs. 42-11–42-16). **B.** Forceps delivery of aftercoming head. Note the direction of movement (*arrow*).

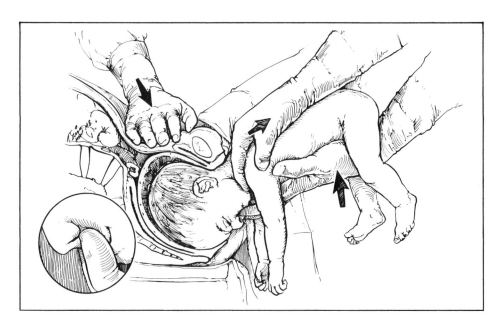

Figure 42-8. Delivery of after-coming head using the Mauriceau maneuver. Note that as the fetal head is being delivered, flexion of the head is maintained by supra-pubic pressure provided by an assistant and simultaneously by pressure on the maxilla (*insert*) by the operator as traction is applied.

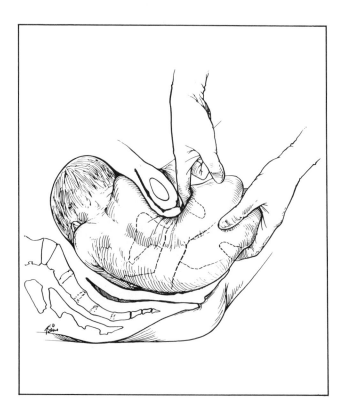

Figure 42-9. Extraction of a frank breech using fingers in groins.

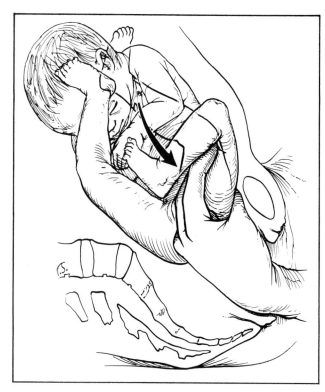

Figure 42-10. Pinard maneuver sometimes used in case of a frank breech presentation to deliver a foot into the vagina.

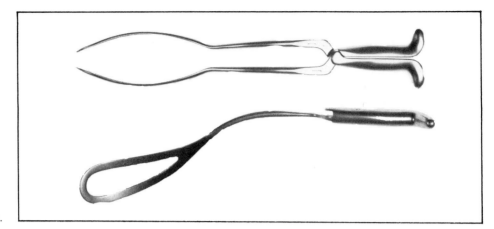

Figure 42-11. Piper forceps.

ginal manipulations that are needed for breech extraction can usually be accomplished with pudendal block and local infiltration of the perineum (see Chapter 18, p. 360). The inhalation of nitrous oxide plus oxygen provides further relief from pain. If for any reason general anesthesia is desired, it can be quickly induced with thiopental plus a muscle relaxant and maintained with nitrous oxide.

Anesthesia for decomposition and extraction must provide sufficient relaxation to allow intrauterine manipulation. Although successful decomposition has been accomplished using epidural, caudal, or spinal anesthesia, increased uterine tone may render the operation difficult. Then, preferably, halothane can be used to relax the uterus, as well as provide pain relief. The safeguards for use of halothane cited in Chapter 18 (p. 355) must be followed.

Prognosis

With complicated breech deliveries, there are increased maternal risks. Manual manipulations within the birth canal increase the risk of maternal infection. Intrauterine maneuvers, especially with a thinned-out lower uterine segment, or delivery of the aftercoming head through an incompletely dilated cervix, may cause rupture of the uterus, lacerations of the cervix, or both. Such manipulations may also lead to extensions of the episiotomy and deep perineal tears. Anesthesia sufficient to induce appreciable uterine relaxation may cause uterine atony and, in turn, postpartum hemorrhage from the placental implantation site. Even so, the prognosis, in general, for *the mother* whose fetus is delivered by breech extraction is probably somewhat better than with cesarean section.

For *the fetus,* the outlook is less favorable and it be-

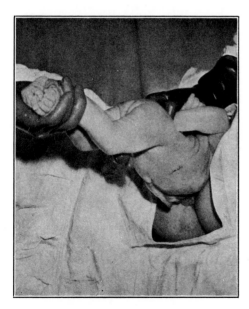

Figure 42-12. Position of infant with head in pelvis prior to application of Piper forceps.

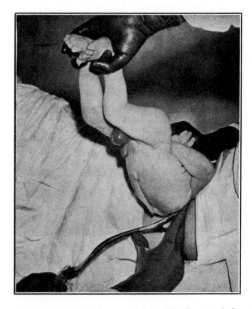

Figure 42-13. Introduction of left blade to left side of pelvis.

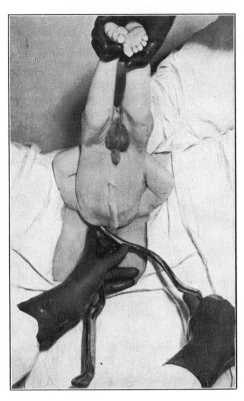

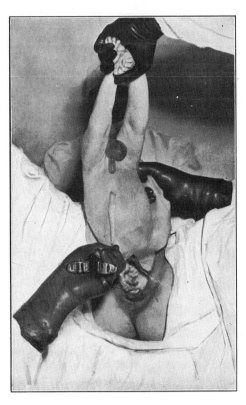

Figure 42-14. Introduction of right blade, completing application.

Figure 42-15. Forceps locked and traction applied; chin, mouth, and nose emerging over perineum.

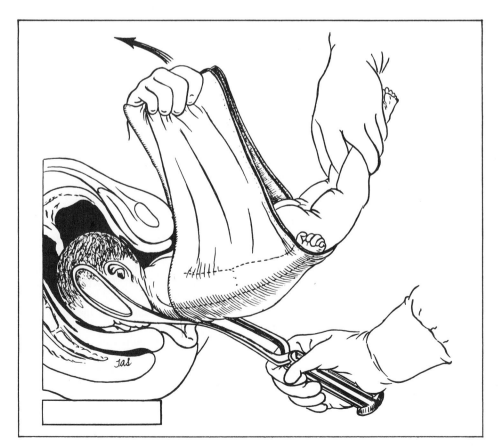

Figure 42-16. Management of fetal arms in breech extraction. (*From Savage: Obstetrics Gynecology 3:55, 1954.*)

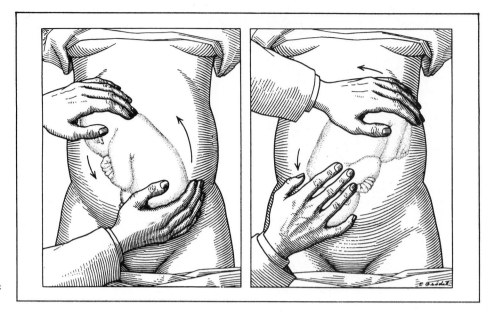

Figure 42-17. External cephalic version.

comes more serious the higher the presenting part is situated at the beginning of the breech extraction. In addition to the increased risk of tentorial tears and intracerebral hemorrhage, which are inherent in breech delivery, the perinatal mortality rate is increased by the greater probability of other trauma during extraction. With incomplete breech presentations, moreover, prolapse of the umbilical cord is much more common than in vertex presentations and this complication further worsens the prognosis for the infant.

Fracture of the humerus and clavicle cannot always be avoided when freeing the arms, and fracture of the femur may occur during difficult frank breech extractions. Hematomas of the sternocleidomastoid muscles occasionally develop after the operation, though they usually disappear spontaneously. More serious problems, however, may follow separation of the epiphyses of the scapula, humerus, or femur. Exceptionally, paralysis of the arm follows pressure upon the brachial plexus by the fingers in exerting traction, but more frequently it is caused by overstretching the neck while freeing the arms. When the fetus is forcibly extracted through a contracted pelvis, spoon-shaped depressions or actual fractures of the skull, generally fatal, may result. Occasionally, even the fetal neck may be broken when great force is employed. Perinatal morbidity and mortality are considered in greater detail in Chapter 30 (p. 652).

VERSION

Version, or turning, is an operation in which the presentation of the fetus is altered artificially, either substituting one pole of a longitudinal presentation for the other, or converting an oblique or transverse lie into a longitudinal presentation.

According to whether the head or breech is made

the presenting part, the operation is designated cephalic or podalic version, respectively. It is also named according to the method by which it is accomplished. Thus, in *external version,* the manipulations are performed exclusively through the abdominal wall; in *internal version,* the entire hand is introduced into the uterine cavity.

External Cephalic Version

The object of the operation is to convert a less favorable presentation to that of a vertex.

Indications. If a breech or shoulder presentation (transverse lie) is diagnosed in the last weeks of pregnancy, its conversion into a vertex may be attempted by external maneuvers, provided there is no marked disproportion between the size of the fetus and the pelvis. Cephalic version is thought by some, but not all, obstetricians to be a frequently successful technique with little morbidity (see Chapter 30, p. 656) and therefore should be attempted in order to avoid the increased perinatal mortality that attends breech delivery. If the fetus lies transversely, a change of presentation is usually the only alternative to cesarean section.

External cephalic version may be attempted only under the following conditions: (1) The presenting part must not be engaged. (2) The abdominal and uterine walls must not be highly irritable. (3) The uterus must contain a sufficient quantity of amnionic fluid to permit easy movement of the fetus. (4) The fetal heart action must be continuously monitored, usually with a doppler sound instrument, so that the obstetrician can continuously hear the fetal heart rate during the procedure. Sonography, immediately available, often proves helpful. Anesthesia should never be used, lest undue force be applied.

In the early stages of labor, before the membranes

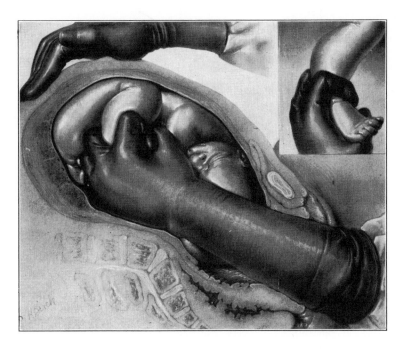

Figure 42-18. Internal podalic version. Note use of long version gloves.

have ruptured, the same indications apply. They may then be extended to oblique presentations as well, although these unstable lies usually convert spontaneously to longitudinal lies as labor progresses. External cephalic version can rarely be effected, however, after the cervix has become fully dilated or the membranes have ruptured.

Method. Cephalic version is performed solely by *external manipulations* (Fig. 42-17) (also see Chapter 30, p. 656). In the technique recommended, the woman's abdo-

men is bared, and the presentation and position of the fetus are carefully ascertained and documented by sonography. Each hand then grasps one of the fetal poles. The pole that is to be converted into the presenting part is then gently stroked toward the pelvic inlet while the other is moved in the opposite direction. This procedure should always be performed with continuous fetal heart rate monitoring and in a labor and delivery unit where a rapid cesarean can be performed should fetal distress develop. After version has been completed, the fetus will tend to return to its original position unless

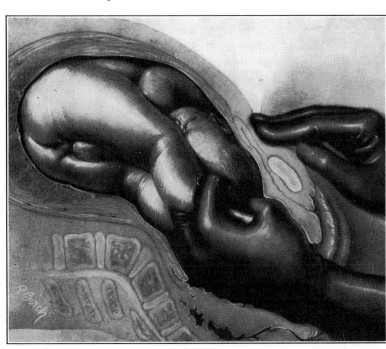

Figure 42-19. Internal podalic version. Upward pressure on head is applied as downward traction is exerted on feet.

the presenting part is fixed in the pelvis. During labor, however, the head may be pressed down into the pelvic inlet and held firmly in position until it becomes fixed under the influence of uterine contractions. With the availability of potent tocolytic agents, several authors now recommend that external version be conducted after uterine relaxation is established with tocolytic agents and especially after failed attempts without tocolytics (Ylikorkala and Hartikainen-Sorri, 1977; Van Dorsten and co-workers, 1981, 1982; Hofmyer, 1983).

Internal Podalic Version

This maneuver consists of turning the fetus by the obstetrician inserting a hand into the uterine cavity, seizing one or both feet, and drawing them through the cervix while pushing transabdominally the upper portion of the fetal body in the opposite direction. The operation is followed by breech extraction.

Indications. There are very few, if any, indications for internal podalic version other than for delivery of the second twin. The technique for delivering the second twin is described in Chapter 26 (p. 520). Very occasionally, this procedure may be justified when the cervix is fully dilated, the membranes are intact, and the fetus in a transverse lie is small or dead. The possibility of serious trauma to the fetus and mother during internal podalic version from a cephalic presentation is apparent from Figures 42-18 and 42-19.

REFERENCES

Bracht E: (Manual aid in breech presentation.) Z Geburthshilfe Gynaekol 112:271, 1936

Hofmyer GJ: Effect of external cephalic version in late pregnancy on breech presentation and cesarean section rate: a controlled trial. Br J Obstet Gynaecol 90:392, 1983

Mauriceau F: (The method of delivering the woman when the infant presents one or two feet first.) Traite des Maladies des Femmes Grosses, 6me ed. 1721, pp 280–285

Pinard A: On version by external maneuvers. Paris, Traite de Palper abdominal, 1889

Plentl AA, Stone RE: Bracht maneuver. Obstet Gynecol Survey 8:313, 1953

VanDorsten JP, Schifrin BS, Wallace RL: Randomized control trial of external cephalic version with tocolysis in late pregnancy. Am J Obstet Gynecol 141:417, 1981

VanDorsten JP: Safe and effective external cephalic version with tocolysis. Contemp Ob/Gyn 19:44, 1982

Ylikorkalo O, Hartikainen-Sorri A: Value of external version in fetal malpresentation in combination with use of ultrasound. Acta Obstet Gynecol Scand 56:63, 1977

43

Cesarean Section and Cesarean Hysterectomy

CESAREAN SECTION

Definition

Cesarean section, or cesarean delivery, is defined as delivery of the fetus through incisions in the abdominal wall (laparotomy) and the uterine wall (hysterotomy). This definition does not include removal of the fetus from the abdominal cavity in case of rupture of the uterus or abdominal pregnancy.

Indications

The indications for cesarean section are discussed in detail throughout the text wherever the fetal or maternal complications that might necessitate cesarean section are presented. The early history of cesarean section is considered at the end of this chapter. In general, cesarean section is used whenever it is believed that further delay in delivery would seriously compromise the fetus, the mother, or both, yet vaginal delivery is unlikely to be accomplished safely.

Frequency

In recent years the use of cesarean delivery has increased at an accelerated rate in large measure because of the widespread emphasis that is given to the recognition of actual or suspected fetal distress. Another possible reason for the increased frequency of cesarean section is the reduction in the parity of most gravidas. Specifically, with up to one half of pregnant women being nulliparas, one would expect an increased number of cesarean sections being done for those conditions that are more common in nulliparous women, especially pregnancy-induced hypertension.

From the mid 1960s to the early 1980s the cesarean delivery rate has increased from less than 5 percent to more than 15 percent nationally (Morrison and co-workers, 1982). The frequency of cesarean delivery at Parkland Memorial Hospital was 4.4 percent in 1964 but 18.3 percent in 1983.

Bottoms and colleagues (1980) described this increase in cesarean section rates as cause for national concern. From a separate analysis of 123,837 births collected from five hospitals that reported indications for cesarean section in a like manner, they classified the reasons for cesarean delivery under five categories: (1) dystocia (33.4 percent), (2) previous cesarean section (23.1 percent), (3) breech presentation (18.8 percent), (4) fetal distress (13.2 percent), and (5) other indications (11.2 percent). The authors stressed that the diagnosis of fetal distress had been minimized due to fetal scalp pH testing. They concluded that the major indications for cesarean section that needed to be considered and possibly reassessed were those relating to dystocia and to previous cesarean section.

Regardless of the indications cited for cesarean section, the increased frequency has been accompanied by an absolute decrease in perinatal mortality. While it is true that the increase in cesarean section rate may have contributed to a lowering of perinatal mortality, many other factors as well may have contributed, for example, better prenatal care, electronic fetal heart rate monitoring, and advances in neonatal care.

In support of the concept that the increased rate of cesarean section was *not* responsible for the observed decrease in perinatal mortality was the report by O'Driscoll and Foley (1983). These authors studied the correlation of decreases in perinatal mortality and the increase in cesarean section rates from 1965 to 1980 in the United States and at the National Maternity Hospital in Dublin, Ireland. They reported that while cesarean section rates were increasing in the United States from less than 5 percent in 1965 to more than 15 percent in 1980, in Dublin among more than 108,000 infants born during the same period of time, the cesarean section rate remained virtually unchanged at 4.2, 4.2, 4.1, and 4.8 percent in 1965, 1970, 1975, and 1980, respectively. Despite the unchanged rate in cesarean sections in Dublin, perinatal mortality fell from 42.1 to 36.5, 24.0, and 16.8 per 1000 infants born during the same years. These authors concluded that these results were compatible with the view that the increased rate of cesarean sections re-

TABLE 43-1. FREQUENCY OF CESAREAN DELIVERIES ACCORDING TO DIAGNOSTIC INDICATION[a]

Indication	United States[b] (1978)	Dublin[c] (1980)
Dystocia	4.7	0.7
Repeat cesarean	4.7	1.1
Breech	1.8	0.6
Fetal Distress	0.8	0.5
Others	3.2	1.9
TOTAL	15.2	4.3

[a] Expressed as percent of all births.
[b] Figures for the United States were calculated from the National Institutes of Health Consensus Statement based on data from New York City.
[c] Figures for Dublin refer to the National Maternity Hospital.
(*From O'Driscoll and Foley, 1983.*)

ported in the United States had not contributed significantly to the simultaneously observed reduction in perinatal mortality.

The lower cesarean section rate in Dublin was attributed to lower frequencies of cesarean section for dystocia, repeat cesarean section, and breech delivery managed in Dublin (Table 43-1).

In summary, O'Driscoll and associates (1969, 1973) attributed their apparent success to a more aggressive management of dystocias with oxytocin in nulliparous patients whose uteri they considered to be "almost immune to rupture except by manipulation," to allowing patients with previous low transverse cesarean sections a trial of labor which proved successful in 60 percent of their patients, and to a liberal trial of labor in breech presentations (Chapter 30).

Although results obtained in Dublin appear impressive, the results pertain to perinatal mortality but not morbidity. Because perinatal morbidity is much more difficult to assess, such results are still to be reported from Europe, Australia, and the United States. Finally, it is unlikely that such low cesarean section rates will be seen in the United States. One reason for this is the prevailing enthusiasm for small families, which likely will result in many women, whose first infants were delivered by cesarean section, electing to have a repeat cesarean section with tubal sterilization. Another possible reason is the reluctance to allow vaginal delivery of breech presentations. Even if the liberal standards recently applied to frank breech presentations and recommended by Collea and associates (1980) were applied, we could expect only a 15 to 30 percent decrease in the cesarean section rate for all breeches. Therefore, if the cesarean delivery rate is to be reduced, the obstetric management of dystocias and of breech presentations must result in many more vaginal deliveries, accompanied by a decrease in the frequency of repeat cesarean deliveries. Is it in the best interests of the mother and the fetus to do so?

Williams and Chen (1982) presented convincing evidence that the reduction in perinatal mortality in new-

borns under 2000 g most likely was attributable directly to the advent of neonatal intensive care *and* the increased rate of cesarean delivery used for these small fetuses. A similar conclusion was reached by Sachs and co-workers (1983), who studied the effects of cesarean delivery on neonatal mortality for breech infants and low birth weight vertex infants using data obtained from the Georgia neonatal surveillance network. This data file contained information on 329,241 singleton deliveries between 1974 and 1978. The risk of neonatal death for breech infants weighing 4000 g or less and delivered vaginally was significantly higher than the risk for infants delivered by cesarean section. *The lower the birth weight, the higher the risk for a vaginal breech delivery.* The risk was 2.5 times greater for breech infants who weighed 1000 to 2500 g and were delivered vaginally compared to those infants delivered by cesarean section. The best outcome for high-risk vertex infants weighing 1000 to 1500 g was achieved in those infants delivered by cesarean in a tertiary perinatal center. Thus increased neonatal survival can be obtained with an increased cesarean delivery rate but at the cost of additional maternal mortality and considerable economic consequences.

The final answers with respect to the frequency, indications, results in terms of safety to the mother and fetus, and the legal, ethical, and economic consequences of cesarean section are unlikely to become apparent for several years. To the credit of the obstetric community, these questions have been addressed by a National Institutes of Health, Child Health and Human Development Task Force. The results reported by this Task Force were then reviewed, and public comment was accepted during a National Institutes of Health Consensus Development Conference held in Bethesda on September 22–24, 1980. The summary (NIH Consensus Development Conference Summary) is concise and is recommended to the reader for additional information concerning this medical, political, social, and economically sensitive issue.

Maternal Mortality

The most remarkable report of the safety of cesarean delivery is that from the Boston Hospital for Women (Frigoletto and associates, 1980). These authors reported a zero maternal mortality rate in 10,231 cases. Certainly, maternal and perinatal mortality and morbidity are typically higher with cesarean delivery than with vaginal delivery, in part because of the complication that led to the cesarean section and in part because of increased risks inherent in the abdominal route of delivery.

Maternal mortality from cesarean section should be less than 1 per 1000. Even this relatively low operative mortality rate must be considered as excessive when one understands that the majority of these deaths occur in young, healthy women undergoing a "normal physiologic process."

The major threats to women undergoing cesarean section have been anesthesia, severe sepsis, and thromboembolic episodes. Each of these areas has been considered earlier in great detail. However, it is worth emphasizing that aspiration pneumonia, which had previously been the leading cause of cesarean section deaths at Parkland Memorial Hospital, has been avoided completely since the routine practice of ingesting 30 ml of milk of magnesia shortly before the induction of anesthesia (Wheatley and co-workers, 1979). Despite such efforts to decrease mortality, it is unlikely that deaths from either cesarean delivery or vaginal delivery can be much reduced in severely compromised women who elect, rightly or not, to pursue pregnancies despite their already tenuous medical status. Therefore, one must consider whether the death was related to a complication of the delivery per se or due at least in part to an underlying factor, such as heart disease. It is reasonable to assume that if the frequency of cesarean deliveries can be reduced without compromising the fetus, significant reductions not only in cesarean section mortality rates but in overall maternal mortality rates as well may be achieved. Thus, a major challenge in obstetrics is to answer correctly the question "Can a significant reduction in cesarean section rate be achieved without increasing perinatal mortality *and* morbidity?"

Maternal Morbidity

Even when morbidity and mortality associated with the problem that led to cesarean section are excluded, maternal morbidity is more frequent and likely to be more severe following cesarean section than following vaginal delivery (Rubin and co-workers, 1981). The common causes of morbidity from cesarean delivery remain infection, hemorrhage, and injury to the urinary tract.

Perinatal Mortality

The frequency of stillbirth and neonatal mortality will depend, of course, on the underlying reason for the cesarean section and the gestational age of the fetus. Although the decreasing perinatal mortality rate observed since the mid-1960s has in many instances been associated with and even been attributed to the marked increase in cesarean section rates in the United States, O'Driscoll and Foley (1983), as mentioned earlier, have questioned this assumption. Specifically, they reported similar and equally dramatic decreases in perinatal mortality rates in patients delivered at the National Maternity Hospital in Dublin without an increase in cesarean section rates (Fig. 43-1).

Perinatal Morbidity

Birth trauma in general is much less likely with cesarean section than with vaginal delivery. However, cesarean section is not a guarantee against fetal injury. For example, the head of a premature breech can be entrapped in a small transverse uterine incision that was judged incorrectly to be large enough for delivery. Such an error

in judgment may result in injury to the fetal spinal cord or brain and may result in either extension of the uterine incision into the uterine vessels or lower uterine segment or both. Finally, the fetus can be wounded during the incision into the uterus.

It is important to emphasize that fetal morbidity has been decreased dramatically with the use of cesarean section in instances of certain breech presentations (Chapter 30, p. 659), transverse lie of the fetus, and placenta previa. Also of importance is the fact that the opportunities for obstetricians-in-training to develop and *maintain* the skills necessary to accomplish successfully a potentially difficult breech delivery or to do an internal podalic version for a second twin have diminished greatly and for sound reasons (Chapter 30, p. 652). Today, and likely for the foreseeable future, such cases will and should be managed by cesarean section.

Although respiratory distress has been claimed to be higher for repeat cesarean section than for vaginal delivery, it is unlikely that there is a significant difference when gestational ages of the fetuses are identical and fetal hypoxia and acidosis are avoided. The methods employed to avoid anesthetic causes of fetal hypoxia and acidosis are discussed in Chapter 18.

Timing of Repeat Cesarean Section

There are advantages to a predetermined time for carrying out repeat cesarean sections. For example, the family can better arrange for assistance in caring for other children while the mother is hospitalized and for the care of the mother and infant after leaving the hospital. Importantly, a competent team can be assembled more easily to provide optimal care, including anesthesia, infant resuscitation if needed, and subsequent care of the newborn. Conversely, with emergency repeat cesarean section, an operating room may not be immediately available, or the mother may have very recently eaten, which increases the anesthetic risk. Of considerable importance when dealing with a gravida with a previous cesarean section is whether a vertical uterine incision was made that might rupture with the onset of labor, resulting in the death of the fetus and serious morbidity or even death of the mother. The likelihood of these disastrous consequences from rupture of a transverse scar in the lower uterine segment is very low.

Iatrogenic Prematurity. Elective termination of pregnancy with the delivery of a premature infant has been a major problem at some institutions. This unfortunate circumstance has led to the strong recommendation by some that amniocentesis with appropriate studies on the amniotic fluid obtained be performed before any elective delivery (Gluck, 1977; Flaksman and co-workers, 1978). This approach is not without complications, however, for, at times, trauma to the placenta or fetus is caused by attempts to obtain amnionic fluid, which may be of scant volume in pregnancies at or near term. Moreover, after an unsuccessful attempt at amniocentesis, the fetus

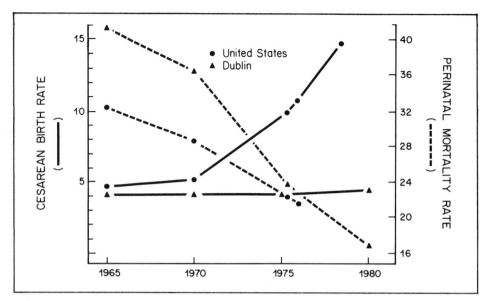

Figure 43-1. Cesarean birth rates per 100 deliveries are represented by solid lines and perinatal mortality rates per 1000 deliveries by broken lines for the United States (*circles*), according to Bottoms and co-workers (1980) and for the National Maternity Hospital Dublin (*triangles*). (*Modified from O'Driscoll and Foley, 1983.*)

has been known to succumb in utero awaiting a subsequent and hopefully successful attempt at aspiration of amnionic fluid. Sonography at the time of amniocentesis diminishes the risk somewhat but adds further to the cost.

The guidelines for timing repeat cesarean section at Parkland Memorial Hospital do not include mandatory amniocentesis to measure the amnionic fluid lecithin/sphingomyelin (L/S) ratio. Instead, the following information is used to identify fetal maturity: (1) the date of onset of the last normal spontaneous menstrual period, (2) results of serial measurements of the height of the uterine fundus above the symphysis initiated in the first half of pregnancy, (3) the time when the fetal heart was first heard with a fetoscope, and (4) the estimated size of the fetus. Delivery is carried out after 38 completed weeks of gestation, based on the last normal menstrual period, without measuring the L/S ratio if the fetal heart was heard at a time when the fundal height was 18 to 20 cm, if the gestational age at that same time calculated from the normal last menstrual period was 18 to 20 weeks, and if the fetus is estimated by each of two experienced examiners to weigh as much as did the previous term infant, or more than 3000 g when the previous infant was premature or growth retarded. Delivery is postponed if there is discordance that implies a lower gestational age and there are no compelling reasons, maternal or fetal, to effect delivery before the onset of labor, such as a previous vertical incision in the uterus or strong suspicion of retarded fetal growth.

With this approach, about 60 percent of repeat cesarean sections have been performed at Parkland Memorial Hospital at a scheduled time, and respiratory distress has not been a problem in those pregnancies terminated by scheduled repeat cesarean section before the onset of labor.

Contraindications

In modern obstetric practice, there are virtually no contraindications to cesarean section. Cesarean section is seldom indicated, however, if the fetus is dead or too premature to survive. Exceptions to this generalization include pelvic contraction of such a degree that vaginal delivery by any means is impossible, most cases of placenta previa, and most cases of neglected transverse lie. Conversely, whenever the maternal coagulation mechanism is seriously impaired, delivery that minimizes incisions—vaginal delivery—is preferable in most instances (Chapter 21).

Vaginal Delivery Subsequent to Cesarean Section

There is no doubt that vaginal delivery most often will prove to be safe following a previous cesarean section. Numerous reports have been published in the past few years that confirm the earlier reports by Riva and Teich (1961), Douglas and co-workers (1963), and McGarry (1969) that attest to the safety and efficacy of vaginal delivery in women who previously had cesarean sections (Gibbs, 1980; Pauerstein, 1981; Merrill and Gibbs, 1978; Saldana and co-workers, 1979; Horowitz and colleagues 1981; O'Sullivan and co-workers, 1981; Lavin and associates, 1982; Benedetti and associates, 1982; Meir and Porreco 1982; Gellman and colleagues, 1983; Martin and co-workers, 1983). It is important, however, to emphasize that all these reports stress that delivery subsequent to cesarean section should be considered only for women who have had a previous low transverse cesarean section.

The issue that has most often prevented physicians from allowing women to undergo a vaginal delivery following a cesarean section has been the fear of uterine rupture or dehiscence. O'Sullivan and co-workers in 1981 reviewed over 8000 deliveries reported in the literature and added several hundred patients of their own. They reported that frank rupture of the uterus or uterine dehiscence, at least, occurred in 1.8 percent of women undergoing cesarean section compared to only 0.5 percent for women undergoing vaginal delivery. In this extensive and excellent review, O'Sullivan and colleagues concluded that vaginal delivery not only was as safe as an elective repeat cesarean section but was in fact the preferred method of management in carefully selected patients.

The issue is not whether a woman can deliver vaginally following a previous cesarean section but rather the criteria that should be applied and rigidly adhered to in order to allow her to labor and attempt a vaginal delivery. Specific guidelines have been established by the American College of Obstetricians and Gynecologists (ACOG Newsletter, 1982). They include the patient's acceptance and understanding of the advantages and risks of both vaginal and repeat cesarean section that have been described above. Moreover, the woman should have undergone but one previous low transverse incision with no extension of the uterine incision, confirmed by written operative report. The issue of whether the previous indication for cesarean section should no longer exist is a highly controversial one. Even though the previous cesarean section may have been performed because of failure of cervical dilatation or lack of descent of the presenting part, these abnormalities are not in and of themselves absolute contraindications to a subsequent vaginal delivery, as pointed out by Seitchik and Ramakrishna (1982). Finally, a judgment must be made as to whether or not the pelvis is adequate for the current pregnancy. If a woman is to undergo a trial of labor following a cesarean section, appropriate technical support must be available in the hospital and should include skilled nursing and an in-house obstetrician, pediatrician, and anesthesiologist. There must be an adequate blood bank staffed 24 hours a day with compatible blood available promptly. Electronic fetal heart rate monitoring is advisable during labor. There must be immediate access to an appropriately staffed operating theater.

The obstetrician in his or her zeal to abandon the old adage "Once a cesarean section, always a cesarean section," should avoid substituting the even more inappropriate motto "Once a cesarean delivery, never again a cesarean delivery!"

TECHNIQUE OF CESAREAN SECTION

Type of Uterine Incision

The so-called classical cesarean incision, a vertical incision into the body of the uterus above the lower uterine segment and reaching the uterine fundus, is seldom used. Most always the incision is made in the lower uterine segment transversely (Kerr technique) or, less often, vertically (Krönig technique). The lower segment transverse incision has the advantage of requiring only modest dissection of the bladder from the underlying myometrium. If the incision extends laterally, the laceration may involve large branches of the uterine artery and vein. The low vertical incision may be extended upward so that in those circumstances where much more room is needed, the incision can be carried into the body of the uterus; otherwise, it is a less desirable incision. More extensive dissection of the bladder is necessary to keep the vertical incision within the lower uterine segment. Moreover, if the vertical incision extends downward, it may tear through the cervix into the vagina and possibly involve the bladder. If, on the other hand, it is extended upward into the body of the uterus, closure, including satisfactory reperitonealization, is more difficult, and the likelihood of rupture in a subsequent pregnancy is increased appreciably. Importantly, it has been the experience of most obstetricians that during the next pregnancy the vertical incision is much more likely to rupture, especially during labor, than is the lower segment transverse incision (Chapter 33, p. 700).

Lower Segment Transverse Incision. For a cephalic presentation, most often a transverse incision through the lower uterine segment is the operation of choice. Generally, the transverse incision (1) results in less blood loss, (2) is easier to repair, (3) is located at a site least likely to rupture with extrusion of the fetus into the abdominal cavity during a subsequent pregnancy, and (4) does not promote adherence of bowel or omentum to the incisional line.

Preparation for Incision. Hair is shaved from the abdominal wall from the level of the mons pubis to somewhat above the umbilicus and laterally to about the level of the iliac crests. The bladder is emptied through an indwelling catheter and continuously drained during and after the procedure. The operative field is thoroughly scrubbed with a suitable detergent, and then all of the abdomen is covered with sterile drapings.

If general anesthesia is to be employed, all of the above steps are carried out and the operating team is fully prepared to operate before induction of anesthesia. If continuous conduction anesthesia is to be used, it is necessary before scrubbing and draping the abdomen to insert the catheter into the epidural or caudal space. If single-dose intrathecal (spinal) anesthesia is to be used, it is injected just before scrubbing and draping the abdomen.

Choice of Abdominal Incisions

An infraumbilical midline vertical incision is quickest to make. The abdominal wall is opened in layers from just above the upper margin of the symphysis to near the umbilicus. The incision should be of sufficient length to allow the infant to be delivered without difficulty, but no

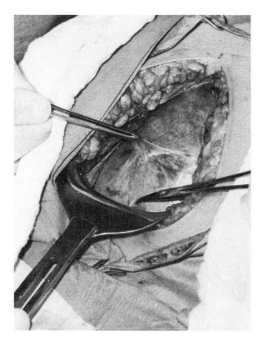

Figure 43-2. The loose vesicouterine serosa is grasped in the forceps. The hemostat tip points to the upper margin of the bladder. The retractor is firm against the symphysis.

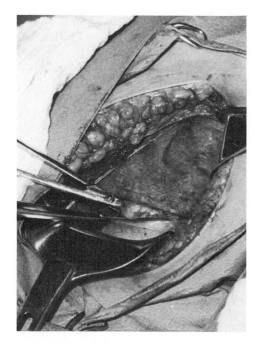

Figure 43-3. The loose serosa above the upper margin of the bladder is being elevated and incised laterally.

longer. Therefore, its length should vary with the estimated size of the fetus. Sharp dissection is performed to the level of the anterior rectus sheath, which is freed of subcutaneous fat to expose a strip of fascia in the midline about 2 cm wide. Some surgeons prefer to incise the rectus sheath with the scalpel throughout the length of the fascial incision. Others prefer to make a small opening and then incise the visualized fascial layer with scissors. There seems to be less bleeding with the latter approach, as well as reduced risk of inadvertently incising underlying structures, especially bowel. The rectus and the pyramidalis muscles are separated in the midline by sharp and blunt dissection to expose transversalis fascia and peritoneum.

The transversalis fascia and properitoneal fat are carefully dissected, beginning near the upper pole of the incision, to reach the underlying peritoneum. The peritoneum near the upper end of the incision is elevated with two hemostats placed about 2 cm apart. The tented fold of peritoneum between the clamps is visualized and palpated to rule out the inclusion of omentum, bowel, or bladder, and only then is the peritoneum carefully opened. In women who have had previous intra-abdominal surgery, including cesarean section, omentum or even bowel may be adherent to the undersurface of the peritoneum. The peritoneum is incised superiorly to the upper pole of the incision and downward to just above the peritoneal reflection over the bladder.

Troublesome bleeding sites anywhere in the abdom-

inal incision are clamped as encountered but are not ligated until later, unless the hemostats are in the way. Bleeding vessels should not be ignored, however, for it is essential that there be no active bleeding when the wound is closed.

With the Pfannenstiel type of incision, the skin and subcutaneous tissue are incised using a lower transverse, slightly curvilinear incision. The incision is made at the level of the pubic hairline and is extended somewhat beyond the lateral borders of the rectus muscles. After the subcutaneous tissue has been separated from the underlying fascia for 1 cm or so on each side, the fascia is incised transversely the full length of the incision. The superior and inferior edges of the fascia are grasped with suitable clamps. First, the inferior margin is elevated by the assistant as the operator separates the fascial sheath from the underlying rectus muscles by blunt dissection with the scalpel handle. Then the superior fascial margin is elevated and the rectus sheath freed from the rectus muscles. Blood vessels coursing between the muscles and fascia are clamped, severed, and ligated. It is imperative that meticulous hemostasis be achieved. The separation is carried to near the umbilicus sufficient to permit an adequate midline longitudinal incision of the peritoneum. The rectus muscles are separated from each other and from the underlying transversalis fascia and peritoneum. The peritoneum is opened as discussed above under the description of the vertical midline incision. Closure in layers is carried out the same as with a vertical incision, except that many operators, in trying to prevent hematoma formation, place beneath the fascia small Penrose drains that exit from each angle of the fascial closure.

The cosmetic advantage of the transverse skin incision is apparent. Moreover, the incision is said to be stronger, with less likelihood of dehiscence or hernia formation. There are, nonetheless, disadvantages in the use of the transverse incision. Exposure of the pregnant uterus and appendages is not as good as with a vertical incision. Whenever more room is needed, the vertical incision can be rapidly extended around and above the umbilicus, whereas the Pfannenstiel incision cannot. If the woman is obese, the operative field is even more restricted. Therefore, Pfannenstiel's incision tends to be used for thin women by operators who have achieved technical expertise, while the vertical incision is used almost to the exclusion of the transverse incision whenever rapid delivery is indicated, the woman is obese, or the operator is developing his skills. It is not appropriate to compare the vertical incision under these more adverse conditions to the transverse incision carried out under much more favorable circumstances. Finally, at the time of repeat cesarean section, reentry through Pfannenstiel's incision is likely to be more time consuming, which, at times, can be detrimental to the fetus.

Uterine Incision

The uterus is quickly but carefully palpated to identify the size and the presenting part of the fetus and to determine the direction and degree of rotation of the uterus. Commonly, the uterus is found to be dextrorotated so that the left round ligament is more anterior and closer to the midline than the right. It may be levorotated, however. Some operators prefer to lay a moistened laparotomy pack in each lateral peritoneal

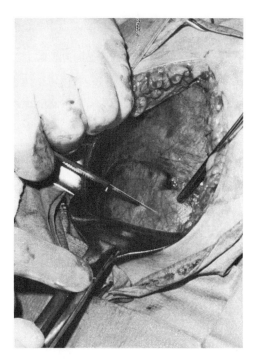

Figure 43-5. The myometrium is being carefully incised to avoid cutting the fetal head.

gutter to absorb amnionic fluid and blood that escape from the opened uterus. This technique is especially valuable in order to help localize the spread of infected amniotic fluid.

The typically rather loose reflection of peritoneum (serosa) above the upper margin of the bladder and overlying the anterior lower uterine segment is grasped in the midline with forceps (Fig. 43-2) and incised with a scalpel or scissors. Scissors, inserted between the serosa and myometrium of the lower uterine segment, are pushed laterally from the midline, while partially opening the blades intermittently, to separate a 2 cm wide strip of serosa, which is then incised. As the lateral margin on each side is approached, the scissors are aimed somewhat more cephalad (Fig. 43-3). The lower flap of peritoneum is elevated and the bladder is gently separated by blunt dissection from the underlying myometrium (Fig. 43-4). In general, the separation of bladder should not exceed 5 cm in depth and usually less. It is possible, especially with an effaced, dilated cervix, to dissect downward so deeply as inadvertently to expose and then enter the underlying vagina rather than the lower uterine segment (Goodlin and co-workers, 1982). The developed bladder flap is held downward beneath the symphysis with a bladder retractor, such as that used with a Balfour self-retaining retractor.

The uterus is opened through the lower uterine segment about 2 cm above the detached bladder. The uterine incision can be made by a variety of techniques. Each is initiated by incising with a scalpel the exposed

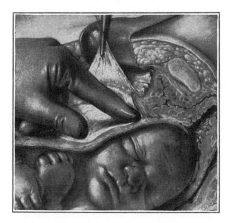

Figure 43-4. Low segment cesarean section. Cross-section showing dissection of bladder off uterus to expose lower uterine segment.

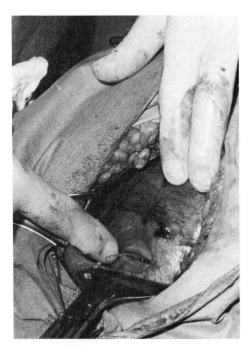

Figure 43-6. The uterine cavity has been entered. Amnionic fluid is escaping through the incision.

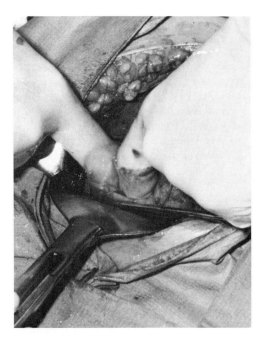

Figure 43-7. The index fingers inserted through the incised lower uterine segment exert moderate pressure laterally to extend the opening in the uterus.

lower uterine segment transversely for 2 cm or so halfway between the lateral margins. This must be done carefully so as to cut completely through the uterine wall but not deeply enough to wound the underlying fetus (Figs. 43-5, 43-6). Suctioning of the operative field by an assistant is especially important. Once the uterus is opened, the incision can be extended by cutting laterally and then slightly upward with bandage scissors, or when the lower uterine segment is thin, the incision of entry can be extended by simply spreading the incision, using lateral pressure applied with each index finger (Fig. 43-7), or a combination of these techniques can be used (Fig. 43-8). Exposure is aided by placement of a Richardson retractor into the wound and retracting the abdominal wall laterally as the incision is extended toward that side. *It is very important to make the uterine incision large enough to allow delivery of the head and trunk of the fetus without either tearing into or having to cut into the uterine arteries and veins that course through the lateral margins of the uterus.* If it appears that the uterine incision is going to be too small, some extra room may be obtained by curving the incision upward bilaterally so as to avoid the lateral uterine vessels. The membranes are incised if this was not done previously. If the placenta is encountered in the line of incision, it must either be detached or incised. Especially when the placenta is incised, fetal hemorrhage may be severe; therefore, the cord should be clamped as soon as possible in such cases.

Delivery of the Infant

The retractors are removed, and if the vertex is presenting, a hand is slipped into the uterine cavity between the symphysis and fetal head, and the head is gently elevated with the fingers and palm through the incision (Fig. 43-9A,B) aided by modest transabdominal fundal pressure. To minimize aspiration by the fetus of amnionic fluid and its contents, the exposed nares and mouth are aspirated with a bulb syringe before the thorax is delivered. The shoulders are then delivered using gentle traction plus fundal pressure. The rest of the body readily follows.

After a long labor with cephalopelvic disproportion, the fetal head may be rather tightly wedged in the birth canal. Upward pressure exerted through the vagina by the sterile-gloved hand of an associate will readily dislodge the head and allow its delivery above the symphysis.

As soon as the shoulders are delivered (Fig. 43-10), an intravenous infusion containing about 20 units of oxytocin per liter is allowed to flow at a brisk rate of 10 ml per minute until the uterus contracts satisfactorily, and then the rate is reduced to 2 to 4 ml per minute. The cord is promptly clamped with the infant at the level of the abdominal wall, and the infant is given to the member of the team who will conduct resuscitative efforts as they are needed. A sample of cord blood is obtained from the placental end of the cord.

If the fetus is not presenting as a vertex, or if there

are multiple fetuses, a longitudinal incision through the lower segment may, at times, prove to be advantageous. The fetal legs must be carefully distinguished from the arms to avoid premature extraction of an arm and a difficult delivery of the rest of the fetus.

The uterine incision is observed for any vigorously bleeding sites. These are promptly clamped, depending upon size and location, with Pean forceps, short-handled ring forceps, or similar instruments. The placenta is promptly removed manually, unless it is separating spontaneously (Fig. 43-11). Fundal massage, begun as soon as the fetus is delivered, reduces bleeding and hastens delivery of the placenta.

Repair of Uterus

After delivery of the placenta, the uterus may be lifted through the incision onto the draped abdominal wall and the fundus covered with a moistened laparotomy pack.*

Immediately after delivery and inspection of the placenta, the uterine cavity is inspected and is wiped out with a gauze pack to remove shreds of membranes, vernix, clots, or other debris. If the cervical canal is not known to be patent, it should be probed with a Pean clamp to assure patency. The contaminated clamp is discarded from the field.

The upper and lower cut edges and each angle of the uterine incision are carefully examined for bleeding vessels. The lower margin of an incision made through a thinned-out lower uterine segment may be so thin as to be ignored inadvertently. At the same time, the posterior wall of the lower uterine segment may occasionally buckle anteriorly in such a way as to suggest that it is the lower margin of the incision. Incorporation of the posterior wall into the closure must be avoided.

The uterine incision may be closed with either one or the more traditional two layers of continuous chromic suture. Individually clamped large vessels are best ligated with a suture ligature. Concern has been expressed by some that sutures through the decidua may lead to

---

* *Extra-abdominal exteriorization of the uterus immediately after delivery of the placenta often has advantages that outweigh the disadvantages. The relaxing uterus can be quickly recognized and fundal massage applied. The uterine incision and bleeding points along its cut margins are more easily visualized and sutured, especially when the incision extended during delivery of the fetus. There is also better exposure of the adnexa, especially the oviducts, which increases the ease and accuracy of tubal sterilization. The disadvantages are discomfort and, less often, vomiting during exteriorization or replacement when epidural or spinal anesthesia is used and possible inadvertent displacement of a ligature from an oviduct at the operative site following tubal ligation and resection. Hershey and Quilligan (1978), in the course of a study of the advantages and disadvantages of exteriorization of the uterus, did not find febrile morbidity to be more common in women whose uteri were exteriorized for closure.*

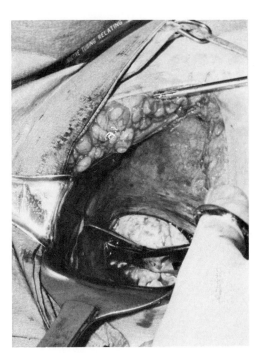

Figure 43-8. Bandage scissors are used to complete the transverse incision when resistance to spreading is encountered.

endometriosis in the scar and a weak scar. In actuality, this is a rare complication. The initial stitch is placed just beyond one angle of the uterine incision. A running-lock suture is then carried out, with each stitch penetrating the full thickness of the myometrium. It is important to select carefully the site of each stitch and, once the needle penetrates the myometrium, not to withdraw it. This minimizes the perforation of unligated vessels and subsequent bleeding from such sites. The running-lock suture is continued just beyond the opposite angle of the incision.

Especially when the lower segment is thin, satisfactory approximation of the cut edges usually can be obtained with one layer of suture. When but one layer of suture is to be used, both hemostasis and closure may be better effected by tying the first running-lock suture at about the middle of the incision, placing a new suture beyond the opposite angle of the uterine incision in the same way as the first, and closing the remainder of the incision with a running-lock stitch. If approximation is not satisfactory after a single-layer continuous closure or if bleeding sites persist, either another layer of suture may be placed so as to achieve approximation and hemostasis, or sites of unsatisfactory approximation or lack of hemostasis can be treated with individual figure-of-eight or mattress sutures.

After the operator is certain that there is no further bleeding after closure of the uterine incision, the cut edges of the serosa overlying the uterus and bladder are

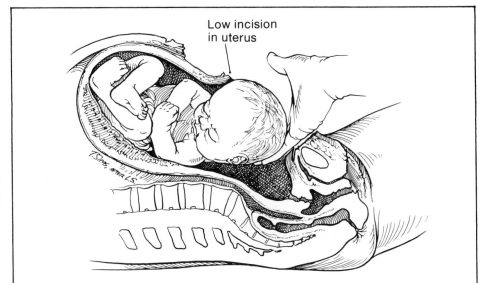

Low incision
in uterus

Figure 43-9. A. Immediately after incising the uterus and fetal membranes, the operator's fingers are insinuated between the symphysis pubis and the fetal head until the posterior surface is reached. The head is carefully lifted anteriorly and, as necessary, superiorly to bring it from beneath the symphysis forward through the uterine and abdominal incisions.

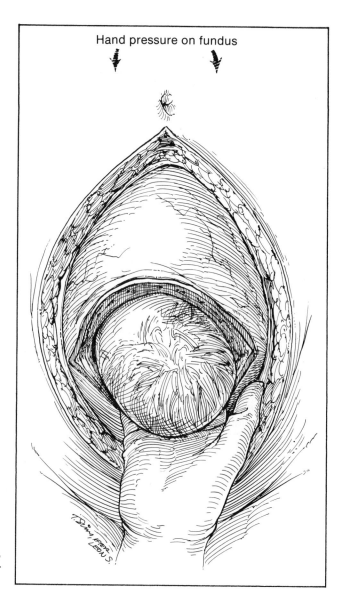

Hand pressure on fundus

Figure 43-9. B. As the fetal head is lifted through the incision, pressure is usually applied to the uterine fundus through the abdominal wall to help expel the fetus.

876

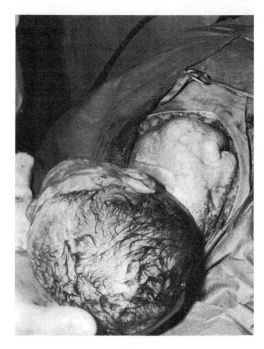

Figure 43-10. Just as the shoulders are delivered, intravenous oxytocin infusion is started.

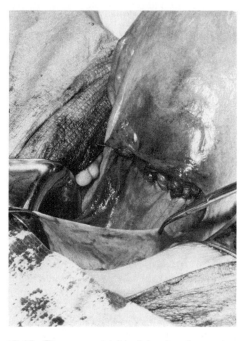

Figure 43-12. The myometrial incision has been closed. The lower edge of the cut serosa is identified in the clamps.

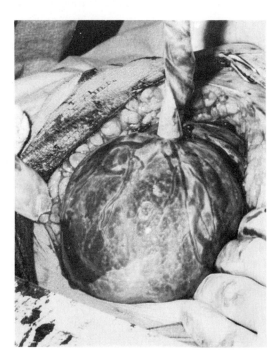

Figure 43-11. Placenta bulging through uterine incision as uterus contracts.

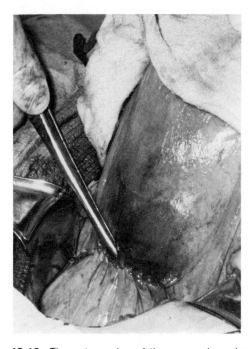

Figure 43-13. The cut margins of the serosa have been approximated to reperitonealize the uterus.

approximated with a continuous 00 chromic catgut suture (Figs. 43-12, 43-13). The lower edge of peritoneum should not be carried above the bladder, especially if the procedure is repeated during subsequent cesarean sections. To do so may lead to bladder discomfort and undue urinary frequency during later pregnancies, as well as difficult dissection of an unusually adherent overlapped peritoneum with subsequent cesarean section or hysterectomy.

Tubal Sterilization

If tubal sterilization is to be performed, it is done now. The failure rate after the following technique is low (Husbands and associates, 1970):

1. Visualize the fallopain tube in its entirety.
2. Grasp the midportion in a Babcock clamp at a site where the mesosalpinx is seen to be free of veins.
3. Perforate the mesosalpinx immediately beneath the fallopian tube with a fine hemostat and then open the jaws to separate the mesosalpinx from the tube for at least 2 cm.
4. Ligate the separated segment proximally and distally with individual pieces of 0 chromic suture so as to isolate a segment of at least 2 cm.
5. Excise the isolated segment, identify it, and submit it for histologic examination.
6. Observe sites of resection for bleeding and, if found, clamp and ligate with fine suture. This technique is described in Chapter 40, p. 827.

Abdominal Closure

Laparotomy packs, if used, are removed, and the gutters and cul-de-sac are emptied of blood and amnionic fluid by gentle suction. If general anesthesia is used, the interior of the abdominal cavity is systematically palpated, as a rule, to evaluate the abdominal contents. With conduction anesthesia, however, this may produce considerable discomfort. The uterus is reexamined and compressed to express any blood within it.

As soon as the sponge and instrument count are found to be correct, the abdominal wall is closed. As each layer is closed, bleeding sites are searched for, clamped, and ligated. Continuous 00 chromic catgut suture is used to close the peritoneum, including the overlying transversalis fascia (Fig. 43-14). It is important to avoid leaving a defect at either end of the incision and to place each suture far enough laterally to ensure a strong closure. The rectus muscles are allowed to fall into place, and the overlying rectus fascia is closed with interrupted 0 nonabsorbable sutures that are placed well lateral to the cut fascial edges and no more than 1 cm apart. The subcutaneous tissue usually need not be closed separately if it is 2 cm or less in thickness, and the skin is closed with vertical mattress sutures of 000 or 0000 silk or equivalent suture. If there is more adipose tissue than this or if clips or subcuticular closure is to be used,

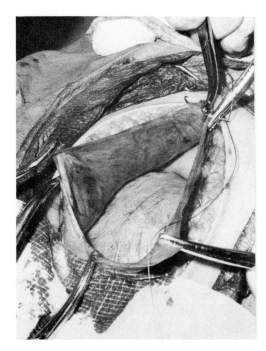

Figure 43-14. The firmly contracted uterus is visible through the uterine incision. The cut margins of the parietal peritoneum are elevated, and closure has been initiated.

a few interrupted 000 plain catgut sutures are used to obliterate dead space and reduce tension on the skin edges.

The abdominal wall in most circumstances need only be covered with a light dressing consisting of three 4 by 4 sponges unfolded once and fastened with three pieces of 1-inch tape.

Classical Cesarean Section

On occasion, it may be necessary to use a classical cesarean section to effect delivery, for example: (1) if the lower uterine segment cannot be exposed or entered safely because the bladder is densely adherent from previous surgery, or if a myoma occupies the lower uterine segment, or if there is invasive carcinoma of the cervix, (2) when there is a transverse lie of a large fetus, especially if the membranes are ruptured and the shoulder is impacted in the birth canal, (3) in some cases of placenta previa with anterior implantation of the placenta, especially if sterilization is to be performed (Chapter 21, p. 441).

Incisions. The abdominal incision usually needs to extend somewhat higher than for a lower segment cesarean section. (Originally the classic incision extended to very near the top of the uterine fundus; therefore, in order to expose the uterus, the abdominal incision typically was made just below, lateral to, and above the umbilicus.) The vertical incision into the uterus is initiated with a scalpel beginning above the level of the attached bladder. It is essential to incise through the uterine wall but not lacerate the fetus. Brisk bleeding during entry may make visualization difficult. Once sufficient room is made with the scalpel, the incision is extended cephalad with bandage scissors until it is sufficiently long to permit delivery of the fetus. Numerous large vessels that bleed profusely are commonly encountered within the myometrium. As soon as the fetus has been removed, these vessels may best be clamped and eventually ligated with sutures of chromic catgut. As soon as the fetus has been delivered, oxytocin is administered and the placenta delivered, as described above under Lower Segment Transverse Incision.

Repair of Uterus. The uterus may be lifted through the incision and placed on the abdominal wall. The uterine incision is closed in such a manner that the cut edges are evenly and completely coapted and hemorrhage is controlled. One method employs a layer of continuous 0 or 1 chromic catgut to approximate the inner halves of the incision. The outer half of the uterine incision is then closed with similar chromic catgut suture, using either a continuous stitch or figure-of-eight sutures. Each stitch should be placed sufficiently deep into the myometrium that it will not pull out. No unnecessary needle tracts should be made lest myometrial vessels be perforated with hemorrhage or hematoma formation. To achieve good approximation and to prevent the suture from tearing through the myometrium, it is essential that an assistant compress the myometrium on each side of the wound medially as each suture is placed and tied. The edges of the uterine serosa, if not already so, are approximated with continuous 00 chromic catgut. The operation is completed as described above under Lower Segment Transverse Incision.

Extraperitoneal Cesarean Section

Early in this century, Frank (1907) and Latzko (1909) recommended extraperitoneal cesarean section rather than cesarean hysterectomy as a method of dealing with pregnancies with infected uterine contents. The goal of the operation was to open the uterus extraperitoneally by dissecting through the space of Retzius and then along one side and beneath the bladder to reach the lower uterine segment. The writings of Waters (1940) and Norton (1946) helped to popularize the operation in this country at midcentury. Enthusiasm for the procedure was transient, however, probably in large part because of the availability of a variety of effective antibacterial agents. The increased frequency in recent years of cesarean section, accompanied by either an actual increase in frequency and intensity of troublesome infections or at least a reawareness of the problem, has rekindled interest in the use of extraperitoneal cesarean section. Perkins (1977), for example, demonstrated some enthusiasm for the procedure but, at the same time, carefully explained the limitations of the procedure as well as the benefits that might be derived from its use. He favors the technique described by Douglas and Stromme (1965), who modified the techniques of Latzko and Norton.

Postmortem Cesarean Section

Both Weber (1970) and Arthur (1978) stressed that a satisfactory outcome for the fetus is dependent upon (1) anticipation of death of the mother, (2) fetal age of more than 28 weeks, (3) personnel and appropriate equipment immediately available, (4) continued postmortem ventilation and cardiac massage for the mother, (5) prompt delivery, and (6) effective resuscitation of the infant. While a few infants have survived with no apparent physical or intellectual compromise, others have not been so fortunate. In more recent years, the capability of life-support systems to maintain some level of vegetative function for long periods of time and the reluctance of physicians to pronounce a patient dead have decreased further the likelihood of delivering an infant that will survive and thrive following a postmortem cesarean section. However, Fogarty and co-workers (1984) reported the successful delivery by cesarean section of an infant whose mother, though brain dead, was maintained for 10 weeks on life-support systems in order for fetal maturation to occur.

CESAREAN HYSTERECTOMY

Indications

The indications for cesarean hysterectomy have been discussed in connection with the various conditions that sometimes require the operation. In summary, intrauterine infection, a grossly defective scar, a markedly hypotonic uterus that does not respond to oxytocics, prostaglandins, and massage, inadvertent laceration of major uterine vessels, significant myomas, severe dysplasia or carcinoma in situ of the cervix, and placenta acreta or increta often may best be treated by immediate hysterectomy if cesarean section is being performed. The major deterrents to use of cesarean hysterectomy are increased blood loss and the frequency of damage to the urinary tract in the form of trauma to the ureters and more commonly to the bladder (Plauché and colleagues, 1981). The merits of cesarean hysterectomy for sterilization, rather than cesarean section plus partial tubal resection, remain the subject of much interest and are discussed in Chapter 40, p. 830.

Technique

After delivery of the infant by either classical or lower segment cesarean section, supracervical or preferably total hysterectomy, usually with retention of adnexa, can be carried out according to standard operative techniques. *Although all vessels to the gravid uterus are appreciably larger than those of the nonpregnant organ,* hysterectomy is usually facilitated by the ease of development of tissue planes. Blood loss commonly is appreciable; however, with cesarean hysterectomy performed primarily for sterilization, blood loss averages about 1500 ml, or about 500 ml more than with cesarean section (Pritchard, 1965).

As the infant's shoulders are delivered, oxytocin is infused intravenously until the uterus is removed. The major bleeding vessels are clamped and ligated quickly. The placenta is removed, and optionally to try to prevent excessive bleeding, a dry laparotomy pack is placed in the cavity over the implantation site before closing the uterine incision with either a continuous suture or a few interrupted sutures.

The uterus is elevated out of the abdominal cavity, and the round ligaments close to the uterus are divided between Heaney or Kocher clamps and doubly ligated. Either size 0 or 1 chromic catgut may be used. The incision in the vesicouterine serosa, made to mobilize the bladder for cesarean section, is extended laterally and upward through the anterior leaf of the broad ligament to reach the incised round ligaments. Any actively bleeding vessels must be clamped and tied to minimize blood loss. The posterior leaf of the broad ligament adjacent to the uterus is perforated just beneath the fallopian tubes, utero-ovarian ligaments, and ovarian vessels, and these are then doubly clamped close to the uterus and severed; the lateral pedicle is doubly ligated. The pedicles adjacent to the uterus may be ligated and the clamps removed from the operative field. The posterior leaf of the broad ligament is next divided inferiorly toward the cardinal ligaments. Again, any bleeding vessels are discretely clamped and ligated. Next, the bladder and attached peritoneal flap are dissected from the lower uterine segment and retracted out of the operative field. Usually this can be accomplished easily with gentle blunt dissection, using gauze over the fingers. If the bladder flap is unusually adherent, as it may be after previous cesarean sections, careful sharp dissection with scissors may be necessary.

Special care is necessary from this point on to avoid injury to the ureters, which pass beneath the uterine arteries. The ascending uterine artery and veins on either side are identified and near their origin are doubly clamped immediately adjacent to the uterus and divided. The vascular pedicle is doubly ligated.

Supracervical Hysterectomy

To perform a subtotal hysterectomy, it is necessary only to amputate the body of the uterus at this level. The cervical stump may be closed with interrupted catgut sutures. If there is persistent oozing of blood or the likelihood of infection, the cervix may be dilated and a drain inserted into the vagina. Reperitonealization is performed as for total hysterectomy.

Total Hysterectomy

To perform a total hysterectomy, it is necessary to mobilize the bladder much more extensively in the midline and laterally. This will help carry the ureters inferiorly as the bladder is retracted beneath the symphysis and will also prevent cutting or suturing of the bladder during excision of the cervix and closure of the vagina. The bladder is dissected free for about 2 cm below the lowest margin of the cervix to expose the uppermost part of the vagina. If the cervix is no more than slightly effaced, the cervical–vaginal junction can be identified by palpation between the fingers of one hand in the cul-de-sac and the fingers of the other hand anteriorly. If the cervix is appreciably effaced and dilated, this maneuver usually cannot be performed satisfactorily. In this circumstance, the uterine cavity may be entered anteriorly in the midline either through the lower pole of the incision made for delivery of the fetus or through a stab wound made at the level of the ligated uterine vessels. A finger is directed inferiorly through the incision to identify the free margin of the dilated, effaced cervix and the anterior vaginal fornix.

The cardinal ligaments, the uterosacral ligaments, and the many large vessels the ligaments contain are systematically doubly clamped with Heaney-type curved clamps, Ochsner-type straight clamps, or similar instruments. The clamps are placed as close to the cervix as possible without including the cervix. It is imperative that not too large a volume of tissue be included in each clamp. The tissue between the pair of clamps is incised, and the lateral pedicle, which invariably is vascular, is ligated appropriately. These steps are repeated until the level of the lateral vaginal fornix is reached. In this way, the descending branches of the uterine vessels are clamped, cut, and ligated as the cervix is dissected from the cardinal ligaments posteriorly.

Immediately below the level of the cervix, a curved clamp is swung in across the lateral vaginal fornix, and the tissue is incised medially to the clamp. The excised lateral vaginal fornix commonly is simultaneously doubly ligated and sutured to the stump of the cardinal ligament. The entire cervix is then excised from the vagina, while an assistant systematically grasps the full thickness of the cut margins of the vagina with straight Ochsner or similar clamps.

The cervix is inspected to insure that it has been completely excised, and the vagina is repaired. Some operators prefer to close the vagina using figure-of-eight chromic catgut sutures. Perhaps the majority prefer to achieve hemostasis by using a running-lock stitch of chromic catgut suture placed through the mucosa and adjacent endopelvic fascia around the circumference of the vagina. The open vagina may promote drainage of the fluids that would otherwise accumulate and contribute to hematoma and abscess formation.

The peritoneal gutters and the cul-de-sac are emptied of blood and other debris. All sites of incision from the upper pedicle (fallopian tube and ovarian ligament) to the vaginal vault and bladder flap are carefully examined for bleeding. Any bleeding sites that are identified are clamped carefully and ligated appropriately. Care is necessary lest the ureter be compromised by such a hemostatic ligature.

The pelvis is reperitonealized. One method employs a continuous chromic suture starting with the tip of the ligated pedicle of fallopian tube and ovarian ligament, which is inverted retroperitoneally. Sutures are then placed continuously so as to approximate the leaves of the broad ligament, to bury the stump of the round ligament, to approximate the cut edge of the vesicouterine peritoneum over the vaginal vault posteriorly to the cut edge of peritoneum above the cul-de-sac, to approximate the leaves of the broad ligament on the opposite side, and to bury the stump of the round ligament and finally the pedicle of fallopian tube and ovarian ligament.

The abdominal wall normally is closed in layers, as previously described under Lower Segment Transverse Incision. In case of sepsis, the abdominal wound may be closed with permanent nonreactive sutures through the peritoneum and fascia in a single layer, while the subcutaneous tissue and skin are not closed until later.

Appendectomy and Oophorectomy. The benefits compared to the risks from incidental appendectomy at the time of cesarean section or hysterectomy continue to be argued. Lacking are results of a study that demonstrate clearly the puerperal morbidity and mortality rates are not increased by appendectomy.

During cesarean hysterectomy, a decision as to the fate of the ovaries has to be made. Should the clamp be placed across the ovarian ligament and fallopian tube medial to the ovary or across the infundibulopelvic ligament just lateral to the ovary and tube? For women who are approaching menopause, the decision is not difficult, but few women who undergo cesarean hysterectomy are approaching the menopause. In general, preservation of the ovaries is favored by most obstetricians unless the ovaries are diseased.

PERIPARTAL MANAGEMENT

Preoperative Care

The woman scheduled for repeat cesarean section typically is admitted the day before surgery and evaluated by the obstetrician who will perform surgery and the anesthesiologist who will provide anesthesia. The hematocrit is rechecked and usually 1000 ml of compatible whole blood or its equivalent in blood fractions is reserved. A sedative, such as secobarbital 0.1 g, may be given at bedtime the night before the operation. In general, no other sedatives, narcotics, or tranquilizers are administered until after the infant is born. Oral intake is stopped at least 8 hours before surgery. An antacid, such as a suspension of magnesium hydroxide (milk of magnesia) 30 ml, given shortly before the induction of a general anesthesia, minimizes the risk of lung destruction from gastric hydrochloric acid should aspiration occur (Chapter 18, p. 357). The authors strongly recommend this be done routinely, even when regional conduction anesthesia will be used; at times it is necessary to switch to, or at least supplement, the regional anesthesia with inhalation anesthesia.

Intravenous Fluids

The requirements for intravenous fluids, including blood during and after cesarean section, can vary considerably. The woman of average size with a hematocrit of 33 or more and a normally expanded blood volume and extracellular fluid volume most often tolerates an actual blood loss of up to 1500 ml without difficulty. The concept that prevailed in some institutions not too long ago that blood loss should be matched milliliter for milliliter by blood transfusion is not tenable, but neither is disregard for excessive bleeding. Careful attention must be paid to blood loss so as to avoid both underestimation and overestimation. Unappreciated bleeding through the vagina during the procedure or bleeding concealed in the uterus after its closure or both commonly lead to underestimation. Blood loss averages about 1 liter but is quite variable (Wilcox and co-workers, 1959; Pritchard, 1965).

Intravenously administered fluids consist of lactated Ringer's solution or similar solution and 5 percent dextrose in water. Typically, 1 to 2 liters that contain electrolyte are infused during and immediately after the operation. As the shoulders of the infant are delivered, oxytocin, 20 units per liter, is added to the infusion, which is then infused for a few minutes at a brisk rate (10 ml per minute) until the uterus is well contracted. Throughout the procedure, and subsequently while in the postoperative recovery area, the blood pressure and urine flow are monitored closely to ascertain that perfusion of vital organs is satisfactory.

Recovery Suite

It is very important that the uterus remain firmly contracted. In the recovery suite, the amount of bleeding from the vagina must be closely monitored, and the uterine fundus must be identified by palpation frequently to assure that the uterus is remaining firmly contracted. Unfortunately, as the patient awakens from general anesthesia or the conduction anesthesia fades, palpation of the abdomen is likely to produce considerable discomfort. This can be made much more tolerable by giving an effective analgesic intramuscularly, such as meperidine (Demerol) 75 mg or morphine 10 mg. A thick dressing with an abundance of adhesive tape over the abdomen interferes with fundal palpation and massage and later causes discomfort as the tape and perhaps skin are removed. Deep breathing and coughing are encouraged.

Once the mother is fully awake, bleeding is minimal, the blood pressure is satisfactory, and urine flow is at least 30 ml per hour, she may be returned to her room.

Subsequent Care

Her subsequent care must include the following.

Analgesia. For the woman of average size, meperidine 75 mg is given intramuscularly as often as every 3 hours as needed for discomfort, or morphine 10 mg is similarly administered. If she is small, 50 mg, or if large, 100 mg of meperidine is more appropriate.

Vital Signs. The patient is now evaluated at least hourly for 4 hours at the minimum, and blood pressure, pulse, urine flow, amount of bleeding, and status of the uterine fundus are checked at these times. Abnormalities are reported immediately. Thereafter, for the first 24 hours, these are checked at intervals of 4 hours, along with the temperature.

Fluid Therapy and Diet. Unless there has been pathologic constriction of the extracellular fluid compartment (diuretics, sodium restriction, vomiting, high fever, prolonged labor without adequate fluid intake), the puerperium is characterized by the excretion of fluid that was retained during pregnancy and became superfluous once delivery was accomplished. Moreover, with the typical cesarean section or uncomplicated cesarean hysterectomy, significant sequestration of extracellular fluid in bowel wall and bowel lumen does not occur, unless it was necessary to pack the bowel away from the operative field or peritonitis develops. Thus, the woman who undergoes cesarean section is rarely a candidate for the development in the fluid compartment of a so-called third space. Quite the contrary, she normally begins surgery with a physiologic third space that she acquired during normal pregnancy, namely, the physiologic edema of pregnancy that she mobilizes and excretes after delivery. Therefore, large volumes of intravenous fluids during and subsequent to surgery are not needed to replace sequestered extracellular fluid. As a generalization, 3 liters of fluid, including lactated Ringer's solution, should prove adequate during surgery and the first 24 hours thereafter. If urine output falls below 30 ml per hour, however, the patient should be reevaluated promptly. The cause of the oliguria may range from unrecognized blood loss to an antidiuretic effect from infused oxytocin (Chapter 17, p. 346). In the absence of extensive intra-abdominal manipulation or sepsis, the woman nearly always should be able to tolerate oral fluids the day after surgery. If not, an intravenous infusion can be continued or restarted. By the second day after surgery, the great majority of women tolerate a general diet.

Bladder and Bowels. The catheter most often can be removed from the bladder by 12 hours after the operation or, more conveniently, the morning after the operation. Subsequent ability to empty the bladder before overdistention develops must be monitored as with a vaginal delivery. Bowel sounds usually are not heard the first day after surgery, they are faint the second day, and they are active the third day. Gas pains from incoordinate bowel action may be troublesome the second and third postoperative days. Frequently, a rectal supposi-

tory followed by defecation or, if that fails, an enema provides appreciable relief.

Ambulation

In most instances, by the first day after surgery the patient should, with assistance, get out of bed briefly at least twice. Ambulation can be timed so that a recently administered analgesic will minimize the discomfort. By the second day she may walk to the bathroom with assistance. With early ambulation, venous thrombosis and pulmonary embolism are uncommon.

Care of Wound

The incision is inspected each day. Thus, a relatively light dressing without an abundance of tape is advantageous. Normally the skin sutures (or skin clips) are removed on the fourth day after surgery. By the third postpartum day, bathing, either by shower or by tub bath, is not harmful to the incision.

Laboratory

The hematocrit is routinely measured the morning after surgery. It is checked sooner when there was unusual blood loss or when there is oliguria or other evidence to suggest hypovolemia. If the hematocrit is significantly decreased from the preoperative level, it is repeated, and a search is instituted to identify the cause of the decrease. If the lower hematocrit is stable, the mother can ambulate without any difficulty, and if there is little likelihood of further blood loss, hematologic repair in response to iron therapy is preferred to transfusion.

Breast Care

Breast-feeding can be initiated by the day after surgery. If the mother elects not to breast-feed, a breast binder that supports the breasts without marked compression will usually minimize discomfort. More recently, bromocriptine has become available in this country for suppression of lactation and has proven to be effective for this purpose. The major disadvantage of bromocriptine remains its high cost. The patient is more comfortable using this drug than using a breast binder, and the suppression of lactation removes one possible source of postpartum fever (Chapter 36, p. 739).

Discharge

Unless there are complications during the puerperium, the mother may be safely discharged from the hospital on the fourth or fifth postpartum day. The mother's activities during the following week should be restricted to self-care and care of her baby with assistance. It is advantageous to perform the initial postpartum evaluation during the third week after delivery rather than at the more traditional time of 6 weeks, for the reasons presented in Chapters 19 and 40.

Prophylactic Antibiotics

Febrile morbidity is rather frequent after cesarean section and appears to be more common among indigent than more affluent women. Since the development of antimicrobial agents, numerous attempts have been made to document the value, if any, of prophylactically administered antibiotics. During the early antibiotic era, various claims for and against such a practice were made. More recently, several reports have appeared in which febrile morbidity was shown to be reduced when antibiotics were administered prophylactically. The issue of prophylactic antibiotics following cesarean section has been addressed by numerous investigators (Gibbs and colleagues, 1973; Gall, 1979; Wong and co-workers, 1978; Green and associates, 1978; and Kreutner and colleagues; 1979).

Cunningham and associates (1978) have developed a plan of management for women at high risk of serious infection if they undergo cesarean delivery. These investigators identified that at Parkland Memorial Hospital, 85 percent of women in labor with membranes ruptured for longer than 6 hours who then underwent cesarean delivery developed troublesome infection. The incidence was much less (29 percent) in women who underwent cesarean section after laboring with membranes intact. Moreover, they noted that wound abscesses and pelvic phlegmons were encountered in less than 1 percent of women with intact membranes, compared to 30 percent of women whose membranes ruptured more than 6 hours before cesarean section. In addition, bacteremia was four times more common in those women whose membranes ruptured longer than 6 hours before surgery and who subsequently demonstrated infection.

Cunningham, DePalma, and their co-workers (1978, 1980, 1982) have evaluated therapeutic intervention in this high risk group of nulliparous women who underwent cesarean delivery because of cephalopelvic disproportion. Since the frequency of pelvic infection was 85 percent without therapy, they considered intervention with antibiotics to be treatment rather than prophylaxis. They observed that the administration of pencillin plus gentamycin or of cefamandole alone as soon as the cord was clamped, followed by two more doses of the same medications given at intervals of 6 hours, resulted in a dramatic reduction in morbidity from infection. Postoperative metritis, for example, was decreased from 85 to 20 percent. Importantly, serious complications, such as pelvic phlegmons, incisional abscesses, and pelvic thrombophlebitis, also decreased dramatically. Currently at Parkland Memorial Hospital, women at extreme risk of morbidity from infection after cesarean delivery receive   antibiotics administered as described above.

HISTORICAL

The origin of the term *cesarean section* is obscure. Three principal explanations have been suggested.

1. According to legend, Julius Caesar was born in this manner, with the result that the procedure became known as the "Caesarean operation." Several circumstances weaken this explanation, however. First, the mother of Julius Caesar lived for many years after his birth. Even as late as the 17th century, the operation was almost invariably fatal, according to the most dependable writers of that period. It is thus improbable that Caesar's mother could have survived the procedure in 100 B.C. Second, the operation, whether performed on the living or dead, is not mentioned by any medical writer before the Middle Ages. Historical details of the origin of the family name Caesar are found in Pickrell's monograph (1935).

2. It has been widely believed that the name of the operation is derived from a Roman law, supposedly created by Numa Pompilius (eighth century BC), ordering that the procedure be performed upon women dying in the last few weeks of pregnancy in the hope of saving the child. This explanation then holds that this *lex regia*, as it was called at first, became the *lex caesarea* under the emperors, and the operation itself became known as the *caesarean* operation. The German term *Kaiserschnitt* reflects this derivation.

3. The word *caesarean*, as applied to the operation, was derived sometime in the Middle Ages from the Latin verb *caedere,* "to cut." An obvious cognate is the word *caesura,* a cutting, or pause, in a line of verse. This explanation of the term *caesarean* seems most logical, but exactly when it was first applied to the operation is uncertain. Since "section" is derived from the Latin verb "seco," which also means "cut," the term "caesarean section" seems tautologic.

It is customary in the United States to replace the "ae" ligature in the first syllable of "caesarean" with the letter "e"; in Great Britain and Australia, however, the "ae" is still retained.

From the time of Virgil's Aeneas to Shakespeare's Macduff, poets have repeatedly referred to persons "untimely ripped" from their mother's womb. Ancient historians, such as Pliny, moreover, say that Scipio Africanus (the conqueror of Hannibal), Martius, and Julius Caesar were all born thus. In regard to Julius Caesar, Pliny adds that it was from this circumstance that the surname(?) rose by which the Roman emperors were known. Birth in this extraordinary manner, as described in ancient mythology and legend, was believed to confer supernatural powers and elevate the heroes so born above ordinary mortals.

In evaluating these references to abdominal delivery in antiquity, it is pertinent that no such operation is even mentioned by Hippocrates, Galen, Celsus, Paulus, Soranus, or any other medical writer of the period. If cesarean section were actually employed at that time, it is particularly surprising that Soranus, whose extensive work written in the second century AD covers all aspects of obstetrics, does not refer to cesarean section. In Genesis (11:21) it is written: "And the Lord God caused a deep sleep to fall upon Adam, and he slept: and he took one of his ribs, and closed up the flesh instead thereof." Are we to conclude from this statement that general anesthesia and thoracic surgery were known in pre-Mosaic times? It would probably be just as logical to draw comparable conclusions about the beginnings of cesarean section from the myths and fantasies that have come down to us.

Several references to abdominal delivery appear in the Talmud, compiled between the second and sixth centuries AD, but whether they had any background in terms of clinical usage is conjectural. There can be no doubt, however, that cesarean section on the dead was first practiced soon after the Christian Church gained dominance, as a measure directed at baptism of the child. Faith in the validity of some of these early reports is rudely shaken, however, when they glibly state that a living, robust child was obtained 8 to 24 *hours* after the death of the mother.

Some of the early reports of cesarean section on the living excite similar skepticism. The case often cited as representing the first cesarean section performed on a living woman is that attributed to a German gelder named Jacob Nufer, who is said to have carried out the operation on his wife in the year 1500. Not only did his wife survive (a miracle in itself) but she lived to give birth to two subsequent children after normal labors, in a period when suturing of the uterine wound during cesarean section was unknown. The case was not reported until almost a hundred years later (1591) by an author who based his description on hearsay handed down through three generations.

Cesarean section on the living was first recommended, and the current name of the operation used, in the celebrated work of Francois Rousset entitled "Traité Nouveau de l'Hystérotomotokie ou l'Enfantement Césarien," published in 1581. Rousset had never performed or witnessed the operation; his information was based chiefly on letters from friends. He reported 14 successful cesarean sections, a fact in itself difficult to accept. When it is further stated that 6 of the 14 operations were performed on the same woman, the credulity of the most gullible is exhausted.

The apocryphal nature of most early reports on cesarean section has been stressed because many of them have been accepted without question. Authoritative statements by dependable obstetricians about early use of the operation, however, did not appear in the literature until the mid-17th century, as for instance in the classic work of the great French obstetrician, François Mauriceau, first published in 1668. These statements show without doubt that the operation was employed on the living in rare and desperate cases during the latter half of the 16th century and that it was usually fatal. Details of the history of cesarean section are to be found in Fasbender's classic text (1906).

The appalling maternal mortality rate of cesarean section continued until the beginning of the 20th century. In Great Britain and Ireland, the maternal death rate from the operation had mounted in 1865 to 85 percent. In Paris, during the 90 years ending in 1876, not a single successful cesarean section had been performed. Harris noted that as late as 1887 cesarean section was actually more successful when performed by the patient herself or when the abdomen was ripped open by the horn of a bull. He collected from the literature 9 such cases with 5 recoveries, and contrasted them with 12 cesarean sections performed in New York City during the same period, with only 1 recovery.

The turning point in the evolution of cesarean section came in 1882, when Max Sänger, then at 28-year-old assistant of Credé in the University Clinic at Leipzig, intro-

duced suturing of the uterine wall. The long neglect of so simple an expedient as uterine suture was not the result of oversight but stemmed from a deeply rooted belief that sutures in the uterus were superfluous as well as harmful by virtue of serving as the site for severe infection. In meeting these objections Sänger, who had himself used sutures in only one case, documented their value, not from the sophisticated medical centers of Europe but from frontier America. There, in outposts from Ohio to Louisiana, 17 cesarean sections had been reported in which silver wire sutures had been used, with the survival of 8 mothers, an extraordinary record in those days. In a table included in his monograph, Sänger gives full credit to these frontier surgeons for providing the supporting data for his hypothesis. The problem of hemorrhage was the first and most serious problem to be solved. Details are found in Eastman's review (1932).

Although the introduction of uterine sutures reduced the mortality rate of the operation from hemorrhage, generalized peritonitis remained the dominant cause of death; hence, various types of operations were devised to meet this scourge. The earliest was the Porro procedure (1876), in use before Sänger's time, that combined subtotal cesarean hysterectomy with marsupialization of the cervical stump. The first extraperitoneal operation was described by Frank in 1907 and, with various modifications, as introduced by Latzko, Sellheim, and by Waters (1940), was employed until recent years.

In 1912, Krönig contended that the main advantage of the extraperitoneal technique consisted not so much in avoiding the peritoneal cavity as in opening the uterus through its thin lower segment and then covering the incision with peritoneum. To accomplish this end, he cut through the vesical reflection of the peritoneum from one round ligament to the other and separated it and the bladder from the lower uterine segment and cervix. The lower portion of the uterus was then opened through a vertical median incision, and the child was extracted by forceps. The uterine incision was then closed and buried under the vesical peritoneum. With minor modifications, this low-segment technique was introduced into the United States by Beck (1919) and popularized by DeLee (1922) and others. A particularly important modification was recommended by Kerr in 1926, who preferred a transverse rather than a longitudinal uterine incision. The Kerr technique is the most commonly employed type of cesarean section today.

A monograph on the history of cesarean section by Trolle (1982) is recommended.

REFERENCES

ACOG Newsletter: Committee reports guidelines for vaginal delivery. 26:1, 1982

Arthur RK: Postmortem cesarean section. Am J Obstet Gynecol 132:175, 1978

Beck AC: Observations on a series of cases of cesarean section done at the Long Island College Hospital during the past six years. Am J Obstet Gynecol 79:197, 1919

Benedetti TJ, Platt L, Druzin M: Vaginal delivery after previous cesarean section for a nonrecurrent cause. Am J Obstet Gynecol 142:358, 1982

Bottoms SF, Rosen MG, Sokol RJ: The increase in the cesarean birth rate. N Engl J Med 302:559, 1980

Collea JV, Chein C, Quilligan EJ: The randomized management of term frank breech presentation: A study of 208 cases. Am J Obstet Gynecol 137:235, 1980

Cunningham FG, Hauth JC, Strong JD, Kappus SS: Infectious morbidity following cesarean section: Comparison of two treatment regimens. Obstet Gynecol 52:656, 1978

DeLee JB, Cornell EL: Low cervical cesarean section (laparotrachelotomy). JAMA 79:109, 1922

DePalma RT, Cunningham FG, Leveno KJ, Roark ML: Continuing investigation of women at high risk for infection following cesarean delivery. The three-dose perioperative antimicrobial therapy. Obstet Gynecol 60:53, 1982

DePalma RT, Leveno KJ, Cunningham FG, Pope T, Kappus SS, Roark ML, Nobles BJ: Identification and management of women at high risk for pelvic infection following cesarean section. Obstet Gynecol 55:185(S), 1980

Douglas RG, Stromme WB: Operative Obstetrics, 2nd ed. New York, Appleton, 1965, pp 449–452

Douglas RG, Birnbaum SJ, MacDonald FA: Pregnancy and labor following cesarean section. Am J Obstet Gynecol 86:961, 1963

Eastman NJ: The role of Frontier America in the development of cesarean section. Am J Obstet Gynecol 24:919, 1932

Fasbender H: Geschichte der Geburlshufe. Jena, 1906, pp 979–1010

Flaksman RS, Vollman JH, Benfield DG: Iatrogenic prematurity due to elective termination of the uncomplicated pregnancy: A major perinatal health care problem. Am J Obstet Gynecol 132:885, 1978

Fogarty M, Creasy R, Laros R, Jonsen A: Life support in maternal brain death during pregnancy. Am J Obstet Gynecol (submitted) 1984

Frank F: Suprasymphysial delivery and its relation to other operations in the presence of contracted pelvis. Arch Gynaekol 81:46, 1907

Frigoletto FD Jr, Ryan KJ, Phillippe M: Maternal mortality rate associated with cesarean section: An appraisal. Am J Obstet Gynecol 136:969, 1980

Gall SA: The efficacy of prophylactic antibiotics in cesarean section. Am J Obstet Gynecol 134:506, 1979

Gellman E, Goldstein MS, Kaplan S, Shapiro WJ: Vaginal delivery after cesarean section: Experience in private practice. JAMA 249:2935, 1983

Gibbs CE: Planned vaginal delivery following cesarean section. Clin Obstet Gynecol 23:507, 1980

Gibbs RS, Hunt JE, Schwarz RJ: A follow-up study on prophylactic antibiotics in cesarean section. Am J Obstet Gynecol 117:419, 1973

Gluck L: Iatrogenic RDS and amniocentesis. Hosp Pract 12:11, 1977

Goodlin RC, Scott JC Jr, Woods RE, Anderson JC: Laparoelytrotomy or abdominal delivery without uterine incision. Am J Obstet Gynecol 144:990, 1982

Green SL, Sarubbi FA, Bishop EH: Prophylactic antibiotics in high-risk cesarean section. Obstet Gynecol 51:569, 1978

Harris RP: Lessons from a study of the caesarean operation in the City and State of New York. Am J Obstet 12:82, 1879

Hershey DW, Quilligan EJ: Extraabdominal uterine exteriorization at cesarean section. Obstet Gynecol 52:189, 1978

Horowitz BJ, Edelstein SW, Lippman L: Once a cesarean . . . always a cesarean. Obstet Gynecol Surv 36:592, 1981

Husbands ME Jr, Pritchard JA, Pritchard SA: Failure of tubal sterilization accompanying cesarean section. Am J Obstet Gynecol 107:966, 1970

Kerr JMM: The technic of cesarean section with special reference to the lower uterine segment incision. Am J Obstet Gynecol 12:729, 1926

Kreutner AK, Del Bene VE, Delamar D, Bodden JL, Loadholt CB: Perioperative cephalosporin prophylaxis in cesarean section: Effect on endometritis in the high-risk patient. Am J Obstet Gynecol 134:925, 1979

Krönig B: Transperitonealer Cervikaler Kaiserschnitt. In Doderlein A, Krönig B (eds): Operative Gynäkologie, 1912, p 879

Latzko W: Ueber den extraperitonealen Kaiserschnitt. Zentralbl Gynaekol 33:275, 1909

Lavin JP, Stephens RJ, Miodovnik M, Barden TP: Vaginal delivery in patients with a prior cesarean section. Obstet Gynecol 59:135, 1982

Martin JN Jr, Harris BA Jr, Huddleston JF, Morrison JC, Propst MG, Wiser WL, Perlis HW, Davidson JT: Vaginal delivery following previous cesarean birth. Am J Obstet Gynecol 146:255, 1983

McGarry JA: The management of patients previously delivered by caesarean section. J Obstet Gynaecol Br Commonw 76:137, 1969

Meir PR, Porreco RP: Trial of labor following cesarean section: A two-year experience. Am J Obstet Gynecol 144:671, 1982

Merrill BS, Gibbs CE: Planned vaginal delivery following cesarean section. Obstet Gynecol 52:50, 1978

Morrison JC, Wiser WL, McKay M, Gookin K, Couvas SG: Cesarean section: What's behind the dramatic rise? Perinatol Neonatol 6:87, 1982

National Institutes of Health: Consensus Development Conference Summary, Vol 3, Number 6, 1980

Norton JF: A paravesical extraperitoneal cesarean section technique. Am J Obstet Gynecol 51:519, 1946

O'Driscoll K, Foley M: Correlation of decrease in perinatal mortality and increase in cesarean section rates. Obstet Gynecol 61:1, 1983

O'Driscoll K, Foley M, MacDonald D: Active management of labor as an alternative to cesarean section for dystocia. Obstet Gynecol 63:485, 1984

O'Driscoll K, Jackson RJA, Gallagher JT: Prevention of prolonged labor. Br Med J 2:477, 1969

O'Driscoll K, Stronge JM, Minogue M: Active management of labour. Br Med J 3:135, 1973

O'Sullivan MJ, Fumia F, Holsinger K, McLeod AGW: Vaginal delivery after cesarean section. Clin Perinatol 8:131, 1981

Pauerstein CJ: Labor after cesarean section: From precept to practice. J Reprod Med 26:409, 1981

Perkins RP: Extraperitoneal section: a viable alternative. Contem Ob/Gyn 9:55, 1977

Pickrell K: An inquiry into the history of cesarean section. Bull Soc Med Hist (Chicago) 4:414, 1935

Plauché WC, Gruich FG, Bourgeois MO: Hysterectomy at the time of cesarean section: Analysis of 108 cases. Obstet Gynecol 58:459, 1981

Pliny the Elder, Natural History, Book VII, Chap IX. Cambridge, Mass, Harvard University Press, 1942. Translated by H. Rackham

Porro E: Della Amputazione Utero-ovarica. Milan, 1876

Pritchard JA: Changes in the blood volume during pregnancy and delivery. Anesthesiology 26:393, 1965

Riva HL, Teich JC: Vaginal delivery after cesarean section. Am J Obstet Gynecol 81:501, 1961

Rousset F: Traité Nouveau de l'Hystérotomotokie ou l'Enfantement Césaerien. Paris, Denys deVal, 1581

Rubin GL, Peterson HB, Rochat RW, McCarthy BJ, Terry JS: Maternal death after cesarean section in Georgia. Am J Obstet Gynecol 139:681, 1981

Sachs BP, McCarthy BJ, Rubin G, Burton A, Terry J, Tyler CW Jr: Cesarean section: Risk and benefits for mother and fetus. JAMA 250:2157, 1983

Saldana LR, Schulman H, Reuss L: Management of pregnancy after cesarean section. Am J Obstet Gynecol 135:555, 1979

Sänger M: Der Kaiserschnitt bei Uterusfibromen. Leipzig, 1882

Seitchik J, Ramakrishna RV: Cesarean delivery in nulliparous women for failed oxytocin-augmented labor: Route of delivery in subsequent pregnancy. Am J Obstet Gynecol 143:393, 1982

Trolle D: The History of Caesarean Section. Copenhagen, Denmark, University Library, CA Reitzel Booksellers, 1982

Waters EG: Supravesical extraperitoneal cesarean section: Presentation of a new technique. Am J Obstet Gynecol 39:423, 1940

Weber CE: Postmortem cesarean section: Review of the literature and case reports. Am J Obstet Gynecol 110:158, 1970

Wheatley RG, Kallus ET, Reynolds RC, Giesecke AH: Milk of magnesia is an effective preinduction antacid in obstetric anesthesia. Anesthesiology 50:514, 1979

Wilcox CF, Hunt AB, Owen CA: The measurement of blood lost during cesarean section. Am J Obstet Gynecol 77:772, 1959

Williams RL, Chen PM: Identifying the sources of the recent decline in perinatal mortality rates in California. N Engl J Med 306:207, 1982

Wong R, Gee CL, Ledger WJ: Prophylactic use of cefazolin in monitoring obstetric patients undergoing cesarean section. Obstet Gynecol 51:407, 1978

Index

H